Problems

Assessment

Diagnosis

PROCESS

Evaluation

Goals

Intervention

McGraw-Hill
Handbook of
Clinical Nursing

McGraw-Hill
Handbook of
Clinical Nursing

EDITORS

Margaret E. Armstrong, R.N., M.S.
Formerly Assistant Professor
School of Nursing and
School of Medicine and Dentistry
University of Rochester

Elizabeth J. Dickason, R.N., M.A.
Associate Professor of Nursing
Queensborough Community College

Jeanne Howe, R.N., Ph.D.
Associate Professor
School of Nursing and Health Sciences
Western Carolina University

Dorothy A. Jones, R.N., M.S.N.
Associate Professor
Graduate Medical-Surgical Nursing
Boston College

M. Josephine Snider, R.N., Ed.D.
Assistant Professor
College of Nursing
University of Florida

McGraw-Hill Book Company
New York   St. Louis   San Francisco   Auckland   Bogotá   Düsseldorf
Johannesburg   London   Madrid   Mexico   Montreal   New Delhi
Panama   Paris   São Paulo   Singapore   Sydney   Tokyo   Toronto

McGraw-Hill Handbook of Clinical Nursing

Copyright © 1979 by McGraw-Hill, Inc. All rights reserved. Printed in the United States of America. No part of this publication may be reproduced, stored in a retrieval system, or transmitted, in any form or by any means, electronic, mechanical, photocopying, recording, or otherwise, without the prior written permission of the publisher.

1234567890   DODO   7832109

This book was set in Souvenir by Monotype Composition Company, Inc.
The editors were Orville W. Haberman, Jr., Richard S. Laufer, and Timothy Armstrong;
the designer was Judith Michael;
the production supervisor was Milton J. Heiberg.
The drawings were done by Educational Media Support Center, Boston University Medical Center.
R. R. Donnelley & Sons Company was printer and binder.

Library of Congress Cataloging in Publication Data
Main entry under title:

McGraw-Hill handbook of clinical nursing.

   Includes index.
   1. Nursing. I. Armstrong, Margaret E.
[DNLM: 1. Medicine—Nursing texts. WY150 M147]
RT41.M18   610.73   78-11612
ISBN 0-07-045020-X

Contents

List of Contributors

Susan Anderson, R.N., M.S.
Assistant Professor, Boston University School of Nursing, Boston, Massachusetts

Margaret E. Armstrong, R.N., M.S.
Formerly Assistant Professor, School of Nursing and School of Medicine and Dentistry, University of Rochester, Rochester, New York

Jacqueline Sicard Baran, R.N., M.S.
Clinical Specialist, Medical-Surgical Nursing, St. John's Mercy Hospital, St. Louis, Missouri

Barbara A. Bihm, R.N., M.S.N.
Instructor of Nursing, Boston University School of Nursing, Boston, Massachusetts

Beverly A. Bowens, R.N., M.N.
Clinical Specialist, Neurosurgery, The Medical Center, University of Alabama at Birmingham, Birmingham, Alabama

Linda M. Burton, R.N., B.S.N., P.N.A.
Continuity of Care Coordinator, Silvain and Arma Wyler Children's Hospital, University of Chicago Hospitals and Clinics, Chicago, Illinois

Ann Cain, R.N., Ph.D.
Professor, School of Nursing, School of Nursing, University of Maryland, Baltimore, Maryland

Mable S. Carlyle, R.N., M.N.
Assistant Professor, School of Nursing and Health Sciences, Western Carolina University, Cullowhee, North Carolina

Meredith Censullo, R.N., M.S.
Nursing Coordinator, Medical Specialty Clinics, Children's Hospital, Boston, Massachusetts

Phyllis L. Collier, R.N., M.S.P.H.
Instructor, School of Nursing, University of Rochester, Rochester, New York

Marilyn de Give, R.N., M.S.
Senior Associate, School of Nursing, University of Rochester, Rochester, New York

Elizabeth J. Dickason, R.N., M.A.
Associate Professor of Nursing, Queensborough Community College, Bayside, New York

Beverley H. Durrett, R.N., M.N.
Formerly Director of Inservice Education, Highland Hospital, Asheville, North Carolina

Mary E. Eddy, R.N., M.S.
Assistant Professor, Medical-Surgical Nursing Program, Yale University School of Nursing, New Haven, Connecticut

Joanne Kelleher Farley R.N., M.S.
Assistant Professor, St. Anselm's College School of Nursing, Manchester, New Hampshire

Helen L. Farrell, R.N., M.S.N.
Supervisor of Adult Health Services, Buncombe County Health Department, Asheville, North Carolina

Annette Crosby Frauman, R.N., M.S.N.
Assistant Professor, College of Nursing, University of Florida, Gainesville, Florida

Phyllis J. Gale, R.N., M.S.
Professor and Director, Nursing Program, Bunker Hill Community College, Charlestown, Massachusetts

Gail Barlow Gall, R.N., B.S.
Adult Nurse Practitioner, Harvard Community Health Plan, Boston, Massachusetts

Cyrena M. Gilman, R.N., M.N., C.H.N.
Pediatric Transplant Coordinator, Shands Teaching Hospital, University of Florida, Gainesville, Florida

Karolyn Lusson Godbey, R.N., M.S.N.
Assistant Professor, College of Nursing, University of Florida, Gainesville, Florida

Patricia E. Greene, R.N., M.S.N.
Clinical Nurse Specialist, Pediatric Oncology, North Carolina Memorial Hospital, Chapel Hill, North Carolina

Diana W. Guthrie, R.N., M.S.P.H., F.A.A.N., C.
Diabetes Nurse Specialist; Assistant Professor, Department of Nursing, Wichita State University, Wichita, Kansas; Assistant Professor and Coordinator of Education and Research, Department of Pediatrics, University of Kansas School of Medicine, Wichita, Kansas

C. Marie Hall, R.N., M.S.N.
Nurse Clinician, Department of Pediatric Hematology-Oncology, Duke University Medical Center, Durham, North Carolina

Faye Gary Harris, R.N., Ed.D.
Associate Professor, College of Nursing, University of Florida, Gainesville, Florida

Patricia Harris, R.N., M.S.N., P.N.P.
Pediatric Nurse Practitioner, Connecticut Health Plan, Bridgeport, Connecticut; Clinical Faculty, Yale University School of Nursing, New Haven, Connecticut

Mary Gorman Hazinski, R.N., M.S.N.
Practitioner-Teacher, Pediatric Intensive Care Unit, Rush–Presbyterian–Saint Luke's Medical Center, Chicago, Illinois, Assistant Professor, Rush University College of Nursing, Chicago, Illinois

Sherry W. Honea, R.N., M.N.
Director of Nursing Service, Highland Hospital, Asheville, North Carolina; Clinical Assistant Professor, Duke University School of Nursing, Durham, North Carolina

Jeanne Howe, R.N., Ph.D.
Associate Professor, School of Nursing and Health Sciences, Western Carolina University, Cullowhee, North Carolina

Mary Bigelow Huntoon, R.N., M.S.N.
Instructor of Nursing, Boston University School of Nursing, Boston, Massachusetts

Mary Marmoll Jirovec, R.N., M.S.
Clinical Instructor, University of Wyoming School of Nursing, Laramie, Wyoming

Dorothy A. Jones, R.N., M.S.N.
Associate Professor, Graduate Medical-Surgical Nursing, Boston College, Chestnut Hill, Massachusetts

Ruth Dailey Knowles, R.N., Ph.D.
Nurse Psychotherapist, Miami, Florida

Hilda Koehler, M.S., C.N.M.
Parent Educator, St. Luke's Hospital Center, New York, New York

Jane Ann LaVigne, R.N., M.S.N.
Formerly Assistant Director of Nurses–Mental Health, Waltham Hospital, Waltham, Massachusetts

Cynthia S. Luke, R.N., M.S.
Instructor, Duke University School of Nursing, Durham, North Carolina

Elizabeth Butler Marren, R.N., B.S., P.N.A.
Assistant Director of Nursing, LaRabida Children's Hospital, Chicago, Illinois

Christine Mitchell, R.N., M.S.
Assistant Professor of Nursing, University of Virginia School of Nursing, Charlottesville, Virginia

Rhoda L. Moyer, R.N., M.N.
Assistant Professor of Nursing, School of Nursing, University of North Carolina, Greensboro, North Carolina

Hazel R. Mummah, R.N., B.A.
Geriatric Nursing Consultant, Japanese Umbrella of Health Care Facilities, Los Angeles, California

Annalee Oakes, R.N., M.A., C.C.R.N.
Associate Professor, Department of Nursing, School of Health Sciences–Nursing, Seattle Pacific University, Seattle, Washington

Sherrilyn S. Passo, R.N., M.S.
Instructor, Indiana University School of Nursing, Indianapolis, Indiana

Rose Pinneo, R.N., M.S.
Associate Professor, School of Nursing, University of Rochester, Rochester, New York

Kathleen Reilly Powderly, M.S.N., C.N.M.
Nurse-Midwifery Educational Program, School of Allied Health Professions, College of Medicine and Dentistry of New Jersey, Newark, New Jersey

Nancy E. Reame, R.N., Ph.D.
Assistant Professor, College of Nursing, School of Medicine, Wayne State University, Detroit, Michigan

Imogene Stewart Rigdon, R.N., M.S.N.
Assistant Professor, College of Nursing, University of Florida, Gainesville, Florida

Dorothy L. Sexton, R.N., Ed.D.
Associate Professor and Chairperson, Medical-Surgical Nursing Program, Yale University School of Nursing, New Haven, Connecticut

Bonnie Silverman, R.N., B.S.N., P.N.C.
Perinatal Nurse Clinician, Booth Memorial Hospital Center, Flushing, New York

Marilyn M. Smith, R.N., M.S., M.B.A.
Associate Professor, College of Nursing, Northeastern University, Boston, Massachusetts

M. Josephine Snider, R.N., Ed.D.
Assistant Professor, College of Nursing, University of Florida, Gainesville, Florida

Janet L. Snow, R.N., M.S.N.
Practitioner-Teacher, Pediatric Special Care Unit, Rush–Presbyterian–Saint Luke's Medical Center, Chicago, Illinois; Assistant Professor, Rush University College of Nursing, Chicago, Illinois

Mackey P. Torbett, R.N., Ph.D.
Associate Professor, School of Nursing, University of Kansas, Kansas City, Kansas

Nora Doherty Tully, R.N., M.A., M.Ed.
Instructor of Nursing, Queensborough Community College, Bayside, New York

Mary P. Wieland, R.N., M.S.N.
Nursing Clinical Instructor, Emergency Medical Services, Honolulu, Hawaii

Lucille Bright Wilson, R.N., Ed.D.
Chairperson, College of Nursing, Albany State College, Albany, Georgia

Preface

Recent trends in nursing education and practice have increased the need for a handbook offering the nurse quick access to information that utilizes the Standards of Nursing Practice and that applies the nursing process to clients with a variety of health problems. The *McGraw-Hill Handbook of Clinical Nursing* has been written to fill this gap.

The *Handbook* is divided into seven separate parts, each of which discusses the specific problems of a particular population. The three chapters in Part 1 orient the reader to the overall use of the *Handbook*. Chapter 1 presents the conceptual framework of the text, Chapter 2 discusses the Standards of Nursing Practice and the components of the nursing process, and Chapter 3 details human growth and development throughout the life span.

Since the Standards of Nursing Practice were developed with a specialty orientation, the editors decided to utilize a similar approach in organizing the remaining parts of the text. Therefore, Parts 2 through 7 focus on the clinical specialties, including maternal-infant, pediatric, medical-surgical, psychiatric, gerontologic, and emergency nursing. The inclusion of separate sections on psychiatric and gerontologic nursing is unique in a handbook of this sort.

Each part opening provides a brief introduction to the specialty covered and a general overview of the content to be discussed in the chapters that follow. In addition, the American Nurses' Association Standards of Practice for that particular specialty area are included for reference and review.

While some variation may exist in the way material is presented within each chapter, they have all been organized according to unifying principles to facilitate the use of the *Handbook*. A definition is given of each problem being addressed; a brief discussion of related pathophysiology follows, as appropriate; and the standards of nursing practice are applied through the vehicle of the nursing process to create the plan of nursing care, i.e., assessment, nursing diagnosis, planning, implementation, and evaluation. Major problems frequently observed in a clinical setting are discussed in depth; those problems observed less frequently are discussed briefly.

The editors believe that the approach to patient care as presented in the *McGraw-Hill Handbook of Clinical Nursing* will (1) provide nurses working within any health setting with specific guidelines to patient care, (2) improve the overall quality of patient care by incorporating the Standards of Nursing Practice into the nursing plan of care, (3) increase accountability and responsibility of nurses to the client by clearly defining expected nursing actions within a specific setting, (4) facilitate the peer review process, and (5) make the unique contributions of nurses to patient care more visible through increased emphasis on the utility and application of the nursing process.

The editors wish to thank the American Nurses' Association for its permission to reprint the Standards of Nursing Practice found throughout the *Handbook,* and also the National Conference Group on the Classification of Nursing Diagnosis. In addition, we would like to thank our families and friends, who have supported us throughout this project. A special word of thanks also goes to the staff at McGraw-Hill, especially Orville Haberman, Richard Laufer, and Timothy Armstrong, who devoted many hours to the successful completion of the *Handbook.*

Margaret E. Armstrong
Elizabeth J. Dickason
Jeanne Howe
Dorothy A. Jones
M. Josephine Snider

Part One

Introduction

1
Purposes, Organizational Framework, and Uses of This Book

Jeanne Howe

This handbook has been prepared to facilitate the planning, implementation, and evaluation of nursing care. The book has been designed primarily for two groups of readers.

STUDENTS AND PRACTICING NURSES

Students and practicing nurses will find here, in an outline form ideal for quick reference, explicit and comprehensive nursing care plans and their rationales for patients with an extensive range of medical-surgical, maternity, psychiatric, pediatric, and gerontologic health conditions. The care plans are presented according to the sequential phases of the nursing process (assessment, nursing diagnosis or problem identification, the establishment of goals of care, intervention, and evaluation), and the content has been carefully arranged for easy location and translation into practice.

QUALITY ASSURANCE EVALUATORS

Secondly, the book has been designed to assist persons involved in quality assurance endeavors, including peer review programs, student and professional staff evaluations, and accreditation-related assessments of nursing service. For this purpose, the American Nurses' Association standards of practice have been included in each patient care section of the book and have been used as the basis for the care plans. By making explicit the methods for using the nursing process to meet ANA standards, this handbook provides a criterion against which care for patients with specific problems can be measured and evaluated.

ORGANIZATIONAL FRAMEWORK

Book Parts

The book is subdivided into seven parts, each composed of several chapters. In Part 1, this first chapter explains the purposes of the manual and describes its organization and uses. Chapter 2 presents the nursing process as it appears throughout subsequent chapters, and introduces an overview of the ANA standards of practice. The final chapter of Part 1 presents growth and development and its incorporation into nursing care for persons of all ages.

Part 2, "Maternity Nursing," applies the nursing process to families with reproductive and genetic concerns, women and their unborn babies throughout pregnancy, and healthy term and preterm infants.

Part 3, "The Nursing Care of Children and Adolescents," details the nursing process as it applies to ill and high-risk infants and to children and adolescents. Health conditions are arranged into chapters according to body systems. Within chapters, content is organized into subcategories such as congenital defects, traumatic injuries, obstructions, inflammations, metabolic disorders, and abnormal cellular proliferations.

Part 4 deals with adult health concerns that fall within the sphere of medical-surgical nursing. Content is organized around body systems and classified into the categories of abnormal cellular growth, cellular metabolic deviation, inflammation, obstruction, trauma, and degeneration. The nursing process is again the vehicle of presentation.

Part 5, "Psychiatric Nursing," outlines the nursing process for children and adults with difficulties related to perception, affect, cognition, interpersonal relationships, societal norms, activities of daily living, and situational crises. Family and group work are given special attention.

Part 6, "The Nursing Care of the Aged," discusses nursing of the aged in relation to normal physiologic, psychologic, and sociocultural effects of aging; significant losses; and health problems seen in atypical responses to aging.

In Part 7, "Emergency Nursing," emergency medical-surgical, pediatric, obstetric, and psychiatric nursing topics are presented, again according to the nursing process and standards of care.

Arrangement of Content to Avoid Overlap

Such a wide-scope reference work requires a good system for coordinating related content areas so that book usability is maximized and repetition is minimized. Nursing care of diabetics, for example, is part of maternity, medical-surgical, pediatric, gerontologic, and emergency practice, but it is obviously undesirable to duplicate information in several different parts of the book. The discussions pertaining to diabetes have been arranged so that the main body of material is presented in the endocrinology chapter of medical-surgical nursing, and information or care approaches which pertain only to other specialty areas are found in those other parts of the book. Thus, information about gestational diabetes and nursing of diabetics during family planning, pregnancy, and delivery is included in the appropriate maternity nursing chapters. Juvenile diabetes, where it differs from adult diabetes in specific ways, is discussed in the pediatric section. The acute crises of insulin shock and diabetic coma are included under emergency nursing. Surgical management and the special aspects of nursing aged diabetics are contained in the medical-surgical and gerontologic sections of the book, respectively.

Cross-reference notations direct the reader from a "specialty" section, such as juvenile diabetes, to the medical-surgical discussion of diabetes for additional information which, since it pertains to both children and adults, needs to be said only once.

The main presentation of each health problem is included in the part of the book that deals with nursing care of the kinds of patients who are most likely to encounter that particular problem. Thus, disorders which most commonly arise during childhood (the acute leukemias, for example, and certain communicable diseases) receive their major discussion in the relevant pediatric nursing chapter. Persons seeking guidelines for the care of adults with those disorders will find in the medical-surgical section only information pertaining to adult care and a reference notation directing them to the pediatric chapter where the principal discussion is contained.

Integration of Content

The psychosocial aspects of care for persons with predominantly physical disorders are not segregated from the discussion of physical care. Anxiety over the possibility of recurring myocardial infarction is dealt with in the same section as the other problems related to the care of a patient with myocardial damage, for example, and grief and body image distortions associated with amputation are integral parts of the discussion of nursing for amputees.

ADDITIONAL REMARKS ABOUT THE BOOK

Authorship

The expansion and deepening of knowledge in nursing and in the related sciences have brought about the end of the single-author broad-scope reference work. This manual has been written by a large number of authors, each selected for the ability to contribute up-to-date accuracy and clinical expertise. In conformity with the editorial board's conviction that the design and evaluation of nursing care are the prerogative and responsibility of nurses, this book has no nonnurse authors.

Applicability to Various Care Settings

While the book was prepared especially with the needs of the acute care practitioner in mind, it is also designed to be useful in other settings. Long-range care, whether in the home and community or in ambulatory care facilities, is discussed as part of each care plan. The nurse working in any setting can to some degree see patients' pasts and futures in this book and should become better able to coordinate care and do patient teaching and long-term planning.

Relationship to Other Literature

The book is not intended to replace texts or to eliminate the need for the other components of the professional's library. On the contrary, each chapter includes a briefly annotated bibliography which supplements the manual's outlines, flowcharts, tables, case studies, and care plans. Most readers will be pleased to note that two large classes of information have been omitted from this book. First, the knowledge and skills which comprise "fundamentals of nursing" were deemed unnecessary for practicing nurses and quality assurance evaluators. Second, because of the widespread availability of procedure manuals and the specificity and individualization among institutions as to how procedures shall be done, minimal book space has been given to instructions for nursing procedures.

2

The Nursing Process and Standards of Nursing Practice

Jeanne Howe

The phrase *nursing process* is relatively recent, and refers to the concept that nursing care consists of an orderly sequence of steps or stages. The identification and description of these subparts of care lends visibility to the logical orderliness underlying the professional practice of nursing.

THE STAGES OF THE NURSING PROCESS

Assessment

In providing professional services, the nurse begins by collecting information about the client or patient.[1] This opening stage of the nursing process is called the *assessment* phase. Through assessment the nurse seeks to determine the person's current health status; to become aware of relevant past experiences, current health practices, and expectations regarding health and the health care system; and to learn what health needs the patient identifies. The methods of gathering this information include interview and history-taking, observation, testing, physical examination, consultation with other professionals who have been involved with the person, and the review of existing health records.

The assessment phase, in addition to initiating the nursing process, is the beginning of the professional relationship between the nurse and the patient (and, often, the patient's relatives and friends). Skilled, sensitive communication is a prerequisite to establishing a trusting relationship in which the patient feels secure about providing relevant personal information.

Diagnosis or Problem Identification

From the data collected during the assessment phase, the nurse compiles a list of the patient's health-related problems. When possible, the nurse next makes certain concise summary statements, called *nursing diagnoses,* to describe the patient's condition.

Nursing diagnosis at the present time continues to be a focus of controversy. One reason is that the word *diagnosis* has traditionally been associated with the practice of medicine. King (1) points out:

Although we may think of diagnosis as the identification of disease, such usage is far too narrow. The word means *to distinguish.* It involves the process of deliberate choice or discrimination, the process whereby we say that *this*—whatever it may represent—is an example of *that*—whatever that may happen to be. If I say, *this* is a *rose,* I am making a diagnosis. . . .

Gordon (2) clarifies the province of the nursing diagnosis:

Nursing diagnoses describe health problems in which the responsibility for therapeutic decisions can be assumed by a professional nurse. In general, these problems encompass potential or actual

[1]The words *patient* and *client* are used interchangeably throughout this book. To some extent, *client* more often refers to an outpatient or other person whose nursing does not include acute care, while hospitalized persons are generally referred to as *patients*. Except where so specified, *client* does not carry the specialized meaning, used by some nurses in private practice, of having a formal contractual agreement for the receipt of nursing services. In no instance does the preferential use of the word *patient* imply that the patient will be manipulated or passive in the nurse-patient relationship.

disturbances in life processes, patterns, functions, or development, *including* those occurring secondary to disease. [Italics added]

The term *nursing diagnosis* makes explicit a distinction between medical and nursing diagnoses. In this book, medical diagnoses, for those patients who have been diagnosed by a physician, are regarded as part of the data pool which the nurse examines during the nursing assessment phase and from which nursing diagnoses or nursing problems are determined.

A second reason why the concept of nursing diagnosis has not been more widely accepted and applied to practice than it yet has been is that there is still no extensive, precise diagnostic language (nomenclature) with which to state and define specific diagnoses. As long as that is the case, nurses will find it difficult to distinguish between a nursing problem and a nursing diagnosis and to rephrase problems as diagnoses. While the profession works to delineate its distinct diagnostic domain and to develop the nomenclature (3) for it, compromise is necessary in the preparation of a book such as this one. Both problems and diagnoses are presented in the second stage of the nursing process outlines throughout the book, with a distinction between the two being made where possible.

Goal Setting

The third phase of the nursing process, the establishment of *goals of care,* builds on assessment and diagnoses or problems. Here the nurse formulates statements describing the outcomes he or she and the patient consider desirable and attainable results of the nursing care to be provided. Both immediate or short-term goals and long-term goals are identified in this book.

The role of the patient (and of family members or others who will participate in working toward attainment of goals) in setting the goals of care is appropriately receiving increasing attention in current practice and literature. This book reflects the growing belief that it is ethically unsound, as well as often futile, for "us" to choose outcomes for "them."

Intervention

Once goals of care are established, the nurse draws up a proposed course of action for achieving the goals and begins the process of carrying out the plan. Nursing activities during this stage of *intervention* may include direct provision of care, counseling, and teaching; referral to other professionals or agencies; and delegation of certain care components to paraprofessionals or others. Interventions need to be highly individualized for each patient. For example, while certain parts of the care of a fracture patient are "standardized," it is obvious that other parts differ depending upon whether the fracture resulted from cancer, accident, child abuse, alcohol abuse, or some other circumstance.

Evaluation

The final stage of the nursing process is the nurse's *evaluation* of the relative success or failure of the nursing care provided. Evaluation consists of comparing the patient's status, after intervention has been going on long enough that changes could be expected to appear, with the desired status as it was described in the goals of care.

It is at this point that the nursing process departs from the tidy, one-step-after-another progression it has previously taken. Evaluation employs the same techniques that were used in the first (assessment) stage—examination, interview, observation, and so forth. Evaluation yields one of two results: either satisfactory progress has been made or it has not. The nurse's subsequent action depends upon which of these results is found.

If the evaluation shows that the patient is moving satisfactorily toward attainment of the goal, or that the goal has been reached, the nurse either continues the nursing care as it has been (when maintenance care is indicated) or updates the problem list or diagnoses, and modifies the goals and proposed interventions to reflect the patient's improved condition. Figure 2-1 is a flowchart of the decisions and actions that follow an evaluation of satisfactory progress or goal attainment.

On the other hand, upon evaluation the nurse may find that the patient is not progressing as had been expected. When outcomes do not conform to expectations, it is necessary to repeat sequentially each phase of the nursing process to discover where things went wrong and to intercede with revisions at the point where error has appeared. This procedure is discussed below and diagramed in Fig. 2-2.

Reassessment may uncover some pertinent information which was not found on first assessment. In this case each subsequent stage of the nursing process—diagnosis, goals, interventions, and evaluation—needs to be repeated and, often, revised to incorporate the new assessment finding. Even when the second assessment reveals nothing different from the first, the nurse may find that restudy of the assessment data suggests an alternative to an original diagnosis. Revised diagnoses lead to revisions in the goals and interventions.

If after reassessment it appears that the original assessment was accurate *and* the initial diagnoses are still appropriate, the nurse must reexamine the goals of care to discover why they have not been attained. Nurse-patient conference may disclose that the patient's resources for moving toward the goals (or commitment to the goals) were more limited than had been thought at first, or that the patient has selected other objectives. The goals of care must be modified to bring them into alignment with the patient's circumstances.

When the original goals are retained, however, the professional's next course of action is to reexamine and revise as necessary the interventions that had been expected to

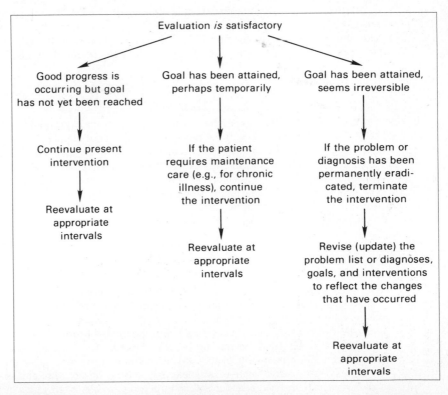

FIGURE 2-1 / Flowchart of the decisions and actions that follow an evaluation of satisfactory progress or goal attainment.

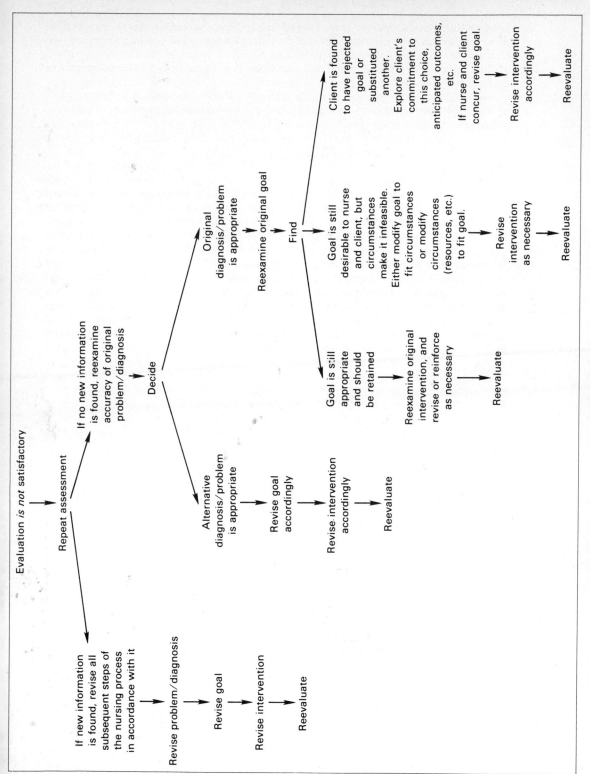

FIGURE 2-2 / Flowchart of the decisions and actions that follow an evaluation of unsatisfactory progress toward goal attainment.

accomplish the goals. Was the patient sufficiently well informed to be able to carry out his or her parts of the interventions? Are staff personnel following the care plan? Have referral recommendations been carried through?

Thus the nursing process commonly goes through repeated cycles from assessment to evaluation and again from reassessment to reevaluation. It is also true that the stages may often run concurrently. Assessment of the patient's condition obviously is an ongoing part of the intervention period, interventions ordinarily continue during evaluation, and new diagnoses may arise at any stage.

STANDARDS OF PRACTICE

Standards of practice are objective criteria, established by the profession, by which nursing practice can be evaluated. Since 1973 the American Nurses' Association Congress for Nursing Practice and the several Divisions on Practice (Medical-Surgical, Gerontological, Maternal-Child, Psychiatric-Mental Health, and Community Health) have published materials setting forth the baselines of acceptable practice, the rationales for the establishment of those standards, and the specific criteria by which practice in any setting can be evaluated to determine whether the standards are being met. Those standards, rationales, and assessment criteria have been incorporated throughout this book to aid practicing nurses in providing care that conforms to professionally accepted criteria of excellence, and to facilitate the evaluation of care. Each book part which deals with clinical nursing (Parts 2 through 7) includes a reproduction of pertinent selections from the relevant ANA publication. In four instances the standards have been further adapted and specified by nurse specialty groups (the Orthopedic Nurses' Association, the Emergency Department Nurses' Association, the Association of Operating Room Nurses, and the American Heart Association Council on Cardiovascular Nursing) in collaboration with the ANA Division on Medical-Surgical Nursing Practice. Those specialty standards are also presented in the appropriate chapters.

The following excerpt from the *American Nurses' Association Standards of Medical-Surgical Nursing Practice* (4) will serve further to introduce standards as they underlie the preparation of this manual.

WHY STANDARDS OF PRACTICE?

"A professional association is an organization of practitioners who judge one another as professionally competent and who have banded together to perform social functions which they cannot perform in their separate capacity as individuals."[2]

A professional association, because of its nature, must provide measures to judge the competency of its membership and to evaluate the quality of its services. Studies show that the tendency for self-organization has been found to be characteristic of professions and the establishment and implementation of standards characteristic of the organization. Mary Follet points out that professional associations have one function above all others: to establish, maintain, and improve standards of practice.[3]

A profession's concern for the quality of its service constitutes the heart of its responsibility to the public. The more expertise required to perform the service, the greater is society's dependence upon those who carry it out. A profession must seek control of its practice in order to guarantee the quality of its service to the public. Behind that guarantee are the standards of the profession which provide the assurance that service of a high quality will be provided. This is essential both for the protection of the public and the profession itself. A profession which does not maintain the confidence of the public will soon cease to be a social force.

In recognition of the importance of standards of professional practice and the need to guarantee quality service, the various Divisions on Nursing Practice of the American Nurses' Association have each formulated standards. The Association recognizes that ongoing revisions of the Standards of

[2]Robert K. Merton, "The Functions of the Professional Association," *American Journal of Nursing,* **58:** 50, January 1958.
[3]*Dynamic Administration,* The collected papers of Mary Follet, edited by Henry C. Metcalf and L. Urwick, Harper & Brothers, New York, 1942, p. 136.

Nursing Practice will be necessary to reflect the enlarging scope of practice as well as the increasingly sharper delineation of the theoretical basis upon which the practice rests.

Congress for Nursing Practice
American Nurses' Association

FINAL COMMENTS ON THE NURSING PROCESS AND STANDARDS OF PRACTICE

Professional nursing care is greater than the sum of the parts that have been described above. The method and order imposed by the nursing process do not diminish the *art* of nursing or discourage personalization of care. Patients bring a nearly infinite range of individuality to their participation in and response to nursing care. Nurses obviously and rightly differ from one another in their ways of applying the nursing process, just as they do in their methods of using other conceptual tools.

Similarly, standards do not undesirably constrain practice or lessen its artistry or innovativeness. Standards are simply criteria for the evaluation of care, and evaluation is not only a component of the nursing process but also a central quality of professionalism and professional responsibility.

REFERENCES

1. L. S. King, "What is a Diagnosis?" *Journal of the American Medical Association,* **202:**714, November 20, 1967.
2. Marjory Gordon, "Nursing Diagnosis and the Diagnostic Process," *American Journal of Nursing,* **76**(8):1298–1300, August 1976.
3. K. M. Gebbie, and M. A. Lavin (eds.), *Classification of Nursing Diagnoses,* C. V. Mosby Company, St. Louis, 1975.
4. *American Nurses' Association Standards of Medical-Surgical Nursing Practice,* American Nurses' Association, Kansas City, Mo., 1974.

3
Human Development through the Life Span

Mable S. Carlyle

Knowledge of human growth and development is basic to nursing practice. Obviously, the assessment phase of the nursing process draws heavily upon the nurse's understanding of norms for physical and behavioral function. Nursing diagnosis and problem identification require that the practitioner be able (1) to recognize deviations beyond the range of effective, normal function, and (2) to anticipate changes that can be expected to occur as time passes and the client's developmental characteristics undergo predictable modifications. The establishment of goals must take into consideration the person's developmental capacities and expected future development. Interventive efforts cannot succeed unless they are geared to the cognitive, affective, and physiologic status and potential of the patient.

To assist the practitioner in understanding the client and his or her potential so that nursing care can be tailored for the individual, this chapter describes major growth and developmental characteristics and milestones for children and adults at various stages of the life span.

Inherent in every discussion of norms is the obvious limitation that a description of "the average person" is inadequate to reveal the richness of human variation. This chapter should in no way be interpreted as implying either what all people *are* like or what people *should* be like. Its purpose, rather, is to serve as a reference point to guide the nurse by identifying commonly occurring human characteristics and sequences of development.

NEONATE (BIRTH TO 1 MONTH OF AGE)

Age-typical Characteristics	*Nursing Implications and Comments*
I. Physical development.	
A. Breathes immediately at birth.	
B. Can yawn, cough, sneeze, swallow, and regurgitate.	Should be turned on side after feeding to prevent aspiration.
C. Blinks and closes eyes. Looks at human face in preference to other visual stimuli.	Presence of the mother (or care provider) and ability to visualize her (e.g., removal of bililight eyepatches during feedings) are important to begin infant-mother bonding.
D. Moves extremities in random and uncoordinated fashion.	
E. Turns head from side to side.	
F. Automatic grasp reflex. Grasp is strong enough for partial lifting of body.	Evaluation of movement and reflex activity indicates neurological status.
G. Hears. Is startled by loud, sudden noises. May show preference for the high-pitched voice of the mother and rhythmic sounds similar to the heartbeat.	Mothers and family members seem intuitively to raise the pitch of the voice when talking to an infant. Rhythmic sounds and movements are soothing.

H. Sucking reflex is strong. The brushing of the cheek elicits rooting behavior (turning of the head and attempting to grasp object with the mouth).

Sucking is pleasurable and apparently a means of releasing tensions.

I. Crying involves the whole body. Character of the cry differs with circumstances. There are no tears.

A young mother may need to learn that the cry can indicate a need other than or in addition to hunger.

J. Lifts head briefly when prone.

K. Temperature regulation mechanism is immature. Sweat glands do not function until about 4 weeks.

A heat source may be needed immediately after birth. Observations should be made for drop or elevation of temperature.

L. Body characteristics:

1. Weighs 6 to 8 lb at birth. Gains about 6 oz per week.

2. Head comprises about one-fourth of the height.

3. Legs and arms are relatively short.

INFANT (AGES 1 TO 12 MONTHS)

Age-typical Characteristics

Nursing Implications and Comments

I. Physical development.

A. Second month:

1. May roll over.

Take precautions to prevent falls from rolling off surfaces.

2. Cries tears.

Often elicits great amount of response from others.

3. Cannot open hand purposefully to grasp toy but will hold it when placed in hand.

B. Third month:

1. Motor coordination development permits purposefully putting hand into mouth.

2. Becomes able to swallow solid foods (extrusion reflex diminishes).

In the interest of preventing allergies and obesity, pediatricians and nutritionists recommend delaying the introduction of solids until 4 to 6 months of age. There is no evidence that adding solids to the diet makes the baby sleep through the night. At whatever age solids are begun, only one new food should be introduced at a time, allowing a week or so before the next new food. Baby seems to respond more to change in texture than taste.

3. Can hold head erect.

4. Can focus eyes on bright objects and follow from side to side.

Brightly colored mobiles are entertaining and provide visual stimulation.

5. Blinking reflex is present.

6. Makes crawling movements when in prone position.

7. Can arch back and hold up head in prone position.

8. Strikes at toy but cannot grasp it.

C. Fourth month:

1. Can seize an object and move it to mouth.

Take precautions to prevent ingestion or aspiration of objects in infant's environment.

2. Turns from back to side.

Prevent falls from rolling off surface.

3. Introduces thumb apposition in grasping.

4. Supports part of weight with legs. Pushes feet against support.

5. Reaches out with hands.

6. Brings hands together, plays with them, and puts them into mouth.

D. Fifth month:

1. No head lag when pulled to sitting position.

2. Rolls from back to side.

3. Can transfer toys from one hand to the other.

4. Doubles birth weight.

E. Sixth month:

1. Can sit alone briefly.

2. Lifts head in anticipation of sitting and pulls into sitting position.

3. Bears a large portion of weight on legs when held in standing position.

4. Bangs objects on table.

5. Holds bottle.

Now is a good time to introduce the cup. Cups designed not to spill are useful.

6. Drops toy from hand to reach when another is offered.

F. Seventh, eighth, and ninth months:

1. Sits alone by eighth month and pulls into standing position by ninth month. Crawls.

2. Completes thumb-finger apposition and learns to pick up small objects.

Caution must be taken that objects small enough to be swallowed or aspirated are removed from play area.

3. Hand-eye coordination is perfected.

4. Two upper and two lower incisors erupt.

Some discomfort, drooling, and low fever may be expected. Begin prevention of "nursing bottle" tooth decay: no sugar-containing liquids (including milk) in bedtime bottle.

G. Tenth, eleventh, and twelfth months:

1. Learns to take a few steps alone.

Soft, flexible shoes or bare feet are best for walking.

2. May try to use spoon but seldom makes it to mouth with food still on it.

Little weight gain is expected at this age.

3. Holds cup alone.

4. Scribbles with crayon.

5. Has tripled birth weight by end of first year.

Rate of weight gain has decreased. Parents need not worry if there is a period of little gain.

II. Psychosocial development.

A. Second month:

1. Tactile stimulation is especially necessary for development during early life.

Holding to feed, diapering, bathing, and other caring activities assist in meeting this need.

2. Smiles in response to stimulation.

3. Coos and squeals.

4. Responds to speaking voice.

B. Third month:

1. Laughs aloud, coos, blows bubbles, squeals, and seems to enjoy the noise.

2. Smiles at mother's face.

3. Cries less.

C. Fourth month:

1. Laughs aloud.

2. Initiates social play.

3. Sleep reaches a pattern of one or two naps and longer periods at night.

D. Fifth month:

1. Lifts arms to be picked up.

      2. Turns head toward voice.

      3. Babbles vowels and "talks" to self.

      4. Splashes in bathwater.

   E. Sixth month:

      1. May develop separation anxiety and fear of strangers.

      2. Begins to act coy.

   F. Seventh, eighth, and ninth months:

      1. Says first words, usually "dada" and "mama."

      2. Responds to "no, no" and cries when scolded.

      3. Is shy with strangers.

      4. Waves bye-bye and plays pat-a-cake.

      5. May feed self finger foods.

   G. Tenth, eleventh, and twelfth months:

      1. Negativism is the general attitude. Tantrums are frequent.

      2. Resists going to bed.

> Setting of limits is expected by the child in spite of tantrums.
>
> A regular bedtime needs to be established and enforced for the benefit of all.

      3. Responds to music and rhythm.

      4. Finds toy where "hidden."

      5. Enjoys simple games.

      6. May say two or three single words correctly.

III. Cognitive development.

   A. Second month:

      1. Repetitiveness in play is enjoyable and necessary for learning.

      2. Begins sucking when placed in feeding position.

   B. Third month:

      1. Behaves as if what he does not see does not exist.

      2. Can wait for brief periods.

   C. Fourth month:

      1. Recognizes mother's face and some familiar objects.

2. Developing a vague idea that unseen objects exist.

D. Fifth month:

1. Recognizes mother from others.

2. Attention span increases and child can play alone for an hour or so.

E. Sixth month:

1. Responds with attentiveness to new stimuli.

2. Beginning to show food likes and dislikes.

F. Seventh through twelfth months:

1. Is aware that objects exist although out of sight.

2. Can associate unfamiliar happenings with familiar ones.

3. Attention span increases.

TODDLER (AGES 1 TO 3)

Age-typical Characteristics	*Nursing Implications and Comments*
I. Physical development.	
A. Developing locomotion skills: can walk, run, jump, slide backwards and sideways, can go down stairs alone, is learning to alternate feet. Can learn to ride tricycle.	Safety must be constantly kept in mind. The child should not be left unsupervised at any time. Mobility is a major means of learning and coping and should not be restricted unnecessarily, especially when child is under stress such as hospitalization.
B. Developing fine motor control. Can build a tower of blocks, feed self, string beads, throw ball, help undress self, and put on simple garments. Turns pages of a book.	
C. Voluntary control of sphincters is developed.	Successful toilet training depends on three factors: 1. Child has experienced discomfort of being soiled. 2. There is motivation to alter the situation. 3. Child recognizes preelimination sensations.
D. Teeth.	Needs to be taught to brush teeth. Foods with concentrated sweets should be avoided. The first visit to the dentist should be made.
1. At 15 months usually has first upper and lower molars.	
2. At 18 months has about 12 teeth.	

3. At 2½ years usually has all 20 deciduous teeth.

E. Probably has discovered genitalia.

Part of the normal process of self-exploration.

F. May sleep about 10 to 14 hours daily.

II. Psychosocial development.

A. Can now spend time away from mother if he or she has met caretaker in mother's presence, and a period of adjustment has been provided.

Several short visits of mother and child with the caretaker before the child is actually left make the transition smoother.

B. Shows pride in independence.

Children need to be permitted to perform tasks they can accomplish, regardless of the fact that this can be time-consuming for the parent and messy.

C. Mostly plays alone when in a group of other children.

Toddlers should not be expected to share toys.

D. Beginning to develop a sense of right and wrong.

Flare-ups of indignation are common. Guilt and shame are developmental hazards.

III. Cognitive development.

A. Demonstrates beginning of memory.

Repetition of learning experiences is necessary for the memory to develop. From this accumulation of experience child can move to new learning experiences.

B. Experiments with environment and activity in order to expand knowledge.

A wide variety of learning experiences can be had with safe objects in the home, such as pots and pans, boxes, colored egg cartons, etc.

C. Language skills are developing.

Bedtime stories are enjoyable and cognitively valuable for toddlers.

1. By age 3, can use a noun, verb, and object in a three-word sentence.

2. Has 300 or more words in vocabulary.

3. Toddlers can comprehend more than they can verbalize.

Simple explanations of events can be understood.

4. Knows own name.

D. Is beginning to think of alternative ways to reach goals without having to act out each one.

PRESCHOOL CHILD (AGES 3 TO 6)

Age-typical Characteristics	*Nursing Implications and Comments*
I. Physical development.	
A. Rate of growth slows.	Parents may worry because appetite decreases or is unpredictable.

B. Birth length has doubled by age 4.

C. Nighttime control of bowel and bladder usually is attained by age 3 or 4.

May have accidents during periods of stress or illness.

D. Learning self-care skills.

Planning the daily schedule to allow time for the child to participate in these activities promotes development of skills and builds self-esteem.

    1. Washes hands by age 3.

    2. Feeds self with some spillage at age 3.

    3. Brushes teeth by self at age 3 or 4.

    4. Undresses self at age 3.

    5. Dresses self at age 5.

E. Ability is limited in judging distance and own strength.

Provide for safety needs:

    1. Provide sturdy, safe toys.

    2. Protect valuable household objects.

    3. Assign a safe play area.

F. Moves with speed and increasing agility.

Watchful supervision is needed.

G. Deciduous dentition is completed and the incisors may be lost.

Child should have already developed a regular habit of brushing teeth and should be making twice yearly visits to dentist.

II. Cognitive development.

  A. Language skills rapidly increase.

Environmental opportunities influence learning.

  B. Learns basic concepts.

    1. Can understand time concepts such as "morning," "evening," etc.

    2. Can count up to 4 or 5.

    3. Knows at least the primary colors.

  C. Fluctuates between reality and fantasy; may have some difficulty distinguishing the two.

Dramatization of experiences by fabrication, exaggeration, or boastfulness is not intentional deceit.

  D. Has belief that whatever moves is alive.

Equipment that moves or makes noise such as hospital equipment may produce fears.

  E. Thinking is concrete. Is unable to analyze or synthesize.

  F. Has own private language and interpretations.

G. Perceives end results of change but may not understand the process.

Preoperative teaching probably has little meaning, but postoperative reteaching of what has happened is now meaningful. The same is true of other experiences: learning and understanding require sensorimotor experience.

H. Focuses on certain details of an object, but usually not the object as a whole.

Is unable to comprehend the whole picture of an event; for example, when about to receive an injection, will focus only on the needle and the anticipated pain, and not the purpose of the injection.

III. Psychosocial development.

A. Learns to distinguish right and wrong and begins to develop a conscience.

The preschool child wants to "do right," and likes kind guidance. Condemns self when things go wrong.

B. Learns sex differences and sexual modesty.

Plays "doctor;" peeking and asking to look at others' bodies are natural.

C. Develops a body image and a body boundary. May masturbate as self-awareness develops.

The child may become greatly concerned about the intactness of his or her body even from the slightest injury or intrusion.

D. Enjoys doing simple chores.

Is proud of accomplishments and enjoys praise.

E. Expands social interests to others outside the immediate family.

Is friendly, likes attention from others, appreciates jokes.

F. Equates death and separation as the same. Thinks that wishing or magical thinking can make a person disappear.

Although death is beyond understanding, the child should be permitted to experience death as it comes naturally within the family or circle of friends or to pets. Give explanations as they are asked for. Reassure the child that fantasies or wishes did not cause the death.

G. Feels more secure when behavioral boundaries are set by adults.

Difficulty in separating fantasy and reality and belief in magical thinking lead to feelings of insecurity.

MIDDLE CHILDHOOD (AGES 6 TO 12)

Age-typical Characteristics

I. Physical development.

A. Growth is less dramatic than during babyhood or later during adolescence.

B. General body configuration changes from childlike and begins to approximate adult proportions.

1. The trunk, head, and extremities more closely approximate adult proportions.

Nursing Implications and Comments

Adults expect behavior also to become more mature. They should guard against overexpectations.

2. The lower portion of the face enlarges as dentition becomes complete.

3. The nose enlarges.

4. Hair becomes coarser and less manageable.

C. Motor skills become refined with practice.

Participation in sports and handicrafts provides both boys and girls opportunity to refine motor skills.

1. Clumsiness, both gross- and fine-motor, and incoordination gradually diminish.

2. Greater muscle strength is gained.

3. Works and plays hard but tires easily.

II. Cognitive development.

A. The child's thinking remains concrete. However, boundaries of knowledge and ability to process information expand at a tremendous rate.

Hobbies, sports, crafts, arts, and other interests may supplement formal schooling in satisfying the need to learn.

1. Develops ability to be reflective.

2. Experience and memories accumulate from which to draw information and understanding.

3. Increases flexibility of thought.

4. Increases use of language.

5. Can consider alternate solutions to a problem.

6. Can consider parts or the whole independently.

7. Can understand and use classification systems.

B. Understands the Piagetian principle of conservation.

C. Develops the Piagetian concept of reversibility.

III. Psychosocial development.

A. Learns to get along with age mates.

1. Chooses a best friend, almost always of the same sex.

B. Learns an appropriate masculine or feminine social role.

    1. Is interested in sex differences.

    2. Plays games that involve male-female roles.

    3. Is interested in the opposite sex but won't admit it.

C. Is developing conscience, morality, and a set of values.

Needs experiences by which to clarify values.

    1. Good sportsmanship becomes important.

    2. Is loyal to friends.

    3. May take a strong stand for ideals.

    4. Develops self-awareness as a growing and developing individual.

This period of curiosity is an ideal time for health teaching. Special effort should be made to eliminate any fears or misinformation about body changes.

        a. Child is curious about body functions and changes that are occurring.

    5. Learns to be independent.

Delegation of tasks supports this learning. Some free time should be provided for introspection and learning about self.

        a. Wants own room.

        b. Will accept responsibility for routine household tasks with occasional reminders.

        c. Likes to participate in family decision making.

    6. Develops attitudes toward social groups and institutions.

        a. Will permit own goals to be subordinate to the group goals.

        b. Likes to belong to clubs.

        c. Puts on "good manners" in social settings.

    7. Family remains the primary agent of socialization, but peer groups are becoming more and more important.

Classroom groups, clubs, and sports groups become very influential in the socialization process.

ADOLESCENCE (AGES 12 TO 20)

Age-typical Characteristics	*Nursing Implications and Comments*
I. Physical development.	
A. A growth spurt takes place be-	Counsel child that final adult height is partly

tween ages 10 and 16. For girls this accelerated growth period begins about 2 years earlier than for boys.

1. Girls gain about 40 lb.

2. Boys gain about 55 lb (weight is attributed mostly to increase in bone and muscle tissue).

3. Girls retain more subcutaneous fat than boys.

4. Muscle development is greater in boys and therefore they are usually stronger.

5. Boys develop large hearts and lungs, have a higher systolic blood pressure, and maintain a slower heart rate at rest.

6. Different body parts reach adult size at different times; extremities grow before the trunk does.

B. Development of primary and secondary sex characteristics.

C. Sequence of development of sexual characteristics for girls.

1. The first visible sign of puberty in girls is usually the appearance of the breast bud. This may begin between the ages of 8 and 13.

2. Growth of pubic hair follows the early breast development. Full growth of pubic hair takes about 3 years.

determined by heredity. Nutritional education:

1. May participate in food fads and unbalanced reducing diets.

2. May overeat as a means of coping with problems.
   a. Loneliness.
   b. Obesity reduces pressures to participate socially or assume a sexual role.
   c. Child may attempt to overcome the feeling of being small and inadequate by becoming big.
   d. Caution both sexes against excessive muscle stress before epiphyses fuse.

This fact explains the gangly appearance and some of the awkwardness typical of adolescence.

The sequential development of these characteristics may be somewhat variable between individuals, but not nearly as variable as the age at which they appear. Puberty usually begins between the ages of 8 and 13 for girls, and 12 and 16 for boys. It can be very reassuring to know that different growth patterns are normal. Education of both sexes about the reproductive process, birth control methods, and prevention and treatment of venereal diseases should be begun at least by the onset of puberty and earlier if interest is shown. Cultural and religious guidelines for handling sexual behavior for both sexes should be discussed early within the family. Masturbation provides release of sexual tension and is not harmful.

3. Axillary hair begins about 1 year after the appearance of pubic hair.

4. Menarche usually occurs just after the growth spurt. The average age for American girls is just under 13.

Menstruation should be fully explained well before the age of onset as a normal and natural occurrence.

5. Menstruation may be irregular and accompanied by a certain amount of discomfort such as backaches or cramps.

Reference to menstruation as an illness should be avoided.

6. Ovulation generally begins a year or so after menarche.

7. The uterus reaches adult size about age 18 or 20.

D. Sequence of development of male sex characteristics.

1. There is increased growth of testes and the scrotum, which becomes redder, coarser, and wrinkled.

2. About this time pubic hair begins to grow.

3. About a year later and at the height of the growth spurt the penis begins to grow in length and circumference. The average age is about 13.

4. The prostate gland and seminal vesicles are maturing.

5. The first ejaculation occurs about a year after the penis begins to grow.

Education well in advance of wet dreams will eliminate unnecessary concern in the young man.

6. A temporary increase of the areola and elevation of the nipple occurs in about one-fourth of boys and is accompanied by breast tenderness. The changes disappear in a year or so.

Learning that this is normal and temporary is reassuring to the adolescent.

7. About 2 years after the beginning of pubic hair growth, facial, axillary, and body hair begins to grow. Body hair continues to spread until adulthood. The mustache comes first in sequence of facial hair.

8. The larynx enlarges and the vocal cords double in length,

causing the voice to deepen in pitch.

9. In both sexes androgen secretion increases. This stimulates the growth of the sebaceous glands and the production of sebum. At the same time developmental changes of the skin, including enlargement of pores, may result in acne.

Continuation of good health practices and in addition frequent cleansing of skin with a mild, nonabrasive soap will appreciably help control acne.

II. Cognitive development.

A. Begins to use formal thought process.

Cause-and-effect relationships are understandable, and expected outcomes of one's behavior can be anticipated, but adolescents are typically very present-oriented and do not take the long view of, for example, preventive health education.

1. Can deal conceptually and logically with abstractions, hypotheses, and hypothetical situations.

2. Considers several solutions to a question.

3. Can problem-solve in a systematic, adult manner.

B. The adolescent searches for new beliefs, resolves inconsistencies of old beliefs, and begins to crystallize a philosophy.

Must learn to deal with strong emotions not previously experienced.

C. The defense mechanisms most often used are asceticism (an attempt to deny entirely the instinctual drives) and intellectualization.

Phases of self-denial and overintellectualizing about self or others are common but may be very brief.

D. Since adolescents' thoughts are primarily about themselves, they assume that they are the center of other people's thought. As a result of this egocentrism negative or positive feelings are magnified, with an "imaginary audience" reflecting these same feelings.

One pimple on the face can become a "serious affliction." The adolescent may feel that everyone on the street is gaping as he or she walks by. Wearing apparel, hair styles, and other fads are of extreme importance.

E. As the result of the body changes taking place, the body image—how a person views the physical self—must undergo similar changes.

The adolescent needs to understand:
1. Body changes normally occur within a wide age range.
2. Changes are not as conspicuous to others as the adolescent thinks.
3. Sexual identity is not dependent on the attainment of a certain size of body parts.

1. The body image is formed from a conglomeration of real and fantasied experiences.

2. Variation in rate of maturation is of real concern to many adolescents.

The adolescent needs objective feedback from others in order to form a realistic body image. Honest feedback is rare and must be handled delicately as the adolescent is

3. Early maturers may have the advantage of being admired by peers and becoming leaders of their age group.

4. They also have the disadvantage of being expected to behave in a more mature way than others in their age group.

5. Late maturers may feel "left out" and unpopular with their peers.

III. Psychosocial development.

A. Achieves a new and more mature relation with age-mates of both sexes.

1. Takes and has good humor.

2. May be highly competitive.

B. Achieves social roles, including sex role. Patterns behavior after role models.

C. Achieves emotional independence from parents and other adults.

1. Becomes independent in schedules and homework.

2. May have employment outside the home.

3. Embarrassed by family in public at age 13 or 14.

4. Relationship with parents begins to improve about age 17 to 18.

D. Begins to consider the possibility of marriage and having a family.

1. Dating may be a major activity.

2. Most experiment with kissing, petting; some engage in intercourse.

3. Often has a fantasy relationship with a movie or television star.

E. Is preparing for economic independence and meaningful work.

1. Begins to explore career possibilities in relation to interest.

2. Ability or inability to set long-range goals influences choice.

already highly sensitive about his or her appearance.

Permission granted by adults for the adolescent to become more independent allows time to practice new behaviors while still in the family setting.

Hobbies, afterschool jobs, career clubs, and role models help with career choice.

3. Aptitude and cultural and parental influence contribute to career choice.

Referral to career guidance counselor or other such persons may be useful.

F. Is acquiring a set of values and an ethical system as a guide to behavior.

Value system is based on the ideal, and the young person may become critical, impatient, and depressed when reality falls short of the ideal.

1. Is developing an ideology.

2. Moral judgment continues to develop in terms of pleasing others and respect for authority.

Later comes to a resolution of conflicting standards and avoids self-condemnation and guilt feelings.

G. Desires and achieves socially responsible behavior.

May serve as junior scout leaders or athletic coaches for younger children, or march for fund drives, etc. Later, "antiestablishment" efforts and experiences help in the formation of a personal value system.

1. Becomes interested in social problems.

2. May become active in service-oriented organizations or, later, in movements promoting social change.

YOUNG ADULT (AGES 20 TO 40)

Age-typical Characteristics	*Nursing Implications and Comments*
I. Physical development.	
A. Fully matured; the rate of physiologic aging begins to overtake the rate of cellular growth.	Cumulative health history should be maintained. Baseline data (ECG, laboratory reports, biorhythm, etc.) should be collected for later reference. Yearly physical and dental exams should be planned to maintain health and check for silent diseases. Good health practices help maintain optimum health. Preventive practices should be taught, such as avoiding obesity and preventing stress-related illnesses.
II. Psychosocial development.	
A. Chooses, prepares for, and practices a vocation.	A multitude of vocational choices make it difficult for the young adult to make a selection.
B. Becomes independent of parents.	This task may be delayed due to the extended period of education required for some vocations.
C. Prepares for and adjusts to marriage or other intimate love relationship.	At the same time may still be a student and dependent financially on parents. Physical maturity has been achieved, but emotional and intellectual maturity may not have been reached yet.
D. Develops a civic consciousness.	

E. Refines own value system.

The continuing examination of values of parents and others, and the lessening of peer influence, permit the formation of an individualized value system. This is more difficult in the present society than previously because of the rapid changes in society, technology, etc., that cause issues to become clouded.

F. Develops a unique personal identity.

The current-day emphasis upon "finding one's self" often produces frustration while this difficult task is being accomplished.

G. Bearing children.

With improved methods of birth control the question is not only the number of children wanted and when to have them, but whether to have children at all. Knowledge about birth control should be available before the person becomes sexually active. Special health care needs of the mother need to be considered.

H. Rearing children.

   1. Reworks patterns of responsibility and accountability.

   2. Adjusts relationships.

   3. Manipulates the budget to meet expanding family needs.

   4. Guides children through their development.

May need education regarding childrearing practices and stages of growth and development. Also, need to know how to provide health care for children as well as the family as a whole.

I. Copes with change and stress. Rapidity of change in all aspects of life compounds the stresses people have traditionally had to cope with.

Needs education about the need for counseling at times when stress is particularly great, with an effort to dispel the stigma attached to seeking counseling. May need to learn new coping mechanisms. Good mental hygiene should be as much a goal as absence of physical stress symptoms.

III. Cognitive development.

   A. Intellectual ability continues to increase if stimulated.

   B. Becomes more serious about schooling.

   C. Interest broadens into community and world affairs.

Because of rapidly changing technology and the growing philosophy toward lifelong learning, the adult may have continued education either on the job or in preparation for a new job if the old one becomes obsolete. Also, the availability of education and shorter work hours permit expansion of interests and hobbies.

MIDDLE AGE (AGES 40 TO 60)

Age-typical Characteristics	Nursing Implications and Comments
I. Physical development.	
A. Progressive physiological changes occur throughout middle life.	The risk factors of aging, stress, and accumulation of environmental influences create a need for annual physical and dental examinations and periodic screening for the diseases most common to this age, such as cancer, hypertension, diabetes, etc.
1. Sensory changes.	
a. Vision: Presbyopia (far-sightedness), and decreases in acuity, night vision, and peripheral vision are all changes frequently associated with aging.	May need to use reading glasses for close work, limit driving to daytime, and learn to shift eyes to maintain wide visual field. Should plan for an eye examination every 1 to 2 years during the period of greatest change (the forties).
b. Hearing: Presbycusis (impaired auditory acuity) is a frequent occurrence. The ability to hear high-frequency sounds is often the first lost.	A suspected hearing loss indicates a need for evaluation and possible fitting for hearing aid. Frequent exams may be indicated if working in noise-polluted area.
c. Taste: There is a decrease in the ability to taste, due to loss of taste buds.	Compensatory behavior of adding additional spices to food may be contraindicated if there is evidence of other health problems.
B. Musculoskeletal changes.	
1. Decrease in bone density and mass permits the body to "shrink."	Mild aches, pains, and soreness may be expected.
2. Muscle tone decreases.	
a. Appearance may be flabbier.	Nutritional teaching should be done to reduce caloric intake without altering other nutritional intake. Supplemental vitamins and minerals are not needed by the healthy adult.
b. Some decrease in muscle strength occurs.	A plan for exercise should be adhered to. Walking is a good form of exercise available to almost everyone.
c. Sleep patterns change.	Decreased need for sleep may create a great deal of worry about insomnia and result in habituation to drugs.
II. Cognitive development.	
A. Little change in cognitive abilities occurs.	
1. Motivation for learning is relative to the importance placed on the task.	

2. The person consciously draws from past experiences in problem solving.

III. Psychosocial development.

A. Assists teenage and young adult offspring to become responsible and happy adults.

1. Works out money matters with teenagers.

2. Establishes a division of labor for sharing the responsibilities of family living.

3. Permits offspring to have affectional relationships and courtship experiences.

4. Keeps communication systems open among family members.

5. Maintains contact with the extended family.

6. Provides financing, if able, for offspring launching a career or continuing their education.

7. Reallocates responsibilities with remaining members of household.

8. Expands the family circle through release of young adults and recruitment of new members by marriage.

9. Tries to reconcile conflicting loyalties and philosophies of life between the generations.

B. Learns and adjusts to role as grandparent.

1. Defines the role of grandparent (e.g., fun-seeking, parent surrogate, reservoir of family wisdom, or distant figure).

2. Maintains a relationship with grandchildren.

C. Achieves adult social and civic responsibility.

1. Significance of friends increases.

2. Significance of relationships with coworkers increases.

3. Participation in civic matters increases.

With the shifting of family structure and additional stresses, additional support systems, including counseling, may be needed.

D. Reaches and maintains satisfactory performance in occupational career.

    1. Heightened productivity.

    2. Redefines vocational aspirations.

        a. Possible job change.

        b. Need for additional education.

        c. Adjusts to having reached the peak.

    3. Reentry into the business world of women who chose earlier to work at home.

Vocational counseling may help with the selection of a new career.

E. Develops adult leisure-time activities.

Teach that physically taxing forms of recreation need not decrease if a pattern of exercise has been maintained. If new activities involving additional stresses are begun, a graduated plan of increased exercise is important.

Susceptibility to anxiety seems to increase with age. Diversity of pleasurable activities assists with coping. Hobbies or sports enjoyed as a child may be a beginning point for persons with no interest at present.

F. Redefines roles in marriage.

    1. Builds a new relationship with spouse.

Marital therapy may be recommended if adjustments are difficult.

    2. Changes marriage partners.

    3. Roles and tasks within the home may change.

G. Adjusts to aging parents or loss of parents.

    1. Reverses the caring and providing roles.

    2. Forgives past hurts and real or perceived inadequacies.

If disabled parents require constant attention, family "vacations" or rest periods may be needed in order for the family to continue with its own developmental tasks.

H. Continues integration of a philosophy of life.

Depression is frequent in this age group.

    1. Learns the meaning of suffering.

    2. Realizes death is inevitable.

    3. Is aware of the philosophical wisdom of the culture.

I. Prepares for retirement.

    1. Makes financial arrangements.

Financial obligations to adult children as well as the primary family may interfere with saving for retirement.

    2. Plans for use of time.

J. Accepts changing body image.

A youth-oriented society may make acceptance of changes difficult.

K. Adapts to changing sexual patterns.

1. The female may experience increased interest due to freedom from fatiguing child care and decreased fear of pregnancy.

Partners need to recognize the change in patterns of sexual functioning as normal.

2. Male may need increased time to produce erection and ejaculation.

Impotence is most likely caused by fear of loss of sexuality rather than by any physical changes.

MATURITY (AGE 60 AND OVER)

Age-typical Characteristics	*Nursing Implications and Comments*
I. Physical development.	
A. General effects of aging.	
1. There is decreased need for sleep.	Four or five hours at night and a short nap in the daytime are probably all that are needed.
2. Decline of functions and abilities may produce safety hazards.	Teaching about preventive safety measures becomes more important at this age. Evaluation of living quarters for hazards may decrease the risk of accidents.
3. Likelihood of degenerative diseases is increased.	
4. Cumulative effect of past illnesses and previous poor health habits increases health risk.	
5. Slowing and fatiguing tendencies may lead to sedentary patterns of behavior.	A regular exercise program helps promote good health and slows the aging process. Excessive fatigue should be avoided.
B. Physiological changes.	
1. General diminution of function.	Many discomforts and functional limitations may result from the aging process, but changes should be evaluated for the presence of some underlying disease process and for appropriate supportive treatment for the symptoms of aging.
2. There may be greater decline in the more complex functions than in simple ones.	
3. Aging takes place at different rates within the individual and also within the individual's tissues and systems.	
4. Vulnerability to disease is increased.	At least yearly physical examinations are part of good health maintenance.
5. Ability to maintain homeostasis is decreased.	Extremes in activity or environment may be less well tolerated than previously.

C. Cell changes.

1. Cells reproduce at a slower rate.

D. Tissue changes.

1. Skeletal changes.

   a. Decrease in bone mass.   Possibility of fractures is increased.

   b. Loss of elasticity of joints.   Movement becomes slower.

   c. Degeneration of cartilage.

E. Systemic changes.

1. Gradual decrease in muscle mass.   Reasonable exercise, determined by past patterns, should be continued.

2. Decrease in efficiency of the nervous system, primarily manifested in increased response time.

3. Increasing loss of sensory functions compounds the effect of other declining functions.   Examination by appropriately prepared person should be done before corrective items such as glasses and hearing aids are purchased. Natural seasonings such as lemon or onion may increase flavor when taste and smell are declining.

4. Alterations in the pulmonary system include: Extra precautions should be taken to avoid respiratory infections. Any illness or disease that directly or indirectly decreases pulmonary functions creates a high-risk situation that demands immediate nursing intervention.

   a. Decreases in breathing capacity, residual lung volume, and total capacity.

   b. Consequent decreases in basal oxygen and metabolic rate.

   c. Decreased bronchoelimination as a result of diminished cough reflex and ciliary mechanism.

5. Changes in digestive system include:

   a. Periodontal disease.   Teeth must function properly so that (1) digestive juices can penetrate the food and (2) the person can ingest roughage foods to stimulate peristalsis. Twice yearly dental examinations are necessary for preventive maintenance of teeth. Dentures should be readjusted for fit as the tissues and structure of the mouth change.

   b. Decrease in digestive juices.

   c. Slowed peristalsis.

d. Interferences with absorption.

Malabsorption is a factor to consider both from a nutritional and pharmacological standpoint.

6. Modifications due to aging in the cardiovascular system include:

Teach the aged person to allow time for adjustment to changes in posture or altitude which temporarily affect blood pressure.

  a. Changes in vessel structure (loss of elasticity and narrowing).

  b. Valvular disease.

  c. Arrhythmias.

7. Renal system:

  a. Renal atrophy contributes to lessening renal function.

  b. Increased risk of lower urinary tract infections.

Maintaining adequate daily fluid intake (2000 to 3000 mL) is often forgotten by the aged.

  c. Involutionary processes affect the renal system.

  d. Extrarenal disease increases with age.

8. Endocrine system.

  a. Hormone production decreases.

  b. There is a decrease in the effect of the hormones produced.

9. Immune system.

  a. Immunologic defenses are diminished.

Extra precautions should be taken to prevent infections.

10. Sexual function is altered.

The libido is generally not reduced until the eighties or so; therefore an active sexual relationship can continue if the mate is able and accepting and if time and privacy are considered. Couples need to know that change in patterns of sexual behavior is a normal process. The possibility of alternative life-styles is being considered by numerous unmarried aged persons.

  a. Tissue changes may reduce the flexibility of the vagina and firmness of the erect penis.

  b. Response time is slowed but is compensated by lengthened arousal period.

II. Psychosocial development.

  A. Adjustment to retirement.

  1. Reduced income.

If previous financial preparation for retirement has not been adequate, additional sources of support may have to be solicited.

  2. Additional time for leisure and other uses.

Satisfactory use of time promotes good mental and physical health. Previous interests of adult life or childhood may be redeveloped at this time. Participation in service-oriented organizations may help fill

3. Readjustments in roles and relationships within the home.

B. Readjusting social roles.

1. Establishes affiliations with own age group.

2. Friendships are no longer focused around the job.

C. There may be a change in living facilities.

1. Present dwelling may be too large, too expensive to maintain, or unsuitable for persons with increasing disabilities.

2. A location previously chosen for convenience to work, schools, etc., may no longer be desirable.

3. A change in climate may be desired.

4. A location in an area with other retired persons may be appealing.

D. Feelings of worth, pride, and usefulness need to be maintained.

E. Deaths of spouse, friends, and acquaintances are realities of the present.

F. Inevitability of own death.

1. Sets goals to achieve before death.

2. Prepares for death through strengthening religious beliefs or other vehicles of self-transcendence.

3. Teaches others how to die through one's own death.

G. Maintains family ties with children, grandchildren, and possibly parents.

III. Cognitive development.

A. There is little change in IQ.

---

this need. Retirement counseling is available at many places of employment.

A spouse who previously spent most of the day at work may now be "underfoot" at home all day.

Participation in clubs and organizations may be one method of developing a new set of friends.

Caution should be recommended concerning changes in residence location. Friends of long standing, the familiar climate, and the variety of people in the community may be more rewarding than recognized at first. A trial period at a new location before cutting the ties from the past may avoid a lot of regrets.

Involvement in activities such as service organizations, volunteer work, consultation, or part-time work may be more rewarding than "play." Feelings of guilt and depression may result if these needs are unfulfilled.

Loss of spouse and friends along with physical losses will result in depression and withdrawal of varying degrees.

Observing others' dying is the only way the next generation can learn about dying.

The slowing or diminution of sensory and motor processes often causes others (and the aged person as well) to conclude that there has been a loss of intellectual ability.

B. Skills and abilities tend to become obsolete rather than lost through deterioration.

The trend toward lifelong learning will tend in the future to prevent this obsolescence from occurring.

C. Intellectual functioning may be somewhat slowed but is compensated for by extra caution and fewer mistakes due to inexperience.

D. Memory losses are for the more recent events, while events of long ago are remembered. Meaningfulness affects what is remembered.

E. Problem-solving ability is decreased because of the loss of recent memory, difficulty in making fine discriminations among stimuli, and a fear of making mistakes.

F. Learning performance may be altered by speed of response, level of motivation, and state of health. A decrease in learning ability has not been proven.

The person should be allowed to pace activities to enhance learning.

BIBLIOGRAPHY

Burnside, Irene Mortenson (ed.): *Nursing and the Aged,* McGraw-Hill Book Company, New York, 1976. A thorough and very helpful exploration of the middle-aged and old person's developmental tasks and vulnerabilities, including health problems, and the nursing process as it applies to maximize the well-being of older persons.

Butler, Robert N., and Myrna I. Lewis: *Aging and Mental Health: Positive Psychosocial Approaches,* 2d ed., The C. V. Mosby Company, St. Louis, 1977. This fine book by the physician-director of the National Institute on Aging and a social worker-gerontologist realistically presents the problems and potentials of the elderly. Assessment and intervention for individuals and groups are presented in a manner that is very helpful to nurses. Government programs, in-service education materials, and social services for the aged and those who assist them are briefly reviewed in the appendixes.

Chinn, Peggy L.: *Child Health Maintenance: Concepts in Family-Centered Care,* The C. V. Mosby Company, St. Louis, 1974. This nursing text provides broad and detailed coverage of growth and development through adolescence. The emphasis is upon health maintenance and developmental assessment and support. Health problems and the care of children with developmental disorders and common illnesses are discussed and interventions are described.

Diekelmann, Nancy: *Primary Health Care of the Well Adult,* McGraw-Hill Book Company, New York, 1977. This book's focus is on the well adult and nursing interventions to meet well-care needs of young, middle-aged, and older adults. Activity, rest, safety, environmental health, and sexuality are among the topics presented.

Erikson, Erik H.: *Childhood and Society,* 2d ed., W. W. Norton & Company, Inc., New York, 1963. This book includes a chapter presenting the classic "eight ages of man," Erikson's *either-or* formulations of developmental tasks throughout the life span.

Havighurst, Robert J.: *Developmental Tasks and Education,* 3d ed., David McKay Company, Inc., New York, 1972. This is the book in which the concept of developmental tasks was first elaborated.

Howard, Rosanne B., and Nancie H. Herbold (eds.): *Nutrition in Clinical Care,* McGraw-Hill Book Company, New York, 1978. Excellent reference about food-related behavior and nutrition throughout the life span and in various states of health and illness.

Howe, Jeanne (ed.): *Nursing Care of Adolescents,* McGraw-Hill Book Company, New York, 1979. This multiauthored book by and for nurses discusses the major substantive topics related to health and health deviations during adolescence (growth and development, response to illness and disability, nutrition, substance abuse, mental retardation, sexuality, health teaching and counseling, crisis, etc.) and describes settings and programs in which adolescents receive health care, including rehabilitation centers, street clinics, women's health clinics, juvenile detention institutions, and others.

Kastenbaum, Robert J.: *Death, Society, and Human Experience,* The C. V. Mosby Company, St. Louis, 1977. This excellent exploration of social and psychological aspects of death and dying includes discussions of "the death system" and the impact of death at various points in the life span.

Manaster, Guy J.: *Adolescent Development and the Life Tasks,* Allyn and Bacon, Inc., Boston, 1977. This readable, current psychology textbook summarizes current thinking about adolescents' physiological, cognitive, moral, sex-role, and personality development and the major developmental tasks—school, work, and interpersonal affiliations.

Murray, Ruth, and Judith Zentner: *Nursing Assessment and Health Promotion through the Life Span,* Prentice-Hall, Inc., Englewood Cliffs, N.J., 1975. Developmental characteristics at each stage of life are described and nursing supports are presented.

Neugarten, Bernice L. (ed.): *Middle Age and Aging: A Reader in Social Psychology,* University of Chicago Press, Chicago, 1968. This valuable collection of readings deals with the psychology of the life cycle and theories of aging. Subtopics include family relationships, work, leisure, retirement, and death.

Scipien, Gladys M., et al. (eds.): *Comprehensive Pediatric Nursing,* 2d ed., McGraw-Hill Book Company, New York, 1979. This exceptionally useful textbook includes chapters about the nursing process as employed in the care of children and about growth and development and effects of illness at each age and stage of childhood.

Sheehy, Gail: *Passages: Predictable Crises of Adult Life,* E. P. Dutton & Co., Inc., New York, 1976. Primarily a journalistic rather than scientific or professional book, this best-seller examines the life tasks and crises of the postadolescent years.

Shneidman, Edwin S. (ed.): *Death: Current Perspectives,* Mayfield Publishing Company, Palo Alto, Calif., 1976. This is a collection of readings from the arts, sciences, and service professions. Intended as a textbook for college students in death and dying courses, it provides an excellent overview of social, demographic, and personal attitudes and practices related to dying.

Woods, Nancy Fugate: *Human Sexuality in Health and Illness,* The C. V. Mosby Company, St. Louis, 1975. This is an excellent nursing reference on the topic of normal human sexual behavior and related nursing care, including care and counseling of ill and handicapped persons.

Part Two

Maternity Nursing

Implementation of the nursing process as a tool in providing family-centered maternity care appears still to be somewhat sporadic. There is, of course, institutional pressure being applied as accreditation review periods arrive. However, it is evident that nursing is still struggling with the responsibility for developing clear nursing plans, goals, and interventions in maternity care.

Although reasons for the difficulty in applying the nursing process will vary from place to place, nurses may recognize the following to be problems common to their setting:

1. There is slow recognition of the rapidly expanding body of knowledge of maternal, paternal, and infant psychologic and physiologic changes during these phases of human life.
2. There is still the inclination to focus only on medically oriented goals, accompanied by some anxiety about disturbing the status quo of hospital routines.
3. There is difficulty identifying, assessing, or considering interventions for normal "problems" facing every childbearing family as parenting begins.
4. The continually changing state of the fetal-maternal unit and the newly born infant make it difficult to plan in detail. This continuum becomes an important, but elusive, modifying factor in all planning during these phases of life.
5. Finally, families are not involved in identifying goals and in decision making in spite of our standards of nursing practice.

In the chapters to follow, these standards of nursing practice guide the writers as they illustrate the use of the nursing process to plan care with the family who is hoping for, rejecting, or achieving pregnancy and parenthood.

Selection of problems was made on the basis of incidence, but basic patterns are applicable, we believe, to most situations encountered in this nursing field.

ANA STANDARDS OF MATERNAL AND CHILD HEALTH NURSING PRACTICE[1]

1. Maternal and child health nursing practice is characterized by the continual questioning of the assumptions upon which practice is based, retaining those which are valid and searching for and using new knowledge.
2. Maternal and child health nursing practice is based upon knowledge of the biophysical and psychosocial development of individuals from conception through the child-rearing phase of development and upon knowledge of the basic needs for optimum development.
3. The collection of data about the health status of the client/patient is systematic and continuous. The data are accessible, communicated, and recorded.
4. Nursing diagnoses are derived from data about the health status of the client/patient.
5. Maternal and child health nursing practice recognizes deviations from expected patterns of physiologic activity and anatomic and psychosocial development.
6. The plan of nursing care includes goals derived from the nursing diagnoses.
7. The plan of nursing care includes priorities and the prescribed nursing approaches or measures to achieve the goals derived from the nursing diagnoses.
8. Nursing actions provide for client/patient participation in health promotion, maintenance, and restoration.
9. Maternal and child health nursing practice provides for the use and coordination of all services that assist individuals to prepare for responsible sexual roles.
10. Nursing actions assist the client/patient to maximize his health capabilities.
11. The client's/patient's progress or lack of progress toward goal achievement is determined by the client/patient and the nurse.

[1]Reprinted with permission from the *American Nurses' Association Standards of Maternal and Child Health Nursing Practice*. Copyright © 1973 by American Nurses' Association.

12. The client's/patient's progress or lack of progress toward goal achievement directs reassessment, reordering of priorities, new goal setting and revision of the plan of nursing care.

13. Maternal and child health nursing practice evidences active participation with others in evaluating the availability, accessibility, and acceptability of services for parents and children and cooperating and/or taking leadership in extending and developing needed services in the community.

4

Family Planning

Phyllis L. Collier

In its broadest sense, *family planning* refers to the process of choosing and planning one's fertility options. For most people this means deciding whether to have children, how many to have, and when to have them.

In the past, children were an economic necessity, natural resources were plentiful, and information was lacking about control over bodily processes. Today, societal needs and attitudes have changed, technology has improved, and natural resources are diminishing. We are now more able to control fertility, and have a greater need to do so. Fortunately, vital statistics for the past several years indicate a steadily declining birth rate. In addition behavioral and attitudinal studies have demonstrated that people from every demographic category—religious, ethnic, socioeconomic—prefer a smaller family.

A range of factors has been influential for this reduced birth rate.

1. In comparison with previous generations, there is improved technology to aid in effective family planning.
2. Abortion has been legalized in the United States and is associated with lower morbidity and mortality rates than childbirth.
3. Improved diagnostic procedures aid in early detection of pregnancy, in prediction of genetic conditions, and in finding the causes of infertility.
4. Less traumatic sterilization techniques have been developed for both males and females.
5. Legal and institutional restrictions for these services have been lessened, particularly those related to age, marital status, parity, and agreement of spouse. Laws and governmental regulations have attempted to ensure that these services are available and accessible to all persons.
6. The role of women is changing. Childbearing and rearing—"motherhood"—is only one of many alternatives now open to women.
7. Finally, it is natural that people who choose to have children wish to offer them the highest quality of life possible. Recent increases in the cost of living make it difficult for many families to provide the basic necessities of life, not to mention higher education and other advantages, to more than a few children.

Every individual is a consumer of health care, with rights and privileges inherent in that role. Optimally, decisions about fertility should be made as follows:

1. Voluntarily, without coercion.
2. With full knowledge of options available, including advantages and disadvantages, effectiveness, side effects, and long-range effects of each method, routine, or procedure.
3. With full access to the alternative chosen.
4. Without intrusion of value judgments or expression of personal preferences by the care provider.
5. With assurance of confidentiality.

One goal of health care is that every child should be planned for and wanted, and that every individual or couple should be able to make fertility decisions which suit their personal desires and ensure their optimum well-being. This goal has been institutionalized into federal regulations and needs to be carefully incorporated into the approach of every family planning care provider.

DEFINITIONS

Contraception involves the use of a method, routine, or procedure to prevent, delay, or space pregnancies. *Temporary methods* prevent conception from occurring during the time they are being used, but provide no obstacle to fertility when they are discontinued. The IUD, diaphragm, foam, condom, rhythm, and oral contraceptives fall into this category. *Permanent methods* of contraception are the surgical procedures (tubal ligation, vasectomy) which end the reproductive capacity. Although there has been some success at reversing these procedures, they should usually be considered permanent.

Categories of Methods and Procedures

I. By mode of action.
  A. Chemical barriers—foam, cream, jelly.
  B. Mechanical barriers—diaphragm, condom.
  C. Hormonal—oral contraceptives, implants, injections.
  D. Natural—rhythm.
  E. Unknown—IUD.
  F. Surgical blockage—sterilization procedures.
II. By ease of accessibility.
  A. Over-the-counter purchase—foam, jelly, cream, condom.
  B. With examination and prescription—IUD, diaphragm, oral contraceptives.
III. By relationship to the time of intercourse.
  A. Used at the time of intercourse—diaphragm, foam, jelly, cream, condom.
  B. Not related to the time of intercourse—IUD, oral contraceptives, surgical sterilization.

Menstrual Cycle

The normal menstrual cycle is altered by oral contraceptives, which inhibit ovulation and frequently cause a lighter menstrual period, and by IUDs, which may cause menstrual flow to be heavier and last longer. Therefore, knowledge of the physiology of the menstrual cycle is essential in evaluating and counseling patients who are choosing a birth control method (see Fig. 4-1).

Contraceptive Methods

For clarity and ease of reference, the temporary and permanent methods of contraception are detailed in Tables 4-1 and 4-2.

Factors Which Influence Contraceptive Use

The choices of whether or not to use a method, which method to use, and how regularly to use it may be influenced by obvious outside factors as well as by complex internal feelings. The decision involves interrelationships, feelings about one's sexuality, and personal or family goals. The following factors frequently have a role in contraceptive decision making:

I. Culture—pregnancy and children seen as a symbol of masculinity or femininity; importance of sons or daughters; pressures from family or friends to have children.
II. Religion—church against some or all artificial methods of birth control; reproductive process viewed as "God's will."
III. Daily activity pattern—sedentary/mobile; regular/irregular hours.

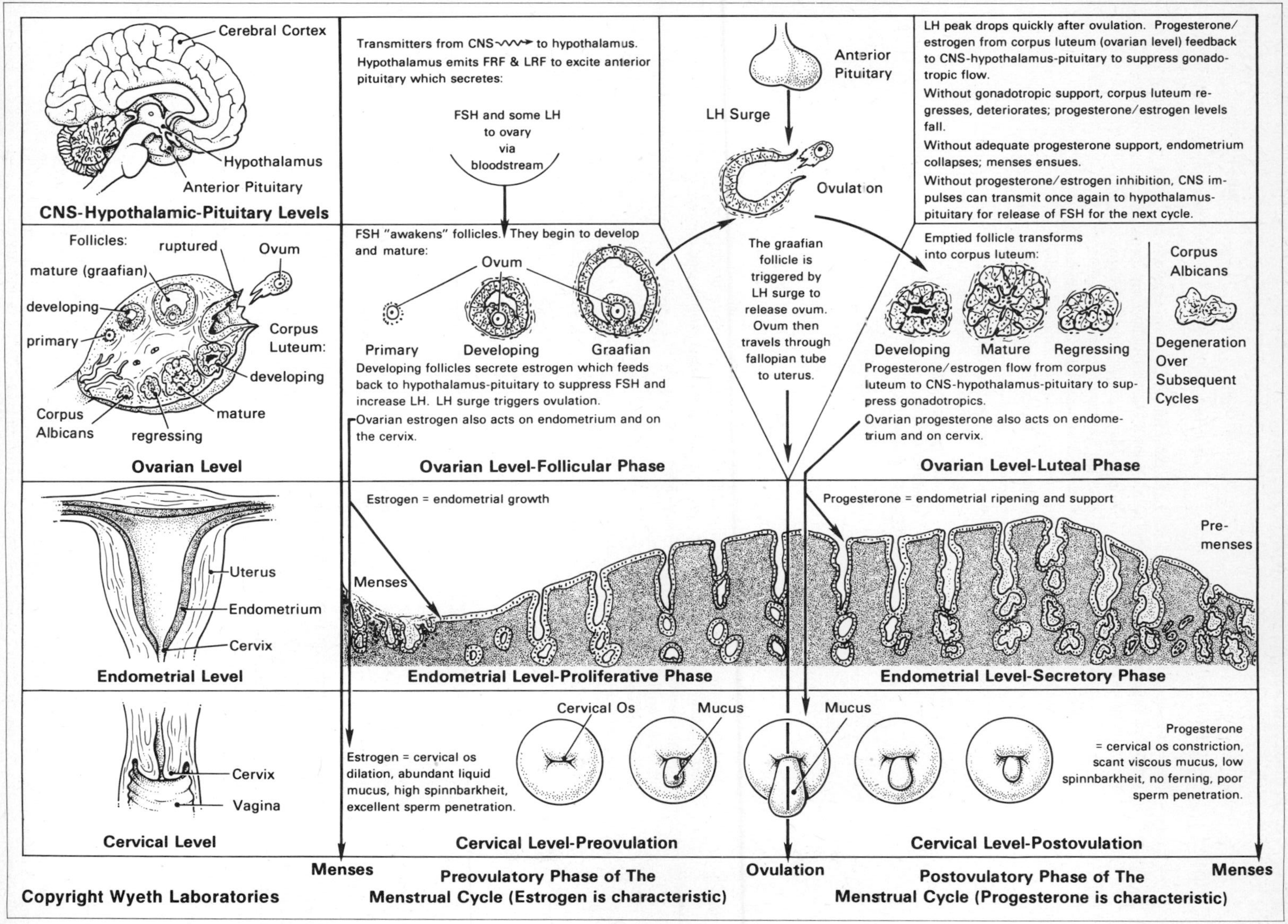

FIGURE 4-1 / The normal menstrual cycle. (Courtesy of Wyeth Laboratories.)

TABLE 4-1 / TEMPORARY METHODS OF CONTRACEPTION

Method	Description of Action	Instructions for Use	Effectiveness* Theoretical	Actual
Oral contraceptives ("the pill")	Tablets containing varying doses of estrogens and progestogens. Main action is suppression of ovulation. They also alter cervical mucus (making it hostile to sperm), and lead to an unfavorable endometrical environment.	1 pill daily for 21 days, at approximately the same time daily. Stop for 7 days. Menses will begin 1–4 days after pill has been stopped. Restart new pack of pills after 28-day cycle has been completed. Some pill packs contain 7 placebo tablets, which can be taken instead of stopping for a week. Start on fifth day of menses; stop at end of pack. For early nausea, take at bedtime or with evening meal. For weight gain, reduce salt and caloric intake.	0.1	0.2
Mini-pill	A tablet form of contraception which contains only low doses of progestogens. Ovulation is probably not inhibited, but hostile cervical mucus and an unfavorable endometrial environment provide contraceptive effect.	1 pill daily, without stopping. Start on first day of menses; stop at end of pack.	1	3
IUD	A plastic or polyethylene device in various shapes and sizes. It is inserted into uterus and usually remains there until user wishes it removed. Action of IUD is unknown, but it is thought to cause a local inflammatory reaction inside uterus, which prevents fertilized ovum from implantation. Copper and progesterone have been added to some IUDs for an extra antifertility effect (Fig. 4-2).	Approximately ½ in of IUD string will be in vagina. Insert finger to check for presence of string. (Can be checked by partner, also.) Notify care-provider if: no string is felt, string feels much longer than after insertion; plastic tip of IUD is felt protruding. Use another method of birth control until reexamined. Insert during menses; remove at any time during the cycle.	2	5
Diaphragm	A dome-shaped rubber cup on a circular metal spring. Used with spermicidal jelly or cream (Fig. 4-3), it fits over cervix and blocks entry of sperm into uterus. Must be fitted by a doctor or trained care-provider.	Prior to insertion put spermicidal jelly in cup and on rim of diaphragm. In lying, standing, or squatting position, ease diaphragm into vagina. Hook rim under symphysis pubis. Check to see that cervix is covered.	3	13

*Number of pregnancies per 100 woman-years of use. Data from S. Romney et al. (eds.), *Gynecology and Obstetrics: The Health Care of Women*, McGraw-Hill Book Company, New York, 1975, p. 552.

Early Changes/Minor Side Effects†	Other Possible Side Effects	Contraindications	Advantages/Disadvantages
Mild nausea; weight gain; breast tenderness; spotting, break-through bleeding; shorter, lighter menses; missed or "silent" periods; mood changes; chloasma	Depression Decreased libido Blood clots Heart attacks Hepatocellular tumors Prolonged amenorrhea after discontinuation	History or present evidence of thromboembolic phenomena Heart disease Hypertension Sickle cell anemia Severe depression Pregnancy Liver dysfunction or disease Impaired cerebrovascular function Known or suspected carcinoma of the breast or genital tracts Migraine headaches Epilepsy Lactation Ovarian dysfunction	Advantages: Nearest to 100% effective Regular menstrual cycle; period predictable Decreased menstrual flow Decreased dysmenorrhea and premenstrual tension Decreased iron-deficiency anemia Not related to intercourse Disadvantages: Increased susceptibility to VD, must take daily even if not having intercourse, must be started at specific time to be effective
Irregularity in amount and duration of menses, spotting between periods, missed periods	None currently known	None currently known	Advantages: No estrogen-related side effects Not related to intercourse Disadvantages: Irregular periods
Heavier and longer periods, cramps, spotting between periods	Spontaneous expulsion Perforation of uterus Embedding of IUD Pelvic inflammatory disease	Pelvic infections (acute, subacute, recurrent) Severe dysmenorrhea Acute cervicitis Uterine abnormalities Allergy to copper Wilson's disease Cervical stenosis Small uterine cavity Abnormal cervical cytology Anemia Congenital or rheumatic heart disease Pregnancy	Advantages: Little maintenance or attention needed after insertion Not related to intercourse Disadvantages: Higher rate of ectopic pregnancy Must be inserted and removed by care-provider (no self-involvement)
None	Allergy to rubber or spermicidal preparation	Damaged pelvic floor or relaxation which prohibits a proper fit Prolapsed uterus Severe cysticele, rectocele Severe retroversion or an-	Advantages: Few side effects Effective for infrequent intercourse Holds back menstrual flow during intercourse

†Usually disappear within 2–3 months.

TABLE 4-1 / TEMPORARY METHODS OF CONTRACEPTION (*Continued*)

Method	Description of Action	Instructions for Use	Effectiveness* Theoretical	Actual
	Diaphragms come in sizes 55–105 mm in gradations of 5 mm, and are inserted and removed by wearer.	If intercourse is repeated, add an applicator of foam or jelly without removing diaphragm. Do not remove diaphragm or douche for 6–8 h after last intercourse. Wash with warm water, dry, and powder with cornstarch. Check for holes or tears periodically.		
Foam, jelly, cream	Spermicidal preparations inserted into the vagina. They slow down and kill entering sperm. Can be used alone or in conjunction with other methods.	Insert an applicator full of foam, cream, or jelly into vagina within 30 min of intercourse. Insert an additional application each time before intercourse is repeated. There is no need to douche; foam or cream is absorbed into skin. If douching is desired, wait 6–8 h after last intercourse. Use with condom for increased effectiveness. Insertion by partner adds to sexual pleasure.	3	20
Condom (rubber prophylactic)	A thin rubber or skin sheath put over an erect penis. Creates a mechanical barrier which prevents sperm from getting into vagina.	Put condom on erect penis *prior to* penetration. If no tip on condom, allow $\frac{1}{2}$ in slack in front to catch semen. Withdraw soon after ejaculation. Semen is more likely to leak out when penis is flaccid. Hold on to condom when withdrawing to prevent slipping off. If condom breaks during intercourse, insert an applicator of foam or jelly immediately. Use with foam for increased effectiveness. Rolling on by partner adds to sexual pleasure.	3	15
Rhythm	A pattern of abstinence from intercourse around the time of ovulation, or greatest time of fertility. Records must be kept of menstrual cycles and calculations made for "safe days." New variations on this method include natural family planning and the Billings method, which add basal body temperature and evaluation of cervical mucus to the traditional rhythm system.	Keep record of menstrual cycles for 3–6 months. Subtract *18* from number of days in shortest cycle; subtract *11* from number of days in longest cycle. For example, cycles ranged from 28–30 days: $28 - 18 = 10$ $30 - 11 = 19$ Fertile or "unsafe" days are days 10–19 of cycle.	14	35–40

*Number of pregnancies per 100 woman-years of use. Data from S. Romney et al. (eds.), *Gynecology and Obstetrics: The Health Care of Women,* McGraw-Hill Book Company, New York, 1975, p. 552.

Early Changes/Minor Side Effects†	Other Possible Side Effects	Contraindications	Advantages/Disadvantages
		teversion of the uterus	Good for learning about female anatomy Disadvantages: Closely precedes sex act May become dislodged during intercourse Can be messy
None	Allergy to spermicidal preparation	Allergy to spermicidal preparation	Advantages: Easily available No prescription needed Helps prevent VD Disadvantages: Can be messy
None	Allergy to rubber	Allergy to rubber	Advantages: Male method, allows for shared contraception Easily available No prescription Increased protection against sexually transmitted diseases Disadvantages: Requires interruption of coitus to put on May reduce sensitivity of glans
None	None	Irregular cycles	Advantages: Acceptable for those with religious or moral objections to artificial birth control methods Promotes learning about bodily systems Disadvantages: Irregular cycles make it difficult to follow successfully Abstinence may cause sexual frustration Problem if partner not cooperative

†Usually disappear within 2–3 months.

TABLE 4-2 / PERMANENT CONTRACEPTIVE METHODS

Method	Description of Procedure	Advantages/Disadvantages	Postoperative Discomforts	Side Effects	Miscellaneous
Tubal ligation by laparotomy	Under general anesthesia an abdominal incision is made. The tubes are cut and tied, and ends may be buried in uterus. Pomeroy, Irving, and Uchida techniques are variations of this procedure.	Advantages: Can be done postpartum. Disadvantages: Must have general anesthesia for procedure. Longer hospital stay, greater cost.	General anesthesia reactions Postsurgical pain	Hemorrhage Infection	If a patient is apprehensive about this procedure, general anesthesia should be used.
Tubal ligation by laparoscopy	Under local or general anesthesia a small incision is made and CO_2 injected. A laparoscope is inserted and tubes are visualized through scope. The tubes are cauterized or clamped, and may be transected. Sometimes called "Band-Aid surgery" because this is frequently used to cover incision.	Advantages: Can be done under local anesthesia; short hospital stay (12–36 hours). Low mortality rate. Disadvantages: If extremely overweight, not eligible for this procedure.	Abdominal fullness and tenderness Shoulder, rib and abdominal soreness from CO_2 gas Constipation and fatigue Tender and itchy incision	Bowel injury Muscle trauma Infection Hemorrhage	
Vasectomy	Under general anesthesia a small incision is made on either side of scrotum. A small piece of vas deferens is removed from each side, and ends tied off. This prohibits sperm from moving beyond the incision point.	Advantages: Can be done under local anesthesia. Inexpensive. Nearly zero mortality rate. Little work time lost. Disadvantages: Not immediately effective.	Tenderness of scrotum	Infection Spermatozoan granulomas Recanalization Immune responses Hematoma	Should continue to use contraceptives until 2 sperm-free specimens have been obtained. 10 to 30 ejaculations are needed to clear genitourinary tract of sperm beyond incision point. Sperm banks are available throughout the United States, where semen can be frozen for several years. Some men have had semen frozen before having a vasectomy performed.

Notes: *Sterilization* refers to a surgical procedure which ends reproductive capability. In the female, sections of the fallopian tube are cut and tied or cauterized (tubal ligation), thus blocking the ovum from reaching the uterine cavity. In the male, the vas deferens is cut and tied (vasectomy), so that sperm are no longer ejaculated. Sterilization does *not* affect physiologic processes such as ovulation, menstruation, production of sperm, and sexual response. All sterilization procedures should be considered permanent, and should be performed only when no more children are desired. The individual or couple considering sterilization should be assisted in evaluating their motivation for this alternative and their feelings about terminating the ability to reproduce. Advantages and disadvantages, risks, and side effects of each procedure should be discussed. Most sterilization procedures have a less than 0.5% failure rate.

IV. Personality—habitual/forgetful; impulsive/methodical.
V. Relationship with partner—monogamous/more than one partner; agreement/disagreement on desirability of pregnancy and who is responsible for contraception; mutual satisfaction with method used; honesty/"gamesmanship."
VI. Feelings about body—like/dislike touching self; sense of control/lack of control over body.
VII. Comfort with sexuality—acceptance of self as a sexual being; freedom/guilt regarding sexual activity.
VIII. Myths and misinformation—all birth control interferes with sexual enjoyment; if you don't have an orgasm you won't get pregnant; birth control pills cause sterility.
IX. Psychological—pregnancy seen as a way of "getting even" with parents or partner, or as punishment for sexual behavior.
X. Balance of gratification and frustration with contraceptive method—ease/difficulty of using method; severity of side effects; degree comforted by or indifferent to effectiveness rates.

Some of this information may be routinely solicited or volunteered during an assessment interview. Because of the nature of these factors, however, their true role in contraceptive decision making may never be fully understood, either by the patient or the care provider.

ASSESSMENT

Initial assessment of the individual or family interested in conception control is done through history-taking, physical examination, laboratory tests, and exploration of goals and motivations. The assessment should be conducted in a setting which ensures privacy and dignity for the patient. The data gathered should be kept confidential. Assuring the patient of this may provide more honest and complete information. An explanation of why the questions are being asked—particularly those questions which some patients may consider intrusive—is important. The assessment can be a learning experience for the individual or couple as well as a source of information for the care provider.

I. Health history.
   A. General health history of the patient, with special attention to conditions which may contraindicate a specific birth control method (see column on contraindications, Table 4-1).
   B. Family history for conditions which may place the patient at higher risk of morbidity or mortality relative to given contraceptive methods.

   Example With a strong family history of breast cancer or diabetes, oral contraceptives may be a questionable method for use.

II. Menstrual history.
   A. Age of menarche, plus interval and length of menses.
   B. Amount of flow—heavy, moderate, light.
   C. Regularity of menses—irregular cycles may be a symptom of various conditions and should be evaluated, particularly before oral contraceptives are prescribed.
   D. Symptoms of premenstrual tension—fatigue, fluid retention, breast tenderness, weight gain, mood changes.
   E. Symptoms of midcycle ovulation—mittelschmerz, mucous viscosity, and higher pH.
   F. Dysmenorrhea—oral contraceptives may help to relieve dysmenorrhea, while an IUD may increase discomfort.
   G. Spotting or bleeding between periods—may be symptomatic of cancer, cervicitis or cervical erosion, vaginitis, traumatic intercourse, or side effects of IUDs and oral contraceptives.
   H. Changes in menstrual cycle while using a given contraceptive method.
   I. Date of onset of most recent menstrual period.

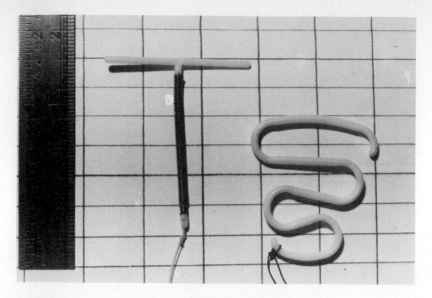

FIGURE 4-2 / Copper T (300L) is reported to have an effectiveness rating of two pregnancies per 100 woman-years, an expulsion rate of 10 percent, and a removal rate of 16 percent, resulting in a continuation rate of 71.4 percent. The Lippes Loop has an effectiveness rating of about two pregnancies per 100 woman-years of use, with a continuation rate of about 75 percent.

1. May influence when a patient can begin a chosen method. IUDs are inserted during a period and oral contraceptives are begun on day 5 of the menses, while other methods can be initiated at any time.
2. If menses is late, evaluate for pregnancy or other conditions prior to prescribing contraception.

III. Obstetric history.
   A. Number of times pregnant.
   B. Pregnancy outcomes—live births, stillbirths, spontaneous abortions, voluntary abortions. Problem patterns can be noted, such as habitual abortions. More than one voluntary interruption of pregnancy may indicate a need for special counseling regarding patient attitudes and practices relating to conception control.
   C. Types of delivery—vaginal, cesarean section.
   D. Complications of pregnancy or delivery.
   E. Birth weight of children: A pattern of high birth weights may indicate a diabetic or prediabetic condition in mother. Evaluate before prescribing oral contraceptives. Low birth weight may be associated with failure-to-thrive syndrome or delayed growth and development.
   F. Number and general health status of living children—provide opportunity for case finding and referral if problems are noted.
   G. Problems with conception—risks of amenorrhea after going off the pill may contraindicate oral contraceptives for a patient who desires a future pregnancy, but who has a history of problem conception.
   H. Number of children desired in the future, and at what intervals.
      1. Discussion may help a patient who is vague or unsure about future conception clarify wishes.
      2. Desired timing for future pregnancies may influence method chosen. If pregnancy is desired within a short period of time, mechanical methods carry less risk of conception-delaying side effects. If no further children are desired,

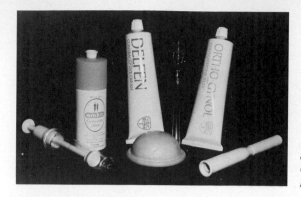

FIGURE 4-3 / Types of foam, jelly, and cream to be used with the diaphragm for chemical contraception. (*From E. J. Dickason and M.O. Schult, Maternal and Infant Care, McGraw-Hill Book Company, New York, 1975.*)

sterilization frees the individual or couple from both the need to use and the cost of temporary contraceptive methods.

IV. Contraceptive history.
  A. Contraceptive method(s) presently or previously used—brand, type, size, or dose. If these are unknown, have the patient describe it by color, shape, type of package, or container.
  B. Satisfaction with method(s).
  C. Length of time used.
  D. Side effects experienced—minor, major.
  E. Reasons for discontinuation.
    1. Planned pregnancy.
    2. Medical complications.
    3. Partner dissatisfaction.
    4. Fear of side effects.
    5. Personal patterns and preferences.
V. Sexual history.
  A. Has patient ever had intercourse? If not, may wish to discuss feelings about becoming sexually active.
  B. Frequency of intercourse.
    1. Patients having infrequent intercourse may not wish to use a method which is active in the body at all times (pills, IUD).
    2. A highly sexually active patient with multiple partners may wish to use a method which is not related to the time of intercourse.
  C. Diversity of sexual contacts.
    1. If in a steady relationship, patient may wish to involve partner in decision making.
    2. If no steady relationship, decision will be more independent.
  D. Presence of pain or bleeding with intercourse may indicate infections, trauma, or psychological factors.
  E. Interference of contraceptive method(s) with sexual pleasure.
    1. Dislike of a method because of interference may cause a patient to use it irregularly or discontinue it altogether.
    2. Partners may not agree about the same contraceptive methods.
  F. Sexual problems.
    1. Lack of communication between partners about sexual satisfaction.
    2. Fear of being "unnatural" or perverted because of sexual experimentation and noncoital intercourse.
    3. Sexual dysfunction—orgasmic impairment, vaginismus, sexual anesthesia, impotence.
VI. Physical examination: The physical examination and laboratory work are geared to maintaining the general health of the patient, ruling out contraindications to specific

birth control methods, and detection of disease. The interval and content of the follow-up visits depend on the contraceptive method being used and the agency providing the service. Initial and annual examinations should include, but not be limited to:

    A. Auscultation of heart and lungs.

    B. Thyroid palpation.

    C. Inspection and palpation of breast and axillary glands, including breast self-examination.

    D. Examination of extremities.

    E. Abdominal and pelvic (bimanual and rectovaginal) examination.

    F. Height, weight, and blood pressure.

VII. Laboratory tests.

    A. Hemoglobin/hematocrit.

    B. Urinalysis for sugar and protein.

    C. Papanicolaou (Pap) smear for detection of cancer, other smears for vaginal infections, evaluation of estrogen level.

    D. Endocervical culture for *Neisseria gonorrhoeae* (rectum and/or throat, if indicated).

    E. Serologic test for syphilis, if appropriate.

    F. Pregnancy test, if indicated.

VIII. Exploration of knowledge and motivation.

    A. What is the patient's knowledge regarding anatomy and physiology, and contraceptive processes?

    B. Stated reasons for desiring contraception.

    C. Personal likes and dislikes regarding methods.

    D. How serious are patient and partner about preventing conception? Definite response, or ambivalence?

    E. Feelings about touching own body.

    F. Cultural and family traditions of childbearing.

    G. Fears about side effects.

    H. Feelings about ability to successfully use selected method of contraception.

    I. Daily activity patterns.

    J. Degree of involvement or influence of partner in decision making.

PROBLEMS

    I. Unplanned or undesired pregnancy may cause stress to an individual or couple, and interfere with attainment of life goals.

    II. Lack of knowledge about anatomy and physiology of the reproductive system is a deterrent to full understanding of a contraceptive routine.

    III. The partner may have preferences, motivations, and fears regarding pregnancy and contraception which differ from those of the patient.

    IV. Contraindications—medical or other—may prohibit a patient from using the contraceptive method most preferred.

    V. The pelvic examination and methods initiated during the examination (IUD insertion, diaphragm fitting) can cause anxiety.

    VI. Reluctance to use any method of birth control may be present if use is perceived as an admission of sexual activity, or if use is seen as destroying the naturalness and spontaneity of sex.

    VII. Ambivalence about pregnancy, one's body, and one's self as a sexual being may influence the ability to control fertility.

DIAGNOSIS

    I. Patient and partner may be highly motivated to initiate and maintain a successful contraceptive regimen.

II. Lack of full information and understanding about contraceptive options available may result in a choice not compatible with the patient's life-style.

III. Client may be unable to use a method because of medical contraindications, both actual or imagined.

GOALS OF CARE

Immediate

I. Physical status of client will be assessed, especially if this is the first entrance into health care.

II. Client will be instructed in methods of contraception so that an informed choice may be made.

III. Client will be oriented to initial procedures and office or clinic routines.

IV. Sexual partner will be involved in decision making when possible.

V. Client will receive support during gynecologic examination.

VI. Client should understand method chosen, and will be able to describe possible side effects to nurse.

Long-range

I. Client is to be advised of follow-up schedule.

II. Client will be referred for other medical or surgical problems as identified in initial visit.

III. Client and nurse will interpret how long-range goals may be reached, after identifying client's contraceptive goals.

IV. Staff will continue to assess correct use on part of client.

Example The highest "dropout" or method discontinuation rates occur during the first 3 months of method use. Much of this is due to poor adjustment to the method, and apprehension regarding minor side effects. Clients who are well informed of these potential changes and minor side effects, who have been given some palliative measures for relief, and who have been encouraged to bear with them while the body adjusts are less likely to discontinue using the method. It is important that the client be seen sometime during the first 3 months to provide encouragement for continuation of the chosen method.

INTERVENTION

I. Orient patient to methods in easily understood language.

A. Initially, emphasize information which will be helpful in decision making, but which will not overwhelm the patient with detail.

Example When presenting preliminary information on oral contraceptives, stress the need to take a pill regularly each day. Save information on when to start the pill, how to take it, what to do if pill is missed, etc., until the patient has actually chosen to use the pill as a contraceptive.

B. Clients should be given background information about anatomy and physiology in relation to contraceptive use.

C. Use of charts, drawings, and models help to make information more realistic and understandable. Actual birth control methods should be available for patients to see and handle.

D. Group education allows a patient to receive information and share experiences with persons in similar circumstances.

II. Prepare client for experience of choosing and being fitted for a contraceptive method.

A. Describe clinic routines—first interview, laboratory work, education and counseling services, fee payment (if appropriate).

B. Explain *who* will do each procedure and *where* in the facility it will be performed.

III. Provide support during gynecologic examination, support which includes the following nursing actions:

A. Explain how a gynecologic examination is done and what procedures are included—speculum insertion, Pap smear, culture, breast and bimanual vaginal, abdominal examinations—especially if it is the patient's first examination.

B. Allow the patient to meet the examiner while sitting in an upright position, *not* while flat on her back with feet in the stirrups.

C. Explain each step of the examination as it is being done.

D. Suggest relaxation measures such as deep breathing if the patient appears to be tense or anxious.

E. Incorporate patient education into the routine; have the patient participate when possible, such as during the breast examination.

F. Inform the patient of her "normality" during the course of the examination; it is more reassuring to hear that "your uterus and ovaries seem to be perfectly normal" than to hear silence.

G. *Ask* the patient if she has any questions about the examination findings, contraceptive methods, etc.; some patients are too shy to ask.

H. If the contraceptive method is initiated during the examination, provide additional care.

    1. Diaphragm fitting—show the patient positions and techniques for reinsertion of the diaphragm. Provide ample time for practice at her pace, without rushing (Fig. 4-4).

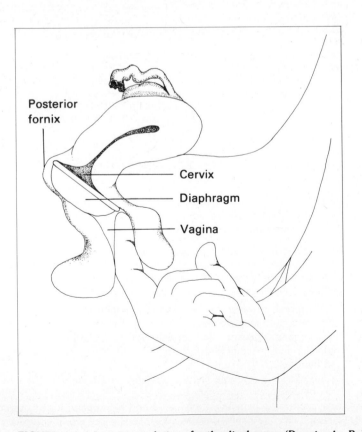

FIGURE 4-4 / Insertion technique for the diaphragm. (*Drawing by P. Rodriguez-Lovink.*)

2. IUD insertion—note signs of tenseness, pain, or fainting during insertion. When there is no discomfort, instruct patient on how to check IUD string. Provide for rest period on table if necessary.

IV. Ensure that client understands the method's use and any side effects.

   A. Demonstrate method, and have patient repeat instructions and information.

   B. Provide literature along with the contraceptive information which the patient can refer to at a later time.

   C. If contraceptive method has been initiated during examination, review previous instructions and add additional details.

   > ***Example*** During the fitting of a diaphragm the emphasis was on learning to handle the diaphragm and insert and remove it. Details on use can now be added, with greater attention from the patient.

   D. If surgical sterilization is chosen, prepare the patient and partner for procedures.

V. Provide homegoing instruction on method satisfaction. For example:

   A. Stress that the patient must give the body time to adjust to the birth control method, and time to become comfortable with it, while incorporating it into the daily routine.

   B. Make sure the patient understands that if she has a continuing problem (longer than 2 to 4 months) with a method, she should ask to try another dose or brand of that method, rather than stopping it altogether. There are 20 to 30 kinds of oral contraceptives on the market, in varying doses. One should be agreeable to the body's system, barring medical contraindications.

   C. Tell her that it is not necessary to continue indefinitely with a method if she or her partner doesn't like it. Motivations, circumstances, and personal preferences change, and she can shift to another method.

   D. Also, stress that patient should not discontinue her method without consulting her care provider. Problems related to contraception can frequently be resolved without discontinuing the method.

   E. And, last, stress that no question related to the process of contraception is too simple to ask. It's her body and her life, and she has the right to ask.

EVALUATION

I. Successful contraception results in absence of conception.

II. Patient returns dissatisfied and requests a new method.

   A. Assess reasons for dissatisfaction.

   B. Assist in obtaining new method.

III. Patient becomes pregnant.

   A. Accepts pregnancy.

   1. Provide beginning prenatal teaching.

   2. Assist in seeking prenatal care.

   3. Promote acceptance of pregnant state.

   B. Seeks abortion.

   1. Provide counseling.

   2. Assist with location of a care facility.

BIBLIOGRAPHY

Boston Women's Health Book Collective: *Our Bodies, Ourselves,* 2d ed., Simon & Schuster, Inc., New York, 1976, chap. 10. Includes detailed information on the menstrual cycle and methods of birth control. Written in lay language; has good diagrams and pictures.

Britt, Sylvia S.: "Fertility Awareness: Four Methods of Natural Family Planning," *Journal of Obstetric, Gynecologic, and Neonatal Nursing* **14:**9–18, March/April, 1977. Describes four types of "natural family planning"—the basal body temperature, calendar rhythm, ovulation, and "sympto-thermal" methods.

Hatcher, Robert, et al.: *Contraceptive Technology 1976–77,* 8th ed., Irvington Publishers, Inc., New York, 1976. Includes detailed information on philosophy and benefits of family planning, the menstrual cycle, contraceptive methods, abortion, sterilization, and sexually transmitted diseases. Incorporates suggestions for teaching and counseling. Updated edition published every 1 to 2 years. An excellent resource book.

Luker, Kristin: *Taking Chances: Abortion and the Decision Not to Contracept,* University of California Press, Berkeley, 1975. Explores the process of contraceptive decision making, with emphasis on social and cultural factors which are influential. Includes implications for care providers.

Manisoff, Mariam: *Family Planning: A Teaching Guide for Nurses,* Planned Parenthood, New York, 1969. Contains a historical view of family planning attitudes, laws, and practices. Speaks especially to the role of the nurse in family planning, in both organization and delivery of services.

Okrent Shirley: *A Clinical Guide to the Intrauterine Device and the Vaginal Diaphragm,* Shirley Okrent, Wantagh, N.Y., 1974.

————: *A Clinical Guide to Oral Contraception,* Shirley Okrent, Wantagh, N.Y., 1971. This booklet and the one preceding it are geared especially to nurse-midwives and nurse-practitioners who are in a position to initiate and manage a contraceptive regimen for patients. Include assessment of a patient for an IUD or oral contraceptive, technical details about those methods, and causes and treatment of minor and major side effects.

Tyrer, Louise: "Advantages and Disadvantages of Nonprescription Contraceptives," *Medical Aspects of Human Sexuality* 11(7):55–56, July 1977. An excellent article for those who counsel patients using diaphragms, foams, jellies, and condoms—methods where high motivation and consistent use are important. Suggestions for history-taking, education, and follow-up are given.

Williams, Juanita: *Psychology of Women: Behavior in a Biosocial Context,* W. W. Norton & Company, Inc., New York, 1977. Includes portions of female growth and development, the menstrual cycle, female sexuality, and birth control.

5

The Infertile Family

Christine Mitchell

Infertility is often a complex life crisis which is psychologically threatening, financially expensive, emotionally stressful, and often physically painful. It involves an individual's feelings about sexuality, self-image, and self-esteem. It necessitates the exploration and assessment of a very sensitive, private area of a couple's relationship. Current emphasis on curbing a rapidly expanding population seems to diminish concern for and interest in the family experiencing infertility. However, family planning in the broadest sense encompasses the choice by a couple regarding whether they will have children, as well as how many children, and at what intervals they are desired. Nurses can play a significant role in assessing, planning, and caring for the infertile family.

DEFINITION

Infertility is a relative term which indicates that a couple has difficulty achieving conception either due to a diagnosed cause which is amenable to treatment or due to unknown factor(s); no sterility having been identified. In contrast, *sterility* indicates the incapacity to conceive and may be the final diagnosis of the infertile man or woman.

Primary infertility is the inability of a couple to conceive after at least 1 year of sexual relations without contraception.

Secondary infertility indicates that a couple has already conceived one or more times (regardless of outcome), but further unrestricted efforts have failed to achieve another conception.

Incidence and Statistics

Information gathered in the United States and other countries keeping reliable records indicates that 15 percent of the population of childbearing age is involuntarily childless (approximately 8.5 million Americans). No cause for infertility can be determined in 5 to 10 percent of all married couples who are medically healthy. Fifty percent of couples seen at large infertility clinics will become pregnant (1, 2).

Normal Factors Which Influence Fertility

I. Age of the female partner: Fertility peaks at approximately 24 years of age, diminishes gradually from 24 to 30, and declines rapidly after the age of 30. Pregnancy rarely occurs after 50 years of age. Normal infertility is coincident with menopause.

II. Age of the male partner: Fertility peaks at approximately 25 years of age, and declines gradually after age 40, but may continue late into old age.

III. Frequency of intercourse: Frequent ejaculation enhances the fertility potential of male semen with respect to degree and quality of motility, and ease of conception (3).

    A. The proportion of conceptions achieved at almost any age level rises with frequency of intercourse.

    B. It is estimated that sexual intercourse averaging four times per week is most likely to produce conception in a 6-month period.

    C. Most married couples report an average of intercourse twice weekly.

IV. Length of exposure: Of average couples not using contraceptive measures, 25 percent conceive the first month, 65 percent conceive in 6 months, 75 percent in 9 months, 80 percent in a year, and 90 percent in 18 months (4).

V. Processes necessary for pregnancy:

  A. The male must produce a sufficient number of normal, motile spermatozoa which have access through patent pathways to be discharged on ejaculation from the urethra.

  B. The female must produce a normal fertilizable ovum which must enter the fallopian tube within a few hours to become fertilized.

  C. Spermatozoa must be deposited in the female in such a way that they reach and penetrate the cervical secretion, and ascend through the uterus to the tube at the time in the cycle appropriate for fertilization of the ovum.

  D. The resulting conceptus must move into the uterus and implant in an adequately developed endometrium, and there undergo normal development.

VI. Causes of fertility disturbance:

  A. Factors causing male fertility disturbance:
    1. Mumps accompanied by orchitis.
    2. Toxoplasmosis.
    3. Syphilis.
    4. Diseases accompanied by high fever (e.g., diphtheria, typhoid).
    5. Occupational exposure to extreme heat (e.g., firefighters).
    6. Injury to testicles.
    7. Hydrocele, varicocele, testicular tumors and/or cysts.
    8. Phimosis.
    9. Hypospadius.
    10. Epispadius.
    11. Cryptorchidism.
    12. Prostatitis.
    13. Epididymitis.
    14. Cystic fibrosis.
    15. Nervous system diseases (e.g., multiple sclerosis).
    16. Spinal injuries.
    17. Retrograde ejaculations.
    18. Autoagglutination of sperm.
    19. Psychological impotence.
    20. Constrictive underclothing.

  B. Factors causing female fertility disturbance:
    1. Severe vaginitis.
    2. Atresia of the hymenal membrane.
    3. Hyperacidity of vaginal secretions.
    4. Chronic cervicitis.
    5. Inadequate cervical mucus.
    6. Cervical stenosis.
    7. Malformations or absence of the uterus.
    8. Tuberculosis endometritis.
    9. Insufficient transformation of the endometrium.
    10. Fibromatous uterus.
    11. Advanced cervical or uterine cancer.
    12. Postabortal infections.
    13. Pelvic inflammatory disease.
    14. Infection and inflammation of the fallopian tubes (salpingitis).
    15. Tubal stenosis or obstruction.
    16. Endometriosis at the uterotubal juncture.
    17. Some ovarian tumors (e.g., arrhenoblastoma).
    18. Stein-Leventhal syndrome (polycystic ovaries).
    19. Ovarian endometriosis.
    20. Production of pathologic ova.

21. "Post-pill amenorrhea."
22. Anovulatory cycles.
23. Antispermatozoan antibody formation.

C. Factors causing fertility disturbance in either the male or female partner or both:
   1. Inadequate or inaccurate sexual knowledge.
   2. Marital maladjustment.
   3. Malnutrition.
   4. Fat, mineral, and/or vitamin deficiency.
   5. Chronic alcoholism.
   6. Nicotine poisoning.
   7. Metal poisoning (e.g., arsenic, lead).
   8. Dye poisoning (e.g., aniline).
   9. Some drug intoxications (morphine, cocaine, quinine, hormones, antineoplastic agents).
   10. Radiation.
   11. Sex chromosomal aberrations (e.g., Klinefelter's syndrome, Turner's syndrome).
   12. Pituitary disturbances.
   13. Thyroid malfunction.
   14. Adrenal dysfunctions.
   15. Gonorrhea with complications.
   16. Severe cardiac disturbances.
   17. Severe chronic nephritis.
   18. Diabetes.
   19. Anemia.
   20. Active tuberculosis.
   21. Extraordinary physical and/or mental stress.
   22. Long-lasting psychic abnormalities.

ASSESSMENT

The purposes of an infertility investigation are to provide a definitive diagnosis if possible, furnish a relative prognosis, and afford a basis for effective intervention. Medical consultation and investigation should be sought after 1 year of undesired infertility in a young couple of childbearing age; earlier for a couple over 30. Both partners should participate in the progressive investigation and subsequent treatment. The length of time required for investigation is usually between 6 and 18 months. The cost is variable but should be estimated and discussed with the couple, both initially and as the investigation proceeds.

Infertility investigation proceeds in progressive steps until a cause(s) has been determined. Most investigations include the following steps: initial interview and general physical exam, basal body temperature (BBT) charting begun and semen specimen analyzed, urinary and blood analyses of both partners, evaluation of genetic status, testing of cervical factors, testing of uterine factors, and testing of testicular factors, not always in this exact sequence.

I. Initial assessment of the infertile family.
   A. Objectives for the first visit: data collection through interview.
      1. Evaluate extent of sexual knowledge.
      2. Determine frequency of intercourse and duration of infertility.
      3. Assess couple's sexual practices influencing fertility.
         a. Note whether coitus regularly occurs in mid cycle.
         b. Collect data regarding libido, douching, and techniques for coitus.
      4. Collect data on past related physical history.
         a. Note relevant sexual history with other partners and/or previous marriage, including contraceptive use.
         b. Gynecologic, menstrual, and obstetric history.
         c. Urogenital history.

5. Appraise environment for possible causative factors (e.g., radiation, heavy metal poisoning, chronic alcoholism, nicotine intoxication).
6. Assess psychosocial status.
   a. Note pertinent sociocultural beliefs and values.
   b. Assess coping mechanisms.
   c. Assess motivations for childbearing.
   d. Note individual's and couple's expectations of infertility investigation.
   e. Identify support system.
B. A general physical exam will also usually be done on each partner during the first visit, noting the following:
   1. General stature and development of secondary sex characteristics.
   2. Size, position, and condition of reproductive organs.
   3. Signs of infection, or any factors related to known causes of infertility.
II. Evaluation of female partner.
   A. Basal body temperature (BBT) chart.
      1. An oral temperature is taken by the female every day before rising, at approximately the same time.
      2. During a normal ovulatory cycle, body temperature usually is low during menses and the first phase, drops to its lowest point at ovulation, rises approximately 1°F during the 24-h ovulatory phase, and maintains that higher temperature level during the final phase of the cycle, until menstruation occurs (see Fig. 5-1).
      3. An anovulatory cycle lacks the characteristic thermal shift and may or may not result in menses (see Fig. 5-2).
      4. BBT charting is usually continued throughout investigation or until pregnancy (see Fig. 5-3).
   B. Postcoital (or Huhner's) test.
      1. Mucus is aspirated from the cervix 3 to 24 h after coitus.

FIGURE 5-1 / Basal body temperature chart illustrating the thermal shift indicative of ovulation in a normal cycle. X = menstruation, O = ovulation.

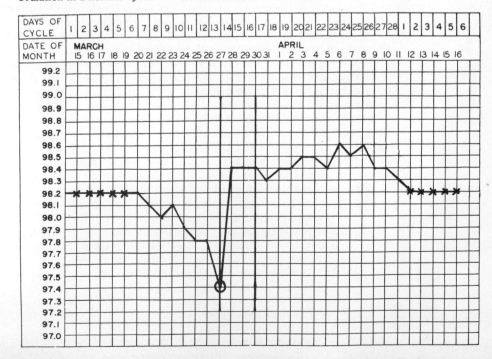

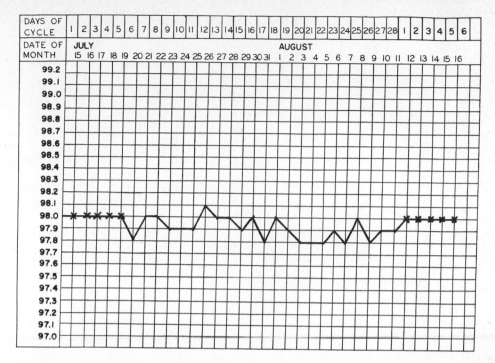

FIGURE 5-2 / **Basal body temperature chart illustrating an anovulatory (monophasic) cycle.** X = menstruation.

2. The test is timed to coincide with ovulation as determined by the BBT chart, and sperm survival is evaluated.
3. Cervical mucus is evaluated for evidence of ovulation.
   a. Spinnbarkeit property: A thin, continuous thread is formed by the cervical mucus as it is pulled apart. The time at which the mucus can be stretched to its maximum length (8 cm or greater) indicates ovulation. This characteristic is a function of increasing levels of estrogen.
   b. Fern test (also called the "arborization phenomenon"): Cervical mucus crystallizes into a fernlike pattern when allowed to dry on a slide; also an indication of the presence of estrogen.
C. Tubal insufflation.
   1. Carbon dioxide is passed through the cervix to the uterus and tubes, while the gas pressure is monitored via a manometer.
   2. At a given pressure carbon dioxide normally passes freely through the fallopian tubes due to peristaltic conditions (causing the manometer needle to fluctuate) and into the abdominal cavity where it is absorbed into the bloodstream (causing a fall in pressure). It is eventually expelled from the body via the respiratory system.
   3. Gas sounds may be heard by placing a stethoscope on the abdomen.
   4. Temporary blockage of gas may be caused by tubal spasm and/or nervousness. After a brief wait, additional attempts are made.
   5. Gas pressure falls even if only one tube is patent.
   6. This relatively painless test is often done in a clinic or physician's office. It may be done at the same time as dilatation and curettage.
D. Hysterosalpingography.
   1. Radiography follows the passage of a water-soluble radiopaque substance (iodine), injected through a cannula which is inserted into the cervix, through the uterus and fallopian tubes with peritoneal spill in 10 to 15 min.

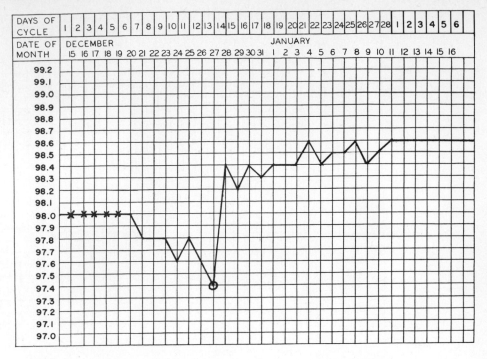

FIGURE 5-3 / Basal body temperature chart illustrating ovulation followed by conception. X = menstruation, O = ovulation.

    2. X-rays are taken at various intervals.
    3. This test is frequently done by the radiology department in a clinic, with light premedication for relaxation.
  E. Endometrial biopsy.
    1. A small piece of endometrium is removed for examination and testing for tuberculosis and progesterone influence on the corpus luteum.
    2. This may be done during dilatation and curettage under general anesthesia, requiring overnight hospitalization, or a specimen may be taken, using a small curette, in an outpatient clinic or physician's office.
    3. The biopsy is taken late in the cycle, just before menstruation, to assess the corpus luteum function, and the state of the endometrium for implantation.
  F. Laparoscopy.
    1. A laparoscope is inserted through a small abdominal incision near the umbilicus.
    2. Simultaneously, methylene blue dye is passed through the cervix, to travel through the uterus, fallopian tubes, and into the peritoneal cavity, if the reproductive tract is patent.
    3. This test detects cysts, endometriosis, adhesions, tumors, and other obstructions or abnormalities.
    4. Overnight hospitalization is necessary. This test is done under general anesthesia.
    5. Ovarian and endometrial biopsies may be taken at the same time.
III. Evaluation of male partner.
  A. Semen analysis.
    1. Total ejaculate.
      a. A specimen is obtained by masturbation (not via condom).
      b. Semen is collected in a clean, dry, glass container after a period of abstinence corresponding to usual coital frequency.
      c. Normal nonuniformity of sperm distribution requires that no part of the ejaculate be lost.

    d. The specimen must be examined as soon after ejaculation as possible. Some require examination within 30 to 60 min; no longer than 3 h after collection.

    e. Ejaculate will be analyzed for:

        (1) Sperm motility—most important factor. At least 40 percent must show good forward progression.

        (2) Sperm count—should be greater than 20 million per milliliter. The norm is 60 to 120 million per milliliter.

        (3) Semen volume—should be greater than 1 mL and less than 4 mL.

        (4) Sperm morphology—60 to 70 percent should have normal appearance.

    f. Frequently three or more specimens will be requested.

  2. Split ejaculate.

    a. The process of seminal emission entails discharge of sequential fractions (i.e., secretion of urethral and bulbourethral (Cowper's) glands, prostatic secretion, testicular and epididymal secretion, and finally vesicle secretion).

    b. Semen is collected as described above, except that the first part of the ejaculate is collected in one container, and the remaining ejaculate in a second (or third) container.

    c. The specimen is evaluated for normal sequence, sperm concentration, citric acid, nucleic acid, acid phosphatase, and fructose.

B. Testicular biopsy.

  1. This involves the surgical removal of a small piece of tissue from one or both testicles for microscopic evaluation.

  2. Bilateral testicular biopsy is indicated in males with azoospermia for the following reasons:

    a. To determine whether spermatogenesis occurs.

    b. To ascertain degree of tubular changes.

    c. To confirm diagnosis of hypogonadism.

    d. To determine suitability for endocrine or surgical therapy.

    e. To confirm prognosis.

  3. The trauma of biopsy may cause permanent damage to spermatogenesis.

C. Less frequently used diagnostic measures include:

  1. Urethral calibration.

  2. Cystourethroscopy.

  3. Vasography.

IV. Diagnostic testing of both partners.

A. Hormone determinations via 24-h urine collection.

  1. Androgen production: normal range is 9 to 22 mg per 24 h in male urine, 6 to 15 mg per 24 h in female urine.

  2. Estrogen production: normal range is 4 to 60 mg per 24 h in female urine (about 45 mg in pregnancy), 4 to 25 mg per 24 h in male urine (5).

B. Evaluation of genetic status.

  1. Buccal smears.

  2. Chromosomal analysis of peripheral blood.

C. When indicated, tests for thyroid function [protein-bound iodine (PBI), T_3 uptake, T_4, ^{131}I, and basal metabolic rate (BMR)], pituitary function, and adrenal function may be performed. Often these are indirect measures, i.e., the test focuses on indicators of a selected hormone's activity, such as abnormal serum sodium levels in adrenal insufficiency.

V. Treatment methods and interventions.

A. Female partner.

  1. Drugs used to stimulate ovulation in the anovulatory woman:

    a. Clomiphene citrate (Clomid) is administered if there is adequate endogenous estrogen and follicular function, but inadequate cyclic stimulation by pituitary gonadotropins. Clomiphene citrate is a nonsteroid estrogen antagonist that stimulates the release of a woman's own endogenously produced gonadotropins.

        (1) The woman should be admitted for endocrine studies, culdoscopy, and lavage of the oviducts prior to clomiphene therapy.

        (2) Use of clomiphene is contraindicated in the presence of an ovarian cyst.

        (3) Side effects include abnormal ovarian enlargement, multiple ovulations (usually double), spontaneous abortions, nausea and vomiting, increased weight gain, mittelschmerz, hot flashes, and visual disturbances.

        (4) Pelvic examination is performed before each course of clomiphene therapy to evaluate the size and consistency of the ovaries.

        (5) The couple should not attempt to conceive during the first treatment cycle because of the increased incidence of abortion.

        (6) Response to clomiphene is measured by BBT charts and/or endometrial biopsy.

        (7) The usual dosage of clomiphene ranges from 50 to 150 mg per day taken during specific days of the menstrual cycle; some authorities recommend days 5 through 10, others recommend administration on days 7 to 14.

        (8) Ovulation generally occurs within 2 to 10 days following the last dose of clomiphene.

        (9) Clomiphene may be prescribed and administered in association with other drug(s) such as human menopausal gonadotropin (HMG, or Pergonal) and/or human chorionic gonadotropin (HCG).

       (10) The safety of long-term administration of clomiphene has not yet been determined. It is currently advised that continuous therapy not exceed 1 year.

    b. Pergonal is administered if there is primary gonadotropin insufficiency.

        (1) A complete gynecologic and endocrinologic evaluation, including uterine curettage, should be done before Pergonal is prescribed.

        (2) Recommended for use only following failure of clomiphene therapy.

2. Surgical interventions indicated in the correction of some causes of female infertility:

    a. The woman with an "incompetent cervix" may be technically fertile but unable to bear children.

        (1) There is usually a history of midtrimester abortions and cervical dilation noted on hysterography.

        (2) The placement of nonabsorbable Dacron mesh (Mersilene) necessitates delivery by cesarean section.

        (3) The placement of temporary polyethylene tubules, which may be severed at the 37th to 38th week of gestation, permits pelvic delivery.

        (4) These procedures should not be done prior to 14 weeks gestation to avoid securing an imperfect ovum.

    b. Congenital abnormalities of the uterus (bicornuate, septate, and double uteri) may necessitate surgical reconstruction.

        (1) Surgery is indicated if no other cause for infertility is discovered and/or there is a history of spontaneous abortions, as well as evidence of a malformed uterus.

        (2) The infertile couple are advised to avoid conception until 8 to 12 months after surgery.

    c. Tuboplasty may be recommended if diagnostic studies reveal normal male fertility and normal female function, except for nonpatent tubes.

        (1) Closed oviducts may be evidenced by insufflation and x-ray (tubograms).

        (2) Lavage of the oviducts by culdoscopy or laparoscopy is usually attempted before proceeding to tuboplasty.

        (3) The general term tuboplasty may be used for several types of reconstructive surgery performed on the oviduct (salpingolysis, salpingoplasty, midsegment reconstruction, and cornual or interstitial resection).

        (4) The formation of adhesions following tuboplasty is a major cause of failure to achieve pregnancy after surgery.

    d. Surgical intervention for the infertile woman diagnosed with Stein-Leventhal syndrome (polycystic ovarian disease) involves an ovarian wedge resection.

        (1) Drug therapy may precede or coincide with surgery.

        (2) This procedure yields widely divergent results; however, average success is high, with restoration of menstrual regularity in 80 percent and attainment of desired pregnancy in 63 percent of infertile women (6).

        (3) If wedge resection does not produce ovulation, the woman's ability to become pregnant is seriously diminished.

    e. Surgical treatment of endometriosis is generally conservative.

        (1) Endometriosis usually progresses slowly over a period of years, is rarely malignant, and regresses at menopause.

        (2) Intervention depends on the severity of endometriosis and the necessity for conserving or promoting childbearing function.

        (3) The incidence of sterility associated with endometriosis is 30 to 40 percent; however, with conservative surgical intervention about one-third of these women subsequently conceive (7).

        (4) Progestational agents may be administered 6 to 12 weeks prior to surgery to soften adhesions.

        (5) Following a successful conception, endometriosis is frequently resolved.

B. Male partner.

  1. Although the male factor is the largest single cause of infertility (8), current understanding and treatment for the infertile male lags behind that for the infertile female. Various drugs may be utilized in an attempt to indirectly or directly influence the quality of the semen.

    a. Improvement of the general health status (as in conditions of obesity, allergy, general or recurrent infection, hypo- or hyperthyroidism) may be assisted by the use of drug therapy.

    b. L-Triiodothyronine (Cytomel) may be used in subfertile men with thyroid dysfunction in an attempt to improve semen quality.

    c. Testosterone propionate may be prescribed to suppress gonadotropin function, seeking subsequent "rebound," or the release of large amounts of gonadotropins, after administration of the drug is discontinued.

    d. Gonadotropin therapy (HMG and/or HCG) may be utilized to stimulate spermatogenesis and increase sperm concentration in oligospermic men.

    e. No presently available drug has been conclusively shown to significantly or consistently improve semen quality.

    f. Potential risks and side effects of drug therapy in the treatment of male infertility must be carefully considered.

  2. Surgical intervention in the treatment of male infertility:

    a. Orchiopexy for undescended testicle, and correction of hypospadius, epispadius, congenital chordee, and other deformities of the penis should be corrected at an early age.

    b. The repair of urethral strictures, fistulas, and diverticuli may be necessary to improve the conduit for the ejaculate.

    c. Varicocelectomy may be performed to improve semen quality, particularly sperm motility. [Approximately 25 percent of infertile males have a varicocele of the left internal spermatic vein (9).]

    d. Vasovasotomies or vasoepididymostomies may be necessary if obstructions are present.

    e. Testicular transplantation and vas deferens grafts are other surgical procedures attempted to improve male fertility.

C. The couple.

  1. Coital technique for promotion of fertility.

      a. Usually the sperm concentration, motility, morphology, and viability are greater in the first portion of ejaculated semen.

      b. The penis is withdrawn from the vagina after coital intravaginal deposition of the better first portion of the ejaculate, depositing remaining semen outside the body.

      c. This coital technique is recommended if analysis of split ejaculate indicates subfertility, high semen volumes, and good quality in the first portion of fractionated semen specimen (10).

      d. Only recommended for use around the fertile period of the menstrual cycle.

2. Artificial insemination (AI).

      a. Semen used for insemination may be fresh or frozen.

         (1) Frozen semen is mixed with a cryopreservative and stored at −80 to −196.5°C in a liquid nitrogen tank.

         (2) Before insemination, frozen semen is thawed for approximately 30 min and sperm are checked for count and motility.

      b. Fresh semen is collected by masturbation into a sterile container.

      c. Methods of artificial insemination (11):

         (1) Cervicovaginal or intracervical: Approximately 0.5 mL of semen is slowly injected into the cervical canal under direct vision. The remainder is allowed to spill onto the cervix and vaginal vault.

         (2) Intravaginal: The entire semen specimen is injected into the vaginal vault.

         (3) Cap technique: Semen is placed in a plastic cap which is fitted over the cervix and left in position for at least 8 h.

         (4) Intrauterine: Approximately 0.1 mL of semen is introduced directly into the uterus. This method is generally reserved for instances where the cervix must be bypassed.

      d. AI is carefully timed to coincide with ovulation as indicated by BBT and spinnbarkeit. If the menstrual cycle is significantly irregular, ovulation may be drug-induced and AI planned.

      e. Two to three inseminations are often done per cycle, usually over a period of time not longer than 12 months.

      f. Ninety percent of women who will become pregnant via AI do so within 6 months, the rest within 12 months (12).

      g. AI practices should be held carefully confidential, and the professional staff should take precautions to ensure confidentiality.

      h. The couple is advised not to discuss AI with family and friends.

      i. Also, it must be noted that artificial insemination is morally unacceptable to many people.

      j. The infertility examination, specifically the semen analysis, determines whether homologous or heterologous insemination is indicated.

         (1) Artificial insemination husband (AIH)—homologous insemination.

            (a) May be recommended in cases where normal coitus is not possible, as with severe vaginismus, vaginal narrowing, marked obesity of partner(s), deformities produced by injury or accident, hypospadius, premature or retrograde ejaculation, impotence, or union of long vagina and short penis.

            (b) AIH is indicated if the sperm count is adequate but the volume of ejaculate is low.

            (c) If the sperm count is low normal, but the volume of ejaculate is adequate, AIH is performed for several cycles before considering AID.

         (2) Artificial insemination donor (AID)—heterologous insemination.

            (a) AID is recommended to couples with infertility secondary to azoospermia, or after unsuccessful AIH with oligospermia; to couples where the male is a carrier of a serious hereditary disease; and to couples with Rh immunologic incompatibility.

(b) Potential donors must be carefully screened and tested with particular attention to inheritable traits, medication and drug habits, blood type and Rh factor, relevant infections, and semen analysis.

(c) Ethnic background and physical characteristics are matched to those of the husband as closely as possible.

(d) The same donor is used, whenever possible, until pregnancy occurs.

(e) The donor and recipient remain anonymous to each other.

(f) There are approximately 10,000 AID children born each year in the United States; approximately 1000 a year in Europe (13).

(g) Some believed advantages of AID over adoption for the infertile family include: the full experience of parenthood, a normal pregnancy, a more private process with less people aware, elimination of the fear that the natural parents might reclaim the child, and donor matching with improved chances that the child will resemble the parents.

(h) The infertile couple must sign a contract indicating that they understand the procedure, its goal, and that any resulting offspring are legitimate legal heirs.

(i) Successful couples may be referred elsewhere for obstetric care to avoid conflict of interest and legal problems (such as perjury with regard to legitimacy in signing the birth certificate).

(3) Adoption.

(a) Adoption may be the only possible or acceptable means for some couples to satisfy the desire to become parents.

(b) The therapeutic value of adoption as a method for stimulating pregnancy in an infertile marriage is speculative and without conclusive evidence (14).

(c) Older children, those with physical and mental deficiencies, and those of non-Caucasian or mixed race are more available for adoption than healthy Caucasian newborns.

(d) Referral should be made to ensure provision of the complex guidance necessary for prospective adopting parents.

PROBLEMS

I. Partner(s) may not desire, or may be ambivalent toward parenthood; may only be seeking confirmation of ability to reproduce.

II. Each partner may have different, possibly conflicting motivations and expectations for the infertility investigation and for childbearing.

III. Partners may lack adequate sexual knowledge, may have inaccurate information, may believe sexual myths, may perceive infertility as a punishment for past sins.

IV. Religious convictions and values may influence the progress of the investigation, cooperation with treatment, and/or selection of secondary alternatives such as artificial insemination.

V. Couple may have difficulty communicating sexual information to each other and/or to professional staff (e.g., sexual needs, concerns, desires, practices, pertinent sexual history).

VI. Couple may be acutely concerned about the potential risks, side effects, and costs of therapy.

VII. Partner(s) may have inadequate support systems during process of investigation.

VIII. Partner(s) may exhibit maladaptive coping mechanisms during the investigation or following a poor prognosis.

IX. In the event of unsuccessful therapy, or diagnosed sterility, partners will need to accept the loss of their reproductive capacity and readjust life plans.

DIAGNOSIS

    I. Undesired infertility has caused increased marital stress.

    II. Difficulty conceiving and repeated frustrations associated with the failures of progressive procedures to result in pregnancy have created alterations in body image and self-concept.

    III. Lack of prior success has generated hostility, shame, guilt, severe anxiety, and/or depression.

GOALS OF CARE

Immediate

    I. Physical and psychosocial problems influencing fertility will be identified.

    II. Rapport with the couple will be established in order to promote open communication.

    III. Couple understands purposes, cost, and course of the infertility investigation.

    IV. Couple understands health care team's expectations of them, as well as what they may expect from the team.

    V. Steps for procedures such as BBT and semen specimen collection are clear.

    VI. Clients and staff together formulate plan for participation in other diagnostic tests and treatment.

Long-range

    I. Couple is supported throughout infertility investigation. Questions are answered, and treatment options and potential risks are made clear.

    II. Individual health is improved where nutritional problems, anemia, poisonings, or intoxications, fatigue, and local infections have existed.

    III. Diagnostic testing, teaching and therapy are done in a coordinated manner by all members of the health team.

    IV. The infertile couple has an opportunity to discuss all the available means of becoming natural parents.

    V. The emotional status of each partner during the lengthy investigation is assessed repeatedly.

    VI. The couple receives appropriate referrals (e.g., for psychologic assessment and/or counseling, for adoption).

    VII. All involved work to resolve conflict and achieve realistic, healthy coping with the diagnosis, treatment, and prognosis.

INTERVENTION

    I. Participate in initial interview to identify patterns of coping with stress, noting any difficulties. Be aware of expressed or unexpressed guilt and fears.

    II. Note partner interaction and communication patterns.

    III. Be aware of nonverbal cues related to anxiety (restlessness, difficulty in maintaining eye contact, posture, sweating).

    IV. Seek to identify source(s) of anxiety, problems, guilt feelings.

    V. Assess adequacy of present support systems.

    VI. Give thorough explanation of specimen collection, procedures, and tests.

    VII. Plan teaching to build on present understanding. Let couple set the pace. Provide literature as appropriate.

VIII. Assist in referrals for other health care, as necessary.
 IX. Provide setting in which sexual questions and practices, myths and inaccurate sexual information can be discussed.
  X. Explore with couples any expressed conflicts arising from religious beliefs, marital stress, ambivalence, and/or poor communication.

EVALUATION

I. Conception occurs.
  A. Provide beginning prenatal teaching.
  B. Promote acceptance and successful adaptation to pregnant state.
  C. Assist in seeking prenatal care.
  D. Refer to or collaborate with prenatal nurse regarding continued care.
II. Conception considered unlikely or impossible.
  A. Assist infertile or sterile family in understanding and discussing prognosis.
  B. Evaluate adequacy of coping methods.
  C. Facilitate healthy grieving and support realistic life adjustments.
  D. Refer for counseling and/or adoption if appropriate.

RELIGIOUS, ETHICAL, AND LEGAL CONSIDERATIONS

Religious convictions frequently influence the infertile couple's attitudes and behavior. For example, masturbation, the most highly recommended method for obtaining semen for analysis or insemination, is considered "unnatural" by Catholic theologians and as "wasting of the seed" by orthodox Jews. It is also discouraged by many Protestant ministers. It thus may be necessary to attempt semen collection via coitus interruptus or coitus condomatosus. The removal of semen from the vagina, after coitus, may be the only acceptable means of obtaining a specimen for analysis.

AIH, except when using semen already deposited in the vagina, and AID are forbidden by the Catholic church; AID is, in fact, considered adultery. The Protestant and Jewish religions have not decreed an official pronouncement regarding AI, but most discourage, and some prohibit, AID. The Lutheran church and most Anglican churches oppose AI, and orthodox Jewish rabbis do not accept AI.

Not all followers of the various religions are aware of or accept the teachings and pronouncements in totality. It is important to help the infertile family anticipate these potential problems, if appropriate, as part of their decision-making process.

Several ethical questions have arisen regarding the treatment of infertility. The following is a cursory, not exhaustive, list:

1. Considering population control goals and problems, should efforts be made to alleviate involuntary childlessness?
2. Is the treatment of infertility contributing to "pollution" of the gene pool?
3. Should the collection of data and statistics regarding AID be encouraged? How should these be used?
4. The opportunity exists for selection of a superior donor, that is, the eugenic use of artificial insemination.
5. The possibility also exists for the proliferation of disease-producing recessive genes through widely used AI donors.
6. Should or can the AID child's genetic identity be revealed? What claim, if any, does the biologic parent have on the AID child?
7. "Innocent incest" is possible if two children produced from the same sperm donor seek to reproduce.

8. When the cost of infertility investigation and treatment exceeds the family's ability to pay, should care proceed, and should cost be borne by the government or other insurance policy holders?

9. Should there be restraints on a woman's desire to go through a normal pregnancy and birth when the situation is such that some form of AI is necessary?

10. The long-term effects on future generations of drug therapy for the infertile couple remain unknown.

11. What are the implications of medical intervention for the infertile family on the natural family structure of society?

12. Anticipated future advances, such as egg transplant, prenatal adoption, and genetic manipulation raise additional ethical dilemmas.

There also has been concern regarding possible legal difficulties related to AID.

1. By legal definition AID does not technically constitute adultery although this question is not completely resolved.

2. Some authorities recommend the pooling of husband and donor semen for artificial insemination, thereby making it difficult to ascertain conclusively which spermatazoa fertilized the ovum.

3. The sperm donor usually signs a document waiving any claim to offspring.

4. The wife, if applicable, of a sperm donor may be requested to give written acknowledgment and consent to the process.

5. Legal questions remain regarding the physician's signature on a birth certificate of the child conceived via AID. The woman's husband, not the donor, is listed as father, despite what the physician may know to be otherwise true.

6. Some advocate maintenance, others destruction of records regarding sperm donors and recipients.

7. As with adoption, there are legal questions regarding the offspring's "right" to know genetic heritage and biologic parent(s).

8. Questions may arise regarding legal heirs, legitimacy, and divorce.

REFERENCES

1. T. H. Green, *Gynecology*, 2d ed., Little, Brown and Company, Boston, 1971, p. 266.
2. R. W. Kistner, "The Infertile Woman," *American Journal of Nursing*, **73**(11):1937, November 1973.
3. R. H. Glass, *Office Gynecology*, The William & Wilkins Company, Baltimore, 1976, p. 249.
4. Kistner, loc. cit.
5. R. M. French, *The Nurse's Guide to Diagnostic Procedures*, McGraw-Hill Book Company, New York, 1971, pp. 46, 146.
6. J. W. Goldzieher, "Polycystic Ovarian Disease," in S.J. Behrman and R. W. Kistner (eds.), *Progress in Infertility*, Little, Brown and Company, Boston, 1975, p. 342.
7. R. W. Kistner, "Endometrosis and Infertility," in S.J. Behrman and R. W. Kistner (eds.), *Progress in Infertility*, Little, Brown and Company, Boston, 1975, p. 442.
8. Glass, op cit., p. 249.
9. Ibid., p. 254.
10. R. D. Amelar and L. Dubin, "A Coital Technical for Promotion of Fertility," *Urology*, **5**(2): 228–232, February 1975.
11. A. Koren and R. Lieberman, "Fifteen Years' Experience with Artificial Insemination," *International Journal of Fertility*, **21**(2):119–122, 1976.
12. Leagans, "Artificial Insemination: Hope for Childless Couples," *Journal of Obstetric, Gynecologic, and Neonatal Nursing*, **3**(4):25, July–August 1974.
13. R. Riquier, "Artificial Reproduction," *Nursing Times*, **70**(13):496, March 28, 1974.
14. G. H. Arronet et al., "The Influence of Adoption on Subsequent Pregnancy in an Infertile Marriage," *International Journal of Fertility*, **19**(3):159, 1974.

BIBLIOGRAPHY

Behrman, S. J., and R. W. Kistner (eds.): *Progress in Infertility,* 2d ed., Little, Brown and Company, Boston, 1975. A carefully organized compilation of articles by leading professionals in the field of fertility and sterility.

Kistner, R. W.: "The Infertile Woman," *American Journal of Nursing,* **73**(11): 1937, 1973. The succinct physical specifics of female infertility.

——— and G. W. Patton: *Atlas of Infertility Surgery,* Little, Brown and Company, Boston, 1975. Helpful illustrations and explanations; useful as a teaching aid.

Rakoff, A. E.: "The Infertility History and Its Evaluation," *Journal of Reproductive Medicine,* **18**(4): 114, 1977. Symposium on diagnosis and treatment of infertility in March and April issues.

Wiehe, V. R.: "Psychological Reactions to Infertility: Implications for Nursing in Resolving Feelings of Disappointment and Inadequacy," *Journal of Obstetric, Gynecologic, and Neonatal Nursing,* **5**(4): 28. August 1976. A perceptive article, especially for insights regarding the feelings of the infertile family.

6

The Family Unready
for Childbearing

Cynthia S. Luke

DEFINITION

Elective abortion is a voluntary means to end an unwanted pregnancy, either during the early period [first trimester from last menstrual period (LMP) through 12th week] or the late period [second trimester from 16th to 24th week]. The early second trimester (13th through 15th week) is a waiting period because methods currently used for uterine evacuations may not be used safely due either to fetal size, thinning and softening of uterine wall, or inadequate amount and poor accessibility of amniotic fluid.

Current Legal Status

The United States Supreme Court decision in 1973 based on the due process clause of the 14th Amendment of the Constitution stated that (1):

1. For the stage prior to approximately the end of the first trimester, the abortion decision and its effectuation must be left to the medical judgment of the pregnant woman's attending physician.
2. For the stage subsequent to approximately the end of the first trimester (12 weeks), the state, in promoting its interest in the health of the mother, may, if it chooses, regulate the abortion procedure in ways that are reasonably related to maternal health.
3. For the stage subsequent to viability (24 weeks) the state, in promoting its interest in the potentiality of human life, may, if it chooses, regulate, and even proscribe, abortion except where it is necessary, in appropriate medical judgment for the preservation of the life or health of the mother.

States and institutions establish policies and procedures in accordance with this decision. Pressure exists on legislatures and hospital administrators to prevent abortion services in some hospitals. Social changes (availability and financing of services, rights of minors, rights of the fetus) and attitudes of professionals are evolving. In this current period, the development of improved techniques for abortions to decrease time involved and to minimize side effects can only result in improved safety.

Methods

For the sake of clarity and ease of reference, methods currently used to achieve abortion are outlined in Table 6-1, with side effects and nursing interventions given.

Long-range Effects

Present studies are inconclusive, with further research required to determine the relationship of abortion to subsequent pregnancy, regarding Rh sensitization, future spontaneous abortion, prematurity, early infant mortality, ectopic pregnancy, placenta previa, secondary sterility, and psychological effects.

ASSESSMENT

I. Data sources.
  A. Health history: Note any asthmatic condition, any renal, cardiovascular, or metabolic disorders, any cervical disorders which may affect dilation, also, drug allergies and usage, and use of contraceptives and failures.
  B. Obstetrical history: Assess prior pregnancies and outcomes, labor and delivery experiences, and previous abortions with circumstances and outcomes.
  C. Physical and pelvic examination: Estimate gestational age of fetus, and determine the last menstrual period date, and expected date of confinement. This assessment will be used to determine the type of abortion possible. This may be in conflict with the woman's estimate and will require explanation and adjustment of her expectations. Cervical and vaginal changes assist in confirming pregnancy.
  D. Laboratory tests: These include the pregnancy test, latex inhibition or agglutination slide tests, or serum radioimmunoassay. Others are the Papanicolaou smear of cervix, gonorrhea smear, hematocrit, white blood count, serologic study, blood group and Rh type (Coombs' test if Rh negative), and urinalysis. Maternal antibody screen for the Rh-negative woman, and explanation of RhoGAM to prevent isoimmunization is needed.
II. Statement of consent must be clearly understood and signed.
III. Caseworker assessment of psychosocial status: The following factors may exist and must be considered: A feeling of ambivalence is natural and the client needs to explore her feelings about abortion—religious, ethical, and motivations resulting in pregnancy. The client must also examine expectations of self, and her perception of the reality of being pregnant. Alternatives, situational supports, coping mechanisms, and financial resources must be considered (2). This may be an opportune time for sex education (anatomy, physiology of menstruation and conception, health teaching about sexual relationships, and contraceptive teaching). Resources are listed (family planning clinics, women's health clinics, health departments, clinics) to assist client maintenance of health in these areas and guidelines are given. Also assessed is any history of seeking help with this abortion decision and any experience with the health care system. It is helpful to offer the name of the head nurse or another caring person in the procedural area to decrease the unknowns.

PROBLEMS

I. The client is emotionally upset.
  A. If there is unusual ambivalence, encourage the client to express her feelings, and then assist her in identifying the reasons for ambivalence. Determine if this is her decision (limit conflicting opinions while she makes her decision); and help her to recognize guilt. Encourage her to talk about her needs that are affected by this decision. Help the client recognize denial as a major defense mechanism, and confront her resulting anger, disappointment, and/or sadness expressed as she gives up denial (3).
  B. Occasionally, the client must be guided in expressing underlying conflicts about femininity, motherhood, and self-control; if necessary, ensure time to consider decision, and provide for group work with other women.
  C. The upset client may express exaggerated fears and anxieties about dying, disgrace, or physical punishment; fears of a future deformed child, or concern about a withdrawal of love or retaliation from loved ones, and isolation and separation. Feelings about destroying living tissue may be present. These feelings may all be normal unless excessive (4). The nurse must enourage expression, and reassure the client that other women experience these feelings. Provide for group work with other women, if necessary.

TABLE 6-1 / METHODS OF ABORTION

Method	Side Effects	Nursing Intervention
5th to 7th Week		
Menstrual extraction (endometrial aspiration, menstrual regulation, mini-abortion, and EUE): Contents of uterus are removed by syringe suction. May or may not require positive pregnancy test.	Mild cramping, minimal vaginal bleeding, systemic and allergic reactions (vertigo, pruritis, hypotension). Incomplete removal of tissue.	Patient should be fasting for 4 h prior to procedure, and with bladder empty. Place in lithotomy position and cleanse vulva with antiseptic solution. Help patient with relaxation techniques when tenaculum is applied to cervix for dilatation. Procedure takes 1–3 min and cervical anesthesia may or may not be used (5–10 mL of 1% lidocaine). Observe supine for 10 min. Monitor vital signs and feeling responses. Blood loss 5–30 mL. Repeat pregnancy test on return visit.
7th to 12th Week		
Vacuum aspiration (suction curettage): Contents of uterus removed by suction. Performed in clinic, hospital, or physician's office with local cervical or general anesthesia. (See Fig. 6-1.)	Mild cramping during procedure. Minimal bleeding, mild cramping after.	As above. Procedure takes 3–5 min and may be followed by curette exploring uterine cavity. Bimanual exam. Observe supine for 10 min. Take vital signs and discharge after 1 h.
Dilatation and curettage (D&C): Contents of uterus scraped out. Performed in clinic or physician's office with local cervical or general anesthesia.	Trauma to uterus and cervix, incomplete evacuation, infection.	Postanesthesia care depending on type. Must be fully responsive for 1–2 h before discharge. Offer food and rest.
13th to 15th Week		
The following procedures are more difficult to perform and involve increasing complications. *Prostaglandin suppository* (PGE$_2$): Inserted in vagina, resulting in mechanical as well as hormonal effect on cervix. Research continues on this method as a means of decreasing cervical trauma.	Vomiting and diarrhea, temperature elevation (CNS reaction). Contractions indicate uterus is emptying.	Give Lomotil $\frac{1}{2}$ h prior to insertion. Prochlorperazine if vomiting occurs. (Not very effective since cause is smooth muscle stimulation.) Repeat insertion may be necessary. IV fluids started. No aspirin as it reduces uterine activity. Assist with relaxation and breathing techniques. Analgesia if necessary.
		Prepare for expulsion of fetus when contractions increase in intensity and frequency. Rupture of membranes may occur several hours to a few minutes before expulsion. Need container for fetus and suture set to clamp and cut cord. Inform client of expulsion.
		Observe vital signs and perineum for bleeding until placenta is expelled; may be few minutes to several hours. (Seek medical assessment after 1 h.) Oxytocin may be used IM or IV to hasten expulsion.

TABLE 6-1 / METHODS OF ABORTION (Continued)

Method	Side Effects	Nursing Intervention
		Increased bleeding may indicate separation of placenta. Have client bear down and push for placental expulsion. Palpate fundus for firm contractibility. Observe vital signs and perineum every 15 min for 1 h. Offer food, fluids, and rest. Give support and reassurance that procedure is completed. Label placenta and fetus for examination by medical staff and send to lab.
16th to 24th Week*		
Prostaglandin intra-amniotic injection (PGF$_{2\alpha}$, 25–40 mg; 15-methyl PGF$_{2\alpha}$, 5 mg): Administered via amniocentesis after test dosage. Contractions may begin within 15 min. Mean abortive time 12–23 h.	Vomiting and diarrhea,† headache.	Treat as above.
	Retained placenta with hemorrhage.	Removal of placenta by manual pelvic exam or D&C, if necessary.
	Cervicovaginal fistula.	With pelvic exam, observe for increased bleeding. Suture repair. IV, oral fluids, and ambulation are encouraged for sense of well-being.
	Allergic reaction with test dosage.	Erythematous at site, fever and shivering. Hypertension, bronchial constriction (mostly with asthmatics). Analgesic and tranquilizer (Demerol, 25 mg, or Valium, 10 mg) for comfort. May slow uterine activity.
	Hypotonic uterus.	Repeat dose of prostaglandin may be necessary if aborting has not occurred within 48 h and membranes are intact. If several hours elapse between rupture of membranes and aborting, IV oxytocin may be started (50 U in 1000 mL Ringer's lactate at 20–30 gtt/min). As above, prepare for expulsion of fetus and placenta.
Urea intra-amniotic injection (80 g per 200 mL solution): Administered via amniocentesis. Mean abortive time 12–36 h. May be used with oxytocin or PGF$_{2\alpha}$ (less commonly used).	Dehydration, alteration in coagulation factors may occur.	Maintain IV fluids, control nausea. Note fibrinogen levels (normal range 160–415 mg per 100 mL) and platelet count changes [normal range 140,000–400,000 per millimeter (Brecher-Cronkite method)].
Saline injection: Administered via amniocentesis. Withdrawal of 250 mL amniotic fluid, test dosage, then injection of 30–40 g of NaCl diluted in 200–240 mL of amniotic fluid. Average abortive time	With infiltration into tissues, hypernatremia is evidenced by increased thirst shortly thereafter.	Note and evaluate symptoms.
	Leakage into vascular system with abdominal pain, severe headache,	Observe for symptoms.

*All methods during this time period are performed in the hospital.
†In the foreseeable future, a type of prostaglandin will be available, the effects of which will be restricted to the uterus, with negligible side effects.

TABLE 6-1 / METHODS OF ABORTION (Continued)

Method	Side Effects	Nursing Intervention
30–36 h. May be used with oxytocin.	backache, tachycardia, confusion, drowsiness, seizures.	
	Infection ascending through vagina with extended rupture of membranes.	Observe for symptoms, request cervical cultures. Maintain perineal cleansing with antiseptic solution and antiseptic technique.
	Coagulation defects leading to hemorrhage.	Observe fibrinogen changes. Be prepared to assist in emptying uterus, administering whole blood, fibrin, or heparin. Vital signs on flow sheet.
	With oxytocin infusion: water intoxication, confusion, drowsiness, headache, cervical tear, uterine rupture.	Accurate infusion rate and observation of urinary output. Treat with Ringer's lactate. Observe for symptoms of bleeding, uterine tenderness and rigidity, abdominal pain. Surgical repair necessary.
Hysterotomy (same procedure as cesarean): Uterine contents removed by abdominal surgery under general anesthesia.	Possible repeat cesarean section necessary for future pregnancies.	Postoperative care.

    D. If the client expresses a feeling of being forced into the abortion, explore the reasons of the person exerting pressure. Encourage discussion with other persons and counselor, and delay decision making until a more satisfactory situation can be worked out.

II. The client is uninformed about procedures.

    A. The nurse must assess the client's knowledge base and expectations (even though information may have been presented, the nurse cannot assume client is informed), and explain the procedure with visual aids.

    B. Areas arousing anxiety must be determined and client should be encouraged to invite a person to be with her.

    C. Provide for continuity of care (primary nursing care is desirable).

III. The client is very young.

    A. Female adolescents (15 to 19 years) in the United States have rates of childbearing among the world's highest. One million U.S. teenagers become pregnant each year, and 30,000 of them are younger than 15 years old. One-third of all women seeking abortions are teenagers. 350,000 teenagers have abortions each year. Between 1973 and 1975 the teenage abortion rate increased by 60 percent (5).

    B. Legal aspects: Federal courts have declared statutory requirements of parental consent for abortion unconstitutional. State legislatures continue to enact restrictive legislation (6). The nurse should determine state law requiring parental consent (case may be appealed to juvenile court if parent refuses to consent).

    C. Decision making: Assess influence of parents and boyfriend on abortion decision and their knowledge about abortion (the client may express acquiescence or blame parents for decision). The nurse must keep in mind that immaturity contributes to ambivalence about decision, and may distort client's perception of procedure (as being dangerous, frightening, punitive, or arousing fears of violence). Mourning from loss is to be expected (7). The nurse must ascertain if client is late in seeking abortion whether it is due to denial, lack of knowledge, or irregular menses. The nurse must also seek to integrate a supportive parent or friend into the client's care.

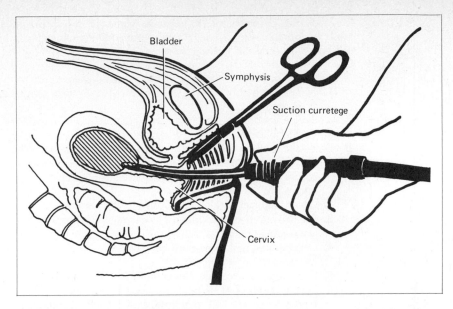

FIGURE 6-1 / Suction method of curettage. (*From E. J. Dickason and M. O. Schult, Maternal and Infant Care, McGraw-Hill Book Company, New York, 1975.*)

D. Sexual and contraceptive teaching: Knowledge base of the young client may be limited despite high school health education, and success depends on the developmental stage. Does the client have the ability to delay impulse gratification, can she understand societal realities, and plan for the future?

E. Signs predictive of contraceptive failure: These will include pregnancy resulting from acting-out tendencies, an overwhelming relationship hunger, magical thinking (it can't happen to me), and precarious self-esteem.

DIAGNOSIS

Client (with identified problem) is seeking termination of a pregnancy of _____ weeks gestation.

GOALS OF CARE

Immediate

I. There should be adequate time for decision making after information is received.

II. Client will be prepared for implications of procedure.

A. Present feelings (what does she know about abortion, what is distressing, what are false beliefs about abortion?)

B. Concerns about future reproductive decisions.

C. Expected reactions during and following procedure.

D. Size and viability of fetus.

E. Time frame.

F. Expected discomforts.

G. Areas for choices (local anesthetic, analgesia, oral fluids, activity, diversional activities).

III. No adverse complication will occur.

    IV. RhoGAM will be given for Rh-negative woman 8 weeks pregnant. For a second trimester abortion woman may require serum antibody screening to determine amount of RhoGAM needed to prevent isoimmunization.

    V. Client must understand instructions for follow-up.

        A. Call clinic or physician for the following unusual signs:

            1. Temperature above 39°C (98.6°F) for 2 days (take temperature twice a day for 4 days).

            2. Severe abdominal pain (but some cramping to be expected).

            3. Vaginal bleeding—soaking a sanitary pad every $\frac{1}{2}$ h for more than 6 h.

        B. Rest—she may be tired for a few days, should drink extra fluids.

            1. Prevent infection—nothing in vagina for 2 weeks (tampons, douching, intercourse, sprays); wipe after toileting from front to back (*E. coli* is major infecting organism).

            2. Client may feel blue for a few days with change in hormones.

            3. Breast care: if breasts feel full, wear tight-fitting bra day and night and drink less liquid.

            4. Observe that next period will be expected in 4 to 10 weeks (client can become pregnant during this time).

            5. Use contraceptives—condoms and foam until follow-up visit.

            6. Follow-up visit will be in 2 to 6 weeks to assess whether cervix, vagina, and uterus have returned to normal state; discuss abortion and contraception at this time.

    VI. Any client with psychosocial problems will be referred to case worker prior to procedure.

    VII. Complete preparation for procedure will be done, including laboratory results and client preparation.

Long-range

    I. Client will understand how to prevent future unwanted pregnancy. Discuss, demonstrate, and supply contraceptive information and refer to clinic for follow-up. (May insert IUD after procedure or begin oral contraceptives 5 days after abortion; diaphragm will be refitted during subsequent checkup.)

    II. If client demonstrates continued emotional problems, counselor's recommendations will be supported.

    III. Family/supportive others will be involved in follow-up. Enlist support of accompanying friend or relative, assist them to listen to concerns, allowing her to relive experience. Encourage contact and other client support.

    IV. Client will be able to discuss sexuality and be assisted to find resources for own exploration (*Our Bodies, Ourselves,* Planned Parenthood pamphlets, Siecus, *Teenage Pregnancy: Prevention and Treatment,* New York, 1971).

    V. Client will be able to explore avenues for meeting health needs, gain entry into system (adolescent clinics).

INTERVENTION

Prior to Abortion

    I. Maintain nonjudgmental approach for therapeutic interaction.

    II. Utilize crisis intervention theory as basis of counseling, recognizing time for potential growth and change.

    III. Allow adequate time for counseling on alternatives to a problem pregnancy.

    IV. Clarify reasoning for decision with client. Provide adequate time between counseling and decision making before procedure.

V. Orient client thoroughly to procedures.
VI. Refer client in conflict to appropriate case worker or religious counselor prior to decision.
VII. Examine feelings of loss of pregnancy.
VIII. Reinforce positive attitudes about self.
IX. Explore interpersonal dynamics leading to pregnancy.

After Abortion

I. Ensure client's understanding of need for follow-up with written instructions.
II. Reinforce decision regarding contraceptive method.
III. Interpret recovery needs to accompanying friend or relative.

EVALUATION

I. Client made informed decision after being clear about options.
II. Referred to counseling for unresolved conflicts.
III. Utilizing family planning successfully for subsequent period.
IV. Normal physical and psychosocial effects noted on subsequent follow-up visits.

REFERENCES

1. H. J. Osofsky and J. D. Osofsky, *The Abortion Experience: Psychological and Medical Impact*, Harper & Row, Hagerstown, Md., 1973.
2. S. Gedan, "Pre-Abortion Emotional Counseling," in *ANA Clinical Sessions*, Appleton Century Crofts, New York, 1972.
3. Ibid.
4. C. Lanahan, "Anxieties and Fears of Patients Seeking Abortion," in L. K. McNall and J. T. Galeenen (eds.), *Current Practice in Obstetric and Gynecologic Nursing*, The C. V. Mosby Company, St. Louis, 1976, p. 201.
5. *Eleven Million Teenagers: What Can Be Done about the Epidemic of Adolescent Pregnancies in the U.S.?*, Alan Guttmacher Institute, New York, 1976.
6. F. W. Paul, H. F. Pipel, and N. F. Wechsler, "Pregnancy, Teenagers and the Law, 1976," *Family Planning Perspectives*, **8**(1):16 January–February 1976.
7. Peter Barlow, "Abortion 1975: The Psychiatric Perspective: With a Discussion of Abortion and Contraception in Adolescence," *Journal of Obstetric and Gynecologic Nursing*, **5**(1):41, January–February 1976.

BIBLIOGRAPHY

Anderson, B., M. E. Comacho, and J. Stark: *Childbearing Family*, vol. II, *Interruptions in Family Health During Pregnancy*, McGraw-Hill Book Company, New York, 1974. Reviews procedures and discusses potential complications with resulting treatment. Includes goals for counseling.

Anderson, C., B. Clancy, and R. Hassanein: "Psychoprophylaxis in Mid-trimester Abortions," *Journal of Obstetric, Gynecologic, and Neonatal Nursing*, **5**(6):29, November–December 1976. Study comparing abortion experiences between women utilizing modified Lamaze techniques and those receiving routine nursing care.

Barlow, Peter: "Abortion 1975: The Psychiatric Perspective: With a Discussion of Abortion and Contraception in Adolescence," *Journal of Obstetric and Gynecologic Nursing*, **5**(1):41, January–February 1976. Discusses behavioral reactions based on developmental needs of adolescents.

Beazley, J. M.: "The Prostaglandin," *Nursing Times*, **72**(16):1800, November 18, 1976. Review of prostaglandins and their physiologic effects on various body systems.

Bolognese, R. J., and S. L. Corson: *Interruption of Pregnancy—Total Patient Approach*, The Williams & Wilkins Company, Baltimore, 1975. Compilation of medical research studies, details of abortion techniques, psychology of abortion and counseling.

Bracken, M., and S. V. Kasl: "Delay in Seeking Induced Abortion: A Review and Theoretical Analysis," *American Journal of Obstetrics and Gynecology,* **121**:1009, April 1975. Examines reasons for delay of women seeking abortions.

Clancy, B.: "The Nurse and the Abortion Patient," *Nursing Clinics of North America,* **8**:469, August 1973. Expands nurses' role in counseling and support.

Easterbrook, B., and B. Rust: "A New Role for Nurses," *The Canadian Nurse,* **73**(1):28, January 1977. Nursing model for pre- and postabortion care utilizing group counseling techniques.

Eleven Million Teenagers: What Can Be Done About The Epidemic of Adolescent Pregnancies in the U.S.? Alan Guttmacher Institute, New York, 1976. Statistical and narrative description of teenagers' (15 to 19 years) need for education, contraception, and abortion.

Evans, J. R., G. Selstal, and W. H. Welcher: "Teenagers: Fertility Control Behavior and Attitudes Before Childbearing or Negative Pregnancy Test," *Family Planning Perspective,* **8**(4):192, July–August 1976. Reports of study indicating use of contraceptives improved markedly after abortion (1972–1975).

Gedan, S.: "Pre-Abortion Emotional Counseling," *ANA Clinical Sessions,* Appleton Century Crofts, New York, 1972. Emphasizes nursing role.

Lanahan, C.: "Anxieties and Fears of Patients Seeking Abortion," *in* L. K. McNall and J. T. Galeenen (eds.), *Current Practice in Obstetric and Gynecologic Nursing,* The C. V. Mosby Company, St. Louis, 1976, p. 201. Approach to abortion clients based on crisis theory and interventions.

Osofsky, H. J., and J. D. Osofsky: *The Abortion Experience: Psychological and Medical Impact,* Harper & Row, Hagerstown, Md., 1973. Extensive research on women's reactions to abortion experience.

Paul, F. W., H. F. Pipel, and N. F. Wechsler: "Pregnancy, Teenagers and the Law, 1976," *Family Planning Perspectives,* **8**(1):16, January–February 1976. Reviews legislative action by states.

Romney, S., M. J. Gray, A. B. Little, J. Merrill, E. S. Quilligan, and R. Stender: *Gynecology and Obstetrics; The Health Care of Women:* McGraw-Hill Book Company, New York, 1975. Reviews techniques with extensive bibliography.

Women's Health Organizing Collective of the Women's Health and Abortion Project: *Saline Abortion,* Healthright, New York, 1973. Frank details of saline abortion in clear terms and language. What to expect.

Woods, N. F.: *Human Sexuality in Health and Illness,* The C. V. Mosby Company, St. Louis, 1975. Considers biologic, psychologic, and sociologic antecedents to abortion. Assists practitioner in dealing with feelings concerning abortion. Reviews questions at end of chapter.

7

Pregnancy: The First, Second, and Third Trimesters

Nora Doherty Tully and Elizabeth J. Dickason

THE FIRST TRIMESTER

Definition

The period from the beginning of the last menstrual period (LMP) until the 14th week (1 to 12 weeks after conception) constitutes the first trimester of pregnancy. It is a period of multiple maternal physical and psychological changes and of fetal organogenesis. It is a crucial time for the developing fetus during which the maternal environment can be beneficial or hazardous. For the mother, it is a time to begin working through developmental tasks which will lead to effective parenting. For details of fetal development during each of the three trimesters, see Table 7-1 and Figs. 7-1 and 7-2. For details of psychophysical changes in the expectant mother during each of these periods, see Table 7-2.

Assessment

I. Health history.
   A. *Family history* should include information about cardiovascular diseases, diabetes mellitus, epilepsy, blood dyscrasias, hereditary diseases, congenital anomalies, tuberculosis, mental illness or emotional problems, and multiple pregnancies.
   B. *Medical history* should include information about her own history of heart disease, diabetes mellitus, epilepsy, rheumatic fever, childhood diseases, blood dyscrasias, tuberculosis, urinary tract disease, drug sensitivity, allergies, immunization, recent viral disease, or exposure to drugs or pollutants.
   C. *Menstrual history* should include information about onset, regularity, duration, and any problems with menses.
   D. *Obstetric history* should include information about number of pregnancies, interrupted pregnancies, abortions, premature deliveries, viable births, any physical or mental problems in these infants, any neonatal complications, stillbirths, previous complications and any problems of infertility, plus experience with success or failure of contraceptive methods.
II. *Determine parity*—refers to deliveries occurring after 20 weeks gestation. (Fig. 7-3).
III. *Establish* estimated date of delivery (EDD).
   A. Usually determined by using Nagele's rule:

   LMP + 7 days − 3 months + 1 year.

   B. Measurement of height of fundus: after 12 weeks, 1 cm per week above symphysis pubis. (Fig. 7-4).
   C. Date of quickening:

   Primigravida = 20 weeks + 2 days after date of quickening

   Multigravida = 21 weeks + 4 days = EDD

IV. Determine the client's present complaints.
V. Medical examination.
   A. General physical examination: eye, ear, nose, and throat (EENT), thyroid, breasts, heart, lungs, abdomen, extremities, baseline weight, blood pressure.

TABLE 7-1 / FETAL DEVELOPMENT DURING EACH TRIMESTER WITH APPLICATION TO PRENATAL CARE AND FETAL STUDIES

Fetal Development	*Application to Prenatal Care and Fetal Studies*
First Trimester	
Days:	
1–7 Cleavage—tubal transport and implantation.	Only affected by substances present or absent from tubal fluid.
8–14 Implantation completed. Primitive placental circulation begins and is functioning by 20 days.	As soon as substances can cross placenta, equilibrium usually occurs between mother and fetus with fetus getting maternal dose.
15 First missed menses.	
20–22 Neural fold develops and heart begins beating.	Brain growth can be inhibited. Heart defects may occur.
27–30 Arm and leg buds begin. Ear and eye development begins.	Phocomelia can occur. Cataracts can be caused. Immunoreactive pregnancy test begins to be positive.
32 Hand plates.	
34 Foot plates.	
36 Oral and nasal cavities contiguous.	Cleft lip and/or palate may result if teratogens are present in maternal system.
38 Upper lip joins.	
40 Palate develops.	
48 Beginnings of all internal and external organs are present.	
Week:	
8 Fetal period begins. External genitalia begin to differentiate. Heartbeat, 40–80 bpm; CR length, 40 mm; weight, 5 g.	Exogenous hormones can affect differentiation of genitalia, gonads.
9 Eyelids close over eyes. Intestine still in proximal umbilical cord.	Ultrasonic B scan can distinguish amniotic sac, fetus.
10 Face looks more "human." Intestines into abdomen. Tooth buds begin. Weight, 14 g.	Calcium becomes more important in maternal diet.
11 Arms bend at elbow. Legs are slower to assume fetal proportions.	
12 Organogenesis almost complete. Sex clearly differentiated. Muscle movements still generalized, but can suck thumb. CR length, 87 mm; weight 45 g.	Heartbeat can be heard with ultrasonic scan at about 120 bpm.
Second Trimester	
Week:	
16 Ears stand out from head. Bones are storing calcium. Sucking, swallowing, respiratory movements are noted on ultrasonic scan (real time). CR length, 140 mm; weight, 200 g.	Diet continues to be very important. Liver is functioning and can metabolize some drugs. Drugs affect fetal systems in same way as in mother's now; i.e., intoxicated mother, drunk baby.
20 Eyebrows, lanugo visible. Vernix because anabolic-catabolic exchange begins. Myelinization in brainstem. Respiratory movements stronger. Liver forming bile. Meconium present. CR length, 190 mm; weight, 460 g; biparietal diameter (BPD) of head, 4.8–5.0 cm.	Preterm infant: 1% viable but immature. Fetus metabolizes some drugs but not others. There is 400 mL amniotic fluid, and castoff fetal cells can be studied: + chromosomes and Barr bodies can determine sex, genetic defects, etc.
24 Fingernails. Eyes begin to reopen. Reacts to light, pain, noise(?). Thick layer of vernix covers body. If born now, high incidence of respiratory failure due to lung immaturity. Now usually called premature infant; 15% rate of premature birth. CR length, 230 mm; weight 650–820 g; BPD, 5.8–6.2 cm.	Maternal emotions and habits are thought to have influence on fetus (studies are incomplete); smoking, excess alcohol, addicting drugs are all negative environmental agents.

Fetal Development	*Application to Prenatal Care and Fetal Studies*
Third Trimester	
Week:	
29 Testes in inguinal canal. Skin translucent. Prominent clitoris; small, separated labia majora. Hypotonic, arms/legs not flexed, do not recoil. No resistance to scarf sign or heel to ear. Wrist shows square window when flexed. Weak suck, swallow. Moro reflexes. CR length, 270 mm; weight, 1000–1300 g; BPD 7.3–7.8 cm.	< 20% survive. Nitrogen, iron, and calcium being stored. Maternal diet very important. Period of most weight gain. All fetal structures develop further ability to function.
32 Vernix all over. No lanugo on face. Hypotonic. Some hip flexion, ear flat, soft cartilage. Creases only over ball of foot. Hair fine, woolly, bunches out from head. Sucking, swallowing stronger. Nails to fingertips. CR length, 300 mm; weight, 1500–2100 g; BPD, 8.0–8.4 cm.	50% survive. Orange-stained fat cells begin to appear in amniotic fluid.
36 Vernix over whole body. Testes in upper scrotum. Rugae only over anterior portion. BPD, 8.9–9.3 cm.	Maternal antibodies stored. Fat developing.
37 Clitoris still exposed, but labia larger. Ear pinna two-thirds incurved. Sole creases two-thirds of foot. Weight of 2500 g usually attained; BPD, 9.0–9.4 cm.	97% survive. *Term period* begins as 38th week of gestation starts.
38 Testes in scrotum. Rugae cover scrotum. Weight, 2600–3600 g; BPD 9.1–9.5 cm or more.	98% survive. Amniotic fluid tests for fetal maturity:
39 Labia majora more prominent. Clitoris nearly covered. Lanugo on shoulders.	1. Optical density, $\Delta OD_{450} = 0.00$. Labor begins within 4 weeks and infant is mature (measures bilirubin in amniotic fluid).
40 Scant vernix. Ear cartilage firm increases.	2. Nile blue stains fetal fat cells orange. When 20% or more of cells in amniotic fluid are orange, baby is mature.
41 Sole crease over heel.	3. Creatinine >2 mg per 100 mL (measures kidney maturity) indicates baby is mature.
42 No vernix or lanugo. Some weight loss. Skin wrinkled, often deeply creased.	4. L/S ratio of 2:1 indicates lung maturity. Correlates with CNS and liver maturity as well (tests may be changed by drugs).
43 Desquamation over most of body. Nails extend well over fingertips. Pendulous scrotum. Deep creases over entire sole of foot.	Post-term infant is one born after the beginning of the 42nd week of gestation (288 days or longer); incidence, 4%. Small-for-gestational-age, large-for-gestational-age, and postmature infants vary in measurements from normals above. Digitalis and aspirinlike drugs delay labor 1–2 weeks. Tests for deteriorating fetal condition:
	1. Estriols, falling.
	2. Oxytocin challenge test, positive.
	3. Meconium in amniotic fluid.
	4. Number of fetal movements on ultrasonic B scan less than normal.

Notes: Average duration of pregnancy from LMP is 280 days, *or 40 weeks, or 10 lunar* months. Pregnancy really lasts 266 ±8 days, *or 38 weeks, or 9½ lunar* months.

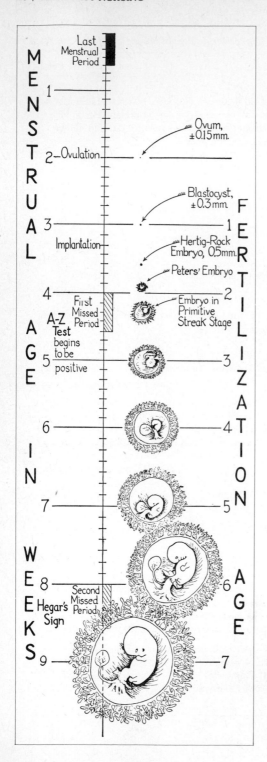

FIGURE 7-1 / Menstrual age compared with fertilization age. Actual size of embryos in relation to mother's menstrual history (*left*) and fertilization age of embryo (*right*). Based on a 28-day cycle. (*From C.E. Corliss, Patton's Human Embryology, McGraw-Hill Book Company, New York, 1976.*)

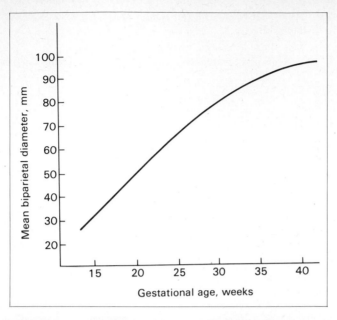

FIGURE 7-2 / Composite curve of mean biparietal diameters as compared to gestational age. (*From S. N. Weiner et al., Radiology, 122:781, 1977.*)

B. Obstetrical exam.
   1. Determine pelvic adequacy for vaginal delivery.
      a. The *diagonal conjugate,* from lower margin of pubic bone to promontory of the sacrum is normally 11.5 cm or larger.
      b. The *biischial diameter,* between both ischial tuberosities, is normally 8 cm or larger.
   2. Estimate fundal location: still a pelvic organ in first trimester; rises to height of symphysis pubis by 12 weeks. Examine for uterine consistency and size.
   3. Cervix is checked for erosion, discharge, color, consistency; Pap and other diagnostic smears may be taken.
   4. Check the vagina for weaknesses in the anterior and posterior walls, or any growths.
   5. Examine the external genitalia, urethral meatus, perineal body, and the anal sphincter.
C. Laboratory tests.
   1. Blood work: complete blood count (CBC), hematocrit (Hct), hemoglobin (Hb), type, Rh factor (potential for isoimmunization in the negative mother), serology, screening for sickle cell, G6PD (glucose 6-phosphate dehydrogenase), and blood glucose in high-risk populations.
   2. Cervical smears: Pap smear, smears for gonorrheal and other infections.
   3. Urinanalysis: glucose, protein, cells, and glucose, protein, on subsequent visits.
   4. Chest x-ray: screening for tuberculosis in high-risk populations.

Problems

    I. Psychological responses are inappropriate for the trimester.
   II. Social problems dominate person's concerns.
  III. Physical signs and symptoms dominate person's concerns.
  IV. Client at an extreme of age range: adolescent or "elderly" gravida.

TABLE 7-2 / DEVELOPMENTAL TASKS, SIGNS AND SYMPTOMS, AND NURSING INTERVENTION DURING FIRST, SECOND, AND THIRD TRIMESTERS

Tasks, Concerns, and Problems	Signs and Symptoms	Nursing Intervention
First Trimester		
Weeks 1–4		
Tasks: Acknowledgment of pregnancy. Acceptance of fetus. Must work through any conflicts with own mother to begin own mothering role. Concerns: Normality of symptoms, future changes in life-style. Changes in relationship with partner. Cost of care and how to manage. Normality of ambivalence to being pregnant. Problems: Exaggerated discomforts such as nausea, sleeplessness. Excessive need for reassurance that she is pregnant. Anger and rejection of idea of pregnancy. Depression, crying, extreme mood swings. Distance from sexual partner.	Subjective: Fatigue, thought to be due to ovarian hormone, relaxin. Nausea, may be due to decreased maternal blood sugar, decreased gastric motility. Peak period from 60 to 100 days after conception. Soreness, tingling of the breasts. Objective: Amenorrhea, but some women may have spotting at time of expected period. Elevated HCG levels Elevated basal body temperature due to presence of corpus luteum.	Teach the importance of adequate sleep, rest periods, sitting while elevating legs, exercise, using good body mechanics. Suggest intake of dry carbohydrate foods before arising; eating small, frequent carbohydrate foods and eliminating greasy, spicy foods. Teaching about avoiding over-the-counter medications for nausea. An early symptom of pregnancy. Instruct on importance of seeking early prenatal care, avoiding any drugs during weeks 1–12 unless prescribed by physician. Isoimmunologic test can be positive 26 days after conception. Client using BBT can see sustained temperature elevation on graph. Pick up client's concerns and begin teaching at those points. Other instruction must wait until anxiety diminishes.
	Weeks 5–8	
	Subjective: Enlarging uterus causes pressure on bladder, frequency of urination. Desire for sexual relations may decrease. Objective: Breasts enlarge, areolas darker. Enlarged Montgomery's tubercles. Mucous plug formation in cervical canal. These signs present by weeks 5–7: Ladin's—softening on anterior side of uterus above uterocervical junction. Goodell's—softening of cervix. Hegar's—softening of lower uterine seg-	In the absence of pain, burning on urination, or hematuria, reassure client that these are due to pressure of the growing uterus. Omit fluids after 6 P.M. to prevent nocturia. Explain that sexual desires vary during pregnancy due to both physical and psychological reasons. Advocate use of a supporting bra, with adjustable cups, wide adjustable straps, and smooth interior to prevent irritation. Lab work at first visit includes type, Rh, CBC, hemoglobin, hematocrit, urinalysis, and often serology. High-risk population are screened for TB, sickle cell disease. Vaginal or cervical smears for gonorrhea, other infections, and a Pap smear may be done. Instruct client to bring first voided speci-

TABLE 7-2 / DEVELOPMENTAL TASKS, SIGNS AND SYMPTOMS, AND NURSING INTERVENTION DURING FIRST, SECOND, AND THIRD TRIMESTERS (*Continued*)

Tasks, Concerns, and Problems	Signs and Symptoms	Nursing Intervention
	ment. Positive pregnancy test for HCG using biologic methods.	men for biologic tests, but obtain freshly voided one for isoimmunologic test.
	Weeks 9–12	
	Subjective: Nausea subsides by 12 weeks.	
	Frequency of urination subsides by 12 weeks.	
	Objective: Gingivitis, hypertrophy of the gums.	Check on intake of vitamin C-rich foods. Advise dental checkup. Use lead apron if dental x-rays needed.
	Weight gain of 0–3 lb. Some may lose weight.	Dietary teaching: weight gain should average 1 lb a month in the first trimester, and 11 lb in each of the second and third trimesters (0.8 lb per week).
	Chadwick's sign a bluish discoloration of the vagina, present at 8 weeks.	
	Height of fundus is at the symphysis, rises about 1 cm per week thereafter.	Teach to report these warning signals of problems in first and second trimester: vaginal bleeding, fever, chills, pain, persistent vomiting, leaking of fluid from vagina.
	12 weeks—fetal pulse detected by ultrasonic techniques.	
	Second Trimester	
	Weeks 13–16	
Tasks: Accepts fetus as a separate being.	Objective: Colostrum is present.	Advise the use of skin cream to soften crusts formed by colostrum. Remove crusts as part of bathing. Avoid soap on nipple.
Manages shifts in dependency from the role of daughter to the role of mother.	Leukorrhea, profuse, thin, white vaginal discharge. Report if pruritis or foul odor develop: *Candida albicans,* trichomonal infections common.	Suggest the external use of a solution of vinegar and water; use of loose, cotton undergarments; vulval pads, changed frequently; tampons are contraindicated.
Continues working through of any conflicts with own parents.	Abdominal appearance of pregnancy.	Advise against tight, constricting clothing or wearing shoes with a heel higher than 1½ in. Reinforce good body mechanics; introduce pelvic rock exercise, body toning exercises.
Mimicry, role playing to help assume the role of mother.	Height of fundus is halfway between symphysis and umbilicus.	
	Weeks 17–20	
Concerns: Nutritional intake.	Subjective: Quickening—maternal perception of first fetal movements.	Instruct client to report any cessation of fetal movement lasting longer than 24 h.
Changing body image.		
Changing life-style and sexual needs.	Often increased sexual desire.	Reinforce concept that variations in sexual interest do occur, that her partner may not understand these variations. Good communication is essential.

TABLE 7-2 / DEVELOPMENTAL TASKS, SIGNS AND SYMPTOMS, AND NURSING INTERVENTION DURING FIRST, SECOND, AND THIRD TRIMESTERS (*Continued*)

Tasks, Concerns, and Problems	Signs and Symptoms	Nursing Intervention
Progression of fetal growth. Warning signs of problems. Problems: Lack of acceptance of pregnancy. Depression, anger, anxiety continue. Numerous physical complaints, and focus on own concerns. Indications of no family support. Indication of inability to plan ahead. Goals: Include siblings in preparation for bith. Prepare to deal with possible sibling rivalry. Buy equipment, baby clothes (unless cultural, socioeconomic restrictions).	Objective: Increase in total blood volume which contributes to lightheadedness or fainting; occurs by 10–14 weeks; peaks at 8½ months (34–36 weeks).	Advise her to get up slowly from a horizontal position.
	The formation of varicosities of the saphenous system, vulva, and rectum.	Avoid constricting bands around legs and long period of sitting and standing. Use of support hose and elevation of legs at a 90° angle at least twice a day may be indicated.
	Headaches.	Report severe headaches—do not take aspirin in large doses. Report visual disturbances; edema of the face, hands, or legs in the morning; scanty, concentrated urine.
	Hemodilution of pregnancy is result of increased plasma (40%) and small RBC increase. Hb of 10.5–12 g, and Hct may be 30–33%.	Include iron-rich foods in diet.
	Fundus is slightly below the umbilicus.	Fetal heart tones are audible with stethoscope.
	Weeks 21–24	
	Subjective: Pelvic joints are relaxing due to hormone relaxin.	Reinforce good body mechanics; use of squatting and tailor position.
	Objective: Possible pigment changes in skin—chloasma of face, linea nigra of abdomen, striae gravidarum.	Reassure patient that while these cannot be prevented, pigmentation will fade after delivery.
	Increased perspiration.	Teach hygiene if necessary.
	Dilation of right ureter due to pressure from dextrorotated uterus.	Since urinary stasis and resultant pyelonephritis may result, reinforce need to report any signs of infection. Lying on side aids kidney efficiency from now on.
	Weeks 25–28	
	Subjective: Leg cramps due to decreased calcium; when there is an increased phosphorus level, fatigue.	Advise exercise, particularly walking, and elevation of legs; as a substitute for milk, calcium tablets may be ordered to achieve Ca:P balance.
	Objective: Hemorrhoids.	Replace if external. Advise use of ice to the part, use of the knee-chest position for up to 15 min. Teach diet to avoid constipation.

TABLE 7-2 / DEVELOPMENTAL TASKS, SIGNS AND SYMPTOMS, AND NURSING INTERVENTION DURING FIRST, SECOND, AND THIRD TRIMESTERS (*Continued*)

Tasks, Concerns, and Problems	Signs and Symptoms	Nursing Intervention
	Braxton Hicks contractions—painless, intermittent contractions.	
	Fetal parts are palpable. Fundus is above umbilicus. Ballotment (the rebound of fetal parts) occurs.	Explain that these occur throughout pregnancy and are not labor contractions.

	Third Trimester	
	Weeks 29–32	
Tasks: Acceptance of pregnancy. Continues to view fetus as a separate individual. Acceptance of physical and psychological changes.	Subjective: Fatigue recurs.	Anticipatory guidance about availabliity of classes in preparation for childbirth. Inform of the signs of labor; be aware of unrealistic attitudes toward labor. Employment will be terminated usually by seventh month. Travel involving trips of over 2–3 h are unwise. If necessary, the woman should be instructed to change position frequently and to walk around.
Concerns: Baby's well-being and factors affecting this. Anxiety over possibility of deformed baby.	May feel faint in supine position, due to pressure on the inferior vena cava, which prevents the return of blood from lower extremities.	Advise a side-lying position such as a modified Sims position.
Expenses. Process of labor and delivery.	Sexual desire again decreases due to physical discomfort.	Counseling about variations in desires, alternative sexual practices, and reassurance that this is normal.
Acceptance of baby by other children. Present discomforts.	Objective: Constipation due to slowed peristalsis, pressure of uterus on lower colon and rectum, and hemorrhoids	Avoidance of constipation by a regular elimination routine, liberal fluid and roughage intake, and exercise is best. Use of home remedies, over-the-counter preparations, and enemas are to be avoided.
Problems: High level of anxiety about self, process of labor.	Heartburn due to pressure of uterus on stomach, causes mild hiatus hernia, regurgitation of stomach acid into esophagus.	Antacids may be ordered by physician. Advise small meals and sitting up after eating. Advise against over-the-counter preparations.
Continued nonacceptance of pregnancy. Behavior which neglects health practices. Lack of support from family or spouse.	Blood pressure returns to prepregnancy level after a slight drop due to vasodilation. Pulse rate has risen to 15 bpm over normal due to increase in cardiac work.	Monitor blood pressure for changes. Blood pressure of 140/90 or an increase of 30 mmHg in the systolic reading or of 15 mmHg in the diastolic reading is considered a symptom of preeclampsia. Reinforce instructions to notify physician of preeclampsia symptoms.
Lack of preparation for or focus on needs of new baby.	Fundus is midway between the umbilicus and the xiphoid.	Prenatal visits will be every 2 weeks until the ninth month, when they will be weekly. If patient plans to breast-feed, teach her to express colostrum. For flat or inverted nipples, teach rolling motion to assist in making them more prominent.

TABLE 7-2 / DEVELOPMENTAL TASKS, SIGNS AND SYMPTOMS, AND NURSING INTERVENTION DURING FIRST, SECOND, AND THIRD TRIMESTERS (*Continued*)

Tasks, Concerns, and Problems	Signs and Symptoms	Nursing Intervention
	Weeks 33–36	
	Subjective: Backache.	Reinforce use of good body mechanics.
	Becomes impatient for ending of pregnancy.	Use of heat, analgesics, and rest as ordered by physician.
	Mood swings occur again as ambivalence about future is demonstrated.	
	Changes in gait.	Use of supportive shoes, sometimes girdle.
	Objective: Shortness of breath and other pressure symptoms increase (heartburn, feeling of fullness after eating, constipation, varicose veins, dependent edema in extremities, hemorrhoids).	Remind patient to limit activities to avoid dyspnea; pillows may be needed at night. Symptoms will disappear when lightening occurs.
	Weeks 37–40	
	Subjective: Lightening—descent of the presenting part into the true pelvis.	Relaxation and breathing techniques, support husband as coach.
	Aching in lower abdomen.	Teach signs of impending labor:
	Objective: Fundus just below the diaphragm until lightening, then appears to tip forward.	1. Contractions increasing in intensity and frequency, which do not stop when walking. 2. Mucous plug, "bloody show," expelled. 3. Membranes may rupture anytime and should be reported to physician.

    V. Presence of a weight problem, under- or overweight.

   VI. Chronic medical or psychological problem that may affect the pregnancy or parenting potential.

Diagnosis

    I. Pregnant woman progressing according to normal pattern.

   II. Woman demonstrating difficulty with:

      A. Psychological adjustment and developmental tasks.

      B. Minor discomforts.

      C. Social or physical adaptation to pregnancy.

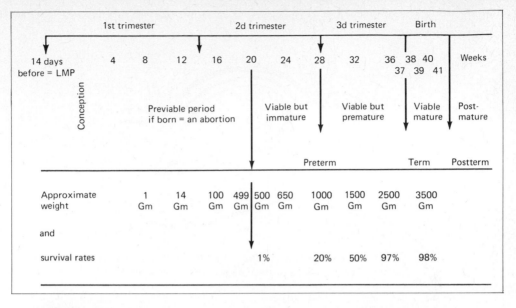

FIGURE 7-3 / Dates, weights, and terminology related to fetal maturity. (*From E. J. Dickason and M. O. Schult, Maternal and Infant Care, McGraw-Hill Book Company, New York, 1975.*)

Goals of Care

Immediate
   I. Physical health status of the woman is assessed.
   II. Status of fetal development and EDD is identified and interpreted to her.
   III. Client is oriented to initial procedures.
   IV. Evaluation of psychosocial response to new pregnancy is based on client's own statements.
   V. Client is assisted to understand psychological and physical changes of trimester.
   VI. Nutrition counseling is applied to client's own food habits.

Long-range
   I. Client understands sequence of follow-up care and referral plans.
   II. She receives referrals as necessary: nutritionist, dentist, or social worker.
   III. Client receives anticipatory guidance according to trimester.
   IV. Client is instructed about adverse over-the-counter drug effects.

Intervention

   I. Elicit history of minor discomforts and answer any questions regarding care and future developments.
   II. Teach nonpharmacologic relief of minor discomforts.
   III. Teach developmental changes in mother and fetus for the next 2 months.
   IV. Interpret physician's instructions, and determine client's level of understanding.
   V. Provide appropriate literature and make suggestions for reading.

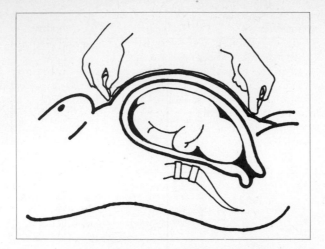

FIGURE 7-4 / **Measuring fundal height.** (*From E. J. Dickason and M.O. Schult, Maternal and Infant Care, McGraw-Hill Book Company, New York, 1975.*)

VI. Alert her to abnormal symptoms of first trimester and what action to take. These symptoms include:
   A. Bleeding.
   B. Urinary infections, other infections.
   C. Severe mood swings, depression.
   D. Protracted vomiting.
VII. Determine her goals and fears for pregnancy period and seek her cooperation in reaching client-determined goals.

Evaluation

I. Woman sequences through first 12 weeks without difficulty.
   A. She accepts being pregnant.
   B. Fetal development seems to be normal.
   C. She is maintaining weight and diet with understanding.
   D. She participates regularly in clinic or physician follow-up.
II. Problems occur in first trimester.
   A. Woman demonstrates poor psychosocial adjustment to pregnancy.
      1. Assessment.
         a. Denial, depression, or regression.
         b. Increased fears or anxiety.
         c. Exaggerated physical discomforts.
      2. Intervention.
         a. Referral for counseling—social service or psychiatric.
         b. Confer about actual obstacles to acceptance; family should be included.
         c. Assistance to reduce physical discomfort.
   B. Woman demonstrates poor physical adjustment to pregnancy.
      1. Vomiting progresses to hyperemesis. *Hyperemesis gravidarum* is constant and excessive vomiting continuing to the 16th week of pregnancy and resulting in loss of 5 percent or more of body weight. Without treatment, it may result in ketosis, ketonuria, neurological disturbances, liver and/or renal damage, death.
         a. Assessment.
            (1) Vomiting throughout day.   (2) Weight loss.

(3) Dehydration. (4) Depression.
  b. Intervention.
    (1) Admission to hospital to maintain fluid and electrolyte balance.
    (2) Psychiatric assessment.
    (3) Medication with antiemetics, tranquilizers, vitamins.
    (4) NPO with IV fluids, then oral nutrition slowly instituted.
2. Vaginal infections occur. During pregnancy higher pH (normally 4.0) and an increase in glucose levels in vaginal tissues support the growth of commonly resident bacteria (see Chap. 30).

Vaginal Infections	Manifestation in Newborn if Untreated
Trichomonas vaginalis	None
Candida albicans (Monilia albicans)	Oral thrush
Herpes progenitalis (herpes simplex, type 2)	Spontaneous abortion; disseminated infection, frequently fatal
Gonorrhea (Neisseria gonorrhoeae)	Conjunctivitis, blindness, septicemia following maternal septicemia
Syphilis (Treponema pallidum) after fifth month of pregnancy	Bone, tooth deformities, progressive nervous system damage

  a. Assessment.
    (1) Vaginal discharge evaluated.
    (2) Vulval irritation, itching, dysuria.
    (3) Painful sexual intercourse, may cause sexual problems.
    (4) Screening for elevated glucose level, may indicate gestational diabetes.
  b. Intervention.
    (1) Medication with specific agent after evaluation of causative organism.
    (2) Provide hygienic information, frequent perineal care, no douches, vinegar wash, use of vaginal pads, no tampons.
    (3) Need to treat partner, provide counseling.
    (4) Follow-up to check for reinfection. Serology may remain positive after treatment for some time (1).
3. Spontaneous abortion occurs: the loss of the conceptus before the end of the 20th completed week after last normal period. When the fetus weighs less than 500 g or measures less than 16.5 cm, crown-rump (CR) length, it is thought to be nonviable. Incidence is 1:15 pregnancies. Spontaneous abortion may be due to a defective embryo or placenta (50 to 60 percent), unknown causes (20 to 30 percent), or maternal disease (15 percent) (2). Early: 8 to 10 weeks. Late: 13 weeks and thereafter.
  a. Threatened abortion.
    (1) Assessment.
      (a) Lower abdominal cramping; spotting, especially when menses is due.
      (b) No advancing cervical dilation.
      (c) Low hormonal levels, estrogen/HCG.
    (2) Intervention.
      (a) Bed rest, observation of possible progression, sedation, fluids, emotional support.
      (b) Abstinence from intercourse.
      (c) 24 h urine for hormone levels: assessment of HCG levels. (1 IU per 100 mL at time of first missed period increasing to 100 IU per 100 mL 60 to 100 days, after LMP, then falls off sharply.) Estriol levels

below 3 to 4 mg per 100 mL in 24-h urine during first trimester indicate fetal death.

b. Inevitable abortion.

   (1) Assessment.

      (a) More severe cramping and bleeding, membranes rupture and progressive dilation takes place (4 to 5 cm).

      (b) Complete: passage of complete conceptus.

      (c) Incomplete: passage of only partial products of conception.

   (2) Intervention.

      (a) Bed rest and replacement of fluids, analgesia if necessary.

      (b) Observation of amount of bleeding, careful check for completeness of aborted fragments.

      (c) Oxytocin upon completion of passage, prn.

      (d) Involution should proceed as after delivery except more rapidly.

      (e) Needs dilatation and curettage (D&C) if incomplete, usually under anesthesia, with IV fluids, oxytocics.

c. Missed abortion: cessation of growth of embryo for a period of 8 weeks without passage of fetus.

   (1) Assessment.

      (a) Absence of fetal heart beat.

      (b) Regression of signs of pregnancy, static uterine size.

   (2) Intervention.

      (a) Depending upon week of gestation: early, dilatation and curettage (D&C); midtrimester, prostaglandin instillation into amniotic fluid.

      (b) Support for grieving, or anxiety about intrauterine fetal death.

d. Habitual abortion: repeated spontaneous abortion, occurring three or more times.

   (1) Assessment.

      (a) Varied symptoms; if incompetent cervix, membranes bulge, dilation takes place after 12 weeks.

      (b) If low hormonal levels, see above.

   (2) Intervention.

      (a) Cerclage procedure.

      (b) Hormonal support.

      (c) Bed rest.

4. Ectopic pregnancy: implantation of fertilized ovum outside the uterus, usually in the fallopian tube. Average incidence of 1:200 pregnancies. Varies widely depending mainly on socioeconomic status and history of health care, as contributing to predisposing factors.

a. Assessment.

   (1) Amenorrhea, followed by spotting, then varying amounts of vaginal bleeding.

   (2) Increasing lower abdominal pressure beginning about 3 to 5 weeks after LMP.

   (3) Syncope, "fainting in bathroom," feels rectal pressure.

   (4) Anemia, fatigue increasing.

   (5) Abdominal pain beginning about 10 to 12 weeks after LMP.

b. Intervention.

   (1) Prepare for culdocentesis, possible laparotomy, blood tests, urinalysis, surgery (obtain surgical consent).

   (2) If hypovolemic, treat symptoms, observe vital signs, provide fluid replacement, keep NPO for surgery.

   (3) Observe after surgery for signs of infection.

   (4) Support in grieving process.

5. The expectant mother is either very young or older. At either end of the childbearing cycle, there is greater risk of delivering infants of low gestational age or of low birth weight, and there is an increased perinatal mortality rate.

a. Adolescents: Pregnancy for them is complicated by immature physical development, interruption of education, and developmental tasks of adolescence not yet achieved. Lack of family acceptance or paternal support often necessitates some difficult decisions about the pregnancy or future of infant such as abortion, adoption, or keeping the infant with grandparent. Incidence rising: 247,000 births to 17-year-olds or less, 30,000 to 15-year-olds or less. Of 1 million pregnancies, 350,000 end in voluntary abortions, 66 percent of which are obtained by unmarried women (3).

(1) Assessment.

    (a) Higher risk of anemia, poor nutrition.

    (b) Increased incidence of preeclampsia, preterm delivery.

    (c) Psychosocial problems—poor adaptation, ambivalence, lack of family support.

    (d) Increased anxiety about labor, parenting.

    (e) Difficulty with developmental tasks, both of adolescence and pregnancy.

(2) Intervention.

    (a) Continuity of care, nutrition counseling, referral to nutritionist.

    (b) Classes in pregnancy, labor, child care more intensive.

    (c) Referral to social service and sometimes psychiatrist.

    (d) Alert labor unit to specific needs of teen and refer for after delivery follow-up.

    (e) Ego strengthening needed, support by family and peers may be lacking.

b. Elderly gravidas are those women having a first baby when over 35 or subsequent children when over 40. They have two times the incidence of maternal mortality, a higher risk of complicating medical problems, a 10 percent incidence of perinatal mortality, and a 3.5 times incidence of placenta previa than younger gravidas. Due to age, delivery is often by cesarean section. Ideally, counseling about childbearing should be done before pregnancy.

(1) Assessment.

    (a) Preexisting health problems, obesity.

    (b) Increased risk of psychosocial problems, anxiety, ambivalence.

    (c) Higher incidence of preeclampsia, hypertension.

    (d) Increased risk of congenital defects (Down's syndrome 1:40 risk).

(2) Intervention.

    (a) Nutritional counseling.

    (b) Assessment of underlying health problems.

    (c) Support, assess difficulties with developmental tasks.

    (d) Monitor physical status.

    (e) Diagnostic amniocentesis.

    (f) Referral for genetic counseling.

    (g) Referral for follow-up to ensure parenting support.

THE SECOND TRIMESTER

Definition

The period 15 to 28 weeks after LMP (13 to 27 weeks after conception) constitutes the second trimester of pregnancy. The uterus enlarges to above the umbilicus and the first fetal movements are felt. During this period fetal organogenesis is completed, but if delivery occurs, chances of survival are slight. (See Tables 7-1 and 7-2.)

Assessment

When client enters the health care system in the second trimester the following information is acquired:
I. Health history.
II. Obstetric course and reason for delay in seeking care.
III. Physical examination—now including abdominal palpation, fundal location, and fetal heart tones.
IV. Laboratory tests.

Problems

I. Presence of dietary problems.
II. Psychological responses inappropriate for the trimester.
III. Changes in body image and physical symptoms dominate client's concern.
IV. Signs of medical problems become overt.

Goals of Care

Immediate
I. With client, adequacy of diet and need for supplemental iron is determined.
II. Client's health status is evaluated.
III. The health status of the fetus, fetal maturity, and EDC, is identified.
IV. Client is oriented to the steps in the health care system.
V. Client understands need for continuing care.

Long-range
I. Determine progress in achieving developmental tasks.
II. Client identifies need for and is supplied with information about sexuality during pregnancy.
III. She receives referrals for psychosocial, nutritional, or dental care as necessary.
IV. Client understands warning signals of pregnancy (see Table 7-2) and action to take.
V. Staff will assess high-risk signals of potential child abuse (see Table 7-4).

Intervention

I. Encourage client to express minor discomforts and ask any questions regarding care and future developments.
II. Teach relief of minor discomforts (see Table 7-2).
III. Reinforce need for good nutrition, and explain side effects if supplemental iron is ordered (Table 7-3).
IV. Interpret physician's instructions while determining patient's level of understanding.
V. Teach developmental changes in mother and fetus during these 3 months.
VI. Counsel client about human sexuality in pregnancy.
VII. Instruct about abnormal signs and symptoms and appropriate action (see Table 7-2).

Evaluation

I. Woman sequences through week 13 to 28 without difficulty and with no adverse environmental factors.
   A. She has achieved second trimester task of identifying the fetus as separate from herself.

TABLE 7-3 / DAILY DIET PLAN IN PREGNANCY

Food	Baseline Diet	Diet during Pregnancy
Milk	Adult: 2 cups	4 cups
	Teenager: 4 cups	4 cups
Meat, fish, poultry, eggs, nuts, dried peas or beans	2 servings (2 oz each)	2 servings (3 oz each)
Vegetable/fruit	4 servings	4 servings
High–vitamin C fruit or vegetable	1 serving daily	1 serving daily
Dark green or deep yellow vegetable	1 serving every other day	1 serving every other day
Bread/cereal, enriched or whole grain	5 servings*	5 servings*

*Four servings if one is a breakfast cereal.
Source: B. Lau Kee and M. O. Schult, "Maternal Development," in E. J. Dickason and M. O. Schult (eds.), *Maternal and Infant Care*, McGraw-Hill Book Company, New York, 1975, chap. 4.

    B. Fetal development appears to be proceeding normally.
    C. She is maintaining weight/diet according to plan.
    D. She can identify warning signals and knows when to call physician or clinic.
    E. She is beginning to prepare for the infant.
    F. She identifies sexual adjustment as satisfactory.
II. Problems occur in second trimester.
    A. Woman demonstrates an excessive weight gain.
        1. Assessment.
            a. Weight gain over 0.8 lb a week.
            b. Diet is high carbohydrate, low protein; she is snacking on junk food.
            c. Is inactive—limited exercise.
            d. No edema, hypertension noted.
        2. Intervention.
            a. Nutrition counseling.
            b. If income is inadequate, refer to social worker.
            c. Encourage exercise in moderation.
    B. Woman demonstrates an inadequate weight gain.
        1. Assessment.
            a. Weight gain is under desired level.
            b. Preoccupation with maintaining "slim" body image.
            c. Control nausea and vomiting as soon as possible.
        2. Intervention.
            a. Nutrition counseling.
            b. Assess psychological status.
            c. Reinforce measures to reduce nausea and vomiting.
    C. Anemia is diagnosed. Reduction in iron-bearing factor or numbers of red blood cells because of (1) inadequate production of erythrocytes, (2) premature destruction of erythrocytes, or (3) blood loss from vascular system. The most common cause is iron deficiency. In pregnancy, about 2 mg additional iron daily must be absorbed to meet requirements of growing fetus, expanded blood volume, and placental growth. In severe cases, blood transfusions and parenteral iron are necessary to restore balance.
        1. Assessment.
            a. Fatigue, poor iron reserve.

        b. Reduced oxygen-carrying capacity.

        c. Increased incidence of infection.

        d. Hb below 11.0 g, and Hct below 33 percent in second trimester.

    2. Intervention.

        a. Teach about balanced diet.

        b. Explain side effects of supplementary iron.

        c. Observe for symptoms of infection.

        d. Recheck lab tests.

        e. If ordered, administer parenteral iron with correct Z-track technique.

D. Hydatidiform mole (hydatid, molar pregnancy): a developmental anomaly of the chorionic syncytium involving degeneration of the villi into fluid-filled grapelike vesicles. In the United States it is thought to occur in 1 out of 2000 pregnancies. Studies indicate it may be more common in women with protein-deficient diets. Lack of, or destruction of, folic acid and amino acids in food preparation may interfere with the developing embryo and be a factor in the development of a mole.

    1. Assessment.

        a. Uterus larger than gestational age would indicate.

        b. Heavy vaginal bleeding which may contain grapelike vesicles.

        c. Anemia.

        d. Hyperemesis may be present.

        e. Early, preeclamptic symptoms—before the 24th week.

        f. Urinary chorionic gonadotropin (UCG) levels to 35,000 IU/mL.

    2. Intervention.

        a. Monitor blood loss.

        b. Prepare for D&C.

        c. Prevent infection.

        d. Psychological support—fear of bleeding to death, loss of "pregnancy."

        e. Follow-up because of possibility of recurrent mole, or choriocarcinoma, a highly malignant cancer.

        f. UCG levels monitored for 6 months to 1 year after operation.

E. Bacteriuria: multiplying bacteria are present in the urine although the client may be asymptomatic. Ascending urinary tract infection may result. Bacteriuria may cause premature labor and has been indicated as a cause of some cases of intrauterine growth retardation (IUGR).

    1. Assessment.

        a. In cystitis—frequency, burning, dysuria.

        b. In pyelonephritis—fever, chills, lumbar pain added.

        c. Urinalysis shows more than 100,000 organisms per milliliter, increased white blood cells, and possibly red blood cells.

    2. Intervention.

        a. Medication with appropriate drugs.

        b. Adequate fluid intake, with acidifying agents; cranberry juice, vitamin C.

        c. Collection of clean, voided specimens for culture and sensitivity.

F. Diabetes mellitus (expanded plan). This inability to metabolize glucose properly is manifested in different degrees of severity. (See classifications in Chap. 24.) The incidence of diabetes mellitus is 1:100 to 1:200 pregnancies. It should be considered for a woman with a family history of diabetes, particularly in a parent or twin; for a woman with a history of spontaneous abortions or infections; for a woman with current symptoms of glycosuria; or for a woman who has delivered an infant weighing 9 lb or more, or a series of infants with increasing birth weights or who have had unexplained congenital anomalies or have died in the perinatal period.

    During pregnancy, a woman with diabetes is five times more prone to develop preeclampsia, and 20 percent of pregnant diabetics have hydramnios. Monilial infections and urinary tract infections are more common as well. As for the fetus, class A (gestational diabetes) infants are often large for gestational age, have a higher risk of respiratory di tress syndrome (RDS) and hypoglycemia in the neonatal period. Infants of diabetic mothers also have a higher incidence of congenital anomalies, RDS, and a higher perinatal mortality rate. There is a 90 percent fetal survival rate with experienced care (4). In severely insulin-dependent diabetics, the infants may have intrauterine growth retardation. Preterm delivery may occur or be planned to rescue a compromised infant.

The quality of metabolic control is most important. Investigators have found that mothers with diabetes mellitus and acetonuria have had offspring with lower IQs than control infants. Dietary control and use of insulin is essential. Oral hypoglycemic agents are not used during pregnancy. They cross the placental barrier and can cause prolonged neonatal hypoglycemia.

1. Assessment.
    a. Family history.
    b. Medical history: detailed history of diabetes onset, control, and evidence of diabetic complications.
    c. Obstetric history.
    d. Laboratory tests; in addition to usual:
        (1) monitor blood glucose levels, fasting blood sugar (FBS), postprandial sugar.
        (2) Urinalysis: glucose, ketone, and protein determinations.
        (3) Blood urea nitrogen.
        (4) 24-h urine for glucose levels to determine how much carbohydrate is lost. If carbohydrate loss is above 20 g of glucose per day, then diet must be supplemented by that amount of carbohydrate (4).
        (5) Possible x-ray studies of the lower extremities to detect vascular calcification.
        (6) Studies of fetal maturity, fetal condition.
    e. Physical exam by obstetrician and/or internist every 2 weeks until the 30th week; thereafter every week.
2. Problems.
    a. Lack of understanding of diabetes mellitus and/or pregnancy.
    b. Overwhelmed by fluctuations in diabetic state.
    c. Expressed fear for self and infant.
    d. Inability to accept diabetes and/or pregnancy.
    e. Concern over cost of complicated pregnancy.
3. Diagnosis.
    a. Pregnant diabetic is in good metabolic control.
    b. Pregnant diabetic is in poor metabolic control.
    c. Pregnant diabetic is in poor metabolic control, denying any problem.
4. Goals of care.
    a. Immediate.
        (1) Educate about diabetes and pregnancy.
        (2) Reinforce diet to control diabetes, discuss importance of normoglycemia.
        (3) Increase client's awareness of adverse symptoms plus importance of early recognition and reporting.
    b. Long-range.
        (1) Intensive instruction and supervision of diet, insulin, and urine testing to achieve normoglycemia.
        (2) Alert client to potential need for repeated hospitalizations during pregnancy for insulin regulation and determinations of fetal status through measurement of estriol levels and oxytocin stress tests.
        (3) Support client through a high-risk pregnancy, maintaining contact.
        (4) Assess potential for effective parenting.
        (5) Prepare for possible early delivery with entry into hospital for evaluation 6 to 8 weeks prior to EDD.

5. Intervention.
   a. Reinforce need for frequent prenatal visits to monitor health status of woman and fetus.
   b. Clarify how diabetes affects her pregnancy and how the pregnancy affects diabetes.
   c. Anticipatory guidance about possible complications.
   d. Ensure client's understanding of dietary control, insulin requirements, urine testing, hygienic measures.
   e. Refer to nutritionist, social worker, or visiting nurse.
   f. Instruct about abnormal signs and symptoms and appropriate action.
6. Evaluation.
   a. Pregnancy of client with diabetes mellitus progressing normally.
   b. Pregnancy of client with diabetes mellitus is complicated by poor metabolic control, superimposed obstetric complications, or psychologic problems.
   c. Pregnancy of client with diabetes mellitus is complicated by progressive vascular, renal disease, with retinopathy.

THE THIRD TRIMESTER

Definition

The period between the end of the 28th completed week of gestation (after LMP) until delivery is a period of rapid fetal growth in size and in ability to function. Every possible week of growth in utero increases the chance of survival for an infant born in this trimester. It is a period of completion of developmental tasks for the mother as well, as she faces taking up the parenting role for 24 h a day. (See Tables 7-1 and 7-2.)

Assessment

Data to be collected if client enters care during the third trimester:
I. Obstetric history and reasons for delay in seeking care.
II. Medical and social history pertinent to pregnancy.
III. Complete physical exam including:
   A. Assessment of gestational age, fetal size, position.
   B. Evaluation of pelvic adequacy.
   C. Laboratory tests to screen for disease.
      1. Pap smear, smear for gonorrhea, other infections.
      2. Complete blood count (CBC), Hct, Hb, serology, plus screening for G6PD, and sickle cell in high-risk populations.
      3. Urinalysis and, if indicated, oral or IV glucose tolerance test.
   D. Breast exam, plus determining if patient wishes to breast-feed.
IV. History of preparation for childbirth, prior feelings about childbirth.
V. Assessment of support system available to client.

Problems

Problems to be surveyed when client delays care until third trimester include the following:

I. Client's behavior indicates noncompliance with prenatal care goals.
II. Psychosocial problems are overwhelming.
   A. Poverty, care of other children, distance from facility.
   B. Drug addiction, prostitution.
   C. Immigrant to country, unfamiliar with availability of health care.

III. Denial of pregnancy can no longer be maintained because of obvious uterine growth.
    A. Highly anxious teenager, delayed seeking care.
    B. Spouse was rejecting pregnancy.
    C. Ambivalence about pregnancy continued past late date for elective abortion.
IV. Physical complications bring patient to seek care.

Diagnosis

  I. Client demonstrating problem which prevented her from seeking early care.
 II. Lack of understanding of need, or resistance to obtaining prenatal care underlies late entry.
III. Client demonstrating poor physical or psychological adjustment to this phase of pregnancy.

Goals of Care

Immediate

   I. Status of fetal health and fetal maturity is identified and interpreted for client.
  II. Client is oriented to steps in health care.
 III. Overall health status of client is assessed and explained to her.
 IV. Client identifies reasons for ignoring health supervision during first two trimesters.

Long-range

    I. She receives referrals to dentist, social worker, or nutritionist as needed.
   II. Client understands need for consistent follow-through on nutrition, clinic visits.
  III. Client attends available classes on prenatal care.
  IV. She can interpret process of labor and warning signals of problems in this trimester in terms adequate for her.
   V. Client begins preparations for infant and infant care, demonstrating achievement of psychologic tasks.
 VI. Staff will assess risks of child abuse (Table 7-4).

Intervention

    I. Determine client's understanding of goals of prenatal care.
      A. Obtain history of pattern with other pregnancies.
      B. Discover if negative experiences govern her choices.
      C. Reassure where possible about unfounded fears.
      D. Explain sequence of the next weeks' plan of care.
   II. Obtain a history of particular discomforts during this pregnancy.
 III. Teach nonpharmacologic methods of alleviation of current problems.
 IV. Determine her goals and fears concerning pregnancy, delivery, and care of infant.
      A. Seek cooperation in reaching client-determined goals.
      B. Encourage health measures she does not yet recognize as important.
   V. Discuss fetal growth, stages of development, and the ways in which the infant's health has been assessed.
 VI. Determine parents' understanding of third trimester developmental tasks and readiness to take up their new role.
VII. Interpret results of physical assessment, needs of this phase of pregnancy, and laboratory tests.
VIII. Interpret physician's instructions. Determine level of understanding, clarify points, and provide appropriate instructional literature.
 IX. Instruct about abnormal signs and symptoms and what action to take:
      A. Bleeding—with/without pain.

TABLE 7-4 / HIGH-RISK SIGNALS IN THE PRENATAL CLINIC SETTING

A high-risk situation is not just any one of the items listed below, but rather varying combinations of these signs, plus the family's degree of emphasis on them, and their inflexibility to changes. The interviewer must take into consideration the patient's age, culture, and education. Many of these signs can be assessed interchangeably throughout the entire perinatal period, but they are listed in the order in which they most often assume significance.

I. Overconcern with the unborn baby's sex.
  A. Reasons why a certain sex is so important—i.e., to fill the parents' or grandparents' needs.
  B. The mother's need to please the father with the baby's sex.
  C. The rigidity of these needs.

II. Expressed high expectations for the baby.
  A. Overconcern with the baby's physical and developmental progress, behavior, and discipline.
  B. The parents' need to have control over the baby's actions and reactions.
  C. Is this child wanted in order to fulfill unmet needs in parents' lives?

III. Is this child going to be one too many?
  A. Is there adequate spacing between this child and the next older child?
  B. During the pregnancy has there been evidence of a disintegrating relationship with the older child(ren), i.e., physical or emotional abuse for the first time?

IV. Evidence of the mother's desire to deny the pregnancy.
  A. Unhappiness with weight gain.
  B. Refusing to talk about the pregnancy in a manner commensurate with the reality of the situation.
  C. Refusing to wear maternity clothes.
  D. No plans made for baby's nursery or layette, etc.

V. Great depression over the pregnancy.
  A. Date of onset of depression to this pregnancy.
  B. Report of sleep disturbance that cannot be related to the physical aspects of pregnancy.
  C. Attempted suicide.

VI. Did either parent formerly ever seriously consider an abortion?
  A. Why didn't they go through with it?
  B. Did they passively delay a decision until medically therapeutic abortion was not feasible?

VII. Did the parents ever seriously consider relinquishment of a baby?
  A. Why did they change their minds?
  B. The reality and quality expressed in the change of decision.

VIII. Who does the mother turn to for support?
  A. How reliable and helpful is this support?
  B. Who accompanies the mother to the clinic?
  C. Are any community agencies involved in a supportive way?

IX. Is the mother alone and/or frightened?
  A. Is this because of lack of education or understanding of pregnancy and delivery?
  B. Is she overly concerned about the physical changes during pregnancy, labor, and delivery?
  C. Do careful explanations, prenatal classes, etc., dissipate these fears?
  D. Does the mother tend to keep the focus of the interview on *her* fears and needs rather than focusing on the new baby?

X. Does the mother have many unscheduled visits to the prenatal clinic or the emergency room?
  A. With exaggerated physical complaints that cannot be substantiated on physical examination or by laboratory tests?
  B. Multiple psychosomatic complaints?
  C. An overdependence on the physician or nurse?

TABLE 7-4 / HIGH-RISK SIGNALS IN THE PRENATAL CLINIC SETTING (*Continued*)

XI. What are the patient's living arrangements?
  A. Are the physical accommodations adequate?
  B. Do they have a telephone?
  C. Is transportation available?
  D. Are there friends or relatives nearby?
XII. The parents can't talk freely on the above topics and avoid eye contact.
XIII. What can you find out about the parents' backgrounds?
  A. Did they grow up in a foster home?
  B. Were they shuffled from one relative to another?
  C. What type of discipline was used?
  D. Do they plan to raise their children the way their parents raised them?

Source: R. E. Helfer and C. H. Kempe (eds.), *Child Abuse and Neglect: The Family and The Community*, The Ballinger Publishing Company, Cambridge, Mass., 1976, with permission.

  B. Urine infection—frequency, pain, burning on urination.
  C. Fluid retention—edema; dark, concentrated, cloudy urine.
  D. Headaches, visual disturbances.
  E. Ruptured membranes.
  F. Premature labor.
  G. Infections elsewhere in the body, URI, thrombophlebitis, vaginitis.
X. Teach process of labor and delivery. Answer patient's questions.

Evaluation

I. The last weeks of pregnancy are uneventful, and resolution of earlier difficulties has occurred.
  A. She has achieved third trimester tasks of being ready to take up parenting and becoming physically separated from infant.
  B. Fetal development appears to be progressing normally.
  C. Weight and diet are being maintained in the normal range.
  D. She understands signs of impending labor and knows when to call the physician or clinic for problems.
  E. She is well involved in preparing for the infant.
  F. She attends the clinic regularly now.
II. Problems occur in third trimester.
  A. Client continues to have unresolved anxieties and is fearful of the delivery process. Appears unable to achieve developmental tasks.
    1. Assessment.
      a. Anxiety demonstrated, and fantasies about death or injuries expressed.
      b. Unable to concentrate on instructions.
      c. Still focusing on self and changed body image rather than focusing on baby and future needs.
    2. Intervention.
      a. Arrange for session with client to express such feelings and fears. May need referral to social worker, psychiatrist.
      b. Make arrangements for orientation to labor unit prior to EDD. Encourage attendance at classes.
      c. Note such a problem for follow-through by labor nurses.
      d. Involve a relative or close friend to attend patient during labor.
      e. Prepare to do intensive postnatal follow-up for adjustment and parenting adaptation.

B. Client is still demonstrating noncompliance with prenatal care goals because of expressed hostility toward pregnancy.

1. Assessment.
   a. Patient's anger at being pregnant has abated somewhat, but she redirects it at the staff. May direct it at infant later.
   b. Demonstrates signs that infant may bear brunt of her diffuse anger.
   c. Blaming behavior seems to diminish when she is accompanied by sister (or friend, boyfriend, or mother).

2. Intervention.
   a. Referral for psychiatric consultation. Recognize displacement and deal firmly with requirements pregnancy places upon her.
   b. Child-abuse alert should continue past neonatal period. Visiting nurse service referral should be planned, and pediatrician notified.
   c. Involve people close to her in steps of education for labor and delivery, and care of infant. Determine how their support can assist woman to cope.

C. Physical complications become more dominant.

1. Varicose veins.
   a. Saphenous system.
      (1) Assessment.
         (a) Dilated, tortuous superficial veins in lower extremities appear in response to increase in femoral venous pressure (18 mmHg), due to obstructed venous return, genetic predisposition.
      (2) Intervention.
         (a) Instruct patient to prevent obstructed venous return by elevating legs when sitting, using sidelying position when resting or sleeping. Have her use elastic support stockings and avoid tight, constricting clothing. Use moderate exercise, especially walking. Check Homans' sign.
   b. Rectal veins.
      (1) Assessment.
         (a) Distended rectal or anal veins, external or internal, may begin early in first trimester but worsen during final months. Aggravated by sitting or standing for long periods, and by constipation. Enlarging uterus obstructs venous return, and aggravates constipation.
      (2) Intervention.
         (a) Treated by preventing constipation with fluids, roughage in diet or stool softener. Passage of stool may be assisted with glycerin suppository. A topical anesthetic spray may alleviate discomfort, as will ice pack to anal area, sitz baths, witch hazel soak to anal area, and frequent perineal care.
         (b) Use same preventive measures as for varicose veins of lower extremities.

2. Thrombophlebitis: inflammation of the vein intima, causing accumulation of fibrin and blood cells to form a clot which is usually attached firmly to the wall and rarely is detached to form emboli. In contrast, deep femoral or pelvic vein thrombus formation takes weeks to develop and may have a long tail which occludes partially or completely the large vein draining venous blood from extremities or pelvic tissues. In time part of this clot may be thrown off to the lungs.
   a. Superficial vein thrombus.
      (1) Assessment.
         (a) Follows preexisting varicose veins especially when there is injury to tissue, or local inflammation. More common in pregnancy and postpartum due to elevated plasma fibrinogen, and occurs more often in women who have had prior history. Clot is quite adherent.
      (2) Intervention.
         (a) Complete bedrest is indicated, with both legs elevated. Application

of dry heat will improve circulation. Use analgesics as necessary and apply elastic stockings before changing to upright position to ambulate.

b. Deep vein thrombophlebitis.

  (1) Assessment.

    (a) Reflex arteriolar spasm causes severe pain, and skin turns pale. Or there may just be deep aching along line of femoral vein. There may be chills, fever, absent popliteal pulse. Leg may be edematous.

    (b) Onset may be within 72 h of traumatic birth, or in presence of postpartum hemorrhage, or infection. May occur as late as 22 days after delivery.

    (c) Emboli can be thrown to lungs. Symptoms of dyspnea, hemoptysis, impending death sensation, pain.

  (2) Intervention.

    (a) Basic treatment is as in superficial phlebitis; however, danger of clot fragmenting into emboli is much more serious.

    (b) Medicated with heparin SC if prior to delivery and Coumadin agent after. Analgesia used for pain. Dose is regulated by bleeding or clotting time.

    (c) Check infant carefully in neonatal period. Breast feeding not recommended if mother is on anticoagulants.

    (d) Absolute bedrest is necessary until clot has been resolved. Heat cradle over bed. Bed kept in Trendelenburg's position to promote superficial draining of venous blood, bypassing femoral vein.

3. Placenta previa: bleeding occurs after 20th week. Placental tissue has been formed by invasion of trophoblastic cells into the uterine endometrium (decidual basalis), rupturing arterioles and venules to form lakes (lacunas) of maternal blood. Into these lakes fetal villi protrude. Any separation by tearing or by the slowly dilating internal cervical os will open a direct line to maternal circulation. Bleeding can be any degree from spotting to massive hemorrhage and is usually only halted by delivery of the fetus and placenta. Incidence of placenta previa is thought to be 1:100 to 1:150, and that of abruptio placentae is (1) complete, 1:500; (2) partial, either concealed or open, 1:85 to 1:139 (5).

a. Assessment.

  (1) Begins as painless spotting, increasing daily.

  (2) Hct and Hb fall; estriols borderline.

  (3) Ultrasound indicates preterm infant.

  (4) Patient most anxious about health of fetus.

  (5) Maternal condition worsens, bleeding increases in spite of treatment (Fig. 7-5).

b. Intervention.

  (1) Admit for observation, assessment of placental function and fetal condition.

  (2) Monitor by serial Hb, Hct, plasma-free estriols, or 24 h urine for estriols qd. Placental localization by ultrasound, plus fetal maturity studies, biparietal diameter (BPD), amniocentesis for lecithin/sphingomyelin (L/S) ratio, creatinine, fat cells in amniotic fluid.

  (3) Complete bed rest is necessary. Take pad count. Monitor maternal-fetal vital signs. Sedation is sometimes necessary. Allow extra time for mother to express fears and to grieve in anticipation of fetal loss.

  (4) Cesarean section with special care for placental location. Blood replacement. Infant to intensive care.

4. Bleeding occurs as labor approaches or during labor.

a. Assessment.

  (1) Open bleeding may first be confused with bloody show, but it is bright or dark red and clots poorly.

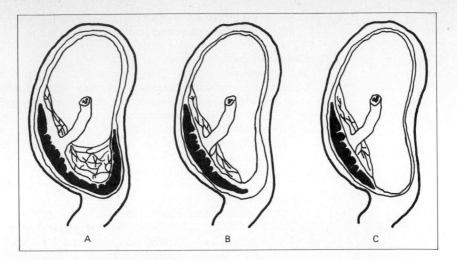

FIGURE 7-5 / Types of placenta previa: (a) total, (b) partial, (c) low-lying. (*From E. J. Dickason and M. O. Schult, Maternal and Infant Care, McGraw-Hill Book Company, New York, 1975.*)

    (2) If concealed bleeding, uterine tonus rises, contractions become erratic or cease, patient complains of severe pain. Fetal distress occurs, late decelerations then bradycardia.

    (3) If complete abruption, maternal shock and fetal death occur. Priority now is on stopping bleeding and correcting shock (Fig. 7-6).

  b. Intervention.

    (1) Careful evaluation without cervical manipulation. If time and equipment are available, use ultrasound localization of placenta.

    (2) Continuous monitoring and support of maternal blood pressure. Oxygen is administered. Type and cross match whole blood. Note clotting time (hypofibrinogenemia may occur).

    (3) Assess fetal jeopardy. Only a fetal scalp electrode is applied for internal monitor. Intervention with cesarean section, unless very near end of second stage and abruption is minor.

5. Cardiac dysfunction: Rheumatic heart disease is becoming increasingly uncommon as rheumatic fever is treated more adequately in childhood. However, women with treated congenital cardiac defects are coming to childbearing age, and the incidence of hypertensive heart disease is increasing. The overall incidence for cardiac disease in pregnancy has been found by Niswonger to be 17:1000. Functional classifications are useful to indicate heart function under the stress of pregnancy. Those women in class I and II given good care can usually go through pregnancy with a minimum of discomfort. Class III and IV patients are at high risk for multiple problems and must be hospitalized in the last trimester, for they are at risk for phlebitis, cardiac failure, preterm delivery, and infection.

  a. Assessment.

    (1) Stress of pregnancy hypervolemia precipitates dyspnea, cardiac arrhythmias, anginal pain, or severe fatigue in patient with underlying cardiac disease.

    (2) Edema without hypertension is present; or

    (3) Hypertensive heart disease is diagnosed.

    (4) Thrombophlebitis may occur, emboli may be thrown.

(5) Preterm labor (1 week early) may occur, labor may be shortened if patient on digitalis-like drugs (6).

(6) Cardiac stress of vaginal delivery equal to stress of operative delivery (7).

b. Interventions.

(1) Cardiac workup: ECG, chest x-ray, renal function studies, electrolytes.

(2) More frequent visits for medical supervision. Low-salt diet, with high protein intake, extra iron. Diuretics may be ordered. Instruct on potassium intake. Prophylactic antibiotics may be ordered. Antiemboli stockings.

(3) Hospitalization at 34 to 35 weeks for evaluation. Encourage bed rest in side-lying position. Curtail activity to what can be done without symptoms. Teach warning signals of increased cardiac stress. Educate patient about labor and delivery to reduce stress of anxiety, fear.

(4) Vaginal delivery with epidural anesthetic, unless obstetric reasons demand cesarean.

6. Preexisting hypertension: in pregnancy this demonstrates as elevated diastolic pressure before the 20th week. This high blood pressure has often not been previously diagnosed and may reflect underlying renal disease. Thus, a workup is essential before any antihypertensive therapy is instituted. These women may have severely elevated pressures without acute symptomatology, therefore, risk of cerebral hemorrhage is present unless treatment modifies pressures. These patients are also at risk for superimposed preeclampsia and abruptio placentae. Placental function is compromised by severe hypertensive states and there is an increased incidence of intrauterine growth retardation (IUGR). In addition, such infants must be observed for lasting drug effects during the transitional period in the nursery.

a. Assessment.

(1) Demonstrates elevated diastolic pressure on entry to prenatal care but no other signs of preeclampsia (8).

	First/Second Trimester	Third Trimester
Mild	80	90
Moderate	90	100
Severe	120	130

(2) Renal function diminished in moderate/severe states to nonpregnancy rate of 200 mL/min or less rather than rate of 750 mL/min (normal).

(3) Fundi, eye grounds show sclerotic changes (moderate) plus occasional hemorrhages, exudates (severe). (Keith-Wagener-Baker classification).

(4) Cardiac enlargement may be evident (moderate) or cardiac symptoms, and ECG evidence of hypertrophy, ischemia (severe).

(5) Fetal growth retardation, small placenta noted, with infarcts.

b. Intervention.

(1) Medication based on prior treatment. If newly diagnosed, cautious induction of treatment, as fetal effects are still unclear, especially in first trimester, and last month. (See Table 7-1).

(2) Bed rest in side-lying position to promote renal function (Fig. 7-7). Renal function studies.

(3) Frequent fundoscopy, vital signs, diet low in salt and high in protein. Intake and output monitored if hospitalized. Daily weights.

(4) ECG, observation of fetal status. OCT, estriols, amniocentesis for fetal maturity. Early delivery if condition deteriorates.

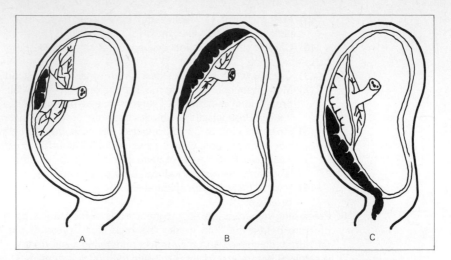

FIGURE 7-6 / Types of abruptio placentae: (a) partial separation (concealed
bleeding), (b) complete separation (concealed bleeding), (c) partial separation
(apparent hemorrhage). (*From E. J. Dickason and M. O. Schult, Maternal and
Infant Care, McGraw-Hill Book Company, New York, 1975.*)

7. Preeclampsia: hypertension occurring after the 20th week accompanied by
edema with rapid weight gain and later by albuminuria, occurs in an incidence
of 6:100 to 7:100. Preventive care has reduced the incidence of severe
preeclampsia and eclampsia, but cases do still occur and are accompanied by
an increased risk of stillbirths, abruptio placentae, chronic fetal distress and
IUGR, and, rarely, maternal death. Although etiology is still incompletely
understood, classic symptoms are those stemming from renal deposits of fibrin
in glomeruli, vasospasm of arterioles and retention of sodium leading to water
retention with increasingly severe edema, retinal arteriolar spasm and papilledema, and finally severe proteinuria and oliguria prior to onset of convulsions.
Symptoms can occur before or after delivery (until 48 h after), and special
observation is needed until pressures return to normal, and renal function is
once more adequate. Treatment has changed markedly over the past few years
with bed rest, fluids, high protein with moderate salt intake diet, being as effective
in the early stages as heavy drug therapy. In severe cases, which have been
unrecognized earlier, sedation and antihypertensive medication will be utilized
in the emergency phase, with early delivery to rescue a compromised infant.
   a. Assessment.
      (1) Edema: more than 0.8 lb per week weight gain, some generalized edema
      evident in the morning (mild).
      (2) Albuminuria: none with mild preeclampsia, +1, +2 (moderate), +3, +4
      (severe).
      (3) Hypertension: 30/15 elevation over base but less than 140/90 (mild),
      may complain of headache, fatigue. 140/90 to 160/110 with severe
      headache, fatigue; estriols may be falling (moderate). Blood pressure
      over 160/110 (severe). Headache more intense, visual disturbances,
      tinnitus, syncope. Amnesia, epigastric distress warning of impending
      convulsions. Hemoconcentration with increased hematocrit. Papilledema,
      with retinal ischemia (Table 7-5).
   b. Intervention.
      (1) Bed rest, side-lying position, increase fluid intake for natural diuresis. If

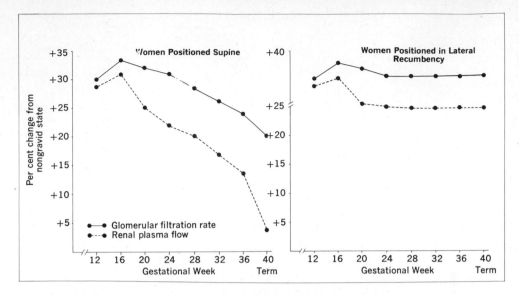

FIGURE 7-7 / Renal hemodynamics in pregnancy. The side-lying position during later pregnancy lifts the heavy uterus off the vessels of the lower abdomen and reduces pressure on the ureters. Increases in glomerular filtration rate and renal plasma flow occur early in pregnancy and are sustained to term if women maintain lateral recumbency position. (*From M. Lindheimer and A. Katz, "Managing the Patient with Renal Disease," Contemporary Ob/Gyn, 3(1) 49, 1974, with permission.*)

    edema severe, patient usually hospitalized, with intake and output monitored hourly, Foley catheter in place.

(2) Increase protein in diet, moderate salt intake, no diuretics or salt restriction for mild hypertension. Moderate to severe may have IV fluids only for intake, at first, or clear fluids. May have diuretic trial only if hospitalized and electrolytes and fluid balance observed closely. Test urine for albumin at every voiding and every 24 h. (See Table 7.5.)

(3) Sedative (phenobarbital), frequent vital signs, quiet room, reduce stress, encourage rest. If severe, continuous observation and monitoring of vital signs. Eclampsia precautions: padded tongue blade, side rails, suction, tracheostomy set at bedside. Serial hematocrit, fundoscopy.

(4) Antihypertensives or magnesium sulfate given IM, IV. Check on level of response of deep tendon reflexes, rate of respiration, and urine output. Calcium gluconate antidote at bedside.

(5) Delivery as soon as symptoms are controlled. Check infant carefully for transitional effect of medications.

TABLE 7-5 / ROLL-OVER TEST*

> **1.** Obtain baseline blood pressure after client has been positioned in the left lateral recumbent position for 5 min and after 15 min.
>
> **2.** Roll over: turn to supine position, to measure blood pressure at once and in 5 min.
>
> **3.** Result: An increase of 20 mmHg diastolic pressure indicates positive roll-over test. Use first and fifth Korotkov sounds (disappearance of sound). Positive is highly indicative of development of pregnancy-induced hypertension.

* Use at 28–32 weeks' gestation. Adapted from (9).

TABLE 7-6 / ADDITIONAL HIGH-RISK CONDITIONS AFFECTING PREGNANCY OUTCOME

Problems	Diagnosis	Intervention
Rh-negative mother with rising antibody titer	No risk to mother. Repeated amniocentesis required to measure bilirubin density, ΔOD_{450}, in amniotic fluid. Fetus may become either hyperbilirubinemic or extremely anemic. Infant may need exchange transfusion or, rarely, intrauterine transfusion.	Antibody titers must be done at regular intervals. Oxygen may be given during labor. Preterm induction may be done to deliver baby in order to do exchange transfusion. No RhoGAM can be given to mother.
Polyhydramnios (hydramnios)	Aggravates all pressure symptoms, severe supine hypotension, pressure on renal vessels. Infant is usually small, often associated with GI or GU anomalies. Preterm labor is common.	Possibly repeated amniocentesis and removal of amniotic fluid. Fetal heart hard to asculate, use ultrasound equipment, try to alleviate maternal anxiety. Expect and prepare for a compromised infant.
Multiple pregnancy[a]	Aggravates all pressure symptoms, causing orthopnea, variocose veins, hemorrhoids, constipation, vena cava syndrome. Anemia, nutritional inadequacy possible. Fetal growth retardation or disproportional growth possible (one fetus larger than other). Preeclampsia, third trimester bleeding from lowlying placenta. Difficulty in labor/delivery, preterm labor, all more common. Involution after delivery delayed. Uterine hypotonia more common.	Bed rest in side-lying position for last 6 weeks of pregnancy to promote renal function. Extra care for other discomforts. Correction of anemia, high protein intake important. Additional iron, folic acid given. Complicated delivery needs advance planning; notification of support personnel. Observe for hemorrhage. Provide extra support for maternal bonding, teaching to cope with more than one infant.
Renal disease[b]	Multiple underlying problems will affect pregnancy by changing renal excretory ability: chronic glomerulonephritis, nephrotic syndrome, solitary kidney, poly-4a1cystic kidney, or severe diabetic renal changes. Proteinuria may be massive, hypertension, edema, vomiting, and accompanying discomforts of nausea, headache, palpitations,, visual disturbances may allow the diagnosis to be confused with severe preeclampsia.	Risk is mainly to fetus unless mother goes into renal failure. Spontaneous abortion, preterm labor, and intrauterine death are possible. High protein, low-salt diet, antihypertensives added, and sometimes diuretics and cardiac glycosides. Bed rest in side-lying position is important. Urine infections are treated vigorously.
Hemoglobinopathies: Folate deficiency anemia[c]	Macrocytic anemia may occur. May underlie conditions such as abruptio placentae, spontaneous abortion, or preeclampsia.	Replacement with folate supplements, accompanying iron supplements. More frequent blood tests. Teach diet with adequate folic acid sources.

TABLE 7-6 / ADDITIONAL HIGH-RISK CONDITIONS AFFECTING PREGNANCY OUTCOME (*Continued*)

Problems	*Diagnosis*	*Intervention*
Thalassemia Major (Cooley's anemia) Minor (heterozygous)	Autosomally transmitted disease. Hemoglobin has altered globin production because of defect in alpha or beta chain.	Screen populations from Mediterranean and Southeast Asian countries.
	Patients with major rarely become pregnant, those with minor have minimal anemia until under stress conditions such as pregnancy.	Supportive care if anemia worsens; blood transfusions.
Sickle cell Disease (SS)[d]	Autosomally transmitted disease. Hemoglobin has poor solubility for oxygen at low oxygen tensions, crystallizes into sickle shape, with sludging of cells, hemolysis, and hypoxia to vital organs.	Treatment of infections, prevention of stress conditions critical.
		High folic acid–bearing foods, iron supplements. Folic acid 1 to 2 mg qd often prescribed.
	25–50:100 pregnancies of sickle disease terminate in abortion, stillbirth, or neonatal death.	Exchange transfusion in pregnancy when crises occur.
	Increased incidence of complications: preeclampsia, infection, premature labor, sickle crises.	
Trait (AS)[e]	Urinary infection, hematuria more common with sickle trait women.	Screen more frequently for bacteriuria.
Hemoglobin C Trait (CA)[f] Disease (SC)[g]	Homozygous state tolerated well with only mild anemia, but pregnancy may precipitate severe crises with maternal mortality 7:100, fetal death 35:100.	Best possible supportive care if homozygous client becomes pregnant.
		Genetic counseling, advise to avoid pregnancy.
Erythrocyte enzyme deficiency: Glucose 6-phosphate dehydrogenase (G6PD) Pyruvate kinase (PK)	May cause chronic hemolytic process or trigger severe hemolytic crises from stress of certain drugs or metabolic stresses such as infection, pregnancy.	Screening of all patients with family history suggesting enzyme deficiency.
		Teach patient to avoid stress conditions which may precipitate hemolytic crises.

[a]Incidence: varied since ovulatory agents in use.
[b]Incidence: varied.
[c]Incidence: 50:100 women show some signs of deficiency before pregnancy ends.
[d]Incidence: 3 to 12:1000 of U.S. blacks.
[e]Incidence: 8 to 10:100 of U.S. blacks. Usually no overt symptoms.
[f]Incidence: 2:100 of U.S. blacks.
[g]Linked with sickle cell.

REFERENCES

1. H. Heineman, "Infections during Pregnancy," in E. J. Dickason and M. O. Schult (eds.), *Maternal and Infant Care,* McGraw-Hill Book Company, New York, 1975, p. 337.
2. N. A. Assali, *Pathophysiology of Gestation,* Academic Press, Inc., New York, 1975, p. 192.
3. *11 Million Teenagers,* Alan Guttmacher Institute, New York, 1976.
4. J. W. Greene, "Diabetes Mellitus in Pregnancy," *Mount Sinai Journal of Medicine,* New York, **42**(5):398, September 10, 1975.

5. R. W. Abdul-Karim, "Antepartum Hemorrhage and Shock," *Clinics in Obstetrics and Gynecology,* **19**(3):533–559, September 1976.
6. J. B. Weaver and J. F. Pearson, "Influence of Digitalis on Time of Onset and Duration of Labor in Women with Cardiac Disease," *British Medical Journal,* **3**:519, 1973.
7. J. W. Niswonger and C. F. Langmade, "Cardiovascular Changes in Vaginal Deliveries and Caesarian Section," *American Journal of Obstetrics and Gynecology,* **107**(3):337, 1970.
8. R. J. Feitleson and M. D. Lindheimer, "Management of Hypertensive Gravidas," *Journal of Reproductive Medicine,* **8**(3):54, 1972.
9. G. W. Marshall and R. L. Newman, "Roll-over Test," *American Journal of Obstetrics and Gynecology,* **127**(6):620, March 15, 1977.

BIBLIOGRAPHY

American College of Obstetricians and Gynecologists, *Obstetric and Gynecologic Terminology,* F. A. Davis Company, Philadelphia, 1972. Complete dictionary of terms as approved by Committee on Terminology. Useful to ensure correct communication.

Barclay, R. L., and M. L. Barclay: "Aspects of the Normal Psychology of Pregnancy, The Mid-Trimester," *American Journal of Obstetrics and Gynecology,* **125**(2):207, May 15, 1976. Introductory study of normal pregnancy.

Blair, C. L., and E. M. Salerno: *The Expanding Family: Childbearing,* Little, Brown and Company, Boston, 1976. Application of systems approach to family-centered nursing care.

Coleman, A., and L. L. Coleman: *Pregnancy, the Psychological Experience,* Herder & Herder, Inc., New York, 1971. Definitive study of phases of pregnancy and their meaning to both partners.

Dickason, E. J., E. M. Morris, and M. O. Schult: *Maternal and Infant Drugs: Nursing Intervention,* McGraw-Hill Book Company, New York, 1978. Identification of drugs thought to be useful and harmful during pregnancy, the first infancy period, and lactation, with discussion of physiologic factors affecting changed responses, nursing interventions, and observations specific to these special patients.

11 Million Teenagers, Alan Guttmacher Institute, New York, 1976. Current statistics and evaluation of approaches to the young client needing family planning or counseling and care during pregnancy.

McFarlane, J.: "Sickle Cell Disorders," *American Journal of Nursing,* **77**(12):1948, December 1977. Clear overview of the various disorders.

Romney, S. L. (ed): *The Health Care of Women: Obstetrics & Gynecology,* McGraw-Hill Book Company, New York, 1975. The first obstetric and gynecologic text to acknowledge wider psychosocial aspects of health care. A storehouse of information, with chapters contributed by many authorities.

Sabbagha, R. E., et. al.: "Sonar BPD Predictive of Three Fetal Growth Patterns," *American Journal of Obstetrics and Gynecology,* **126**:485, 1976. Comprehensive discussion of small-for-date infants and average growth rates based on biparietal measurements.

8
Labor and Delivery

Susan Anderson

Labor is the physiologic process by which the uterus expels, or attempts to expel, the fetus and placenta at 20 weeks or more of gestation. It is a complex process during which the nurse plays a major role in assessing, planning, and intervening to meet the physical and psychosocial needs of the mother, fetus, and family.

Labor is divided into three stages. The first stage is the period from the onset of labor through complete dilatation of the cervix. The second stage is the period from complete dilatation of the cervix through the birth of the fetus. The third stage is the period from the birth of the fetus through expulsion or extraction of the placenta and membranes. For the purpose of this chapter there is added a fourth stage, which is the first hour after the birth of the fetus.

FIRST STAGE OF LABOR

Definition

The *first stage of labor* is divided into phases (Table 8-1). The *latent phase* (Fig. 8-1) is the period from the onset of labor to 2 to 3 cm dilatation. The *active phase* is the period from 2 to 3 cm to complete dilatation of the cervix (Table 8-1). According to Friedman (1) the active phase is further divided into an acceleration phase, a phase of maximum slope, and a deceleration phase. The *acceleration phase* is the "get going" phase; it is a period when contractions begin to increase in frequency and intensity, and dilatation increases. The *phase of maximum slope* (Fig. 8-2) is a period when the greatest dilatation is made in the shortest period of time. The *deceleration phase* (Fig. 8-3) is a period from 9 to 10 cm when contractions decrease in frequency, but remain the same in intensity.

Assessment

I. Psychosocial assessment.
   A. Assess preparation for childbirth.
      1. Clients may have attended prenatal classes of varying natures.
         a. Psychoprophylactic techniques involve a conditioning of the response to pain which helps the client block pain by focusing on another stimulus. Exercises, breathing and alternative activities are included.
         b. Relaxation techniques are based upon alleviation of fear, apprehension, and tension through controlled breathing and relaxation exercises.
      2. Clients may have had no prior preparation.
         a. Controlled breathing and relaxation techniques can be taught in early first stage of labor.
         b. Charts and pictures should be used to provide explanations of the physiology of labor.
   B. Assess support system available to client.
      1. Labor can be a very anxious period for a woman and she should not be alone.
         a. The support system may be provided by the client's husband or another close person.
         b. Support may be provided by a trained labor coach, or monatrice.
         c. Support must be provided by the nursing staff (2).

TABLE 8-1 / CHANGES DURING THE FIRST STAGE OF LABOR

Stage	Physical Changes	Behavioral Changes
Latent phase (see Fig. 8-1)	Contractions: mild Duration: 20–40 s Frequency: 5–10 min Dilatation: 0–3 cm, early effacement Primipara: 8–10 h or more Multipara: 3–5 h	Eager to be in labor but apprehensive and ambivalent. Receptive to teaching. Low pelvic cramps or backache.
Active phase: Acceleration	Contractions: moderate pressure, 50 mmHg Duration: 40–60 s Frequency: 3–5 min Dilatation: 3–4 cm, effacement continues Primipara: 2 h Multipara: 0.5–1 h	Contractions require attention. Must begin breathing and relaxation techniques. Desires supportive contact. Pain is perceived as contraction rises above pain threshold.
Maximum slope (see Fig. 8-2)	Contractions: moderate to strong pressure, 75 mmHg Duration: 50–60 s Frequency: 3–5 min Dilatation: 4–9 cm, effacement usually completed Primipara: 1.5 h Multipara: 1 h	Increasingly tense and fearful. Restless with contractions. Frequent demands for attention, support, medication. Pain becomes increasingly strong. Decreased response to environment.
Deceleration (see Fig. 8-3)	Contractions: strong pressure, 50–100 mmHg Duration: 60–90 s Frequency: 2–3 min Dilatation: 9–10 cm, effacement complete Primipara: 1.5 h Multipara: 0.5–1 h	Irritable, anxious, wants to go home. Withdraws from environment. May be nauseated, perspire, legs tremble.

    C. Assess client's emotional response to labor.
        1. Client may have unrealistic expectations regarding length of labor, degree of discomfort, outcome of labor, and her own behavior.
        2. Client may have unrealistic perceptions of environment, body image, discomfort, and behavior of others.
  II. Physical assessment.
    A. Data must be gathered regarding pregnancy in order to anticipate progress and outcome of labor.
        1. Date of last menstrual period (LMP).
        2. Expected date of delivery (EDD).
        3. Parity.
            a. Abortions: less than 20 weeks.
            b. Premature birth: 20 weeks or more.
            c. Stillbirths: after 20 weeks.
            d. Multiple births: count as one delivery regardless of number of babies.

Term	Preterm	Abortion	Living

B. Data on last food intake are gathered to determine eligibility for anesthesia and to anticipate nutritional needs during labor.
    1. Time of last food intake.   **2.** Amount and type of food ingested.
C. A client's medical status can be antagonized by labor and delivery and may create additional risks to mother and fetus. It is important to note the presence or history of the following:

1. Diabetes.	**6.** Allergies.
2. Epilepsy.	**7.** Varicosities.
3. Heart disease.	**8.** Hypertension.
4. Asthma.	**9.** Accidents.
5. Urinary tract infections.	**10.** Surgery.

D. Vital signs need to be taken on admission and compared with prenatal values in order to establish baseline data.

FIGURE 8-1 / Prelabor and latent phase of labor. (*a*) Cervical status. (*b*) Fetal position: head in left occipitotransverse (LOT) position. (*c*) Contraction intensity. [(*a*) *From Ross Clinical Educational Aid, "The Phenomena of Normal Labor"; (b) from "The Birth Atlas," Maternity Center Association, with permission.*]

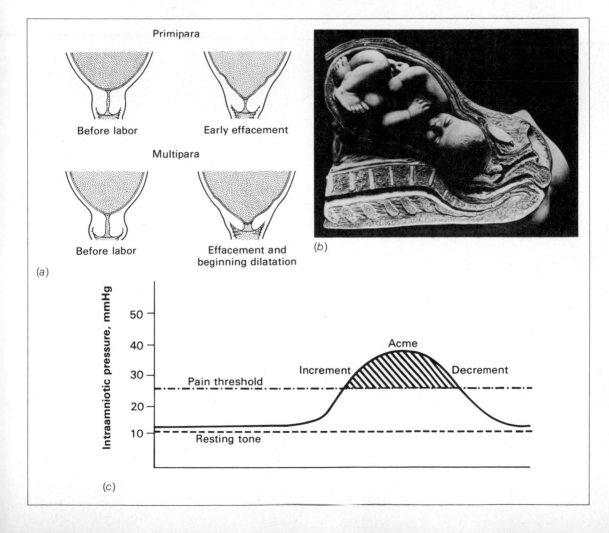

E. An abdominal exam should be performed to determine the following:
1. Leopold's maneuver is performed to determine lie, presenting part, position, and engagement.
2. Measurement of the height of the fundus may be done to determine gestational age.
F. Evaluation of labor status is done on admission to determine onset of labor and stage of progress.
1. An external perineal exam is done for:
a. Varicosities which may cause excessive bleeding during the second stage.
b. Warts.
c. Discharge.

FIGURE 8-2 / Active phase of labor. (a) Cervical status. (b) Fetal position: contraction and flexion completed. (c) Contraction intensity, acceleration phase: duration, 40 to 60 s; recurrence, every 3 to 5 min. [(a) From Ross Clinical Educational Aid, "The Phenomena of Normal Labor;" (b) from "The Birth Atlas," Maternity Center Association, with permission.]

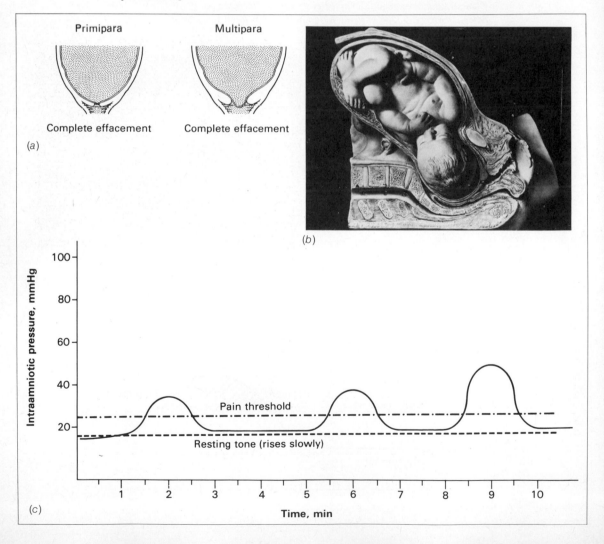

(1) Bloody show, which indicates that cervical dilatation has begun.

(2) Leukorrhea, which may indicate a vaginal infection and should be cultured.

d. Signs of laceration scars.

e. Ulcerations and lesions should be cultured for possible venereal disease.

2. An internal exam is done to determine the status of:

a. Membranes.

(1) If they are intact note whether they are tense or bulging.

(2) If ruptured, note time, color of amniotic fluid, amount of fluid expelled, odor of fluid, and engagement of presenting part.

(3) If there is a question as to whether or not the membranes have ruptured, test with Nitrazine paper. The alkalinity of the amniotic fluid will turn the paper dark blue.

FIGURE 8-3 / Deceleration phase of labor. (*a*) Cervical status: dilatation completed. (*b*) Fetal position: internal rotation in progress. (*c*) Contraction intensity: duration, 60 to 90 s; recurrence, every 2 to 3 min. [(*a*) *From Ross Clinical Educational Aid,* "*The Phenomena of Normal Labor;*" (*b*) *from* "*The Birth Atlas,*" *Maternity Center Association, with permission.*]

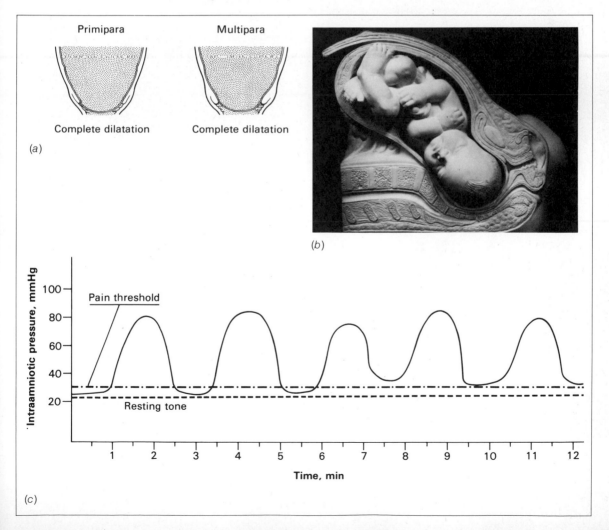

  b. Cervical condition.
   (1) A firm posterior cervix may prolong labor or indicate false labor.
   (2) If the cervix is soft and anterior, it indicates a readiness of the cervix for dilatation and effacement.
   (3) Dilatation of the cervix is recorded in centimeters (0 to 10).
   (4) Effacement determines the degree to which the cervix has been incorporated into the lower uterine segment. It is recorded in percentages (0 to 100).
 3. The presenting part should be assessed for the following:
  a. Presentation is determined by the presenting part (see Fig. 8-4 for less common presentations).
  b. Position is the relationship of the presenting part to the maternal pelvis and is determined by location of suture lines and fontanels in cephalic presentations, and by the position of the sacrum in breech presentations (see Fig. 8-5).
  c. Station is the degree of descent of the presenting part into the pelvis relative to the ischial spines (Fig. 8-6).
   (1) 0 station is at the spines.
   (2) Minus stations indicate levels above the spines, −1, −2, −3.
   (3) Positive stations indicate levels below the spines, +1, +2, +3.

FIGURE 8-4 / Less common types of presentation: (*a*) shoulder presentation; (*b*) frank breech; (*c*) incomplete breech; (*d*) left sacroanterior (LSA); (*e*) left sacroposterior (LSP); (*f*) brow presentation; (*g*) prolapse of cord. (*From Ross Clinical Educational Aid No. 18.*)

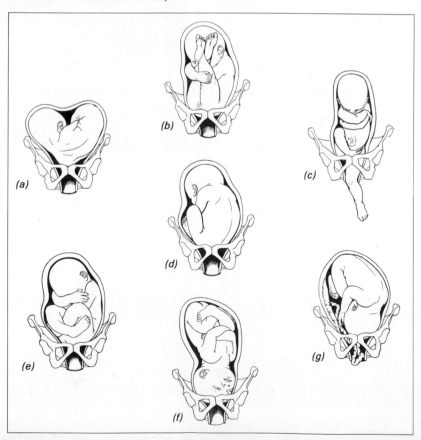

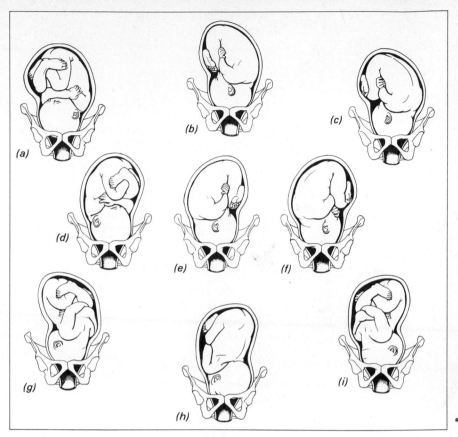

FIGURE 8-5 / Positions of the fetus in cephalic presentation: (*a*) left occipitoposterior (LOP); (*b*) left occipitotransverse (LOT); (*c*) left occipitoanterior (LOA); (*d*) right occipitoposterior (ROP); (*e*) right occipitotransverse (ROT); (*f*) right occipitoanterior (ROA); (*g*) left mentoanterior (LMA); (*h*) right mentoposterior (RMP); (*i*) right mentoanterior (RMA). (*From Ross Clinical Educational Aid No. 18.*)

4. Contractions must be evaluated with regard to the following:
    a. Time of onset of regular contractions.
    b. Frequency of contractions.
        (1) Regular contractions increasing in frequency and intensity usually indicate true labor.
        (2) Irregular contractions indicate false labor, very early first stage, or a posterior position.
    c. Duration of contractions—normally from 20 to 60 s by palpation, but are often longer by monitor record.
    d. The client's description of the location and intensity of discomfort.
        (1) Discomfort which is located in the lower abdomen or groin usually indicates false labor.
        (2) Fundal region pain radiating to the back usually indicates true labor.
        (3) Sacral region discomfort is common with a posterior position.
        (4) Intensity of discomfort usually increases as labor progresses.
G. Laboratory data may be available from antepartum records and if not should be gathered at the time of admission.
    1. Blood type and Rh, cross-match tube held.
    2. Urinalysis, including sugar and albumin.

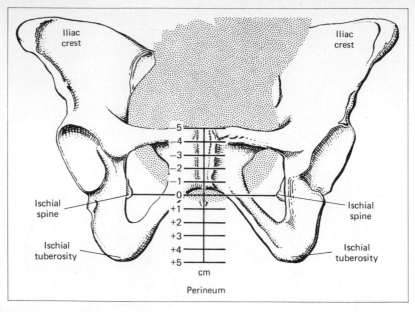

FIGURE 8-6 / **Stations of the presenting part. (*From Ross Clinical Educational Aid, "The Phenomena of Labor."*)**

3. Serology.
4. Hb and Hct.
5. Rubella titer.

Problems

I. Psychosocial problems.
   A. Patient may display excessive anxiety.
      1. Patient may lack knowledge of the labor process.
      2. There may be unrealistic perceptions of current labor status.
      3. Patient may be fearful of bodily harm or death.
      4. Expectations for pain relief may be unmet.
      5. Expectations of hospital staff may be unmet.
   B. Patient may be lacking a support system.
      1. A supportive person may be available, but is not effective.
      2. A supportive person may not be available, as in cases of single parents.
II. Physical problems.
   A. Patient experiences excessive discomfort.
   B. Labor progress may indicate an abnormal labor curve (see Fig. 8-7). Lack of progress is indicated by:
      1. Lack of dilatation.
      2. Lack of descent of presenting part.
      3. Excessive molding of presenting part.
   C. Fetal distress may be indicated by:
      1. Abnormal fetal heart rates.
         a. Tachycardia, rate above 160 beats per minute (bpm).
         b. Bradycardia, rate below 120 bpm.
         c. Loss of beat-to-beat, or less than 5-bpm variation.
         d. Deceleration patterns as seen on fetal monitor.
      2. Meconium-stained fluid in absence of breech presentation.

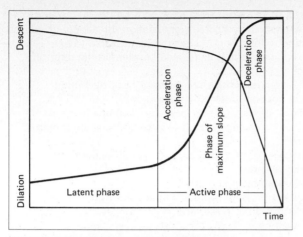

FIGURE 8-7 / Dilatation and descent, normal curve.
(From E. Friedman and J. P. Greenhill, Biological Principles and Modern Practice of Obstetrics, W. B. Saunders Company, Philadelphia, 1974.)

Diagnosis

I. Decreased coping ability due to physical stress of labor.
II. Decreased coping ability due to anxiety associated with the labor process.
III. Threat to physical well-being of mother and fetus due to labor process.

Goals of Care

I. Immediate.
   A. The needs of patient for information will be met at her level of understanding.
   B. Appropriate data for physical and psychosocial assessment will be collected promptly on admission.
   C. A relationship of trust with patient and family will be sought so that support can be offered.
   D. The patient will be informed of progress in labor and will receive explanations of any procedures.
   E. The patient will be encouraged to verbalize fears and concerns in order to reduce anxiety.
   F. Discomfort will be alleviated as much as possible.
II. Long-range.
   A. Physical and behavioral changes will be assessed as labor progresses and the patient's changing needs met.
   B. The patient will be provided an environment that will promote the best possible outcome for mother and fetus.

Intervention

I. Decrease anxiety associated with labor by explaining:
   A. Physiological processes of labor.
   B. Changes in physical sensations as labor progresses.
   C. Approximate time parameters of labor progression.

   D. Procedures such as enema, perineal prep, vaginal exams.

   E. Review method of childbirth preparation, breathing, or relaxation techniques.

  II. Provide support for client if there is none available to her.

 III. Provide comfort measures as needed by client in the form of:

   A. Positioning.

    1. Knee-to-chest position to alleviate back discomfort.

    2. Sims position to promote relaxation.

   B. Back rubs, especially in sacral area; effleurage.

   C. Hard candy, ice chips, or a wet washcloth for dry mouth.

   D. Hygiene:

    1. Changing of bed linen to keep client clean and dry.

    2. Perineal care.

 IV. Monitor physical status of mother.

   A. Take blood pressure every 4 h unless not in normal range, then every $\frac{1}{2}$ to 1 h.

   B. Take temperature, pulse, and respiration every 4 h unless membranes ruptured, then every hour.

   C. Note frequency and duration of contractions every 30 min; in advanced labor, every 15 min.

   D. Note progress in cervical dilatation every hour.

   E. Note type and amount of vaginal discharge every 30 min.

  V. Monitor physical status of fetus.

   A. Utilize doptone or fetoscope to assess fetal heart rate and record every 15 min in active labor, then every 5 min in second stage.

   B. Apply the fetal monitor, either internal or external, and observe for the following patterns (see Fig. 8-8):

    1. Variable decelerations caused by cord compression.

     a. These patterns are variable in shape and onset with regard to the contractions, and may dip as low as 60 bpm.

     b. A change in maternal position may relieve the cord compression by moving fetal head off cord.

    2. Early decelerations are caused by head compression.

     a. These patterns have their onset at the time of beginning contraction and reflect the symmetrical curve of a contraction.

     b. The patterns are innocuous and do not lead to fetal distress.

    3. Late decelerations are caused by uteroplacental insufficiency.

     a. These patterns have their origin after the beginning of a contraction and are symmetrical in shape.

     b. Such patterns require immediate nursing action to allow optimum maternal-fetal exchange via the placenta.

      (1) Increase isotonic intravenous fluid to increase circulating volume.

      (2) Relieve maternal hypotension by positioning on left or right side.

      (3) Administer oxygen.

      (4) Cut off oxytocin drip until cause can be evaluated.

     c. These patterns may be caused by placental separation or any condition reducing oxygen exchange at the placenta: abruptio placentae, placenta previa, oxytocin drip with hypertonic uterine contractions, and epidural anesthesia with hypotensive response in patient.

Evaluation

   I. Patient's psychosocial and physical status is consistent with stage of labor.

  II. Patient is unable to utilize adequate coping mechanisms to deal with the stress of labor.

   A. Reinforce patient teaching.

   B. Reassess psychosocial history for possible reasons (separated from husband, unplanned pregnancy, or complications with other pregnancies).

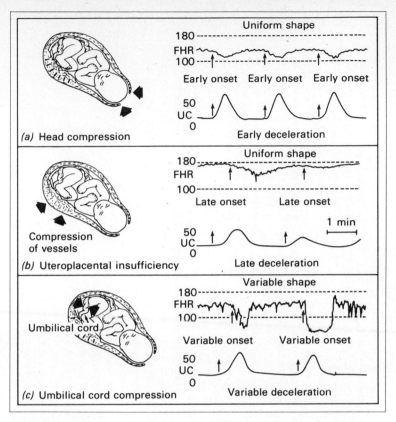

FIGURE 8-8 / Types of deceleration seen on fetal monitor. (a) This fetal heart rate (FHR, beats per minute) deceleration pattern is thought to be due to fetal head compression. It is of uniform shape, reflects the shape of the associated intrauterine pressure curve (mmHg), and has its onset early in the contracting phase of the uterus. Hence, it has been labeled *early deceleration*. (b) This FHR deceleration pattern is thought to be due to acute uteroplacental insufficiency (UPI) as the result of decreased intervillous space blood flow during uterine contractions. It is also of uniform shape and also reflects the shape of the associated intrauterine pressure curve. In this case, however, in contradistinction to the uniform deceleration pattern of (a), its onset occurs late in the contracting phase of the uterus. Hence, it has been labeled *late deceleration*. (c) This FHR pattern is thought to be due to umbilical cord occlusion. It is of variable shape, does not reflect the shape of the associated intrauterine pressure curve, and its onset occurs at a variable time during the contracting phase of the uterus. Hence, it has been labeled *variable deceleration*. (From E. Hon, An Introduction to Fetal Heart Monitoring, Harty Press Inc., New Haven, Conn., 1968.)

III. Decreased ability to cope with discomforts of labor.
   A. Proceed to next level of breathing exercises.
   B. Use more direct commands to patient when coaching.
   C. Administer appropriate analgesics, observe for adverse reactions, and assess degree of relief (see Table 8-2).
   D. Prepare for administration of anesthetics.
IV. Physical findings are not consistent with stage of labor.
   A. Cervical dilatation not progressing because of quality of contractions.

TABLE 8-2 / NARCOTICS, BARBITURATES, AND TRANQUILIZERS USED IN LABOR

Agent	Dosage	Onset	Duration	Maternal Effects	Fetal Effects
Narcotics					
Meperidine (Demerol, Pethidine)	30–100 mg IM 25 mg IV diluted in 5 mL normal saline* SC not advised	10–20 min 3–5 min	2–3 h 1.5–2 h	70–90% relief of pain, and sedation. Delays labor if dose excessive, but may enhance labor for some. Nausea and vomiting, hypotension, some respiratory depression, urine retention.	Rapid placental transmission. Possible CNS depression, respiratory depression. In newborn, large doses result in lowered oxygen saturation. Metabolites hinder adaptation to stimuli for more than 1 month.
Alphaprodine (Nisentil)	40–50 mg SC 15–20 mg IV	10 min 3–5 min	2–3 h 1.5–2 h	70–90% relief of pain, and sedation. Delays labor if given too early or in excessive dose. Enhances labor for some. Similar to meperidine in effect, but *shorter* duration.	Rapid placental transmission. Since shorter duration of action in mother, if dose/time interval observed, may not affect infant as much in newborn period. Studies incomplete.
Anileridine (Leritine)	30–40 mg SC 20–40 mg IM 15–20 mg IV	15–30 min 10–20 min 3–5 min	4–5 h 2.5–4 h 2–3 h	Similar to meperidine, but less sedation and sleep and short duration of side effects: respiratory depression, hypotension. Some antiemetic and antitussive effects.	Depressant effects on fetus may be more severe than for meperidine in equigesic doses. Must have Narcan available.
Morphine	8–10 mg SC 3–5 mg IV diluted in 5 mL normal saline†	15–30 min 3–5 min	4–5 h 1.5–2 h	Given in equigesic doses, morphine is no more depressing than other narcotics. Time/dose interval before birth is critical; therefore not commonly used subcutaneously. Side effects: nausea and vomiting; slower respirations; hypotension; urinary retention, which may require intervention.	Rapid placental transmission. CNS depression in high doses. Respiratory depression counteracted by Narcan. Observe infant 2–3 h after delivery because of short action of Narcan.
Oxymorphone (Numorphan)	0.75–1.5 mg SC‡ 0.5–1.0 mg IM 0.5–0.75 mg IV	15–30 min 10–20 min 3–5 min	4–5 h 2.5–4 h 1.5–2 h	Pain relief and sedation. Similar effects as morphine. Maternal respiratory depressant. May delay labor if given too early or in too large doses. Note that subcutaneous doses are not recommended during active labor since the duration is so long.	Similar to morphine effects.
Barbiturates§					
Secobarbital (Seconal)	50–200 mg PO	20–30 min	4–5 h	Sleep and sedation, but no analgesic or amnesia action. No effects on	Attention depressed for 2–4 days after birth. Enhances microsomal liver

Drug	Dose	Onset	Duration	Maternal Effects	Fetal/Neonatal Effects
Pentobarbital (Nembutal)	50–200 mg PO	20–30 min	4–5 h	progress of labor, but must be given so that drug is completely metabolized before birth. Depressive effect on respiratory and circulatory systems with higher doses. Sleep and sedation, but no analgesic or amnesic action. No effects on progress of labor. Drug must be completely metabolized before birth.	metabolic rate. May affect action of other drugs. Attention depressed for 2–4 days after birth. Enhances microsomal liver function, thus metabolizing other drugs faster.

Tranquilizers

Drug	Dose	Onset	Duration	Maternal Effects	Fetal/Neonatal Effects
Promethazine (Phenergan)	25–50 mg IM 25 mg IV	15–20 min 3–5 min	3–4 h 2–3 h	Antihistaminic action adds extra sedation with narcotic. Potentiates narcotic; reduce dosage. Stimulates respirations, decreases nausea and vomiting. Some disorientation, hypotension, tachycardia may occur. No effect on labor progress.	CNS depression; equilibrates with maternal level within 15 min (intravenous route). Transitional effects depend on level/time of dose.
Promazine (Sparine)	25–50 mg IM 25 mg IV	15–20 min 3–5 min	3–4 h 2–3 h	Effective in combination with narcotic. Labile hypotension may occur. Other effects same as for promethazine.	CNS depression. Into fetal circulation within 4 min (intravenous route). Transitional effects depend on level/time of dose.
Hydroxyzine hydrochloride (Vistaril)	50–100 mg IM	15–20 min	3–4 h	Reduces nausea. Some sedation. Potentiates narcotic; reduce dose by 50%.	CNS depression. In high doses, observe for infant sedation.
Propiomazine (Largon)	20–40 mg IM 20–40 mg IV	15–20 min 3–5 min	2–4 h 2–3 h	Avoid combination in syringe with other drugs. May cause hypotension, some respiratory depression in adult.	Minimal CNS depression.
Diazepam (Valium)	5–10 mg IM 5–10 mg IV diluted in 5 mL normal saline¶	10–15 min 2–3 min	5–7 h 5–6 h	Not used during labor. May be given intravenously during delivery only. Will potentiate any analgesic. Not recommended if mother is to breast-feed.	Into fetus in 4–6 min. Higher doses concentrate. Affects thermoregulation and responses, for up to 1 week after delivery. May affect pulse, respiration for 24 h.

*Dose reduced if given with tranquilizer.
†Give slowly over 2–3 min.
‡For postoperative use only.
§Used only in very early labor to provide sleep.
¶Give over 5-min period.

1. Mild, irregular contractions may be Braxton-Hicks, in which case patient should be prepared for discharge.
2. If contractions are strong and regular but not effecting any cervical changes, the following should be assessed:
    a. If the fetal position is left occipitoposterior (LOP; see Fig. 8-5), a change in position to the right side may facilitate rotation of the fetus and promote more effective contractions.
    b. If vaginal and abdominal exams are inconclusive regarding fetal presentation (see Fig. 8-4) and adequacy of pelvis, the physician may order a flat plate of the abdomen.
        (1) Prepare client for x-ray with explanation of procedure.
        (2) Transport client to x-ray via wheelchair or stretcher depending on phase of labor.
        (3) Allow a relative or close friend to accompany client.
        (4) Carry an emergency delivery kit.
    c. If a malpresentation or pelvic inadequacy is present, prepare for possible cesarean section.
        (1) Obtain consent forms.
        (2) Check lab work for complete blood count (CBC), Hb, and Hct, and type and cross match.
        (3) Abdominal prep.
        (4) Insert Foley catheter.
        (5) Establish intravenous system.
        (6) Reassure client and family with explanation of procedures.
3. If contractions are mild and ineffective, the client may require stimulation of labor.
    a. The following criteria are necessary for stimulation of labor.
        (1) Adequate pelvis.
        (2) Cervical dilatation of 2 to 3 cm.
        (3) Cervical effacement of more than 50 percent.
        (4) Engagement of presenting part.
    b. Nursing care involves:
        (1) Careful monitoring of flow rate.
        (2) Observing for uterine hyperactivity and discontinuing IV fluid if hyperactivity occurs (3).
        (3) Monitoring the fetal heart rate, preferably with the fetal monitor observing for late decelerations.
B. If bleeding occurs, it is necessary to assess:
    1. The time of onset.
    2. Color and amount.
        a. A pad count may help to determine the amount of vaginal bleeding.
        b. A change in body position may have a tamponade effect by the presenting part and decrease bleeding.
    3. Monitor vital signs, noting signs of shock.
    4. Assess fetal well-being, preferably with external fetal monitor observing for late decelerations.
    5. Do not perform vaginal exams at risk of increasing bleeding.
    6. Prepare patient for ultrasound procedure to determine the location of the placenta. Alleviate anxiety by explaining the procedure and give reassurances that it is not harmful to mother or fetus.
    7. Maintain bed rest and decreased activity.
C. A finding of pain other than that associated with uterine contractions is not consistent with normal labor.
    1. Assess tone of abdomen; if it is rigid it may indicate abruptio placentae.
    2. Monitor vital signs for signs of shock due to hemorrhage at placental site.

3. Apply fetal monitor, observing for late decelerations.
4. Arrange lab work for Hb, Hct, and clotting factors, and type and cross match for several units of blood.
5. Prepare for cesarean section if fetus is viable.
6. Observe for development of clotting defect.
   - *a.* Bleeding without clotting.
   - *b.* Unusual bruisability.
   - *c.* Oozing at IV site.
   - *d.* Hematuria.
   - *e.* Bleeding from gums.
7. Reassure patient and family, keeping them informed of status of fetus and mother.

D. An elevation of blood pressure over 140/90 is considered pathologic; however, an elevated blood pressure should be determined from baseline data.
1. If blood pressure is elevated:
   - *a.* Test urine for albumin.
   - *b.* Examine client for edema, especially of hands and face.
   - *c.* Assess for hyperreflexia.
2. If the above findings are positive:
   - *a.* Monitor vital signs every 10 to 15 min.
   - *b.* Restrict activity and sensory input.
   - *c.* Place on strict intake and output.
   - *d.* Employ seizure precautions.
   - *e.* Apply fetal monitor.

E. If physical assessment reveals an elevated temperature:
1. Assess fluid balance, noting last food and fluid intake to determine possibility of dehydration.
2. Monitor fetal heart rate, observing for tachycardia and decreased variability as seen on internal monitor patterns and indicating maternal infection.
3. Assess status and time of rupture of membranes, noting any odor.
4. Monitor administration of intravenous fluids and antibiotics as ordered.
5. Evaluate temperature every hour.
6. If membranes are ruptured for over 24 h, induction or cesarean section may be performed, since ascending infection is hazardous to mother and infant.

F. Inappropriate EDD, indicating the following conditions:
1. Postmaturity, 42 weeks or more gestation.
   - *a.* Assess size of fetus.
     - (1) Height of fundus.
     - (2) Use ultrasound to determine biparietal diameters.
   - *b.* Assess placental function.
     - (1) Collect 24-h urine for estriols.
   - *c.* Assess fetal well-being.
     - (1) Prepare for oxytocin challenge or stress test.
       - (*a*) Set up piggyback intravenous system.
       - (*b*) Apply external fetal monitor.
       - (*c*) Titrate oxytocin drip until contractions occur at a rate of three in 10 min.
       - (*d*) Observe fetal heart rate pattern for late decelerations.
   - *d.* Prepare client for possible induction or cesarean section, depending on results of tests.
2. Prematurity, 37 weeks or less gestation.
   - *a.* Assess size of fetus.
     - (1) Height of fundus.
     - (2) Use ultrasound to determine biparietal diameters.
   - *b.* Assess fetal maturity.
     - (1) Prepare client for amniocentesis.
       - (*a*) Use ultrasound to locate placenta and fetal position.

        (b) Remain with client for emotional support as well as monitoring of fetal heart and vital signs.

  c. Note laboratory results.

     (1) The L/S ratio reflects lung maturity of fetus, with a ratio of 2:1 indicating maturity.

     (2) Creatinine levels reflect kidney maturity, with 1.5 mg per 100 mL usually indicating maturity.

  d. Assess labor status.

     (1) If in labor provide bed rest and decreased activity.

     (2) Client may receive intravenous alcohol (4).

        (a) Assure client it is not harmful to her or the fetus.

        (b) Explain that she may feel dizzy and inebriated; provide safety measures.

  e. Notify nursery of possible premature infant.

  f. If client has ruptured membranes and no signs of labor:

     (1) Provide bed rest, monitor temperature especially.

     (2) Administer antibiotics as ordered.

     (3) Assess vaginal discharge for odor.

     (4) Observe for onset of labor.

G. The presence of chronic disease requires special observation and intervention by the nurse.

  1. Cardiac complications.

    a. Observe for signs of cardiac insufficiency.

     (1) Rales.

     (2) Edema.

     (3) Respiratory rate over 28 with dyspnea.

     (4) Pulse rate over 100 with palpitations.

    b. Promote rest and decreased activity.

    c. Position patient in a high semi-Fowler's position.

    d. Administer antibiotics as prescribed.

    e. Monitor pulse and respirations every 15 min, use cardiac monitor.

    f. Prepare client for epidural anesthesia.

    g. Ensure availability of oxygen, morphine, digitalis, and diuretics if cardiac failure occurs.

  2. Diabetes

    a. Definition (see Chap. 7).

    b. Assess for hypoglycemia characterized by:

     (1) Pallor, sweating, weakness, shallow respirations.

     (2) Test urine for sugar and acetone every 4 h.

    c. Prepare for possible premature infant since fetal size may not be indicative of gestational age.

    d. Prepare client for induction or cesarean section depending on fetal size.

    e. Administer insulin subcutaneously to cover glucose in IV fluids (do not add to IV solution).

  3. Rh sensitization.

    a. Definition.

     (1) Rh sensitization occurs when an Rh-negative mother carries an Rh-positive fetus. The passage of red blood cells from the mother provokes antibody formation against the positive Rh factor of the fetus, leading to hemolysis of red blood cells in the fetus with resultant anemia, fetal edema, and congestive heart failure. The fetus is usually delivered prematurely, then prepared for exchange transfusion.

    b. Fetal well-being must be carefully monitored.

     (1) Amniocentesis will determine fetal bilirubin level.

     (2) Apply fetal monitor.

c. Patient should be prepared for possible induction dependent on status of fetus in utero.
  (1) Support grieving mother.
  (2) Keep patient informed of fetal status.

SECOND STAGE OF LABOR

Definition

The *second stage of labor* is the period of labor from full dilatation to complete delivery of the fetus. It is the period of fetal descent through the vaginal canal. (See Table 8-3 and Fig. 8-9.)

Assessment

I. Psychosocial assessment should reveal client:
  A. Totally preoccupied with contractions.
  B. Withdrawn from environment.
  C. Irritable and exhausted.
II. Physical assessment.
  A. Vaginal exam should reveal complete dilatation of the cervix.
  B. Presenting part should be engaged and descending.
  C. Fetal heart should be monitored every 5 min. Early decelerations may be observed as head compression occurs.
  D. Monitor contractions for frequency and duration, telling patient when to bear down.

Problems

I. Psychosocial problems.
  A. Patient may be unable to cope with loss of control imposed by second stage of labor.
    1. Patient may be exhausted and fearful.
    2. Patient may display aggressive behavior toward nurse or family.
  B. Patient's need for constant emotional support and coaching may interfere with her need for privacy.
II. Physical problems.
  A. Patient experiences excessive discomfort or back labor.
  B. Lack of descent, abnormal length of second stage.
  C. Fetal distress occurs.

TABLE 8-3 / CHANGES DURING THE SECOND STAGE OF LABOR (SEE FIG. 8-9)

Physical Changes	Behavioral Changes
Cervix: effacement complete Contractions: strong with several acmes Duration: 90–110 s Frequency: 3–5 min Dilatation: completed; internal rotation completed; extension begins Strong rectal pressure: perineum bulges, crowning, head born, external rotation, then shoulders, anterior then posterior, and body follows.	May be nauseated and exhausted. If conditioned to push, may feel it as a relief. Fearful of losing control. Amnesia between contractions, needs steady coaching.

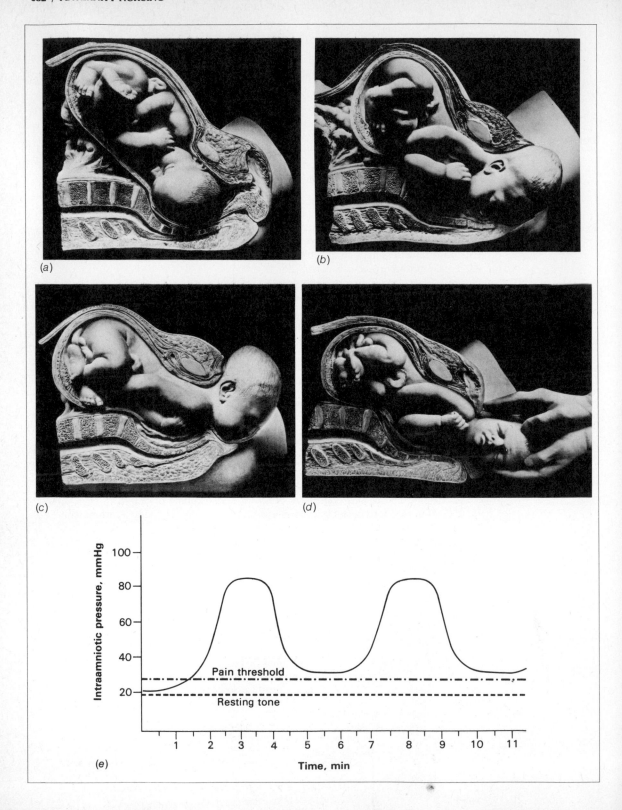

(a)

(b)

(c)

(d)

(e)

Diagnosis

I. Ability to push is decreased due to:
  A. Inappropriate positioning.
  B. Excessive fear of physical harm.
  C. Exhaustion, analgesia, or anesthesia.
II. Ability to cope with discomfort is decreased.
III. Physical well-being of mother and fetus is threatened by:
  A. Infection due to fecal contamination.
  B. Lacerations caused by uncontrolled pushing.

Goals of Care

I. Patient receives encouragement of effective pushing in order to shorten second stage.
II. Patient is given emotional support and privacy.
III. A safe environment is maintained.

Intervention

I. Position patient for effective pushing.
  A. Place in semi-Fowler's position with legs abducted, chin on chest, and hands grasping legs behind the knees.
  B. May push in Sims position if fetus is in a posterior position.
II. Encourage effective pushing.
  A. Utilize breathing techniques.
  B. Coach patient continually.
III. Provide emotional support for her and the coach.
  A. Explain patient's behavior to husband.
  B. Encourage and praise patient's effort.
IV. Provide privacy.
  A. Drape client properly while she is pushing.
  B. Draw curtains.
V. Minimize chances of infection.
  A. Keep bed linen clean and dry.
  B. Cleanse perineum to prevent fecal contamination.
  C. Maintain aseptic technique in the delivery room.
VI. Minimize physical complications.
  A. Observe for perineal bulging and crowning of presenting part.
  B. Monitor fetal heart every 5 min or after each contraction.
VII. Decrease anxiety regarding delivery process.
  A. Explain delivery room procedures.
    1. Method of administration of anesthesia (Tables 8-4 and 8-5).
    2. Use of stirrups, restraints.
  B. Provide mirror in which parents can view the delivery.
VIII. Provide immediate newborn care.
  A. Maintain patent airway.
    1. Position on side or in Trendelenburg's position.
    2. Use bulb or nasogastric suction.
    3. Provide necessary equipment if resuscitation is needed.

FIGURE 8-9 / Second stage of labor. (*a* to *d*) Fetal positions: (*a*) internal rotation completed; (*b*) extension and crowning; (*c*) extension completed; (*d*) delivery of head and external rotation. (*e*) Contraction intensity: duration, 90 to 110 s; recurrence, every 3 to 5 min. [(*a* to *d*) *From "The Birth Atlas," Maternity Center Association, with permission.*]

TABLE 8-4 / REGIONAL ANESTHETICS USED DURING LABOR

Anesthetics	Period of Labor	Location of Injection	Comments	Precautions
Paracervical block (uterosacral block)	First stage: active dilatation, phase of maximum slope	Hypogastric nerve plexis and ganglia beside cervix in each lateral fornix. Anesthesia to second, third, and fourth sacral nerves and to eleventh and twelfth thoracic nerves.	Relieves pain of dilatation but not perineal pain. Effective for 1–2 h. Does not inhibit uterine contractions. Because of direct absorption of local anesthetic into maternal system and transfer across placenta, a paracervical block has a negative inotropic, chromotropic, and dromotropic effect on fetal heart. Not used in any case of chronic fetal distress or prematurity.	Check fetal heart tone prior to and frequently after administration. Monitor closely for 30 min. Check fetal scalp vein pH whenever bradycardia persists. (Bradycardia and late decelerations occur in 30–70% of cases.) Recovery usually without any lasting effect, but cesarean section necessary if longer than 15–18 min or if pH fails. Uterine hypertonicity may result if myometrium is infiltrated.
Prudendal block	Second stage: expulsive phase	Pudendal nerves above and behind ischial spines. Anesthesia to second, third, and fourth sacral nerves.	Blocks sensation to entire perineum but not to uterus. Must allow 5–10 min for anesthetic to take full effect. Additional local to site of episiotomy. Does not cover pain of manual extraction of placenta or midforceps delivery. Recovery takes place within 1 h.	May have one-sided effect if placement is incorrect. Aspiration for blood is important since area is very vascular. Usually quite safe for mother and infant.
Peridural block: Caudal (continuous)	First stage: active labor, phase of maximum slope through second stage	Insertion into sacral cornua low block to second, third, and fourth sacral nerves, higher block to tenth thoracic and fifth sacral. Blocks cervical and perineal pain, depending on dose and location of catheter.	Patient in knee-chest position or lateral decubitus. Test dose always administered with 5-min wait for response. Plastic cannula taped in place for future additional doses. When each dose is administered, check for bilateral anesthesia, vasodilation in legs, and toe temperature. Patient will not have sensation to bear down. Must be coached. Recovery complete by 2–3 h, depending on dose and type of medication.	After dose is given, patient is moved into supine position to distribute medication to both sides. Then semi-Fowler's position may be assumed. Check that catheter taping is secure. Watch for hypotension in first adjustment period; elevate legs to correct. Watch for vena cava compression. During recovery, no urge to void. Delayed recovery of sphincter control may persist after full recovery or leg movement. Watch for bladder distension.
Lumbar epidural (continuous) for vaginal delivery	First stage: active labor through second stage	Insertion at interspace between second, third, or fourth lumbar, depending	Lateral decubitus position with neck flexed. Contractions are not impaired, but	After the catheter has been inserted and taped, move patient into semi-sitting position while

section		catheter. Anesthesia for cesarean section to sixth and seventh thoracic by insertion of catheter up toward first lumbar.	...terated. Check effectiveness of anesthesia and signs for hypotension every 5 min for first 20 min.	...-mL test dose is inserted. Observe for vena cava compression and hypotension (see above for caudal). Administer IV fluids and oxygen to prevent further hypotension and hypoxia in infant. Postural hypotension possible during recovery as well as voiding problems (see above).
Subarachnoid block:	Second stage or just prior to delivery	Insertion of needle at fourth lumbar through dura into spinal fluid.	Does not block contractions, but no urge to push. Must be coached.	Hypotension most common complication due to vena cava compression. Must position uterus with a lateral tilt.
Saddle block (low spinal)		Hyperbaric solution used to allow anesthetic to gravitate down toward sacral area. Anesthesia to tenth thoracic and to fifth sacral at level of umbilicus.	Administered in a sitting position; remain upright 90–120 s for solution to descend, then place supine with neck flexed on pillow. Must be well hydrated with IV fluids to alleviate hypotension. Postoperative: Usually quick recovery but keep flat 6–8 h as precaution against spinal headache. Watch for postural hypotension when first ambulatory.	
Spinal	Just prior to cesarean section or difficult delivery	Insertion of needle at fourth lumbar through dura and into spinal fluid. Blocks to sixth, seventh, and eighth thoracic nerves.	Patient in side-lying position with neck and knees flexed. Usually obliterates contractions, so forceps and fundal pressure may be necessary for vaginal delivery.	Hypotension is most common complication. Other adverse effects: (1) back pain from muscle trauma; (2) postpuncture headache from loss of spinal fluid and stretching of meninges (patient kept flat until hydration by IV fluids restores CSF); (3) postural hypotension when first ambulatory; (4) inability to void; (5) very rare, respiratory paralysis from medication rising in cord to affect nerves to thorax.

Source: From E. J. Dickason, M. O. Schult, and E. M. Morris, *Maternal and Infant Drugs and Nursing Intervention*, McGraw-Hill Book Company, New York, 1978.

TABLE 8-5 / GENERAL ANESTHETICS AND PRECAUTIONS FOR USE IN DELIVERY

Anesthetic	Absorption, Fate, Excretion	Effect	Comments
Inhalation Anesthetics			
Diethyl ether, ether	Absorbed through pulmonary epithelium. Slow induction, but well marked planes of anesthesia. Eliminated unchanged by lungs with very small amount metabolized (<10%).	Depresses CNS on all levels with excellent muscle relaxation. Stimulates secretions and increases respiratory rate and heart rate. Supraventricular arrhythmias may occur. Decreases renal function. Toxicity: Respiratory arrest with overdose.	Irritating to respiratory tract; patient may gag, cough, and have laryngospasm. May increase secretions from upper respiratory tract. Usually given with preoperative atropine. Watch urine output. Artificial ventilation removes ether from system and restores respiration. Postoperative: Nausea and vomiting common after ether anesthesia persisting into recovery period.
Halothane (Fluothane)	Administered with nitrous oxide to obtain quicker analgesia and hasten anesthesia. 80% pulmonary exchange with 20% excreted through urine; however, may be stored in body tissue for long periods, and metabolites may have some toxicity.	Produces stage IV anesthesia without oxygen loss. Causes mild cerebral vasodilation and also causes arterial hypotension because of generalized vasodilation. Alterations in cardiac rhythm may occur. Toxicity: Acute hypotension; fetal toxicity occurs with prolonged anesthesia; ventricular arrhythmias may occur if catecholamines are injected.	Rarely used in obstetrics. Used when uterine relaxation is desired effect. Not used with cardiac, renal, or liver disease. Profound hypotension must be prevented. Must be used with adjunct medication and neuromuscular blockers because does not cause adequate muscle relaxation. Since has smooth muscle dilatation effect, strongly inhibits uterine tonus and reduces responses to oxytocins. Nonirritating to respiratory tract. Causes bronchiolar dilatation; therefore useful with asthmatic patients. Postoperative: Shivering may occur to increase body temperature. Provide blankets. Nausea and vomiting rare in recovery. Watch for hypotension. Observe for delayed awakening. Observe for extra bleeding. Check fundal contraction after delivery.

Agent			
Fluoroxene (Fluoromar)	Similar to halothane but less potent. Does not appear to affect infant adversely if given less than 10 min before delivery.	Excites sympathetic activity; produces cardiac stability. Does not cause vasodilatation.	Flammable but not explosive. Can be used when patient is in hemorrhagic shock or for central or peripheral circulatory failure. After 10 min, look for depression of infant.
Methoxyflurane (Penthrane)	Used with nitrous oxide and muscle relaxants or barbiturates. Extensively metabolized and excreted slowly.	Most potent inhalation agent with good muscle relaxation, but because of slow induction (up to 20 min) other agents are added. Depresses respiration and causes mild hypotension and sometimes bradycardia. Some question of toxicity of metabolites and longlasting neurobehavioral effect on infants. Delirium during induction not uncommon.	Nausea and vomiting infrequent. Nonirritating to respiratory tract. Does not cause laryngospasm. Tolerated well by asthmatics. Exercise special care with obstetric patients with regard to time/dose interval because 70% of maternal level is in fetal system by 10–15 min. Some very low Apgar scores after prolonged administration. In very low doses, has been used for inhalational analgesia throughout active labor, without apparent adverse effect on Apgar score. Postoperative: Very slow recovery since slowly metabolized.
Enflurane (Enthrane)	Very little metabolized; 85% expired. Therefore, less danger of toxic metabolites than with halothane.	Anesthesia similar to that obtained with halothane with some respiratory depression. Arterial hypotension common. Sensitizes myocardium to catecholamines, and if used with them, may cause ventricular extrasystoles. Temporary depression of kidney, liver function.	Nonflammable, chemically stable. Occasional seizure-like EEG patterns noted, plus involuntary muscle movements. Newly introduced anesthetic (1973). Information incomplete about fetal response. Postoperative: Observe for hypotension. Check urine output. Observe for involuntary muscle movements.
Nitrous oxide	Low solubility in blood. Excreted unchanged through lungs; small amount through skin.	Cannot produce deep planes of anesthesia; therefore, used most often with IV barbiturates and supplemented with other agents. In subanesthetic doses, provides extensive	Nonflammable, but supports a flame. Caution must be taken to prevent hypoxia. Few side effects with normal doses, but

TABLE 8-5 / GENERAL ANESTHETICS AND PRECAUTIONS FOR USE IN DELIVERY (Continued)

Anesthetic	Absorption, Fate, Excretion	Effect	Comments
Inhalation Anesthetics			
		analgesia, especially useful during second stage of labor. Does not provide muscular relaxation.	nausea and vomiting may occur. Nonirritating to respiratory tract. Postoperative: Quick recovery depending on adjunct medication.
Cyclopropane	Must be given with anticholinergic preoperatively. Absorbed and eliminated through lungs. Recovery very rapid, with only traces left 3 h after delivery.	Can produce any desired level of anesthesia with muscular relaxation. Some respiratory depression but spontaneous respiration can be maintained during anesthesia. Some increase in blood pressure due to increased peripheral resistance. Stimulation of sympathetic nerves to myocardium; cardiac rate slows. Arrhythmias may occur if catecholamines are added during administration. Smooth muscle constriction is expected, and blood flow to renal and hepatic tissue is reduced. Incidence and magnitude of fetal depression is directly related to depth and duration of cyclopropane administration.	Flammable and explosive. Rapid induction of 2–3 min. Minimal irritation to respiratory tract, but some salivation unless given atropine-like medication preoperatively. Laryngospasm possible; sometimes delirium. Not used for asthmatics. Increased blood flow to skin and muscles; therefore, some extra bleeding at wound may occur. Enhances intestinal muscle tone and maintains uterine tone. Postoperative: Nausea and vomiting frequent during recovery. Some recovery delirium unless narcotic administered IV prior to termination of anesthesia. Prepare to give narcotic in half-dose fairly soon in recovery room. Hypotension and headache fairly common. Observe wound for oozing. Check urine output.
Intravenous Anesthetics			
Thio barbiturates: thiopental (Pentothal), thamylal (Surital)	Penetrates all body tissues, so initial high effect on brain is diminished quickly as drug diffuses and distributes to fat and lean tissue. Final elimination after many hours.	Very short-acting; blocks brain stem core. Does not provide analgesia until higher doses administered. Usually used for induction hypnosis accompanied by inhalation anesthetics.	Laryngospasm or bronchospasm may occur, especially in asthmatics. Cold clammy skin due to peripheral vasoconstriction may be seen.

Drug	Administration	Effects	Comments
	Crosses placenta rapidly but does not depress infant unless dose larger than 6.3 mg/kg is used (total dose greater than 250–300 mg).		Depresses respiration, reduces cardiac output, but increases total peripheral resistance. Depresses aortic and carotid chemoreceptors as well as respiratory center. Postoperative: Recovery may include restlessness because of pain. Shivering may occur due to hypothermia. Vomiting is minimal.
Ketamine hydrochloride (Ketaject, Ketalar)	Given IV or IM. May be used for rapid induction, followed by nitrous oxide for anesthesia.	Causes "dissociative" anesthesia. Patient is awake and without respiratory depression. Elevates heart rate 10–25%, and elevates cardiac output. Has antiarrhythmic effect. Traverses placenta rapidly. If 5–10 min elapse, infant is depressed and newborn is hyper-tonic, so that resuscitation is difficult.	Not used in delivery situations. Valuable for procedures about the head and neck. Analgesia and anesthesia good, but muscle relaxation is poor. Cough reflex is depressed however, and aspiration occurs. Postoperative: Nausea and vomiting infrequent. Prolonged recovery period, sometimes with bad dreams. In some patients, these dream episodes recur for days or weeks.
Nonbarbiturates (neuroleptic-narcotic combinations): droperidol (Inapsine) plus fentanyl citrate (Sublimaze) as Innovar	Intravenous injection over a period of 5–10 min. Administered with atropine as preoperative medication and accompanied by nitrous oxide if anesthesia desired. Also can be administered IM as a preoperative preparation for difficult procedures.	Anesthetic effect evident after 3–5 min. Produces mild to moderate arteriolar hypotension and bradycardia. Respiratory depression may occur.	Too rapid injection causes chest wall spasm. Given alone without nitrous oxide, provides a state of psychic indifference to difficult procedures. Patient remains awake. Postoperative: Nausea and vomiting. Grogginess may persist for 24 h.

Source: From E. J. Dickason, M. O. Schult, and E. M. Morris, *Maternal and Infant Drugs and Nursing Intervention*, McGraw-Hill Book Company, New York, 1978.

    B. Provide warmth.
        1. Dry infant immediately.
        2. Place in heated crib, cover with blanket.
    C. Physical assessment of newborn.
        1. Apgar score.
        2. Weight, length, head and chest circumferences.
        3. General appearance.
    D. Promote bonding by allowing mother and father adequate time with infant.
    E. Prevent physical complications.
        1. Administer vitamin K, 1 mg intramuscularly to prevent neonatal hemorrhage.
        2. After mother has held infant, instill silver nitrate drops in each eye and rinse (depending on hospital routine orders).

Evaluation

    I. Patient progresses through second stage without complications.
   II. Patient exhibits difficulty progressing through second stage.
    A. The presenting part does not descend despite strong contractions and effective pushing.
        1. Nursing observations should include evaluation of position of presenting part and increased molding.
        2. Prepare for forceps delivery with possible Scanzoni rotation if fetal position is posterior.
        3. If pelvis is inadequate or a malpresentation is present prepare for cesarean section.
    B. Hypotension may result from use of anesthetics.
        1. Change position to alleviate pressure of gravid uterus on inferior vena cava.
        2. If unable to change position then move uterus to left side of body.
        3. Administer oxygen.
    C. Fetal distress.
        1. Fetus may demonstrate variable decelerations associated with cord compression.
            a. Prepare resuscitation equipment.
            b. Provide suction and oxygen for infant.
            c. Have available sodium bicarbonate and calcium gluconate.

THIRD STAGE OF LABOR

Definition

The *third stage of labor* includes the period of time from the delivery of the infant to delivery of the placenta and membranes. (See Table 8-6 and Fig. 8-10.)

Assessment

    I. Psychosocial assessment.
    A. Reaction to infant may be excited, laughing, crying, angry, or rejecting.
    B. Reaction to delivery may be one of relief or one of guilt regarding behavior and performance in labor, or shock and disbelief that it is over.
   II. Physical assessment.
    A. Observe for separation of the placenta characterized by:
        1. Fundus rising in abdomen.
        2. Gush of blood from vaginal canal.

TABLE 8-6 / CHANGES DURING THE THIRD STAGE OF LABOR (SEE FIG. 8-10)

Physical Changes	*Behavioral Changes*
Contractions: strong Duration: 120 s Frequency: 3–5 min Delivery of placenta completed	Must be asked to push, since relief of pressure diminishes sensation of contraction. Patient may laugh or cry and ask about infant. May be excited or exhausted.

    3. Lenthening of umbilical cord.
  B. Note time and type of placental delivery.
    1. Spontaneous expulsion.
      a. Duncan mechanism: the maternal surface presents first.
      b. Schultz mechanism: the fetal surface presents first.
    2. Manual removal by the physician.
  C. Monitor vital signs every 10 min to assess changes precipitated by hemorrhage or complication of anesthesia.
  D. Palpate fundus to determine degree of contraction. Fundus should be firm and located at the level of the umbilicus.

FIGURE 8-10 / Third stage of labor: delivery of the placenta. *Left,* separation of the placenta from the uterine wall; *right,* contraction of the uterus after placental delivery. (*From "The Birth Atlas," Maternity Center Association, with permission.*)

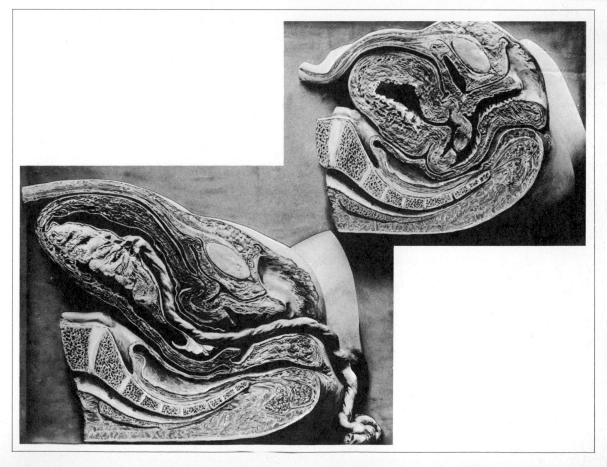

Problems

I. Client may reject infant, expressing anger or disappointment (see Table 8-7).

II. Close monitoring of vital signs and contractility of fundus is necessary.

Diagnosis

I. Patient is unable to deal with reality of delivery.

II. Patient is unable to cope with adjustment to newborn.

III. Physical well-being is threatened by:

 A. Uterine atony.

 B. Retained placenta.

 C. Vaginal or cervical lacerations.

Goals of Care

I. Parents will have contact with newborn as soon as possible.

II. Physical complications of the third stage will be prevented.

III. Safe, immediate newborn care will be provided.

Intervention

I. Allow parents to see and touch infant as soon as possible and breast feed, if mother wishes.

II. Encourage discussion of fears and anxieties regarding infant.

III. Monitor vital signs every 10 min.

TABLE 8-7 / HIGH-RISK SIGNALS IN THE DELIVERY ROOM

1. Written form with baby's chart concerning parents' reactions at birth.
    a. How do the parents *look?*
    b. What do the parents *say?*
    c. What do the parents *do?*
2. The following phrases may help in the organization of information regarding observations for the above-mentioned form.
    a. Do the parents appear sad, happy, apathetic, disappointed, angry, exhausted, frightened, ambivalent?
    b. Do the parents talk to the baby, talk to each other, use baby's name, establish eye contact, touch, cuddle, examine?
    c. Do the parents (and significant others) offer each other support, criticism, rejection, ambivalence?
3. If this interaction seems dubious, further evaluation should be initiated.
4. Reactions of concern at time of delivery include:
    a. Lack of interest in the baby, ambivalence, passive reaction.
    b. Parent keeps the focus of attention on self.
    c. Unwillingness or refusal to hold the baby, when offered.
    d. Mother directs hostility toward father, who put her "through all this."
    e. Inappropriate verbalizations, glances directed at baby, with definite hostility expressed.
    f. Disparaging remarks about the baby's sex or physical characteristics.

Source: From R. E. Helfer, and C. H. Kempe (eds.), *Child Abuse and Neglect: The Family and the Community,* The Bullinger Publishing Co., Cambridge, Mass., 1976.

IV. Assess location and contractility of fundus.
V. Administer oxytocins as ordered.
VI. After care of newborn is complete, provide time for baby and parents in recovery room.

Evaluation

I. Patient has no physical problems regarding expulsion of placenta and reactions to newborn are within normal limits.
II. Patient demonstrates signs of impaired physical state.
  A. Excessive bleeding and boggy fundus indicates uterine atony.
    1. Massage fundus with palm of hand.
    2. Administer oxytocin as ordered.
    3. Prepare for reexamination of perineal area, vagina, and cervix.
    4. Be sure bladder has been emptied.
  B. If cervical and/or vaginal lacerations characterized by bright red bleeding are present in spite of a firmly contracted uterus, notify physician and prepare for suturing of lacerations.

FOURTH STAGE OF LABOR

Definition

For the purposes of this chapter, the *fourth stage of labor* is the period of 1 h after delivery of the fetus. (See Table 8-8 and Fig. 8-11.)

Assessment

I. Psychosocial assessment.
  A. Patient may be sleeping after having seen and held infant.
  B. Patient may be excited and talkative regarding her labor and delivery experience or about the appearance and well-being of her child.
II. Physical assessment.
  A. Perineum should be intact with some edema present.
  B. Fundus should be firm and located between the symphysis pubis and the umbilicus.
  C. Lochia may be heavy rubra with some small clots.
  D. Vital signs should reflect admission baseline data.

Problems

I. Patient needs rest after the stress of labor and delivery.

TABLE 8-8 / CHANGES DURING THE FOURTH STAGE OF LABOR (SEE FIG. 8-11)

Physical Changes	Behavioral Changes
Uterus contracts Duration: 100 s Frequency: 5 min, unless receives oxytocins; then stays contracted until IV absorbed Infant suckling will promote contraction Mother may shiver and have chills	Seeks reassurance of performance. Usually fatigued. Preoccupied with labor experience; needs to talk about it. Father of child or other family member should be with mother during this time, plus infant if possible.

II. Patient must come to terms with experience of labor and delivery and accept the reality of having given birth.

III. Patient needs safety and comfort.

Diagnosis

I. Patient may be unable to rest due to excitement and concern regarding her infant or herself.

II. She may have difficulty coping with the reality of delivery.

III. Patient may not react favorably to infant (Table 8-7).

IV. There may be physical complications of fourth stage.

    A. Perineal hematoma.   D. Perineal discomfort.

    B. Trembling.   E. Bladder distension.

    C. Dehydration.

Goals of Care

I. Immediate.

    A. An environment conducive to rest will be maintained.

    B. Adjustment to newborn and to new maternal role will be promoted by supporting father and allowing time together.

    C. Physical complications of the fourth stage will be prevented or managed.

FIGURE 8-11 / Uterine contractions in the fourth stage. (Montevideo unit = product of frequency and intensity of uterine contractions in each 10-min period.) The initially high pressures after delivery are required for hemostasis. Within 24 h the myometrial activity declines rapidly. [*From H. Vorherr, in N. Assali (ed.), Pathophysiology of Gestation, vol. I, Maternal Disorders, Academic Press, Inc., New York, 1972, chap. 3.*]

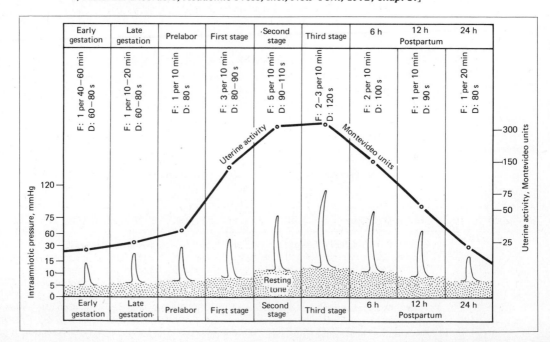

II. Long-range.
   A. The mother will recover from labor and delivery without physical or psychosocial handicaps.
   B. Acceptance of new roles and the newborn will take place.

Intervention

   I. Promote comfort by clean linen, changing pads as necessary, use of warm blanket to decrease trembling, and giving partial bed bath and clean hospital gown.
  II. Promote rest by decreasing environmental stimuli.
 III. Reassure mother as to health of newborn and her performance in labor and delivery.
 IV. Monitor fundus, vaginal flow, and vital signs every 10 min.
  V. Allow parents to hold and examine newborn. Provide time for quiet holding and touching in the recovery room if possible.
 VI. Encourage mother to talk about labor and delivery.
VII. Provide food and fluid as tolerated.

Evaluation

  I. Patient progresses through fourth stage within normal limits.
 II. Patient displays evidence of:
   A. Bladder distension as indicated by displacement of fundus above and to one side of the umbilicus.
     1. Provide bed pan and privacy.
     2. Catheterize if patient is unable to empty bladder.
   B. Patient demonstrates difficulty in accepting newborn.
     1. Encourage patient to express anger and disappointment.
     2. Assess her ability to deal with newborn based on past coping abilities and support system.
     3. Allow her to grieve any unfulfilled expectations—of sex, weight, well-being, or appearance.

REFERENCES

1. Emmanuel Friedman, *Labor: Clinical Evaluation and Management,* Appleton-Century-Crofts, New York, 1967.
2. C. Anderson, "Operational Definition of 'Support,'" *Journal of Obstetric, Gynecologic, and Neonatal Nursing,* **5**(1):17, January/February 1976.
3. E. J. Dickason, M. O. Schultz, and E. M. Morris, *Maternal and Infant Drugs and Nursing Intervention,* McGraw-Hill Book Company, New York, 1978, pp. 222–229.
4. J. C. Hyo, "Arresting Premature Labor," *American Journal of Nursing,* **76**(5):810, May 1976.

BIBLIOGRAPHY

Anderson, S. F.: "Childbirth as a Pathological Process: An American Perspective," *The American Journal of Maternal and Child Health,* **2**(4):240, July 1977. Challenges routine obstetrics and gives positive methods of returning control to parents.
Bean, C.: *Methods of Childbirth Preparation,* Dolphin Books/Doubleday & Company, Inc., Garden City, N.Y., 1972. A comparison of Lamaze, Read, Kitzinger, and Wright.
Friedman, Emmanuel: *Labor: Clinical Evaluation and Management,* Appleton-Century-Crofts, New York, 1967. An in-depth discussion of normal and dysfunctional labor patterns.
"Intrapartum Evaluation of the Fetus," *Journal of Obstetric, Gynecologic, and Neonatal Nursing,*

5(5/suppl.), September/October 1976. A collection of articles on intrapartum fetal evaluation covering the physiologic basis, clinical application, and societal issues regarding fetal monitoring.

Pritchard, J., and P. MacDonald: *Williams Obstetrics,* Appleton-Century-Crofts, New York, 1976. A comprehensive medical text covering the medical aspects of childbearing.

Tepperman, H. M., S. N. Beydown, and R. W. Abdul-Karim: "Drugs Affecting Myometrial Contractility in Pregnancy," *Clinical Obstetrics and Gynecology,* **20**(2):423, June 1977. Thorough discussion of all methods of induction and stimulation.

Whitley, A.: "Uterine Contractile Physiology: Applications in Nursing Care and Patient Teaching," *Journal of Obstetric, Gynecologic,and Neonatal Nursing,* **4**:54, September 1975. Nursing care is properly based on the physiologic changes which the patient is experiencing. Article useful to correct customs.

9
Recovery: The Fourth Trimester

Hilda Koehler

DEFINITION

The *postpartum period* includes the time from giving birth until the woman's physical recovery 6 to 8 weeks later. In addition to the bodily changes with which she must cope, a postpartum woman is undergoing significant psychosocial stress; she is in the process of adjusting her relationship to herself, to her mate, to her new baby, and to any other children or residents in her household. A term synonymous with postpartum is *puerperium,* from the Latin *puer,* "child," and *parere,* "to bring forth."

ASSESSMENT

Data needed for planning care are:
  I. Age, marital status, religion.
  II. Expected date of delivery (EDD), parity.
  III. Antepartum course and preparation for birth.
  IV. Description of labor process (e.g., length, medications, support received).
  V. Description of birth experience (e.g., length, forceps, anesthesia, cesarean section, or precipitate).
  VI. Recovery room events.
  VII. Baby's condition.
  VIII. Laboratory results (complete blood count, type, Rh, bilirubin, Coombs', rubella).
  IX. Home environment and support system.
  X. Expectations for baby (e.g., family care, adoption, institution).

PROBLEMS

  I. Physical recovery prolonged or disrupted.
  II. Maternal-infant bond faulty.
  III. Relationship to family and friends impaired.
  IV. Anxiety regarding new role and status.

DIAGNOSIS

  I. Recovery.
    A. Proceeding according to accepted norms.
    B. Complication preventing full recovery.
  II. Maternal-infant bonding.
    A. Mother and infant ecstatic with each other.
    B. Barrier to effective attachment between mother and infant.
  III. Relationship with family and friends.
    A. Relationship with mate and others warm and supportive.
    B. Tension exists between mother and others.

IV. Task development.
  A. Mother growing in ability to perform new role and tasks.
  B. Complication interfering with nurturing skills.

GOALS OF CARE

I. Immediate.
  A. Recovery from birth will proceed without complications.
  B. Nursing care will be based on individualized priorities established with each patient.
  C. Infant bonding will be sought and supported in every possible way.
  D. The patient will have the opportunity for supervised care of self and baby.
  E. Both mother and father will participate in defining and seeking family health goals.
II. Long-range.
  A. Anticipatory guidance will be available: teaching will be based on the patient's need for information.
  B. The family will receive referrals as indicated [visiting nurse service (VNS), social worker, family planning clinic, pediatrician, La Leche League, Parents of Twins club, food assistance programs, etc.].
  C. The patient will understand the need for follow-up care for herself and her baby, and can describe her plans to the nurse.
  D. The patient will understand the available methods of contraception and will seek assistance before the next menses if pregnancy is not desired.
  E. The patient will understand infant growth and development for period of the next few months, and be able to base care on infant's needs.
  F. The staff will assess risks of child abuse (see Table 9-4) and make appropriate preventive referrals as well as provide therapeutic intervention in the form of counseling, teaching, etc.

FIGURE 9-1 / Descent of the uterus (involution). (*From E. J. Dickason and M. O. Schult, Maternal and Infant Care, McGraw-Hill Book Company, New York, 1975.*)

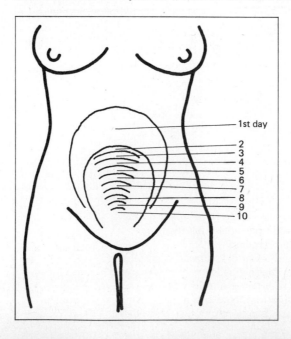

INTERVENTION

For clarity and ease of reference, physical and psychologic changes during the puerperium are presented with nursing interventions in Table 9-1.

TABLE 9-1 / NURSING INTERVENTIONS BASED UPON PUERPERAL CHANGES

Factors for Consideration	Physiology and/or Psychology	Intervention
1. Uterine complications **a.** Involution	1. Oxytocin, endogenous and/or exogenous, contracts uterus to prepregnant state (see Fig. 9-1). 2. Breast-feeding promotes excretion of oxytocin.	1. Check progressive involution of fundus, and massage if "boggy." 2. Empty bladder promotes involution. 3. Massage stimulates contraction. Prepare mother for discomfort when nurse does massage. Teach her to check and stimulate own fundus. 4. Prone position with pillow under abdomen and hips anteverts uterus (see Fig. 9-2).
b. Cramps or "afterpains"	1. Increases with each pregnancy. 2. Give anticipatory guidance to mother if she is breast-feeding.	1. Keep bladder empty. 2. Use position in Fig. 9-2 to lessen cramps. 3. Ensure warmth. 4. Give analgesia as ordered, if necessary. 5. Assure mother discomfort will lessen as involution is accomplished.
c. Lochia	1. Placental site sloughs off, and then much of endometrium is regenerated. 2. Lochia consists of blood, decidual tissue, epithelial cells from vagina, mucus, bacteria, and occasionally membranes and blood clots. 3. Lochia bright red for about 4 days (*lochia rubra*), then for about 4 more days is brownish pink (*lochia serosa*), then becomes whitish yellow (*lochia alba*), and may continue as such until the woman resumes her menstrual cycle.	1. Teach proper perineal care, as in factor 2. 2. Teach signs of infections or complication: bright red bleeding beyond fourth postpartum day; foul odor; absence of lochia in first 2 weeks after birth; clots or tissue in lochia; bright bleeding recurring after lochia alba begins. 3. Breast-feeding promotes uterine contractions which accelerate resolution of lochia from placental site. 4. Remind her not to douche as long as lochia persists.

FIGURE 9-2 / Prone position favors uterine descent.

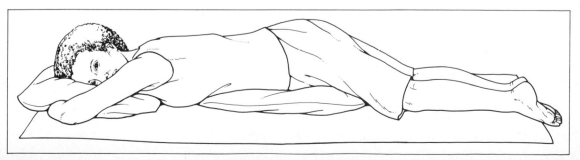

TABLE 9-1 / NURSING INTERVENTIONS BASED UPON PUERPERAL CHANGES (Continued)

Factors for Consideration	Physiology and/or Psychology	Intervention
2. Care of perineum	1. Birth greatly stretches perineal muscles; additionally, may have episiotomy and/or laceration(s) repaired. 2. Expulsion of baby may have simultaneously pushed out previously known or unknown hemorrhoids ("piles"), which developed during pregnancy from increased distension of rectal veins and pressure of uterine contents on the vein, and may have been aggravated by constipation.	1. Prevent infection: change pads from front to back always; irrigate using warm water after each voiding or bowel movement. Inspect carefully. 2. Teach perineal care. 3. Teach signs of complication or infection: edema, inflammation, increased pain, distended area, sense of fullness, dragging sensation in vagina. 4. Advise to refrain from wearing a panty girdle (keeps out air and light, which encourage healing). 5. Give analgesia if ordered and if needed. 6. Administer other treatments as ordered and needed: sitz bath, witch hazel compresses, heat lamp, analgesic spray. Rubber ring for sitting. 7. Teach Kegel exercises (see factor 11). 8. Teach how to sit properly; uncushioned chair, approached directly rather than at an angle, perineum and buttocks contracted; sit upright in back of chair.

3. Vital signs	1. Temperature should remain within normal limits throughout. Puerperal morbidity from fever exists when temperature is over 100.4°F (38°C) for 48 h after the first 24 h in consecutive readings.
	2. Pulse is often slower than usual, averaging between 60 and 70. Very slow pulse is transient and no cause for concern. Tachycardia suggests need for investigation of cause.
	3. Respirations should be within normal limits.
	4. Blood pressure varies according to course and management of labor. Often temporarily slightly elevated after birth from physical exertion, excitement; then slight drop from blood loss, medication, decrease in circulating blood volume.
	5. Increased blood pressure may indicate postpartum preeclampsia, pain, or distress. Evaluate and provide remedy or consultation.
	6. Lowered blood pressure indicates possible bleeding, reaction to medications, delayed involution. Correlate with other vital signs and condition of whole patient.
		1. Readings:
		  a. Take temperature every 4 h for 24 h, then qid as long as normal.
		  b. Take pulse and respiration every 15 min for 1 h, every ½ h for 3 h, every then 1 h for 3 h, then qid.
		  c. Take blood pressure on same schedule as pulse and respiration, except when stable take bid until discharge.
		2. Mother may experience some chills right after birth, with trembling and shivering, from stress and fatigue. Provide warmth (covering, beverage, supportive presence).
		3. Slight temperature elevation may indicate excitement, anxiety, dehydration, or beginning morbidity. Consider all data and supply corrective intervention.
		4. Temporary temperature elevation on third postpartum day usually signals accompanying signs of filling of the breasts with milk. See factor 8 for actions.
		5. Elevated pulse and respirations may indicate excitement, anxiety, dehydration, infection, bleeding, anemia, pain.

TABLE 9-1 / NURSING INTERVENTIONS BASED UPON PUERPERAL CHANGES (*Continued*)

Factors for Consideration	Physiology and/or Psychology	Intervention
		Assess and provide remedy and/or get consultation.
		6. If patient is excited or anxious, find most helpful resource to share or decrease impact—mate, other family, spiritual counselor, obstetrician, pediatrician, social worker, nurse.
		7. If there are signs of infection, get consultation, cultures/specimens, give medications and treatments as ordered, use isolation technique if needed.
		8. If woman in pain, provide pharmacologic and nursing measures that are appropriate.
		9. If signs of hemorrhage or shock, try to stop bleeding, get consultation, monitor signs carefully, provide warmth, fluids, position change, oxygen, reassurance.
4. Bladder function	1. Stress of labor and/or trauma from forceps may have caused edema, urethral spasm with pain. 2. Diuresis follows loss of hormones of pregnancy. Is delayed if woman receives antilactation medication.	1. Ambulate to bathroom if mother's condition will allow this safely. 2. Provide privacy for voiding. 3. Adequate fluid intake. 4. If difficulty voiding: warm bedpan, giving sitz bath, warm perineal shower, listening to water run may promote micturition. Ice to perineum may reduce edema enough for voluntary voiding. 5. Urecholine-type drugs may be ordered. 6. Catheterize if all else fails.
5. Weight loss, nutrition, diaphoresis (see Table 9–2)	1. Weight loss of products of conception approximately 12 lb; continued catabolism over 3- to 6-week period approximately an additional 12 lb. 2. Loss of hormones of pregnancy responsible for diaphoresis, and diuresis.	1. Review maternal nutrition in light of plan to breast- or bottle-feed. 2. Supervise and guide eating pattern. 3. Encourage fluids ad libitum (see also factors 4 and 6). 4. Assure woman as to normality of heavy perspiration. 5. Encourage showers/skin care. Provide for linen and garment changes. (If she uses hospital rather than own gowns, her laundry chores will be minimal.)
6. Bowel function	1. During late pregnancy there was considerable pressure on bowel; now pressure is off, and pelvic muscles may be quite stretched and lax. 2. The prospect of the first bowel move-	1. Early ambulation stimulates function. 2. Adequate fluid intake; hot drinks. 3. High-fiber diet (prune juice, dried fruits, bran and/or whole grain products, raw fruits and vegetables).

TABLE 9-1 / NURSING INTERVENTIONS BASED UPON PUERPERAL CHANGES (*Continued*)

Factors for Consideration	Physiology and/or Psychology	Intervention
	ment after giving birth may elicit anxiety if the mother has a sore perineum.	4. Give laxative or stool softener if ordered and if necessary. 5. Encourage relaxation and assurance that if feces are soft there will be little if any discomfort. 6. Give enema if ordered and if necessary.
7. Skin care	1. Effort of birth, diaphoresis, and intensified emotions lead to need for consistent hygienic measures. 2. Some cultures prescribe against showers, shampoo for 40 days postpartum.	1. Provide sponge bath as soon as possible after birth unless woman's weariness contraindicates. 2. Continue to give sponge bath until mother is able to care for herself (e.g., new cesarean section, recuperating from prolonged, difficult labor). 3. Encourage daily shower, and shampoo when desired. 4. Review perineal hygiene, breast care.
8. Need for rest and sleep	1. The birth experience drains physical and emotional energy, but excitement immediately postpartum masks weariness. 2. Alteration in life-style with new baby will entail disruption in sleep habits.	1. Provide privacy for mother, father, and baby when possible. 2. Group nursing activities for minimal disturbance. 3. Encourage frequent rest periods. 4. Provide back rub, warm drink, conversation, darkness and quiet, disconnected telephone, and if necessary, sedation as indicated. 5. Prepare mother for rest needs at home. 6. Assess plan for help at home, and provide advice and referral.
9. Circulation	1. Increased progesterone during pregnancy predisposes women to blood-clotting problems. 2. 20–50 percent of gravidas develop varicosities, increasing potential for problems postpartum.	1. Assess status of veins from prenatal chart and personal observation. 2. Encourage ambulation as early as policy and woman's condition allows. 3. Check Homans' sign daily (use one hand to keep knee extended, flex foot pointing toes toward knee). Pain in calf indicates possible clot. 4. Apply elastic stockings or Ace bandages in those particularly at risk (cesarean section patients, history of prior phlebitis or moderate to severe varicosities, extended general or spinal anesthesia used for delivery, traumatic birth, multiple birth). 5. Remind mother to elevate legs. 6. Give moist or dry heat to legs if ordered.

TABLE 9-1 / NURSING INTERVENTIONS BASED UPON PUERPERAL CHANGES (*Continued*)

Factors for Consideration	Physiology and/or Psychology	Intervention
10. Breast care	1. Lactation usually begins 48 h after birth. 2. Stimulation (nursing) increases milk supply; lack of stimulation will promote milk supply to "dry up." 3. Not only the lactating lobes, acini, and lactiferous ducts become full at the beginning of milk production, but the surrounding lymph and blood vessels become distended. 4. The hormone oxytocin prompts the "let-down" reflex, contracting myoepithelial cells around the collecting milk sinuses under the areola of the nipple. 5. Many obstetricians no longer order hormones to suppress lactation.	1. Determine what breast care mother has been using during pregnancy; nipple rolling, massage, nipple cream. 2. Teach mother to keep breasts and nipples clean by careful cleanliness of her own hands whenever she handles breasts, using fresh washcloth for breasts during care. No soap used on nipples (too drying). Remove plastic liners from bras. Fresh bra used daily, ensuring good support. Fresh nursing pads (commercial, or men's handkerchiefs, or cut-up perineal pads or "Swedish milk cups") as woman prefers. 3. Exposing nipples to air and light helps keep them in good condition. 4. Limit and gradually increase nursing time so that nipples become accustomed to suckling. (3–5 min first day, 5–7 min second day, 7–10 min third day; lower number applicable to fair, or sensitive-skinned women.) 5. Alternate breast on which feeding begins each time, to keep breast size balanced. 6. Teach method of "breaking" suction (press nipple away from baby's mouth, put clean little finger between nipple and mouth, hold baby's nose) to minimize trauma to nipples. 7. Use nipple cream or nipple guard if needed. 8. If breast-feeding, when milk first comes in: liberal fluid intake, baby to breast ad libitum, very warm showers or/and compresses to breast before feeding, accompanied by exercises to remove lymph and blood engorgement (see Fig. 9-3). If more than moderate fullness: apply ice packs to axilla for 15 min and on top of breasts for 15 min after feeding (see Table 9–2). 9. If bottle-feeding: moderate fluid intake, warm shower to breasts with exercises shown in Fig. 9-3; ice packs as above every 3–4 h. Give hormones and analgesia if ordered. 10. Teach mother to be alert to symptoms of nipple cracking or breast abscess.

TABLE 9-1 / NURSING INTERVENTIONS BASED UPON PUERPERAL CHANGES (*Continued*)

Factors for Consideration	Physiology and/or Psychology	Intervention
11. Recovery or enhancement of abdominal and perineal tone	1. Expulsion of products of conception leaves the abdominal muscles stretched and loose, in need of exercise to restore or improve from prepregnancy state (see Fig. 9-4). 2. Diastasis of rectus abdominis muscles is common after pregnancy. 3. Pregnancy and birth leave perineal muscles stretched (see Fig. 9-5).	1. Remind mother of correct posture; contract abdominal muscles while in bed, at least 3 times a day, 5 times each, even if she has had a cesarean. 2. Abdominal toning: (a) Lay flat on back on bed (on floor on carpet or blanket at home) with ankles crossed and hands palms down resting lightly across lower abdomen, elbows on bed

FIGURE 9-3 / Exercises to relieve breast fullness. (*a*) With bra off, place hands on shoulders, raise elbows to shoulder height, and slowly rotate in wide circles. (*b*) Place left hand on hip, raise right arm over head, bend at the waist to left, and return. Repeat on other side. (*c*) Place both hands on rib cage, thumbs front; "wing" elbows as far as possible. Return elbows to sides and repeat.

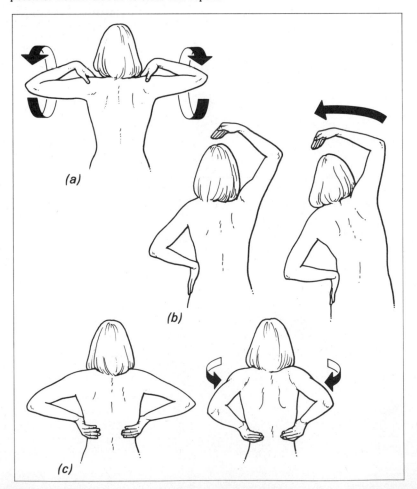

(a)

(b)

(c)

TABLE 9-1 / NURSING INTERVENTIONS BASED UPON PUERPERAL CHANGES (*Continued*)

Factors for Consideration	Physiology and/or Psychology	Intervention
		but not using elbows for support. (*b*) Inhale deeply through nose. (*c*) In deliberate sequence, tighten abdominal, then buttocks, then perineal muscles; hold. (*d*) Very slowly (to slow count of 8) raise head (not shoulders) as though lifting head to look at toes; at same time very slowly blow air out as though making a candle flame flicker. (*e*) Very slowly lower head back to bed, continuing to blow out air unless supply depleted. (*f*) Release all muscles. (*g*) Repeat to total of 5, morning and evening first day, 6 twice a day the second day, 7 twice a day the third, working up to 10 bid. (For additional exercises see Fig. 9-6.) 3. Kegel exercise (also called pelvic floor or perineal tightening): (1) (Easiest to learn when passing urine)—start stream of urine, then voluntarily stop stream before voiding completely. (2) Start and stop stream until sure of the sensation of releasing and tightening muscles around urethra, vagina, rectum. (3) Remind mother to practice Kegel every time she visits bathroom,

FIGURE 9-4 / Abdominal musculature may need toning exercises.

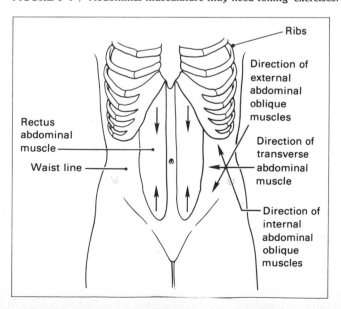

TABLE 9-1 / NURSING INTERVENTIONS BASED UPON PUERPERAL CHANGES (*Continued*)

Factors for Consideration	Physiology and/or Psychology	Intervention
		and at least 3 times a day for 5 times the rest of her life! (4) Impress on her that faithful attention to perineal muscles, keeps swelling and therefore soreness at a minimum around sutures, increases blood supply for healing, ensures good pelvic floor support as prevention of incontinence problems as an older woman, and provides the basis for maximum pleasure during sexual stimulation and intercourse.
12. Parental-infant bonding	**1.** Klaus and Kennell* have identified the following seven principles crucial to the process of attachment: **a.** "There is a sensitive period in the first minutes and hours of life during which it is necessary that the mother and father have close contact with	**1.** Provide privacy and time for parents to hold baby, ensuring warmth for infant and comfort to all, preferably at least the first hour after birth. **2.** Encourage parents to participate as fully in care of baby as both can manage.

*From Klaus, Marshall H., and Kennell, John H.: *Maternal-Infant Bonding,* St. Louis, 1976, The C. V. Mosby Co.

FIGURE 9-5 / Perineal muscles will respond to Kegel exercises.

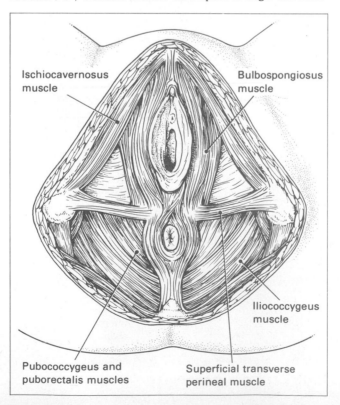

TABLE 9-1 / NURSING INTERVENTIONS BASED UPON PUERPERAL CHANGES (*Continued*)

Factors for Consideration	Physiology and/or Psychology	Intervention
	their neonate for later development to be optimal. *b.* "There appear to be species-specific responses to the infant in the human mother and father that are exhibited when they are first given the infant. *c.* "The process of the attachment is structured so that the father and mother will become attached optimally to only one infant at a time. Bowlby (1958)† earlier stated this principle of the attachment process in the other direction and termed it *monotropy.* *d.* "During the process of the mother's attachment to her infant, it is necessary that the infant respond to the mother by some signal such as body or eye movements. We have sometimes described this, 'you can't love a dishrag'. *e.* "People who witness the birth process become strongly attached to the infant. *f.* "For some adults it is difficult simultaneously to go through processes of attachment and detachment, that is to develop an attachment to one person while mourning the loss or threatened loss of the same or another person. *g.* "Some early events have long-lasting effects. Anxieties about the wellbeing of the baby with a temporary disorder in the first day may result in long-lasting concerns that may adversely shape the development of the child (Kennell and Rolnick, 1960)."‡	3. Observe interaction among all three, affirming positive elements. 4. When teaching, avoid any methods or language that would imply professional staff is "expert" and new parents are inadequate. 5. Strive for consistency among staff in example and teaching. 6. Arrange for group interaction among parents on maternity unit. 7. Refer to parenthood workshops in community if available. 8. Seek consultation if attachment process delayed or faulty.
13. "Taking in, taking hold, letting go"	1. Reva Rubin has described the behavior of new mothers in three phases: *a. Taking in* lasts 2 or 3 days and indicates the mother is trying to absorb her experience. *b. Taking hold* lasts about 10 days and indicates the mother is exercising initiative in responsibility for caring for herself and her baby.	1. Be sensitive to period of adjustment that mother and father are in, and tailor care according to phase of puerperium. 2. Seek consultation if delay in resolution of any phase.

†J. Bowlby, "Nature of a Child's Tie to His Mother," *International Journal of Psychoanalysis,* **39:**350–373, 1958.
‡J.H. Kennell and A. Rolnick, "Discussing Problems in Newborn Babies with Their Parents," *Pediatrics,* **26:**832–838, 1960.

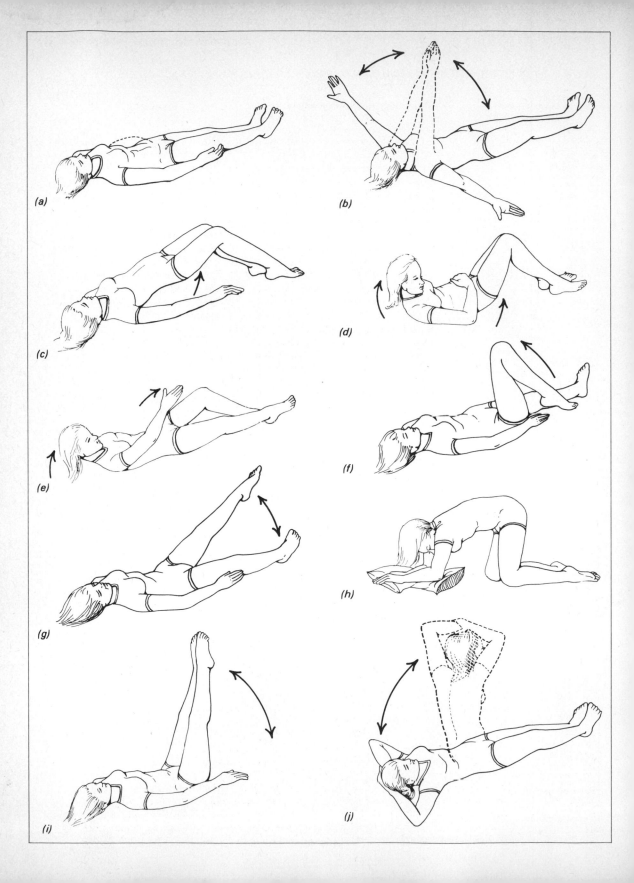

(a)

(b)

(c)

(d)

(e)

(f)

(g)

(h)

(i)

(j)

TABLE 9-1 / NURSING INTERVENTIONS BASED UPON PUERPERAL CHANGES (*Continued*)

Factors for Consideration	Physiology and/or Psychology	Intervention
	c. Letting go occurs when mother indicates she is ready to regard the new baby as truly a separate person.§	
14. Postpartum blues	1. Losing the hormones of pregnancy, physical adjustments (milk coming in, first bowel movement, hemorrhoids), anticipation of coping with baby 24 h a day, 7 days a week, plus the change from exaltation and euphoria immediately after birth may leave mother unreasonably weepy and bewildered by emotions. 2. May be unconsciously or consciously "grieving" over shattered unrealistic expectations of themselves, family, or hopes for birth experience, or over this less than ideal baby.	1. Provide anticipatory guidance. 2. Enlist understanding and support of significant others. 3. Urge mother to get help if feelings of depression are extended or severe at home. 4. Explore plans for assistance during first days at home. Make suggestions or referrals as appropriate.
15. Relationship to relatives and friends *a.* Baby's father	1. Mother's preoccupation with baby's needs may inspire surprising (to him) jealousy. 2. Father may center attention on baby and seemingly ignore mother. 3. Father may be threatened by male child, or need reassurance as to his ability to provide for family.	1. Encourage parents to freely share joys, fears, frustrations, hopes, and to listen to each other. 2. Affirm primary wisdom of taking care of their own relationship first. 3. Urge mother to help father to develop his own relationship with the infant by being alone regularly with the baby, unmonitored by mother.

§R. Rubin, "Basic Maternal Behavior," *Nursing Outlook*, 9:683, 1961.

FIGURE 9-6 / Postpartal exercises. (Note: Each exercise is to be repeated four times, twice daily, with a new exercise added each day.) (*a*) *First day:* Breathe in deeply; expand the abdomen. Exhale slowly, hissing; draw in abdominal muscles forcibly. (*b*) *Second day:* Lie flat on the back with the legs slightly apart. Hold arms at right angles to the body; slowly raise the arms, keeping the elbows stiff. Touch hands together and gradually return arms to their original position. (*c*) *Third day:* Lie flat on the back with the arms at the sides. Draw the knees up slightly. Arch the back. (*d*) *Fourth day:* Lie flat on the back with the knees and hips flexed. Tilt the pelvis inward and contract the buttocks tightly. Lift the head while contracting the abdominal muscles. (*e*) *Fifth day:* Lie flat on back with the legs straight. Raise the head and one knee slightly. Then reach for, but do not touch, the knee with the opposite hand. Alternate with the right and left hand. (*f*) *Sixth day:* Slowly flex the knee and then the thigh on the abdomen. Lower the foot to the buttock. Straighten and lower the leg to the floor. (*g*) *Seventh day:* Raise first the right and then the left leg as high as possible. Keep the toes pointed and the knee straight. Lower the leg gradually, using the abdominal muscles but not the hands. (*h*) *Eighth day:* Rest on the elbows and knees, keeping the upper arms and legs perpendicular with the body. Hump the back upward. Contract the buttocks and draw the abdomen in vigorously. Relax, breathe deeply. (*i*) *Ninth day:* Same as seventh day, but raise both legs at the same time, etc. (*j*) *Tenth day:* Lie flat on the back with the arms clasped behind the head. Then sit up slowly. (If necessary, hook feet under furniture.) Slowly lie back. (*Reproduced with permission from R. C. Benson, Handbook of Obstetrics and Gynecology, 5th ed., Lange Medical Publications, Los Altos, Calif., 1974.*)

TABLE 9-1 / NURSING INTERVENTIONS BASED UPON PUERPERAL CHANGES *(Continued)*

Factors for Consideration	*Physiology and/or Psychology*	*Intervention*
b. Other children	1. A new baby is usually a threat to older children, for they are never sure there will be enough love left for them when the newcomer is included. 2. Toddlers will tend to act out distress in physical terms. 3. In units without sibling visiting privileges, a 2- or 3-year-old can come to the conclusion that "mother has abandoned me purposely."	1. Inform parents of ways to prevent or minimize trauma. 2. If unit has sibling visiting privileges, encourage parents to use them. 3. If sibling cannot visit, give anticipatory guidance, in particular regarding the "cold shoulder" the mother will get when she first sees 2- or 3-year-old.
c. Grandparents or other household members	1. Unresolved conflicts between older parents and their children of childbearing age may be intensified at grandchild's arrival. 2. Grandmothers may unconciously (or consciously) need to demonstrate that they are the expert in child care.	1. Explore potential disagreement areas. 2. Include all family members in teaching of baby care skills in hospital and/or at home. 3. Encourage parents to present a unified plan of child care to grandparents, and to support each other if resistance is met.
d. Pets	1. Pets frequently exhibit jealousy regarding newborn and may require restraint and extra attention.	1. Provide anticipatory guidance.
16. Visitors	1. See factor 8.	1. Monitor effect of visitors on mother in hospital; intervene if mother unable to recognize own limitations of energy or be "impolite" to guests. 2. Establish plan with parents for receiving visitors at home.
17. Help at home	1. The pattern of the nuclear family often means the couple with a newborn is isolated. 2. The physical weariness of the new mother and constancy of responsibility for baby care can strain personal resources. 3. Multiple births greatly increase the need for household assistance.	1. Encourage father to take advantage of paternity leave plan if available. 2. Explore resources for securing help with cooking, shopping, cleaning, laundry. Be financially realistic but urge parents to think of arrangements as an investment. 3. Delineate clearly what can be expected from relatives or "baby nurse" so that any friction that might develop can be kept to a minimum. 4. See Table 9-3.
18. Sexual activity	1. Trauma and/or changes in the woman's genitalia lead to concern over resuming intercourse. 2. The stress and newness of adjusting to an altered life-style may decrease or increase libido in either partner. 3. Pregnancy is possible before the woman resumes menstrual functioning. 4. Until lochia has ceased there is increased possibility of vaginal infection.	1. Many women hesitate to initiate questions about this subject; do not hesitate in providing information. 2. Suggest possibility that couple may find it helpful to plan, when ready to express love sexually, to physically "pleasure" each other and see if events continue to penetration and intercourse. This can disperse the tension of "we must have coitus tonight."

TABLE 9-1 / NURSING INTERVENTIONS BASED UPON PUERPERAL CHANGES (*Continued*)

Factors for Consideration	Physiology and/or Psychology	Intervention
		3. Prepare couple that new father may have temporary erection problems. **4.** Assist in selection of family planning method or appointment for follow-up care (see Chap. 4).
19. Postpartum/inter-conceptional care	**1.** The woman's total well-being as well as the return of reproductive organs to their prepregnancy state, is assessed by the obstetric team. **2.** Many women tend to neglect keeping their postpartum appointment, and receiving interconceptional health supervision, unless they have a presenting problem (obvious difficulty as a sequel to giving birth, need for prescription refill for contraceptive pills, etc.).	**1.** Encourage patient to keep appointment, whatever her own assessment of condition. **2.** Answer questions as they arise. **3.** Determine need for learning breast self-examination, and provide information as needed.

TABLE 9-2 / SUGGESTED MEAL PLAN DURING LACTATION

Milk	4 cups
Meat and meat substitutes	6 oz daily, 2 to 3 servings
Vegetables, fruits	4 servings
Dark green or yellow	1 serving daily
Vitamin C source	1 serving daily
Bread or cereal	4 or 5 servings
Fluids	6 to 8 cups daily in addition to milk

EVALUATION

I. Adaptation uneventful, no difficulties encountered.

II. Physical state appears normal, but psychosocial elements require further assessment and intervention.

   A. Bonding is not proceeding normally.

      1. Assessment.

         a. Mother does not maintain closeness, there is infrequent eye contact, little talk with infant.

         b. Attention focused on own discomforts, needs.

         c. Watches TV while feeding infant.

         d. Has not named infant.

         e. Often absent from room during feeding time.

         f. Home-going plans unformed.

      2. Intervention.

         a. Stay with and observe feeding behavior, pick up teaching points. Find out where mother's concerns are (see Table 9-4).

         b. Provide analgesia if patient uncomfortable.

         c. Give praise for positive interaction.

TABLE 9-3 / HELPFUL SUGGESTIONS FOR NEW PARENTS

1. The responsibilities of parenthood are learned; become informed, and do not hesitate to get help and advice.
2. Make friends of other couples who are experienced with young children.
3. Don't overload yourself with unimportant tasks.
4. Don't move soon after the baby arrives.
5. Don't be overconcerned with keeping up appearances.
6. Get plenty of rest and sleep. Try to rest when the baby sleeps during the day to make up for your broken night's sleep the first few months.
7. Men: reduce your outside activities for a time after the baby comes so you can be more available at home. Perhaps you could take some vacation time.
8. Don't be a nurse to elderly relatives at this period.
9. Plan ahead to find a good babysitter so you will be able to take time off occasionally without worry.
10. Don't give up outside interests, but cut down on responsibilities and rearrange schedules.
11. Get a family doctor or pediatrician early.
12. Confer and consult with each other, family, and experienced friends; discuss your plans and worries.

Source: Adapted from R. E. Gordon, E. E. Kapostins, and K. K. Gordon, "Factors in Postpartum Emotional Adjustment," *Obstetrics and Gynecology,* **25**(2):158–66, February 1965.

    d. Involve other members of the family in infant care.
    e. Refer for social worker assessment of home support system, reasons behind indifference toward infant.
    f. Note problem for referral and follow-up.
B. Anxiety about ability to cope continues.
    1. Assessment.
      a. Crying, expresses fears.
      b. Asks nurse to feed infant at bedside, expresses fears that baby is fragile.
      c. Family support appears missing, or fragmentary, few visitors.
      d. No prior experience with infant care.
    2. Intervention.
      a. Provide time for therapeutic listening, to "hear" what real problem is.
      b. Work with mother on her own feeding techniques. Teach growth and development of infant and how needs are expressed. Provide literature.
      c. Refer to social worker for family assessment of strengths, financial needs.
      d. Refer to VNS for close follow-up. Note problem for clinic nurses' attention.
      e. Set up postpartum mothers' support group, meeting weekly with additional phone-in assistance.
C. Depression occurs.
    1. Assessment.
      a. Turns away from help or conversation.
      b. Body language indicates depression; poor hygiene, grooming, posture.
      c. Crying, not eating well.
      d. Expresses more than normal inadequacy about parenting, seems in despair about coping.
    2. Intervention.
      a. Assess responses to infant, staff, family.
      b. Alert physician for possible psychiatric referral.
      c. Remind patient of reality, work with her on infant care. Be sure she can return satisfactory demonstration of basic infant care.
      d. Refer to VNS for close follow-up.
      e. Refer to social worker for family involvement, in supportive approach.
      f. Involve in weekly mothers' group.

TABLE 9-4 / HIGH-RISK SIGNALS IN THE POSTPARTUM PERIOD (ON POST-PARTUM WARD AND IN WELL BABY CLINIC)

1. Does the family remain disappointed over sex of baby?
2. What is the child's name?
   a. Who is baby named for/after?
   b. Who picked the name and when was the named picked?
   c. Is the name used when talking to or about the baby?
3. What was/is the husband's and/or family's reaction to the new baby?
   a. Are they supportive? Are they critical?
   b. Do they attempt to take over and control the situation?
   c. Is the husband jealous of the baby's drain on the mother's time and energy?
4. What kind of support, other than family, is the mother receiving?
5. Are there sibling rivalry problems? Do parents think there will be any? How do they plan to handle them? Or do they deny that a new baby will change existing family relationships?
6. Is the mother or father bothered by the baby's crying? How does it make them feel? Angry? Inadequate?
7. Feedings
   a. Does the mother or father view the baby's needs to eat as too demanding?
   b. Are the baby's demands frequently ignored?
   c. Is either repulsed by infant's messiness, spitting up, and sucking noises?
8. How do parents view changing diapers? Is either repulsed by the messiness, smells, etc.?
9. Are the developmental expectations for the child far beyond his or her capabilities?
10. Mother's (or father's) control or lack of control during clinic visit:
    a. Is there involvement and control over baby's needs and fears while in the waiting room and during the exam?
    b. Is control relinquished to the physician, nurse, etc. (undressing, holding, allowing the child to express fears, etc.?)
11. Can either mother or father express that they are having fun with their baby?
    a. Can they view infant as a separate individual?
    b. Are parents proud of attention focused on the baby, or do they seem jealous, or threatened by it?
12. Can parents establish and maintain eye-to-eye, direct contact, en face position, with the baby?
13. Do they talk with the baby?
14. Do the parents talk about the child negatively?
15. Is the baby comforted when she or he cries?
16. Are there complaints about the child that cannot be verified?
    a. Multiple emergency calls for very minor complaints, not major issues.
    b. Calling all the time for small problems, things that to you seem unimportant, but could be very major for mother.
    c. The baby does things "on purpose" just to aggravate the parents.
    d. In your presence the mother describes a characteristic you can't verify, such as baby crying continually.
    e. Mother tells you unbelievable stories about the baby—e.g., not breathing, or turning colors for the past 30 min—but it seems fine "now that the nurse is looking."
17. Is there manipulation of professionals working with the family by pitting nurse against lay therapist, for example, or physician against social worker through complaints, stories, and miscommunicating information?

Source: Adapted from R. E. Helfer and C. H. Kempe, *Child Abuse and Neglect: The Family and the Community,* Ballinger Publishing Co., Cambridge, Mass., 1976.

TABLE 9-5 / HYPOVOLEMIC SHOCK

Physiologic Changes	Patient's Symptoms	Intervention
Cardiac/Circulatory Status		
Decreased venous pressure, cardiac output, pulse pressure, arterial pressure	Feels weak, dizzy; may feel rapid heartbeat.	Record vital signs, if necessary take apical pulse. Monitor CVP; if severe hypotension persists, line should be inserted by physician. Support blood volume with plasma expanders, whole blood, Ringer's lactate.
Adrenal medulla stimulated to produce catecholamines, adding to vasoconstriction	Feels cold, peripheral tissues are pale, nails blanch slowly.	Keep patient warm, check skin color, turgor, mucous membrane moisture, temperature.
	Feels restless, anxious, fearful.	Reassure patient, stay with her. Record expressed statements, observations.
Respiratory Status		
Tachypnea, respiratory center stimulated by hypoxia	Complains of "air hunger," shortness of breath.	Note rate, rhythm, depth of respirations. Administer oxygen by mask (do not use Trendelenburg's position during pregnancy; instead, place patient in side-lying position).
Gastrointestinal Status		
Fluid shift from interstitial tissues and intestinal tract to vascular compartment (takes several hours to shift)	Sensation of thirst increases.	Drop in hematocrit observed after shift. Draw blood for serial Hb/Hct. Keep NPO if returning to operating or delivery room for correction of bleeding.
Decreased parasympathetic activity = reduced GI motility, secretions	Nausea may occur.	
Renal Status		
Conservation of fluids and salts stimulated by vasoconstriction of renal arterioles (needs 70 mmHg pressure to filtrate blood effectively)	May have no sensation of need to void.	Observe closely for oliguria (lower limit of normal 30 mL/h). Record hourly output and specific gravity, from Foley catheter.

III. Physical condition requires further assessment and intervention.

 A. Hemorrhage occurs. Early postpartum hemorrhage may be due, in order, to (1) atonic uterine muscle, (2) laceration with open or concealed bleeding, hematoma formation, (3) retained placental fragments, or (4) rarely, bleeding and clotting problems. Loss of blood of 500 mL or more places the patient in danger of shock if uncorrected, since the open placental site will continue to bleed until the cause is corrected and uterine muscle can be firmly contracted, or the laceration repaired.

  Late postpartum hemorrhage is usually the result of retained placental fragments or of infection causing delayed involution. Such hemorrhage usually does not begin until 1 to 2 weeks after birth.

  1. Assessment.

   a. Bleeding observed, soaking vaginal and bed pad.

   b. Vital signs change with elevated pulse, lowered blood pressure.

   c. Uterus boggy, bladder distended (atonic uterus).

   d. Uterus firm, but bright red bleeding continues (laceration).

      e. Patient complains of weakness, dizziness, is anxious, and may be thirsty (see Table 9-5).

  2. Intervention.

      a. Begin noting amount of bleeding, frequency of change of pad. Save and measure any clots.

      b. Frequent check of vital signs.

      c. Have patient empty bladder or catheterize her before massaging fundus.

      d. Speed up IV fluids if already in use. Begin IV fluids if not in use with large-bore catheter.

      e. Work with physician to identify source of bleeding.

      f. Prepare for return to delivery room or OR as necessary to correct cause.

B. Infection occurs. Postpartum infection is that occurring in the reproductive tract within the first 48 days after birth. Symptoms are usually a fever over 100.4°F (38°C) after the first 24 h, accompanied by signs of wound infection of site of laceration repair of episiotomy, pelvic cellulitis or endometritis.

    Routes can be from autoinfections of normally resident bacteria, from poor asepsis, or be a result of ascending infection from premature rupture of membranes. Bacteria are of three main types: (1) hemolytic streptococci, (2) mixed anaerobic-aerobic bacteria normally present in the vagina, and (3) anaerobic bacteria present in GI tract (clostridial or *E. coli* infections.)

    Differential diagnosis takes time, and treatment is usually initiated with broad-spectrum antibiotics, after blood and wound cultures have been obtained.

  1. Assessment.

      a. Change in character of lochia, or absent flow.

      b. Pain and tenderness upon palpation of lower abdomen or at episiotomy site.

      c. Chills, fever.

  2. Intervention.

      a. Obtain wound, lochial, and cervical cultures at once, before beginning antibiotics.

      b. Obtain blood culture, send at once to lab.

      c. Record more frequent vital signs.

      d. Prepare for IV antibiotic regimen.

      e. Depending on organisms, maintain wound isolation precautions.

      f. Encourage fluids, high protein diet.

      g. Give extra support, as infant may not be allowed in room with mother.

BIBLIOGRAPHY

Boston Women's Health Collective: *Our Bodies, Ourselves,* Simon & Schuster, Inc., New York, 1976. Complete guide to gynecologic and obstetric care written for lay women.

Brazelton, T. B.: "Anticipatory Guidance," *Pediatric Clinics of North America,* **22:**533, 1975. Guidance for new parents.

————: "The Parent-Infant Attachment," *Clinical Obstetrics and Gynecology* **19**(2):373, June 1976. Comprehensive review of research in bonding.

Gruis, M.: "Beyond Maternity: Postpartum Concerns of Mothers," *Maternal and Child Nursing,* **2**(3): 182, May–June 1977. Identification of women's concerns about their own recovery.

Haight, J.: "Steadying Parents as They Go: By Phone," *Maternal and Child Nursing,* **2**(5):311, September–October 1977. Recommendations for follow-up after delivery.

Klaus, M. H., and J. H. Kennell: *Maternal-Infant Bonding,* The C. V. Mosby Company, St. Louis, 1976. The now-classic work on maternal-infant bonding, including ways of assisting grieving parents.

Lozoff, B., et al.: The "Mother-Newborn Relationship: Limits of Adaptability," *Journal of Pediatrics,* **91**(1):1–12, July 1977. A fine summary of all the work on bonding by members of Klaus's group.

"The Postpartum Period," *American Journal of Nursing,* **77:**1170–80, July 1977. A series of five articles.

Salk, L.: *Preparing for Parenthood,* Bantam Books, Inc., New York, 1975. Readily understood, balanced discussion of the factors and tasks of parenting.

10

The Full-Term Newborn

Kathleen Reilly Powderly

The newborn infant is an amazing human being. Not too long ago, medical science believed the newborn to be a tiny, helpless individual who could not contribute much to the surrounding family or environment. Through the work of such individuals as T. Berry Brazelton (1) and Marshall Klaus and John Kennell (2) we now know this is not so. Indeed, the infant can see and hear and does interact with its surroundings, and in particular with its significant caretakers. It is obvious that we have much to learn about all newborns. It is also obvious that we are only now beginning to realize the impact of this crucial period.

Many health care professionals consider work in the newborn nursery to be a rather routine assignment. However, when we consider the possible impact of this period, we must realize what an awesome challenge it is. The future physical, mental, and emotional development of this tiny human being can be greatly helped or hindered by the kind of care given in the first few days of life, and by the quality of the education given to the parents before discharge from the hospital.

I. Data base.
  A. Delivery room preparation.
    1. Maintain asepsis and prevent infection.
    2. Maintain environmental temperature.
        a. Minimize *evaporative* loss by providing a dry towel for infant.
        b. Minimize *conductive* loss by placing infant on a warm, dry surface.
        c. Minimize *convective* loss by utilizing a warm delivery room with no drafts.
        d. Minimize *radiant* heat loss by having an open bed with a radiant overhead heat source available.
    3. Supplies should be available for resuscitation, identification, and eye care.
  B. Maternal history.
    1. Review records to determine any problems identified with history or prenatal course. Especially note the blood type and Rh, serology, presence of any chronic disease, hemoglobin, hematocrit, expected date of delivery (ultrasound evaluations), and oxytocin challenge test evaluations. In addition, note carefully any medications taken in recent weeks.
    2. Review the course of labor by determining the duration of the first and second stages, and the presence of any signs of fetal distress. Evaluate the fetal monitoring record, the type, amount, and timing of any analgesia and anesthesia given. Establish when the membranes ruptured and whether any signs and symptoms of infection or problems with hypertension or bleeding are present.
II. Care of infant in the delivery room.
  A. Delivery room assessment.
    1. Apgar score at 1 and 5 min after birth is determined by nurse (see Tables 10-1 and 10-2).
    2. Note length of umbilical cord and presence of any abnormalities: e.g., nuchal cord, true knots. Determine number of umbilical vessels (two arteries, one vein).
    3. Observe for any gross deformities or anomalies in infant. Note general condition. Give special attention to:
        a. Dimples, skin tags, birth marks (Table 10-3).
        b. Fontanels and sutures: Check for openness and presence of bulging. Check for caput.
        c. Eyes: Note presence of cataracts and opacities.
        d. Nose: Check for patency of passage and appearance of septum.
        e. Ears: Determine location of pinna, eye line, and patency of external opening of canals.

TABLE 10-1 / APGAR NEWBORN SCORING SYSTEM

	Sign	Score		
		0	1	2
A (appearance)	Heart rate	Not detectable	Below 100	Above 100
P (pulse)	Respiratory effort	Absent	Slow, irregular	Good, crying
G (grimace)	Muscle tone	Flaccid, limp	Some flexion of extremities	Active motion
A (attitude, tone)	Reflex irritability	No response	Grimace*	Cough, sneeze*
R (respiration)	Color†	Blue, pale	Extremities blue, body pink	Completely pink

*When stimulated by suction in nose.
†If the natural skin color of the child is dark, alternative tests for color are applied, such as the color of the mucous membranes of the mouth and conjunctiva, the color of the lips, palms, and soles of the feet.

    f. Mouth: Look for cleft lip and/or palate, presence of teeth, and symmetry of movement of facial muscles.
    g. Neck: Check for full range of motion; no masses.
    h. Chest: Inspect for equal expansion, no barreling, or retractions. Find heartbeat on left side.
    i. Abdomen: Determine that it is rounded, and not scaphoid or flaccid. Omphalocele and umbilical hernia are absent.
    j. Genitalia: Check for normal configurations for gestational age, and determine that there are no hernias in the inguinal area.
    k. Anus: Inspect for imperforate anus.
    l. Back: Look for meningomyelocele, meningocele, and/or spina bifida.
    m. Extremities: Note numbers of fingers and toes, range of motion, and any positional abnormalities.
  B. Maintain an adequate airway and assist respiratory function.
    1. Suctioning—10 to 15 mL fluid will be expelled with squeezing of chest during birth. Gentle suctioning of mouth and then nose with bulb syringe is usually adequate. Deeper suctioning may sometimes be necessary, then only gentle negative pressure with DeLee or wall suction (3).
    2. Positioning—place in a 15° Trendelenburg's position in crib or on mother's abdomen for early minutes. Observe for respiratory rate, retractions, nasal flaring, or grunting.
    3. Resuscitation—will be necessary if infant is depressed by drugs or hypoxia. Provide oxygen by mask and bag. Prepare for intermittent positive pressure, deep tracheal suctioning by pediatrician. Gastric suctioning and administration of medication may be necessary.
  C. Maintain temperature.
    1. Dry infant completely as soon as possible [a wet newborn can drop rectal (core) temperature at the rate of 0.1°C/min].

TABLE 10-2 / CORRELATION BETWEEN APGAR SCORE AT 1 min AND BLOOD pH

Apgar Score	pH
1–3	6.9–7.0
4–7	7.0–7.20
8–10	≥ 7.25

Source: Adapted from P.A.M. Dawes, "Resuscitation of the Newborn," *American Journal of Nursing,* **74**(1):68, January 1974.

TABLE 10-3 / MINOR BIRTH INJURIES AND COMMON BIRTHMARKS

	Onset	Characteristics	Resolution
Cephalohematoma	Appears after birth, within 24–48 h.	Sometimes overlaid by caput swelling. May be bluish color. Bleeding occurs between skull bone and periosteum, usually over parietal bones. Does not cross suture line. Sometimes associated with skull fracture.	Complete resolution in 6 weeks to 2 months. May cause elevation of bilirubin levels.
Molding	Apparent at birth, especially in infants of primigravidas or infants that are large for gestational age.	Shifting of fetal skull bones, parietal moves up and back, occipital down and forward.	Resolves within several days if infant is placed prone and on side to sleep.
Vacuum extraction	Marks apparent at birth and may worsen within first few hours.	Traumatic, circular ecchymotic area over presenting aspect of head. May have some lacerations as well.	Usually resolves within a few weeks. If bruise is large, bilirubin levels may be slightly elevated.
Internal monitor (fetal electrode)	Occurs during attachment of electrode.	Small wound on scalp. May become infected if care is not taken.	Resolves with wound healing.
Forceps marks	Apparent at birth and may worsen within first few hours.	Ecchymoses. There may be lacerated skin over cheeks or ears if forceps are placed wrongly or if delivery is difficult.	Usually begin to fade several days after birth.
Mongolian spots	Apparent at birth and may become more pronounced within a few days.	Blue-black (slate-gray) pigmentation on back, buttocks, and sometimes extremities. Seen in 90% of babies of Asian, African, Southern European, and American Indian ancestry.	Begins to fade within 3–4 years.
Stork's beak mark (nevus simplex)	Seen at birth or soon after.	Red areas often present on nape of neck, bridge of nose, glabella, or eyelids. Whiten on pressure. Common (30–50%) in infants of Northern European ancestry.	Usually fades within first year, but may remain throughout life.
Strawberry mark (strawberry hemangioma)	Seen at birth or appears within 2–3 weeks.	Raised, red area. Texture similar to a strawberry.	Grows until 3 months, when regression begins. Parents become alarmed. Takes several years to disappear. No treatment.

2. Place under radiant warmer, or next to skin of mother (4).
3. Attach temperature probe if infant is under radiant heater (Fig. 10-1).
4. As soon as initial procedures are complete, wrap baby in blankets and allow mother to hold. (See point III under "Intervention.")

D. Maintain safety.
  1. Identification:
     a. Identification of baby must take place before mother and infant are separated. Take footprints, mother's forefinger print, and establish sex, verified by mother. Identification bands are attached to mother and infant and read by mother.
     b. All charting is done with correct identification.
  2. Prevent infection and potential hemorrhage:
     a. Eye prophylaxis is necessary to prevent gonorrheal infections. This protection usually is provided by one or two drops of 1% silver nitrate in each conjunctival sac. The eye may then be rinsed with sterile water. Delay doing this until mother has seen infant, as eyes will become somewhat inflamed in 90 percent of babies in the subsequent 24 h (5).
     b. Observe for abrasions and signs of infection, especially if there was premature rupture of membranes.
     c. Administer vitamin K, water-soluble preparation, 0.5 to 1.0 mg intramuscularly, either in delivery room or in nursery.
     d. Observe for developing cephalohematoma, and continue observations of vital signs, color, cry, and activity.

E. Initiate parent–infant bonding.
  1. Parents must be allowed to hold or touch infant while mother is still on delivery table.
  2. As soon as initial procedures are finished and baby's condition is stable, mother may hold and breast-feed infant. (Be sure infant is kept warm.)
  3. Baby can accompany mother and father to the recovery room until ready to enter the first sleep period (20 to 40 min after birth).
  4. Do the initial evaluation of infant at bedside, and later assessment for gestational age may be done at bedside, also.
  5. Explain all minor variations and all procedures (6).

F. Transport to the nursery.
  1. The infant is moved to the nursery or to rooming-in location while wrapped in a blanket and in a warm portable crib. Contact with staff, patients, and visitors from outside the obstetrical unit should be avoided en route.

DEFINITION

Any newborn infant who is born within the 38th and 42d week of gestation is considered a full-term infant. Assessment for maturity paralleling estimated age should be done as soon as practical. In addition to determining maturity, the infant must be evaluated for size. An infant may be small for its gestational age (SGA), appropriate for its gestational age (AGA), or large for its gestational age (LGA). Gestational age is *related to but not dependent upon* weight at birth. Since complications of the neonatal period vary greatly with the degree of maturity and with weight, both parameters are important to measure. Once gestational age has been determined, it should be plotted against the weight on a graph similar to the one in Fig. 10-2.

Lubchenco (7) states:

The estimation of gestational age is usually made by the nurse admitting the infant. She gives each sign a gestational age, interpolating the age if necessary. If the ages assigned are fairly uniform, she records the clinical estimate as the observed mean or gives the age as a range—37 weeks or 36 to 37 weeks. If there are discrepancies between items, the admitting nurse should note them, and if there is a clear

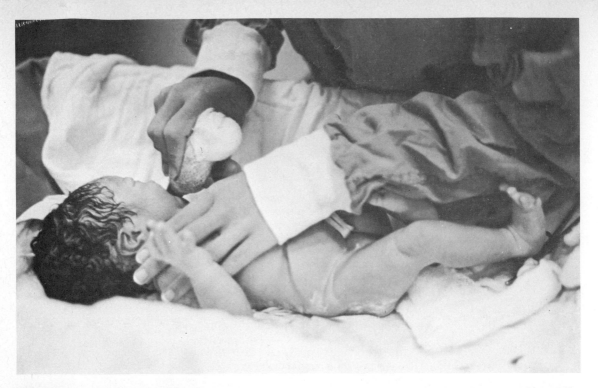

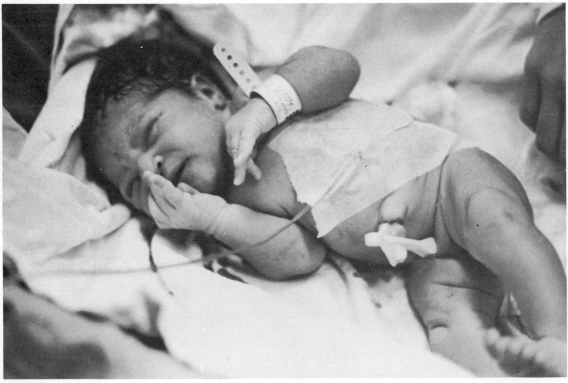

FIGURE 10-1 / *Top,* oropharyngeal suctioning. *Bottom,* newborn with temperature probe attached to abdomen to monitor temperature constantly. (*Courtesy of Mary Olsen Johnson, M.D.*)

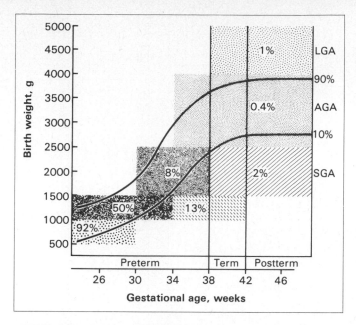

FIGURE 10-2 / Neonatal mortality risk based on birth weight and gestational age (Colorado data, 1958 to 1968). LGA, AGA, SGA = large, appropriate, small for gestational age, respectively. [*From C. H. Kempe, H. K. Silver, and D. O'Brien* (eds.), *Current Pediatric Diagnosis and Treatment, 2d ed., Lange Medical Publications, Los Altos, Calif., 1972, with permission.*]

difference between her assessment and the gestational age calculated from the mother's dates, she records both. The infant with a discrepancy . . . is classified as a high risk infant and is observed for the morbidity suggested by the findings.

Using the Lubchenco (University of Colorado) scoring system found in Fig. 10-3, the physical characteristics should be assessed fairly soon after birth, as there may be a few changes after interaction with the environment. Nicolopoulous (8) noted that the following nine physical signs yield a high (0.878) correlation with gestational age. When there is any question, or when discrepancies arise, the neurologic examination after 24 h should be added (with 0.85 correlation).

Physical Criteria (Nine Keys)	*Neurologic Criteria (Eight Keys)*
Skin texture, color, opacity	Posture
Amount of lanugo	Square window, dorsiflexion of foot
Nipple form and breast size	Popliteal angle, heel-to-ear degree of
Ear formation and firmness	flexion
Plantar creases	Scarf sign
	Head lag and ventral suspension

ASSESSMENT

    I. The following is a summary of the physical characteristics one would expect to find in a full-term infant.

        A. Breast nodule: average, 7 mm; nipple raised.

        B. Earlobe: firm; folds are prominent; there is instant recoil from folding.

Weeks of gestation

Week scale: 20 21 22 23 24 25 26 27 28 29 30 31 32 33 34 35 36 37 38 39 40 41 42 43 44 45 46 47 48

Physical findings		Findings (by approximate week of gestation)
Vernix		Appears (~21); Covers body, thick layer (25–34); On back, scalp, in creases (38); Scant, in creases (40); No vernix (45)
Breast tissue and areola		Areola and nipple barely visible, no palpable breast tissue (22); Areola raised (35); 1–2 mm nodule (36); 3–5 mm (38); 5–6 mm (39); 7–10 mm (41); ?12 mm (46)
Ear	Form	Flat, shapeless (24–27); Beginning incurving superior (34); Incurving upper two-thirds pinnae (36–37); Well-defined incurving to lobe (42–45)
	Cartilage	Pinna soft, stays folded (23–26); Cartilage scant, returns slowly from folding (32–33); Thin cartilage, springs back from folding (37–38); Pinna firm, remains erect from head (43–44)
Sole creases		Smooth soles without creases (24–28); 1–2 anterior creases (32–33); 2–3 anterior creases (35); Creases anterior two-thirds of sole (36–37); Creases involving heel (39–40); Deeper creases over entire sole (43–45)
Skin	Thickness and appearance	Thin, translucent skin, plethoric, venules over abdomen, edema (24–30); Smooth, thicker, no edema (33–34); Pink (36); Few vessels (39); Some desquamation, pale pink (40–41); Thick, pale, desquamation over entire body (44–45)
	Nail plates	Appear (20–21); Nails to fingertips (33); Nails extend well beyond fingertips (43)
Hair		Appears on head (20–21); Eyebrows and lashes (25–26); Fine, woolly, bunches out from heat (29–30); Silky, single strands, lays flat (38); ?Receding hairline or loss of baby hair, short, fine underneath (44)
Lanugo		Appears (20); Covers entire body (26); Vanishes from face (34); Present on shoulders (40); No lanugo (45)
Genitalia	Testes	Testes palpable in inguinal canal (28–30); In upper scrotum (37); In lower scrotum (44)
	Scrotum	Few rugae (32); Rugae, anterior portion (37); Rugae cover (41); Pendulous (44)
	Labia and clitoris	Prominent clitoris, labia majora small, widely separated (31–33); Labia majora larger, nearly covered clitoris (37–38); Labia minora and clitoris covered (43)
Skull firmness		Bones are soft (24–27); Soft to 1 in from anterior fontanelle (30–31); Spongy at edges of fontanelle, center firm (36); Bones hard, sutures easily displaced (39–40); Bones hard, cannot be displaced (44)
Posture	Resting	Hypotonic, lateral decubitus (23); Hypotonic (28); Beginning flexion, thigh (30–31); Stronger hip flexion (32); Frog-like (34); Flexion, all limbs (36); Hypertonic (39); Very hypertonic (44)
Recoil	Leg	No recoil (26); Partial recoil (34); Prompt recoil (42)
	Arm	No recoil (24); Begin flexion, no recoil (34); Prompt recoil, may be inhibited (37); Prompt recoil after 30 s inhibition (41)

Weeks of gestation

	Physical findings	20	21	22	23	24	25	26	27	28	29	30	31	32	33	34	35	36	37	38	39	40	41	42	43	44	45	46	47	48
Tone	Heel to ear								No resistance					Some resistance	Impossible														
	Scarf sign			No resistance											Elbow passes midline			Elbow at midline				Elbow does not reach midline							
	Neck flexors (head lag)							Absent												Head in plane of body					Holds head				
	Neck extensors													Head begins to right itself from flexed position			Good righting, cannot hold it		Holds head few seconds		Keeps head in line with trunk 40s			Turns head from side to side			
	Body extensors													Straightening of legs			Straightening of trunk		Straightening of head and trunk together								
	Vertical positions										When held under arms, body slips through hands					Arms hold baby, legs extended			Legs flexed, good support with arms								
	Horizontal positions										Hypotonic, arms and legs straight							Arms and legs flexed		Head and back even, flexed extremities			Head above back					
Flexion angles	Popliteal			No resistance							150°			110°		100°			90°		80°				A preterm who has reached 40 weeks still has a 40° angle			
	Ankle													45°				20°		30°		0°						
	Wrist (square window)										90°			60°				45°		30°		0°							
Reflexes	Sucking							Weak, not synchronized with swallowing						Stronger, synchronized		Perfect			Perfect, hand to mouth					Perfect				
	Rooting							Long latency period, slow, imperfect			Hand to mouth			Hand to mouth		Brisk, complete, durable								Complete				
	Grasp							Finger grasp is good, strength is poor									Stronger			Can lift baby off bed, involves arms						Hands open		
	Moro				Barely apparent			Weak, not elicited every time						Stronger		Complete with arm extension, open fingers, cry		Arm adduction added							?Begins to lose Moro	
	Crossed extension							Flexion and extension in a random, purposeless pattern						Extension but no adduction		Still incomplete		Extension, adduction, fanning of toes						Complete			
	Automatic walk											Minimal		Begins tiptoeing, good support on sole			Fast tiptoeing		Heel-toe progression, whole sole of foot				A preterm who has reached 40 weeks walks on toes			?Begins to lose automatic walk	
	Pupillary reflex	Absent					Appears							Present															
	Glabellar tap	Absent						Absent				Appears									Present								
	Tonic neck reflex				Absent							Appears					Appears				Present								
	Neckrighting					Absent											Appears		Present after 37 weeks										
		20	21	22	23	24	25	26	27	28	29	30	31	32	33	34	35	36	37	38	39	40	41	42	43	44	45	46	47	48

FIGURE 10-3 / Clinical estimation of gestational age. *Top,* examination to be completed in first hours after birth. *Bottom,* confirmatory neurologic examination to be completed 24 h after birth. [From J. V. Brazie and L. O. Lubchenco, "The Estimation of Gestational Age," in C. H. Kempe, H. K. Silver, and D. O'Brien (eds.), *Current Pediatric Diagnosis and Treatment, 5th ed., Lange Medical Publications, Los Altos, Calif., 1977, with permission.*]

    C. Sole creases: creases throughout, especially over ball of foot.

    D. Hair: Silky, thickening in texture, one can distinguish strands laying flat to head.

    E. Male genitalia: enlarged scrotum with descended testes; anterior aspect, at least, covered with rugae.

    F. Female genitalia: labia minora and clitoris completely or almost completely covered by labia majora.

II. The following is a summary of the neurologic characteristics one would expect to see in a full-term infant after 24 h.

    A. Posture: hypertonic, flexion of all limbs at rest.

    B. Arms and legs: prompt recoil from extension.

    C. Heel to ear: impossible, heel will not go past umbilical level.

    D. Scarf sign: elbow does not reach midline.

    E. Head lag (neck flexors): hold head in plane of body.

    F. Neck extensors: hold head a few seconds.

    G. Body extensors: straightening of trunk and possibly straightening of head and trunk together.

    H. Vertical positions: legs flexed, good support with arms.

    I. Horizontal positions: head and back even, flexed extremities.

    J. Popliteal (flexion) angle: 80 to 90°.

    K. Ankle flexion angle: 0 to 20°.

    L. Wrist flexion angle (square window): 0 to 30°.

    M. Newborn infant reflexes: see Table 10-4.

PROBLEMS

I. Transition to extrauterine life may be hindered by drugs, anesthesia, or fetal distress during labor.

II. Infant falls into SGA or LGA categories.

III. Infant is assessed as premature or postmature.

IV. Birth injuries or anomalies may have occurred.

V. Mother's chronic medical or psychologic problems may affect the potential for parenting and bonding.

VI. Infection, respiratory difficulty, or jaundice may develop during recovery.

DIAGNOSIS

I. The full-term infant adapts to extrauterine life without any apparent difficulty.

II. The full-term infant with minor birth defects adjusts well and parents accept the situation.

III. The parents of a full-term infant are unable to or are hindered in bonding by psychologic or physical problems.

IV. The full-term infant has developed residual problems in the adjustment period. These may include drug withdrawal, jaundice, infection, respiratory difficulty, hypoglycemia, etc.

GOALS OF CARE

I. Immediate.

    A. The infant will recover from the trauma of birth without residual difficulties.

    B. Assessment of adequacy of weight and maturity will take place.

    C. Body temperature will be maintained within the normal range.

    D. Adequate fluid and caloric intake will be established.

    E. Normal bowel and bladder function will be established.

    F. Skin integrity will be maintained.

TABLE 10-4 / DEVELOPMENTAL REFLEXES

Reflex	Testing Technique	Normal Response	Indications of Abnormality	Disappearance of Reflex
Moro reflex	Lift the head of the crib about 2 in and drop it. This method is less traumatic on the baby's back and neck than lifting the head and shoulders and dropping them. (Making a loud noise to elicit this reflex tests hearing.)	Abduction and extension of the arms; extension of at least fingers 3–5 followed by adduction and flexion of upper extremities. Lower extremities may be extended. Infant may be startled and cry.	Asymmetrical reaction may indicate hemiparesis, fractured humerus or clavicle, or brachial plexus injury. Sluggish reaction may indicate hypotonia.	After 4 months of age.
Tonic neck reflex (fencing position)	Turn the infant's head to the left.	The left arm and leg will show extension and increased tone, while the right arm and leg will flex and show a decrease in tone.	The infant who is not able to break this posture a few seconds after it is elicited is exhibiting an obligatory response, which is abnormal.	After 4 months of age.
Stepping reflex	Hold the infant upright and place one foot in contact with the bed.	The leg in contact with the bed extends while the other leg flexes.	Hypertonia may be indicated if both legs are held in extension. Hypotonia may be indicated if the infant is not able to bear any weight.	After 3–4 months of age.
Palmar grasp	Apply pressure to the palm of the hand.	Flexion of the fingers and grasp of the object. The grasp is strong enough to allow the infant to be lifted from the bed by placing traction on the object.	Lethargy: illness will cause hypotonia.	?
Plantar grasp	Press your thumb to the infant's sole just below the toes.	The toes should flex around your thumb.	Absence of this reflex is seen in infants with hypotonia, spinal cord injury, or injury to the lumbosacral plexus.	After 10 months of age.
Rooting reflex	Touch the infant's cheek.	Infant will turn head toward the stimulus and begin to suck.	Weak in infants with decreased alertness or in those who have just been fed.	After 6 months of age.

Source: Adapted from B. Silverman, "Assessment of the Newborn," in E. J. Dickason and M. O. Schult (eds.), *Maternal and Infant Care*, 2d ed., McGraw-Hill Book Company, New York, 1979, chap. 14.

II. Long-range.
  A. Bonding will be established.
  B. Adequate fluid and caloric balance will be maintained and parents will understand the infant's nutritional needs.
  C. Anticipatory guidance will be given to the mother regarding all aspects of infant care (see Chap. 9).
  D. The infant will receive follow-up care at 2 to 4 weeks of age, in a pediatrician's office or a well-baby clinic.
  E. The infant will receive immunizations at appropriate intervals (see Table 22-1).
  F. The infant's growth and development will proceed at an optimal level and parental care (especially in the first month after birth) will be based upon understanding of the infant's growth pattern.
  G. Appropriate referrals will be made as necessary.

INTERVENTION

I. Support recovery and infants' transition to extrauterine life so that it occurs without difficulties.
  A. Place the infant in a warmed crib or Isolette for the first sleep period until temperature stabilizes (2 to 4 h).
  B. Observe for any lasting effects of anesthesia and transitional drugs.
  C. Observe vital signs, color, posture, activity, and cry (see Table 10-5).
  D. Suction with bulb syringe as often as necessary. Expect extra mucus within 12 h of birth, depending upon maternal drugs.
  E. Always position infant on side or abdomen to prevent aspiration of secretions or gastric contents. Prone position for sleep (see Table 10-6) promotes longer, quieter sleep (9).
  F. Do not bathe baby until temperature is stable.
  G. Observe for hypoglycemia and hyperbilirubinemia (see Chap. 11).
II. Assess adequacy of weight gain, and maturity.
  A. Do early physical assessment using Lubchenco score. If there are discrepancies, note and report. Follow through with neurologic assessment when infant is 24 h old (see Fig. 10-3).
  B. Weigh on admission and then every day or every other day until discharge. Calculate weight loss as a percentage of birth weight. Evaluate intake.
III. Support temperature and maintain in normal range.
  A. Nursery should be warm enough, at least 23.8°C (75°F) (10). Circulating air input should be near top of room, with outflow near bottom, and heat sources should be shielded. Babies must be protected from the radiant heat of strong sunlight or radiators.
  B. Axillary or skin temperatures should be maintained in range of 36.1 to 36.4°C (97.2 to 97.6°F) to maintain desirable core (rectal) temperature of 36.5 to 37.0°C (98 to 98.6°F). Otherwise, infant must utilize *nonshivering thermogenesis,* burning up fat stores and using calories and oxygen to provide additional heat (11).
  C. Dehydration due to poor fluid intake, increased evaporative losses, or diarrhea and vomiting may raise temperature. Heat radiating from environment may raise temperature. Infant becomes flushed, has tachypnea, and perspires on face and hands.
  D. Use radiant heaters cautiously, with skin temperature probes attached to abdominal skin correctly. Do not expose infant unnecessarily.
IV. Maintain adequate fluid and caloric intake (see Table 10-7).
  A. Infant should be given nothing orally (NPO) until stable, then should be offered sterile water for one feeding.

TABLE 10-5 / NORMAL CHARACTERISTICS OF A FULL-TERM INFANT

	Normal Values	*Comments*
Temperature:		
Rectal	36.5–37°C (97.7–98.6°F); not below 36°C (97°F)	If the infant is kept nude in an environment colder than 70–73°F, its body temperature will not be able to adjust adequately.
Axillary (skin)	36.1–36.5°C (97–97.6°F)*	Clothing and blankets help, but the environment must be kept warm enough.
Respiratory rate:		
During first hour after birth	40–50 breaths per minute	May have some periodic breathing, and 5–10 s of apnea in first period; later these episodes decrease.
Afterward	30–50 breaths per minute	A rate of respiratory above 60 breaths per minute may indicate that some problem is present. There should be no retraction of the lips, grunting, flaring of nostrils, circumoral cyanosis, or other respiratory noise. Infant is already hypoxic when cyanosis becomes evident.
Pulse (apical rate)	110–130 beats per minute	Pulse may be 90 beats per minute if deeply asleep or up to 160–180 beats per minute if crying. A low pulse should accelerate with stimulation. Slight early murmurs are common until cardiovascular changes are complete.
Blood pressure	80/60 (average)	Blood pressure varies, depending upon size, gestational age, and amount of placental transfusion. If infant is held above level of placenta for any length of time during delivery, i.e., with cesarean section, there is a possibility of its being hypovolemic. Hypovolemia may be associated with RDS.
Weight	2500–4100 g†	Term infants above (LGA) or below (SGA) weights are of higher risk (see Fig. 10-4).
Length	44–55 cm‡	Crown-heel measurements. Allow for caput and cephalohematoma. Measure when infant is relaxed (drowsy or asleep).
Head circumference	32–38 cm§	Allow for changes in head (of molding) and remeasure before discharge from unit.
Chest circumference	2 cm less than head circumference¶	Allow for breast engorgement.

*0.4–0.5°C (0.8–1.0°F) below core (rectal) temperature.
†Mean = 3400 g (7.5 lb).
‡Mean = 50 cm (20 in).
§Mean = 33 cm (13 in).
¶Ranges from 7 cm less to 5 cm more than the head circumference.

B. Begin milk feedings:
  1. Breast:
   a. Every 3 to 4 h.
   b. Offer sterile water after each feeding until milk comes in.
   c. Offer sterile water freely if baby cries between feedings.
   d. No supplementary feeding of formula unless ordered by pediatrician for good reason; e.g., mother is NPO for tubal ligation.

TABLE 10-6 / INFANT STATES

State	Characteristics
Quiet sleep	Regular respirations and heart rate; absence of body or eye movements; very little will disturb infant in this phase.
Active sleep (REM sleep)	Phasic limb movements; irregular respiration; eye movement; startles spontaneously; can be awakened, usually to cry.
Drowsy	Activity level varied; appears to be dozing; delayed neurologic response if being tested; responds to repeated stimuli by becoming more awake.
Quietly awake	Quiet motor activity of arms and legs; opens and closes eyes; reacts to noises with startles; intermittent fussing.
Actively awake	Alert; focuses attention on stimuli; interested in communication with care given.
Crying	Tachycardia; flushed; active motion of all limbs; not paying much attention to attempts to soothe.

Source: Adapted from H.F.R. Prechtl et al., "Behavioral State Cycles in Abnormal Infants," *Developmental Medicine and Child Neurology* **15**:606, October 1973.

   2. Bottle:
      a. Every 4 h unless pediatrician orders "on demand," or every 3 h for smaller babies.
      b. Offer 20 cal per 30 mL of formula. Give ½ oz (15 mL) every 4 h for 12 h, then 1 oz (30 mL) every 4 h for 24 h. Increase by ½ oz per day up to 3 oz (90 mL).
      c. Offer sterile water freely if baby cries between feedings (12).
   C. Assess stool and urine quality, looking for signs of under- or overfeeding.
   D. Assess weight gain pattern.
   E. Assess mother's skill at bottle feeding and her knowledge of home care techniques:
      1. Teach formula preparation. Discuss cost and prevention of infection.
      2. Discuss fluid needs and weight gain pattern. Discuss overfeeding.
   F. Assess breast-feeding mother's skill and teach self-care and infant care.
      1. Anatomy and physiology of lactation.
      2. Treatment for engorgement, e.g., supportive bra, warm showers, compresses, analgesia, increased feeding, and manual expression of milk.
      3. Advise on schedule to begin lactation: Give both breasts at each feeding. Alternate the breast on which feeding is begun. Nurse initially for short (3 to 5 min) periods, increase time each day until up to 10 to 15 min per side.
      4. Feed on demand with no supplementation. There may be an exception of one bottle per day to accustom infant to nipple. Bottle may be water, later juice, or occasionally formula to allow mother time away from infant.
      5. Provide anticipatory guidance for common problems. Give phone number of La Leche League.
V. Observe for establishment of normal bowel and bladder function.
   A. The newborn should begin voiding by 24 h of age. There should be at least four to six wet diapers a day. (During the first 48 h, 30 to 60 mL should be voided, depending on intake and placental transfusion influence on blood volume.)
   B. An admission urinalysis is usually done: specific gravity should measure 1.004 to 1.018 with no protein or RBC; sometimes there may be urate crystals appearing as "brick dust" on diaper.
   C. Stools: Meconium should be passed by 24 h and lasts 24 to 48 h; transitional stool

depends on milk intake. Typical bottle-fed stool appears by 48 to 72 h; typical breast milk stool, after milk comes in.

D. New cystic fibrosis meconium strip test may be ordered for susceptible babies. Other abnormalities may be a meconium plug, constipated stools, or diarrhea.

VI. Maintain skin integrity.

  A. Skin care for newborns:

   1. Depending on setting, newborn should be bathed in nursery with bacteriostatic soap, or *dry skin care* may be used. This means to wash with water only the parts needing cleaning, such as the perineum and creases. *No* bathing will be done in either case *until* temperature is stable.

      a. At home, any mild soap may be used, but not on face. Lotions, oils, and powders should be used minimally but not on face.

  B. Cord care.

   1. Current methods include drying cord with no application of medication, with application of triple dye, and with application of alcohol.

FIGURE 10-4 / Classification of newborns based on maturity and intrauterine growth. (*After L. O. Lubchenco, C. Hansman, and E. Boyd, Pediatrics, 37:403, 1966, and F. C. Battaglia and L. O. Lubchenco, Journal of Pediatrics, 71:159, 1967.*)

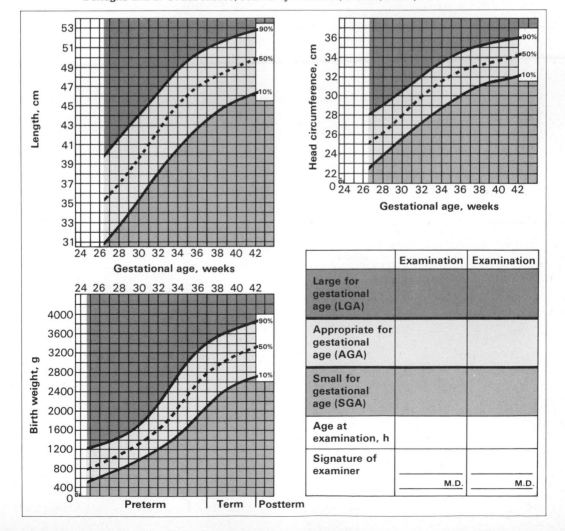

TABLE 10-7 / INFANT FLUID AND NUTRIENT REQUIREMENTS

Requirements	Birth to 6 Months
Kilocalories	117 kcal/kg
Protein	2.2 g/kg
Fluid intake	165 mL/kg

2. Remove clamp when cord appears dry, usually after 24 h. Expose cord to air. When it separates from navel, apply alcohol to stump as often as necessary.

C. Circumcision care.

   1. Depending on technique used—Hollister Plastibell or Gomco clamp—a petroleum-jelly impregnated gauze is wrapped around circumsized penis for 12 to 24 h. After this, A and D ointment on sterile gauze may be placed between penis and diaper for several days until area appears less sore.

   2. Instruct mother carefully if circumcision is done on day of discharge.

VII. Foster bonding.

A. Assess quality of initial periods of time with infant. Provide for extra time, according to parental wishes.

TABLE 10-8 / LABORATORY TESTS WHICH MAY BE DONE BEFORE DISCHARGE

Laboratory Test	Normal Result	Comments
Cord blood:		
Blood type and Rh	A, B, AB, O	Check on incompatibility if jaundice occurs.
Direct Coombs' test	Negative	Detects sensitized RBC. Does not define blocking agent.
Serology	Negative	If positive, check time of treatment of mother since some time must elapse after treatment for her test to show negative.
Bilirubin	1.0–1.8 mg/dL	Detects intrauterine hemolysis.
Urinalysis	1.004–1.018 (specific gravity); no protein or RBC	Detects rare renal problems or infection.
Heel-stick capillary sample:		
Screening for inborn errors of metabolism	Negative	Detects phenylketonuria (PKU) and several other inborn errors of metabolism. Needs to be repeated later if milk intake is not adequate or if infant is discharged early.
Screening for hypothyroidism (T_4 level)		
Sickle cell disease	Negative	
Bilirubin	At 3–4 days an elevation of 4–6 mg/dL	See Chap. 11 for discussion of treatment.
Meconium:		
Cystic fibrosis test	No elevated albumin in meconium	Test strip changes to deep blue if 4a1positive.
Cultures of body orifices, cord, urine	Negative	Use varies; done especially if infant's mother had prematur rupture of the membranes or if there is a problem in the nursery with chronic infections.

      B. Involve parents in care of infant, especially if infant has to be in Isolette for warmth or oxygen.

      C. Interpret each procedure for parents and prepare them for discharge.

      D. See Chap. 11 for signs of poor bonding, and Tables 7-4, 8-7 and 9-4 for clues to potential child abuse.

VIII. Make referrals and prepare parents for follow-up for well-baby care.

      A. Refer any baby with even minor problems of adaptation, jaundice, any congenital anomaly, or poor intrauterine growth for care. Refer babies whose mothers have problems connected with pregnancy or psychosocial problems, also.

      B. Provide literature for parents detailing the immunization schedules, feeding schedules, and schedules for visits to the pediatrician. Provide literature describing expected growth and development for period before first pediatrician sees infant. (Remember that the neonatal period is the most important time for infant, and yet it is most often the time when parents have the least guidance.)

      C. Be sure all lab tests are completed before discharge (Table 10-8).

EVALUATION

I. Adaptation to extrauterine life is completed with no residual difficulties.

II. Family relationships appear to have been established.

III. Infant's course did not proceed normally, and baby was transferred to high-risk nursery or acute care pediatrics (see Chap. 11 and Part 3).

REFERENCES

1. T. Berry Brazelton, *Infants and Mothers: Differences in Development,* Dell Publishing Company, Inc., New York, 1969.
2. Marshall Klaus and John Kennell, *Maternal-Infant Bonding,* The C. V. Mosby Company, St. Louis, 1976.
3. J. Roberts, "Suctioning the Newborn," *American Journal of Nursing,* **73**:63, January 1973.
4. C. Phillips, "Neonatal Heat Loss in Heated Cribs and Mothers' Arms," *Journal of Obstetric, Gynecologic and Neonatal Nursing,* **3**:11, November–December 1974.
5. H. Nishida, and R. M. Risenberg, "Silver Nitrate Ophthalmic Solution and Chemical Conjunctivitis," *Pediatrics,* **56**(3):368, September 1975.
6. P. deChateau, "The Importance of the Neonatal Period for the Development of Synchrony in the Mother-Infant Dyad: A Review," *Birth and the Family Journal,* **4**(1):11, Spring 1977.
7. L. O. Lubchenco, *The High Risk Infant,* W. B. Saunders Company, Philadelphia, 1976, p. 61.
8. D. Nicolopoulous et al., "Estimation of Gestational Age in the Neonate, *American Journal of Diseases of Children,* **130**(5): 480, May 1976.
9. Y. Brackbill, T. C. Douthitt, and H. West, "Psychophysiologic Effects in the Neonate of Prone versus Supine Placement," *Journal of Pediatrics,* **82**:82, January 1973.
10. N. A. DeLue, "Climate and Environmental Concepts," *Clinics in Perinatology,* **3**(2):426, September 1976.
11. M. H. Klaus, and A. A. Fanaroff, *Care of the High-Risk Neonate,* W. B. Saunders Company, Philadelphia, 1973, pp. 59–67.
12. S. Fomon, *Infant Nutrition,* W. B. Saunders Company, Philadelphia, 1977, p. 1038.

BIBLIOGRAPHY

Avery, Gordon B.: *Neonatology—Pathophysiology and Management of the Newborn,* J. B. Lippincott Company, Philadelphia, 1975. Good source for pathology; includes antepartum and intrapartum management where appropriate.

Barness, Lewis A.: *Manual of Pediatric Physical Diagnosis,* 4th ed., Year Book Medical Publisher, Inc., Chicago, 1972. Good chapter on newborn physical assessment.

Bates, Barbara: *A Guide To Physical Examination,* J. B. Lippincott Company, Philadelphia, 1974. Good chapter on newborn physical assessment.

Boston Children's Medical Center and Richard Feinbloom: *Child Health Encyclopedia,* Delacorte Press, Boston, 1975. Good reference book for parents.

Brazelton, T. Berry: *Infants and Mothers: Differences in Development,* Dell Publishing Company, Inc., New York, 1969. Excellent description of normal variations in newborn behavior; good reference book for parents.

Caplan, Frank (ed.): *The First Twelve Months of Life,* Grosset & Dunlap, Inc., New York, 1973. Contains tables of expected developmental milestones, yet is flexible enough to allow for normal variations. Good reference for parents.

Clark, A., and F. Affonso: *Childbearing: A Nursing Perspective,* F. A. Davis Company, Philadelphia, 1976. Good reference for the nursing process.

Clausen, J., et al.: *Maternity Nursing Today,* 2d ed., McGraw-Hill Book Company, New York, 1977. Good nursing text with detail on newborn.

Eiger, M., and S. Olds: *The Complete Book of Breast-Feeding,* Workman Publishing Company, Inc., New York, 1972. Valuable reference for breast-feeding mothers.

Fraiberg, Selma: *The Magic Years,* Charles Scribner's Sons, New York, 1959. A classic on the wonders of the growing infant; good reference for parents.

Klaus, Marshall, and John Kennell: *Maternal-Infant Bonding,* The C. V. Mosby Company, St. Louis, 1976. A compilation of much of the original research on maternal-infant bonding.

Kübler-Ross, Elisabeth: *On Death and Dying,* The Macmillan Company, New York, 1969. Useful preparation for dealing with grieving parents.

————: *Lactation: A Programmed Review,* Merrill-National Lab, Ohio, 1967. Good review on endrocrinology of lactation.

La Leche League: *The Womanly Art of Breastfeeding,* The Interstate Printers & Publishers, Inc., Danville, Ill., 1963. Excellent practical reference for breast-feeding mothers.

McBride, Angela Barron: *The Growth and Development of Mothers,* Harper & Row, Publishers, Inc., New York, 1973. Discusses ups and downs of motherhood. An excellent reference book for mothers.

Overbach, Arvin M., and Morton J. Rodman: *Drugs Used with Neonates and during Pregnancy,* Medical Economics Company Book Division, Oradell, N.J., 1975. Good outline of drugs and their effects on fetus and newborn.

Pryor, Karen: *Nursing Your Baby,* Harper & Row, Publishers, Inc., New York, 1963. Good reference book for breast-feeding mothers.

Schaffer, Alexander J., and Mary Ellen Avery: *Diseases of the Newborn,* 4th ed., W. B. Saunders Company, Philadelphia, 1977. Good textbook for newborn pathology.

Spock, Benjamin: *Baby and Child Care,* Pocket Books, New York, 1968. Classic reference for practical information on infant care.

Vulliamy, D. G.: *The Newborn Child,* 4th ed., Churchill Livingstone, Edinburgh, 1977. Inexpensive paperback reference with much valuable information on the normal newborn.

11

The Preterm Newborn[1]

Elizabeth J. Dickason

GENERAL CONSIDERATIONS

Premature labor continues to be the major cause of infant mortality. The outcome of a birth occurring before 37 completed weeks of gestation depends in large measure on the management of the intrapartum period by the perinatal team. Success in delaying labor will allow a few more hours or days for maturation of processes necessary to support extrauterine life, and careful delivery management will further protect the fragile infant.

Definition

It is important to differentiate between weight and maturity, two parameters which influence birth outcome in different ways. A *low-birth-weight infant* is any infant whose weight at birth falls between 500 and 2500 g. A *premature infant* is any infant born after the beginning of the 20th week of gestation and before the end of the 37th week. Within the parameters of weight and age, further distinctions are necessary. Using the graph in Fig. 11-1, an infant who is plotted below the 10th percentile in expected weight is identified as being *small for gestational age* (SGA). Such an infant has been affected by intrauterine factors which decrease nourishment to the fetus, or by an inability to use the nutrients present. This can be the result of preeclampsia, kidney disease, severe diabetes (classes D, E, and F), smoking, and chronic hypertension, as all may cause reduced placental blood flow. Nutrients can be reduced because of poor maternal intake, alcoholism, and maternal gastrointestinal diseases. Fetal ability to use normal supplies of nutrients can be inhibited by congenital anomalies in the fetus. As a result of these varied factors, any SGA infant can be considered to have suffered intrauterine stress of some kind, and to have an increased risk of extrauterine problems.

The infant whose weight is plotted above the 90th percentile is termed a *large for gestational age infant* (LGA). Larger-than-average infants almost universally are born of women with mild to moderate diabetes (classes A, B, and C) and have grown in response to an extra glucose and insulin supply. Such an infant is often premature in development and has difficulty with extrauterine adaptation, although appearing to be full size.

Assessment

The infant's maturity at birth will affect respiratory and metabolic adaptation especially. The less mature the infant, the more severe the problems. In recent years mortality has been sharply curtailed with the establishment of regional intensive care centers. AGA preterm infants between 1000 and 1500 g have had a 90 percent survival rate in one center (1). In another center, infants under 1000 g have had a survival rate of 47.6 percent (2). Causes of death in infants under 1500 g in the past have been respiratory distress, pneumonia, and intracranial hemorrhage. Currently, the pattern is shifting. Major causes of death are, in some measure, attributed to the effects of the extraordinary procedures used to sustain life in small infants; e.g., mechanical ventilation and methods of supplying nutrients. Causes of death which are assuming more prominence are necrotizing enterocolitis, pneumothorax,

[1]The author acknowledges discussions with and advice freely given by Beatrice Holland, R.N., M.S., Neonatal Intensive Care Unit, Long Island Jewish–Hillside Medical Center, New York.

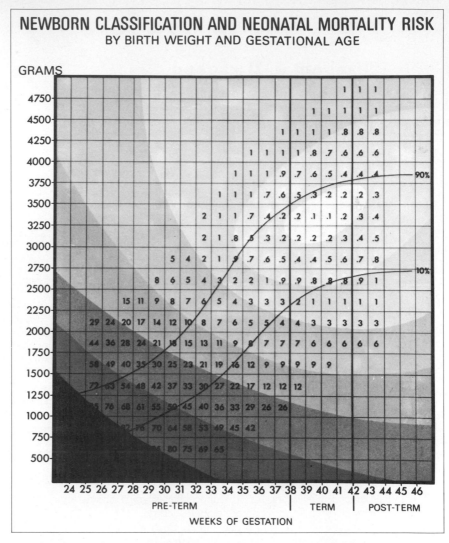

NEWBORN CLASSIFICATION AND NEONATAL MORTALITY RISK
BY BIRTH WEIGHT AND GESTATIONAL AGE

FIGURE 11-1 / Newborn classification and neonatal mortality risk by birth weight and gestational age. Interpolated data based on mathematical fit from original data gathered in University of Colorado Medical Center newborn study, July 1, 1958, to July 1, 1969. (*From L. O. Lubchenco, D. T. Searles, and J. V. Brazie, "Neonatal Mortality Rate: Relationship to Birth Weight and Gestational Age," Journal of Pediatrics, 81:814, 1972.*)

and bronchopulmonary dysplasia. In addition, congenital anomalies, respiratory distress, and pulmonary and intracranial hemorrhage continue to be causes of death (3).

Sequelae of neurologic and pulmonary problems have been reduced. Of surviving infants under 1300 g, it is estimated that with excellent care 65 to 79 percent are normal, and those with handicaps are left with less severe problems than was formerly the case (4).

To improve these statistics and to increase the possibility of a better quality of survival, regionalization of care for such babies appears to be necessary. Adequate care for these infants demands specialization. Regionalization brings with it problems of transport of the tiny baby during the period when early adjustment to extrauterine life is occurring. To reduce transport problems, high-risk mothers should be moved to the regional hospital for delivery, and transport teams need to develop precise techniques (5).

Transport to a Regional Center[2]

I. Preparation by the referring hospital to be ready for transport team's arrival.
   A. Prepare copies of prenatal and labor records, and recovery records of the mother.
   B. List names, addresses, and telephone numbers of physicians responsible for prenatal care, delivery, and follow-up.
   C. Provide record of infant responses (Apgar score, respiratory efforts, temperature) and initial treatment in the delivery room (such as administration of vitamin K and eye prophylaxis, and resuscitative measures).
   D. Provide laboratory reports of acid-base status during labor and after delivery; indicate glucose levels, electrolytes, hematocrit, and bilirubin.
   E. Have tubes of maternal blood and cord blood ready. In some instances placental blood is extracted by the blood bank and prepared for autotransfusion, if deemed necessary.
   F. Provide x-rays if any disease entities are present.
   G. Note if baptism was administered.
   H. Provide copies of consent for transfer, and obtain consents for treatment. If a parent was not able to sign before transport, ensure that father arrives promptly at regional center.

II. Communication with transport team.
   A. Report status of infant. Include status of all attached equipment, amount of oxygen, current glucose level, vital signs, and respiratory status.
   B. Note equipment function, e.g., temperature setting and oxygen levels in incubator.
   C. Take directions by phone as to other supportive measures.

III. Preparation for transport by the team.
   A. Obtain vital signs, and evaluate temperature stability and current glucose level.
   B. Evaluate immediate needs of baby for respiratory stabilization; e.g., whether oxygen, intubation, or bag breathing is necessary.
   C. Secure ECG monitor.
   D. Call center and report findings and stability of patient, with approximate time of departure.

IV. Preparation of parents.
   A. Check identification and verify information as to address, parity, and religion. Obtain telephone numbers in case of emergency.
   B. Permit mother to see baby in transport incubator. Allow parents to touch and hold infant if condition permits.
   C. Explain plan of care at the center. Review telephone and visiting opportunities. Obtain consents if not already done.
   D. Ask father to visit center as soon as possible. Some transport units ask father to accompany infant to center (Fig. 11-2).

V. Admission to center.
   A. Report infant status and any unusual findings during transit.
   B. Check identification of infant with primary nurse receiving patient.
   C. Determine vital signs once infant is placed in warm environment. (Take temperature before removing from transport incubator.)
   D. Obtain complete lab work as ordered, but do not let infant become extremely fatigued.
      1. Tests should include a complete blood count with differential, platelets, reticulocytes, hemoglobin, hematocrit, and bilirubin (if not already done).
      2. Acid-base tests should indicate pH, Pa_{CO_2}, Pa_{O_2}, base deficit.
      3. Include septic workup if membranes were ruptured for more than 12 to 24 h before birth; and culture of throat, blood, urine, cord, skin, and stool.
   E. X-ray location of umbilical line, of position of any tubes in place, and of lung should be done if indicated. Protect infant from chilling (Fig. 11-3).

[2]Angela Venitt and Katherine Rasasco participated in formulating the transport procedures and "Goals of Care."

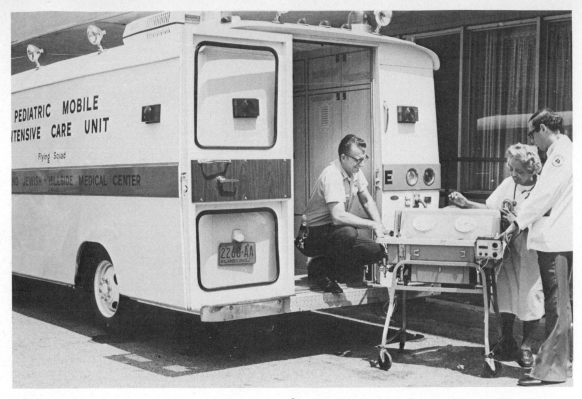

A

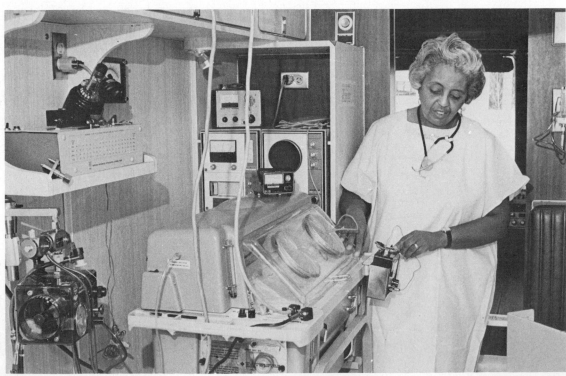

B

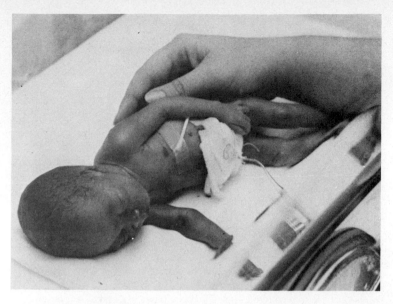

FIGURE 11-3 / A 1300-g infant with estimated gestational age of 31 weeks. Note arterial catheter via umbilical vessel and temperature-sensing probe attached to skin. (*Courtesy of Long Island Jewish–Hillside Medical Center, New York.*)

Problems

I. Labile temperature will need support.
II. Unstable respiratory function will need stimulation and perhaps oxygen and mechanical assistance.
III. Cardiovascular function may be jeopardized by hypovolemia or patent ductus arteriosus.
IV. Glucose and electrolyte balance may be upset.
V. Nutritional and fluid needs and method of intake will vary with status.
VI. Neurologic status may demonstrate immaturity with bradycardia and periodic apnea, or it may be affected by birth trauma.
VII. Skin integrity may be jeopardized by equipment attached to the skin and by lack of movement.
VIII. Bowel and bladder function may be impaired.
IX. There may be barriers to parental bonding.
X. Lack of stimulation or inappropriate stimulation for growth may be a problem.
XI. Congenital anomalies or intrauterine growth retardation may influence status and recovery.

Diagnosis

I. Low-birth-weight preterm infant who recovers without apparent problems.
II. Low-birth-weight infant who is also small for dates (or large for dates, or postmature).

FIGURE 11-2 / Pediatric mobile intensive care unit. (*a*) Preparing to move transport incubator into ambulance. (*b*) Internal view of equipment. (*Courtesy of Long Island Jewish–Hillside Medical Center, New York. Photograph by Herbert Bennett.*)

III. Low-birth-weight infant who has extra risk factors of respiratory distress (or hypovolemia, patent ductus arteriosus, hypoglycemia, etc.).

IV. Parents of low-birth-weight infant are having difficulty with bonding.

Goals of Care

I. Immediate.
   A. Maintain a thermoneutral environment.
   B. Monitor and support respiratory status.
   C. Assess maturity.
   D. Maintain fluid and electrolyte balance.
   E. Assess nutritional intake daily. It must support the rapid growth rate with adjustments made according to infant's condition.
   F. Maintain skin integrity.
   G. Promote normal bowel and bladder function.
   H. Prevent infection.

II. Long-range.
   A. The infant will have a weight gain in line with the normal curve.
   B. Neurologic development will not be impaired.
   C. Bonding with parents will take place as soon as possible. Parents will be kept informed of the infant's status.
   D. Parents will be prepared for the infant's discharge and for infant care.
   E. Appropriate referrals will be made for supportive services.

Intervention

I. Maintain a thermoneutral environment.
   A. A thermoneutral environment is that ambient temperature within which an infant's metabolic rate remains stable, and no extra effort to stabilize core temperature is demanded (6).
   B. Desirable *core* (rectal) temperature is 36.5 to 37°C (98 to 98.6°F), and is not below 36°C (97°F). To achieve this, an environment which maintains a skin temperature of 36.3 to 36.5°C may be necessary for the small premature baby. [A detailed table for the varying amounts of ambient requirements based on weight and age can be found in Klaus and Fanaroff (7).]
   C. Brown adipose tissue (BAT) is metabolized to release energy. Stores can be quickly depleted. In cold stress, kilocalories are used and weight loss occurs, accompanied by hypoxia, fatigue, and acidosis.
   D. The *temperature gradient* (differences between body core and skin temperature, and that of skin temperature and surrounding environment) is critical.
   E. Nursing interventions include:
      1. Hourly monitoring of temperature of baby and environment until condition is stable, and then every 4 h.
      2. Careful adjustment and monitoring of radiant heaters, temperature, humidity, and airflow in controlled environment cribs (Fig. 11-4).
      3. Prevention of increased temperature gradient during treatments and examinations.

II. Monitor and support respiratory status.
   A. Average respiratory rate is 40 to 60 breaths per minute. Support will be needed if respirations are too shallow or irregular, fast or slow, or if apneic episodes occur.
      1. Tachypnea (over 100 breaths per minute): Breathe by bag with mask for 5 min each 30 min.
      2. If respirations are under 30 breaths per minute, breathe by bag continuously until mechanical assistance can be set up.

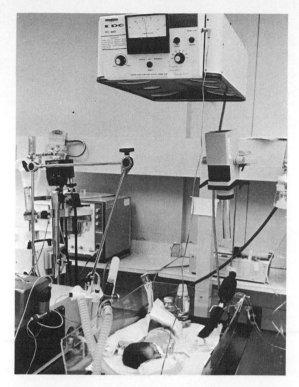

FIGURE 11-4 / Radiant heat crib for infant receiving frequent therapy and needing continuous monitoring. (*Courtesy of the Long Island Jewish–Hillside Medical Center, New York. Photograph by Herbert Bennett.*)

    3. Apnea (no breaths for more then 15 to 20 s) with bradycardia and cyanosis: Check environmental temperature, airway, and glucose level. Gently stimulate, suction briefly, then breathe by bag (8).

B. Many small infants will require respiratory assistance because of rising arterial P_{CO_2}, falling arterial P_{O_2}, and falling pH. Cyanosis may appear when P_{O_2} levels fall below 50 mmHg, but hypoxemia can begin before that point.

C. Other signs of respiratory difficulty are increasing periods of apnea, bradypnea, or tachypnea, lethargy, retractions, flaring nares, and respiratory sounds.

D. Methods of respiratory assistance:

    1. Hand-operated bag with mask is utilized, applying intermittent positive pressure (IPPB).

    2. Mechanically assisted intermittent positive pressure is maintained through an endotracheal tube (there are many varieties of machines and functions available).

    3. Continuous positive airway pressure (CPAP) is obtained by means of application to endotracheal tube, application to nasal prongs, or use of head box or pressurized plastic bag (Fig. 11-5).

    4. Continuous negative pressure (CNP) on parts of body provides continuous positive airway pressure in respiratory tract. Negative pressure on infant's trunk is maintained while head is at atmospheric pressure through use of a plastic body chamber to apply negative pressure to trunk.

    5. Intermittent negative pressure ventilation (INPV) applies negative pressure to trunk while head is at atmospheric pressure, but cycles in rhythmic breathing rate.

    6. Positive pressure is applied with residual end expiratory pressure (PEEP).

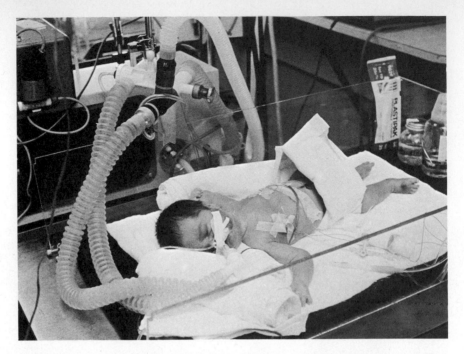

FIGURE 11-5 / Infant receiving continuous positive airway pressure via nasal cannulas. (Courtesy of Long Island Jewish–Hillside Medical Center, New York. Photograph by Herbert Bennett.)

    E. Goals for respiratory support.
        1. Maintain the following readings:
            a. Pa_{O_2} = 60 to 90 mmHg.
            b. Pa_{CO_2} = 35 to 40 mmHg.
            c. pH = 7.30 to 7.45.
        2. Prevent hyperoxemia (110 mmHg for more than 1 to 2 h) and avoid eye damage and bronchopulmonary dysplasia (9). Monitor oxygen levels in environment (every 1 to 2 h) and assess Pa_{O_2} levels frequently (at least every 4 h) during assisted respiration.
    F. Nursing interventions during assisted ventilation include:
        1. Suctioning at least every 2 h, gently and briefly, while maintaining strict aseptic technique.
        2. Preventing injury to mucous membranes of nose and mouth.
        3. Good skin care necessary to prevent breakdown; repositioning baby at least every 3 h.
        4. Maintaining body temperature.
        5. Maintaining caloric intake, and fluid and electrolyte balance.
III. Assess maturity.
    A. Characteristics of the preterm infant can be evaluated by physical observations and neurologic testing. Figure 11-6 illustrates major criteria indicating prematurity.
    B. The Dubowitz scoring system (10) for evaluation of gestational age uses 11 physical criteria and 10 neurologic criteria. A weighted score is calculated using Fig. 11-7. Such a score has a 1.02-week error of prediction if all 21 items are evaluated. (See Tables 11-1 and 11-2 and Fig. 11-8 to complete the test.)
    C. In addition, weight, length, and head circumference should be measured, and weight-length ratios determined.

IV. Maintain fluid and electrolyte balance (see Table 11-3).
   A. Fluid needs are calculated individually and daily depending on condition and environmental factors (e.g., assisted ventilation, phototherapy, degree of respiratory difficulty, and other stress).
   B. Adequate replacement must be given for insensible water losses. Figures must be

FIGURE 11-6 / **Characteristics of the preterm infant.** (*a*) **Preterm infant lying supine; note lack of muscle tone, resulting in froglike position with extremities flat on the bed.** (*b*) **Preterm infant facies; note lack of subcutaneous fat.** (*c*) **Head turned beyond the point of the shoulder.** (*d*) **Scarf sign; the arm can be pulled around the neck much farther than the arm of a full-term infant.** (*e*) **Ventral suspension; the preterm infant hangs limply with straight legs and arms when tested for strength of back and neck muscles.** (*Courtesy of Kenneth Holt, M.D., from tape-slide program "Neurologic Examination of the Newborn," London, 1970.*)

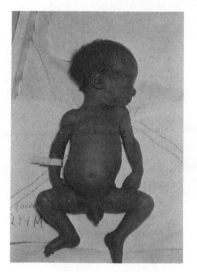

A

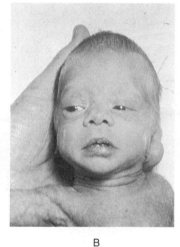

B

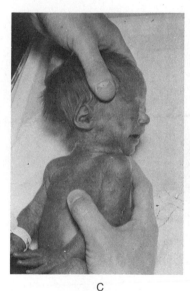

C

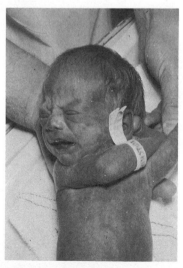

D

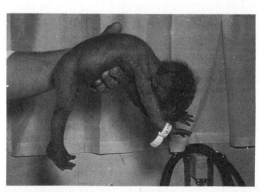

E

TABLE 11-1 / SCORING SYSTEM FOR EXTERNAL PHYSICAL CHARACTERISTICS

External Sign	Score*				
	0	1	2	3	4
Edema	Obvious edema of hands and feet; pitting over tibia	No obvious edema of hands and feet; pitting over tibia	No edema		
Skin texture	Very thin, gelatinous	Thin and smooth	Smooth; medium thickness. Rash or superficial peeling	Slight thickening	Thick and parchmentlike; superficial or deep cracking
Skin color	Dark red	Uniformly pink	Pale pink; variable over body	Pale; only pink over ears, lips, palms, or soles	
Skin opacity (trunk)	Numerous veins and venules clearly seen, especially over abdomen	Veins and tributaries seen	A few large vessels clearly seen over abdomen	A few large vessels seen indistinctly over abdomen	No blood vessels seen
Lanugo (over back)	No lanugo	Abundant; long and thick over lower part of back	Hair thinning	Small amount of lanugo and bald areas	At least half of back devoid of lanugo
Plantar creases	No skin creases	Faint red marks over anterior half of sole	Definite red marks over more than anterior half; indentations over less than anterior third	Indentations over more than anterior third	Definite deep indentations over more than anterior third

Nipple formation	Nipple barely visible; no areola	Nipple well defined; areola smooth and flat, diameter less than 0.75 cm	Areola stippled, edge not raised, diameter less than 0.75 cm	Areola stippled, edge raised, diameter less than 0.75 cm
Breast size	No breast tissue palpable	Breast tissue on one or both sides, 0.5-cm diameter	Breast tissue both sides; one or both 0.5–1.0 cm	Breast tissue both sides; one or both less than 1 cm
Ear form	Pinna flat and shapeless, little or no incurving of edge	Incurving of part of edge of pinna	Partial incurving of whole of upper pinna	Well-defined incurving of whole of upper pinna
Ear firmness	Pinna soft, easily folded, no recoil	Pinna soft, easily folded, slow recoil	Cartilage to edge of pinna, but soft in places, ready recoil	Pinna firm, cartilage to edge; instant recoil
Genitals: Male	Neither testis in scrotum	At least one testis high in scrotum	At least one testis right down	
Female (with hips half abducted)	Labia majora widely separated, labia minora protruding	Labia majora completely cover labia minora		

*If score differs on two sides, take the mean.

Source: Adapted from Farr et al., "Developmental Medicine and Child Neurology," **8**:507, 1966; and reproduced from Dubowitz et al., "Clinical Assessment of Gestational Age in the Newborn Infant," *Journal of Pediatrics,* **77**:1–10, 1970.

TABLE 11-2 / SOME NOTES ON TECHNIQUES OF ASSESSMENT OF NEUROLOGICAL CRITERIA

1. Posture: Observed with infant quiet and in supine position. Score 0—arms and legs extended; 1—beginning of flexion of hips and knees, arms extended; 2—stronger flexion of legs, arms extended; 3—arms slightly flexed, legs flexed and abducted; 4—full flexion of arms and legs (Fig. 11-6a).

2. Square window: The hand is flexed on the forearm between the thumb and index finger of the examiner. Enough pressure is applied to get as full a flexion as possible, and the angle between the hypothenar eminence and the ventral aspect of the forearm is measured and graded according to diagram. (Care is taken not to rotate the infant's wrist while doing this maneuver.)

3. Ankle dorsiflexion: The foot is dorsiflexed onto the anterior aspect of the leg, with the examiner's thumb on the sole of the foot and other fingers behind the leg. Enough pressure is applied to get as full flexion as possible, and the angle between the dorsum of the foot and the anterior aspect of the leg is measured.

4. Arm recoil: With the infant in the supine position the forearms are first flexed for 5 s, then fully extended by pulling on the hands, and then released. The sign is fully positive if the arms return briskly to full flexion (score 2). If the arms return to incomplete flexion or the response is sluggish, it is graded as score 1. If they remain extended or are followed only by random movements, the score is 0.

5. Leg recoil: With the infant supine, the hips and knees are fully flexed for 5 s, then extended by traction on the feet, and released. A maximal response is one of full flexion of the hips and knees (score 2). A partial flexion scores 1, and minimal or no movement scores 0.

6. Popliteal angle: With the infant supine and the pelvis flat on the examining couch, the thigh is held in the knee-chest position by the examiner's left index finger and thumb supporting the knee. The leg is then extended by gentle pressure from the examiner's right index finger behind the ankle and the popliteal angle is measured.

7. Heel-to-ear maneuver: With the baby supine, draw the baby's foot as near to the head as it will go without forcing it. Observe the distance between the foot and the head as well as the degree of extension at the knee. Grade according to diagram. Note that the knee is left free and may draw down alongside the abdomen.

8. Scarf sign: With the baby supine, take the infant's hand and try to put it around the neck and as far posteriorly as possible around the opposite shoulder. Assist this maneuver by lifting the elbow across the body. See how far the elbow will go across, and grade according to illustrations. Score 0—elbow reaches opposite axillary line; 1—elbow between midline and opposite axillary line; 2—elbow reaches midline; 3—elbow will not reach midline (Fig. 11-6d).

9. Head lag: With the baby lying supine, grasp the hands (or the arms if the infant is very small) and pull baby slowly toward the sitting position. Observe the position of the head in relation to the trunk, and grade accordingly. In a small infant the head may initially be supported by one hand. Score 0—complete lag; 1—partial head control; 2—able to maintain head in line with body; 3—brings head anterior to body.

10. Ventral suspension: The infant is suspended in the prone position, with examiner's hand under the infant's chest (one hand in a small infant, two in a large infant). Observe the degree of extension of the back and the amount of flexion of the arms and legs. Also note the relation of the head to the trunk. Grade according to diagrams (Fig. 11-6e). If score differs on the two sides, take the mean.

Source: Adapted from C. Amiel-Tison, "Neurologic Evaluation of the Maturity of Newborn Infants," *Archives of Diseases of Children,* **43**:89, 1968; reproduced from Dubowitz et al., "Clinical Assessment of Gestational Age in the Newborn Infant," *Journal of Pediatrics,* **77**:1–10, 1970.

increased from amounts in Table 11-4 if radiant heaters are in use, or if any of above factors are present.

C. Measurement of urine output is helpful but not always accurately possible. Normal

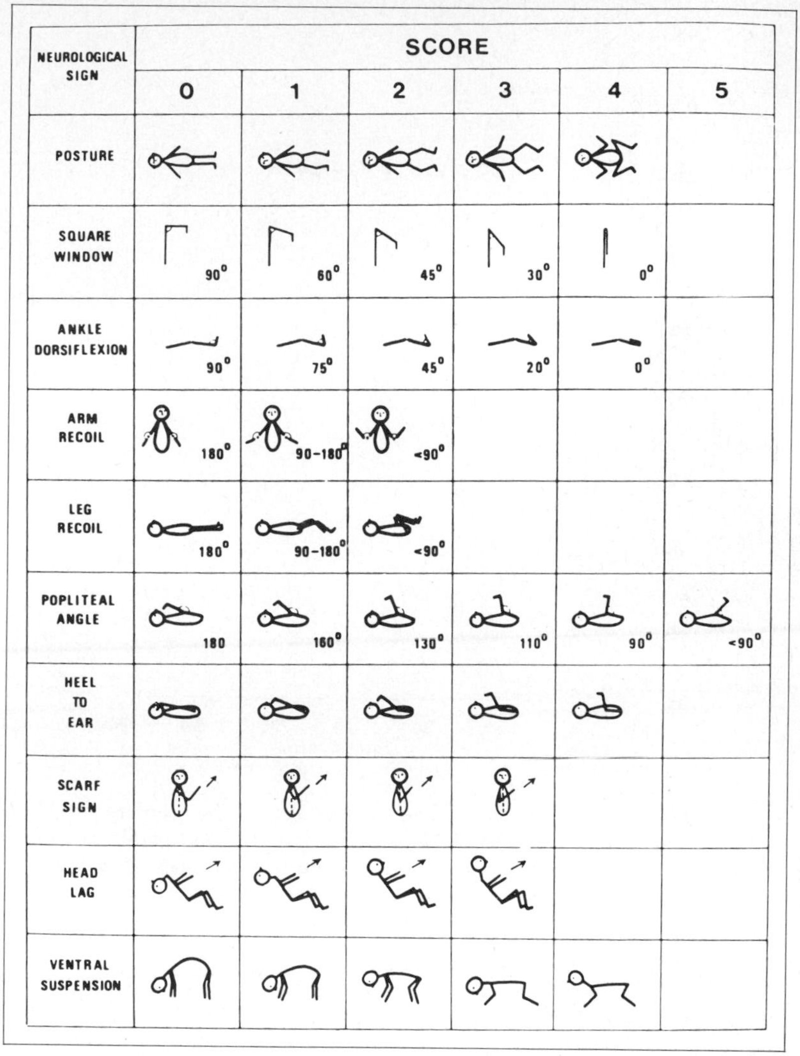

NEUROLOGICAL SIGN	SCORE					
	0	1	2	3	4	5
POSTURE						
SQUARE WINDOW	90°	60°	45°	30°	0°	
ANKLE DORSIFLEXION	90°	75°	45°	20°	0°	
ARM RECOIL	180°	90–180°	<90°			
LEG RECOIL	180°	90–180°	<90°			
POPLITEAL ANGLE	180	160°	130°	110°	90°	<90°
HEEL TO EAR						
SCARF SIGN						
HEAD LAG						
VENTRAL SUSPENSION						

FIGURE 11-7 / Scoring system of neurological signs for assessment of gestational age. (*From V. Dubowitz et al., "Clinical Assessment of Gestational Age in the Newborn Infant," Journal of Pediatrics, 77:1, 1970.*)

hydration will yield a volume of 35 to 100 mL/kg per day, with a specific gravity of 1.005 to 1.012 and an osmolality of 75 to 300 mosmol/kg (11).

D. Weight loss or gain guides therapy. The period of active growth should begin by 1 week unless infant is very unstable. Growth should then assume normal curves.

V. Maintain adequate fluid and nutrient intake.

A. The infant is given nothing orally (NPO) until stable. However, when possible, early feeding is important to reduce hypoglycemia.

B. The method of feeding is dependent upon infant condition. See Table 11-5 for relative advantages and disadvantages of different methods of enteral feeding.

C. Vigorous infants are fed sterile water for the first two feedings and then water and formula in a 1:1 mixture for 72 h. Afterward, if the condition is stable, full-strength milk feedings are begun (12). Some authorities recommend sterile water for the first several feedings while administering 10% dextrose and water parenterally. Undiluted formula is begun as soon as condition permits (13).

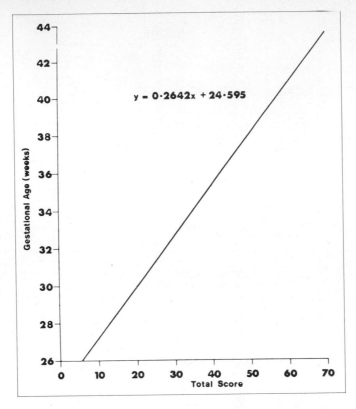

$$y = 0 \cdot 2642x + 24 \cdot 595$$

FIGURE 11-8 / Graph for reading gestational age. The score from Table 11-2 is added to the score from Fig. 11-7. A line is drawn from the horizontal axis to the diagonal line; then from the intersecting point, a line to the perpendicular axis will indicate the age in weeks. (*From V. Dubowitz et al., "Clinical Assessment of Gestational Age in the Newborn Infant," Journal of Pediatrics, 77:2, 1970.*)

TABLE 11-3 / RANGE OF BLOOD VALUES IN THE FETUS AND NEWBORN INFANT

	Fetus (Last Trimester) or Preterm Infant of 1500–2000 g	Term Newborn Weighing More than 2500 g (Cord Blood)	7 Days Later
Red blood cells, millions per cubic millimeter	4.5–6.5	5.5–6	4–5
Reticulocytes, %	6	3–5	0–1
Hemoglobin, g/dL	17–20 (90–95% Hb F, 5–10% Hb A)	17–19 (80% Hb F, 20% Hb A)	14–17 (rising % of Hb A)
Hematocrit, %	45–60 (others state 53–65)	48–60 (average capillary blood 5–10% higher)	50
White blood cells, per cubic millimeter		up to 18,000	11,000–12,000
Blood volume, ml/kg	100–108	85–90 (higher if cord clamped late)	75–80 by 2 months

TABLE 11-3 / RANGE OF BLOOD VALUES IN THE FETUS AND NEWBORN INFANT (*Continued*)

	Fetus (Last Trimester) or Preterm Infant of 1500–2000 g	Term Newborn Weighing More than 2500 g (Cord Blood)	7 Days Later
Platelets,* thousands per cubic millimeter	290±70 (lower than newborn)	310±68 (below 150 is abnormal)	280±56
Prothrombin time,* s	17 (12–21)	16 (13–20) (prolonged until 4 days unless vitamin K is given)	Adult values by 1 week
Partial thromboplastin time,* s	70	55±10	Adult values by 2–9 months
Bilirubin, mg/dL	Preterm values rise higher than full-term usually	1.8–2.0	After rising to 4–8 mg/dL, reduces slowly to adult levels of 1–2 mg/dL
pH	0.15 pH units less than maternal pH (fetal); soon assumes full-term level	7.28 (rising to 7.34–7.45 soon after birth if there is no respiratory difficulty)	7.34–7.45
Pa_{O_2}, mmHg	35 (rises to 50–70 soon after birth)	35 [umbilical venous blood (rises to 50–70 soon after birth)]	50–70
Pa_{CO_2}, mmHg	40–50 (35–40 after birth)	48 (50–55)	35–40
HCO_3, meq/L		17.5	19–22
Base excess		−4 to +4	−4 to +4
Glucose, mg/dL†	In utero reflects maternal levels; after birth 40–50 (severe hypoglycemia when below 20 mg)	Varies widely; averages 60–83 [cord (severe hypoglycemia when below 30 mg during first 72 h)]	45–115, then quickly assumes adult range (severe hypoglycemia if below 40 mg/dL)
Electrolytes: Na, meq/L	134–140, depending on birth weight	147–149	147–149
K, meq/L	5.6–6.4	7.8 (5.6–12)	5.9 (5.0–7.7)
Cl, meq/L	100–105	103 (98–110)	103 (98–112)
Ca, mg/dL	7.0–7.5 (preterm infant)	8–10 or 4–5 meq/L (hypocalcemia if below 7.0–7.5)	Imbalance of Ca/P ratio can develop at 7–10 days in formula-fed infants
Mg, meq/L		0.9–2.6, depending on maternal levels	1.4–1.7

*Data from W. E. Hathaway, "The Bleeding Newborn," *Seminars in Hematology*, **12:**175, 1975.

†Some authorities state that a glucose value below 40 mg/dL at any time indicates hypoglycemia.

Note: It should be noted that readings vary widely, depending on laboratory methods in a particular setting. It is most valid for each hospital to have listings of blood values agreed upon by its particular laboratory.

Sources: I. Stave, *Physiology of the Perinatal Period*, Appleton-Century-Crofts, Inc., New York, 1970; C. A. Smith and N. M. Nelson, *The Physiology of the Newborn Infant*, Thomas Publishing Company, Inc., Springfield, Ill., 1976; M. H. Klaus and A. A. Fanaroff, *Care of the High-Risk Neonate*, W. B. Saunders Company, Philadelphia, 1973; S. B. Korones, *High-Risk Newborn Infants*, The C. V. Mosby Company, St. Louis, 1973.

TABLE 11-4 / TWENTY-FOUR HOUR NUTRIENT NEEDS OF LOW-BIRTH-WEIGHT INFANTS

	First Week	*Period of Active Growth*
Calories	50–100 kcal/kg	120 kcal/kg (110–150 kcal/kg*)
Protein	Amount depends on intake and concentration of formula (parenteral amino acid hydrolysate may be ordered)	2.5–5 g/kg (using modified cow's milk formula) 1.7–1.8 g/kg (using breast milk)†
Fluids	60–100 mL/kg (80–120 mL/kg). Often provided intravenously as 5–10% dextrose in water for first 48 h	150 mL/kg (150–200 mL/kg per day).‡ 1.8% NaCl in 4.3% dextrose and water, or 2% NaCl in 5% dextrose and water, given intravenously to make up total fluid requirements
Fat	Amount depends on intake of formula; unsaturated fats are absorbed best (may be provided as IV Intralipid, a soybean preparation)	40–50% of caloric intake with at least 3% made up of linoleic acid

*SGA infants have a higher basal metabolic rate than AGA infants of the same weight and may need more calories (17).
†With adequate intake, the lower protein of breast milk may still support desired growth because of the unique distribution of amino acids (18). Breast milk also confers other benefits because of ideal protein and fat quantity and quality, immune factors, and osmolar factors suited to human infants (19).
‡Higher fluid needs are present when the infant is under a radiant heater, receiving phototherapy, or has diarrhea, vomiting, or cold stress.

    D. Formula choices (see Table 11-6):
        1. 20 cal/oz or 67 cal/dL (tolerated best by very low-birth-weight infants).
        2. 24 cal/oz or 81 cal/dL (provides correct calorie and water balance).
        3. 27 cal/oz or 91 cal/dL (solute load often is too high; then supplemental water must be given, usually intravenously).
    E. Breast milk is recommended for its balance of protein, carbohydrates, and fats (see Table 11-6) for comparison between breast milk and formula).
    F. Feeding volumes are ordered every day depending on infant's response. Retention of more than one-fourth of the last feeding indicates a reduction of volume by that amount or omission of oral feedings until stomach is empty (13). Milk retention may signal developing illness.
    G. There are varying regimens for administering vitamins. Vitamin K is always administered at birth in amounts of 1 mg intramuscularly. Some centers repeat this dose every week if baby is not on formula. If baby is taking oral fluids, some centers include vitamin C, beginning at 2 to 3 days of life. Multivitamins are administered also in varying proportions. Some recommend vitamins A, D, E, and all of the B group from the first week. Water-soluble vitamin E is considered important if iron-fortified formula is started after several weeks of life (14). Other centers do not administer vitamins since formulas are enriched.
    H. "Iron deficiency usually concides with a doubling of the birth weight (preterm in 1 to 2 months)" (15). Iron is not routinely given, therefore, during the first few weeks of life.
    I. "The optimal diet for the low birth weight infant may be defined as one that supports a rate of growth approximating that of the third trimester of intrauterine life, without imposing stress on the developing metabolic or excretory systems"

TABLE 11-5 / SOME ADVANTAGES AND DISADVANTAGES OF THE VARIOUS METHODS OF ENTERAL FEEDING

| Method | Advantages | | Disadvantages | |
	Intermittent	Indwelling	Intermittent	Indwelling
Orogastric	Can use larger diameter catheter than with na- sogastric	No vagal stimulation	Danger of tracheal intu- bation and possible as- piration	Nasal erosion
Nasogastric	Less chance of aspiration Can aspirate for residual before feeding Can use with endotra- cheal tube in place Conserves energy and prevents fatigue Easy and quick to pass catheter Can be quickly taught	No vagal stimulation	Vagal stimulation Gagging and possible vomiting on introduc- ing catheter Vagal stimulation with rapid infusion	Nasal erosion Nasal airway obstruction Rhinorrhea Otitis media Conjunctivitis
Nasojejunal	Less chance of aspiration Less nursing time for feed- ing Conserves energy and prevents fatigue Possibly greater fluid and calorie intake in early neonatal period		Danger of perforation with polyvinyl and polyethylene catheters Can use only isosmolar or hypoosmolar feedings Causes change in duodenal microflora It may take hours for tube to pass pylorus Vomiting and/or diarrhea Gagging on introducing catheter Clogging of catheter	
Gastrostomy	Less chance of aspiration Not for routine neonatal feeding			Utilizes calories Infection
Dropper	No vagal stimulation ?Allows baby to use some swallowing function		Staphylococcal enterocol- itis Considerable skill re- quired Aspiration, gagging, vom- iting, air swallowing	
Nipple	Physiologic (32–34 weeks) No vagal stimulation		Utilizes calories Aspiration, gagging, vom- iting, air swallowing	

Source: From H. S. Dweck, "Feeding the Prematurely Born Infant," Clinics in Perinatology, 2(1):194, 1975.

(16). Other workers feel that this growth rate is too high an expectation for the tiny baby.

J. Later, growth rates will be calculated best if weight and length at EDD are compared with the average full-term weight and length. Then comparisons can be made about adequate growth in the first year of life.

VI. Support normal bowel and bladder function.

   A. The preterm infant usually voids within 12 to 16 h after birth (20). The quantity is usually small and dependent on early or late cord clamping, as affecting blood volume.

   B. Specific gravity is usually low, 1.004 to 1.018. No protein or red blood corpuscles should be present.

TABLE 11-6 / NUTRIENT COMPOSITION OF HUMAN MILK AND PROPRIETARY INFANT FORMULAS AND RECOMMENDED LEVELS FOR FULL-TERM AND LOW-BIRTH-WEIGHT INFANTS[a]

Nutrient	Minimum Level Recommended[b]	Human Milk	Enfamil	PM 60/40	Premature Formula	Similac	SMA	Similac (13, 24, or 27 kcal/oz)
Protein, g	1.8[c]	1.3–1.6	2.3	2.3	2.8	2.3	2.3	2.7
Fat, g	3.3[d]	5	5.5	5.2	5.1	5.3	5.3	5.3
Carbohydrate, g	—	10.3	10.3	11.1	11.5	10.6	10.7	10.3
Ash, mg	—	300	530	320	680	530	370	580
Vitamin A, IU	250	250	250	370	250	370	390	370
Vitamin D, IU	40	3	63	60	63	60	63	60
Vitamin E, IU	0.3 (0.7)[e]	0.3	1.9	2.2	1.9	2.2	1.4	2.2
Vitamin K, μg	4	2	9	4	9	14	9	4
Vitamin C, mg	8	7.8	8.1	8.1	8.0	8.1	8.6	8.1
Thiamin, μg	40	25	78	96	78	96	105	96
Riboflavin, μg	60	60	94	147	94	147	156	147
Niacin, μg	250	250	1250	1074	1250	1030	780	1000
Vitamin B_6, μg	35[f]	15	63	49	63	60	63	60
Folic acid, μg	4	4	16	7.3	16	7.3	8	7.3
Pantothenic acid, μg	300	300	470	440	470	440	310	440
Vitamin B_{12}, μg	0.15	0.15	0.3	0.22	0.3	0.22	0.16	0.22
Biotin, μg	1.5	1.0	2.5	1.7	2.5	1.5	3.0	1.5
Inositol, mg	4	20	5	7.5	6	5.0	5.5	—
Choline, mg	7	13	7	18.8	7	15	13	25
Calcium, mg	50	50	80	60	156	75	66	102
Phosphorus, mg	25[g]	25	70	30	78	57	49	79
Magnesium, mg	6	6	7	6	10	6	8	6
Iron, mg	0.15[h]	0.1	0.2[i]	0.4	0.2	Trace[i]	1.9	Trace[i]
Iodine, μg	5	4–9	10	6	8	15	10	15
Copper, μg	60	60	100	62	100	60	70	60
Zinc, mg	0.5	0.5	0.65	0.59	0.65	0.74	0.55	0.74
Manganese, μg	5	1.5	160	5	160	5	23	5
Sodium:								
mg	20[g]	24	42	23	40	32	24	38
meq	0.9[g]	1.0	1.8	1.0	1.7	1.6	1.0	1.7
Potassium:								
mg	80	81	102	85	110	103	83	126
meq	2.1	2.1	2.6	2.2	2.8	2.5	2.1	3.2
Chloride:								
mg	55	55	80	66	85	79	55	94
meq	1.6	1.6	2.3	2.0	2.4	2.3	1.6	2.7
Renal solute load,[j] mosmol	—	11.3	16	14.3	18.1	16.2	13.6	18.4

[a] Per 100 kcal.
[b] Committee on Nutrition recommendations for formula for full-term infants per 100 kcal.
[c] Protein of a nutritional quality equivalent to casein.
[d] Including a minimum of 300 mg of essential fatty acids.
[e] Committee on Nutrition recommendation different for low-birth-weight infants; also 1.0 IU/g linoleic acid.
[f] Minimum of 15 μg of vitamin B_6 per gram of protein
[g] Some evidence for higher requirement for low-birth-weight infant.

[h] 1.0 mg in iron-fortified formula.
[i] 1.5 mg in iron-fortified formula.
[j] Calculated by the method of Ziegler and Fomon.

Source: From the Committee on Nutrition, American Academy of Pediatrics, "Nutritional Needs of Low Birth Weight Infants," *Pediatrics,* **60**(4):523, October 1977.

C. The first meconium stool is usually passed within 12 to 16 h by about 65 percent of infants. If delayed 16 to 48 h beyond that time, there may be increased enterohepatic recycling of bilirubin and slightly higher jaundice levels. Most infants usually pass stool within 36 h (20).

D. Assessment of patency of urethra and anus is included in early evaluation.

VII. Maintain skin integrity.

A. The smaller the infant, the more fragile the skin. Abrasions, pressure areas, and skin breakdown can threaten skin integrity.

1. Infants must be positioned in correct body alignment, protecting skin surfaces. Protect skin from numerous attachments for monitoring and infusions.

2. Turn infant every 3 h as a minimum to prevent pressure, stasis.

3. Use protective lamb's wool for vulnerable spots.

4. Keep bathing to a minimum. Use nondrying soaps or plain water.

VIII. Prevent infection.

A. Host defenses in the preterm infant are still maturing (21). Among other deficiencies there is limited phagocytosis and delayed inflammatory response, incomplete transfer of placentally acquired immunoglobulins, and immaturity of intestinal tract with vulnerability to gastrointestinal infections.

B. Perform adequate handwashing before and after working with each infant. Use individual gown technique if infant is out of a closed crib; e.g., for treatments under radiant warmer, or being fed out of crib.

C. Prevention of infection at umbilical cord site is especially important. Umbilical catheters and exchange transfusions may make infection more probable. Observe carefully for signs of local inflammation.

D. Isolation policies will vary according to hospital policies. Follow policy meticulously.

E. See "Infection" for treatment of infections.

IX. Encourage bonding.

A. Note parental reactions to initial contacts.

B. Involve parents from the outset by discussing progress, treatments, and prognosis. Answer all questions and provide updated status reports by telephone when parents are unable to visit.

C. Involve parents in the care of infant as soon as possible; e.g., by bottle feeding, or having mother provide breast milk. Encourage parents to come into nursery to touch, stroke, and talk to infant as soon as possible.

D. Observe for clues to poor parental adjustment to birth of preterm infant.

E. Make referrals and prepare parents for homegoing.

F. Explain expected growth patterns of first year, and ensure a continuation of evaluation of infant's progress.

Evaluation

I. Baby progressed without any problems in the usual pattern of growth and maturation of neurologic function.

II. No apparent disturbances occurred in bonding to parents.

III. Problems occurred in bonding or adaptation.

FAULTY PARENTAL-INFANT BONDING

Definition

Parents of vulnerable infants (22) may demonstrate excessive anxiety, protectiveness, or hidden hostility toward a child who is imperfect. Feelings of failure to produce a normal full-term infant or one without defects may lead to blame, guilt, and inability to deal with the situation (23, 24).

Assessment

I. Mother or father cannot admit their anxiety, and are afraid to question the doctor or nurse.

II. Mother does not receive much help from family or friends. Mother-father communication seems inhibited.

III. Blame directed at others, or at irrelevant factors.

IV. Mother or father does not go through anticipatory grieving (when contact with hospital regarding infant's progress is limited for fear of hearing that infant has died). This behavior for a short period is not indifference or rejection.

V. On infant's beginning recovery, parents have difficulty believing baby is getting well, and remain fearful. They cannot prepare for homegoing (25).

Interventions

I. Initiate simple explanations of all procedures. Therapeutic listening is important. Assign one staff person to relate in depth. Work out communication plans with premature center.

II. Explore briefly what supports are available. Work with social service.

III. Do not return hostility, as behavior stems from struggle to accept reality, and is a stress response. Recognize maternal resentment that nurses can care for her baby better than she can at this point.

IV. Hospital staff must keep communication open. Provide reports to parents on the reality of the situation.

V. As soon as possible, parents should be able to touch, hold, and feed infant in the nursery.

VI. There should be careful exploration of parental feelings of guilt, utilizing several counseling sessions if necessary.

VII. Refer to visiting nurse service for home visit follow-up if necessary.

RESPIRATORY DISTRESS SYNDROME (HYALINE MEMBRANE DISEASE)

Definition

The respiratory distress syndrome (RDS) encompasses a group of signs and symptoms, the etiology of which appear to stem from immaturity of all the processes involved with oxygen exchange in the lung. There is a primary lack of *surfactant,* a substance needed to maintain a low surface tension at the oxygen-fluid interface of the alveolus. Such a lack contributes to alveolar collapse with each breath and results in areas of lung atelectasis; in severe cases, up to 60 percent of the lung area may show atelectasis (26). Atelectasis reduces residual capacity, and each breath requires higher than normal pressures in an attempt to reinflate the collapsed alveoli. Grunting respirations (from forced expiration against a partially closed glottis) are the classic early signs of such a syndrome.

In addition, there may be a persistent high pulmonary vascular resistance which hinders the progression to neonatal circulation. There may be a persistent right-to-left shunt through a patent ductus arteriosus, a condition which commonly occurs in infants of less than 34 weeks' gestational age. The result is a reduction in oxygenation in spite of tachypnea and an adequate supplemental oxygen supply.

Respiratory distress syndrome occurs in about 10 percent of all preterm infants and is seen most commonly in babies born of diabetic mothers, in infants who have suffered perinatal asphyxia or who are hypovolemic, and in those who weigh between 1000 and 1500 g (up to 50 percent). However, infants weighing below 1200 g have the highest mortality rate (50 to 80 percent) (27). Lung maturation proceeds rapidly in the neonatal period, and if the infant is well supported in the initial crisis, survival is often ensured. There may be accompanying sequelae of the extreme measures to support life, e.g., broncho-pulmonary dysplasia, and interstitial emphysema (28).

Assessment

I. Note lecithin/sphingomyelin (L/S) ratio if done prior to birth (lung maturity with ratio of 2).

II. Respiratory rate rises above 60 after first hour of adaptation. The first hour is often difficult.

III. Accessory muscles of respiration are used. Expiratory grunting or whining is evident in early hours.

IV. Cyanosis, first circumoral, periorbital, and in nail beds, progresses to general facial and body cyanosis as hypoxemia increases.

V. Umbilical cord pulsations still may be present 20 min after birth (29).

VI. Increased acidosis and hypoxia is noted, with decreased air entry.

VII. Hypovolemia may be present. A right-to-left shunt through a patent ductus arteriosus may be evident. Characteristic cardiac sounds become more evident after the first 24 to 48 h.

Intervention

I. Provide some form of assisted ventilation with either CPAP or PEEP to prevent alveolar collapse with each breath.

II. Provide a thermoneutral environment with adequate humidity.

III. Monitor color, crying, temperature, blood pressure, and oxygen levels every hour, and respirations and heart rate continuously.

IV. Obtain blood for biochemical monitoring every 4 h.

V. Monitor blood volume so that hypovolemia can be prevented. Restoration of blood volume may be ordered.

VI. Exchange transfusion may be ordered to restore albumin and plasminogen levels, to correct hypovolemia and provide blood with normal 2,3-DPG concentrations which support better tissue oxygenation (30).

VII. Provide skilled, organized, and gentle care which disturbs infant as little as possible.

VIII. Set up and monitor parenteral infusion. RDS is usually accompanied by poor gastric motility. (See Table 11-7 for parenteral nutrition.)

HYPOGLYCEMIA

Definition

Hypoglycemia is a state of low serum glucose levels. In the first 3 days of life, levels of 30 mg per 100 mL in the full-term infant and 20 mg per 100 mL in the preterm infant have been identified as hypoglycemia. After 3 days, a level of 40 mg per 100 mL or below is considered indicative of hypoglycemia for any infant. Other workers indicate that levels below 40 mg per 100 mL at any time in any infant should be considered a problem (31). Uncorrected low glucose levels lead to irreversible cell damage.

Infants of diabetic mothers are often hypoglycemic (50 percent) within the first 4 to 6 h after birth. Infants of any age who are small for date and postmature infants are especially susceptible to hypoglycemia. Asphyxia, birth stress, respiratory distress, and hypothermia particularly contribute to rapid depletion of any glycogen stores in the newborn. Numerous other hypoglycemic syndromes exist, making differential diagnosis difficult.

TABLE 11-7 / COMPOSITION OF INFUSATE FOR TOTAL PARENTERAL ALIMENTATION*

Constituent	Amount per day
Nitrogen source†	2.5 g/kg
Glucose	25–30 g/kg
Sodium (NaCl)	3–4 meq/kg
Potassium‡	2–3 meq/kg
Calcium (calcium gluconate)	0.5 meq/kg
Magnesium (MgSO₄)	0.25 meq/kg
Vitamins:	
Multivitamin infusion (MVI)	1 mL
Vitamin B₁₂	5–10 μg
Folic acid	50–75 μg
Vitamin K₁	250–500 μg
Total volume	130 mL/kg

*The composition of nutrients is not uniformly agreed upon and varies from institution to institution and for individual infants. (Currently, Intralipid is also being administered for nutrition.)
†Either protein hydrolysate or a mixture of crystalline amino acids.
‡2 meq/kg is provided as KH₂PO₄; remainder is provided as KCl.
Source: From W. C. Heird and J. M. Driscoll, Jr., "Newer Methods for Feeding Low Birth Weight Infants," *Clinics in Perinatology,* **2**(2):312, September 1975.

Assessment

I. Infant is under stress from numerous factors, shows signs of fatigue and lethargy, and has poor cry or none at all.
II. Respiratory effort appears to tire infant and cyanosis is present in spite of ambient oxygen. Breathing rates are irregular and apnea and bradycardia continue.
III. There is an inability to suck well, and intake is inadequate.
IV. Tremors are increasing.
V. The infant is large for gestational age, born of a diabetic mother (IDM).
VI. The infant is small for gestational age, has little body fat, and appears hungry, weak, and listless.
VII. The infant is postmature, and shows signs of recent weight loss and intrauterine stress.
VIII. Assessed blood glucose levels are at or below normal.

Intervention

I. Reduce external stress as much as possible and keep handling to a minimum.
II. Provide ambient thermoneutral temperature, adequate humidity, and adequate oxygen levels to supply an optimum environment in an effort to minimize respiratory distress.
III. Initiate prompt testing for hypoglycemia when any symptoms appear in infants who are not high risk. Do regular preventive screening (Dextrostix) on all high-risk infants.
IV. When Dextrostix (Ames) are used, warm the heel first. Test the validity of surface material of a test stick from the same bottle. To do this apply a drop of 5% glucose and water to the stick for a strong glucose reading. (The enzyme on the stick decomposes with light and humidity.)
V. Always send a lab specimen if the Dextrostix reading is below 45 mg. Avoid false readings by sending iced lab specimens promptly.
VI. Initiate early oral feedings whenever possible, especially for infants of diabetic mothers.
VII. Parenteral dextrose and water should be administered in conjunction with oral feedings

to high-risk infants. Glucose is calculated in grams per kilogram in 24 h. Such IV dextrose must be tapered off, rather than abruptly discontinued, or rebound hypoglycemia may occur.

VIII. For persistent hypoglycemia, in spite of parenteral glucose or oral feedings, steroids and/or glucagon may be ordered.

HYPOCALCEMIA

Definition

Hypocalcemia is a state of depleted calcium; levels fall to or below 7.0 to 7.5 mg per 100 mL. Low levels of serum calcium commonly follow a drop in glucose, partially since glucagon is activated, which in turn promotes calcium excretion. Depletion can occur after episodes of resuscitation, especially if sodium bicarbonate has been used, and after exchange transfusion. In some infants, several days after formula has been instituted, a calcium-phosphorous imbalance may develop. Symptoms are never specific and are often confused with other problems. They present mainly as jitteriness, high-pitched crying, vomiting, cyanosis, or more severely as tetany and convulsions. Preferred therapy is the administration of calcium parenterally or orally.

Assessment

See "Hypoglycemia."

Intervention

I. Serum calcium measurements guide therapy. Serum magnesium must also be measured.
II. Recognize that after exchange transfusion, citrate may combine with calcium and, even though extra calcium gluconate is given, hypocalcemia may be present.
III. Prevent extravasation of parenteral calcium injection. Monitor flow carefully.
IV. Monitor vital signs, especially the heart rate, while calcium is being administered.
V. Low-phosphorous formula should be ordered for Ca/P imbalance, PM 60/40 (Ross).

NECROTIZING ENTEROCOLITIS

Definition

Still of unknown etiology, this severe complication occurs most often in infants under 1500 g who have had episodes of asphyxia, respiratory distress, acidosis, hypovolemia, shock, and patent ductus arteriosus, or obstruction of blood flow to mesenteric arteries because of an umbilical line. Hyperosmolar feedings, especially by nasojejunal route, have been implicated. Inflammation and ulceration of ileum or proximal colon may occur, progressing to perforation. Time of onset is between 8 and 44 days (32).

Assessment

I. Any of above risk factors are present.
II. There is poor enteral feeding with residuals in stomach.
III. Vomiting and diarrhea are present.
IV. Blood may appear in the stool (guaiac-positive).

V. Abdominal distension, lethargy, hypothermia, pallor and shock occur (33).

VI. Pneumoperitoneum, and/or gas in the bowel wall (pneumatosis intestinalis) defined upon x-ray.

Intervention

I. Abdominal x-ray is necessary for evaluation.

II. Septic workup must be done.

III. Antibiotic therapy is begun.

IV. Enteral feedings are discontinued, and parenteral feedings begun.

V. Dextran as a volume expander may be administered if hypovolemia is present.

VI. Nasogastric tube is inserted and attached to low suction.

VII. Prepare for abdominal surgical intervention if perforation is suspected.

HYPERBILIRUBINEMIA

Definition

The newborn infant has a normal increase in bilirubin after birth because of rapid destruction of extra fetal hemoglobin. (See Table 11-3 for levels at birth and after 7 days.) The immature liver is unable to effectively metabolize the extra bilirubin and indirect (unconjugated) levels rise to 4 to 8 mg per 100 mL by the third or fourth day of life in the full-term infant. If levels rise to 16 to 18 mg per 100 mL, the bilirubin pigment crosses the blood-brain barrier to settle in the nuclear areas of the brain. High levels therefore lead to *kernicterus,* with varying degrees of brain damage causing mental retardation and/or cerebral palsy, deafness, and in less severe cases, "minimal brain dysfunction."

The younger the infant, the more difficulty there will be, because (1) liver function is less mature, (2) there are smaller amounts of serum albumin to bind the bilirubin, and (3) there is a lack of intestinal bacteria to aid in the reduction of bilirubin to urobilinogen. A number of other factors are involved: e.g., time of meconium passage, state of illness, presence of competing drugs, and presence of any inherited defect or metabolic deficiency. Kernicterus can occur at lower levels in the preterm infant and at even lower levels (as low as 10.5 mg per 100 mL) if there is acidosis, hypoxia, or infection (34). The obvious sign of elevated levels is a yellow color in the skin and sclera, and a change in color of stool and urine. Jaundice is merely a symptom of multiple possible causes of delayed metabolism or excretion of bilirubin.

Phototherapy has largely replaced exchange transfusion as the treatment of choice, but in severe cases where bilirubin levels are elevated within the first 48 h or rise very rapidly, exchange transfusion is usually carried out. Long-term effects of phototherapy are not yet clearly described, and careful monitoring is in order, with judicious use (35).

Assessment

I. A high-risk infant shows signs of rising bilirubin levels (over 5 to 8 mg per 100 mL in the first 24 h after birth or over 9 mg per 100 mL after 24 h). The earlier the increase, the more serious the problem. Causes are multiple:

A. Episodes of asphyxia, or acidosis.

B. Protracted periods of induction of labor with oxytocin. "The incidence rises sharply when oxytocin total dosage exceeds 20 units" (36).

C. Rh incompatibility, with positive direct Coombs' test (peak of jaundice usually occurs by 48 h).

D. ABO incompatibility with type O mother, especially (peak of jaundice usually is delayed to 72 h).

    E. Concealed hemorrhage; cerebral hemorrhage, hematoma, bruising, vacuum extraction (reabsorption of extra RBC results in peak of jaundice, usually at 48 h).

    F. Enzyme deficiency (G6PD, pyruvate kinase).

    G. Congenitally deficient systems to metabolize or excrete bilirubin (metabolic and intestinal disorders).

    H. Polycythemia with a hematocrit over 60 percent.

    I. Infection or dehydration.

    J. Maternal diabetes or drug ingestion.

    K. Certain infants receiving breast milk. (0.5 to 1.0 percent must temporarily receive formula for 3 to 7 days until initial jaundice levels fall. Breast milk can then be resumed.)

II. Indirect levels are elevated but direct levels are usually within normal limits if the problem is immaturity of function.

III. Toxic symptoms are seen in diminished Moro response, poor sucking, vomiting, hypotonia, and high-pitched cry (37). However, in small premature babies, increasing apneic spells may be the only sign.

Intervention

I. Laboratory evaluations will include:

    A. Coombs' test, direct and indirect.

    B. Retyping of maternal blood and cross-matching of maternal serum with newborn blood.

    C. Indirect and direct bilirubin levels at regular intervals.

    D. Complete blood count, hemoglobin, hematocrit, and reticulocytes.

    E. Serum proteins plus bilirubin protein-binding capacity (HABA, salicylates, and Sephadex).

    F. pH.

II. Note and report any maternal drugs which could be passed to infant and could occupy neonatal albumin binding sites (38). Note neonatal drugs.

III. Evaluate meconium passage (time and amount). A delay in meconium passage will result in increased enterohepatic reabsorption and higher levels may be present.

IV. Choice of phototherapy or exchange transfusion will depend upon guidelines set in individual institutions (39).

    A. Phototherapy:

        1. Levels of 5 to 9 mg per 100 mL in first 24 h.

        2. Levels of 10 to 14 mg per 100 mL in 24 to 72 h.

        3. Levels of 15 to 19 mg per 100 mL in 48 to 72 h.

    B. Exchange transfusion:

        1. Levels over 10 mg per 100 mL in first 24 h.

        2. Levels of 15 to 19 mg per 100 mL in 24 to 48 h.

        3. All levels over 20 mg per 100 mL.

    C. Regimen is modified whenever respiratory distress, acidosis, hypothermia, immaturity, and low serum albumin are present and exchange is indicated earlier.

V. Support infant during phototherapy.

    A. Lights must be monitored for wavelength, not brightness. "Brightness of light is *not* the key, but rather the amount of energy output at wavelengths close to 460." Energy output must be monitored by hospital engineer (40).

    B. Side effects of diarrhea and increased insensible water loss can be treated with lactose-free formula, and extra fluid intake. Careful observation of intake and output is important. Some infants develop a rash for which there is no specific treatment.

    C. Skin must be uncovered as much as possible while correct ambient temperature is maintained. Monitor temperature. Do not allow hypothermia or hyperthermia to develop.

    D. Eyes must be completely covered with an opaque mask over soft cotton eye patches. Both mask and patches should be removed for feedings to observe eyes for signs of irritation or infection and for cleansing purposes.

    E. Give careful explanation to parents of reasons for and progress of treatment. Mother should feed infant whenever possible.

HEMORRHAGE

Definition

Hemorrhage accounts for about 10 percent of mortality in small infants. Subdural, subarachnoid, intraventricular, and pulmonary hemorrhage are most frequently seen on autopsy. Usually there are other accompanying problems.

Intracranial hemorrhage is often the result of severe asphyxia with accompanying acidosis, and frequently is seen in infants dying of respiratory distress syndrome. It is thought that the bleeding results from the anoxic insult (41).

Pulmonary hemorrhage usually develops in the first few days of life. Periods of bradycardia, apnea, or very slow respirations, and peripheral vasoconstriction are accompanied by pulmonary edema. The bloody fluid bubbling from the trachea is edema fluid mixed with a small amount of blood [such edema is thought to be a result of acute left heart failure precipitated by hypoxia (42)]. Treatment is not usually successful.

Assessment

    I. Infant has periods of distress from hypoxia, birth injury, or respiratory distress.

    II. Symptoms can develop gradually or may be precipitated suddenly, as in subarachnoid or intraventricular hemorrhage.

    III. Increasing anemia, pallor, shock, cyanosis, and mottled skin may be ascertained. Neurologic signs of disturbed function will vary from apnea and tremors to seizures.

    IV. Infant with pulmonary hemorrhage will show bradycardia, gasping breaths, peripheral vasoconstriction, and bloody tracheal fluid.

Intervention

    I. Prevent hypoxia.

    II. Handle gently and protect during the birth process.

    III. Assist ventilation early if there are periods of bradycardia.

    IV. Monitor blood pressure, volume, and hematocrit carefully.

    V. Perform exchange transfusion of whole fresh blood, especially if disseminated intravascular coagulation is demonstrated.

    VI. Lumbar puncture may be necessary for diagnosis.

    VII. Perform serial head measurements (43).

    VIII. Maintain supportive ambient warmth, humidity, fluids, nutrition, oxygen.

INFECTION

Definition

Infection in the preterm infant may seriously jeopardize recovery since host defenses are immature. Incidence varies depending upon the aggregation of risk factors, the particular infant's condition, and the quality of care given during recovery. Prolonged ruptured membranes associated with ascending infection from a colonized vagina, birth trauma, or asphyxia with resuscitative measures predispose the infant to early onset (48 to 72 h) of symptoms. Procedures necessary in nursery care such as placement of parenteral lines for nutrition and fluids, intubation, assisted respiration, and surgical procedures, and finally and perhaps most importantly, poor handwashing by personnel may lead to later onset of infection (after 48 to 72 h) (44).

Signs and symptoms may at first be nonspecific and an infant may look well while infection becomes established. The baby may then appear not to be gaining or feeding well. There may be vomiting, diarrhea, or abdominal distension. Lethargy or irritability may increase. If septicemia or meningitis occurs, tremors, seizures, bulging fontanels, and abnormal eye movements may be present. Respiratory effort will increase, especially if infection is localized in the lung. Tachycardia, cyanosis, hypothermia, hypotension, jaundice, purpura, rashes, and edema may develop. Other associated signs and symptoms accompany severe infection, depending on the site.

Assessment

   I. Review maternal history, time of membrane rupture, and presence of other infections.
  II. Review delivery history for trauma, asphyxia, or resuscitation.
 III. Note trend in baby's vital signs, weight gain, alertness, and respiratory adjustment.
 IV. Observe for external signs of infection.

Intervention

     I. Obtain cultures of all body fluids and orifices, including cord.
    II. Obtain smears from any lesions and stool (Gram's stain).
   III. Send blood specimen to lab.
   IV. Chest x-ray will be ordered.
    V. Do serology, immunoglobulins, and coagulation studies.
   VI. Begin antibiotic parenteral therapy after cultures have been taken. Maintain therapy for 1 to 3 weeks. Observe carefully for adverse effects of the drugs (45). Infusion sites may develop inflammation. Change sites on a regular basis.
  VII. Maintain a supportive environment, providing adequate oxygen, heat, and humidity.
 VIII. Parenteral nutrition is preferred to oral feedings in early stages of infection. Gradually return to oral feedings after condition stabilizes.
   IX. Exchange transfusion may be ordered to support host defenses and to correct anemia or shock.
    X. Lumbar puncture may be ordered.
   XI. Observe umbilical area; keep clean and dry.

REFERENCES

1. A. A. Fanaroff and I. R. Merkatz, "Modern Obstetric Management of Low-Birth-Weight Infants," *Clinics in Perinatology,* **4**(1):215, March 1977.
2. C. Sarasohn, "Care of the Very Small Premature Infant," *Pediatric Clinics of North America,* **24**(3):615, August 1977.
3. A. J. Aballi, F. Costales, and H. Aces, "Variations in Findings from Neonatal Autopsies," *Pediatric Resident,* **11**:530, 1977.
4. H. S. Dweck, "The Tiny Baby: Past, Present, and Future," *Clinics in Perinatology,* **4**:(1):425, August 1977.

5. M. Johnson and J. Gash, "Transport of Neonates: A Matter of Prevention," *The Canadian Nurse,* May 1976, p. 20.
6. E. Hey, "Thermal Neutrality," *British Medical Bulletin,* **11**(1):69, 1977.
7. M. H. Klaus and A. A. Fanaroff, *Care of the High-Risk Neonate,* W. B. Saunders Company, Philadelphia, 1973, p. 68.
8. Johnson and Gash, op. cit., p. 22.
9. Klaus and Fanaroff, op. cit., p. 140.
10. L. M. S. Dubowitz, V. Dubowitz, and C. Goldberg, "Clinical Assessment of Gestational Age in the Newborn Infant," *Journal of Pediatrics,* **77**:1–10, 1970.
11. A. J. Schaeffer and M. E. Avery, *Diseases of the Newborn,* 4th ed., W. B. Saunders Company, Philadelphia, 1977, p. 27.
12. Ibid., p. 1039.
13. L. A. Barness, "Nutrition for the Low-Birth-Weight Infant," *Clinics in Perinatology,* **2**(2):347–349, September 1975.
14. Schaeffer and Avery, op. cit., p. 1040.
15. J. A. Stockman, III, "Anemia of Prematurity," *Clinics in Perinatology,* **4**(2):239, September 1977.
16. American Academy of Pediatrics, Committee on Nutrition, "Nutritional Needs of Low-Birth-Weight Infants," *Pediatrics,* **60**(4):524, October 1977.
17. Ibid., p. 519.
18. Ibid., p. 526.
19. Barness, op. cit., p. 351.
20. D. A. Clark, "Times of First Void and First Stool in 500 Newborns," *Pediatrics,* **60**(4):458, October 1977.
21. M. E. Miller, "Host Defenses in the Human Neonate," *Pediatric Clinics of North America,* **24**:43, 1977.
22. M. Green and A. J. Solnit, "Reactions to the Threatened Loss of a Child: A Vulnerable Child Syndrome," *Pediatrics,* **34**:58, 1964.
23. D. R. Dubois, "Indications of an Unhealthy Relationship Between Parents and Premature Infants," *Journal of Obstetric, Gynecologic, and Neonatal Nursing,* **4**(3):21, 1975.
24. M. Klein and L. Stern, "Low Birth Weight and the Battered Child Syndrome," *American Journal of Diseases of Children,* **122**:15, 1971.
25. C. R. Barnett, P. H. Leiderman, R. Grobstein, and M. H. Klaus, "Neonatal Separation: The Maternal Side of Interactional Deprivation," *Pediatrics,* **45**:197, 1970.
26. Klaus and Fanaroff, op. cit., p. 129.
27. W. A. Fawcett and L. Gluck, "RDS in the Tiny Baby," *Clinics in Perinatology,* **4**(2):411, September 1977.
28. Ibid., p. 414.
29. Klaus and Fanaroff, op. cit., p. 129.
30. M. A. Gottusco et al., "Exchange Transfusions in Low-Birth-Weight Infants with RDS," *Journal of Pediatrics,* **89**(2):279, August 1976.
31. L. E. V. Mirandes and H. S. Dweck, "Perinatal Glucose Homeostatis," *Clinics in Perinatology,* **4**(2):351, September 1977.
32. Sarasohn, op. cit., p. 619.
33. Schaeffer and Avery, op. cit., p. 384.
34. G. B. Odell, R. L. Poland, and E. M. Ostrea, "Neonatal Hyperbilirubinemia," in M. H. Klaus and A. A. Fanaroff (eds.), *Care of the High-Risk Neonate,* W. B. Saunders Company, Philadelphia, 1973, pp. 191–193.
35. J. W. Seligman, "Recent and Changing Concepts of Hyperbilirubinemia and Its Management in the Newborn," *Pediatric Clinics of North America,* **24**(3):509, August 1977.
36. Ibid., p. 515.
37. Klaus and Fanaroff, op. cit., p. 190.
38. E. J. Dickason, M. O. Schult, and E. M. Morris, *Maternal and Infant Drugs and Nursing Intervention,* McGraw-Hill Book Company, New York, 1978, p. 238.
39. Klaus and Fanaroff, op. cit., p. 197.
40. Seligman, op. cit., p. 515.
41. S. J. Gross and M. J. Stuart, "Hemostasis in the Premature Infant," *Clinics in Perinatology,* **4**(2): 283, September 1977.
42. Klaus and Fanaroff, op. cit., p. 142.
43. Ibid.

44. V. Schauf and D. Vidyasagar, "Critical Care Problems of the Newborn: Bacterial Colonization and Infection in the Intensive Care Unit," *Critical Care Medicine,* **4**(1):15, 1976.

45. Dickason et al., op. cit., pp. 283–288.

BIBLIOGRAPHY

Amiel-Tison, C.: "Neurologic Evaluation of the Maturity of Newborn Infants," *Archives of Diseases of Children,* **43**:89, 1968. Foundational work for gestational age evaluations.

Avery, G. B. (ed.): *Neonatology: Pathophysiology and Management of the Newborn,* J. B. Lippincott Company, Philadelphia, 1975. A reference book with many contributors who are authorities in the field of neonatology.

Cornell, E. H., and A. W. Gottfried: "Intervention with Premature Infants," *Child Development,* **47**:32, 1976. A critical review of the literature dealing with the effects of psychological intervention in the development of premature infants. Questions most methods of intervention and makes recommendations for future studies.

Fitzhardinge, P. M.: "Early Growth and Development in Low Birthweight Infants following Treatment in an Intensive Care Nursery," *Pediatrics,* **56**(2):162, August 1975. Recent survivors of intensive care are not really comparable with those in studies of 5 or 10 years ago. Methods to delineate the differences are outlined.

Harper, R. G., M. M. Sokol, and C. G. Sia: "Mothers in the Neonatal Intensive Care Unit: An Examination of Some Problems and Consequences of Modern Intensive Care on Mother-Infant Interaction," *Clinics in Perinatology,* **3**(2):441, September 1976. Facets of how to allow maternal-infant interactions during intensive neonatal care are explored.

Heird, W. C., et al.: "Newer Methods for Feeding Low Birth Weight Infants," *Clinics in Perinatology,* **2**(2):393, September 1975. A comprehensive review of methods of parenteral alimentation, precautions, and possibilities for growth.

Hull, D.: "Temperature Regulation and Disturbance in the Newborn," *Clinics in Endocrinology and Metabolism,* **5**(1): 39, March 1976. A classic review of the problem of providing thermoneutrality for the small infant.

Hunt, J. V.: "Mental Development of Preterm Infants during the First Year," *Child Development,* **48**(1):204, March 1977. A fairly complex article concerning ways of studying mental development without bias.

Kennell, J. H., H. Slyter, and M. H. Klaus: "The Mourning of Parents to the Death of a Newborn Infant," *New England Journal of Medicine,* **283**(7):344, 1970. Basic work which is included in later book, but spells out grieving process.

Korones, S. B.: *High-Risk Newborn Infants,* The C. V. Mosby Company, St. Louis, 1973. Very useful nursing reference on the newborn infant.

Luchenco, L. O.: *The High-Risk Infant,* W. B. Saunders Company, Philadelphia, 1976. Comprehensive, concise text on identification of high-risk factors with excellent descriptions of characteristics of SGA, AGA, and LGA infants, both term and preterm.

Nalepka, C. D.: "Understanding Thermoregulation in Newborns," *Journal of Obstetric, Gynecologic, and Neonatal Nursing,* **5**(6):17, December 1976. Clear description of problem with application of principles to clinical situation.

Smith, C. A., and N. M. Nelson: *The Physiology of the Newborn Infant,* Thomas, Springfield, Ill., 1976.

Stave, I.: *Physiology of the Perinatal Period,* Appleton-Century-Crofts, Inc., New York, 1970. Both this and Smith and Nelson's text are fairly complex references but are thorough in their treatment of the newborn adjustment phase.

Vulliamy, D. C.: *The Newborn Child,* Churchill-Livingstone, Longman, Inc., New York, 1977. A text-handbook of all aspects of newborn care.

12

Birth Defects: The Infant and the Family

Bonnie Silverman and Elizabeth J. Dickason

DEFINITION

Birth defects are the result of disturbances in structure or biochemical function during the preconception, pregnancy, or birth periods. They result in structural defects, growth retardation, and biochemical and behavioral effects often lasting a lifetime. It is estimated that 3 in 100 babies are born with some form of defect. Fortunately, most are minor in nature or are correctable by surgery. However, mental retardation continues to be a severe, uncorrectable result of genetic or teratogenic insults to the fragile human fetus.

Birth defects are divided into three categories: (1) genetic disorders caused by chromosomal, single-gene, or polygenic defects; (2) congenital disorders, which are the result of teratogenic or disease interference with the growth and development of the fetus in utero; (3) disorders due to birth injuries which are the result of anoxic or drug insult during labor and delivery, or due to trauma to the infant during the birth process.

Disorders Due to Genetic Defects

Chromosomal Defects[1]

I. Monosomy: absence of one of a pair of chromosomes.
   A. Autosomal monosomy.
      1. Mortality: 100 percent.
   B. Sex chromosome monosomy (Turner's syndrome): 45, XO.
      1. Incidence: 1:2500.
      2. Characteristics: short stature, shield chest, web neck, infertility, lack of secondary sex characteristics, mild mental retardation.
      3. Mortality: 98 percent abort spontaneously; 2 percent survive (2).
II. Trisomy: presence of a third chromosome, usually due to nondisjunction either at first or second meiotic division. Translocation can also occur if one or more chromosomes break and recombine in various ways.
   A. Autosomal trisomy.
      1. Trisomy 21 (Down's) syndrome: 47, XX or XY, +21.
         a. Nondisjunction, 95 percent; mosaicism, 2 to 3 percent; translocation (D/g or G/G), 2 percent.
         b. Incidence: 1:600 (1:100 among women over 40).
         c. Characteristics: mental retardation, multiple defects, macroglossia, low-set ears, epicanthal fold over eye, flat bridge on nose, simian crease in palm, abnormal hand- and footprints.
         d. Mortality: 30 percent die in first month; 60 percent by 10 years of age (3).
      2. Trisomy 18 (Edwards') syndrome: 47, XX or XY, +18.
         a. Incidence: 1:4500.
         b. Characteristics: cardiac defects, severe mental retardation, small chin, low-set ears, strangely flexed fingers, failure to thrive.
         c. Mortality: 90 percent die by 1 year of age.
      3. Trisomy 13 (Patau's) syndrome: 47, XX or XY, +13.
         a. Incidence: 1:5500.

[1] All reports of incidence are from Porter (1).

       b. Characteristics: mental retardation, microphthalmus, cleft lip and palate, polydactyly, rocker bottom feet.

       c. Mortality: rare survival after infancy.

B. Sex chromosome trisomy: extra X chromosomes do not accentuate sexual characteristics, but may contribute to mental retardation and systemic malfunctions.

   1. Triple-X syndrome: 47, XXX.

       a. Incidence: 1:1200.

       b. Characteristics: physical characteristics rarely are overt; fertility is unaffected; abnormality may pass on to offspring; mild mental retardation, but more severe with tetrasomy (XXXX) or pentasomy (XXXXX).

   2. Klinefelter's syndrome: 47, XXY.

       a. Incidence: 1:600 to 1:1000.

       b. Characteristics: IQ is affected to varying degrees, sometimes there is mild mental retardation; infertility results because of low testosterone levels and lack of testicular growth in puberty, but not usually impotence; lack of development of secondary sex characteristics in puberty may be first indication of syndrome (4).

   3. XYY syndrome: 47, XYY.

       a. Incidence: 1:1000.

       b. Characteristics: no mental retardation; fertile; very tall; muscular; aggressive; acne may continue into adulthood; appearance normal otherwise.

III. Mosaicism: due to mitotic nondisjunction, there occurs a mixed karyotype with some cells normal and some abnormal. Symptoms of above disorders are muted by the presence of cells with normal chromosome configurations. Gonadal dysgenesis may occur, resulting in infants who appear to have a male-female phenotype. Often the mosaicism occurs with XO (Turner's) syndrome.

IV. Double fertilization (true hermaphroditism): "Origin is probably double fertilization of a binucleate egg since such patients have two distinct sets of blood groups" (5). Fifty percent have only XX cells present, 25 percent have only XY cells present, and 25 percent are mosaics. At birth, infant is seen to have ambiguous genitalia or cryptorchidism, hypospadias, and failure of labioscrotal fusion.

V. Abnormal structure: deletions or translocations of parts of an individual chromosome can lead to extensive effects in the infant. Mental retardation is universal, and cardiac disease occurs often.

A. Cri-du-chat syndrome: 46, XX or XY, 5p−.

   1. Characteristics: mental retardation, microcephaly, weak cat cry, cardiac defects, failure to thrive, short stature, low-set ears, simian crease in palm, and many more possible anomalies.

B. Deletions are also possible at chromosomes 4, 9, 13, 18, 21, and 22.

Single-gene Defects[2]

I. Autosomal gene defects.

A. Autosomal dominant and recessive disorders affect males and females with equal frequency.

B. Each person carries five to eight recessive, deleterious genes (one gene–one function).

C. If a child is conceived by parents, each of whom carry the same defective autosomal recessive gene, there is a 1:4 chance of overt disease in the child.

D. A defective autosomal dominant gene is passed directly to the next generation. A child has a 1:2 chance of inheriting a disease when one parent has such a dominant gene.

E. There are over 1200 dominant gene defects that contribute to disease. For example:

   1. Genetic hyperlipidemia: contributes to premature coronary artery disease.

   2. Gastrointestinal polyposis: predisposes to cancer of the gastrointestinal tract.

[2]All reports of incidence are from Erbe (6).

3. Multiple neurofibromatosis (von Recklinghausen's disease): multiple skin tumors, CNS involvement, hypertension, lower fertility.
4. Achondroplasia (Marfan's syndrome): failure of long bone growth, ocular lens dislocation.
5. Retinoblastoma: tumor of eye in young infant; fatal if untreated.

F. There are over 900 recessive gene defects. These tend to follow racial lines, but intermarriage and migration reduce the number of individuals with homozygous genes needed for the passage of these diseases. For example:
   1. Most inborn errors of metabolism. Major examples (7) are:
      a. Phenylketonuria: 1:10,000 incidence in those of Northern European ancestry. Diet restrictions can allow normal growth and development. Precautions must be taken during the childbearing period.
      b. Tay-Sachs disease: 1:6000 incidence in those of Eastern European Ashkenazi Jewish ancestry. Carriers occur with an incidence of 1:30. Infants with Tay-Sachs disease do not survive past 2 to 3 years of age.
   2. Cystic fibrosis: 1:2000 incidence in newborns of Middle European ancestry. Life expectancy now extends past puberty.
   3. Sickle cell anemia: 1:625 incidence in newborns of African or Mediterranean ancestry. Follows geographic lines of high incidence of malaria.

II. Sex-linked gene defects.
   A. A normal X chromosome can dominate ("Lyonize") an abnormal gene on a second X chromosome; therefore, females can carry trait or have only mild to moderate symptoms. Males always show disease if they have the abnormal X chromosome, since the Y chromosome does not counterbalance the effect. The most common diseases include the following (8):
      1. Glucose 6-phosphate dehydrogenase (G6PD): predisposes individuals to hemolytic disease on exposure to certain foods and drugs. 12:100 incidence among black males, 1:140 incidence among black females, 24:100 black females are carriers. G6PD follows the same worldwide geographic distribution as do sickling diseases.
      2. Duchenne's muscular dystrophy: 1:10,000 incidence among males; rarely survive teenage period.
      3. Hemophilia: 1:8000 incidence among males, mostly from Northern European ancestry. Only recently have they survived the teenage period.
      4. Red-green color blindness: 10:100 incidence among males of Arab, Caucasian, or Ashkenazi Jewish ancestry. Lower rates exist in other groups studied, but the disorder is very widespread throughout the world.

Polygenic Defects and Multifactorial Disorders

A combination of genes and environment affects all inherited characteristics. Polygenic inheritance underlies the predisposition for certain diseases passed on in families. This predisposition, when combined with unfavorable environmental factors, may result in overt signs of the disease. The risk of inheritance is difficult to calculate and is much smaller than with single-gene defects. Among the major disorders thought to be due to polygenic inheritance are those listed below, categorized as appearing either at birth and in infancy, or later in childhood and adult life (9).

Infancy	*Childhood and Later*
Anencephaly	Coronary artery disease
Spina bifida	Diabetes mellitus
Congenital dislocation of hip	Gout
Congenital heart disease (some types)	Hypertension
Cleft lip, plus cleft palate	Schizophrenia
Pyloric stenosis	

Congenital Disorders Due to Environmental Factors

Teratogenic agents (teratogens) are "one or more mechanisms that cause cells to die, change their rate of proliferation or biosynthesis, or otherwise fail to follow their prescribed course in development" (10). Genetic susceptibility, dosage level and duration, and the specific day of embryonic development that coincides with drug intake are major factors influencing drug effect. In addition, maternal health and nutrition, placental functioning, and numerous other factors will be influential in whether or not a specific teratogenic agent does in fact have an injurious effect on the developing human. Such agents are thought to be the cause of 2 to 3 percent of birth defects and to contribute to a large number of unknown causes for disability or dysfunction in the developing human (see Table 12-1).

TABLE 12-1 / POSITIVELY ASSOCIATED TERATOGENIC AGENTS

Agents	*Adverse Effects*
Radiation:	
Low dose	Increased incidence of leukemia in prepubertal child, genetic mutations
High dose	Early abortion, microcephaly
Antimetabolites:	Inhibited cell proliferation, early abortion, multiple anomalies
Alkylating agents	
Folic acid antagonists	
Antibiotics:	
Streptomycin	Injury to eighth cranial nerve
Tetracycline	Long bone and tooth deposits, some bone growth inhibition
Steroid hormones:	
Androgenic agents	Masculinization of female fetus
Estrogenic agents	Abortion (high doses)
Nonsteroid hormones:	Vaginal adenosis with possibility of adenocarcinoma when female approaches puberty; effect on male shows higher rate of gonadal dysfunction
Estrogenic agents (DES)	
Heavy metals:	Abortion, multiple deformities
Lead	
Mercury	
Infectious agents:	
Chickenpox	CNS damage, skin lesions, fetal death
Coxsackie virus B	Infection of fetal cardiac and CNS tissue
Cytomegalovirus	Microcephaly, cerebral calcification, jaundice, stunted growth
Herpes simplex	Disseminated infection, residual CNS damage
Mumps	Sometimes early embryo death
Rubella	Cardiac defects, cataracts, deafness, microcephaly, mental retardation, persisting neonatal infection
Smallpox	Fetal smallpox, death
Vaccinia (smallpox vaccination)	Fetal infection, death(?)
Syphilis	Bone and tooth deformities, progressive CNS damage
Toxoplasma	Microcephaly, cerebral calcifications, chorioretinitis

Source: After J. G. Wilson, "Environmental Effects on Developmental Teratology," N. Assali and C. R. Brinkman (eds.), *Pathophysiology of Gestation: Fetal Disorders,* vol. 2, Academic Press, Inc., New York, 1972.

Disorders Due to Drug Effects and Birth Trauma

The transitional period before birth is a highly sensitive one, since any drugs in the maternal system usually reach the fetus. After birth, without the maternal excretory mechanisms, the infant must metabolize and excrete dosages near to or higher than maternal levels. Immaturity of body functions will result in extended periods before drugs are finally excreted from the infant's body. Drugs used during labor are especially implicated, but chronic drug intake (addiction) or drugs given for maternal disease may also have adverse effects. All resulting effects of maternal drugs in the newborn should be thought of like "withdrawal" effects, and careful monitoring of signs and symptoms is necessary. Supportive therapy is of course supplied if needed. Anoxic trauma and mechanical injury are prevented by careful perinatal monitoring and judicious use of oxytocics, analgesics, and anesthetics (see Chap. 8).

ASSESSMENT

I. Take health history, seeking similar defects in extended family.
II. Determine karyotype and test for carrier state of parents and any siblings. Amniocentesis may be recommended to a known family of carriers, but is only advised if abortion is an option, since currently no treatment is available (see Fig. 12-1).
III. Physical examination of child and parents is needed.
IV. Assess family strength and support system.

PROBLEMS

I. Family response to defect may be any combination of fear, shock, grief, confusion, and anxiety.
II. Difficulties in care will be presented by problems of infant.

DIAGNOSIS

I. Family faces adjustment to an imperfect infant.
II. Family is grieving and does/does not have adequate support.
III. Infant is in need of special care and services.

GOALS OF CARE

I. Immediate.
  A. The family will receive supportive care after delivery.
  B. The staff will adopt a unified approach to the family.
  C. The staff will recognize and support normal grief (Fig. 12-2).
  D. The need for therapeutic intervention may be indicated by signs of reduced coping, increased hostility, and guilt.
  E. Parents will be included as soon as possible in care of infant.
II. Long-range.
  A. Parents and staff will identify problems facing the family in home care of infant.
  B. Planning will be done together for such care.
  C. Parents will understand nutrition and techniques of feeding.
  D. Referrals will be made to appropriate agencies and the visiting nurse service.
  E. The family will be assisted in considerations about therapy to correct defect, if possible.

F. When parents are ready, repeat pregnancies, genetic counseling, and future amniocentesis will be considered.

INTERVENTION

I. Provide for continuity of care by the same staff.
II. Provide parents a quiet time to grieve and offer support.
III. Assess grief and possible depression; refer when necessary.
IV. Assess responses to information given by physician and include family in this assessment.

FIGURE 12-1 / Amniocentesis: (a) needle placement; (b) sites of insertion. Ultrasound evaluation of placental location and fetal position precedes all amniocentesis attempts. (*From E. J. Dickason and M. O. Schult, Maternal and Infant Care, McGraw-Hill Book Company, New York, 1975.*)

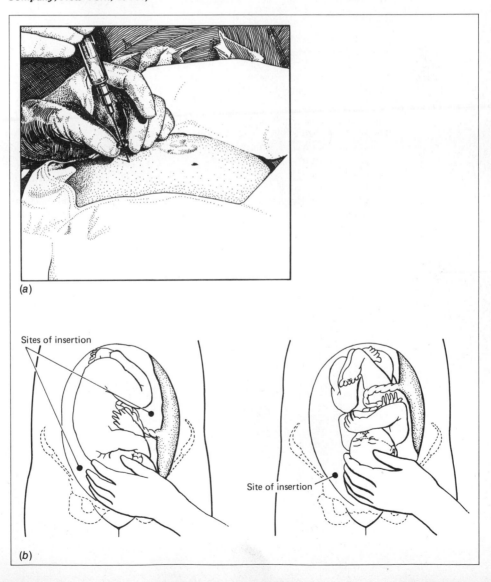

V. Teach home care of infant, providing time to practice and for confidence to develop.
VI. Teach growth and developmental guidelines for next period before return to clinic.
VII. Assist mother and father in problems of meeting family expectations.
VIII. Refer to agencies that can assist in home care if necessary, and participate in referrals to agencies for children with defects.
IX. Refer to social service for financial assistance if necessary.
X. Follow through on evaluation of adjustment in 4 to 6 weeks (see Table 12-2).

EVALUATION

I. Evaluate follow-through on homegoing plans. Check with the visiting nurse service or clinic, and make a home visit whenever possible.
II. Assess acceptance of infant and parenting responsibility and assess ability to cope with physical care.
III. Reevaluate infant's status regularly and work toward alleviation of problems using team approach.

CASE STUDY

Assessment

Health History   *Name:* Joan Brown   *Age:* 17

PSYCHOSOCIAL ASSESSMENT
Home situation   Lives with 27-year-old husband who is a waiter in local restaurant. Couple lives in a three-room apartment, but plans to move soon. Parents are divorced, and she has one married sister. Husband's family is in Ecuador.

FIGURE 12-2 / **Hypothetical model of sequence of normal parental reactions to birth of a child with congenital malformations. (*After D. Drotar, A. Baskiewicz, N. Irvin, J. H. Kennell, and M. H. Klaus, Pediatrics, 56:710–717, November 1975.*)**

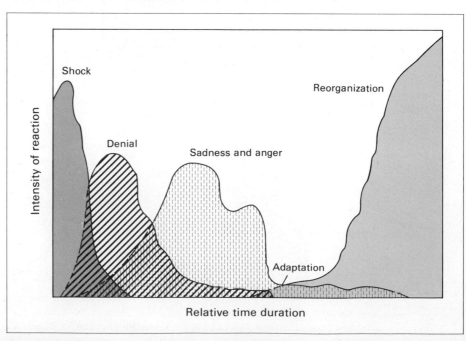

TABLE 12-2 / CONGENITAL ANOMALY QUESTIONNAIRE FORMAT

I. Parental perception of the child's deformity.
  A. When did you first suspect your baby had a problem?
  B. How did you find out?
  C. What were you told?
  D. When?
  E. How did you feel?
II. Parental feelings.
  A. What has happened since then with the baby?
  B. With both of you?
III. Assessment of parental attachment.
  A. Does it seem like the baby is yours? When?
  B. Do you feel close to the baby?
  C. When did you start to feel close to the baby?
  D. Do you consider your baby cuddly?
  E. How did you go about naming the baby?
IV. Effects of the anomaly.
  A. Could you go back to the time of the baby's birth and say how each of you had adapted to the situation?
  B. Have you shared your feelings together?
  C. How much have you cried?
  D. Do you find yourself very blue? Very angry? Irritable?
  E. Have you found yourself doing unusual things? Having unusual thoughts?
  F. Has there been a change in your health?
  G. Your outlook for the future?
  H. Your eating? Sleeping? Dreaming? Mood?
  I. What changes have you noticed in each other, in your friends, and in your relatives?
  J. Could you compare your family life since the baby was born with the way it was before?
V. Parental attitudes toward handling of the situation.
  A. To review, could you tell me again what stages you remember going through since the baby was born?
  B. What helped?
  C. What didn't help?
  D. What suggestions would you have for other families in the same situation?
  E. What could doctors or nurses do that would be helpful?

Source: D. Drotar, A. Baskiewicz, N. Irvin, J. Kennell, and M. Klaus: "The Adaptation of Parents to the Birth of an Infant with a Congenital Malformation: A Hypothetical Model," *Pediatrics,* **56**(5):712, November 1975.

Education Patient has 11th grade education. Began secretarial school; wants to work after pregnancy.

Economic status Adequate income for support of family and new baby. Husband has medical coverage. Ms. Brown's father contributes each month to family's income.

Support system Good. Wife's parents, although divorced, offer help and demonstrate interest in couple. Husband is actively involved with Ms. Brown's family and seems happy.

Reactions to pregnancy *Activities of daily living* (**ADL**) Feels nauseated in morning and has increased fatigue.
  Marital/sexual Has been having unprotected intercourse for past 6 to 8 months. Used condoms for awhile but feels they are "too messy." No plans for future methods of contraception. Frequency of relations now decreasing due to fatigue.

Behavior during interview Slow to warm up. Answers questions adequately without volunteering additional information. Avoids eye contact at times.

Assessment of child abuse potential Antepartum assessment at this time indicates low risk (see Table 7-4).

Appearance Wearing clean jeans and T-shirt. Hair, makeup, and appearance are appropriate for age. Well developed, well nourished, in no distress.

Drugs, alcohol, tobacco Smokes one pack of cigarettes per day. No other intake.

GENETIC ASSESSMENT
See family tree (Fig. 12-3).

PAST HEALTH HISTORY

Obstetric history Para: 0. LMP: 8/10. EDD: 5/18.

Menstrual history Onset: 11 years. Frequency: every 28 days. Duration: 5 days. Moderate dysmenorrhea.

Medical history Childhood illnesses: measles, rubella, mumps, chickenpox. Vaccinations: up to date. Allergies: none known. Hospitalizations: at 7 years for diagnosis of diabetes.

Present health problems Class D diabetes. Approximately 10 weeks pregnant.

Medications 40 U NPH, once daily in morning.

Physical Assessment

Vital signs Temperature: 37°C. Pulse: 87 beats per minute. Respiration: 24 breaths per minute. Blood pressure: 98/74.

Height and weight 5 ft 3 in, 105½ lb (usually 103 lb).

General appearance WDWN white female in no apparent distress.

Chief complaint Amenorrhea for one cycle, "tingly" breasts, nausea, fatigue.

Review of systems HEENT: within normal limits (WNL). Heart: RSR, 87 bpm, no murmurs. Chest: clear to P&A. Breasts: glandular, no masses or discharge. Abdomen: soft. Orthopedics: WNL. Extremities and skin: WNL; no edema, varicosities, or lesions. Pelvis: adequate, no prominent spines. Uterus: approximately 10 weeks pregnant. Cervix: nulliparous.

Problems

Active Date	*Medical Problems*	*Nursing Problems*
10/14 (admission to obstetric clinic)	1. Class D diabetes mellitus.	1. Pregnant teenager demonstrates lack of understanding of physical condition and denies diabetic needs.
	2. Intrauterine pregnancy of 10 weeks' duration.	
11/16 (second trimester clinic visit)	3. Unexplained albuminuria.	
3/22 (admission to hospital for regulation)	4. Discharged against advice.	2. Noncompliance with health care goals.
4/21 (delivery and recovery period)	5. Birth of LGA infant with cleft lip and palate.	3. Grieving parents.
		4. Acceptance of infant with defect, and care of infant.
		5. Family planning information is needed.

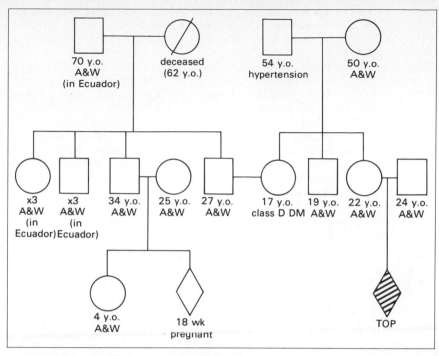

FIGURE 12-3 / The Brown family genetic history.

Diagnosis

I. 10/14: Pregnant 17-year-old has poorly controlled diabetes mellitus and lack of understanding of both diabetes mellitus and pregnancy.

II. 11/15: Patient demonstrates noncompliance with medical and nursing goals and denies existence of any problems.

III. 4/22: Family is grieving after birth of infant with cleft lip and palate.

Goals of Care

I. Immediate.
   A. Patient will be educated about diabetes and pregnancy.
   B. Diabetes will be controlled and regular clinic visits continued.
   C. Trust will be sought between patient and staff to facilitate these goals.
II. Long-range.
   A. The safest possible delivery will be sought.
   B. Recovery will occur without complications.
   C. Positive parent-infant bonding will occur.
   D. Parent education for family planning will be provided.
   E. Parent education for care for an infant with a defect will be provided.
   F. Follow-up will be planned for the infant.
   G. Evaluation of team support of family during grief and resolution of grief and of family's recovery process will be done by perinatal staff.

Intervention and Evaluation

In this patient, diabetes and pregnancy are affected by behavior normally present in adolescence. Resistance to authority and problems following a strict diet and exercise regimen are accompanied by a lack of knowledge about her condition and a tendency to focus on the present (11). In addition, she tends to concentrate on her own physical feelings, demonstrating some problem with progressing through the developmental tasks of pregnancy.

Many teenage mothers show lack of understanding of child care and the needs of the baby. Some conceive with the hope that "the baby will love me and I'll have someone to live for" (12). Interventions for such an adolescent with pregnancy complicated by diabetes will include the following.

    I. Immediate intervention.

        A. Reassess behavior periodically to note progression through developmental tasks.

        B. Give education about diabetes and pregnancy in terms she can comprehend. Find other, more mature diabetic who has gone successfully through a pregnancy to share how she managed.

        C. Medical plan will include:

            1. Weekly clinic visits with regulation in hospital once or twice during the pregnancy (this was refused by patient). (See Table 12-3.)

            2. Baseline studies: ultrasound, blood work, urinalysis, ophthalmologic evaluation. After 32 weeks, estriols, urine culture, and oxytocin challenge test (OCT) will be added.

            3. Weekly checks on weight, glucose, acetone, and albumin in urine. Vital signs, fundal height, and fetal heart evaluation will be included.

            4. Evaluation of diabetes with fasting blood sugar (FBS), insulin, and diet counseling. FBS may be 60 to 80 mg per 100 mL, and random blood sugar should be under 120 mg per 100 mL. Sugar in urine may spill to 1+ without concern.

TABLE 12-3 / SUMMARY OF PRENATAL PROGRESS AT FIRST HOSPITAL ADMISSION (3/22)

Medical Problems	Note
Problem 1	*Subjective:* "Feels fine." *Objective:* No symptoms of hypo- or hyperglycemia. FBS, 65–70% 4 P.M. blood sugar, 180. Fractional urines: glucose, 2+ to negative; acetone, negative. Receiving NPH 42 U and regular insulin 8 U at 7 A.M., plus 5 U NPH at 10 P.M. followed by snack. Weight, 115–120 lb. *Assessment:* Stable but requires observation to maintain control. *Plan:* Continue insulin as above; recommend hospitalization until delivery. Put on 2500-cal diet and take daily weights.
Problem 2	*Subjective:* Feels baby move. *Objective:* Fetal heart rate, 140–150 bpm (left lower quadrant). Ultrasound monitoring and uterine size are consistent with date. Estriols are 15.8 and rising. Oxytocin challenge test 1 is negative. *Assessment:* No uteroplacental insufficiency at present. Condition stable but needs continued assessment. *Plan:* Delivery timed to OCTs, estriols, L/S ratio, and progress of diabetes. Measure estriols daily and OCTs weekly. Employ ultrasound for placental location and then amniocentesis for L/S by 36 weeks.
Problem 3	*Subjective:* No headaches, blurred vision, or fainting. *Objective:* 3+ albuminuria since 15th week of pregnancy; 1+ since admission. Blood pressure is within normal range. Deep-tendon reflexes (DTR), 2+ with no edema. Weight decreased with bed rest. *Assessment:* Renal consultation indicates that preeclampsia or renal disease cannot be determined at present. *Plan:* Monitor albuminuria, blood pressure, edema, and reflexes. Re-evaluate kidney status after delivery.

TABLE 12-3 / SUMMARY OF PRENATAL PROGRESS AT FIRST HOSPITAL ADMISSION (3/22) *(Continued)*

Medical Problems	Note
Problem 4	*Subjective:* Feels fine; cannot understand reason for "fuss." *Objective:* Patient refuses continued hospitalization until delivery; signed release against medical advice. *Assessment:* Patient continues to deny any problems of diabetes or pregnancy and needs primary care follow-up. *Plan:* Refer to perinatal nurse clinician (PNC). Patient promises to return weekly to clinic.

Nursing Problems	Note
Problem 1	*Subjective:* She states, "I've had diabetes for 10 years and can take care of myself. I don't have problems with insulin or testing urine." *Objective:* Does not rotate insulin sites; uses only upper arms and thighs. Has lipodystrophy in these areas. Cannot describe diet. Injection technique is correct, yet uses fixed insulin amount regardless of carbohydrate intake or physical symptoms. Not sure what to do with facts about ketoacidosis or hypoglycemia. Foot care adequate. *Assessment:* Appears to resent any supervision, yet lacks knowledge in several important areas. *Plan:* Diabetic nurse specialist will teach insulin administration, urine testing, dietary needs, and rationale for care. Encourage patient to talk with nurse about her condition. Reinforce strengths. Set limits for behavior affecting health of pregnancy.
Problem 2	*Subjective:* "Pregnancy is nothing to worry about. I just wish the baby would come out. I'm tired of these pregnancy clothes." *Objective:* Signed a release for discharge against medical advice. No one can ascertain why she is so adamant about leaving. *Assessment:* Lack of understanding of pregnancy continues; attempts to educate have not been successful. *Plan:* To be seen by PNC who will make new plan with patient and follow with primary care through rest of pregnancy, labor, and delivery and with baby in nursery.

D. After hospital admission the nursing plan of care will include:
1. Once referred to perinatal nurse clinician (PNC) for primary care, patient, physician, and nurse will agree on goals.
2. The following plans were agreed upon after Ms. Brown was discharged against advice on 3/25. She agreed to new plans.
   a. Weekly visits for evaluation of pregnancy and diabetes.
   b. At least one visit with diabetic nurse specialist and nutritionist.
   c. Conference with PNC at each weekly visit to learn about labor, delivery, child care, and birth control methods.
   d. Visits will include measurement of OCTs and estriols as per medical plan. OCTs will be done by PNC (Fig. 12-4).
3. These learning objectives were set for Ms. Brown:
   a. By 4/21 she will be able to explain in lay terms why estriols, determining the lecithin/spingomyelin (L/S) ratio, and OCTs are necessary for her care.
   b. She will be able to name three signs of impending labor and will know how to obtain help.

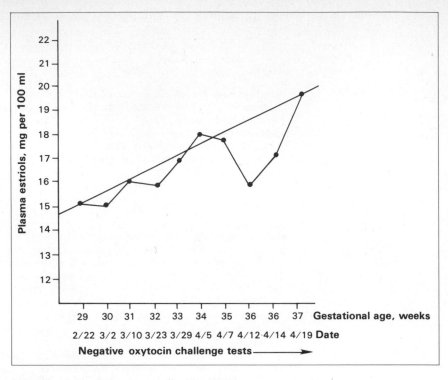

FIGURE 12-4 / General trend of rising estriols.

   c. She will be able to describe three methods of birth control and have some
      idea of which method she may choose.
II. Evaluation of immediate intervention.
   A. Perinatal nurse clinician has seen patient weekly since 3/29. Diabetic and nutritional
      counseling has been accomplished. She has met learning objectives identified on
      3/29.
   B. Patient continues to spill 2+ to 3+ sugar in the urine but has considerably expanded
      her knowledge of diabetes. She has learned to rotate injection sites.
   C. Amniocentesis performed for L/S ratio on 4/19 showed L/S = 1.5:1, creatinine = 1.8
      percent, and nile blue staining = 1 percent of cells. Ms. Brown realizes that this
      means the infant is still immature at this time (see Table 12-4).
III. Long-range intervention admission No. 2: (delivery and follow-up care of mother and
   baby).
   A. The safest possible delivery will be sought. Monitoring was carried out continuously,
      no oxytocin was given, and very low doses of analgesia were given within the
      guidelines of the age, anxiety, and preparation of the mother. Fetal gestational age
      was assessed at 36 weeks, with an estimated weight of 6 to 7 lb. Diabetic status was
      under control, but unexplained proteinuria continued.
      1. After one episode of sustained bradycardia, oxygen at 6 L was administered and
         patient positioned on left side. Bradycardia was not greatly improved and
         delivery intervention began.
      2. Under regional anesthesia, a LOA, midforceps delivery of a viable female infant
         took place. Apgar score was 5 at 1 min, and 8 at 5 min. Infant weighing 7 lb
         14 oz has complete unilateral (left side) cleft lip and palate. Infant required
         suctioning only and was taken to special care nursery in fairly good condition.
   B. Recovery will occur without complications. Ms. Brown was transferred in good
      condition. An intravenous infusion of 5% dextrose and one-third normal saline and

20 U of oxytocin was discontinued when absorbed. Insulin was given only by coverage after fractional urines: for 3+ sugar, 5 U; for 4+, 10 U. Insulin requirements will be adjusted before discharge. Involution proceeded without complication.

C. Positive maternal-infant bonding will occur. Ms. Brown was told of her baby's cleft lip and palate when she arrived in the recovery room. Her initial responses were: "Can you fix it?" and "Will she be all right?" Mr. Brown was told when the baby was brought to the nursery. He asked to see the baby and then began to cry. The following recommendations for care (13) were used as a guide to intervention in this crisis:

1. Initial contact was made as soon as possible. Baby Brown was shown to her parents shortly after the deformity was explained to them. Ms. Brown's reaction was, "It's not as bad as I thought."

2. Positive emphasis was stressed. The fact that the defect was not life-threatening was emphasized, as was the baby's initially successful adjustment to extrauterine life.

3. Tranquilizers were avoided. The Brown family suffered bouts of crying and restlessness during the first stage (shock) of their grieving. A mild sedative was given to Ms. Brown at bedtime, but other emotion-blunting drugs were not used.

4. Special caretaking was necessary during this period. It was advisable to have one nurse available to the family for the whole period of their stay. The PNC spent long periods of time allowing the family to ventilate emotions, encouraging parent-infant contact, answering questions, and teaching infant care.

5. Prolonged contact was emphasized. "The mother of the normal infant goes through a period of one to three days in which she gradually realigns the image in her mind of the baby she expected with the image of the actual baby she delivered" (14). Increased contact between mother and infant was allowed to compensate for this adjustment of images.

6. Visiting periods need flexibility. Mr. Brown spent long periods with his wife and child. Grandparents visited, saw and held baby, and were present at feeding times, when teaching was done.

7. Progression was at the parents' pace. By asking the parents questions, such as "How does the baby look to you?", the understanding, emotional reactions, and coping mechanisms could be assessed. Plans could be altered to meet the needs of the family.

D. Parent education for family planning will be provided.

1. Perinatal nurse clinician taught methods of family planning prior to delivery, and mother attended postpartum classes. She has elected to use an IUD.

2. Appointment for family planning clinic set for 4 weeks from discharge. Caution given about use of alternate method if intercourse occurs before clinic visit.

E. Parent education is given for care of infant with defect.

1. Perinatal nurse clinician taught methods of general infant care prior to delivery.

2. After delivery, both parents participated in care. There were several home visits by PNC and telephone counseling.

3. Appropriate literature was provided on growth and development.

F. Follow-up will be planned for infant.

1. Parents will be encouraged to join a parent's group at hospital where infant has surgery. Support during this process is important.

2. Plans for surgery and immediate and long-range recovery care will be discussed in detail with parents.

3. Genetic counseling will be encouraged.

4. Referrals to the visiting nurse service will be made.

5. Regular returns to well-baby clinic will be encouraged with contact made with PNC for encouragement and liaison with pediatric-obstetric team.

G. Evaluation of team support of family during grief and resolution of grief and of family's recovery process will be done by perinatal staff (see Table 12-2).

TABLE 12-4 / SUMMARY OF CLINIC RECORD

Dates	Estimated Duration of Gestation, Weeks	Weight, lb	Blood Pressure	Fetal Status		
				Fundal Height, cm	Fetal Heart Rate*	Ultrasound Monitoring
10/14	10	105	98/74	10	—	Agrees with date
11/23	16	106	120/70	16	—	—
11/30†						
12/4†						
12/14	19	108	120/68	17	—	—
3/3	30	118	120/70	28	+/Vtx	—
3/29	34	120	120/90	30	+/Vtx	Agrees with date
4/14	36	130	125/95	33	+/Vtx	Agrees with date

*+/Vtx = heart beat heard; infant in vertex position.
†Did not show up for scheduled visits at clinic. Phone disconnected.

IV. Evaluation of long-range intervention.
  A. At 1 month, infant is being fed correctly and is gaining weight.
  B. Family displays warmth and affection toward infant.
  C. Plans are complete for surgical repair. Parents have been referred to CL/CP Parents support group.
  D. Mother continues to struggle with taking responsibility for own diabetic control. She is keeping clinic appointments, however.
  E. Transfer conference with pediatric clinic and diabetic clinic initiated by physician and PNC.

REFERENCES

1. I. H. Porter, "The Clinical Side of Cytogenetics," *Journal of Reproductive Medicine,* **17**(1):3–15, July 1976.
2. Ibid., p. 10.
3. Ibid., p. 5.
4. P. S. Gerald, "Sex Chromosome Disorders," *New England Journal of Medicine,* **294**:706, 1976.
5. Porter, op. cit, p. 14.
6. R. W. Erbe, "Principles of Medical Genetics," *New England Journal of Medicine,* **294**:281, 480, 1976.
7. Ibid., p. 480.
8. Ibid., p. 381.
9. Ibid., p. 481.
10. J. G. Wilson, "Environmental Effects on Developmental Teratology," in N. Assali and C. R. Brinkman (eds.), *Pathophysiology of Gestation: Fetal Disorders,* vol. II, Academic Press, Inc., New York, 1972, p. 271.

	Maternal Status							
	Urinalysis			Blood Sugar			Daily Caloric Intake	Daily Insulin Dosage‡
Estriols	Fractional Sugar	Acetone	Albumin	Fasting	2 h	5 h		
—	N	N	N	—	111	—	2300	40 U NPH
—	N	N	2+	65	136	40	—	45 U NPH + 5 U reg
—	3+	N	3+	—	—	—	—	42 U NPH + 4 U reg
15.1	3+	N	3+	—	—	—	—	42 U NPH + 4 U reg
16.9	2+	N	2+	70	—	180§	2500	42 U NPH + 8 U reg, 5 U NPH at 5 P.M.
17.4	2+	N	2+	—	—	—	—	42 U NPH + 8 U reg, 5 U NPH at 5 P.M.

‡Administered in morning, unless specified otherwise.
§At 4 P.M.

11. J. McFarlane and C. C. Hames, "Children with Diabetes: Learning Self-care At Camp," *American Journal of Nursing,* **73**(8):1362, 1973.
12. L. Fosburgh, "The Make-believe World of Teen-age Maternity," *The New York Times Magazine,* August 7, 1976.
13. M. H. Klaus and J. H. Kennell, *Maternal-Infant Bonding,* The C. V. Mosby Company, St. Louis, 1976, pp. 203–208.
14. D. Drotar, A. Baskiewicz, N. Irvin, J. H. Kennell, and M. H. Klaus, "The Adaptation of Parents to the Birth of an Infant with a Congenital Malformation: A Hypothetical Model," *Pediatrics,* **56**(5): 710, November 1975.

BIBLIOGRAPHY

Dunn, P. E.: "Pregnancy Complicated by Diabetes," unpublished case presentation, Adelphi University, Perinatal Nurse Clinician Program, November 18, 1976.
Eppink, H.: "Genetic Causes of Abnormal Fetal Development and Inherited Disease," *Journal of Obstetrics and Gynecologic Nursing,* **6**:14, September–October 1977. A review of the technical principles of genetics and inherited disease with basic terms defined and genetic history (pedigree) illustrated and explained.
Erbe, R. W.: "Principles of Medical Genetics," *New England Journal of Medicine,* **294**:281, 480, 1976. Current review in clearly described language.
Floyd, C. C.: "A Defective Child is Born: A Study of Newborns with Spina Bifida and Hydrocephalus," *Journal of Obstetric, Gynecologic, and Neonatal Nursing,* **6**(4):56, 1977. Study of 11 mothers during the process of grieving in the first week, with suggestions for intervention.
Gerald, P. S.: "Sex Chromosome Disorders," *New England Journal of Medicine,* **294**(7):706, March 25, 1976. Concise survey of topic for practitioners.
Miller, K. L.: *Before We Are Born: Basic Embryology and Birth Defects,* W. B. Saunders Company, Philadelphia, 1974. Well-illustrated explanation of origins of birth defects due to genetic or congenital causes.

White, Priscilla: "Diabetes in Pregnancy," *Clinics in Perinatology,* **1**(2):331, September 1975. Complete overview of care.

Wilson, J. G., and F. C. Frazer (eds.): Handbook of Teratology, Plenum Publishing Corporation, New York, 1977. Up-to-date compilation of results of environmental effects on the human infant.

Young, R. K.: "Chronic Sorrow: Parents' Response to the Birth of a Child with a Defect," *Journal of Maternal and Child Nursing,* **2**:38, January–February 1977. Describes continuing support needed by such a family.

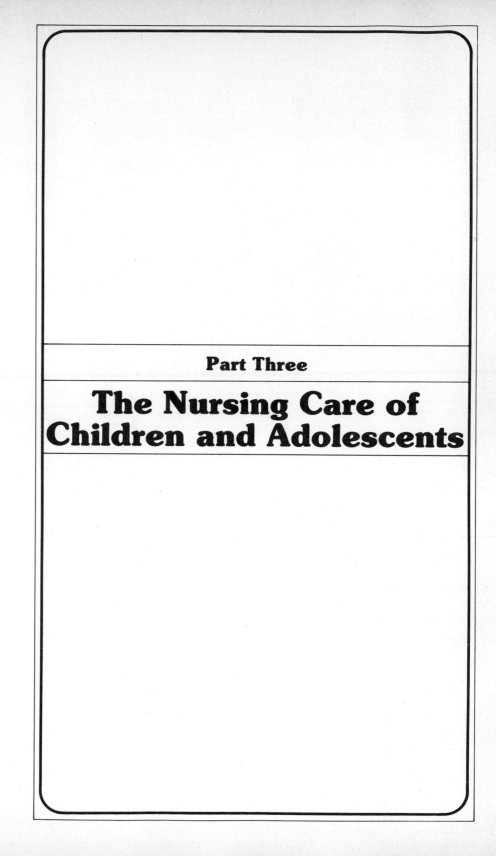

Part Three

The Nursing Care of Children and Adolescents

In the following chapters, nurses selected for excellence in their respective pediatric clinical practice specialties present essential child and family care information arranged according to the steps of the nursing process. Most of the chapters open with an overview of nursing assessment as it pertains to children who may have some health problem related to the body system under discussion in the chapter. The complete nursing process is then presented for specific health disorders; that is, the authors list focuses and techniques of assessment, identify problems, state goals, recommend interventions, and specify evaluation criteria.

In preparing their chapters, the authors have been guided by the standards of care developed by the American Nurses' Association Division on Maternal-Child Health Nursing Practice. Those standards are listed at the beginning of Part 2, "Maternity Nursing."

13
The Cardiovascular System
Mary Gorman Hazinski

GENERAL ASSESSMENT

General Comments

I. Procedure of assessment.
- A. Children must often be assessed in an informal way.
  1. Consider child's physical and emotional tolerance levels.
  2. First obtain any resting vital signs or measurements (e.g., observation of color at rest, respiratory rate and effort during sleep, auscultation of heart sounds) *before* disturbing child. Reserve most uncomfortable or intrusive procedures until later in exam.
  3. Consider developmental level of patient.
     - a. Infants may be distracted by faces, gentle voices, or brightly colored objects.
     - b. Toddlers may feel extremely threatened by exam (especially if forced into a reclining position). Try to perform assessment on primary caretaker's lap.
     - c. Preschool and school-age children often enjoy participating in exam. Provide reasonable choices and appropriate explanations, and allow them to play with equipment and examine you.
     - d. Adolescents may become extremely self-conscious during examination. Ensure privacy (as for any child) and drape parts of body not being examined.
- B. Perform as much of the assessment as possible during play.
  1. Observe psychomotor, cognitive, and psychosocial skills demonstrated.
  2. Note physical tolerance of activity.
  3. Observe child-family interaction.
  4. Obtain resting level vital signs.
- C. Include child *and* family in assessment.
  1. Take cues from them to discover areas of concern.
  2. Mother may feel frustrated or guilty about illness—she may feel she has "failed" to keep child healthy.
  3. Presence of congenital lesion may cause parents to feel guilty for conceiving and giving birth to a less than perfect infant.
     - a. Mourning process may result (grief at loss of a perfect child cannot be completely resolved, as condition is chronic).
     - b. Parents may feel they caused the heart disease.
  4. Parents will need reassurance, support, and understanding.
  5. Explore emotional responses of child and family to health and illness.
  6. If parent(s) are not the primary caretaker(s), health history must also be obtained from that caretaker.

II. Assess cardiac and respiratory systems.
- A. Often symptoms of heart disease have noncardiac manifestations. Watch for nonspecific symptoms (e.g., feeding or play patterns may be affected first).
- B. Respiratory or cardiac pathology may cause symptoms in both systems (assess both together).

Child's Health History

I. General health.
- A. Ask parent to describe child's health in word or phrase (days of school missed may help to define this).

B. Separate the physical limitations placed by parents from those self-imposed by child.

C. Determine exercise tolerance.

    1. Note daily sleep patterns.

    2. Determine whether fatigue interferes with play.

D. Emotional health and significance of illness to child must be ascertained.

E. Ascertain current medications, diets.

    1. Daily diet and favorite foods should be noted.

    2. Purpose, dosage, schedule of medications, and response to them must be determined.

II. Gestational and neonatal health history.

    A. Maternal exposure to some viruses (the virus causing rubella, the Coxsackie virus) during pregnancy (especially during the third through the seventh weeks, when most cardiac development is occurring) has been linked with some forms of congenital heart disease.

    B. Maternal use of *some* drugs (thalidomide, stilbestrol, tranquilizers, smallpox vaccine) has been associated with congenital heart disease in offspring.

    C. Increased incidence of congenital heart disease has been noted in offspring of insulin-dependent diabetic mothers.

    D. Note: Most congenital heart disease is of unknown etiology—be careful to avoid speculation about causes.

    E. Determine maternal and family response to the pregnancy.

        1. If pregnancy is unplanned and the child is born with congenital disease, parental anger and guilt may be magnified.

        2. Assess any emotional, cultural, or financial problems the family may be experiencing as a result of the birth.

III. Perinatal health history.

    A. A low birth weight may be associated with an increased incidence of some congenital heart defects in premature infants.

    B. Resuscitation or need for oxygen at birth may indicate cardiac or respiratory distress.

    C. Murmur: Determine whether the heart murmur was present at birth (often, murmurs do not appear until later).

IV. History of growth and development through infancy.

    A. Feeding patterns during infancy:

        1. Feeding difficulties are most often the first symptoms of cardiac distress in infant.

        2. Poor suck, prolonged feeding times, frequent vomiting, and rapid tiring during feeding may be the result of cardiorespiratory distress (infant has difficulty coordinating breathing, sucking, and swallowing).

        3. Determine maternal response to any feeding difficulties (frustration may be transmitted between mother and baby).

    B. Weight gain during infancy:

        1. Poor weight gain may reflect feeding difficulties.

        2. Explore daily diet (ensure that adequate nutrition *is* being offered).

    C. Respiratory patterns during infancy:

        1. Rapid, labored breathing may occur as a result of cardiac compromise.

        2. Frequent upper respiratory infections may result from pulmonary complications of some heart defects.

    D. Cardiovascular status during infancy:

        1. Heart murmur.

            a. Age at time of appearance of murmur may help determine type of defect present (reliable only if medical follow-up is regular and thorough).

            b. Many children have "innocent murmurs" (not associated with pathology) noted between birth and 10 years; most disappear with child's growth.

      2. Cyanosis.

         a. Circumoral or acrocyanosis may be normal in neonates.

         b. Cyanosis relieved by crying may indicate respiratory cause of hypoxemia (lung aeration improves with cry, and results in improved respiratory function and decreased cyanosis).

         c. Cyanosis aggravated by crying may indicate cardiovascular disease (resistance to pulmonary blood flow is increased during expiratory phase of cry, and causes decreased pulmonary blood flow and increased cyanosis).

         d. If cyanosis has been noted, obtain information regarding:

            (1) Onset.

            (2) Precipitating and alleviating factors.

            (3) Severity.

            (4) Distribution.

E. Illnesses during infancy.

    1. Frequent upper respiratory infections may occur as a complication of congenital heart disease.

    2. Solicit child's and family's response to hospitalizations and to health care personnel.

F. Activity patterns.

    1. Determine whether baby interrupts play to rest.

    2. Ask mother to describe posture most frequently assumed by infant at play and at rest (Fowler's or semi-Fowler's position is usually preferred by infants with cardiorespiratory distress).

G. Achievement of developmental milestones in infancy.

    1. Frequent hospitalizations introduce the baby to multiple caretakers and added stress which may result in delay in achievement of developmental milestones.

    2. Determine maternal response to baby's progress.

V. History of growth and development through preschool and school years.

A. Nutritional patterns.

B. Weight gain.

    1. Rapid weight gain occurs with edema, but may also be part of normal growth pattern.

    2. Always graph weight on growth chart and consider in terms of percentiles. Longitudinal records are valuable.

    3. Chronically ill children may be smaller than healthy children (explore child's body image).

C. Respiratory patterns (as above; *see* point IV C above).

D. Cardiovascular status (as above; *see* point IV D above).

E. Illness.

    1. Frequent upper respiratory infections may be symptomatic of respiratory complications of congenital heart disease.

    2. Group A beta-hemolytic streptococcus pharyngitis always precedes the development of rheumatic fever and resultant rheumatic carditis (though acute infection may be difficult to document).

    3. Children with heart lesions resulting in turbulent intracardiac blood flow are especially prone to development of bacterial endocarditis as complication of bacteremia (bacteria tend to lodge around disfigured valves, prosthetic patches, or abnormal orifices).

    4. Determine child's and family's concepts of health and medical care (child may feel that imperfect heart makes one "bad").

F. Activity patterns.

    1. Mother may compare child's development and activity level to that of other children in family.

      a. This may be a source of stress if children differ in play preferences.

      b. Consider individual variation and social and sexual norms when attempting to interpret any comparisons.

2. Frequent squatting during play may be the cyanotic child's instinctive attempt to relieve hypoxemia of tetralogy of Fallot (squatting helps to increase pulmonary blood flow in these children).

G. Onset of nocturia or oliguria may indicate presence of congestive heart failure.

H. Central nervous system symptoms.

1. An increased incidence of thrombus, embolus, and brain abscess may be noted in children with cyanotic heart disease and resultant polycythemia (blood increases in viscosity due to increased red blood cell formation, so clots form more easily).

2. Note presence (and details) of any syncopal episodes.

3. Cyanosis does *not* cause mental retardation.

VI. History of growth and development during adolescence (see points IV and V above, but the following factors deserve special emphasis).

A. Nutritional patterns:

1. Determine the child's response to and compliance with any diets ordered by physician.

2. "Fad foods" are usually not allowed in salt-free or low-cholesterol diets.

B. Growth and weight gain:

1. Note presence or absence of prepubescent growth spurt (delay or absence of this spurt may occur as result of chronic illness and/or chronic hypoxemia resulting from cyanotic heart disease).

2. Onset and regularity of menses may be delayed if girl is chronically ill.

3. Attempt to discover adolescent's feelings about his or her heart disease (explore body image).

C. Current therapy and medication:

1. Determine the child's comprehension, physical and emotional response, and compliance with therapeutic regimen.

2. Adolescent may frequently "test" regimen by attempting to "do without" medications or special diets.

3. Determine whether drugs, diets, or therapy are still producing desired results (e.g., diuretics). Medication dose adjustment, or some change in regimen may be indicated.

D. Activity pattern:

1. Determine importance of physical activity to the adolescent.

2. If activity restrictions are recommended, determine the teenager's comprehension, physical and emotional response, and compliance with restrictions.

VII. Family health history.

A. Ascertain family history of heart disease, hypertension, or congenital anomalies.

1. Family's previous experience with heart disease may affect their responses to illness.

2. Some forms of congenital heart disease have familial tendencies and are associated with inherited diseases or syndromes (see Table 13-1).

3. The occurrence of any unexplained infant deaths in the family may be the result of congenital heart lesion.

B. Explore the impact of illness on the child and family.

1. Do parents have adequate health insurance and adequate financial resources to support hospitalizations, tests, special medical equipment, diets, and medications required?

2. Explore importance of health to family.

3. Coping strategies.

a. Parents of a chronically ill child may demonstrate chronic grief, guilt, extreme anxiety, or anticipatory mourning (anticipating death).

b. Assess coping strategies and family support systems already developed.

4. Include patients' interpretations of and feelings about health care (especially during school years, there may be feelings that heart disease occurred as punishment for wrongdoing).

TABLE 13-1 / CARDIAC ANOMALIES COMMONLY ASSOCIATED WITH CONGENITAL DISEASES OR SYNDROMES

Disease or Syndrome	Associated Cardiac Anomaly
Trisomy 13 (Patau's) syndrome	Patent ductus arteriosus and/or ventricular septal defect with pulmonary hypertension
Trisomy 18 (Edwards') syndrome	Ventricular septal defect
Trisomy 21 (Down's) syndrome	Endocardial cushion defect
Turner's syndrome	Coarctation of the aorta
Mosaic Turner's syndrome (XO/XY)	Pulmonic stenosis
Marfan's syndrome	Aortic or mitral valve abnormalities, dissecting aortic aneurysms, myocardial disease
Holt-Oram syndrome	Atrial septal defect or single atrium, severe pulmonary vascular disease, total anomalous pulmonary venous return, or arrhythmias
Ellis–van Creveld syndrome	Single atrium or atrial septal defect
William's syndrome	Aortic stenosis, peripheral pulmonary stenosis
Laurence-Moon-Biedl syndrome	Aortic or pulmonary valvular stenosis
Hunter's and Hurler's syndromes	Abnormalities of the mitral or tricuspid valves, or coronary artery obstruction
Friedreich's ataxia	Myocarditis
Neurofibromatosis	Pulmonary valvular stenosis

Physical Examination

I. General appearance.
   A. Decreased activity or irritability may suggest the presence of hypoxemia or congestive heart failure.
   B. Body build and weight.
      1. Note percentiles on growth chart.
      2. Be alert for unusual physical characteristics which may be associated with congenital syndromes.
   C. Preferred posture.
      1. Child with cardiorespiratory distress may prefer head elevated.
      2. Child with tetralogy of Fallot may interrupt play to squat, or may prefer a knee-chest position when reclining.
   D. Color.
      1. Compare patient's color when at rest to color when active.
      2. Cyanosis may be difficult to perceive with concurrent anemia or jaundice.
      3. Cyanosis is most readily discernible in mucous membranes or nail beds. Note:
         a. Onset.
         b. Precipitating or alleviating factors.
         c. Severity.
         d. Distribution.
      4. Pallor may indicate anemia, shock, pain, fever, or anxiety.
      5. Diaphoresis (excessive sweating) may be caused by the sympathetic nervous system's stress response to heart failure.

    6. Compare color of upper extremities to that of lower extremities. In some congenital heart lesions (coarctation of the aorta, patent ductus arteriosus), disparity may exist.

II. Skin.

    A. Turgor: Assess hydration, as circulating blood volume may affect cardiac output.

        1. "Tenting" of skin when pinched occurs with dehydration.

        2. Pitting or nonpitting edema with shiny, taut skin may result from heart failure (in children, periorbital edema is often seen first).

    B. Color (see also point I D above).

        1. *Erythema marginatum* (sharply circumscribed, reddened, flat, or slightly raised lesions) or subcutaneous nodules (firm, nonreddened, nontender lumps) may occur with rheumatic fever. If present, either one requires assessment for rheumatic carditis.

        2. *Petechiae* (reddish-purple subcutaneous lesions) may be associated with bacterial endocarditis.

    C. Temperature of extremities must be assessed. Coolness may indicate inadequate circulation (consider environmental temperature, however).

III. Head and neck.

    A. Face: Some asymmetry of features can be caused by chromosomal disorders (their presence would lead you to assess for specific, commonly associated heart defects).

    B. Neck.

        1. Observe for jugular vein distension, which usually indicates systemic venous congestion; this is usually difficult to see in infants (jugular vein prominence when baby cries vigorously is normal).

        2. Observe and palpate for any *thrills* (palpable vibrations caused by turbulent blood flow) or *bruits* (abnormal sounds auscultated over areas of turbulent blood flow).

            a. Arterial pulsations, thrills, or bruits in the neck usually indicate abnormalities of aortic blood flow (aortic stenosis or coarctation of the aorta).

            b. Suprasternal thrills usually indicate abnormalities of aortic (stenosis or coarctation) or pulmonary blood flow (pulmonic stenosis or patent ductus arteriosus).

IV. Eyes, ears, nose, and throat. (Examine all these structures for signs of infection which may accompany heart disease or complicate it.)

    A. Eyes.

        1. Periorbital edema often indicates congestive heart failure (especially in infants and preschoolers).

        2. Check conjunctiva for pallor of anemia or blueness of cyanosis (report these to physician).

    B. Nose.

        1. Epistaxis (nosebleed) may occur with increased frequency or severity when hypertension or polycythemia (increased red blood cell number) is present.

        2. Flaring of nares usually indicates increased respiratory effort.

    C. Mouth and throat.

        1. Color (note presence of cyanosis).

        2. Dental caries.

            a. Caries may be seen with increased frequency in cyanotic children.

            b. They can serve as a source of bacterial infection which, if allowed to invade the bloodstream, can cause bacterial endocarditis in child with heart disease.

        3. Check for presence of reddened and/or sore throat, which may indicate presence of group A beta-hemolytic streptococcus pharyngitis.

        4. Hoarseness occurs with compression of the recurrent laryngeal nerve and/or trachea by a dilated aorta, pulmonary artery, or vascular ring.

V. Chest.

    A. Inspect configuration and appearance of chest.

1. Abnormalities of the chest may occur as the result of a congenital thoracic malformation or cardiorespiratory disease.
2. Prominence of the sternum may be due to right ventricular enlargement (because this structure lies just below the sternum).
3. Left chest prominence may be due to left ventricular hypertrophy.
4. Observe for size and location of any operative scars which would indicate previous cardiac surgery.

B. Observe respirations.
   1. Observe quality, rate, and depth.
   2. Accessory muscle involvement indicates increased respiratory effort.
      a. Note pattern of respirations: Infants are normally abdominal breathers, children 2 to 3 years of age are normally costal breathers (any variation from this pattern may be significant).
      b. Determine rate of respiration. Normal rates are infant, 40 per minute; child, 20 to 30 per minute.
      c. Nasal flaring and chest retractions indicate distress.
      d. Gasping and grunting with increased respiratory effort usually indicate severe distress.

C. Palpate chest.
   1. Thrills in the supraclavicular area are often present with abnormalities of aortic or pulmonary blood flow.
   2. Thrills in the pericostal areas often appear with large (turbulent) intercostal artery flow (usually as a collateral circulation due to congenital heart lesion).

D. Percuss chest.
   1. Dullness is heard over fluid-filled areas (e.g., consolidated lung, area of pleural effusion).
   2. Hyperresonance is heard in chest areas with high air density (e.g., suggesting emphysema, pneumothorax).

E. Auscultate lung fields.
   1. Congestive heart failure usually does not produce rales in infants or young children except very late in the clinical course.
   2. Rales usually indicate respiratory infection. Children with congestive heart failure or certain congenital heart defects have high pulmonary venous pressures. This causes pulmonary changes which make patient more susceptible to development of respiratory infections.

VI. Heart (see Fig. 13-1).
   A. Inspection.
      1. Look for *point of maximal impulse* (PMI), seen as chest vibration with each heartbeat.
         a. The PMI normally is located in approximately the fifth intercostal space at the midclavicular line.
         b. If one ventricle is enlarged, the PMI shifts in the direction of that ventricle.
      2. Observe for any additional pulsations present over the heart.
   B. Palpation.
      1. Palpate the PMI and note whether localized or diffuse.
      2. Presence of thrills over cardiac areas indicate *very* turbulent blood flow and would lead you to expect the presence of a murmur of at least grade IV to VI intensity. Establish location.
      3. If the sternum lifts (or taps) against your hand, right ventricular enlargement is present (this sign is called *sternal lift*).
      4. If the left chest is felt to "heave" under your fingertips, left ventricular hypertrophy is present (this sign is called *left ventricular heave*).
   C. Auscultation (performed when patient is supine, sitting, and lying on left side).
      1. Determine rate and rhythm by apical auscultation for a full minute. Compare apical rate to peripheral pulse rate and note any disparity (this should be reported to the physician).

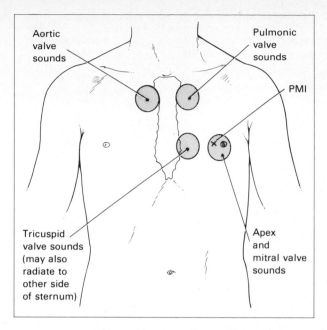

Aortic valve sounds

Pulmonic valve sounds

PMI

Tricuspid valve sounds (may also radiate to other side of sternum)

Apex and mitral valve sounds

FIGURE 13-1 / Major auscultatory areas of the chest.

2. Heart rate increases approximately 8 to 10 beats per min with each degree Farenheit elevation in child's temperature.
3. There is normally a slight variation in cardiac rhythm with each respiration (called sinus arrhythmia).
4. Locate areas where S_1 and S_2 are heard best (S_1 is usually heard best at the apex, S_2 is usually best auscultated in the pulmonic area).
5. Observe for any unusual sounds (murmurs, clicks, S_3, or S_4).
   a. Record where these sounds are heard best, and where they radiate, and localize these sounds in the cardiac cycle (note whether they occur during systole, diastole, or throughout cycle).
   b. A *murmur* is an abnormal sound usually caused by turbulent flow within the heart or great vessels (unless of great intensity, murmurs can't be heard without stethoscope).
   c. "Innocent" murmurs are not associated with pathology, and may be temporarily present in children from birth through 10 years of age. These are usually systolic murmurs heard best over the pulmonic area of the heart.
   d. *Pericardial friction rub* ("squeaky door" sound heard with each heartbeat) is always abnormal, and usually indicates the presence of pericarditis.
   e. *Clicks* may be auscultated over valvular areas when valve anomalies are present.
   f. A third heart sound (S_3) may be normal in children, but is often indicative of turbulent or forceful ventricular filling (may be present if child is in congestive heart failure).
   g. A fourth heart sound (S_4) is always abnormal, and usually indicates atrial enlargement.
VII. Blood pressure and peripheral pulses.
   A. Take into consideration child's age and emotional state (see Table 13-2).
   B. General guidelines.
      1. Take blood pressure in all four extremities if any abnormality is suspected (if at all possible, do so when child is under same conditions of rest).

TABLE 13-2 / NORMAL BLOOD PRESSURES FOR CHILDREN

Child's Age, years	Systolic Range, mmHg*	Diastolic Range, mmHg*
2–6	82–112	50–78
6–8	84–116	54–78
8–10	88–120	58–80
10–12	94–130	62–82
12–14	100–134	62–84
14–16	104–140	64–86
16–18	108–142	64–88

*Ranges indicate those blood pressures falling between the 10th and 90th percentiles of results obtained in the task force study. (Therefore, 80 percent of children tested fell within the ranges indicated.)
Source: This table was compiled from charts prepared by the National Heart, Lung, and Blood Institute's Task Force on Blood Pressure Control in Children.

     a. During infancy, arm and leg blood pressures usually are equal, but beyond 1 year of age, leg blood pressures are usually 10 to 40 mmHg *higher* than arm blood pressures (absence or reversal of this relationship should be reported to the physician).

     b. Use proper size cuff—bladder of cuff should not cover more than two-thirds of upper arm or thigh, and should not be wrapped more than 1¼ times around extremity.

  2. If any abnormal blood pressure is obtained, deflate cuff, allow child to rest, and remeasure blood pressure in a few minutes (anxiety may cause elevation in blood pressure). If blood pressure measurement is difficult to obtain in the extremities of an infant by using conventional methods, the "flush" technique may be used. The extremity is wrapped with a blood pressure cuff of appropriate size and elevated at a 90° angle. The extremity is "milked" white and the cuff is inflated. As you *deflate* the cuff, note the pressure at which the extremity returns to a pink color. This pressure corresponds to the child's *mean arterial pressure.*

C. Decreased systolic blood pressure.

  1. Decreased systolic pressure most often is due to shock and low cardiac output (an emergency situation).

  2. Shock may be present despite a "normal" measured blood pressure if sympathetic nervous system discharge is increasing arterial wall tone (evaluate all clinical aspects).

D. Elevated systolic blood pressure.

  1. An elevated systolic pressure may indicate hypertension (often seen in upper extremities when coarctation of the aorta is present).

  2. It may also indicate high-output cardiac states.

E. Low diastolic blood pressure.

  1. Low diastolic pressure is often present when cardiovascular defects (aortic insufficiency, patent ductus arteriosus) allow aortic "runoff" (diversion of some aortic blood flow to other than systemic arteries).

  2. It may indicate shock.

F. Widened pulse pressure (greater than 55 mmHg difference between systolic and diastolic readings).

  1. This situation may occur with fever, anemia, exercise, or heart block.

  2. It may also result from any condition causing increased systolic and/or decreased diastolic components.

G. *Pulsus alternans* (alternating strong and weak beats heard while deflating cuff during blood pressure reading) usually indicates left ventricular failure, myocardial weakness, or premature ventricular contractions.

H. *Pulsus paradoxus* is the disappearance of pulses during blood pressure cuff deflation for 10 mmHg or more during inspiration. It indicates pericardial effusion, constrictive cardiac anomalies, myocardial disease, or airway obstruction (notify physician).

I. Note quality of peripheral pulses.

    1. A *bounding pulse* (*"water-hammer"* pulse) is usually symptomatic of cardiovascular disorders causing aortic runoff.

    2. A *biphasic pulse* may be due to aortic stenosis.

    3. Palpate all major peripheral pulses and note absence of any pulses (if an artery from an extremity has been used for palliative cardiac surgery, corresponding pulse will be absent).

    4. Discrepancies between right and left radial pulses or between upper and lower extremity pulses are abnormal, and may be due to coarctation of aorta or congenital aortic stenosis.

VIII. Abdomen.

  A. Observe for any pulsations. Epigastric pulsations may be present normally in children.

  B. Auscultate.

    1. *Paralytic ileus* may be symptomatic of low serum potassium (which may be responsible for cardiac arrhythmias).

    2. *Abdominal bruits* may be normal in children but may also indicate an abdominal aortic aneurysm.

  C. Palpate liver for hepatomegaly.

    1. *Hepatomegaly* (enlarged liver) is one of the *first* signs of congestive heart failure in children.

      a. Hepatomegaly occurs long before generalized edema as a sign of right heart failure in infants.

      b. It is also symptomatic of right ventricular failure in older children.

      c. A liver palpable 1 to 2 cm below right costal margin is normal in newborns and in infants and pathologic if palpable beyond 2 cm below costal margin.

      d. After 6 months of age, the liver normally is not palpable below costal margin. If it is, this sign indicates liver inflammation or venous engorgement due to congestive heart failure.

    2. *Splenomegaly* (enlarged spleen) often indicates presence of bacterial endocarditis or hemolytic disorder in neonate.

      a. The spleen usually is not palpable below left costal margin.

      b. If spleen enlargement *is* verified, *do not palpate further,* as spleen is easily ruptured.

IX. Examination of extremities.

  A. Assess color, muscle tone, activity, skin turgor, and temperature (including presence or absence of cyanosis and edema).

  B. Check *capillary filling time.* Press on nail bed or area of skin and count seconds it takes for skin or nail to return from white to pink (should be no more than a few seconds). A delay indicates decreased perfusion.

  C. *Clubbing* (rounding of tips of fingers and toes) occurs beyond 6 months of age in children subjected to chronic peripheral tissue hypoxia accompanying cyanotic congenital heart disease or respiratory disorders.

  D. Swollen, painful joints often occur with rheumatic fever.

HEMODYNAMIC PRINCIPLES

I. Pressure, flow, and resistance relationship (pressure = flow × resistance).

  A. Blood will flow in path of *least resistance; resistance* (opposition to blood flow) is largely determined by the diameter of the outflow tract or vessel.

  B. If increased resistance is offered to flow, increased pressure must be generated to maintain the same amount of blood flow.

II. Development of pulmonary vasculature.
   A. During fetal life, lungs are collapsed and the pulmonary arteries are thick-walled and offer high resistance, so little flow occurs through pulmonary arteries.
   B. At birth, pulmonary arterial walls begin to thin out and offer less resistance to flow, thus flow occurs through these vessels.
      1. Pulmonary vascular resistance normally continues to decrease as vessel walls thin out over the next 6 weeks to 3 months, but may fall more quickly or slowly in premature infants.
      2. After 3 months, pulmonary vessels offer approximately one-sixth the resistance offered by the systemic vessels.
      3. If an *intracardiac shunt* (abnormal route of blood flow) is present, blood will have a greater tendency to flow into the pulmonary circuit (*least resistance*) if pulmonary vascular resistance is low.
   C. If pulmonary vessels are subjected to high flow, their walls begin to thicken again and they offer more resistance to flow.
      1. If high pulmonary flow occurs under *high* pressures, walls thicken quickly and will offer more resistance in a few years.
      2. If high flow occurs under *low* pressures, resistance increases slowly over decades.
      3. With increased pulmonary resistance, blood has *less* tendency to flow into pulmonary circuit.

CONGESTIVE HEART FAILURE

Definition

I. *Congestive heart failure* is a term used to describe a set of clinical findings which occur when cardiac output is insufficient to meet the metabolic demands of the body.
II. There are many causes of heart failure:
   A. Congenital heart disease is the most frequent cause, especially in infants.
   B. Surgery for congenital heart disease can alter cardiac function and result in congestive heart failure.
   C. Arrhythmias may seriously impair ventricular filling or contraction.
   D. Rheumatic carditis or other inflammatory diseases of the heart may interfere with myocardial or valvular function.
   E. Metabolic disease can cause heart failure if overwhelming demands are placed on the heart or if the myocardial cellular environment is altered.
   F. Respiratory disease.
      1. Prolonged alveolar hypoxia may cause severe increase in pulmonary vascular resistance, resulting in eventual right ventricular failure (*cor pulmonale*).
      2. Severe hypoxia depresses cardiac function.
III. Pathophysiology of heart failure: metabolic aspects.
   A. Cardiac output is decreased.
   B. Diminished cardiac output stimulates sympathetic nervous system compensatory mechanisms (increased heart rate and contractility, increased vasomotor tone, and peripheral vasoconstriction).
   C. Renal compensatory mechanisms stimulate sodium and water retention, resulting in increased blood volume.
      1. Renal perfusion is decreased due to decreased cardiac output and sympathetic vasoconstriction, so renin release is stimulated.
         a. This process results in sodium and water retention (through the release of aldosterone).
         b. It may also cause increased arterial constriction (through the action of angiotensin).
IV. Pathophysiology of heart failure: hemodynamic mechanisms.
   A. Heart rate and contractility are immediately increased with fall in cardiac output (sympathetic nervous system response).

    B. As cardiac output falls, intraventricular diastolic and filling pressures increase and ventricular hypertrophy may occur. If output continues to fall, the heart dilates in an attempt to receive and pump more blood.

    C. Increased circulating blood volume and increased intraventricular pressures cause elevated systemic and pulmonary venous pressures leading to *venous engorgement*. Increased pulmonary venous pressures can also occur if a congenital heart defect causes high pulmonary blood flow under high pressures.

        1. Hepatomegaly and, later, peripheral edema, result from systemic venous engorgement.

        2. With pulmonary venous engorgement, the lungs become less compliant, so tachypnea and hyperventilation result as respiratory compensatory mechanisms are stimulated.

  V. Either ventricle may fail, but in children symptoms of combined ventricular failure usually coexist.

Assessment

  I. Four main signs of congestive heart failure are observable in children:

    A. Tachycardia.

    B. Decreased urine output.

    C. Tachypnea.

    D. Hepatomegaly.

  II. Evidence of decreased cardiac output and resultant cardiac and sympathetic compensatory mechanisms will be noted:

    A. Tachycardia.

    B. Cardiomegaly: Active precordium may be observed, and cardiac silhouette will be enlarged on x-ray.

    C. Decreased urine output (less than 1 mL per kilogram of body weight per hour) or *oliguria,* will occur *despite* adequate fluid intake.

    D. Peripheral vasoconstriction will exist, and extremities may be cool.

    E. Diaphoresis will be seen, especially in infants.

  III. Pulmonary venous engorgement will produce respiratory symptoms.

    A. Tachypnea.

    B. There will be evidence of increased respiratory effort (retractions will be present in infants, or nasal flaring or use of accessory muscles of respiration may be observed).

    C. Infants will have feeding difficulties, finding it hard to coordinate rapid breathing with sucking and swallowing.

    D. Rales occur only as late sign of pulmonary venous engorgement in children; they may indicate, however, the presence of concurrent respiratory infection.

  IV. Signs of systemic venous engorgement will also be present.

    A. Hepatomegaly will usually be the first symptom observed in children.

    B. Periorbital edema.

    C. Jugular venous distension, difficult to detect in infants, will exist.

    D. Edema of the hands and feet may be noted in infants but is usually not seen in older children.

    E. Dependent (sacral) edema or ascites are only very late signs of chronic or severe heart failure in children.

  V. With continued severe reduction in cardiac output, evidence of severe compromise of systemic perfusion will be apparent:

    A. Altered level of consciousness (child may be "fussy" or lethargic).

    B. Weak, thready pulses (hypotension will appear if sympathetic compensation is inadequate).

    C. Metabolic acidosis (the result of anaerobic metabolism).

Problems

  I. Patient has tendency to develop circulatory compromise.

  II. There is respiratory distress related to congestive heart failure and possible concurrent respiratory infection.

III. Child has tendency to develop fluid retention and possible edema due to heart failure.

IV. Nutritional compromise may develop.

> *Note* The following problems (V to VII) are common to most children with any type of heart disease and to their families or primary caretakers. These will be discussed here, but should be a part of care for all children.

V. Patient may experience extreme anxiety related to his or her illness or cardiorespiratory distress (or hospitalization).

VI. Parents or primary caretaker may experience anxiety related to illness and prognosis.

VII. Child and primary caretaker(s) require specific teaching about medical regimen and home care.

Goals of Care

I. Restore, promote, and/or maintain optimal circulatory function.

II. Reduce respiratory distress and promote optimal respiratory function.

III. Promote optimal fluid balance.

IV. Prevent skin breakdown.

V. Promote optimal nutritional status.

VI. Assist child in developing and/or mobilizing adequate coping mechanisms.

VII. Support family's coping attempts.

VIII. Provide adequate information to and supervision of child and primary caretaker to ensure successful continuation of medical regimen, and early detection and/or prevention of further deterioration of cardiac function.

Intervention

I. Circulatory compromise.

 A. Monitor carefully for signs of decreased cardiac output and severe compromise of systemic perfusion. If signs of severe deterioration in child's condition occur, notify physician immediately.

 B. Administer digitalis derivative if prescribed.
   1. Check dosage appropriate for child's age and weight (Table 13-3).
   2. Monitor cardiovascular response to digitalis (heart rate should slow and cardiac output should increase).
     a. Arrhythmias are usually the first sign of digitalis toxicity in children (vomiting occurs only as a late sign, or in older children).
     b. Confer with physician if heart rate slows significantly: (Consider child's previous rate, also.)
       (1) Less than 110 beats per minute (bpm) in infants.
       (2) Less than 90 bpm in toddlers.
       (3) Less than 80 bpm in school-age children.
       (4) Less than 60 bpm in adolescents.
   3. Teach adolescent, or younger child's primary caretaker to administer digitalis, and provide teaching to ensure detection of digitalis toxicity.
     a. If caretakers are sensitive and observant, merely request that they notify physician if child becomes ill, or fatigues more easily.
     b. Some health care facilities require that caretakers be taught to take patient's pulse prior to administration of digitalis. Focusing on any firm range of heart rate must be avoided, however (tell caretaker to allow for rate increase with exercise, or decrease during sleep).

 C. Monitor electrolyte values (if child is hospitalized), as low serum potassium can make patient more susceptible to digitalis toxicity (ingestion of a glass of orange juice or a banana in the morning should prevent hypokalemia).

 D. If child is in moderate distress, attempt to decrease the physical and emotional stress which may increase cardiovascular requirements.
   1. Ensure adequate rest periods without examinations and procedures for child.
   2. Prevent rapid or frequent fluctuations in body or environmental temperature

TABLE 13-3 / TOTAL DIGITALIZING DOSES FOR CHILDREN (DIGOXIN)

Child's Age	Dosage of Digoxin*
Neonate	0.044–0.066 mg/kg (0.02–0.03 mg/lb)
2 weeks to 2 years	0.066–0.088 mg/kg (0.03–0.04 mg/lb)
2–10 years	0.044–0.066 mg/kg (0.02–0.03 mg/lb)
10 years to adult	2–3 mg (average)

*Intravenous dosage should be two-thirds of given dosages.
Note: Above doses should be given in divided doses approximately as follows (may be slight variation in various institutions): For digitalization: $\frac{1}{2}$ of digitalizing dose given initially; $\frac{1}{4}$ of digitalizing dose given 6–8 h later; last $\frac{1}{4}$ of digitalizing dose given after 6–8 h more. For maintenance: $\frac{1}{8}$ of digitalizing dose given 12 h later and every 12 h thereafter.

(especially in neonatal period, when thermoregulatory mechanisms are immature).

3. Ensure adequate nutritional intake.
4. Provide soothing, sensitive nursing care.

II. Respiratory distress.
A. Assess carefully for signs of increased respiratory distress. If severe respiratory distress is present, maintenance of adequate ventilation has priority.
B. Provide adequate pulmonary toilet to a degree appropriate to child's distress.
1. If oxygen therapy is required to maintain acceptable blood P_{O_2}, monitor inspired oxygen levels carefully (to prevent oxygen toxicity), and monitor response to therapy. Note child's tolerance of brief periods away from oxygen.
2. If oxygen therapy is required, or if there is pulmonary congestion, humidification of inspired air (using hood, high humidity tent, or home vaporizer) is necessary; monitor response to and tolerance of humidity.
3. If concurrent respiratory infection is present, provide chest physiotherapy (postural drainage, percussion, vibration, or suctioning) to facilitate removal of respiratory secretions. Enlist child's participation.
   a. Encourage child to cough vigorously, and to take deep breaths.
   b. *Slight* pressure on the trachea, just above sternum, will usually stimulate cough (if absolutely necessary).
   c. Ask child to blow inverted paper cup across counter top, or to pretend to blow out birthday candles.
   d. Child may enjoy blowing soap bubbles.
C. Attempt to minimize oxygen requirements. If severe distress is present place child in a comfortable position.

III. Fluid retention.
A. Monitor patient's fluid balance.
1. If there is associated respiratory distress, oral fluid intake may be decreased, as patient's appetite or energy probably is decreased.
2. If supplemental intravenous therapy is ordered, verify the amount ordered. It should not exceed the patient's daily fluid requirements, and should be reduced if urine output is decreased.
3. Daily weights and records of 24-h intake and output may be necessary to determine fluid balance during hospitalization (rarely needed when child is at home).
4. Infant's diapers should be weighed before and after infant wears them if accurate measurement of urine output is required (only in hospital).

  B. Diuretics may be necessary to maintain urine output.

   1. Ensure appropriate dosage for age and weight.

   2. Teach adolescent or younger child's primary caretaker how to administer dosage and note renal response.

   3. If patient is receiving concurrent digitalis and diuretic therapy, ensure adequate electrolyte (potassium) replacement if necessary.

  C. A low-sodium diet may be prescribed by physician in order to decrease probability of fluid retention.

   1. Child and primary caretaker should be taught which foods to avoid.

   2. Attempt to provide palatable, yet appropriate diet; since most "fad" foods (potato chips, pizza, some soft drinks) are not compatible with a low-sodium diet, school-age child or adolescent may be expected to "test" diet (and break it).

   3. It is *nearly always* physically and emotionally healthier for patient if health team manipulates diuretic dosage and allows child to eat regular diet. (It is usually impractical and unsafe to rely on child's strict adherence to diet.)

  D. If fluid restriction is required, discuss this with patient and primary caretaker, and attempt to formulate what is the most reasonable distribution of fluids throughout the day.

  E. Provide thorough mouth care. Hard candy may provide effective route for caloric intake while relieving dryness of mouth (lemon and glycerine swabs only increase dryness).

  F. Provide thorough skin care (keep skin dry, and improve circulation with massage); child will usually turn often.

  G. Maintain adequate nutritional intake.

   1. Calculate the daily fluid and nutritional requirements and divide into individual feedings.

   2. Small, frequent feedings are usually better tolerated by children with respiratory distress.

   3. If infant is unable to suck strongly enough to obtain adequate nutrition through the nipple, supplementation of oral intake with gavage or nasojejunal feedings or parenteral nutrition may be required temporarily. Continue to reinforce child's suck, however.

   4. Assess weight gain, skin turgor, and hair and fingernail texture to ensure adequate nutritional intake.

IV. The following interventions are common to most children with any type of heart disease and to their families or primary caretakers. These will be discussed here, but should be a part of care for all children.

  A. A child with congenital heart disease may be hospitalized frequently, so it is important that hospitalizations be as positive an experience as possible under the circumstances.

  B. Assess any sources of anxiety (nightmares, fantasies, medical treatments, hospital environment, family crisis, separation from family). Much assessment may be accomplished with play.

   1. Provide medical equipment and nonmedical toys, allowing patient to play freely. Watch and listen for clues to fears, concerns, opinions.

   2. Request school-age child to draw a self-portrait and then discuss this with you.

   3. It may be helpful to ask patient to "name one thing that is scary" (children often respond better to specific rather than vague or broad questions).

  C. Determine child's interpretation of the illness and severity of his or her condition (school-age children often feel illness or pain is a punishment for their wrongdoings). Child may need support in working through these feelings.

  D. Determine any concurrent psychosocial or developmental stresses patient may be experiencing.

  E. Reinforce patient's discussion of fears if this helps child cope with them; if discussion is too threatening, use other, nonverbal modes of communication.

F. Assist child in developing plan to eliminate sources of unwarranted fear, and to deal with those that remain.

    1. Some imagined sources of fear may be eliminated through discussion and carefully worded explanations.

    2. Remaining sources of fear may be mastered through use of therapeutic play, and by patient's participation in care whenever possible (offer child reasonable choices and some control over scheduling of treatments).

G. Provide child with the same health team members whenever possible (at home or in hospital), and a consistent schedule to increase child's familiarity with environment and care regimen.

H. Assist caretakers or parents with planning adequate rest periods.

I. Include parents or primary caretakers in care.

J. Provide appropriate preparation for any procedures or treatments.

K. Help child maintain emotional bond with family (telephone calls home while child is hospitalized may help).

L. Assess sources of parental anxiety, and family structure and support systems (see discussion of family health history under "Child's Health History").

M. Determine meaning of illness to family.

    1. Note parents' (or primary caretaker's) descriptions of child's health; note any misconceptions present and correct these.

    2. Assess family's interpretation of severity of illness and prognosis.

    3. Note any concurrent stresses (financial or emotional) which may interfere with family support at this time.

N. Allow family to discuss fears and frustrations; correction of minor misconceptions is usually more appropriate when parents have more energy available to assimilate new information.

O. Encourage family to participate in child's care (to a degree comfortable to them) but maintain integrity of the parental role. Do not attempt to make nurses out of parents, as the child needs a "safe" person who does not give painful treatments.

P. Familiarize the family with patient's care schedules, the health team members and health care regimen (include parents in planning health care), and provide appropriate teaching.

Q. Assess learning needs of child and caretaker.

    1. Provide child and caretaker with sufficient opportunity to ask questions. Availability and sensitivity of a nurse often ensures effective communication between family and health team.

    2. Be aware that information *you'd* like to give patient and primary caretaker is not always consistent with amount or type of information actually *needed* to care for child (don't overwhelm them with useless information).

    3. Child's and caretaker's comprehension, interpretation, and support of care regimen must be assessed.

R. Assess child's and family's ability and willingness to learn.

    1. Assess importance of health to child and caretaker.

    2. Identify economic, cultural, or social factors which may hinder learning of or compliance with therapy (eliminate these or incorporate them into teaching plan).

S. Provide teaching regarding assessment of child's condition.

    1. If patient has congestive heart failure, primary caretaker should be aware that child is more susceptible to upper respiratory infections.

    2. Child and family should be urged to seek medical care whenever child demonstrates evidence of upper respiratory congestion.

    3. When parent or primary caretaker is sensitive and observant, determination of child's health status becomes instinctive and accurate.

        a. Parent will bring child to physician with complaint that "something's not right." This is often a most sensitive indicator of child's health status.

        b. Teaching should then center on reinforcement of this feeling by assisting caretaker to clarify associated symptoms (e.g., when "something's not right," child may breathe more rapidly).

4. If caretaker is less observant, or demonstrates more difficulty appreciating patient's symptoms of disease, teaching should include simple observational tasks and more frequent visits with health care personnel.

T. Provide teaching regarding child's activity.

1. In the majority of cardiac conditions, few if any restrictions must be placed on activity (child will usually tire long before there will be stress on cardiac function).

2. If acute rheumatic carditis is cause of congestive failure or heart disease, child's activity may often need to be restricted (the extent of inflammatory damage to the heart may increase with exercise).

3. Adolescents and school-age children may frequently test restrictions on activity due to peer pressure; when children have congestive heart failure, they usually tire and limit their own activity before any serious compromise of cardiac function occurs.

Evaluation

I. Circulatory function is optimized; circulatory compromise is quickly detected and appropriate interventions made.

II. Respiratory function is adequate; respiratory distress is quickly detected and appropriate interventions made.

III. Fluid balance is maintained.

IV. Skin breakdown is avoided.

V. Nutritional status is optimized.

VI. Child copes well and is well adjusted at an age-appropriate level.

VII. Family copes well.

VIII. Child and family are adequately informed.

IX. Child and family demonstrate cooperative participation in care regime.

Case Study

Jenny S., 2 months old, has been brought to the clinic by her mother because of failure to gain weight. Birth weight was 3 kg, and Jenny was pronounced healthy by her pediatrician at the time of birth. Her mother reports that Jenny has been "fussy" lately and "doesn't like any of the baby formulas" and "doesn't eat much" (approximately 40 mL every 2 to 3 h). The mother has noticed that Jenny "breathes heavy" at night. She has not had a fever.

Physical examination reveals a slender, acyanotic, diaphoretic infant who weighs 3.2 kg and is in moderate respiratory distress. She is most comfortable when held over her mother's shoulder. Respiratory rate is 52 with moderate intercostal retractions and nasal flaring. Lungs are clear to auscultation. Jenny's precordium is very active, her heart rate is 156 and regular, and a harsh, systolic murmur is heard at the left lower sternal border (accompanied by a thrill). Jenny's liver can be palpated 3 cm below her costal margin. Extremities are cool, peripheral pulses unremarkable.

Jenny is admitted to the pediatric ward with a diagnosis of congestive heart failure and probable congenital heart disease. Ms. S. is crying as Jenny is admitted.

ASSESSMENT

Jenny has demonstrated vague signs of distress (poor feeding, fussiness) and failure to gain weight. She has tachycardia, tachypnea, increased respiratory effort, and hepatomegaly. She also demonstrates a possible predisposing factor: she has a cardiac murmur which may be indicative of a congenital heart lesion, probably ventricular septal defect.

PROBLEMS

I. Tendency toward circulatory compromise.

II. Respiratory distress.

III. Nutritional compromise.

IV. Maternal anxiety.

V. Developmental needs of 2-month-old.

GOALS OF CARE

I. Maintain optimal cardiovascular function.

II. Decrease distress.

III. Promote optimal nutritional status.

IV. Reduce anxiety and support maternal-child relationship.

V. Promote normal development without increasing fatigue.

VI. Preparation of family for Jenny's future treatments and care and eventual homegoing.

INTERVENTION

I. Monitor child carefully for evidence of increased cardiac compromise.

II. Attempt to decrease cardiac workload.

    A. Maintain constant environmental temperature.

    B. Monitor fluid balance to prevent fluid overload.

        1. Jenny's daily fluid requirement is approximately 320 to 480 mL per 24 h (100 to 150 mL/kg per day).

        2. Jenny's urine output should be approximately 144 mL per day and *no less* than 72 mL per day [minimum of 1 mL/(kg·h)].

    C. Administer digitalis derivative if ordered (digitalizing dose should be approximately 0.21 to 0.28 mg given in divided doses). Monitor drug effects.

    D. Administer diuretics as ordered.

III. Monitor for evidence of systemic venous engorgement (measure hepatomegaly, peripheral edema).

IV. Assess degree of distress and monitor for changes.

V. Assess child for evidence of concurrent respiratory infection and keep child away from people with respiratory infections.

VI. Decrease oxygen requirements.

    A. Organize care to provide rest periods for infant.

    B. Maintain constant environmental temperature.

    C. Place child in comfortable position.

VII. Jenny requires approximately 320 to 480 cal per 24 h (100 to 150 cal/kg per day). If oral intake is insufficient to meet these requirements, meet with the health team to consider advisability of gavage or nasojejunal feedings temporarily.

VIII. Monitor Jenny's state of hydration.

IX. Assess Ms. S.'s sources of anxiety.

X. Orient her to pediatric unit and health team and Jenny's care routine.

XI. Encourage her to discuss Jenny's illness.

XII. Reinforce Ms. S.'s positive feelings about Jenny and her interactions with her (e.g., note that she is a "good" mother and that Jenny knows she is there).

XIII. Provide age-appropriate stimulation (voices, tactile, and visual stimulation) within Jenny's energy limits.

EVALUATION

I. Has heart rate increased or decreased?

II. Is child still fussy?

III. Are fluid intake and output appropriate?

IV. Has hepatomegaly decreased? Are there other signs of systemic venous engorgement?

V. Has respiratory rate decreased?

VI. Have retractions and nasal flaring decreased?

VII. Are lungs still clear?

VIII. Is child still afebrile?

IX. Does child still tire rapidly during feeding?
X. Is Jenny gaining weight (not due to edema)?
XI. Is she receiving adequate caloric intake?
XII. Is her skin turgor good?
XIII. Is mother familiar with Jenny's routine and the health team?
XIV. Is she still able to relate to Jenny (note eye-to-eye contact between them)?
XV. Is Ms. S. demonstrating stress behavior?
XVI. Is development at age level?

CONGENITAL CARDIOVASCULAR DISORDERS

Patent Ductus Arteriosus (PDA)

Definition (See Fig. 13-2)

I. The *ductus arteriosus* is a necessary, normal fetal vessel which provides the pathway for diversion of blood from pulmonary arteries into the aorta; it normally constricts within 72 h after birth, and eventually becomes a ligament (the *ligamentum arteriosum*).
II. *Patent ductus arteriosus* (a ductus which fails to constrict after birth) is responsible for approximately 8 percent of congenital heart disease in children.
   A. Cause of continued patency of ductus is not established.
   B. This condition is seen with increased frequency in premature infants with respiratory distress syndrome (also seen, however, in otherwise healthy children).
III. Hemodynamic effects.
   A. With a shunt between the aorta and the pulmonary artery, blood will follow the path of *least resistance*.

FIGURE 13-2 / Patent ductus arteriosus.

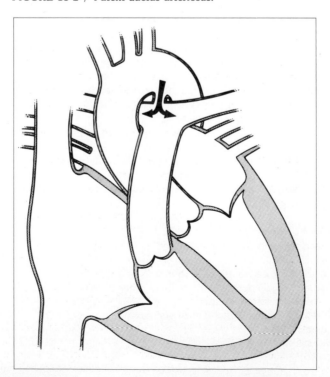

     1. Little flow occurs through the ductus while pulmonary vascular resistance is still high (early infancy).

     2. Once pulmonary vascular resistance drops, blood flows preferentially from the aorta to the pulmonary artery (occurs normally in infants 6 weeks to 3 months of age, but may occur earlier in premature infants).

     3. Flow through shunt initially occurs only during systole (as pulmonary vascular resistance begins to fall), then becomes continuous.

   B. With an aortic to pulmonary artery shunt, the pulmonary vessels are exposed to high blood flow under high pressures. This is not well tolerated, and congestive heart failure may result.

   C. If defect is unrepaired, over several years the child's pulmonary arteriole walls hypertrophy and pulmonary vascular resistance increases, and the shunt may become bidirectional.

IV. Closure of patent ductus.

   A. Administration of prostaglandin inhibitors such as indomethacin in one or two small doses has been shown to close the ductus arteriosus in some premature infants.

   B. Surgical ligation does not involve the use of cardiopulmonary bypass, and is accomplished through a left thoracotomy incision.

V. If the child has a second cardiac lesion causing *decreased* pulmonary blood flow, the child may be dependent on the aorta-to-pulmonary artery shunting provided by a patent ductus arteriosus. In such an instance the ductus is not closed either medically or surgically.

Assessment

I. Children with patent ductus arteriosus defect may remain asymptomatic, with a cardiac murmur as the only abnormal finding (especially children beyond infancy).

II. Pulmonary congestion and congestive heart failure may occur, however, as a result of abnormal pulmonary blood flow (especially during infancy, if the baby was premature).

   A. Refer to assessment in congestive heart failure.

   B. Children may be brought to health care facility with complaints of frequent upper respiratory infections.

III. Cyanosis is rare.

IV. A continuous, machinery-like murmur, heard best in the second intercostal space at the midclavicular line is usually present (may be accompanied by thrill).

V. Peripheral pulses are often bounding (including pedal pulses).

   A. They are called *"water-hammer"* pulses due to pounding quality.

   B. Widened pulse pressure is usually present (due to aortic runoff into pulmonary artery).

Problems

I. If child has congestive heart failure, refer also to the preceding section, "Congestive Heart Failure."

II. Preparation for child's cardiac catheterization and surgery is needed by both patient and family.

III. Child and family require thorough care following cardiac catheterization.

IV. Thorough postoperative care following ductal ligation is required.

V. Child and parents experience anxiety and need teaching about the care regimen and home care.

Goals of Care

I. Provide adequate information and psychological support to promote successful coping with stress of hospitalization and surgery.

II. Foster a positive relationship between family and health team members to aid communication and minimize stress for family and child.

III. Restore and maintain optimal cardiovascular function after catheterization.

IV. Restore and maintain adequate cardiorespiratory function following surgery.

Intervention

I. If congestive heart failure is present, refer also to the preceding section, "Congestive Heart Failure," for discussion of interventions.

II. Since the child has a cardiovascular defect causing turbulent blood flow, he or she is susceptible (if bacteremia is present) to development of aggregations of bacteria around site of turbulent flow, which may cause bacterial emboli or bacterial endocarditis (children are especially susceptible during and beyond school years, when dental caries and frequent infections may occur).

    A. If the child is diagnosed as having patent ductus, this defect is usually surgically repaired before school age, so the possibility of development of carditis is eliminated.

    B. If the defect is not repaired by school years, the child should receive antibiotic prophylaxis 1 or 2 days before and 3 days after dental or surgical procedures (antibiotic prophylaxis may also be provided in one large dose). The drug of choice is a penicillin derivative.

    C. The child and parents or primary caretaker should be familiar with this precaution.

III. Preoperative instruction.

    A. Assess the child's and family's precatheterization and preoperative learning needs and abilities and develop appropriate teaching plan.

    B. To decrease the fear of unknown aspects of care, it is often helpful to familiarize the patient and family with some of the equipment and procedures involved in the postcatheterization and/or postoperative care.

        1. Avoid overwhelming the family with useless (and potentially threatening) information.

        2. Be sensitive to what the patient and family *hear* (not always the same as what you may be saying).

        3. Children often fear mutilation when they anticipate surgical procedures—nursing care should support the patient so he or she feels comfortable enough to express these fears and/or work through them (e.g., through play).

        4. Consider patient's age and cognitive development when determining appropriate timing for preparatory teaching.

            a. If the child does not yet understand the concept of future events, early preparation may only provide excessive time for fears to build up (or may only confuse child). Prepare patient immediately prior to event.

            b. If patient is of school age or older, he or she can usually comprehend future events, and preparation should be planned to allow sufficient time for mobilization of emotional defenses before the procedure.

        5. Usually, younger patients are more concerned with what they will *feel;* older ones are often more curious about *why* and *how* things are done.

        6. If child and family have sufficient energy and emotional strength, familiarize them with the postcatheterization or postoperative care unit, unit visiting hours, unit routines (briefly), and, especially, child's nurse.

    C. Attempt to provide child and family with timetable of procedures that will involve them.

    D. Familiarize all members of the health team with particular concerns of child and family.

IV. Postcatheterization care.

    A. Monitor cardiac output, as cardiac arrhythmias and irritability may follow angiocardiography. If arrhythmia is present, determine whether it compromises cardiac output, and notify physician.

    B. Monitor urine output: Contrast media can act as an osmotic diuretic (causing increased urine volume as kidneys attempt to excrete hypertonic solution), but children may not void immediately if still sedated.

    C. If an artery is used for catheterization, ensure maintenance of adequate arterial perfusion to extremity distal to catheterization site.

        1. The patient is usually kept in bed for several hours after catheterization to decrease possibility of hemorrhage.

        2. Peripheral pulses should be present and the extremity should remain warm and

pink—notify physician *immediately* if extremity becomes cool, mottled, or pale in color.

   3. If artery develops spasms, thrombus formation can quickly occur along length of artery, causing severe compromise of circulation to extremity (if this occurs acutely, collateral circulation will not develop rapidly enough to maintain perfusion to extremity), and severe tissue necrosis may occur.

   a. If arterial circulation is compromised, application of heat to the *opposite* extremity may cause reflex arterial vasodilatation to affected extremity. *Do not apply heat to affected extremity,* as that increases metabolic demands of already compromised tissue.

   b. Intravenous infusion of heparin may arrest progression of thrombus formation, if begun as soon as compromise of arterial perfusion is noted.

   D. *If a vein is used for catheterization,* ensure maintenance of adequate venous return from extremity.

   1. Veins used for catheterization are usually tied off after the procedure, so venous return from extremity must be accomplished by other veins and by newly developed collateral circulation.

   2. Bed rest following catheterization usually is less restrictive than if an artery is used.

   3. The extremity may become edematous and cyanotic, because venous return is impeded (unoxygenated blood remains in capillaries in extremity). Notify physician if edema interferes with arterial perfusion (evidenced by decreased pulse).

   a. Elevation of the extremity will promote venous return.

   b. Provide thorough skin care and gentle handling of the extremity—as it can be very painful.

   E. Monitor catheterization site for evidence of bleeding or hematoma; apply pressure and ice if bleeding is present, and notify physician immediately if bleeding is prolonged or severe.

   F. Continue to support child's and family's coping mechanisms.

V. Postoperative care.

   A. Surgical mortality following ligation of patent ductus is very low, but is increased for premature infants and children in congestive heart failure at time of surgery.

   B. Respiratory distress and hemothorax (bleeding into chest cavity) are the most frequent postoperative complications.

   1. Monitor closely for signs of increased respiratory rate and effort.

   2. Child may "splint" incision, breathing more shallowly due to pain of left thoracotomy incision. This may cause decreased lung aeration and make the child more susceptible to development of respiratory infection.

   a. Provide vigorous chest physiotherapy (if needed) and encourage child to cough and take deep breaths.

   b. Child may cough more effectively if pain medications are administered (if ordered) prior to chest physiotherapy.

   c. Holding pillow or pressed hands against incision site may decrease pain of coughing.

   3. Increased respiratory distress, accompanied by decreased breath sounds and dullness to percussion over a lung field may indicate hemothorax, or consolidation, atelectasis, or pleural effusion (see also assessment of the chest under "General Assessment").

   a. Chest tube insertion is necessary if large hemothorax is present (performed by physician).

   b. Monitor closely for signs of cardiovascular compromise due to hemorrhage.

   C. If the patient's condition deteriorates rapidly following ductal ligation, the child may well have another congenital heart lesion which made him or her dependent on blood flow through the ductus for survival (e.g., transposition of great vessels).

   D. Ensure maintenance of a clean, nonstressed suture line.

1. Keep incision dry and intact.
2. Observe for signs of inflammation of suture line (pain or tenderness, erythema, heat, or drainage).
3. Encourage patient to move left arm slowly at first, then more frequently.
4. Child and primary caretaker should be taught appropriate wound care upon discharge.

VI. Monitor and support child's and family's coping and adjustment. (See "Intervention," point IV, under "Congestive Heart Failure," above.)

Evaluation

I. See "Evaluation" section under "Congestive Heart Failure" for information related to that condition.
II. Child and family are adequately prepared for cardiac catherization and surgery.
III. Child and family cope well with hospitalization and treatment.
IV. Postcatheterization care is adequate.
V. Postoperative care is adequate.

Aorticopulmonary Window

This unusual defect, caused by incomplete division of the common great artery trunk, results in the presence of a hole (and associated shunt) between the aorta and the pulmonary artery at a place where they share a common wall. Hemodynamic consequences and nursing care are the same as those involved in care of a child with patent ductus arteriosus. The surgical intervention carries a slightly higher risk, as cardiopulmonary bypass is used. Postoperative complications are similar.

Coarctation of the Aorta

Definition (See Fig. 13-3)

I. *Coarctation* means narrowing of the aorta; this defect arises during fetal life or at birth and is caused by an infolding of the wall of the aorta. This narrowing usually involves the area of the aorta near its junction with the ductus arteriosus but sometimes involves the thoracic aorta.
II. Coarctation of the aorta is responsible for approximately 8 percent of congenital heart disease in children; however, if often occurs in association with other congenital heart lesions (especially other anomalies of the aorta, defects of the left side of the heart, and ventricular septal defects).
III. Hemodynamic effects.
   A. Preductal coarctation:
      1. If coarctation is a *true* preductal coarctation, the aortic arch is hypoplastic, and the narrowing of the aorta occurs in the arch—the arch may be interrupted.
      2. Children with this defect always have distress early in life, as coarctation provides severe obstruction to left ventricular outflow and systemic perfusion (and no alternative flow patterns exist).
      3. Less severe coarctation *immediately* before the ductus causes symptoms virtually identical to those produced by postductal coarctation, once the ductus closes.
   B. Postductal coarctation:
      1. When coarctation is distal to the ductus arteriosus, collateral circulation often develops during fetal life, to maintain blood supply to tissues supplied by the descending aorta.
      2. The child's tolerance of this defect depends on the severity of the aortic narrowing. If the aorta is extremely narrow, there will be distress within the first months of life; if less narrow, the defect may be tolerated well for a few years.

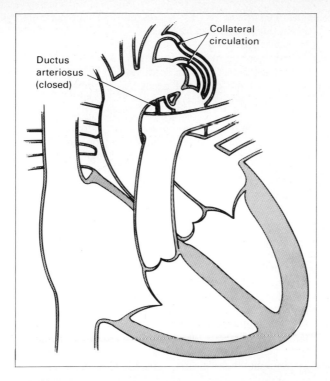

FIGURE 13-3 / **Postductal coarctation of the aorta with formation of collateral circulation.**

    C. A bicuspid aortic valve and consequent aortic valvular stenosis is present in approximately half of children with coarctation.

  IV. Any type of coarctation causes decreased blood flow to the descending aorta and lower extremities, so renal (renin-angiotensin) and neural (vasomotor) antihypotensive mechanisms are activated (exact etiology of involvement of these mechanisms is unclear).

    A. These mechanisms result in *hypertension* of the upper extremities, without significant increase in blood pressure in the lower extremities.

    B. Hypertension of the upper extremities may remain even after the coarctation is surgically repaired, especially if defect is not repaired until adolescence. The mechanisms of this are unclear.

   V. Diminished blood flow to lower extremities may cause child to experience pain and cramping during exercise, as blood flow is inadequate to meet metabolic demands of exercise.

  VI. The left ventricle hypertrophies in an attempt to generate sufficient pressure to overcome aortic flow obstruction.

 VII. If congestive heart failure is present, medical management (usually digitalis, diuretics) is required. If coarctation is severe and causes severe distress, immediate surgical resection of narrowed aortic segment is necessary. Surgery is always recommended before child's fifteenth year and is usually accomplished without cardiopulmonary bypass.

Assessment
   I. Clinical findings depend on the severity of the coarctation.

  II. Congestive heart failure and extreme cardiorespiratory distress may occur within the first weeks of life if the coarctation is severe, or if an associated cardiac lesion is present (congestive heart failure was discussed earlier).

    III. Left ventricular hypertrophy is usually present (right ventricular enlargement is present only if a patent ductus arteriosus exists).

    IV. Cyanosis is usually absent.

    V. A systolic aortic murmur may be present if blood is passing through the area of coarctation. Systolic bruits, possibly accompanied by thrills, may be heard along the ribs and chest if a large collateral circulation is present (usually involving dilated intercostal and mammary arteries).

    VI. Peripheral pulses.

        A. Generally, hypertension is found in the upper extremities, and hypotension in the lower extremities (lower extremity pulses may be diminished or absent).

        B. With coarctation or aortic stenosis, "streamlining" of aortic blood flow (creation of preferential flow patterns) may result in increased blood flow into the innominate artery (first branch off aorta) and, consequently, higher blood pressure in right arm than in left arm.

    VII. Child may complain of leg pain or cramping with exercise (due to diminished lower extremity blood flow).

Problems

    I. If child has congestive heart failure, refer to "Congestive Heart Failure," above, for identification of problems.

    II. If cardiac catheterization is required, child and family require preparation and aftercare.

    III. If surgical resection of coarctation is performed, child and family require preparation and aftercare.

    IV. Child and family experience anxiety.

    V. Child and family need teaching about the care regime, including home care.

Goals of Care

    I. If child has congestive heart failure, refer to "Congestive Heart Failure," above, for identification of goals of care.

    II. Child and family will be adequately prepared for catheterization.

    III. There will be adequate postcatheterization care.

    IV. Patient and family will be adequately prepared for surgery.

    V. Adequate postoperative care will be given.

    VI. Anxiety will be minimal.

    VII. Child and family will be well informed so they can cooperatively participate in the care regime.

Intervention

    I. If patient has congestive heart failure, see "Intervention" section under "Congestive Heart Failure," above.

    II. Refer to point IV in "Intervention" section under "Congestive Heart Failure" for anxiety-reducing and informative actions.

    III. Usually, fatigue or leg pain will limit the patient's activity, so no restrictions are required.

    IV. No particular diet is required.

    V. Physician should be consulted whenever child develops infectious illnesses, as risk of bacterial endocarditis is present (as was discussed under "Patent Ductus Arteriosus").

    VI. Antibiotic prophylaxis is extremely important prior to and following any surgical or dental procedures, and its importance should be stressed to those caring for the patient.

    VII. Usually, hypertension in the upper extremities recedes once coarctation is resected; however, severe or persistent hypertension is cause for concern.

        A. Generally, hypertension is not treated prior to child's reparative surgery, as surgical repair *is* the treatment for the problem.

        B. Antihypertensive drugs are usually ordered only if severe hypertension is present after surgery and/or it persists into young adulthood.

1. It is usually necessary to assist the child and family to *avoid* focusing on blood pressure (stress itself may cause elevation in blood pressure).
2. If antihypertensive medication is required, teaching regarding medications (therapeutic and side effects, dosage, and schedule of administration) will be necessary.

VIII. If cardiac catheterization is required, see previous discussion under "Patent Ductus Arteriosus" for child and family preparation, and for postcatheterization care of child and family.

IX. Refer to "Patent Ductus Arteriosus" for discussion of preoperative preparation.

X. Monitor closely for signs of congestive heart failure. Mortality following repair of coarctation is low but may be increased if child is in congestive failure at the time of surgery or if severe preductal coarctation is present. *The most frequent cause of postoperative death is cardiac failure.*

XI. Monitor lower extremity pulses and perfusion to ensure adequate circulation.

XII. Respiratory distress or hemothorax may occur, so monitor respiratory rate and effort carefully (see also "General Assessment" in the early part of this chapter).

XIII. Chylothorax (lymph fluid in the thoracic cavity) may occur if thoracic duct is injured during surgery (this structure lies near the thoracic aorta).
  A. Child will demonstrate signs of increased respiratory distress, decreased aeration of lung on involved side, and dullness to chest percussion (evidence of fluid in thoracic cavity will be noted on x-ray).
  B. Chest tubes should be inserted, and milky drainage (lymph fluid) should occur.
  C. Patient will require adequate replacements of fats and fat-soluble vitamins in diet.

XIV. Abdominal pain may be present postoperatively. Exact etiology is unknown, but it is postulated that decreased preoperative aortic blood flow causes mesenteric arteries to develop into fragile vessels which cannot tolerate the high-pressure blood flow they receive once coarctation is repaired.
  A. Monitor bowel sounds carefully for evidence of decreased motility of bowel.
  B. If abdomen becomes extremely tender, or if fever or elevated white cell count is present, notify physician (bowel necrosis may be present).
  C. Complaints of "tummy" pain may also signify that there is discomfort in the chest (ask patient to point to the area that hurts).

XV. Hypertension may be present in upper extremities, as was discussed earlier; if so, attempt to provide quiet, soothing environment (prevent excessive stimulation), and administer analgesics for headache.

XVI. If much dissection is required along the thoracic aorta to resect the coarctation, injury of the blood supply to the spinal cord may result. Monitor lower extremity movement and sensation.

XVII. If a patch is required to rejoin segments of the aorta during surgical repair of coarctation, the child becomes susceptible to infection around the patch if bacteremia is present.
  A. Obtain blood cultures if patient has high or persistent fever, and monitor white blood count.
  B. Observe closely for signs of cardiovascular compromise (see "Assessment" section under "Congestive Heart Failure").
  C. Antibiotic prophylaxis will be necessary prior to and following any surgical or dental procedure, even after discharge from the hospital—it is important to teach the child and primary caretaker about this. Refer to "Intervention" under "Patent Ductus Arteriosus" for more information.

XVIII. If coarctation is surgically corrected during infancy, surgical site of resection and resewing of aorta may become fibrotic and fail to grow adequately with child. Coarctation (and associated symptoms) can recur, and reoperation will be necessary.

XIX. Maintain a clean, dry incision, and monitor for inflammation.

Evaluation

I. If child has congestive heart failure, refer to "Evaluation" section under "Congestive Heart Failure," above.

II. Child and family are adequately prepared for catheterization and surgery and cope well.

III. Postcatheterization and postoperative care are adequate.

IV. Child and family are well-informed participants in the care regime.

Congenital Aortic Stenosis

Definition

I. *Aortic stenosis* refers to several forms of obstruction to the left ventricular outflow; these comprise nearly 4 percent of all forms of congenital heart disease in children.

II. There are three main types of aortic stenosis:

A. *Valvular* (most common form): This type results from incomplete separation of valve leaflets during embryologic development. A bicuspid valve is usually present (this form is often associated with coarctation of the aorta).

B. *Subvalvular* stenosis usually results from the formation of a membranous web below the aortic valve. Idiopathic hypertrophic subaortic stenosis (IHSS) is an unusual form of subvalvular stenosis caused by thickening of the left side of the ventricular septum.

C. *Supravalvular* (least common) form is usually caused by formation of a fibrous ring just above the aortic valve (may be seen in conjunction with hypertelorism, mental retardation, and unusual facial characteristics in those afflicted).

III. Hemodynamic effects: a wide range of severity.

A. As with any aortic obstruction, the left ventricle must generate sufficient pressure to maintain adequate flow through the stenotic area (left ventricular hypertrophy occurs).

   1. If stenosis is *extreme*, the left ventricle may be unable to generate sufficient pressure to maintain cardiac output, and congestive heart failure occurs within the first weeks of life. This form of aortic stenosis is generally associated with extremely high mortality.

   2. In most forms of congenital aortic stenosis, the left ventricle is able to sustain aortic flow sufficient for child's resting requirements, but is unable to sustain maximum cardiac output during exercise.

   3. With subvalvular aortic stenosis, aortic valvular insufficiency is often also present.

B. The pressure gradient across the stenotic area determines the gravity of the child's defect. (The pressure gradient is the pressure in aorta measured distal to the stenosis subtracted from pressure measured in the left ventricle and is obtained during cardiac catheterization.)

   1. If less than a 50 mmHg gradient exists between left ventricle and arch of the aorta, the child usually tolerates this defect well (without evidence of cardiac compromise).

   2. If greater than a 50 mmHg gradient exists, the left ventricle is subjected to an enormous pressure load, and decompensation is more likely.

      a. Congestive heart failure indicates decompensation.

      b. Appearance of left ventricular strain patterns noted by ST segment changes on the electrocardiogram indicate great risk of decompensation.

      c. Once the limits of the patient's cardiac compensation are reached, increased activity or demands on cardiac output can cause sudden and fatal arrhythmias, syncope (indicating insufficient cerebral perfusion), or sudden death. To prevent this, activity must be restricted.

C. Arterial oxygen saturation is usually normal.

IV. If congestive heart failure is present, medical management (digitalis and diuretics) is necessary, but surgical intervention must also be performed. Surgery is also required if the gradient across stenotic area is 50 mmHg or greater, and is essential if signs of left ventricular strain are noted on the electrocardiogram.

    A. Cardiopulmonary bypass is required (hypothermia may be used if patient is an infant).

    B. Resection of the stenotic web, fibrous ring, or membrane is sometimes accomplished through an aortic incision, but a ventricular incision may be required.

    C. If supravalvular aortic stenosis is severe, a patch may be placed in the wall of the aorta, to increase its size.

Assessment

    I. The majority of patients with aortic stenosis are asymptomatic.

    II. If congestive heart failure is present, see "Congestive Heart Failure" for appropriate assessments.

    III. Cyanosis is rare.

    IV. Left ventricular heave may be palpated due to left ventricular hypertrophy. Check electrocardiogram for signs of left ventricular strain.

    V. Heart sounds.

        A. With all forms of aortic stenosis, an ejection systolic murmur is present and is usually heard best at the aortic area (may be accompanied by a thrill).

        B. With valvular aortic stenosis, a click may be noted in the fourth intercostal space at the left sternal border.

        C. If aortic valvular insufficiency coexists, an aortic diastolic murmur will be present.

    VI. Peripheral pulses.

        A. Peripheral pulses may be unremarkable if stenosis is mild.

        B. With moderate stenosis, decreased systolic blood pressure and a narrow pulse pressure are usually present (if aortic insufficiency is also present, pulse pressure may be normal).

        C. With severe stenosis and congestive heart failure, peripheral pulses may be diminished.

        D. "Streamlining" of blood flow into the innominate artery (first branch off the aortic arch) may cause higher blood pressure measurements in right than in left arm.

    VII. Question child and primary caretaker about child's exercise tolerance, and notify physician immediately of any history of syncopal episodes. Also determine if any restrictions are placed on activity (and extent of child's compliance).

Problems

    I. If child has congestive heart failure, see "Problems" under "Congestive Heart Failure."

    II. Child and family are likely to be anxious about illness, treatment, and prognosis.

    III. Child and family may need instruction and information.

    IV. Cardiac catheterization may be necessary. See previous section, "Patent Ductus Arteriosus," for nursing problems related to precatheterization preparation and postcatheterization care.

    V. Surgical intervention may be necessary.

Goals of Care

    I. If child has congestive heart failure, see "Goals of Care" under "Congestive Heart Failure."

    II. Reduce anxiety and provide needed information.

    III. Provide preparation and aftercare for catheterization and surgery.

Intervention

    I. If child has congestive heart failure, see "Congestive Heart Failure" for interventions.

    II. Refer to point IV in "Intervention" section under "Congestive Heart Failure" for anxiety-reducing actions. In addition:

        A. If child has severe aortic stenosis, and physician has discussed activity restriction and possibility of child's sudden death with family, extreme anxiety would be family's normal response.

        B. It will be difficult, but the health team must attempt to prevent family from focusing abnormal attention on child's cardiac function.

            1. If a specific plan of activity restriction is provided by physician, attempt to make this more acceptable by suggesting or supplying quiet, diversional activities.

       2. Activity restriction will be especially difficult during adolescence, when peer pressure may cause the teenager to test activity restrictions. (Surgery should be scheduled as soon as evidence of stenosis requiring activity restriction is discovered.)

       3. Family may be comforted to know that health team members are available to answer questions or provide assistance if necessary.

III. Turbulent blood flow around aortic valve makes patient especially susceptible to development of bacterial thrombus and embolus and to endocarditis (described more fully under "Intervention" in "Patent Ductus Arteriosus." Child and primary caretaker should be taught about antibiotic prophylaxis. This will be required even after surgery, as turbulent blood flow will still be present.

IV. No fluid restriction or special diets are necessary (unless congestive heart failure is present).

V. If stenosis is severe, activity restriction may be required until surgical repair is accomplished.

    A. Health team should confer with patient and parents and determine specific activities child is to avoid.

    B. Health care follow-up must be frequent and thorough; physician should be notified immediately if there are any syncopal episodes or further deterioration in health status.

    C. Attempt (if possible) to help family avoid focusing on child's health status (discussed above).

VI. Usually a digitalis derivative is not helpful in improving cardiac output, as increased cardiac contractility will not change the amount of resistance offered by the stenotic outflow area of left ventricle or aorta (digitalis may be required if child has congestive heart failure pre- or postoperatively).

VII. If cardiac catheterization is performed, see "Interventions" under "Patent Ductus Arteriosus" for a discussion of preparation of child and family and postcatheterization care.

VIII. If surgical intervention is necessary, see "Intervention" under "Patent Ductus Arteriosus" for a discussion of preoperative preparation of child and family.

IX. Monitor cardiac rate and rhythm carefully for evidence of arrhythmia; sudden arrhythmia is the commonest reported cause of postoperative death.

    A. If irregularity exists in the cardiac rhythm, notify physician, and determine if irregularity is causing compromise of the systemic perfusion (see "Assessment" section of "Congestive Heart Failure").

    B. Attempt to determine if any precipitating factors (such as electrolyte imbalance) or alleviating factors (such as administration of antiarrhythmic drugs) exist, so further arrhythmias may be prevented.

    C. Administer antiarrhythmic drugs as ordered (ensure proper dosage, and monitor for therapeutic, side, and toxic effects).

    D. Monitor electrolyte values, especially potassium and calcium; imbalance may result from use of cardiopulmonary bypass, and may precipitate arrhythmias.

    E. If the child is stable, continue to monitor, but avoid obviously focusing attention on auscultation of the chest or on observation of the cardiac monitor, as this may magnify child's and family's anxiety.

X. Assess for signs of congestive heart failure or systemic circulatory compromise and provide appropriate therapy if present (see "Assessment" and "Intervention" under "Congestive Heart Failure").

XI. Monitor child's fluid balance.

    A. Child's intake of fluid should not exceed daily fluid requirement plus urine output (if urine output is adequate).

    B. Cell lysis occurs with use of cardiopulmonary bypass, so monitor urine for evidence of hemoglobinuria or decreased urine output (if output is decreased, decrease intake).

XII. Provide adequate pulmonary toilet (discussed under "Congestive Heart Failure" and under "Patent Ductus Arteriosus"). Child will have median sternotomy incision.

XIII. Monitor for signs of postoperative hemorrhage.

    A. Watch for signs of decreased systemic perfusion.

    B. Increased systemic venous congestion with simultaneous acute decrease in cardiac output may indicate *cardiac tamponade* (bleeding around the heart, usually within the pericardium, which exerts pressure on the myocardium, decreasing the ability of ventricles to fill and pump effectively).

XIV. Support child's and family's coping mechanisms. (See "Intervention," point IV, under "Congestive Heart Failure.")

XV. Maintain a clean, dry incision line—observe for and report any signs of inflammation.

Evaluation

I. If child has congestive heart failure, refer to "Evaluation" section under "Congestive Heart Failure."

II. Anxiety is minimal and both child and parents cope adequately.

III. Child and parents are well-informed participants in the care regime.

IV. Postcatheterization and postoperative care are adequate.

Vascular Rings

Definition (See Fig. 13-4)

I. Anomalies of aortic arch development during fetal life can result in the formation of a variety of anomalous vessels which encircle the trachea and esophagus—these are referred to as *vascular rings*. They may be produced by anomalies or remnants of the following vessels:

    A. Double aortic arch.

    B. Right (instead of left) aortic arch with left-sided ductus arteriosus.

    C. Anomalous subclavian or innominate artery.

II. Vascular rings usually cause compression of the soft, cartilaginous trachea and the esophagus.

    A. Compression of the trachea reduces airway size, causing respiratory distress and predisposing child to frequent upper respiratory infections.

    B. Compression of the esophagus interferes with swallowing.

    C. Occasionally, vascular rings cause few or no symptoms (if compression of the trachea or esophagus is minimal).

III. Surgical ligation of anomalous vessels and medical treatment of respiratory infections is necessary.

Assessment

I. If slight or no compression of the trachea or esophagus occurs, child will remain asymptomatic.

II. If child is symptomatic, distress will usually be present soon after birth and increase with age (the trachea and esophagus grow with the child, so increased constriction occurs).

III. With compression of the trachea, symptoms of upper airway obstruction occur.

    A. Respirations are noisy, and child demonstrates increased respiratory effort.

        1. Coarse rhonchi heard equally over entire chest wall are indicative of upper airway obstruction.

        2. Stridor (high-pitched wheeze heard with inspiration) may be audible.

    B. Child has frequent upper respiratory infections, which cause severe respiratory distress by further compromising respiratory function.

IV. With compression of the esophagus, feeding difficulties occur.

    A. Child has difficulty swallowing and may vomit frequently.

    B. Child tires easily during feedings.

V. Presence of vascular ring should be suspected when any child exhibits a combination of upper airway obstruction and feeding difficulties.

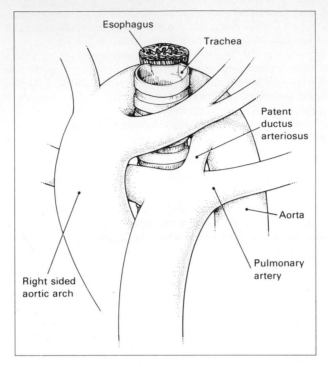

FIGURE 13-4 / **Vascular ring.**

VI. Cardiovascular findings are usually negative, though cardiac catheterization is usually required to establish diagnosis. Murmur (possibly accompanied by a thrill) may be auscultated over area of aortic arch. A murmur characteristic of a patent ductus arteriosus may be noted if this structure is part of vascular ring.

Problems

I. Child has extreme respiratory distress.
II. Nutritional status is compromised.
III. Parent(s) or primary caretaker(s) may experience extreme anxiety related to child's respiratory distress, feeding difficulties, frequent illness, or surgery.
IV. Child is candidate for cardiac catheterization and surgery.

Goals of Care

I. Reduce respiratory distress and promote optimal respiratory function.
II. Ensure adequate nutritional intake and promote child's optimal growth.
III. Support family's coping mechanisms and provide appropriate information to decrease anxiety.
IV. Prepare child and family for catheterization and surgery, and provide aftercare.

Intervention

I. Monitor respiratory rate, effort, and function (see "General Assessment" at beginning of this chapter).
II. Provide appropriate pulmonary toilet (discussed in "Intervention" section under "Congestive Heart Failure.")
III. Provide quiet environment and minimize noxious stimuli (see "Intervention" section under "Congestive Heart Failure").
IV. Provide for nutritional needs (see related intervention under "Congestive Heart Failure").

V. Alleviate parental anxiety and need for information and instruction.
   A. See "Intervention," point IV, under "Congestive Heart Failure."
   B. Parent(s) or primary caretaker will be frustrated in their attempts to nurture child; it may help them to realize that feeding and respiratory difficulties could not have been avoided.
   C. Include parent(s) and caretaker(s) in care as much as possible (ask their advice about ways they have found to comfort child).
VI. For nursing interventions regarding child's catheterization and postoperative care, refer to related interventions under "Patent Ductus Arteriosus."
   A. Surgical complications are infrequent and resemble those encountered following ligation of ductus arteriosus.
   B. Development of congestive heart failure pre- or postoperatively is rare.

Evaluation
I. Respiratory distress is minimal; respiratory function is optimal.
II. Nutritional intake is adequate and supports growth.
III. Family copes adequately and is well informed to participate in care regime.
IV. Pre- and postcatheterization care and pre- and postoperative care are adequate.

Atrial Septal Defect (ASD)

Definition (See Fig. 13-5)
I. *Atrial septal defect* results from improper embryologic development of atrial septum, and accounts for approximately 12 percent of congenital heart disease in children.
II. Many varieties of ASD exist:
   A. *Ostium secundum:* Defect is high in the atrial septum (most common form). Well-tolerated.
   B. *Ostium primum:* Defect is low in the atrial septum, and involves the endocardial

FIGURE 13-5 / Secundum atrial septal defect.

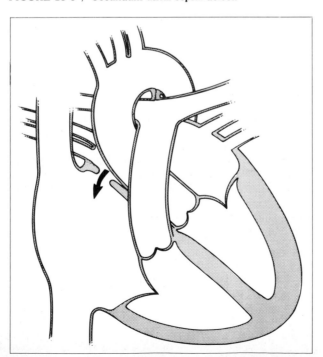

cushions and atrioventricular valves to a variable degree (see "Endocardial Cushion Defects" in this chapter).

    C. *Sinus venosus:* Improper development of the septum results in unequal division of atria; some of the pulmonary veins empty into the *right* atrium.

    D. Reopening of (fetal) foramen ovale may occur as a result of a defect which greatly increases resistance to right atrial or right ventricular outflow (e.g., tricuspid atresia, pulmonary valvular stenosis); right-to-left shunting then occurs between the atria.

III. Hemodynamic effects: ostium secundum malformation (see "Endocardial Cushion Defects" for discussion of ostium primum).

    A. With a defect in the atrial septum, blood will flow through defect in path of *least resistance* (into right atrium to right ventricle and into pulmonary outflow tract once pulmonary vascular resistance has dropped, usually by 6 weeks to 3 months of age).

    B. Pulmonary arterioles receive increased blood flow, but under *low* pressures generated by right ventricle, so pulmonary vascular resistance (due to pulmonary arterial wall hypertrophy) increases only slowly over 20 to 40 years (see "Hemo-dynamic Principles" near beginning of this chapter).

    C. The right atrium and right ventricle hypertrophy with volume load; congestive heart failure almost never occurs.

    D. Defect must be closed surgically with sutures or patch (cardiopulmonary bypass is required).

Assessment

I. Children with secundum atrial septal defect are generally asymptomatic (see "Endo-cardial Cushion Defects" for discussion of assessment of child with ostium primum defect).

II. Pulmonary congestion and heart failure are rare in childhood.

III. Right ventricular hypertrophy may cause sternal lift, and ripple may be noted along middle of chest as large blood flow enters right ventricle.

IV. Heart sounds:

    A. Soft, pulmonic systolic murmur is present due to greatly increased pulmonary blood flow; fixed, wide splitting of the S_2 sound occurs (pulmonary valve closes late with high flow).

    B. With a large shunt, a tricuspid diastolic murmur may appear and may be accompanied by a thrill due to large flow through this valve into the right ventricle.

    C. Atrial fibrillation or flutter may appear if the right atrium becomes very large.

Problems

I. Child and family require preparation for cardiac catheterization and surgery.

II. Thorough care following cardiac catheterization and surgery is required.

III. Child and family experience anxiety and need teaching about the care regimen, including home care.

Goals of Care

I. Provide adequate information and psychological support to promote successful coping with stress of hospitalization and surgery.

II. Promote positive relationship between family and health team members to foster effective communication and minimize stress for family and child.

III. Restore and maintain optimal cardiovascular function after catheterization.

IV. Restore and maintain adequate cardiorespiratory function following surgery.

Intervention

I. Interventions for child's and parents' anxiety and teaching needs are presented in detail in "Intervention," point IV, under "Congestive Heart Failure."

II. Since children with secundum atrial septal defect are rarely symptomatic, no restrictions are placed on diet or activity.

III. It is recommended that parents seek medical attention if child becomes ill, and that antibiotic prophylaxis be administered before and after any surgical or dental procedures because there is a small possibility of developing endocarditis until the defect (source of turbulent blood flow) is closed. See "Intervention" section under "Patent Ductus Arteriosus" for further discussion.

IV. Interventions related to cardiac catheterization and surgery are discussed above under patent ductus arteriosus and congenital aortic stenosis. Surgical mortality for closure of atrial septal defect is low; arrhythmias are the most frequent complication. Development of congestive heart failure following surgery is rare.

Evaluation
I. Child and family cope adequately and are well-informed participants in the care regime.
II. Child and family are adequately prepared for catheterization and surgery.
III. Care following catheterization and surgery is adequate.

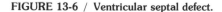

Ventricular Septal Defect (VSD)

Definition (See Fig. 13-6)

I. VSD is the most common form of congenital heart disease, responsible for approximately 30 percent of all congenital heart disease in children.

II. It is a result of improper embryologic formation of the ventricular septum; thus, blood is allowed to flow between ventricles, following the path of *least* resistance.

A. Little or no shunting of blood occurs during neonatal period (when pulmonary vascular resistance is high), but left-to-right shunting will occur once pulmonary vascular resistance drops (usually when child is 6 weeks to 3 months of age), as pulmonary outflow tract offers the path of least resistance.

B. Size of shunt is proportional to size of defect (large defect allows large shunt) if no other cardiac abnormalities are present.

C. Many small ventricular septal defects close spontaneously; all septal defects become

FIGURE 13-6 / **Ventricular septal defect.**

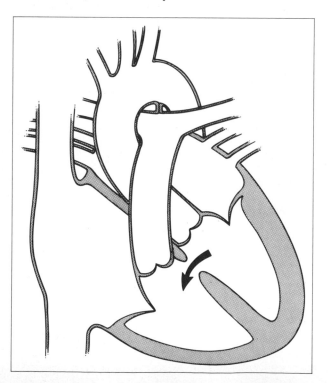

proportionally smaller with growth. As a result, many children with small ventricular defects are followed closely for years, with hopes that the defect will close (or continue to cause no problems).

   D. A small defect allows only a small shunt, and this results in only slightly increased pulmonary blood flow under low pressure (the small diameter of the defect dampens out much of the pressure head of blood shunting from the left to the right ventricle). This defect is better tolerated and the child may remain asymptomatic.

   E. If the defect is large, equalization of pressures between ventricles occurs, and increased pulmonary blood flow occurs under *high* pressures (once pulmonary vascular resistance falls).

   1. This is not well tolerated by pulmonary vascularity, and congestive heart failure frequently occurs at this time (6 weeks to 3 months of age, if pulmonary vascular resistance falls normally).

   2. With this pulmonary flow, pulmonary vascular resistance soon increases as pulmonary arterial walls hypertrophy; if increased pulmonary resistance is allowed to progress, the shunt may become bidirectional after several years.

   F. When a large defect causes congestive heart failure, medical management (with digitalis and diuretics) is necessary; if the child remains in severe congestive heart failure, surgical intervention is necessary.

   1. A palliative procedure known as *pulmonary banding*, which consists of placement of a band around the pulmonary artery, will decrease pulmonary blood flow (and prevent pulmonary vascular changes).

   2. Open-heart closure of the septal defect may be accomplished through use of cardiopulmonary bypass in children, and with use of *hypothermia* in infants.

   a. Defect may be closed through use of sutures or a patch, using an atrial or ventricular incision.

   b. Hypothermia involves cooling of infant's core body temperature to reduce metabolic rate and, hence, child's circulatory demands—heart may then be stopped for several minutes to permit surgical repair without adverse effect on vital organs.

Assessment

   I. Child may remain asymptomatic if defect is small or if child is a neonate (and pulmonary vascular resistance is still high).

   II. Symptoms of congestive heart failure and respiratory distress may be present in infant beyond 6 weeks of age.

   III. Cyanosis is unusual; it may occur during crying or late in the clinical course (due to development of increased pulmonary vascular resistance and consequent reversal of shunt).

   IV. The "classic" VSD murmur is a harsh, systolic murmur heard best at the left lower sternal border and radiating over much of the chest (it may be accompanied by a thrill). If shunt is large, causing *large* pulmonary blood flow, a diastolic mitral murmur may be heard over the apex when large pulmonary venous return moves into the left ventricle.

Problems

   I. If child has congestive heart failure, refer to "Problems" section under "Congestive Heart Failure."

   II. Child and family require preparation for child's cardiac catheterization and surgery.

   III. Postcatheterization and postoperative care will be necessary.

   IV. Child and parents experience anxiety and need teaching about the care regime and home care.

Goals of Care

   I. If congestive heart failure is present, refer to "Goals of Care" section under "Congestive Heart Failure."

   II. Provide adequate information and psychological support to promote successful coping with stress of hospitalization and surgery.

III. Restore, promote, and maintain optimal cardiovascular function following catheterization.

IV. Promote, restore, and maintain adequate cardiorespiratory function following surgery.

Intervention

I. If child has congestive heart failure, refer to "Intervention" section under "Congestive Heart Failure."

II. See "Intervention," point IV, under "Congestive Heart Failure" regarding child's and parents' anxiety and teaching needs.

III. Since child possesses intracardiac defect causing turbulent blood flow, antibiotic prophylaxis is required before and after any surgical or dental procedures, as explained in the "Intervention" section under "Patent Ductus Arteriosus." Counsel child and primary caretaker to seek medical care if child becomes ill or has a fever.

IV. Prepare child and family for catheterization and surgery. Interventions are those given under "Patent Ductus Arteriosus."

V. Provide postcatheterization and postoperative care. Interventions are those given under "Patent Ductus Arteriosus."

VI. Since congestive heart failure is the most frequent postoperative complication, monitor for signs of congestive heart failure (see "Assessment" section under "Congestive Heart Failure") and provide appropriate care as described in interventions for congestive heart failure.

VII. Monitor the cardiac rate and rhythm carefully for arrhythmia.

    A. If irregularity exists in the cardiac rhythm, notify physician, and determine whether irregularity is causing compromise of child's systemic perfusion (see "Assessment" section under "Congestive Heart Failure").

    B. Attempt to determine whether any precipitating factors (such as electrolyte imbalance) or alleviating factors (such as administration of antiarrhythmic drugs) exists, so further arrhythmias may be prevented.

    C. Administer antiarrhythmic drugs as ordered (ensure proper dosage, and monitor for therapeutic, side, and toxic effects).

    D. Monitor electrolyte values, especially potassium and calcium—imbalance may result from use of cardiopulmonary bypass and may precipitate arrhythmias.

    E. If child is stable, continue to monitor but avoid obviously focusing attention on auscultation of chest or observation of cardiac monitor—this may magnify child's and family's anxiety.

VIII. Monitor fluid balance:

    A. Fluid intake should not exceed daily fluid requirement plus urine output (if urine output is adequate).

    B. Cell lysis occurs with use of cardiopulmonary bypass, so monitor urine for evidence of hemoglobinuria or decreased urine output (if output is decreased, decrease intake).

IX. Provide adequate pulmonary toilet (discussed under "Congestive Heart Failure" and under "Patent Ductus Arteriosus").

X. Monitor for signs of postoperative hemorrhage:

    A. Watch for signs of decreased systemic perfusion.

    B. Increased systemic venous congestion with simultaneous acute decrease in cardiac output may indicate cardiac tamponade (bleeding around the heart, usually within the pericardium, which exerts pressure on the myocardium and decreases the ability of the ventricles to fill and pump effectively).

XI. Support child's and family's coping mechanisms (see "Intervention," point IV, under "Congestive Heart Failure").

XII. Maintain a clean, dry incision line—observe for and report any signs of inflammation.

XIII. Surgical mortality for repair of VSD or for pulmonary banding is low if either is done electively; if child is in congestive heart failure or has severely increased pulmonary vascular resistance at the time of surgery, mortality is higher.

Evaluation

    I. If child has congestive heart failure, refer to evaluations under the section on congestive heart failure.

    II. Anxiety is minimized and both child and parents cope adequately.

    III. Child and parents are well-informed participants in the care regime.

    IV. Postcatheterization and postoperative care are adequate.

Endocardial Cushion Defects

Definition (See Fig. 13-7)

    I. *Endocardial cushion defects* represent approximately 2 percent of all congenital heart disease in children, but account for nearly 40 percent of the congenital heart lesions found in children with Down's (trisomy 21) syndrome.

    II. This defect results from improper fusion of endocardial cushions during fetal development, and results in some combination of the following defects:

        A. Atrial septal defect (low in atrial septum—ostium primum).

        B. Ventricular septal defect.

        C. Abnormalities of the artrioventricular (especially mitral) valves.

    III. Hemodynamic effects: There is a wide range of severity of defects.

        A. The milder form consists largely of an ostium primum atrial septal defect with only a cleft in the mitral valve.

            1. Hemodynamic effects are very similar to those of an ostium secundum atrial septal defect.

            2. Mitral cleft may cause mitral insufficiency and result in pulmonary venous congestion (pre- or postoperatively).

        B. The most severe form (complete atrioventricular canal) consists of combined atrial and ventricular septal defect and severe mitral insufficiency; the large common

FIGURE 13-7 / **Endocardial cushion defect with complete atrioventricular canal.**

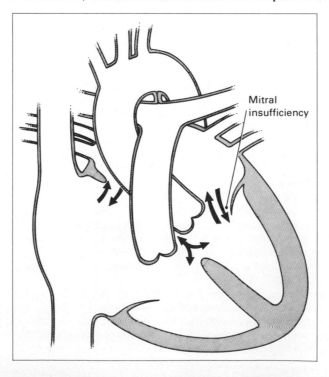

Mitral insufficiency

    defect allows mixing of oxygenated and deoxygenated blood throughout the chambers, and equalization of ventricular pressures.

    1. Pulmonary blood flow is similar to that caused by large ventricular septal defect.

    2. Severe mitral insufficiency may cause pulmonary edema.

  C. Congestive heart failure requires medical treatment. If severe congestive heart failure continues, surgical palliative or reparative intervention is necessary:

    1. Pulmonary artery banding (described in "Definition" under "Ventricular Septal Defect") may be performed as a palliative procedure to restrict some pulmonary blood flow.

    2. Total repair is electively performed when child is 18 months to 4 years old, but may be performed with use of hypothermia in infancy.

    3. Total correction consists of closure of atrial and ventricular septal defects (one patch used) and suturing of cleft in mitral valve (if valve is too deformed to repair, insertion of a prosthetic mitral valve is performed).

IV. A child with cyanotic heart disease (due to right-to-left cardiac shunt and consequent mixing of deoxygenated with oxygenated blood within the heart) may develop several systemic complications:

  A. Polycythemia (increased numbers of red cells in blood) occurs in response to chronic arterial oxygen desaturation; with polycythemia, blood viscosity increases, so the child becomes more susceptible to thrombus and embolus formation and has an increased risk of sustaining a cerebral vascular accident.

  B. Pulmonary capillary macrophages phagocytize bacteria. If systemic venous blood bypasses the lungs and enters the aorta, bacteria may enter the systemic circulation and may cause brain abscess.

  C. Because child has turbulent intracardiac blood flow, there is an increased risk of developing endocarditis (see "Intervention" section under "Patent Ductus Arteriosus" for discussion).

Assessment

I. Congestive heart failure may be noted (see "Assessment" section under "Congestive Heart Failure").

II. Cyanosis:

  A. May be absent, if child's defect consists primarily of an atrial septal defect.

  B. Will be present if much mixing of arterial and venous blood occurs within the heart.

  C. Clubbing of tips of fingers or toes may occur with cyanosis (due to chronic peripheral hypoxia).

III. Heart sounds include those found when atrial septal defect is present (see "Assessment" section under "Atrial Septal Defect") and when ventricular septal defect is present (see "Assessment" section under "Ventricular Septal Defect"). A systolic murmur is noted over the mitral area if mitral insufficiency is present.

IV. Right bundle branch block is often noted on electrocardiogram.

Problems

I. If child is to have cardiac catheterization or surgery, child and family need thorough preparation and aftercare.

II. Child and family experience anxiety and need teaching about the care regime, including home care.

III. If patient has congestive heart failure, refer to the earlier section on congestive heart failure for identification of problems.

IV. If child has severe cyanosis, he or she is at risk for the consequences of polycythemia and hypoxemia.

Goals of Care

I. Provide adequate information and psychological support to promote successful coping with stress of illness, hospitalization, and treatment.

II. Promote positive relationship between family and health team members to foster effective communication and minimize stress for family and child.

III. Restore, promote, and maintain optimal cardiovascular function following catheterization.

    IV. Promote, restore, and maintain adequate cardiorespiratory function following surgery.
    V. If child has congestive heart failure, refer to goals of care in "Congestive Heart Failure."
    VI. Minimize consequences of polycythemia and hypoxemia.

Intervention

    I. If congestive heart failure is present, see "Intervention" section under "Congestive Heart Failure."
    II. Refer to "Intervention," point IV, under "Congestive Heart Failure" for anxiety-reducing and informative actions.
    III. If there is severe cyanosis, refer to related interventions under "Tetralogy of Fallot."
    IV. Usually, child's fatigue will limit activity, so enforced restriction is not required.
    V. Salt or fluid restrictions may be necessary if severe heart failure or mitral insufficiency (and pulmonary edema) are present before or after surgery.
    VI. A patient with cyanosis and compensatory polycythemia cannot tolerate dehydration (especially an infant), so parents or primary caretaker must be instructed to notify physician if prolonged or recurrent fever, vomiting, or diarrhea are present.
    VII. Child should receive well-balanced diet.
    VIII. Antibiotic prophylaxis is extremely important to reduce risk of endocarditis (refer to related interventions under "Patent Ductus Arteriosus").
    IX. If catheterization or surgery is to be done, prepare child and parents. Interventions are given under "Patent Ductus Arteriosus."
    X. Provide postcatheterization care. Interventions are given under "Patent Ductus Arteriosus."
    XI. Provide postoperative care.
        A. Note: If mixing of deoxygenated with oxygenated blood is still present, *any* air allowed to pass intravenously may enter the aorta and cause cerebral air embolus (stroke)—*absolutely no air bubbles are allowed in intravenous line.*
        B. There is a wide range of surgical morbidity and mortality following complete repair of this defect; if severe mitral insufficiency is present postoperatively, mortality is high. Development of pulmonary edema (due to mitral insufficiency) and congestive heart failure are the most frequent postoperative complications.
            1. Auscultate chest for mitral insufficiency murmur.
            2. Auscultate chest and check chest x-ray for evidence of pulmonary edema.
            3. Monitor child carefully for the development of congestive heart failure (see "Assessment" section under "Congestive Heart Failure") and respiratory distress (see "General Assessment" at beginning of chapter).
                a. If heart failure or pulmonary edema is present, scrupulous management of intravenous therapy is required.
                b. Aggressive chest physiotherapy is required.
                c. See "Congestive Heart Failure" for further nursing interventions for child with congestive heart failure.
        C. Arrhythmias also occur frequently following repair of endocardial cushion defects (see "Intervention" section under "Aortic Stenosis" for assessment and interventions related to arrhythmias).
        D. Assess child carefully for any evidence of thrombus or embolus formation, especially cerebral and pulmonary emboli.
        E. Children with cyanotic heart disease and polycythemia often have abnormalities of platelet function, and have an increased risk of hemorrhage postoperatively.
        F. Monitor fluid balance:
            1. Intake should not exceed daily fluid requirement plus urine output (if output is adequate).
            2. Cell lysis occurs with use of cardiopulmonary bypass, so monitor for hemoglobinuria or decreased urine output (if output is decreased, decrease intake).
        G. Provide adequate pulmonary toilet (discussed under "Congestive Heart Failure" and "Patent Ductus Arteriosus").
        H. Monitor for signs of postoperative hemorrhage:
            1. Watch for signs of decreased systemic perfusion.

2. Increased systemic venous congestion with simultaneous acute decrease in cardiac output may indicate cardiac tamponade (bleeding around the heart, usually within the pericardium, which compresses the heart and decreases the ability of the ventricles to fill and pump effectively).

  I. Maintain a clean, dry incision line—observe for and report any signs of inflammation.

Evaluation

  I. Child and parents are adequately informed participants in care regime.
  II. Child and parents cope adequately.
  III. Preparation and aftercare related to catheterization and surgery are adequate.
  IV. Complications due to polycythemia and hypoxemia are minimized.
  V. If child has congestive heart failure, refer to evaluations under that heading.

Tetralogy of Fallot

Definition (See Fig. 13-8)

  I. *Tetralogy of Fallot* is responsible for approximately 8 percent of congenital heart disease in children. It consists of an association of four abnormalities:

  A. Pulmonary infundibular stenosis (stenosis of the muscular band just below the pulmonary valve). If pulmonary infundibular stenosis is extremely severe, the pulmonary artery may be extremely small; this defect is often called *pseudotruncus,* as the output of both ventricles enters the aorta and the majority of pulmonary artery blood flow must occur through collateral circulation developed from the descending aorta (see "Definition" section under "Truncus Arteriosus").

  B. Ventricular septal defect (membranous ventricular septum fails to fuse properly).

FIGURE 13-8 / Tetralogy of Fallot.

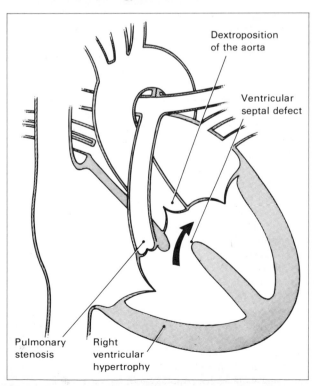

Dextroposition of the aorta

Ventricular septal defect

Pulmonary stenosis

Right ventricular hypertrophy

      C. Overriding aorta (since pulmonary infundibulum and artery are underdeveloped, the aorta grows more anterior and to the right than normal and consequently rests immediately over the ventricular septal defect).

      D. Hypertrophy of right ventricle (occurs with *any* obstruction to pulmonary outflow).

II. Hemodynamic effects.

      A. With mild infundibular stenosis, pulmonary blood flow may be maintained.

      B. If infundibular stenosis is moderate, blood flows through the ventricular septal defect (right to left), and almost directly into the aorta (this becomes the path of least resistance).

      C. Right ventricular hypertrophy occurs, because the pulmonary artery and aorta both offer much resistance to right ventricular outflow.

      D. The left ventricle is smaller than normal, as it only pumps the small amount of blood returning from the lungs (blood shunting from right ventricle through ventricular septal defect usually enters the aorta directly and does not circulate through the lungs.)

III. Congestive heart failure is rare.

IV. A child with cyanotic heart disease (due to right-to-left cardiac shunt and consequent mixing of deoxygenated with oxygenated blood within the heart) may develop several systemic complications. These complications frequently occur in tetralogy of Fallot.

      A. Polycythemia (increased numbers of red cells in the blood) occurs in response to chronic arterial oxygen desaturation; with polycythemia, blood viscosity increases, so child becomes more susceptible to thrombus and embolus formation and has an increased risk of sustaining a cerebral vascular accident.

      B. Pulmonary capillary macrophages phagocytize bacteria. If systemic venous blood bypasses the lungs and enters the aorta, bacteria may enter the systemic circulation and may cause brain abscess.

      C. Because child has turbulent intracardiac blood flow, there is an increased risk of endocarditis (see "Intervention" under "Patent Ductus Arteriosus" for discussion).

V. The infundibular muscle may go into spasm, causing an acute, *severe* decrease in pulmonary blood flow (often causes syncope); this is called a *tet spell*.

      A. Relief may be obtained by placement of child in knee-chest position (this increases venous return, increases systemic arterial resistance, and thereby decreases the right-to-left shunt through the ventricular septal defect, increasing pulmonary blood flow).

      B. Beta-adrenergic blocking agents may help to relieve muscle spasm.

VI. If stenosis causes severe hypoxemia and distress, palliative surgery may be performed. Surgical correction is also necessary whenever tetralogy is present.

      A. All forms of palliative surgery provide increased pulmonary blood flow without use of cardiopulmonary bypass (often used to relieve distress of child until big enough for complete repair). Some medical centers prefer complete repair of tetralogy during infancy, instead of palliation.

           1. The aorta to pulmonary artery anastomosis (called the Waterston or the Potts procedure, depending on whether the anastomosis is performed on the ascending or the descending aorta, respectively) creates a shunt between these arteries (the aorta and pulmonary artery are sewn together side to side, at areas of normal overlap, and a hole is created in their common wall). The Waterston procedure is often used in neonates.

           2. The subclavian to pulmonary artery anastomosis (called the Blalock-Taussig procedure) is utilized in infants beyond 2 months of age (the subclavian artery is detached peripherally, and joined to the pulmonary artery).

      B. Reparative surgery for tetralogy of Fallot is accomplished with use of cardiopulmonary bypass, and with use of hypothermia during infancy.

           1. The ventricular septal defect is closed with a patch.

           2. The area of pulmonary infundibular stenosis is incised.

           3. A patch may be placed in the pulmonary artery wall to enlarge this artery.

           4. Any previous palliative shunts are closed or tied off.

Assessment

I. A child with tetralogy generally demonstrates few symptoms at birth but becomes progressively more distressed during later infancy.

II. Development of congestive heart failure is rare.

III. Cyanosis is usually present.

    A. Degree of cyanosis is proportional to severity of pulmonary stenosis and usually becomes more severe as child grows.

    B. The child may experience periodic cyanotic episodes, and may instinctively squat during play to decrease hypoxemia (serves as knee-chest position, the effect of which is explained in point V under "Definition," above).

    C. Clubbing of tips of fingers and toes may be present.

IV. Heart sounds.

    A. Child will have pulmonic systolic murmur (caused by turbulent flow around the stenotic area).

    B. A harsh, systolic murmur is noted at the left lower sternal border due to ventricular septal defect.

Problems

I. Child has arterial oxygen desaturation (with tendency toward hypoxemia) and polycythemia.

II. Patient and family require preparation for cardiac catheterization and surgery.

III. Thorough care following catheterization and surgery is required.

IV. Child and parents experience anxiety and need teaching about the care regimen, including home care.

Goals of Care

I. Promote and maintain optimal cardiorespiratory function.

II. Minimize systemic consequences of polycythemia.

III. Provide preparation for and aftercare following catheterization and surgery.

IV. Provide adequate information and psychological support to promote successful coping by child and family.

Intervention

I. Monitor carefully for signs of increased cardiorespiratory distress.

    A. Monitor color—watch for deepening of cyanosis.

    B. Monitor heart rate and rhythm (severe hypoxemia may compromise cardiac function).

    C. Note respiratory rate and effort; monitor for evidence of increased respiratory distress or fatigue.

    D. Look for signs of an altered level of consciousness.

    E. Monitor blood gas values if condition warrants.

II. Observe tolerance of activity; child will usually rest when fatigued (note if child squats).

III. If child should demonstrate signs of severe cyanosis or cardiorespiratory distress (*tet spell*), priority intervention is maintenance of adequate cardiopulmonary function.

    A. Placing in knee-chest position may relieve cyanotic episode; parents or primary caretaker should be taught this position.

    B. Increased inspired oxygen usually does not relieve periodic hypoxic episode.

    C. Administration of beta-adrenergic blocking agents may relieve infundibular spasm (if this is the source of distress).

IV. Monitor fluid balance.

    A. Child cannot tolerate dehydration (dehydration of polycythemic child increases risk of thrombus and embolus formation).

    B. Parents or primary caretaker must be instructed to notify physician if child has prolonged or recurrent fever, vomiting, or diarrhea.

V. Monitor neurologic status for evidence of cerebral embolus or brain abscess; parents should notify physician if child is irritable and febrile.

VI. While right-to-left shunt is present, *there must not be air in intravenous lines.* Air bubbles introduced into the venous circulation may be shunted into the aorta, causing cerebral air embolus (stroke).

    VII. Reduce anxiety. Cyanosis serves as constant reminder that child is ill; this can become focus of family's and others' attention. See "Intervention," point IV A to P, under "Congestive Heart Failure" for ways to reduce anxiety.

   VIII. Teach child and primary caretakers about care. Refer to "Intervention," point IV Q to T, under "Congestive Heart Failure."

      A. Fluid restriction is rarely required preoperatively as child is not prone to congestive heart failure, but may be required postoperatively.

      B. Child's activity is usually self-restricted; if syncopal episode occurs, physician should be notified and surgery should be scheduled.

    IX. Prepare child and family for catheterization and surgery. Interventions are given under "Patent Ductus Arteriosus."

     X. Provide postcatheterization and postoperative care.

      A. Interventions following catheterization are described in "Intervention" section under "Patent Ductus Arteriosus."

      B. Congestive heart failure may occur following reparative surgery (see "Congestive Heart Failure" for assessment and intervention).

      C. Arrhythmias may occur following reparative surgery (see "Intervention" section under "Congenital Aortic Stenosis").

      D. Postoperatively, monitor for arrhythmias, congestive heart failure, fluid imbalance, and hemorrhage; and provide pulmonary toilet, support for coping, and suture line care. Interventions for all these are described under "Congenital Aortic Stenosis."

Evaluation

      I. Optimal cardiorespiratory function is maintained.

    II. Consequences of polycythemia are minimized.

   III. Preparation of child and family for catheterization and surgery is adequate.

   IV. Postcatheterization and postoperative care are adequate.

    V. Child and family cope adequately and are informed participants in child's care regime.

Pulmonary Stenosis

Definition

      I. Isolated *pulmonary stenosis* is responsible for approximately 7 percent of congenital heart disease in children; it usually results from improper formation of the pulmonary valve leaflets.

      A. If the commissures fail to form in the pulmonary valve, a membrane may totally prevent flow into the pulmonary artery (called pulmonary valvular atresia).

      B. Pulmonary stenosis can also result from thickened walls of the peripheral pulmonary arteries (called peripheral pulmonary stenosis).

    II. Hemodynamic effects.

      A. With obstruction to the right ventricular outflow, the right ventricle hypertrophies (degree of hypertrophy is proportional to degree of stenosis).

      B. With *severe* stenosis, the right ventricle may become unable to maintain flow into the pulmonary artery, and right ventricular, then right atrial engorgement occurs. If the atrium is stretched sufficiently, the foramen ovale may reopen, and right-to-left atrial shunting then occurs.

   III. If pulmonary valvular atresia is present, emergency surgery is required immediately (within hours of birth). If stenosis is moderate, child will require surgery later but does not usually need emergency surgery early in life).

      A. The Brock procedure is performed for the neonate with pulmonary valvular atresia or severe pulmonary valvular stenosis (a curved blade is inserted into the right ventricle—which is surrounded by "purse-string" sutures to avoid bleeding—and the fused cusps of the pulmonary valve are cut apart. Cardiopulmonary bypass is not required.

B. Reparative surgery for pulmonary valvular stenosis requires use of cardiopulmonary bypass or hypothermia and involves incising of fused cusps under direct visualization.

C. There is no reparative surgery for peripheral pulmonary stenosis.

Assessment

I. Severity of symptoms is proportional to severity of stenosis.

II. Congestive heart failure is unusual, unless stenosis is severe (or pulmonary valvular atresia is present), then signs of systemic venous engorgement will be present (see "Assessment" section under "Congestive Heart Failure").

III. Signs of right ventricular hypertrophy are usually present.

IV. A systolic pulmonic murmur is heard due to stenosis if stenosis is very severe, and due to thickening of cusps a "click" may be noted.

V. Cyanosis is absent unless pulmonary stenosis is so severe that right-to-left shunting occurs between atria.

VI. If pulmonary valvular atresia is present, symptoms will be similar to those of a child with tricuspid atresia.

Problems

I. Child and parents experience anxiety and need teaching about the care regime, including home care.

II. Preparation for and care following cardiac catheterization is required.

III. If there is cyanosis, arterial oxygen desaturation (with tendency toward hypoxemia) and polycythemia will be present.

IV. If child is to have surgery, preparation for it and care afterward is required.

Goals of Care

I. Provide adequate information and psychological support to promote successful coping by child and family.

II. Provide preparation for and aftercare following catheterization and surgery.

III. Minimize systemic consequences of polycythemia.

Intervention

I. If child is asymptomatic, nursing interventions center around reduction of anxiety (see "Intervention," point IV A to P, under "Congestive Heart Failure).

II. See "Intervention," point IV Q to T, under "Congestive Heart Failure" for discussion of teaching child and primary caretaker about care regime. In addition:

A. No diet or activity restrictions are required (if congestive heart failure is present due to severe pulmonary stenosis, surgery is necessary).

B. Child should be treated as normally as possible.

C. Antibiotic prophylaxis is required before and after any surgical or dental procedures (see related intervention under "Patent Ductus Arteriosus" for discussion).

D. If stenosis is mild, caretaker should be instructed to notify physician if child becomes ill, febrile, or cyanotic.

E. If child is cyanotic, instruct caretaker to notify physician if there is prolonged or recurrent fever, vomiting, or diarrhea (child with cyanosis and compensatory polycythemia cannot tolerate dehydration because of risk of thrombus and embolus formation).

III. If catheterization is performed, refer to related interventions under "Patent Ductus Arteriosus."

IV. If surgery is performed, see "Congenital Aortic Stenosis" for interventions.

Evaluation

I. Child and family are well-informed participants in the care regime.

II. Child and parents cope adequately and are well adjusted.

III. Preparation and aftercare for catheterization and surgery are adequate.

IV. Consequences of polycythemia are minimized.

Tricuspid Atresia

Definition (See Fig. 13-9)

I. *Tricuspid atresia* accounts for approximately 1 percent of congenital heart disease in children, and occurs as a result of failure of normal reabsorption of tricuspid tissue during fetal life. Thus, no opening exists between the right atrium and right ventricle (valve cusps remain fused).

    A. Child must have a patent foramen ovale and some other left-to-right shunt to survive; tricuspid atresia is usually associated with an atrial septal defect (foramen ovale), a small ventricular septal defect, an underdeveloped right ventricle, and slight pulmonic stenosis.

    B. If ventricular septal defect is absent, a patent ductus must be present for child to survive.

    C. Transposition of the great vessels is sometimes associated.

II. Hemodynamic effects.

    A. Right atrial engorgement occurs, and blood must flow (from right to left) through the patent foramen ovale into the left side of the heart; pulmonary blood flow is then accomplished by left-to-right flow through the ventricular septal defect into the pulmonary artery (blood may also flow from left to right through the patent ductus arteriosus and into the pulmonary artery).

      1. Systemic venous engorgement occurs.

      2. Arterial oxygen desaturation is present, as the left side of the heart becomes a common mixing chamber (see "Definition" section under "Tetralogy of Fallot" for systemic consequences of cyanotic heart disease).

      3. Pulmonary blood flow may be increased or decreased (it is decreased if left-to-right shunt is small).

    B. Left ventricular hypertrophy occurs, and right ventricle is usually underdeveloped (therefore, the PMI shifts to the left).

Assessment

I. Children with tricuspid atresia usually have severe distress within the first weeks of life.

II. Evidence of systemic venous engorgement and left ventricular hypertrophy is present.

III. Cyanosis is present from birth.

    A. Child usually has severe cyanosis (unless transposition of the great arteries is present, then cyanosis is moderate); there may be periodic hypoxic episodes.

    B. Clubbing of tips of fingers and toes is noted.

    C. See "Definition" section under "Tetralogy of Fallot" for systemic consequences of cyanotic heart disease.

IV. Heart sounds: No distinctive murmur is noted with tricuspid atresia; associated defects such as ventricular septal defect or pulmonary stenosis produce their characteristic murmurs.

V. Severe hypoxemia, due to decreased pulmonary blood flow necessitates surgical palliation or reparative surgery.

    A. The Waterston, Potts, and Blalock-Taussig shunts (all increase pulmonary blood flow) are discussed in the "Definition" section of "Tetralogy of Fallot."

    B. The Glenn shunt (anastomosis between superior vena cava and right pulmonary artery) may be performed to increase pulmonary blood flow.

    C. Reparative surgery for tricuspid atresia is called the Fontan procedure. It makes the right atrium function as the right heart pumping chamber.

      1. A valved tube graft is sewn between the right atrium and pulmonary artery.

      2. The ventricular septal defect is closed.

Problems   See "Pulmonary Stenosis," above.

Goals of Care   See "Pulmonary Stenosis," above.

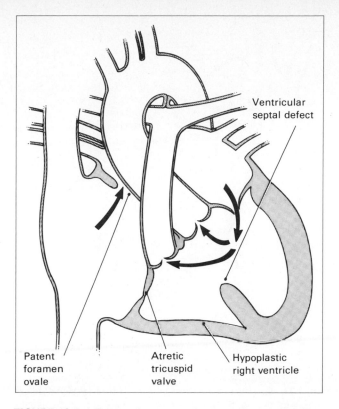

Patent foramen ovale

Atretic tricuspid valve

Hypoplastic right ventricle

Ventricular septal defect

FIGURE 13-9 / Tricuspid atresia with ventricular septal defect.

Intervention   See "Pulmonary Stenosis," above.

Evaluation   See "Pulmonary Stenosis," above.

Transposition of the Great Vessels

Definition (See Fig. 13-10)

  I. The many forms of transposition of the great vessels account for nearly 4 percent of congenital heart lesions in children.
 II. *Transposition* means that the normal relationship of the ventricles to the great vessels is reversed; abnormal division of the common great artery trunk during fetal development causes the aorta to arise from the right ventricle and the pulmonary artery to arise from the left ventricle.
III. Hemodynamic effects.
   A. Without the presence of a shunt, unoxygenated systemic venous blood enters the right heart and returns to the systemic circulation via the aorta; oxygenated pulmonary venous blood enters the left heart and is returned to the lungs via the pulmonary artery. Thus, two parallel circulations exist, a situation which is incompatible with life.
   B. Lifesaving shunts may exist (or be created) at several levels: patent ductus arteriosus, atrial septal defect, or ventricular septal defect.
     1. When shunt exists, blood will follow path of *least* resistance (once the newborn's pulmonary vascular resistance falls), so the propensity of shunt is usually right to left, to pulmonary artery.

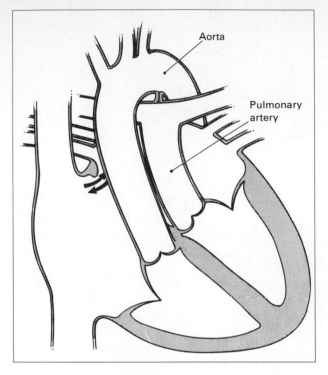

FIGURE 13-10 / Transposition of the great vessels with atrial septal defect. This hemodynamic pattern may exist naturally or occur as a result of Rashkind or Blalock-Hanlon procedures.

      a. Pressures of pulmonary blood flow are determined by the location of the shunt.

      b. A right-to-left shunt does not improve systemic oxygen saturation (aortic blood is still deoxygenated).

   2. Usually, there is some bidirectional flow through each shunt, so some mixing of oxygenated and deoxygenated blood occurs. This slightly improves the oxygen saturation of aortic blood.

  C. A large atrial septal defect is the ideal associated lesion, as it allows good mixing of oxygenated and deoxygenated blood, which may decrease cyanosis considerably (also, high pulmonary blood flow will be under low pressures, which are better tolerated by lungs, and there will be less risk of congestive heart failure).

  D. A ventricular septal defect or patent ductus arteriosus does not allow good mixing, and each causes high pulmonary blood flow under high pressures; congestive heart failure is likely to result.

  E. Pulmonary valvular stenosis is frequently present with ventricular septal defect, so pulmonary blood flow may also be decreased.

 IV. See relevant part of "Definition" section under "Tetralogy of Fallot" for systemic consequences of cyanotic heart defect.

 V. If cyanosis is severe in neonatal period, surgical creation of a shunt is vital. Since a shunt at the atrial level is ideal, this is usually created.

  A. During cardiac catheterization, a balloon-tipped catheter may be used to create a hole in the atrial septum (Rashkind procedure).

  B. A Blalock-Hanlon atrial septectomy may be performed. This procedure involves clamping of the atrium at the area of the septum, incision within the clamped area, and removal of a portion of the atrial septum.

       1. This procedure does not require use of cardiopulmonary bypass.

       2. It usually allows for creation of a large septal defect (larger than Rashkind procedure).

VI. If congestive heart failure is present due to increased pulmonary blood flow under high pressures, medical management is attempted. If failure persists, pulmonary artery banding may be considered as a palliative measure or complete surgical repair may be performed.

VII. Total repair of the transposition defect is called the Mustard procedure (though some other procedures are presently used, this is most widely accepted).

    A. The Mustard procedure is performed with a cardiopulmonary bypass, and hypothermia in infancy.

    B. A common atrium is made for total repair (the atrial septum is excised).

    C. A pericardial baffle is sewn in atria to provide a tunnel, so systemic venous return flows under the tunnel to the left ventricle (and into the pulmonary artery), and pulmonary venous return flows on top of the tunnel to the right ventricle (and into the aorta).

    D. Any associated cardiac defects are usually corrected at this time.

Assessment

I. Child may have little distress at birth, especially if ductus arteriosus is patent. Cyanosis and distress usually become progressive within hours to days. If child has no associated lesion allowing mixing of oxygenated and deoxygenated blood, progressive and severe distress will be present immediately after birth.

II. Congestive heart failure is often present (see "Assessment" section under "Congestive Heart Failure") and biventricular hypertrophy is noted.

III. Cyanosis is expected (unless other defects allow extremely good mixing of arterial and venous blood).

    A. Cyanosis may be mild at birth and increase as the ductus arteriosus closes.

    B. Compensatory polycythemia and elevation of hemoglobin and hematocrit are expected; with polycythemia, cyanosis is more noticeable, and with anemia, cyanosis is less readily apparent.

    C. Clubbing of tips of extremities is seen after child is 6 months of age.

    D. Cyanosis should improve following palliative procedure (Rashkind or Blalock-Hanlon procedure).

IV. Heart sounds.

    A. Murmurs are generally absent if no associated lesions are present.

    B. Murmurs typical of ventricular septal defect or patent ductus arteriosus are noted if these defects are present.

    C. Systolic pulmonic murmur may be present due to pulmonary stenosis or secondary to large pulmonary blood flow caused by shunt (once neonate's pulmonary vascular resistance has dropped).

V. Neurological exam should be performed to rule out possibility of cerebral embolus or brain abscess if child has symptoms of neurological irritability.

Problems

I. Child and parents experience anxiety and need teaching about the care regime, including home care.

II. Preparation for and care following cardiac catheterization and surgery is required.

III. Child has arterial oxygen desaturation (with tendency toward hypoxemia) and polycythemia.

Goals of Care

I. Promote and maintain optimal cardiorespiratory function.

II. Minimize systemic consequences of polycythemia.

III. Provide preparation for and aftercare following catheterization and surgery.

IV. Provide adequate information and psychological support to promote successful coping by child and family.

Intervention

I. Refer to "Intervention" section under "Tetralogy of Fallot" for care of child with arterial oxygen desaturation. Child with transposition of the great vessels should not have periodic hypoxic episodes, and oxygen therapy may relieve cyanosis slightly.

   A. Child with unrepaired transposition of the great vessels will generally not have arterial oxygen saturation above 60 percent (normal saturation is 95 to 100 percent), even after palliative surgical procedure. This low oxygen saturation may be tolerated fairly well, but with compensatory polycythemia, increased risk of thrombus and embolus formation, and risk of cerebral abscess.

II. If child has congestive heart failure, see "Intervention" section under "Congestive Heart Failure."

III. See "Intervention," point IV, under "Congestive Heart Failure" for reduction of anxiety and provision for teaching needs.

   A. Child with severe cyanosis and compensatory polycythemia cannot tolerate dehydration (especially an infant), so parents or primary caretaker must be instructed to notify physician if there is prolonged or recurrent fever, vomiting, or diarrhea.

IV. See "Intervention" section under "Patent Ductus Arteriosus" for preparation for cardiac catheterization and care following it. If the Rashkind procedure is performed, monitor for atrial arrhythmias. Interventions for arrhythmias are discussed under "Congenital Aortic Stenosis."

V. Postoperatively, monitor for arrhythmias and congestive heart failure, which are the most common complications following repair of transposition. Arrhythmias can also occur after the Blalock-Hanlon procedure.

VI. Systemic or pulmonary venous engorgement may occur if the pericardial baffle causes obstruction to the venous return (see "Assessment" section under "Congestive Heart Failure"). Notify physician if these occur.

VII. *Strict management of fluid balance is essential:* Fluid overload predisposes child to congestive heart failure, and dehydration predisposes him or her to thrombus or embolus formation.

VIII. Assess carefully for any evidence of thrombus or embolus formation, especially cerebral and pulmonary emboli.

IX. Monitor child for postoperative hemorrhage. Children with cyanotic heart disease and polycythemia often have abnormalities of platelet function, and thus an increased risk of postoperative hemorrhage.

Evaluation   See "Tetralogy of Fallot," above.

Case Study   Timmy L. is a 4-kg newborn with transposition of the great vessels, admitted to the pediatric unit following an emergency atrial septostomy performed during a venous cardiac catheterization. He is a very cyanotic infant in moderate distress. Admitting vital signs include heart rate of 164, respiratory rate of 68 with moderate retractions, and palpable blood pressure of 80 mmHg. Arterial blood gases obtained at the end of his cardiac catheterization are pH 7.35, P_{O_2} 38, P_{CO_2} 20. Timmy's left leg below the catheterization site is cyanotic and slightly edematous, but pulses are strong. His liver is palpable 1 cm below the costal margin.

Timmy's father is at his isolette, looking very worried. He states that their last infant died of heart disease and that Timmy is their only other child.

ASSESSMENT

Timmy demonstrates evidence of a cyanotic heart defect and respiratory distress (tachypnea and increased respiratory effort). There are no signs of systemic venous engorgement, and the catheterization site looks good.

Hemodynamic pathology   The aorta receives *deoxygenated* blood from the *right* ventricle and cycles it repeatedly to the body without its going to the lungs for oxygen; the pulmonary artery arises from the *left* ventricle and cycles *oxygenated* blood repeatedly into the pulmonary circulation. The Rashkind procedure created an atrial septal defect to allow some mixing of oxygenated with deoxygenated blood within the heart so aortic blood flow has a slightly improved oxygen saturation.

PROBLEMS
I. Arterial oxygen desaturation.
II. Respiratory distress.
III. Paternal anxiety.
IV. Incision.

GOALS OF CARE
I. Maintain optimal cardiorespiratory function and minimize effects of polycythemia.
II. Reduce distress.
III. Reduce anxiety and support coping mechanisms.
IV. Maintain clean catheterization incision to prevent infection.
V. Monitor for bleeding.

INTERVENTION
I. Minimize oxygen requirement.
   A. Maintain constant environmental temperature.
   B. Maintain adequate fluid intake to prevent dehydration (approximately 400 to 600 mL per day is Timmy's fluid requirement) yet prevent fluid overload. *No air in IV line!*
II. Administer digitalis derivative as ordered (digitalizing dose will be approximately 0.18 to 0.26 mg to be given in divided doses).
III. Monitor for evidence of congestive heart failure.
IV. Have resuscitation breathing bag and infant airway ready (can be out of sight) in case of cardiorespiratory deterioration. Monitor systemic circulation.
V. Assess degree of distress.
VI. Decrease oxygen requirements (see above).
VII. Confer with health team about increasing Timmy's inspired oxygen.
VIII. Obtain blood gases if Timmy demonstrates increased distress.
IX. Encourage Mr. L. to discuss fears, questions, concerns.
X. Orient Mr. L. to the unit and equipment if he indicates an interest in these or if he seems to be worried about the equipment (don't overwhelm him with information that doesn't concern him).
XI. Encourage Mr. L. to touch Timmy and be involved in caring for him if this would help him deal with his fears of Timmy's death. (Mr. L. may cope by remaining detached from Timmy temporarily.)
XII. Provide encouragement to Mr. L. when Timmy shows signs of improvement by pointing them out to him—but be realistic.
XIII. Keep incision clean and dry.
XIV. Monitor for evidence of inflammation.
XV. Monitor for any swelling or bleeding from site.
XVI. Provide for adequate caloric intake.
XVII. Include parents in care as soon as possible.
XVIII. Plan with family for homegoing as soon as condition stabilizes and discharge date can be anticipated.

EVALUATION
I. Has heart rate decreased?
II. Has cyanosis decreased?
III. Is there evidence of congestive heart failure?
IV. Are Timmy's intake and output appropriate?
V. Is his skin turgor good and is his fontanel flat?
VI. Has Timmy's respiratory rate decreased?
VII. Has his cyanosis deepened?

VIII. Are blood gases improved? (Evidence of acidosis requires immediate intervention.)
IX. Is Mr. L. able to cope with his feelings of anxiety (can he relate to his surroundings and to people appropriately) or is he showing signs of increasing stress?
X. Is Mr. L. able to discuss his fears for Timmy and to comprehend information given to him?
XI. Does inflammation occur? (If so, culture wound and notify physician.)
XII. Does bleeding occur? (If so, apply pressure to incision and notify physician if bleeding doesn't stop.)

Truncus Arteriosus

Definition (See Figs. 13-11 and 13-12)

I. This defect accounts for approximately 1.5 percent of congenital heart disease in children.
II. The truncus is a fetal structure which serves as a common great artery early in fetal life; it normally develops into the aorta and pulmonary artery. Failure of this division results in a single vessel arising from both ventricles.
   A. A ventricular septal defect is present.
   B. Pulmonary blood flow is supplied by branches off this main trunk.
      1. If pulmonary branches are big and arise from the proximal aorta, the pulmonary blood flow is large and under high pressure once the newborn's pulmonary vascular resistance has dropped (see Fig. 13-11).
      2. If no main branches of the trunk supply the pulmonary arteries, blood flow to the pulmonary arteries is achieved only through development of collateral

FIGURE 13-11 / Truncus arteriosus.

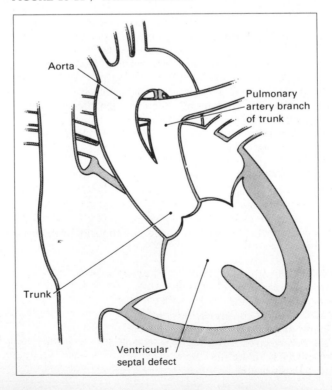

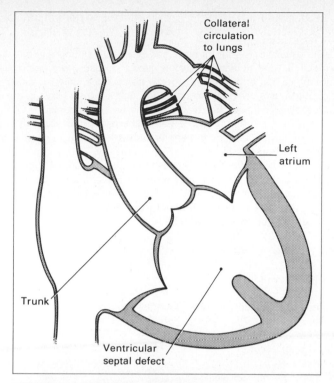

Collateral circulation to lungs

Left atrium

Trunk

Ventricular septal defect

FIGURE 13-12 / Truncus arteriosus, type IV.

circulation, usually from enlarged bronchial and mammary arteries from the descending aorta (see Fig. 13-12).

III. Hemodynamic effects.

   A. If there are big pulmonary branches supplying a large flow to the pulmonary vessels under high pressure, hemodynamic consequences are similar to those encountered with complete atrioventricular canal defect (see "Definition" section under "Endocardial Cushion Defect").

   B. If pulmonary blood flow is low, hemodynamic consequences are similar to those encountered in children with severe tetralogy of Fallot.

   C. Since the ventricles become a common chamber with common outflow (mixed oxygenated and deoxygenated blood), pressures equalize between ventricles, and arterial oxygen desaturation occurs.

   D. When pulmonary blood flow is reduced, development of collateral circulation is stimulated; over long periods of time this collateral circulation may proliferate so that pulmonary blood flow is *increased*. Congestive heart failure may then result from this increased pulmonary blood flow under high (aortic) pressures.

IV. The systemic consequences of cyanotic heart disease include polycythemia, bacteremia, brain abscess, and endocarditis. (See "Definition," point IV, under "Tetralogy of Fallot" for discussion.)

V. If child is extremely cyanotic, palliative surgery may be performed to increase pulmonary blood flow. Palliative procedures are discussed in "Definition" section under "Tetralogy of Fallot." Reparative surgery involves the following:

   A. Patch closure of ventricular septal defect, so that left ventricular output enters the common trunk.

   B. Ligation (and oversewing) of anomalous or collateral pulmonary circulation.

   C. Insertion of a tube graft between right ventricle and distal pulmonary arteries to allow flow into lungs.

Assessment
    I. Child is generally in severe distress (death during infancy is common).
    II. Congestive heart failure is noted with some forms of this defect (see "Congestive Heart Failure" for assessments).
    III. Cyanosis is usually present from birth, and is severe if pulmonary blood flow is reduced.
        A. Hemoglobin and hematocrit are elevated (compensatory polycythemia).
        B. Clubbing of tips of fingers and toes is noted once child reaches 6 months of age.
    IV. A systolic murmur is generally present. Although it is heard best at the left lower sternal border, it radiates all over the chest and may be accompanied by a thrill.
        A. If high pulmonary blood flow is present, a mitral diastolic murmur may be heard due to a large pulmonary venous return entering the left atrium, sometimes accompanied by a thrill.
        B. If pulmonary blood flow is accomplished only by collateral circulation, systolic bruits are heard along the anterior and posterior chest, often accompanied by thrills.
        C. An S_3 sound may be present if child is in congestive heart failure.
    V. Peripheral pulses are usually bounding, with rapid upstroke; widened pulse pressure may be present (due to aortic runoff).

Problems
    See "Tetralogy of Fallot," above.

Goals of Care
    See "Tetralogy of Fallot," above.

Intervention
    I. See "Intervention" section under "Congestive Heart Failure" if child has congestive heart failure.
    II. Interventions are the same as for tetralogy of Fallot except that periodic cyanotic episodes do not occur.

Evaluation
    See "Tetralogy of Fallot," above.

Total Anomalous Pulmonary Venous Return (TAPVR)

Definition
    I. This defect, which accounts for approximately 1 percent of all congenital heart defects in children, results from failure of the pulmonary veins to join with the left atrium during fetal development. An atrial septal defect is usually also present (or infant will expire immediately).
    II. Hemodynamic effects.
        A. The pulmonary veins empty into anomalous connecting veins; these anomalous veins enter the systemic venous circulation—thus, pulmonary venous blood is eventually returned to the *right* atrium (this chamber receives a mixture of oxygenated and deoxygenated blood).
            1. Most of the anomalous veins empty into the systemic venous circulation near the heart.
            2. Some anomalous vessels enter the systemic venous circulation below the diaphragm (mortality highest).
        B. Anomalous vessels often produce obstruction to flow, resulting in increased pulmonary venous pressure and pulmonary edema (this obstruction is most severe if the anomalous vessels enter the systemic circulation *below* the diaphragm).
        C. If anomalous connecting veins provide less obstruction to flow (this may occur if these veins empty almost directly into the right atrium), pulmonary edema may be less severe, and these infants will demonstrate less distress.
    III. Virtually all children with total anomalous pulmonary venous return demonstrate signs of cyanosis and congestive heart failure within the first days or weeks of life.
        A. Both pulmonary and systemic venous blood returns to the right atrium, so pulmonary blood flow is usually high.
        B. Mixed oxygenated and deoxygenated blood is shunted into the left atrium through an atrial septal defect (this supplies the systemic circulation).

C. The systemic consequences of cyanotic heart disease include polycythemia, bacteremia, brain abscess, and endocarditis. (See "Definition," point IV, under "Tetralogy of Fallot" for discussion.)

IV. Surgery is necessary, usually within the first days or weeks of life.
   A. Hypothermia is required for surgical repair in infancy.
   B. Pulmonary veins are joined to the left atrium at the point where they pass behind the atrium.

Assessment

I. Child usually presents with severe distress within first days of life (especially if pulmonary venous obstruction is present).

II. Congestive heart failure (with symptoms of pulmonary edema and respiratory distress) is usually present within the first days of life.
   A. Biventricular enlargement is present.
   B. See "Assessment" section under "Congestive Heart Failure."

III. Cyanosis is present in virtually all children with this defect, and may become progressively severe as pulmonary edema produces respiratory compromise.

IV. No distinctive murmur is present with total anomalous pulmonary venous return. An S_3 sound may be noted in association with congestive heart failure. A systolic pulmonary sound may be present due to increased pulmonary blood flow.

Problems

I. Congestive heart failure is usually present and continues to some degree for several months after surgery.

II. Cardiac catheterization and surgery are usually required.

III. Child has arterial oxygen desaturation.

Goals of Care

I. See "Congestive Heart Failure" for related goals.

II. Prepare child and parents for catheterization and surgery, and provide aftercare.

III. Minimize consequences of arterial oxygen desaturation.

Intervention

I. Assess child frequently for evidence of cardiac or respiratory distress (see "General Assessment" at beginning of this chapter).

II. Interventions for child with congestive heart failure and for child's parents are presented under "Congestive Heart Failure."

III. Strict monitoring of fluid balance is required. Fluid overload worsens predisposition to congestive heart failure, dehydration predisposes to thrombus and embolus formation. *There must be no air bubbles in the intravenous line,* because some venous blood enters the aorta and air may cause cerebral air embolus (stroke).

IV. Interventions for child with arterial oxygen desaturation are presented under "Tetralogy of Fallot." Knee-chest position will not relieve cyanosis in child with TAPVR.

V. Pre- and postcatheterization interventions are discussed in the section "Patent Ductus Arteriosus."

VI. Postoperatively, monitor for arrhythmias, thrombus or embolus formation, hemorrhage, and wound infection. Refer to "Intervention" section under "Ventricular Septal Defect" for discussion of all these.

Evaluation

I. Optimal cardiorespiratory function is maintained.

II. Consequences of polycythemia are minimized.

III. Preparation for and care following catheterization and surgery are adequate.

IV. Parents cope adequately and are informed participants in child's care.

Hypoplastic Left Heart Syndrome

Definition

I. Incomplete or inadequate development of the mitral valve, aorta, or aortic arch during fetal life may result in an underdeveloped left ventricle.

II. Hemodynamic effects.
   A. The right ventricle is the only pumping chamber, so extreme compromise of systemic circulation results.
   B. Aortic blood flow is markedly decreased (though it may be supplemented with flow through a patent ductus arteriosus).
   C. Pulmonary venous blood may encounter much resistance in left atrium; some of this blood may shunt through a stretched foramen ovale into the right atrium.
III. This defect generally results in death.

Assessment

I. Child is generally in extreme distress within first hours of life; evidence of systemic venous engorgement and decreased systemic perfusion (described in "Assessment" section under "Congestive Heart Failure") are the rule unless a *large* patent ductus arteriosus is present.
II. Child may be cyanotic, but pallor is often present.

Problems,
Goals of Care,
Intervention,
and Evaluation

The major consideration here is that the child has a congenital cardiac lesion that results in death. The objective is to support the parents during the child's deterioration and make the infant as comfortable as possible. Interventions and evaluation are based on this goal.

   Occasionally an infant may have an interrupted aortic arch with a viable left ventricle (then symptoms include a combination of the above symptoms and those of severe coarctation of the aorta). Early surgical intervention may result in successful patching of the aortic arch, but mortality is still extremely high (see "Coarctation of the Aorta").

RHEUMATIC HEART DISEASE

Definition

I. *Rheumatic heart disease* is the major acquired heart disease in children; it results from inflammatory changes occurring within the heart in association with rheumatic fever.
   A. Rheumatic fever follows a group A beta-hemolytic streptococcal infection, and is most prevalent in children 5 to 15 years of age.
   B. Carditis occurs in approximately half of the children during the acute phase of rheumatic fever.
      1. Presence of carditis is documented by any of the following symptoms: cardiomegaly, appearance of a *new* cardiac murmur, pericarditis, onset of congestive heart failure, and certain changes in the electrocardiogram (evidence of cardiac chamber hypertrophy).
      2. Marked cardiomegaly and/or congestive heart failure at the time of acute rheumatic fever are the most consistent precursors of later rheumatic heart disease.
II. Pathophysiology of rheumatic carditis involves an inflammatory (possibly autoimmune) process which causes temporary or permanent damage to any of the three layers of the heart.
   A. Endocardial involvement usually is restricted to the valves.
      1. Edema and inflammatory erosion of valve tissue occurs acutely.
      2. Scarring of valve leaflets, fusion of valve cusps, or fibrosis and shortening of papillary muscles may produce valvular stenosis or insufficiency.
   B. Myocardial and pericardial involvement is usually transient and mild (pericardial effusion may occur).
III. Rapid treatment of rheumatic fever and minimization of associated inflammation of cardiac tissue may prevent permanent cardiac damage.
   A. Penicillin is usually used to treat the streptococcal infection (therapy is continued indefinitely to prevent recurrence of rheumatic fever and repeated risk of cardiac damage).
   B. Salicylates (and possibly corticosteroids) are administered to decrease inflammatory reaction.

    C. Bed rest is usually encouraged to reduce cardiac workload (it is sometimes thought this will decrease cardiac damage), especially if child has congestive heart failure.

IV. If acute inflammation progresses or recurs, scar formation occurs, and valvular damage may become permanent. Mitral insufficiency is the most common rheumatic heart lesion seen in children; aortic insufficiency also occurs, but less frequently.

    A. With mitral insufficiency, the left ventricle hypertrophies in an attempt to maintain systemic output despite regurgitation of blood into the left atrium.

        1. Mitral insufficiency is usually minor, causing slight left ventricular hypertrophy and left atrial enlargement.

        2. If the mitral insufficiency is severe, left atrial, then pulmonary venous engorgement occurs; pulmonary edema may result.

    B. Aortic insufficiency also causes left ventricular dilatation and hypertrophy (pulmonary edema and congestive heart failure rarely occur during childhood).

    C. Aortic stenosis may also occur (see "Definition" section under "Congenital Aortic Stenosis" for discussion of hemodynamic effects of aortic valvular stenosis).

    D. As a result of valvular malformation, child has increased risk of developing bacterial endocarditis.

V. If severe valvular damage is sustained (indicated by development of congestive heart failure or evidence of left ventricular strain on electrocardiogram), surgical treatment is required.

    A. Cardiopulmonary bypass is necessary.

    B. If fused valve cusps are causing valvular stenosis, separation of valve cusps (commissurotomy) is performed.

    C. If valve is severely damaged, insertion of a prosthetic valve may be performed.

Assessment

I. Child may have a wide range of cardiovascular symptoms.

II. Acute phase of rheumatic carditis.

    A. Murmurs of aortic and mitral valvular insufficiency may be present (apical systolic murmur is nearly always noted).

    B. Heart sounds are usually muffled and child's precordium is very active (symptoms of biventricular enlargement are present).

    C. Pericardial friction rub will be present if pericarditis occurs.

    D. Symptoms of congestive heart failure are less common, but they may occur (usually indicating more serious cardiac involvement).

    E. Child will also demonstrate some of the other manifestations of rheumatic fever such as: fever, arthritis (or arthralgia), rash, rheumatic nodules, or abdominal pain (chorea usually does not appear at same time carditis is present).

III. Rheumatic heart disease (late valve involvement).

    A. Mitral insufficiency.

        1. Apical (mitral) systolic murmur is usually present (thrill may be palpable).

        2. Evidence of left ventricular hypertrophy will be present.

        3. Child often is asymptomatic. (Congestive heart failure occurs only if insufficiency is severe, in which case surgery is required.)

    B. Aortic insufficiency.

        1. Diastolic aortic murmur usually is noted and may be accompanied by a thrill.

        2. Widened pulse pressure.

        3. If *severe* aortic insufficiency is present, evidence of left ventricular strain on electrocardiogram indicates that surgery is necessary.

    C. Child may develop accumulation of vegetations (bacteria, fibrin) on damaged valves—this may cause emboli to form. Child also is prone to development of bacterial endocarditis (monitor for evidence of these complications).

Problems

I. Child has rheumatic carditis.

II. Child and parents experience anxiety and require instruction and information about child's care.

III. Congestive heart failure may occur.

IV. Cardiac catheterization and/or surgery may be required.

Goals of Care

I. Maintain and promote optimal cardiovascular function.

II. Promote child's comfort.

III. Reduce anxiety and provide information and support to promote child's and family's cooperative participation in care regime.

Intervention

I. Monitor child's cardiovascular status.
   A. Assess for signs of congestive heart failure (see "Assessment" section under "Congestive Heart Failure").
   B. Monitor for symptoms of carditis (given under "Definition," above).

II. Maintain bed rest if ordered (child may be hospitalized or remain at home).
   A. Position child comfortably and carefully (especially if arthralgia is present).
   B. Attempt to make bed rest as tolerable as possible.
      1. Provide patient with companionship (visit often, and encourage visits by friends and family).
      2. Design quiet, age-appropriate activities.
      3. Allow child to participate in planning care.
   C. Keep skin dry (this is difficult if fever is present).
   D. If child is extremely frustrated by continued bed rest, brief periods up in a wheelchair will often place less stress on cardiac function than bed rest under conditions of anxiety and frustration.

III. Administer penicillin (and salicylates and/or corticosteroids) as ordered.
   A. Check dosage and observe child carefully for therapeutic, side, and toxic effects. Large doses of penicillin may be given.
   B. If congestive heart failure is present (and fluid restriction is required), monitor amounts of sodium and potassium that are present in the penicillin (if sodium or potassium penicillin is administered).
   C. If corticosteroids are administered, monitor child closely for side effects. If salicylates are administered concurrently, gastrointestinal bleeding may occur.

IV. Teach child and primary caretaker about care regimen.
   A. During acute phase of rheumatic fever, child may be placed on complete bed rest—importance of this should be stressed to child and caretaker.
   B. Administration of antibiotic therapy for the duration of the acute phase, and indefinitely continued administration of antibiotic prophylaxis should be taught to child's primary caretaker, and their importance emphasized.
   C. If child has congestive heart failure, see "Congestive Heart Failure" for references to appropriate teaching.
   D. See "Intervention" section under "Congestive Heart Failure" for general teaching information.
   E. Since child may sustain further deterioration of cardiovascular status, after the acute stage, the family should receive careful medical and nursing follow-up and should be urged to seek medical care whenever child becomes ill.

V. Alleviate child's anxiety, which may be extreme.
   A. See "Intervention," point IV A to K, under "Congestive Heart Failure."
   B. Anxiety may be compounded by child's discomfort and frustration about bed rest (sensitive, gentle care is required).
   C. If child becomes demanding, consider whether this is evidence that child would like more attention or is extremely anxious. It will be extremely difficult for the child to understand and cooperate with strict bed rest if he or she does not feel ill or in pain when out of bed. It does not help to explain that you are trying to prevent cardiac problems later.

VI. Alleviate parents' anxiety about child's condition or prognosis.
   A. See "Intervention," point IV L to P, under "Congestive Heart Failure."

   B. Teaching parents about child's home care (and medications) may help alleviate some anxiety.

   C. If it is difficult for parents to maintain child on bed rest during the day, hospital admission may be indicated during the acute phase of rheumatic fever (however, this should not be made to sound like a punishment).

  VII. If cardiac catheterization or surgery is required:

   A. See "Intervention" section under "Patent Ductus Arteriosus" for child and family preparation.

   B. See "Intervention" section under "Patent Ductus Arteriosus" for care of child and family after child's catheterization.

   C. See "Intervention," points IX to XV, under "Congenital Aortic Stenosis" for care of child following open-heart surgery.

Evaluation

  I. Is child's cardiovascular status stable (decreased evidence of carditis, or evidence of improved cardiovascular function)?

  II. Is child emotionally tolerating bed rest?

  III. Are medications producing desired results without side effects?

  IV. Are parents or primary caretaker coping with the illness?

BIBLIOGRAPHY

ASSESSMENT

Fink, Burton W.: *Congenital Heart Disease: A Deductive Approach to Its Diagnosis,* Year Book Medical Publishers, Chicago, 1975. Excellent paperback reference which discusses embryology, hemodynamic principles, and clinical presentation for all the major congenital heart defects. Very helpful for nurses. Small bibliography provided.

CARDIOLOGY

Heymann, Michael A., Abraham M. Rudolph, and Norman H. Silverman: "Closure of the Ductus Arteriosus in Premature Infants by Inhibition of Prostaglandin Synthesis," *The New England Journal of Medicine,* **295:**530–533, September 1976. Describes recent medical advance for pharmacologic treatment of patent ductus arteriosus. Findings have since been substantiated at other medical centers.

Nadas, Alexander S., and Donald C. Fyler: *Pediatric Cardiology,* 3d ed., W. B. Saunders Company, Philadelphia, 1972. A classic text on the subject. Provides a good basis for understanding heart disease in children.

PSYCHOSOCIAL FACTORS

Linde, Leonard M., and Shirley D. Linde: "Emotional Factors of Pediatric Patients in Cardiac Surgery," *American Operating Room Nurse,* **18:**95–99, July 1973. Very good article which considers psychosocial factors of heart disease in children (applicable to both surgical and nonsurgical pediatric cardiac patients).

Reif, Kerry: "A Heart Makes You Live," *The American Journal of Nursing,* **72:**1085, June 1972. Brief, interesting summary describing the progression of a child's concepts about the function of the heart (based on interviews and art from a small group of children).

SURGERY

Cooley, Denton A., and Grady L. Hallman: *Surgical Treatment of Congenital Heart Disease,* Lea & Febiger, Philadelphia, 1975. Excellent reference for anyone involved in caring for children undergoing cardiac surgery. These authors have compiled information regarding the embryology, clinical manifestations, surgery (and surgical techniques), and postoperative complications for major congenital heart defects. Bibliography not current. Morbidity and mortality statistics are based on the authors' own considerable patient population.

King, Ouida M.: *Care of the Cardiac Surgical Patient,* The C. V. Mosby Company, St. Louis, 1975. This is an excellent nursing text which should prove to be quite useful for the nurse involved in caring for the cardiac surgical patient of any age. Ms. King has included a very good chapter on congenital heart disease, which briefly includes some of the major postoperative complications associated with the more common defects. A review of postoperative complications is also elaborated in a chapter of the same name.

14

The Respiratory System

Janet L. Snow

GENERAL ASSESSMENT

I. Data sources.
- **A.** Parents—to obtain necessary information, the examiner must work through a spokesperson, such as a parent or principal caretaker.
- **B.** Child.
  1. A child over 7 years old can contribute to a health history.
  2. The child may provide important clues to a situation described by the parent.
- **C.** Others.
  1. Grandparents.
  2. Babysitter.
  3. Schoolteachers.
- **D.** Old records.
  1. Past clinic and hospital records can provide important information regarding the child's health status.
  2. Previous hospitalizations, illnesses, and immunizations are part of the past records.

II. Health history.
- **A.** General notes on interviewing the parent and child.
  1. Whenever possible, the interview should be conducted in a relaxed, private setting.
  2. The child should be included in the interview when possible by asking questions appropriate for his or her age and language development.
  3. Always remember that the spokesperson is translating the child's behavior and problems for you; therefore, it is important to ask specifically what actually happened in any described situation.
  4. Parents of an ill child often feel anxious, helpless, or guilty when they must seek medical care for their child.
  5. Parents often need reassurance and a concerned but nonjudgmental attitude on the part of the nurse.
  6. Never assume you know the meaning of a statement until you have clarified the details in terms that both you and the parent can understand.
  7. Provide time for parents to ask questions and obtain information.
- **B.** General health status.
  1. Ask parents to describe general status in one short phrase.
  2. Days of school missed should be assessed.
  3. Assess general emotional health.
  4. Current medications and diet.
  5. Physical limitations, either self-imposed by the child or set by parents.
- **C.** Neonatal health status—approximately 30 percent of infants with insulin-dependent mothers have respiratory distress syndrome.
- **D.** Perinatal health.
  1. Birth weight—premature infants are the population mainly at risk for respiratory distress syndrome.
  2. Resuscitation or the need for prolonged oxygen at birth is a clue to early respiratory problems.
- **E.** Growth and development considerations.
  1. Achievement of normal developmental milestones—obtain history.
  2. Poor weight gain in infancy may reflect a feeding problem or a need for increased

calories if oxygen consumption is increased due to respiratory disease. Assess what the child is offered and what is eaten.

3. Assess rapid weight gain or loss in an older child.

4. Assess need for naps.

5. Feeding patterns.

    a. Feeding difficulties at birth may indicate a congenital respiratory problem, e.g., tracheoesophageal fistula.

    b. Vomiting, rapid tiring during feeding, poor suck response, and long feeding time should be noted as possible signs of respiratory disease.

F. Family history.

  1. Some respiratory diseases are transmitted genetically, e.g., cystic fibrosis.

  2. Cardiac malformations should be noted because a close association always exists between the respiratory and cardiac systems.

  3. Family response to illness.

    a. Socioeconomic and cultural considerations.

    b. Religious considerations.

    c. Assess family's interrelationships, note whether child receives emotional support from one particular family member.

    d. Assess family's and child's perceptions of the illness.

    e. Assess current coping mechanisms of child and family.

    f. Family may exhibit guilt, frustration, and anxiety in response to an ill child.

  4. Assess home environment—may give clues to an allergy. Common household irritants include house dust, tobacco smoke, molds, strong odors and fumes, pets, and upholstered furniture.

G. Sleep habits—the child may prefer an upright position when sleeping. This may indicate that respiratory maneuvers are performed more comfortably in this position and respiratory disease may be present.

H. Emotional status—a respiratory condition such as asthma may have an emotional component.

III. Pediatric chest examination.

A. General considerations.

  1. Depending, of course, upon their age, children generally have shorter attention spans, less comprehension of verbal instructions, and a different perception of objects and events than adults.

  2. Encourage the parents to remain with the child during the examination.

  3. The same basic maneuvers of inspection, palpation, percussion, and auscultation are performed in the child as in the adult, but some maneuvers must be modified to accommodate the young child's size and ability to follow verbal instructions.

  4. Stethoscopes should have a small diaphragm and bell with rubber margin to obtain adequate contact with the thin, bony chest wall. Keep stethoscope in plain sight and allow the child to touch or play with it prior to the examination.

  5. Perform the least distressing parts of the exam first.

B. General clues in interpretation of findings.

  1. A child's chest wall is thin; therefore, breath sounds will be louder, more intense, and easily transmitted throughout the chest.

  2. Upper airway sounds are easily confused with lower airway sounds.

  3. A child's head should be in straight alignment with the body as turning the head to one side may cause decreased breath sounds in the opposite side of the chest.

C. Developmental considerations that may affect physical findings.

  1. Mouth breathing—newborn infants are obligatory nose breathers and do not breathe through their mouths (except when crying) until after approximately 6 weeks of age; therefore, any narrowing or blockage in the nasal airway of an infant will make respiratory maneuvers difficult.

  2. Increased amount of lymphoid tissue—children up to the age of puberty have an abundance of lymphoid tissue located in the pharyngeal area: the tonsils and adenoids. This tissue serves as the first line of defense against respiratory

infections and it hypertrophies in response to infections. The adenoids, in particular, can enlarge to such a degree that they completely occlude the nasopharyngeal area, obstructing breathing and swallowing.

3. Diaphragmatic breathing—the intercostal muscles of respiration are immature and not well developed until age 6 or 7; therefore, the diaphragm is the major muscle of respiration in younger children and diaphragmatic breathing is a normal finding.

4. Middle ear infection—middle ear infections are more common in young children because their eustachian tubes are short, straight, distended tubes with the nasopharyngeal orifice in close proximity to the adenoids. As the child grows, the tubes become longer, more twisted and narrow, providing anatomic protection against infection.

5. Foreign body aspiration—foreign bodies are most often aspirated into the right lung because the right main bronchus is wider and more directly in line with the axis of the trachea than the left main bronchus.

6. Accessory muscles of respiration—the muscles of the neck should be developed for head control between 2 and 3 months of age. When these muscles stabilize the head and neck, the scalene and sternomastoid muscles will function efficiently when recruited as accessory muscles of respiration.

IV. Physical examination.
  A. General appearance.
    1. Color.
       a. Assess color at rest *and* when active or during crying.
       b. Note presence of pallor—this may indicate anemia or fever.
       c. Note presence of cyanosis—check mucous membranes and nailbeds. The detection of cyanosis involves subjective color perception. Skin thickness and lighting as well as the child's pigmentation affect its recognition.
    2. Skin.
       a. Note state of hydration—check skin turgor.
       b. Pitting or nonpitting edema may indicate accompanying heart disease.
  B. Head and neck.
    1. Face—an anxious facies may be present in moderate to severe respiratory distress.
    2. Nose.
       a. Flaring of nares often accompanies respiratory distress.
       b. Polyps often occur with cystic fibrosis.
       c. Presence of foreign bodies.
       d. Discharge from nose.
       e. Color of mucosa—pale, boggy nasal mucosa occurs in children with allergies.
       f. The "allergic salute" (a characteristic gesture of rubbing the nose) may cause a crease across the bridge of the nose and is commonly found in children with allergies.
    3. Mouth.
       a. Color—circumoral pallor or cyanosis of lips and mucous membranes (central cyanosis) often accompanies severe respiratory or cardiac defects.
       b. Odors—halitosis can be attributed to infection of the teeth, sinuses, adenoids and tonsils, allergic rhinitis, foreign bodies, and poor oral hygiene.
       c. Assess moistness of tongue and mucous membranes.
       d. Retropharyngeal exam for postnasal drip, color, edema, and exudate.
    4. Neck—cervical nodes greater than 1 cm in diameter constitute enlargement. These nodes drain the sinuses, ears, mouth, and pharynx, and enlargement may indicate infection in any of these areas.
  C. Chest.
    1. Inspection.
       a. Chest configuration.
          (1) Developmental considerations—In children under $3\frac{1}{2}$ years, the thorax

is normally round with the anteroposterior diameter equal to the transverse diameter. After this age, the transverse diameter enlarges and is greater than the anteroposterior diameter.

(2) A barrel-shaped chest indicates overinflation of the lungs.

(3) Pectus carinatum (pigeon breast) is a congenital abnormality in which the sternum protrudes.

(4) Pectus excavatum (funnel chest) is characterized by sternal depression.

(5) Kyphosis and scoliosis: S-shaped curvature of the spine with a hump over the scapular area.

(6) Precordial bulge is a left-sided anterior chest bulge due to cardiac enlargement.

   b. Chest movements.

(1) Retractions of the chest: note location and magnitude.

(2) Use of accessory muscles.

(3) Inspiratory–expiratory time ratio is normally 1:2.

   c. Respirations—best to evaluate when child is asleep or resting.

(1) Rate of respirations (Table 14-1).

   (*a*) Rapid rate (*tachypnea*)—common in respiratory disorders, particularly lower airway obstruction, fever, anxiety, and heart failure.

   (*b*) Slower rate (*bradypnea*)—suggests central respiratory depression, increased intracranial pressure, alkalosis of long duration.

(2) Depth—deep (*hyperpnea*) indicates degree of anoxia present, the presence of acidosis or possible upper airway obstruction.

(3) Quality—gasping, grunting respirations as well as dyspnea, orthopnea, and restlessness may indicate respiratory distress.

2. Palpation.

   a. Symmetry of movement.

(1) Asymmetric chest movements may indicate pneumothorax or a chronic localized chest disease.

(2) Precordial bulging may indicate cardiac disease.

   b. Position of trachea (Fig. 14-1)—a shift from midline may occur with diseased lung tissue or pleura, or abnormality of the bony chest cage or diaphragm.

   c. Tactile fremitus—normally felt over the entire chest as a tingling sensation when the child speaks or cries.

(1) Fremitus increases when underlying lung tissue is dense as a result of a disease process, e.g., pulmonary consolidation.

(2) Fremitus decreases when either fluid or air is present in the pleural space or in the presence of airway obstruction.

3. Percussion—the chest wall is thin and the muscles small; therefore, the chest of a child is hyperresonant as compared to an adult's. Percussion is not usually a valuable maneuver in the child for diagnostic purposes.

4. Auscultation.

   a. This maneuver can be performed on a crying infant, as inspiration can be heard between cries.

   b. The infant's head should be in straight alignment with the body—turning of

TABLE 14-1 / NORMAL RESPIRATORY RATES FOR CHILDREN

Age	Normal Respiratory Rates
Newborn	30–50 per minute
6 Months	20–30 per minute
2 Years	20–30 per minute
Adolescent	12–20 per minute

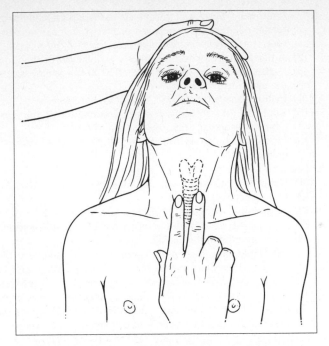

FIGURE 14-1 / Technique for ascertaining tracheal position. The relative size of the fossae located between the sternocleidomastoid muscles and the trachea is determined by the fingers. In this figure, the index finger fits well in the right fossa, but on the left the middle finger is too large for the fossa, indicating that the trachea has shifted to the left.

the head to one side may cause decreased breath sounds in the opposite side of the chest.

  c. Allow the child to handle the stethoscope prior to its use; grasping the stethoscope tubing during the exam distorts the sounds.

  d. An older child can listen with the stethoscope to alleviate anxiety; deep breathing during auscultation can be elicited by playing a game such as "take a deep breath and blow out all the candles on a birthday cake."

  e. Bronchovesicular and even bronchial breath sounds are considered a normal finding in infants and small children. The thin chest wall and lack of muscle mass accounts for sounds that are louder and harsher-sounding than in older children and adults.

  f. Normal breath sounds are easily transmitted to all parts of the chest. An infant with a pneumothorax may have seemingly normal breath sounds.

  g. Auscultation over various lobes of the lung.
    (1) Anterior chest (Fig. 14-2).
      (a) Ribs 1 to 6 = upper lobe, left side.
      (b) Ribs 1 to 4 = upper lobe, right side.
      (c) Ribs 4 to 6 = upper middle lobe, right side.
      (d) Note: only a wedge of the lower lobe is present in the anterior chest.
    (2) Posterior chest.
      (a) Clavicular area to 4th rib = upper lobe, right and left sides.
      (b) Ribs 4 to 10 = lower lobes, right and left sides.

  h. Crackling sounds (*rales*) may be heard scattered over the chest in infants and children with bronchiolitis, bronchopneumonia, atelectasis, and edema.

  i. Coarse sounds (*rhonchi*) may be heard in children with airway obstruction.

      j. Wheezing may be heard in children with laryngeal edema, foreign body, asthma, or bronchiolitis.

      k. Inspiratory stridor may be heard without the stethoscope, and usually indicates upper airway obstruction.

D. Heart—respiratory distress and failure can occur due to a cardiac defect or congestive heart failure.

E. Extremities—assess for cyanosis and presence of clubbing.

V. General assessment of respiratory distress (Fig. 14-3).

    A. Signs and symptoms of respiratory distress in infants and young children.

      1. Flaring nares—a bilateral widening of the nares during inspiratory efforts, which accompanies labored breathing.

      2. Head bobbing—observed as a subtle flexion of the head accompanying each inspiratory effort during episodes of increased work of breathing in an infant under 3 months of age.

      3. Expiratory grunting—occurs when an infant exhales against a partially closed glottis. This maneuver retards expiratory flow of air, producing a back-pressure which is transmitted from the glottis to the alveoli. This expiratory retard maintains an increased functional residual capacity and therefore increases arterial oxygen tension.

      4. Abnormal retractions of the chest—the soft tissues of the chest wall are not fully developed in the young child and ossification of the sternum and anterior ribs is incomplete. These pliable structures readily yield and pull inward when abnormally low intrathoracic pressures are required for ventilation.

      5. Intercostal bulging—this sign indicates that an increased muscular effort is required to force air out of the lungs, as, for example, in asthma. The result is an exaggeration in intrapleural pressure, causing it to exceed atmospheric pressure, and resulting in flattening or bulging out of the soft tissues of the intercostal spaces.

FIGURE 14-2 / Anterior view of the chest showing lung lobes (shaded areas) in relative location to the ribs. Note that the right lung has three lobes, and the left has two lobes.

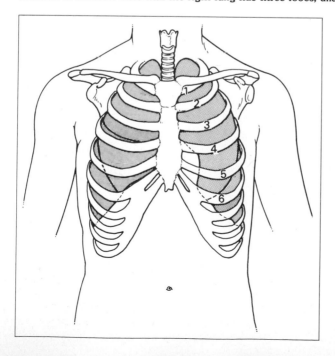

6. Inability to suckle.
7. Inspiratory stridor—this sign is observed as a high-pitched, harsh sound that is produced by obstruction to the flow of air through the larynx. Obstruction of the larynx or of the epiglottic or hypopharyngeal regions causes stridor during inspiration because the extrathoracic airways normally constrict during inspiration. Any additional reduction of the diameter of the airway results in stridor.

B. Signs and symptoms of distress in older children.
1. Shortness of breath.
2. Recurrent cough.
3. Lung congestion.
4. Nasal congestion.
5. Orthopnea.
6. Sneezing.
7. Possible chest pain.

C. Nonspecific signs and symptoms of respiratory distress.
1. Anorexia—often the first sign of illness in a child.
2. Irritability.
3. Vomiting and diarrhea—early sign of an infectious process in a child. Toxins appear to affect the immature nervous system of children by stimulating the medullary area of the brain where the centers for vomiting and defecation are located.

FIGURE 14-3 / Observation of respiratory distress. (*From W. A. Bauman, "The Respiratory Distress Syndrome and Its Significance in Premature Infants," Pediatrics, 24(2):194–204, August 1959.*)

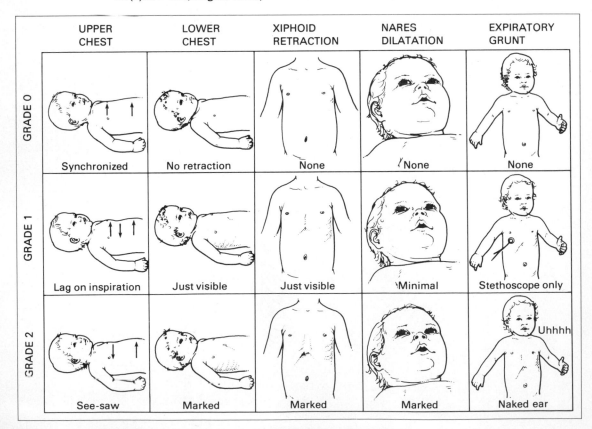

	UPPER CHEST	LOWER CHEST	XIPHOID RETRACTION	NARES DILATATION	EXPIRATORY GRUNT
GRADE 0	Synchronized	No retraction	None	None	None
GRADE 1	Lag on inspiration	Just visible	Just visible	Minimal	Stethoscope only
GRADE 2	See-saw	Marked	Marked	Marked	Naked ear

CONGENITAL MALFORMATIONS

Diaphragmatic Hernia

Definition

Diaphragmatic hernia is a free communication between the thoracic and abdominal cavities with the abdominal contents displaced into the chest. Because of the resultant respiratory distress, diaphragmatic hernia is a surgical emergency of the perinatal period. The condition occurs about once in 2200 live births and shows no predilection for race or sex. The most common site for the diaphragm defect is the posterolateral segment, which normally fuses by the sixth week of fetal life to separate the pleural cavity from the peritoneal cavity. The defect occurs five times more often on the left side than on the right. The homolateral lung is usually completely collapsed and may be hypoplastic. The mediastinal structures are shifted to the contralateral side of the chest. The contralateral lung is often partially compressed and may be hypoplastic. The treatment is surgical. This disorder carries a mortality rate of 25 to 40 percent; the lower limits of these figures are associated with early diagnosis and treatment.

Assessment

I. Large barrel chest in comparison with small abdomen.
II. Tachypnea—respiratory rate may be as high as 120 per minute.
III. Nasal flaring.
IV. Severe chest retractions usually becoming more prominent with crying.
V. Cyanosis.
VI. Absent breath sounds, particularly on the left side of the chest.
VII. Heart sounds may be displaced to the right.
VIII. Difficulty in feeding.

Problems

I. The child has severe respiratory distress with resultant hypoxemia due to compression of the thoracic contents by the abdominal organs.
II. The child may exhibit signs of intestinal obstruction.
III. The parents may exhibit severe anxiety.

Goals of Care

I. Reduce respiratory distress and prevent respiratory complications.
II. Facilitate the maintenance of a supply of oxygen to all body cells.
III. Facilitate nutrition and fluid and electrolyte balance.
IV. Prevent aspiration and other complications of GI obstruction.
V. Reduce stresses on the family and maintain effective communication with the parents.

Intervention

I. Preoperative.
    A. Monitor vital signs, especially respirations.
    B. Monitor child's color.
    C. Monitor breath sounds frequently to detect further respiratory compromise.
    D. Monitor blood gases—an increased P_{CO_2} and a decreased P_{O_2} occur with hypoxemia.
    E. Provide supplemental oxygen and humidity.
    F. Assess child's level of activity—increased restlessness may indicate increasing fatigue.
    G. A semi-Fowler's position will help alleviate pressure of the abdominal contents upon the thorax.
    H. Placing the child on the affected side will help the unaffected lung expand more fully.
    I. Help the family establish realistic goals in view of the high mortality.
    J. Parenteral therapy.
    K. Keep NPO.
    L. Use nasogastric tube to decompress the stomach.
    M. Establish a support system for parents.
    N. Provide explanations to parents concerning mechanical aids that may be present postoperatively; e.g., monitoring, chest tube.

II. Postoperative.
  A. Monitor vital signs closely.
  B. Maintain water-seal chest suction for 2 to 3 days postoperatively.
  C. Utilize semi-Fowler's position to aid ventilatory maneuvers.
  D. Monitor blood gases.
  E. Provide supplemental oxygen if necessary.
  F. Provide respiratory assistance if necessary.
  G. Use nasogastric tube.
  H. Keep NPO status until peristalsis resumes.
  I. Maintain accurate intake and output record.
  J. Observe for bleeding, distension of abdomen, and alterations in intake and output.
  K. Utilize small, frequent feedings with frequent burping and maintain semi-Fowler's position when feeding.
  L. Restore mother-child relationship.
  M. Teach newborn care and feeding techniques to parents.

Evaluation

I. Preoperative.
  A. Respiratory effort and retractions decrease, respiratory rate stabilizes.
  B. Nasogastric tube works well to decompress gastrointestinal organs in the chest and prevent vomiting and aspiration.
  C. Proper hydration and electrolyte balance are maintained.
  D. Parents cope adequately and are prepared for surgery.
II. Postoperative.
  A. There is no cyanosis or other evidence of respiratory distress.
  B. Water-seal drainage functions properly.
  C. Gastrointestinal function is restored.
  D. Hydration, electrolyte balance, and nutrition are adequate.
  E. A good parent-child interaction exists.

Laryngotracheal Malacia

Definition

Malacia refers to softening and resultant loss of support in the area. *Laryngeal malacia* is flabbiness of the epiglottis and/or supraglottic area; *tracheal malacia* is weakening of a section of tracheal cartilage resulting in collapse of the area during inspiration (the extrathoracic airways normally constrict on inspiration). Noisy respirations may cause concern, but treatment is seldom necessary. The condition is usually self-limiting.

Assessment

I. Stridor on inspiration.
II. Retractions of the chest wall.
III. Difficulty or inability to suckle.
IV. Difficulty breathing.

Problems

I. The child exhibits mild to moderate respiratory distress shortly after birth.
II. Normal sucking and nutritional intake are curtailed due to respiratory distress.
III. The parents and child may exhibit increased anxiety when the child's respiratory distress increases.

Goals of Care

I. Reduce respiratory distress.
II. Prevent respiratory infections.
III. Promote adequate nutrition.
IV. Reduce anxiety and stress for the child and parent.
V. Teach parents specific interventions to alleviate respiratory distress in the child at home.

Intervention

I. Assess degree of respiratory distress and provide assistance as needed.
II. Prevent respiratory infections.
III. Maintain semi-Fowler's position during distress.
IV. Provide high humidity in environment.

     V. Provide slow, careful feedings.
     VI. Allow frequent rest periods if respiratory distress is present.
     VII. Promote parent participation in care of the child.
     VIII. Teach parents:
       A. Health maintenance of child.
       B. Prevention of respiratory infections.
       C. Assessment of degree of respiratory stridor and distress.
       D. Feeding technique (slow feedings, rest periods as necessary).
     IX. Reassure parents that most children outgrow symptoms in several months or a few years.
     X. Encourage parents to promote normal developmental patterns.

Evaluation
     I. There is good respiratory exchange.
     II. Parents cope well and are prepared for home care.

OBSTRUCTIONS

Foreign Body Aspiration

Definition
Toddlers are particularly prone to aspiration of objects and food. The severity of respiratory distress and the treatment depend on the type of object aspirated, the location of the object, and the degree of obstruction. Aspirated objects commonly lodge in the laryngotracheal area, but they can also pass into a main stem bronchus or further down into a segmental bronchus.

Assessment
     I. Immediate signs.
       A. Choking.   **C.** Coughing.
       B. Gagging.   **D.** Aphonia.
     II. Later signs.
       A. Hoarseness.   **D.** Dyspnea.
       B. Coughing.   **E.** Possible fever.
       C. Cyanosis.   **F.** Retractions of the chest.

Problems
     I. The child may exhibit mild to severe respiratory distress with oxygen deprivation.
     II. The child may be frightened and anxious; the parents may also be anxious.
     III. The child may or may not experience pain and/or discomfort at the site of the foreign body.
     IV. The child and parent will require teaching related to the technique and postoperative care for a laryngoscopy or bronchoscopy.

Goals of Care
     I. Immediate.
       A. Reduce respiratory distress and maintain oxygen supply to all body cells.
       B. Reduce anxiety and provide a quiet environment.
       C. Provide reassurance for child and parents.
       D. See that the foreign body is promptly removed.
     II. Postoperative.
       A. Assess child for respiratory complications and prevent their occurrence.
       B. Resume adequate nutritional intake.
       C. Provide preventive teaching to avoid subsequent aspiration.

Intervention
     I. Immediate.
       A. Monitor vital signs.
       B. Assess degree of respiratory distress and oxygenation.
         1. Check color, note any cyanosis.
         2. Note retractions of chest.

          C. Administer oxygen if necessary.
          D. Provide high humidity.
          E. Prevent eating and drinking until after laryngoscopy or bronchoscopy.
          F. Allow parents to be with child to reduce anxiety.
          G. Assess need for sedation.
          H. Provide a quiet, restful environment.
      II. Postoperative.
          A. Assess return of swallowing reflex after laryngoscopy or bronchoscopy.
          B. Provide clear liquids and gradually advance diet.
          C. Assess presence of laryngeal edema.
             1. Note presence of inspiratory stridor.
             2. Monitor degree of respiratory distress.
          D. Monitor vital signs and signs of increased respiratory distress.
          E. Provide oxygen and high humidity.
          F. Prevent aspiration by teaching parents to keep small objects out of the reach of children.
          G. Teach parents the Heimlich maneuver for removal of aspirated foreign bodies: The Heimlich maneuver consists of standing behind the victim, putting your arms around the victim's chest area under the diaphragm, and applying a sharp "hug" with the fists clenched to dislodge the foreign object.

Evaluation
      I. Respiratory distress is resolved.
      II. Infection responds to treatment.
      III. Postoperative complications are avoided.
      IV. Parents know how to avoid recurrence of aspiration.
      V. Parents know how to apply the Heimlich maneuver.

Foreign Body in the Nose

Definition
Foreign bodies such as nuts, beads, fruit seeds, small stones, and erasers may be pushed into the nares. They may be pushed back farther if an unskilled person attempts to remove them. Hygroscopic substances, such as peas or a cotton wad, may increase in size as they absorb fluid and further promote nasal obstruction.

Assessment
      I. Discomfort or soreness in the nose.
      II. Sneezing.
      III. Bloody discharge.
      IV. Purulent discharge if infected.
      V. Nasal obstruction.

Problems
      I. The child may exhibit mild to severe nasal obstruction.
      II. The foreign body may be aspirated into the lungs.
      III. The foreign body may cause mucosal irritation and localized infection.
      IV. The parents and child may need preventive teaching.

Goals of Care
      I. Reduce respiratory distress.
      II. Prevent manipulation of foreign body by unskilled person.
      III. Assess child for presence of localized infection even after foreign body has been removed.
      IV. Provide child and parents with information concerning the prevention of recurrence.

Intervention
      I. Have object removed promptly by a physician.
      II. Avoid manipulation of the object by an unskilled person.
      III. Parents should know the signs that indicate that a foreign body is present and should realize the importance of having a skilled person remove the object.
      IV. Instruct parents and child about prevention.

Evaluation	**I.** Foreign body is removed without complication.
	II. Residual infection responds to treatment.
	III. Parents and child are instructed about prevention of recurrence.

Foreign Body in the Ear

Definition Foreign bodies such as beads, stones, food, and insects may be pushed into the external auditory canal by young children. An object may be hygroscopic or rough-edged and cause damage within the ear. Objects may remain in the ear canal for weeks before their presence is known. A foreign body in the ear canal may cause obstruction, infection, and possible deafness in the affected ear.

Assessment
I. Discomfort in the affected ear.
II. Deafness.
III. Cellulitis.

Problems
I. The foreign object within the ear may result in temporary deafness.
II. The child may exhibit anxiety due to the sudden deafness or discomfort.
III. The parents and child may require instruction to prevent a recurrence.

Goals of Care
I. Promote prompt removal of the foreign object.
II. Prevent an unskilled person from manipulating the object.
III. Provide a quiet environment for the child.
IV. Allow parents to stay with the child.
V. Child and parents should be aware that objects should not be placed in the auditory canal and that if an object accidentally or deliberately is placed in the canal, a skilled person should remove it.

Intervention
I. Reassure parents and child.
II. Identify the object prior to removal, as different objects require different methods of removal (see point III).
III. Instill appropriate irrigant or lubricant solution (except for a hygroscopic object, which requires no irrigant): e.g., removal of wax is facilitated by hydrogen peroxide instillation; beads can be lubricated with oil or a soap solution.
IV. Have object removed promptly by a physician.
V. Consider that the child may have a temporary hearing deficit; approach the child with this in mind.
VI. Assess external ear for edema and/or a break in the skin.
VII. Monitor ear canal for signs of infection.
VIII. Provide parents and child with information about foreign body removal and prevention of recurrence.

Evaluation
I. Foreign body is removed without complication.
II. Residual infection responds to treatment.
III. Parents and child are instructed about prevention of recurrence.

Bronchiolitis

Definition *Bronchiolitis* is an acute viral illness which is usually caused by the respiratory syncytial or parainfluenza viruses. It is characterized by widespread lower airway obstruction. Bronchioles become partially or totally occluded by the inflamed, edematous bronchiolar mucosa. The tenacious exudate made up of mucus and cellular debris causes hyperinflation and atelectasis of the alveoli. Bronchiolitis occurs almost exclusively in children under 2 years of age, with the peak incidence around 6 months. Several factors contribute to the occurrence at this age:

I. The short distance between the upper and lower airway, which facilitates rapid spreading of the viral infection and inflammation from the upper airway along the continuous respiratory membrane to the lower airways.

II. Low levels of antibodies during the first year of life (prenatally acquired antibodies are largely destroyed by the third month of life).

III. Very small lumen diameters of the bronchioles.

IV. Rapid respiratory rates produce more turbulent airflow, increased airway resistance, and increased effort for breathing.

Assessment

I. Expiratory wheezing.
II. Nasal flaring.
III. Overdistended chest.
IV. Retractions of the chest.
V. Cyanosis.
VI. Restlessness.
VII. Hacking cough.
VIII. Tachypnea.
IX. Fever may or may not be present.

Problems

I. The child may exhibit severe respiratory distress with resulting hypoxia.
II. The child may exhibit restlessness and possibly fatigue as the work of breathing increases.
III. The child may be unable to take fluids by mouth due to extreme respiratory distress.
IV. There may be an elevation in body temperature.
V. Respiratory acidosis may develop due to inadequate ventilation.

Goals of Care

I. Reduce respiratory distress.
II. Assess progression of respiratory distress.
III. Facilitate the maintenance of a supply of oxygen to all body cells.
IV. Provide for rest and sleep.
V. Provide for adequate fluid and nutrition.
VI. Assess state of hydration.
VII. Maintain normal body temperature.
VIII. Maintain normal body pH.

Intervention

I. Respiratory distress.
   A. Provide humidified oxygen.
   B. Reposition frequently to allow increased ventilation of affected lung.
   C. Assess degree of respiratory distress.
   D. Provide chest physiotherapy.
II. Restlessness and fatigue.
   A. Reduce stresses in the environment.
   B. Encourage parents to stay with child.
   C. Provide frequent rest periods.
   D. Observe for cardiac arrhythmias—most cardiac arrhythmias are the result of hypoxia.
III. Dehydration.
   A. Monitor intake and output.
   B. Assess for signs of dehydration—daily water loss may be increased because insensible water loss (that lost through skin and lungs) increases with increased respiratory rate.
   C. Parenteral therapy when in severe distress.
   D. Encourage oral intake of fluids when not in acute distress.
   E. Prevent overhydration.
IV. Fever.
   A. Monitor temperature.
   B. Administer antipyretic as prescribed.
   C. Sponge with tepid water as needed.
   D. Observe for febrile convulsions.

    E. Administer antibiotics as prescribed.

    F. Monitor blood gases if child is in severe distress.

Evaluation

    I. Respiratory distress resolves.

    II. There is good hydration, nutrition, and electrolyte balance.

    III. Body temperature rturns to normal.

Case Study

Timmy is an 18-month-old boy admitted to the pediatric ward with respiratory distress and a diagnosis of bronchiolitis. Timmy's mother states he was well until 2 weeks ago when he developed a "mild head cold" and a fever. Tylenol and fluids were given on the doctor's advice. The cold appeared to get better, but 3 days prior to admission Timmy became irritable and anorectic. Two days ago he developed diarrhea and a fever of 38.9°C (102°F). Upon admission Timmy's temperature is 37.9°C (100.2°F), his pulse is 124, and his respiratory rate is 40 per minute. He is lethargic and pale. He has substernal and intercostal retractions and nasal flaring. Upon auscultation, wheezing and rales are heard.

PROBLEMS

    I. Respiratory distress

    II. Elevated body temperature.

    III. Fluid imbalance.

GOALS OF CARE

    I. Reduce distress.

    II. Maintain normal body temperature.

    III. Maintain adequate fluid balance.

INTERVENTION

    I. Provide humidified oxygen via tent.

    II. Change position frequently.

    III. Chest physiotherapy.

    IV. Remove secretions as often as necessary.

    V. Monitor temperature closely.

    VI. Administer antipyretics as prescribed.

    VII. Observe for febrile convulsions.

    VIII. Monitor intake and output of liquids closely.

    IX. Assess for signs of dehydration.

    X. Encourage clear liquids if not in respiratory distress.

    XI. Give fluids intravenously if in severe distress.

EVALUATION

    I. Assess progression of distress.

    II. Does supportive care alleviate severe respiratory distress?

    III. Does body temperature return to normal?

    IV. Does child manifest normal hydration?

Croup

Definition

Croup is a general term which refers to the clinical syndrome of *laryngitis* and *laryngotracheobronchitis* (LTB). The vocal cords, subglottic tissue, trachea, bronchi, and bronchioles can be involved. The infectious type of croup can be either of viral or bacterial origin. *Viral croup:* (85 percent of reported cases) occurs mostly in chidren between the ages of 3 months and 4 years. *Bacterial croup* (caused by *Hemophilus influenzae* type B) occurs in children aged 2 to 12 years. Croup caused by *Corynebacterium diphtheriae* is rare but is always a possibility in a child who has not received the series of DPT immunizations. *Noninfectious croup* may result from asthma or may follow endotracheal intubation or foreign body aspiration.

In response to either mechanical or infectious processes occurring in the laryngeal area, the tissues become inflamed and edematous, and partial or total obstruction of the airway results. With the child under 2 years of age, the glottic opening is small and the mucous membrane of the laryngeal airway is highly vascular and apt to become rapidly edematous in response to inflammation.

Assessment

I. Health history.
    A. Recent upper respiratory infection.
    B. Recent sore throat.
II. Physical assessment.
    A. Hoarse, barking cough.
    B. Inspiratory stridor.
    C. Restlessness, anxiety.
    D. Chest retractions.
    E. Diminished breath sounds with rales and rhonchi.
    F. Intermittent cyanosis.
    G. Possible fever.
    H. Possible hypercapnia and hypoxia.
    I. Tachycardia.

Problems

I. The child will exhibit some degree of respiratory distress with possible hypoxemia and hypercarbia.
II. The child will exhibit moderate to severe anxiety.
III. The child may exhibit some degree of fatigue.
IV. There will be an elevation in body temperature.
V. The child and parents may require teaching prior to discharge.

Goals of Care

I. Maintain patency of the airway and adequate oxygenation.
II. Reduce anxiety and stresses in the environment.
III. Promote rest and sleep.
IV. Maintain normal body temperature.
V. Maintain adequate hydration.
VI. Teach parents about use of humidification at home if recurrence threatens.

Interventions

I. Respiratory distress.
    A. Provide humidified oxygen.
    B. Assess degree of airway obstruction.
    C. Monitor vital signs.
    D. Monitor blood gases.
    E. Administer antibiotics as prescribed.
    F. Have intubation and tracheostomy equipment of the proper size ready at bedside for possible use.
II. Anxiety.
    A. Provide reassurance for child and parent.
    B. Explain nursing actions prior to care.
    C. Assist the older child in communicating his or her needs.
    D. Anticipate the child's needs.
III. Fatigue.
    A. Provide a quiet environment that allows for physical and emotional rest.
    B. Try not to disturb the child except for necessary nursing care.
IV. Fever.
    A. Monitor temperature.
    B. Administer prescribed antipyretics.
    C. Administer sponge bath with tepid water as necessary.
    D. Maintain parenteral fluids at prescribed rate.
    E. Prevent eating and drinking in acute phase.

   F. Maintain accurate intake and output records.

   G. Check specific gravity of urine.

  V. Discharge care.

   A. Teach care of tracheostomy if child goes home with tube in place (rare).

   B. Provide information to parent concerning croup and the possibility of its recurrence.

Evaluation

  I. Respiratory distress responds to treatment.

  II. Temperature returns to normal without complications.

  III. Good hydration is reestablished.

  IV. Parents have been instructed in home care.

   A. Avoidance of respiratory infections.

   B. Recognition and treatment of early signs of recurrence.

Epiglottitis

Definition

Epiglottitis is an inflammatory response (to an infectious agent) which causes swelling of the epiglottis, false cords, and aryepiglottic folds. The bacterial agents most often responsible are *Hemophilus influenzae, pneumococci, staphylococcus aureus,* and beta-hemolytic streptococci. The epiglottis is a long, narrow structure which closes off the narrow glottis during swallowing. Edema of the epiglottis and surrounding tissues can completely occlude the laryngeal airway in a matter of minutes or hours.

Assessment

  I. Severe inspiratory stridor.

  II. Marked retractions of the chest and supraclavicular area.

  III. Hoarseness.

  IV. Acute anxiety.

  V. Restlessness.

  VI. Abrupt onset of high fever; 39 to 40°C (102 to 104°F).

  VII. Dysphagia and drooling of saliva may occur—the patient usually prefers a sitting position with mouth open, tongue protruding.

  VIII. Cyanosis.

  IX. Breath sounds may be diminished.

  X. Possible hypercapnia and/or hypoxia.

  XI. Cherry-red epiglottis.

  XII. Fatigue.

  XIII. Impaired consciousness.

Problems See "Croup."

Goals of Care See "Croup."

Intervention See "Croup."

Evaluation See "Croup."

Bronchial Asthma

Definition

Bronchial asthma is a recurrent generalized airway obstruction characterized by dyspnea and wheezing which in the early stages are paroxysmal and reversible. A severe form, *status asthmaticus,* exists in which the patient deteriorates in spite of treatment. Asthma is rare in infancy but increases in incidence in children over 2 years of age. Most cases are thought to be precipitated by allergy. Common irritants that can cause bronchial asthma include pollen, mold spores, feathers, house dust, certain foods, air pollutants, psychological or emotional factors, cold weather and exercise, and respiratory infections.

An attack of asthma begins with an *antigen-antibody reaction* that causes the release of *histamine* and the slow-reacting substance of anaphylaxis (SRS-A). This results in dilatation of blood vessels, excess production of mucus, development of edema, and contraction of the small muscles in the airways. The lungs become emphysematous because inspired air cannot be fully exhaled.

Pulmonary function studies show:

1. Increased airway resistance.
2. Decreased forced expiratory volume within 1 s.
3. Increased total lung volume.
4. Increased functional residual capacity.
5. Uneven ventilation/perfusion ratios.

Assessment

I. Family history—may be evidence of other family members having asthma.
II. Emotional history—emotional status should be assessed.
III. Physical assessment.
    A. Early signs and symptoms.
        1. Gradual onset with nasal congestion and sneezing.
        2. Wheezing on expiration.
        3. Anxiety and restlessness.
        4. Altered vital signs—increased heart rate, increased respiratory rate.
        5. Diaphoresis.
        6. Coughing.
    B. Late signs and symptoms.
        1. Increased wheezing.
        2. Thick, tenacious mucus.
        3. Nasal flaring.
        4. Use of accessory muscles of respiration.
        5. Cyanosis.
        6. Extreme fatigue.
        7. Altered blood gases.
        8. Vomiting.

Problems

I. The child may exhibit mild to severe respiratory distress with hypoxemia.
II. The child may be unable to take adequate fluids.
III. Both parents and child will need information about medications used in the treatment of asthma.
IV. There may be severe anxiety during an attack.
V. The child and parents may need assistance to develop a healthy, realistic attitude toward the illness.
VI. Both also will need information concerning measures which will help maintain optimal health.
VII. The child and parents will need information concerning environmental control of the offending material.

Goals of Care

I. Respiration.
    A. Reduce respiratory distress.
    B. Maintain oxygen supply to all body cells.
    C. Teach child and parent appropriate breathing exercises.
    D. Provide adequate hydration to liquefy secretions in respiratory tract.
II. Medication.
    A. Administer prescribed medications on a regular schedule.
    B. Teach child and parents drug information, i.e., action, dosage, and side effects of the drugs used in the treatment of asthma.
III. Anxiety.
    A. Reduce stresses in the treatment environment.
    B. Secure psychological counseling for child and family if necessary.

      C. Assist child and parents in developing a therapeutic attitude toward the child's illness.

      D. Teach child and parents proper habits necessary to maintain and assure optimal health.

IV. Environmental control.

      A. Remove offending substance from the treatment environment.

      B. Provide clean environment.

      C. Teach child and parent to avoid environmental settings and conditions that expose child to contact with an offending allergen.

Intervention

I. Respiratory distress.

      A. Assess degree and progression of respiratory distress.

            1. Observe for nasal flaring, chest retractions, presence of wheezing, and presence of cyanosis.

            2. Note any increase in restlessness and/or anxiety.

      B. Monitor vital signs, especially during an attack and when drugs are being administered.

      C. Position child in Fowler's position with arms extended over bed table to allow for maximum lung expansion.

      D. Administer oxygen and provide mist tent.

      E. Monitor blood gases—treat acidosis if present.

      F. Administer medications and vaporized inhalations as prescribed (Table 14-2).

      G. Reduce stresses in environment and give sedation if necessary.

      H. Teach chest physiotherapy and proper breathing habits.

            1. General considerations:

                  a. Breathing exercises provide for maximum use of the respiratory muscles, especially the diaphragm.

                  b. Have the child remove secretions from nasal passages prior to beginning exercises.

            2. Abdominal breathing (Fig. 14-4*a*):

                  a. Have child lie on back with knees bent and feet flat on the floor.

                  b. Have child inflate lungs by taking a series of short inspirations through nose without allowing chest to rise.

                  c. Then have child exhale through mouth with pursed lips very slowly and completely until all the air is out.

                  d. Repeat 10 times.

            3. Forward bending (Fig. 14-4*b*):

                  a. Sit, leaning forward with a straight back and arms resting on the knees.

                  b. Breathe in through nose, expanding upper abdomen, and blow all the air out slowly through the mouth while keeping the chest still and remaining erect.

            4. Side expansion (Fig. 14-4*c*):

                  a. Sit in a chair with palms of hands on each side of the lower ribs.

                  b. Inhale, expanding lower ribs, then exhale through mouth, contracting upper part of the thorax and lower ribs.

                  c. Compress hands against ribs and expel air from the base of the lungs.

                  d. Repeat 10 times.

      I. Assess response to present therapy, including drugs.

      J. Assess need for further hyposensitization.

II. Hydration.

      A. Maintain parenteral fluid administration in acute phase.

      B. Encourage oral fluid intake.

            1. Determine fluid preferences.

            2. Avoid iced fluids as they may stimulate bronchospasm.

      C. Observe for signs of dehydration.

            1. Lack of tears.

TABLE 14-2 / BRONCHODILATORS FOR ASTHMATIC CHILDREN

Drug	Rationale	Action	Method	Dosage	Side Effects
Ephedrine	Prophylactic relief of nocturnal paroxysms and wheezing induced by exercise	Slow; prolonged duration; bronchodilation	Oral	Varies from 8 mg for preschooler to 25 mg for older children	Tachycardia, central nervous system stimulation, vomiting
Pseudoephedrine	Same as ephedrine	Same as ephedrine	Oral	About twice the dose of ephedrine	Relatively free of side effects
Epinephrine	Severe asthma: relief of paroxysm	Rapid; short duration; bronchodilation	1:1000 solution SC 1:100 solution by inhalation. *Never used for injection*	Small doses at 20- to 30-min intervals: 0.05 mL for infant; 0.2–0.3 mL for older child	Pallor, tachycardia, and palpitation
Epinephrine aqueous suspension	Relief of paroxysms, especially frequent ones	Rapid; sustained (8–10 h)	1:200 aqueous suspension SC	Maximum single dose 0.15 mL (0.005 mL/kg)	Anxiety, restlessness, tremor, headache, dizziness, pallor, respiratory weakness, and palpitation
Ethylhorepinephrine	Same as epinephrine	Same as epinephrine	SC or IV	Same as epinephrine	Relatively free of side effects
Isopropylnorepinephrine	Relief of paroxysm	Same as epinephrine	Aerosol: Use must be supervised by an adult.	1–2 "puffs" or sprays at ½- to 1-h intervals (4–6 total daily "puffs")	Status asthmaticus with prolonged use: overdose (hypotension and cardiac arrest) with daily use
Aminophylline*	Relief of paroxysm when ephedrine has failed	Slow; prolonged; bronchodilation	Suppository: drug is unevenly distributed in suppository, so fractional doses are unreliable Oral IV in a 2.5% solution *slowly* to avoid cardiac arrythmias or hypertension	3–4 mg/kg every 8 h (total daily dose by all routes should not exceed 12 mg/kg)	Initial signs of toxicity: increasing restlessness, irritability, and vomiting Life-threatening signs of toxicity: increasing excitement or delirium, vomiting of blood, and convulsions

*Never given in conjunction with epinephrine or ephedrine unless aminophylline dosage reduced. Otherwise, toxic effects potentiated.

Source: Adapted from M. Chard and G. M. Scipien, "The Respiratory System," in G. M. Scipien et al. (eds.), *Comprehensive Pediatric Nursing,* McGraw-Hill Book Company, New York, 1975, p. 531.

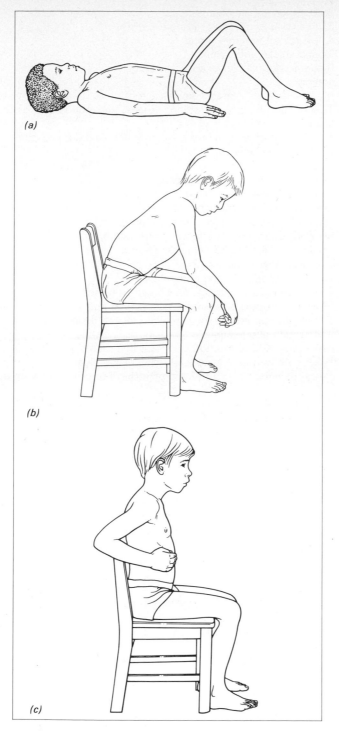

FIGURE 14-4 / (a) Abdominal breathing position. (b) Forward-bending breathing position. (c) Side expansion breathing position.

   2. Dry mucous membranes.
   3. Poor skin turgor.
   4. Decreased urinary output.
   D. Monitor intake and output.
   E. Return to normal diet as soon as feasible.
III. Medication.
   A. Assess child's and parents' knowledge of drugs used in treatment.
   B. Teach child and parents action, dosage, and side effects of drugs used in the treatment of asthma.
   C. Encourage child and parents to administer only drugs prescribed by the physician.
IV. Anxiety and apprehension.
   A. Assess child's level of anxiety.
   B. Provide child maximal reassurance.
   C. Provide a quiet, clean environment.
   D. Evaluate need for sedation.
   E. Arrange for psychiatric counseling if necessary.
   F. In hospital, organize care so as not to disturb child.
   G. Discuss plan of care with child and parent.
V. Child's and parent's attitudes toward illness.
   A. Avoid overprotection and dependence.
   B. Encourage child to manage for himself or herself.
   C. Promote an open, accepting atmosphere at home and in the hospital.
   D. Provide an opportunity for parents to discuss their frustrations.
VI. Environmental considerations.
   A. Avoid any physical exertion or irritant that causes wheezing or dyspnea.
   B. Teach child and parents to avoid offending antigens.
VII. Encourage parent and child to keep physician's or clinic follow-up appointments.

Evaluation
I. Respiratory distress is relieved.
II. Physiologic status is optimized (nutrition, hydration, rest, and acid-base balance).
III. Parents (and child, if old enough) understand and cooperatively participate in the treatment regime, including home care.
IV. Parents and child cope adequately with the illness.
V. Child develops appropriately for age.

Case Study
John, a 9-year-old, is admitted to the hospital with severe asthma of 3 days' duration which has not responded to three injections of epinephrine. John is an acutely ill, dyspneic child with severe audible wheezing, a respiratory rate of 32 per minute, and pulse at 130 per minute. Other presenting signs include circumoral cyanosis, severe supraclavicular and substernal chest retractions, episodes of paroxysmal coughing, and severe anxiety. Auscultation reveals that breath sounds are diminished bilaterally. Arterial blood gas analysis reveals P_{O_2} 62 mmHg, P_{CO_2} 55 mmHg, and pH 7.30, indicating hypoxemia, hypercapnia, and metabolic acidosis. An IV solution with isoproterenol has been started by the physician.

PROBLEMS
I. Severe respiratory distress.
II. Metabolic acidosis combined with respiratory acidosis.
III. Acute anxiety.
IV. Fluid balance: inability to take oral fluids.

GOALS OF CARE
I. Alleviate distress.
II. Ensure oxygenation to all body cells.
III. Restore normal pH.
IV. Reduce anxiety.
V. Maintain fluid and electrolyte balance.

INTERVENTION

I. Monitor degree of respiratory failure and have intubation equipment ready.

II. Monitor vital signs, especially respirations.

III. Administer oxygen.

IV. Monitor arterial blood gases closely.

V. Administer medications.

    A. Aminophylline.   **D.** Sympathomimetic agents.

    B. Isoproterenol.   **E.** Antibiotics.

    C. Corticosteroids.

VI. Engage in intermittent positive pressure breathing (IPPB) as prescribed.

VII. Monitor blood gases.

VIII. Administer sodium bicarbonate as prescribed.

IX. Assess need for assisted ventilation.

X. Reassure patient.

XI. Allow parents to stay with John.

XII. Assess need for sedation.

XIII. Keep NPO in severe distress.

XIV. Monitor intake and output of fluids carefully.

XV. Give fluids intravenously as prescribed.

EVALUATION

I. Has degree of distress been reduced?

II. Do clinical signs and blood gases indicate increasing respiratory failure?

III. Does John need assisted ventilation?

IV. Is he responding to medications?

V. Assess for side effects from various medications (cardiac arrhythmias, hypertension).

VI. Has pH returned to normal?

VII. Does he need intubation and assisted ventilation?

VIII. Is he less anxious? If not, is he more hypoxic?

IX. Is he getting an increased amount of fluids to compensate for increased insensible water loss through respiration and thick respiratory secretions?

X. Is patient showing signs of dehydration or overhydration?

Cystic Fibrosis

Definition

Cystic fibrosis is a recessive hereditary disorder of the exocrine glands. Its incidence is approximately 1 in every 2000 live births, with males and females equally afflicted. About 50 percent of children with cystic fibrosis survive to the age of 10 years; approximately 20 percent may live to be 30 years of age.

Five to ten percent of children with cystic fibrosis have meconium ileus as newborns. With pancreatic insufficiency, present in about 80 percent of children with cystic fibrosis, symptoms of intestinal malabsorption arise as the pancreatic ducts become clogged with abnormally tenacious mucus and are unable to secrete enzymes which are essential to digestion of food. Pulmonary involvement is progressive as the thick secretions cause obstruction and permanent dilatation of the smaller airways. The result is lobar atelectasis, fibrotic changes, hypoxemia, pulmonary hypertension, and possible cor pulmonale.

Assessment

I. General characteristics.

    A. May be irritable.

    B. Has thin extremities with a protruding abdomen.

    C. Tires easily.

    D. History of sibling or parent with the disease.

II. Pancreatic insufficiency.

    A. Voracious appetite.   **C.** Frequent fatty stools (steatorrhea).

    B. Distended abdomen.   **D.** Fat-soluble vitamin deficiency.

III. Pulmonary manifestations—onset may be within weeks or years after birth.
   A. Dry, nonproductive cough progressing to a productive cough.
   B. Cyanosis.
   C. Barrel chest.
   D. Chest retractions.
   E. Clubbing of fingers and toes.
   F. Chronic hypoxemia.
   G. Recurrent respiratory infections.
IV. Specific diagnostic tests.
   A. Absence of pancreatic enzymes—trypsin is absent in over 80 percent of affected children.
   B. Excessive amount of fat in the stools.
   C. Increased sweat electrolytes—particularly chloride (normal sweat chloride is below 60 meq/L).
   D. Pulmonary function tests.
      1. Increased airway resistance.
      2. Uneven ventilation/perfusion ratios.
      3. Increased residual lung volume.

Problems

I. The child will manifest nutritional problems.
II. The child will manifest progressive respiratory problems.
III. The child and family may exhibit social and psychological problems related to the disease.

Goals of Care

I. Maintain an adequate fluid and nutritional state.
II. Promote good respiratory hygiene.
III. Delay progression of the respiratory lesion.
IV. Assist family in dealing with the social and psychological problems of a chronic disorder.
V. Make genetic counseling available to family.

Intervention

I. Pancreatic deficiency.
   A. Provide pancreatic extracts such as Cotazym or Viokase. The dosage is dependent on the preparation selected and the child's response. It can be sprinkled on the food directly or ingested as a tablet. The preparation is given with each meal and snack in a dose appropriate to the amount of food taken.
   B. Medium-chain triglycerides may be given as a dietary supplement.
II. Vitamin deficiency—administer supplemental fat-soluble vitamins (A, D, E, and K) as prescribed. (Children with cystic fibrosis require a water-miscible vitamin preparation, usually administered in double the usual recommended dose because of poor absorption by the intestine.)
III. The child may require sodium chloride tablets in hot weather when perspiring excessively.
IV. Evacuation of mucopurulent secretions.
   A. Use clapping, cupping, deep breathing, assisted coughing, and vibration techniques as part of chest physiotherapy.
   B. Use aerosol therapy to hydrate bronchial secretions.
   C. A mist tent is helpful; mucolytic agents may be given via mist treatment.
   D. Give expectorants.
   E. Employ bronchial lavage.
V. Prevention and treatment of respiratory infections.
   A. Antibiotic therapy—drug of choice depends on the organism.
   B. Pulmonary lavage.
VI. Oyxgen therapy.
VII. Provide emotional support to the child and family with the assistance of other health team members.
VIII. Provide an opportunity for the family to discuss concerns and frustrations.

IX. Assist family with appropriate referrals.
  A. Social worker.
  B. Psychologist.
  C. Community resources, e.g., American Lung Association, state crippled children's services, home health agency.
  D. Genetic counseling.

Evaluation

I. Parents (and child, if old enough) understand and cooperatively participate in the treatment regime, including home care.
II. Nutritional and respiratory maintenance regimens are effective in bringing about optimal health and function.
III. Family members, including child, cope and adjust adequately.
IV. Family members are informed about genetic transmission risks.

INFLAMMATORY DISORDERS

Respiratory Distress Syndrome (RDS)

Definition

Respiratory distress syndrome, a syndrome of premature newborn infants, is characterized by inadequate pulmonary exchange of oxygen and carbon dioxide, frequently progressing to respiratory failure and death. RDS is the most common cause of death in premature infants with the infant whose birth weight falls at approximately 1 to 1.5 kg being at greatest risk. Signs appear by 6 to 8 h of age. Maternal problems such as bleeding and diabetes can play a major etiologic role.

RDS is characterized physiologically by formation of a hyaline membrane composed of fibrin in the alveoli and bronchioles. The exact cause of the membrane is not known but may be increased capillary permeability which permits effusion from the pulmonary capillary into the alveoli. Deficiency in surfactant results in decreased surface tension in the affected alveoli and atelectatic areas in the lung. Large inflation pressures are needed to achieve volume expansion of the lungs. There is an instability at low lung volumes and atelectasis results. Peripheral vasoconstriction and systemic hypotension accompany the pulmonary disorder.

Bidirectional shunting of blood flow may occur through the ductus arteriosus as well as right-to-left shunting at the pulmonary level due to atelectasis.

Assessment

I. Physical assessment.
  A. Tachypnea—rate is usually above 60 per minute.
  B. Retractions of the chest with chest lag.
  C. Nasal flaring.
  D. Grunting on expiration.
  E. Progressive cyanosis.
  F. Fine rales on auscultation.
  G. Metabolic acidosis.
  H. Hypotension.
  I. Hypothermia.
II. Laboratory tests.
  A. Blood chemistry.
    1. Serum bilirubin tends to be elevated.
    2. Total serum protein is usually below 5 g per 100 mL in severe RDS.
  B. Blood gas determinations.
    1. pH—decreased, usually less than 7.30.
    2. P_{CO_2}—increased, usually above 60 mmHg.
    3. P_{O_2}—decreased, usually below 40 mmHg.
  C. Pulmonary function.
    1. Frequency—increased, 70 to 120 respirations per minute.

2. Work of breathing—increased.
3. Tidal volume—decreased.
4. Functional residual capacity—decreased.
5. Ventilation/perfusion imbalance—increased.
6. Shunting—increased, up to two-thirds cardiac output through patent ductus arteriosus.

Problems

I. The child will exhibit moderate to severe respiratory distress.
II. The child may have metabolic acidosis.
III. There may be severe fatigue.
IV. Hypothermia must be prevented.
V. Adequate fluids, calories, and electrolytes will be needed.
VI. The child will need to be monitored for possible complications.
VII. The parents may exhibit anxiety about the child's condition.

Goals of Care

I. Reduce respiratory distress and facilitate the maintenance of a supply of oxygen to all body cells.
II. Maintain normal body pH.
III. Provide an environment that promotes maximum rest.
IV. Keep environment warm enough to maintain normal body temperature.
V. Provide adequate fluid, calories, and electrolytes.
VI. Prevent and/or reduce the incidence of complications.
VII. Reduce parental anxiety.

Intervention

I. Respiratory distress.
   A. Provide humidified oxygen.
      1. Measure concentration every hour.
      2. Note and record child's response to oxygen.
      3. Administer oxygen with a plastic hood or by incubator.
      4. Have emergency intubation equipment ready at the bedside for possible use.
   B. Monitor arterial blood gases closely; keep arterial P_{O_2} between 50 and 70 mmHg.
   C. Monitor respirations and heart rate, and observe for apnea.
   D. Have prescribed ventilator ready for possible use.
II. Metabolic acidosis.
   A. Monitor arterial blood gases.
   B. Administer sodium bicarbonate as prescribed.
III. Hypothermia.
   A. Maintain body temperature between 36.5 and 37°C (97 to 98°F).
   B. Check temperature of isolette every hour.
   C. If radiant warmer is used, monitor temperature closely.
IV. Fluids, calories, and electrolytes.
   A. Monitor intravenous fluid intake carefully (10 percent glucose is usually used to spare protein catabolism).
   B. Monitor serum electrolytes; in metabolic acidosis, serum potassium may be elevated.
   C. If an umbilical artery catheter is being used, monitor for bleeding.
V. Complications and anxiety.
   A. Monitor for complications: retrolental fibroplasia, blocked endotracheal tubes, pneumothorax, pneumomediastinum, and bronchopulmonary dysplasia (BPD).
   B. Provide realistic reassurance for parents.
   C. Allow parents to visit child.

Evaluation

I. Avoidable complications do not occur; others are promptly detected and recognized.
II. Infant's needs for oxygenation, hydration, nutrition, rest, and body warmth are adequately provided for.
III. Parents are kept well informed and are given adequate emotional support.

Bronchopulmonary Dysplasia (BPD)

Definition *Bronchopulmonary dysplasia* is a syndrome of infancy similar to adult pulmonary oxygen toxicity. BPD occurs in some infants who survive respiratory distress syndrome (RDS). The cause is postulated to be a combination of high oxygen concentrations during treatment for RDS and respirator therapy.

Physiologic features include:

1. Hyalin membranes form in proximal bronchioles.
2. Areas of pulmonary hemorrhage and fibrosis develop.
3. Capillaries and alveolar membranes sustain damage and show evidence of increased permeability.
4. The infant suffers chronic hypoxia, decreased pulmonary perfusion, pulmonary vascular disease, pulmonary hypertension, and resultant cor pulmonale (right-sided heart failure as blood cannot enter the pulmonary system as well due to the fibrosis).
5. Pulmonary damage is reversible, but healing may take months or years.

Assessment The child with BPD essentially has chronic lung disease. The specific findings are general to all children with a chronic lung disorder.
  I. Signs of increased work of breathing.
    A. Tachypnea.
    B. Cyanosis.
    C. Shortness of breath.
    D. Irritability.
    E. Barrel-shaped chest from lung hyperinflation.
  II. Chronic hypoxemia.
  III. Possible hypercapnia.
  IV. Clubbing of fingers and toes.
  V. Possible delayed physical development.
  VI. Chronic respiratory infection.
  VII. Signs of heart failure (see Chap. 13).

Problems I. The child exhibits increased difficulty in breathing.
  II. The child has mild to severe hypoxemia which may progress to respiratory failure.
  III. The child is susceptible to recurrent respiratory infections.
  IV. Physical development may be delayed.
  V. Heart failure may develop secondary to respiratory disease.
  VI. The parents will need teaching regarding the child's home care.
  VII. The parents may have anxiety and frustration related to the chronicity of the disease.

Goals of Care I. Respiratory distress.
    A. Decrease work of breathing.
    B. Ensure a patent airway.
    C. Maintain an adequate supply of oxygen to all body cells.
    D. Prevent respiratory infection.
  II. Monitor child's cardiac status and detect early signs of heart failure.
  III. General.
    A. Promote growth and development.
    B. Assure adequate caloric and fluid intake.
    C. Provide parents with necessary information regarding health maintenance and home care.
    D. Reduce parents' anxiety and fristration.

Intervention I. Respiratory distress.
    A. Administer oxygen and humidity therapy.
    B. Chest physiotherapy methods should be utilized.
    C. Clear out respiratory secretions.

     D. Use bronchodilators and antibiotics as prescribed.
     E. Tracheostomy may be necessary.
     F. Assisted ventilation may be necessary.
  II. General.
     A. Advise parents to keep child away from others with infections.
     B. Encourage regular medical follow-up.
     C. Monitor growth and development—take weekly weights during infancy; keep a growth chart.
     D. Provide rest periods for child during day, depending on level of activity.
     E. Encourage parents to treat child as normally as possible.
  III. Monitor for signs of heart failure:
     A. Hepatomegaly.   *D.* Edema.
     B. Anorexia.   *E.* Decreased urine output.
     C. Abdominal pain.   *F.* Diaphoresis.
  IV. Home care—instruct parents in the following:
     A. Oxygen therapy.
     B. Chest physiotherapy and removal of secretions.
     C. Diet therapy: furnishing a diet high in protein and calories.
     D. Importance of prevention of respiratory infections.
     E. Monitoring for complications.
       1. Respiratory infections.
       2. Heart failure.
     F. Assist parents to develop a realistic attitude toward the child's illness.
     G. Encourage parents to ask questions and discuss frustrations.
     H. Assist with referrals.
       1. Home health nurse. 3. American Lung Association.
       2. Social service. 4. State crippled children's association.

Evaluation

  I. Maximal respiratory function is attained and maintained.
  II. Parents understand and participate in the therapeutic regime, including home care.
  III. Family members, including child, cope well and adjust adequately to chronic illness.

Bronchopneumonia

Definition

Bronchopneumonia is an inflammation of the lungs in which there are scattered areas of consolidation and inflammation of the interstitial mucosa. Bronchopneumonia can be caused by a viral or bacterial agent. Affected areas of the lung cannot be ventilated properly and ventilation/perfusion mismatching occurs. The alveoli become congested with red blood cells and fibrin exudate.

  Bronchopneumonia is prevalent in children in the first 4 years of life. It differs from the kind of pneumonia that older children or adults get, in which only one or more lobes are involved.

Assessment

  I. Health history.
     A. Upper respiratory infection of several days' duration prior to pneumonia.
     B. Decrease in appetite prior to diagnosis.
     C. Possible vomiting and diarrhea.
  II. Physical assessment.
     A. Abrupt onset of fever. *D.* Cough.
     B. Nasal flaring. *E.* Tachypnea and tachycardia.
     C. Retractions of chest. *F.* Rales.

Problems

  I. The child may exhibit mild to severe respiratory distress.
  II. The child may have an elevated body temperature.
  III. There may be signs of dehydration and fatigue.
  IV. The child may develop gastrointestinal or respiratory complications.

Goals of Care
    I. Reduce respiratory distress and improve oxygenation.
    II. Maintain normal body temperature.
    III. Provide adequate hydration and nutrition.
    IV. Promote rest and avoid unnecessary disturbances.
    V. Assess child for possible complications.

Intervention
    I. Respiratory distress.
      A. Monitor vital signs closely.
      B. Assess degree of distress.
      C. Provide humidified oxygen.
      D. Remove respiratory secretions.
      E. Provide frequent position changes.
      F. Chest physiotherapy.
      G. Administer antibiotic therapy as prescribed.
    II. Fever.
      A. Monitor body temperature closely.
      B. Administer antipyretics as prescribed.
      C. Give sponge baths as necessary.
      D. Observe for febrile convulsions.
    III. Hydration and nutrition.
      A. Administer parenteral therapy when in acute distress.
      B. Keep accurate intake and output records.
      C. Encourage oral fluid intake.
      D. Offer child small, frequent feedings except when in acute distress.
      E. Provide quiet, restful environment.
      F. Allow for frequent rest periods.
      G. Try not to disturb child unless necessary.
    IV. Complications.
      A. Assess for possible respiratory complications.
        1. Aspiration of feeding.
        2. Tension pneumothorax due to empyema in staph pneumonia.
      B. Assess for possible GI complications.
        1. Distended abdomen.
        2. Paralytic ileus.
        3. Constipation.

Evaluation
    I. Respiratory distress is alleviated.
    II. Child's needs for hydration, nutrition, rest, and body temperature regulation are met.
    III. Avoidable complications do not occur; others are promptly detected and treated.

Case Study
Jane is a 3-month-old infant admitted from the emergency room to the pediatric unit with a flushed face, circumoral cyanosis, nasal flaring, grunting respirations, substernal and intercostal retractions, a respiratory rate of 86 per minute, a heart rate of 160 per minute, and a rectal temperature of 39.4°C (103°F).

The mother says Jane has been fretful and has had a decreased appetite for about 3 days. Tracheal aspiration reveals *Diplococcus pneumoniae,* and a chest x-ray shows widespread infiltration of both lung fields.

PROBLEMS
    I. Respiratory distress.   **III.** Elevated body temperature.
    II. Infection.   **IV.** Possible dehydration.

GOALS OF CARE
    I. Reduce distress.   **III.** Maintain normal body temperature.
    II. Treat infection.   **IV.** Maintain normal fluids and electrolytes.

INTERVENTION
I. Monitor vital signs carefully.
II. Provide humidified oxygen.
III. Change position often.
IV. Chest physiotherapy.
V. Remove accumulated secretions.
VI. Administer antibiotic as prescribed (penicillin G intravenously or penicillin V orally are the drugs of choice).
VII. Monitor temperature closely.
VIII. Administer antipyretic as prescribed.
IX. Observe for febrile convulsion.
X. Monitor intake and output of fluids carefully.
XI. Encourage fluids or administer fluids intravenously if in distress.

EVALUATION
I. Does supportive care alleviate respiratory distress?
II. Repeat tracheal aspirate study. Is the antibiotic appropriate for the organism?
III. Has body temperature returned to normal?
IV. Does chest x-ray show clearing?
V. Assess antibiotic used in treatment for possible allergic reaction or for nonsensitivity.
VI. Assess state of hydration.
VII. Are intake and output of fluids adequate for child's weight?

Chemical Pneumonia

Definition   Ingestion (as well as direct aspiration) of lipid and hydrocarbon substances can cause *chemical pneumonia,* depending on the amount and type of material ingested. Common agents include kerosene, gasoline, turpentine, and vegetable oils. Oil-base vitamin preparations and oily nose drops must not be administered to a crying child because of the danger of oil aspiration, which results in chronic fibrosis of the affected lung tissue. Ingested petroleum distillates (kerosene, charcoal starter, gasoline, etc.), because of their low surface tension, easily spread along the esophageal mucosa to enter the respiratory tract where they can set up a stubborn pneumonia. Petroleum distillate ingestion and aspiration are serious and potentially fatal, both because of the pulmonary sequelae and because of their metabolic and neurological consequences. Emergency treatment is dealt with in Part 7.

Assessment   See "Bronchopneumonia." Additional considerations may be warranted by neurological status.

Problems   See "Bronchopneumonia." Additional considerations may be warranted by neurological status.

Goals of Care   See "Bronchopneumonia." Additional considerations may be warranted by neurological status.

Intervention   See "Bronchopneumonia." Additional considerations may be warranted by neurological status.

Evaluation   See "Bronchopneumonia." Additional considerations may be warranted by neurological status.

Tonsillitis

Definition   Also referred to as *pharyngitis,* tonsillitis is an infectious invasion of the lymphatic tissue called the *faucial tonsils* located on either side of the pharynx. An acute as well as a chronic form of the condition exists. About 85 percent of all cases are caused by viruses, while 15 percent are caused by group A beta-hemolytic streptococcus. The peak incidence is between 4 and 6 years of age.

The faucial tonsils are part of Waldeyer's ring, a circle of lymph tissue that surrounds the pharynx. The tissue filters microorganisms and protects against infection of the respiratory and gastrointestinal tracts. Invasion by microorganisms causes the tissues to swell and potentially obstruct the airways. The lymphoid tissues are normally largest in children under 5 years of age and gradually decrease in size until puberty. Chronic tonsillitis may require tonsillectomy.

Assessment	I. Acute tonsillitis.
	   A. Fever.
	   B. Malaise.
	   C. Pharyngeal erythema.
	   D. Moderately enlarged lymph nodes (cervical).
	   E. Elevated WBC level, increased to 40,000 per cubic millimeter.
	   F. Sore throat, difficulty swallowing.
	   G. Possible pharyngeal exudate.
	II. Chronic tonsillitis.
	   A. Persistent sore throats.
	   B. May have offensive breath odor.
	   C. Chronic enlargement of cervical lymph nodes.

Problems	I. The child will exhibit some degree of tonsillar enlargement and discomfort. II. There may be an elevated body temperature. III. The child should be observed for an allergic reaction to penicillin if he or she is receiving the antibiotic. IV. Tonsillectomy may be indicated.
Goals of Care	I. Maintain patency of airway. II. Maintain normal body temperature. III. Detect allergic reaction to penicillin early. IV. Prepare child for surgery if surgical intervention is planned. V. Effective postoperative care is needed if surgery is performed.

Intervention	I. Immediate.
	   A. Give warm saline gargles.
	   B. Apply hot or cold packs to neck area.
	   C. Give aspirin as prescribed for pain.
	   D. Avoid hot foods or liquids—administer cool, bland liquids only.
	   E. Administer antipyretic as prescribed.
	   F. Give patient sponge bath with tepid water as needed for fever.
	   G. Have patient drink fluids as tolerated.
	   H. Observe for signs of penicillin allergy: increased heart rate, increased respiratory rate, decreased blood pressure, skin rash, difficulty breathing.
	   I. If surgery is planned, prepare child and parents.
	II. Postoperative.
	   A. Keep in semiprone position until recovered from anesthesia (to facilitate drainage and detection of bleeding).
	   B. Observe for excessive bleeding (frequent swallowing, bloody emesis, vital signs changes, postanesthetic restlessness).
	   C. Give fluids and a soft diet.
	   D. Apply ice collar (if tolerated) and give aspirin as prescribed for pain.
	   E. Instruct parents regarding home care (give soft diet, avoid overactivity, and observe for bleeding, all for 1 week).

Evaluation	**I.** Respiratory distress and infection are alleviated.
	II. Allergy to antibiotics is promptly detected and treated.
	III. Surgical course is uncomplicated.

Otitis Media

Definition   *Otitis media* is an infection of the middle ear which usually occurs secondary to a recent upper respiratory infection. About two-thirds of cases are of viral origin and one-third are bacterial. Common bacterial pathogens are pneumococci, *Hemophilus influenzae,* beta-hemolytic streptococcus, *Staphylococcus aureus,* and *Escherichia coli.* The microorganisms that infect the middle ear usually are transmitted from the pharyngeal area via the eustachian tube. Infants and young children are especially prone to otitis media because their eustachian tubes are relatively wide, straight, and short, and thus allow pathogens easy access to the middle ear.

Assessment
    I. Irritability and restlessness.
    II. Infant may rub or pull at ear.
    III. Older child may have pain, headache, and dizziness.
    IV. Fever.
    V. Eardrum may be bulging or retracted and red or yellow in color instead of normal pearl-gray.
    VI. If tympanic membrane has ruptured, there may be discharge from the ear, i.e., pus or serous fluid.
    VII. There may be hearing loss.

Problems
    I. The child may have discomfort or pain in the ear with or without hearing loss.
    II. The child may have a fever.
    III. Complications may develop from the initial upper respiratory infection.

Goals of Care
    I. Reduce pain and discomfort.
    II. Treat infection.
    III. Maintain normal body temperature.
    IV. Observe for potential complications.

Intervention
    I. Administer prescribed antibiotic—penicillin for 10 days is the drug of choice for streptococcal or pneumococcal otitis.
    II. Give analgesic as prescribed to reduce discomfort.
    III. Surgery (myringotomy) is indicated when there is inadequate response to antibiotic.
    IV. Monitor temperature closely.
    V. Administer antipyretic as prescribed.
    VI. Encourage oral fluids.
    VII. Give sponge bath with tepid water if necessary.
    VIII. Observe for perforation of eardrum, febrile convulsions, and development of chronic otitis media, mastoiditis, brain abscess, and reaction to penicillin.
    IX. Provide follow-up evaluation for hearing loss.

Evaluation
    I. Pain and fever are controlled.
    II. Infection resolves without sequelae.
    III. Hearing evaluation referral is arranged in the event of residual hearing deficit.

BIBLIOGRAPHY

Alexander, M., and M. Brown: *Pediatric Physical Diagnosis for Nurses,* McGraw-Hill Book Company, New York, 1974. This book provides a detailed guide for the nurse learning the skills of physical assessment. The chest, lungs, and heart are covered in two chapters. A bibliography, glossary, and list of resources are presented at the end of each chapter.

Avery, Mary Ellen: *The Lung and Its Disorders in the Newborn,* W. B. Saunders Company, Philadelphia, 1974. This monograph is specifically devoted to the lung and its disorders in the newborn infant. Normal development and physiology of the fetal and neonatal lung, disorders of respiration, and artificial respiration are described in detail.

Kendig, Edmund: *Pulmonary Disorders,* vol. I, W. B. Saunders Company, Philadelphia, 1972. This book serves as a complete reference for anatomy, physiology, development, and diseases of the respiratory system in children.

Korones, S.: *High-Risk Newborn Infants: The Basis for Intensive Nursing Care,* The C. V. Mosby Company, St. Louis, 1972. In this book written for nurses caring for high-risk newborn infants, Korones presents all aspects of nursing care. Respiratory distress syndrome is well covered.

Lough, M., C. Doershuk, and R. Stern: *Pediatric Respiratory Therapy,* Yearbook Medical Publishing Company, Chicago, 1974. Writing for nurses, respiratory therapists, physical therapists, and physicians interested in pulmonary diseases in children, Lough and other contributors present development and physiology of the respiratory system, respiratory diseases in the newborn, respiratory therapy techniques, respiratory physical therapy, and pulmonary function testing. A bibliography follows each chapter.

Northway, W., R. Rosan, and D. Porter: "Pulmonary Disease Following Respiratory Therapy of Hyaline Membrane Disease," *New England Journal of Medicine,* **276**:357–367, February 16, 1967. In this classic journal article that first described bronchopulmonary dysplasia, early statistics are presented as well as significant pathologic stages of the disease and healing process.

Scipien, Gladys M., et al. (eds.): *Comprehensive Pediatric Nursing,* McGraw-Hill Book Company, 2d ed., New York, 1979. This comprehensive and current pediatric nursing textbook includes chapters on the nursing process and an extensive chapter dealing in detail with the care of children with respiratory problems.

15
The Hematologic System

Patricia E. Greene and C. Marie Hall

APLASTIC ANEMIA

Definition

The bone marrow is the primary site of the production of erythrocytes, leukocytes, and platelets. Severe hypoplasia or absence of their precursors in the marrow is termed *aplastic anemia*. A viral illness may precipitate an aplastic state with the most severe instance of the disease occurring after a viral hepatitis. Certain drugs such as chloramphenicol and the sulfonamides have been implicated as causing aplastic anemia. Toxic chemicals such as aromatic hydrocarbons are known causative agents. Aplastic anemia may present with signs of anemia, infection secondary to leukopenia, or bruising and bleeding secondary to thrombocytopenia. The patient's course is highly variable, and the outcome is closely related to the initial cause and severity of aplasia. Diagnosis is confirmed by a bone marrow biopsy which is hypocellular. Treatment may include steroids and possibly androgens, but the response is unpredictable. Supportive measures consist of antibiotics, although transfusions are frequently required.

Assessment

Data sources are parents, the patient, schoolteachers, and the previous medical history.
  I. Health history.
    A. Recent infection: viral hepatitis, etc.
    B. Exposure to toxic chemicals: insecticides, toluene, aromatic hydrocarbons.
    C. Recent doses of toxic drugs: chloramphenicol, sulfonamides, anticonvulsants.
    D. Weakness.
    E. Pallor.
  II. Physical assessment.
    A. Tachycardia.
    B. Fever.
    C. Skin and mucous membranes: pallor, bleeding, bruises, petechiae; "waxen complexion."
    D. Cardiac exam: flow murmur.
    E. Abdominal exam: no hepatosplenomegaly.

Problems

  I. Lack of defense against infection.
  II. Increased susceptibility to serious bleeding.
  III. Anemia.
  IV. Potential complications from therapy: bone marrow stimulatory agent (steroids, androgens), transfusion.

Goals of Care

I. Maximum protection from exogenous and endogenous infectious agents.
II. Prevention of bleeding.
III. Modifying activity by degree of anemia.
IV. Education of patient/parents regarding side effects of steroid and/or androgen therapy.
V. Maximum protection from complications of transfusions.
VI. Parental teaching regarding the avoidance of reexposure of child to causative agent, if identifiable.

Intervention

I. Maximum protection from exogenous and endogenous organisms—see leukopenia guidelines under "Neutropenia."
II. Prevention of bleeding.
   A. With a platelet count of 10,000, recommend sedentary activity with bathroom privileges.
   B. With a platelet count greater than 10,000 but less than 50,000, suggest moderate exercise, i.e., walking, swimming (not diving).
      1. Consult physical therapist for suggested exercises.
      2. Encourage patient not to overexert or sweat as this may precipitate petechial bleeding.
   C. With a platelet count of 50,000, but less than 100,000, suggest participation in more active sports, discouraging contact sports such as football, basketball, soccer, and wrestling, as well as skateboards and climbing trees.
   D. Consider any ecchymoses or petechiae as an indication to stop activity.
   E. Maintain pressure over intravenous and finger sticks until bleeding stops.
   F. Evaluate carefully the need for intramuscular injections.
   G. Observe carefully for signs of intracranial bleeding and for altered neurologic status.
   H. Evaluate the need for gastrointestinal or mucosal irritants (i.e., nasogastric tube, suctioning, catheters).
   I. For mouth care, use only soft bristles, cotton swabs or products such as toothettes when platelet count is below 50,000.
   J. Monitor stools for occult blood.
   K. Observe for and report bleeding from mucosal membranes.
   L. Avoid the use of salicylates (aspirin), which interfere with platelet aggregation.
III. Modify activity by degree of anemia.
   A. For hemoglobin value less than 5 g, suggest:
      1. Bed rest with bathroom privileges.
      2. Monitor pulse and respiration every 2 h, temperature and blood pressure every 4 h.
   B. For hemoglobin values between 5 and 7 or 8 g per 100 mL, suggest:
      1. Moderate activity.
      2. Frequent rest periods during the day.
IV. Teach patient/parents regarding side effects of steroid therapy.
   A. Fluid retention with concomitant weight gain and Cushingoid appearance.
   B. Hypertension—suggest low-salt diet.
   C. Increased diaphoresis and night sweats.
   D. Increased urinary frequency (bed-wetting).
   E. Transient increase in appetite.
   F. Gastrointestinal irritability—suggest giving steroids with milk or meals.
   G. Masked infections.

      H. Acne, especially in teenagers.

      I. Possibility of striae with long-term use.

      J. Mood changes—depression, euphoria.

      K. Maintain dosage of steroids once therapy is instigated, as a precipitous decrease can lead to shock.

      L. Consider contraindications if used concomitantly with diuretics, antibiotics.

   V. Teach patient/parents about side effects of androgen therapy.

      A. Increased hair growth over body: face, axillae, groin.

      B. Lowering of voice.

      C. Increased muscle mass.

      D. Transient weight gain.

   VI. Provide maximum protection from complications of transfusions (see "Hemolytic Disease of the Newborn").

   VII. Teach parents regarding reexposure of child to causative agent, if identifiable.

      A. Counsel parents, schoolteacher to prevent reexposure of child to causative agent.

      B. Consider obtaining Medic-Alert necklace.

      C. See "Neutropenia."

Evaluation

   I. Infections are prevented or controlled.

   II. Traumatic bleeding does not occur.

   III. Activity is adjusted to degree of anemia and well tolerated.

   IV. Parents (and child, if old enough) can describe and recognize side effects of hormone therapy and cope well with them.

   V. Transfusion reactions are avoided or immediately recognized and treated.

   VI. Causative agent, if identifiable, is subsequently avoided.

ACQUIRED HEMOLYTIC ANEMIA

Definition

The lowered red blood cell population in *acquired hemolytic anemia* may be due to radiation therapy, chemicals, drugs, or infections. The mechanism for destroying red blood cells can be attributable to phenomena such as complement fixation, an autoimmune mechanism which facilitates destruction of the red blood cell. The drugs which are implicated in red cell aplasia are quinidine, quinine, salicylic acid, phenacetin, aminopyrine, streptomycin, penicillin, cephalosporins, methyldopa, and stibophen. Compounds with benzene rings, and sulfa and chloro compounds are the general categories of causative agents. Implicated in acquired red cell aplasia are the Coxsackie virus, measles, varicella, cytomegalovirus, and encephalitis. Although normal red cell production may recover with time, steroids may be used to stimulate marrow activity. The condition should not recur except in the presence of the causative agent.

Assessment

The data sources are the patient, parents, and schoolteachers.

   I. Health history.

      A. Recent infection.

      B. Recent drug ingestion.

      C. Recent exposure to toxic chemicals—has the home been sprayed for insects?

      D. Previous occurrence of a similar incident.

      E. Weakness.

      F. Pallor.

II. Physical assessment.
   A. Skin—pallor.
   B. Mucous membranes—pale.
   C. Cardiac exam—flow murmur secondary to anemia.
   D. Weakness.

Problems

See "Aplastic Anemia."

Goals of Care

See "Aplastic Anemia."

Intervention

See "Aplastic Anemia."

Evaluation

See "Aplastic Anemia."

IRON-DEFICIENCY ANEMIA

Definition

Iron deficiency, the most common cause of anemia, occurs as a result of decreased available iron stores. The iron shortage may be caused by insufficient dietary intake and absorption, or by loss of blood and subsequent depletion of reusable iron from the hemoglobin of the lost red cells. Inadequate dietary intake is the usual cause of iron deficiency anemia. Dietary iron insufficiency is most common between 6 months and 3 years of age, and is again prevalent in adolescence. Gastrointestinal malabsorption syndromes can produce iron-deficiency anemia because iron, although available in the diet, is not absorbed by the gut.

Assessment

I. Health history.
   A. Weakness, reduced exercise tolerance.
   B. Pallor.
   C. Abdominal complaints.
   D. Recent infection.
   E. Pica.
   F. Cow's milk intolerance.
   G. Irritability.
   H. Thorough diet history.
II. Physical assessment.
   A. Obesity in infants and toddlers secondary to excessive milk intake (milk is a very poor source of iron and, when taken in large quantities, displaces iron-rich foods from the diet).
   B. Possible abdominal pain on palpation.
   C. Pallor.

Problems

    I. Dietary practices need revision.
    II. Anemia.

Goals of Care

    I. Promote normal iron stores.
    II. Modify daily activity by degree of anemia.

Intervention

    I. Provide prescribed iron replacement.
        A. If oral, counsel parents regarding possible side effects: diarrhea, constipation, nausea, black stools. Suggest that iron supplement be given with meals to minimize gastric irritation. Liquid iron preparation can stain teeth if allowed to contact them: use a straw.
        B. If intramuscular or intravenous, counsel parents regarding side effects: soreness at intramuscular injection site, soreness along the vein when given intravenously (rarely necessary), and possibility of stain in skin at injection site. Use the Z-track method to administer iron intramuscularly.
    II. Educate patient/parents regarding natural sources of iron (consult dietitian for a complete list): fortified cereals and breads, green vegetables and some yellow vegetables, organ meats, lean meats, egg yolks.
    III. Suggest modified levels of activity with rest periods until hemoglobin value returns to normal.

Evaluation

    I. Recommended dietary modifications are carried out.
    II. Supplementary iron is given as prescribed without needless side effects.
    III. Activity does not exceed tolerance.
    IV. Hemoglobin and hematocrit are markedly improved after 4 weeks.

MEGALOBLASTIC NUTRITIONAL ANEMIAS (VITAMIN B_{12} AND FOLIC ACID DEFICIENCY ANEMIAS)

Definition

Vitamin B_{12} deficiency anemia is a megaloblastic anemia rarely seen in children and usually associated with neurologic sequelae. Vitamin B_{12} absorption is dependent on an intrinsic factor (IF) secreted by the stomach and then transported to the terminal ilium where the IF and B_{12} are absorbed into the bloodstream. In conditions where there is little IF available, as in the atrophic gastritis of pernicious anemia, B_{12} deficiency is predictable.

    Neurologic manifestations are the hallmarks of the deficiency when occuring with anemia. Paresthesias in the extremities, ataxia, irritability, and alterations in sight, smell, and taste are attributable to the lack of B_{12}. Smoking may exacerbate and aggravate visual symptoms progressing to amblyopia. The hematologic picture is comprised of a megaloblastic hyperchromic anemia with hypersegmented polymorphonuclear cells.

    In the juvenile form of the disease, there may be a congenital deficiency of IF. A thorough family history is helpful, as the deficiency can be hereditary. A complete dietary history is another necessary aspect of the assessment. B_{12} deficiency is ameliorated by supplemental B_{12}.

Folic acid deficiency anemia is a rare deficiency in U.S. infants, as adequate doses of folic acid are contained in cow's milk and commercially available formulas. Goat's milk and dry milk may contain less folic acid.

Folic acid levels are known to decrease with diarrhea, infections, and scurvy. Folates are absorbed by bacteria in the gut. Diarrhea does not allow time for absorption of the ingested folates. Presence of weakness, pallor, lethargy with diarrhea or infection should be a challenge to examine for nutritional deficiencies, one of them being folic acid. Folic acid deficits are associated with other anemias such as sickle cell anemia. Findings that support the diagnosis of folate deficiencies are glossitis and mouth or mucous membrane ulceration. A history of malabsorption, malnutrition and alcoholism are predisposing factors. High-dose methotrexate, used in the treatment of various malignancies, is a cause of folic acid deficiency and is used therefore in conjunction with folic acid replacement.

Folate may be supplemented whenever the production of red blood cells is increased, as in sickle cell anemia. Folic acid deficiency has been linked with B_{12} deficiency, as both are megaloblastic anemias; however, only B_{12} deficiency may cause neurologic sequelae. With folate supplements, there is an observable improvement over a few days.

Assessment

Data sources are parents, the patient, and the extended family (B_{12} deficiency).
I. Health history.
   A. Gastric complaints—hematemesis, diarrhea.
   B. Recent infection.
   C. Pallor.
   D. Weakness.
   E. Dietary history (strict vegetarians can be deficient in B_{12}).
   F. History regarding recent abdominal surgery (B_{12} deficiency).
   G. Alcoholism, teenage (folic acid deficiency).
   H. Recent methotrexate therapy (folic acid deficiency).
   I. Sickle cell disease or other high red cell production states (folic acid deficiency).
II. Physical assessment.
   A. Skin—pallor.
   B. Neurologic manifestations—irritability, amblyopia, paresthesias, ataxia, alterations in sight, taste, smell (B_{12} deficiency only).
   C. Mucous membranes (folic acid deficiency).
      1. Mouth—presence of ulcers, glossitis.
      2. Rectum—character of mucosa.

Problems

I. Altered nutritional status secondary to B_{12} and folic acid deficiencies.
II. Anemia.
III. Potentially altered neurologic status (B_{12} deficiency).

Goals of Care

I. Promote normal B_{12} and folic acid levels to provide for hematologic homeostasis.
II. Modify activities by degree of anemia.
III. Monitor neurologic status.

Intervention

I. Folic acid:
   A. Provide prescribed folate supplement.

    B. Educate patient/parent regarding natural sources of folates: asparagus, broccoli, spinach, lettuce, kidney, liver, yeast, mushrooms.

II. Vitamin B_{12}:

    A. Provide prescribed B_{12} supplement.

    B. If given intramuscularly, rotate sites.

    C. Educate patient/parent regarding natural sources of B_{12}: meats, cheese, eggs, milk, *not* vegetables.

III. Suggest modified levels of activity with rest periods, until hemoglobin value returns to normal.

IV. Report paresthesias, kinesthetic disturbances, ataxia.

V. Provide protective environment as necessary to prevent injury.

Evaluation

I. Folic acid or vitamin B_{12} supplements are taken as prescribed.

II. Dietary modifications as recommended are followed.

III. Activity does not exceed tolerance.

IV. Anemia improves markedly within a few weeks.

V. Injuries due to altered neurological status are avoided.

BLACKFAN-DIAMOND SYNDROME (CONGENITAL HYPOPLASTIC ANEMIA)

Definition

Blackfan-Diamond syndrome (BDS) is an aplasia or hypoplasia of red cells. The condition may be a transient phenomenon and resolve, or it may require long-term management of the anemia. One of the first observable signs is pallor which becomes apparent by 6 months of age.

If the anemia associated with BDS is severe, compensatory tachycardia and congestive heart failure may result. There may be an increase in liver and spleen size due to the cardiac alterations. As many as one-fifth of the patients have skeletal abnormalities.

Numerous other anomalies become apparent in chronic management of the disease and are related to the therapy necessary. Steroids and androgens may be helpful bone marrow stimulatory agents. Repeated red cell transfusions may be necessary during stress for the patient, or for long-term management of the anemia. As red cells from transfusions are broken down, the products are excreted, with the exception of iron, which is stored in the bone marrow and components of the reticuloendothelial system. Organs which may evidence deposits of iron during chronic treatment are the kidney, liver, spleen, heart, and gastrointestinal tract. The toxic deposition of iron is termed *hemosiderosis*. Other phenomena accompanying the iron deposition are a bronzed-dusky skin color, a retardation of bone growth (short stature), and eventual cirrhosis. The iron deposits in the heart can alter cardiac function significantly. The hazards of iron deposition are minimized by the administration of an iron chelating agent, deferoxamine, which binds the iron and aids its excretion. Persons with congenital hypoplastic anemia, such as Fanconi's anemia, experience complications from the disease *and* its treatment.

Assessment

See "Fanconi's anemia," but references to leukopenia, thrombocytopenia, and causative agents do not apply.

Problems

See "Fanconi's anemia," but references to leukopenia, thrombocytopenia, and causative agents do not apply.

Goals of Care

See "Fanconi's anemia," but references to leukopenia, thrombocytopenia, and causative agents do not apply.

Intervention

See "Aplastic Anemia," but references to leukopenia, thrombocytopenia, and causative agents do not apply.

Evaluation

See "Aplastic Anemia," but references to leukopenia, thrombocytopenia, and causative agents do not apply.

FANCONI'S ANEMIA (CONGENITAL APLASTIC ANEMIA)

Definition

Fanconi's anemia, characterized by a pancytopenia and concomitant decrease of precursor blood elements in the bone marrow, is often associated with a variety of congenital anomalies which may include dwarfism, microcephaly, strabismus, outer and inner ear anomalies, skeletal changes (abnormalities of thumb and radius), small genitalia, hyperpigmentation of the skin, kidney abnormalities, and mental retardation. The anemia is usually noticed between the ages of 4 and 12 years. The trait for Fanconi's anemia is autosomal recessive and may or may not be clinically apparent in other family members.

The treatment consists of steroids and androgens used separately or together to stimulate the bone marrow. The remainder of the therapy is supportive. (If the child is not responsive to standard treatment, the supportive therapy becomes the maintenance therapy.) If there is poor bone marrow response to the drugs, the patient may be maintained on blood transfusions. Persons with Fanconi's anemia may develop complications secondary to treatment (see "Blackfan-Diamond Syndrome") of the anemia, and have a propensity to develop leukemia later in life.

Assessment

Data sources are the parents, the patient, the extended family, and the previous medical record.
  I. Health history.
  A. Presence of other congenital anomalies in patient or extended family.
  B. Pallor.
  C. Weakness, fatigue.
  II. Physical assessment.
  A. Height and weight—dwarfism.

B. Skin and mucous membranes—pallor, pigmentation.

C. Head—microcephaly.

D. Eyes—strabismus.

E. Ears—inner and outer ear abnormalities.

F. Cardiac exam—possible increased size, murmurs associated with decreased cardiac output, decreased stroke volume.

G. Abdomen—possible increased liver and spleen size.

H. Extremities—skeletal changes, thumb and radial abnormalities.

I. Kidneys—malformations in genitourinary tract.

J. Neurologic exam—possible neurologic deficits, mental retardation.

K. Genitalia—delayed puberty.

Problems

I. Anemia.

II. Susceptibility to infections.

III. Susceptibility to bleeding.

IV. Potential complications from therapy—transfusion or hormones.

V. Altered self-concept secondary to disease and treatment.

Goals of Care

I. Modify activity by degree of anemia.

II. Maximum protection against overwhelming infection.

III. Prevention of bleeding.

IV. Maximum protection from complications of transfusion therapy.

V. Education of patient/parents regarding side effects of steroid and/or androgen therapy.

VI. Encourage positive self-concept and activities appropriate for growth and development.

Intervention

See "Aplastic Anemia."

Evaluation

See "Aplastic Anemia."

HEMOLYTIC DISEASE OF THE NEWBORN

Definition

Hemolytic disease of the newborn is a neonatal disorder characterized by increased hemolysis of red blood cells as a result of maternal sensitization by the fetal erythrocyte antigens (e.g., Rh, A, B). ABO incompatibility cannot be prevented, and maternal sensitization may lead to hemolysis, anemia, and elevated bilirubin levels in newborns. Most cases of the Rh disease, including erythroblastosis fetalis, can be prevented by the administration of Rh immune globulin, to mothers at risk, immediately after each pregnancy (including abortions and miscarriages). The Rh immune globulin is indicated if the mother is Rh antigen and antibody negative, and the child is Rh-positive. A Coombs' test on the newborn's blood (cord blood) as well as blood typing of the mother and child are helpful in determining the presence of maternal antibodies against fetal blood.

Elevated bilirubin levels result from increased destruction of red cells and consequent release of hemoglobin. The hemoglobin is converted to bilirubin and excreted by the liver. Increased bilirubin levels of 10 mg or less per 100 mL of blood can occur in newborns secondary to hemolysis in conjunction with hepatic enzymatic immaturity. Bilirubin levels greater than 10 mg per 100 mL result from brisk hemolysis. Levels above 15 mg in the premature and above 20 mg per 100 mL in the full-term infant can cause kernicterus, a form of brain damage.

Phototherapy increases the degradation and excretion of bilirubin and constitutes a part of the accepted regimen of therapy. If the bilirubin level becomes dangerously high, one or more exchange transfusions may be indicated to rapidly lower the blood levels of bilirubin. Even though the jaundice resolves, a low-grade hemolysis continues for several weeks, which necessitates evaluating the child for late anemia.

Assessment

Data sources are the mother and the mother's past medical record.
I. Health history.
   A. Maternal blood type and Rh.
   B. Previous pregnancies (children, stillbirths, miscarriages).
   C. Previous RhoGAM (Rh immunoglobulin) injections, when administered in relation to previous pregnancy.
II. Physical assessment.
   A. General—irritable, cries continuously, presence of other anomalies, is edematous.
   B. Skin—jaundice apparent especially on hands, feet, and with blanching in other areas; yellow-tinged sclerae.
   C. Abdomen—increased liver and spleen size.
   D. Neurological—seizure activity; high-pitched cry; poor suck reflex; hypo- or hyper-reflexia; irritability; opisthotonus.
   E. Urine—dark amber.
   F. Feces—green, squirty stools.

Problems

I. Metabolic alteration secondary to phototherapy and/or exchange transfusion.
II. Altered sensorium.
III. Altered nutritional and fluid-electrolyte balance secondary to the disease.

Goals of Care

I. Maximum protection from complications of exchange transfusion.
II. Protection from side effects of phototherapy.
III. Minimal noxious stimuli (irritable infant).
IV. Monitor neurologic status.
V. Adequate nutrition, fluid and electrolyte balance.
VI. Assist parents, teach them about prevention of recurrence with subsequent pregnancies.

Intervention

I. Prevent, observe for, and immediately treat complications of transfusion.
   A. Check infant and blood-donor blood type compatibility.
   B. Monitor vital signs before, during, and after transfusion; suggest cardiac monitor during transfusion.

C. Observe for signs of circulatory overload (dyspnea, cough, cyanosis).

D. If signs of circulatory overload appear, stop the transfusion, position patient with head and chest elevated and legs dependent, prepare to administer oxygen.

E. Have normal saline hung and ready to attach to the infusion tubing in the event signs of transfusion reaction appear. Do not substitute glucose solutions, which cause hemolysis and clogging of the tubing.

F. Have drugs ready for immediate treatment of transfusion reaction (e.g., epinephrine, Benadryl).

G. Observe for indications of transfusion reaction (itching, urticaria, chills, fever, wheezing, dyspnea, hypotension, nausea and vomiting, flushing, tachycardia, pain in kidney region).

H. If signs of transfusion reaction occur, immediately stop the transfusion. Administer epinephrine or antihistamine as prescribed. Monitor vital signs and temperature. Measure intake and output and check urine for hemoglobin (renal tubular obstruction as a result of hemolysis is a potential serious complication of transfusion reaction). Prepare to administer plasma expander, vasopressor, and/or corticosteroid as prescribed (to counteract shock and protect kidneys).

II. Protect infant from side effects of phototherapy.

   A. Eyes must be covered with eye shields (commercially manufactured shields or cotton balls and hypoallergenic tape). Explain shield use to parents. Change at regular intervals. Light can be turned off and shields removed for parental visits (eye contact is an important part of parent-infant bonding).

   B. Monitor for hypothermia or hyperthermia, since infant must be undressed and uncovered for maximal exposure to light.

   C. Protect diaper area from skin irritation caused by therapy-induced diarrhea. (Water-insoluble creams, sunlamp, no urine bags.)

   D. Turn every 2 h to minimize skin irritation as well as to maximize skin exposure to light.

III. Minimize upsetting stimuli to infant.

   A. Organize care to allow for frequent rest periods.

   B. Minimize noise, noxious stimuli.

   C. Neurologic excitation: observe and report increases in irritability, high shrill cry, opisthotonus, hypertonia, seizure activity.

   D. Neurologic depression: observe and report hyporeflexia, absence of Moro, root, and suck reflexes.

IV. Provide adequate nutrition and fluid-electrolyte balance.

   A. Accurately record intake and output, daily weights.

   B. Evaluate the need for altered feeding regimens—may need nasogastric feeding secondary to altered neurologic status (severe disease).

   C. Consider increased fluid and caloric needs of infants under phototherapy.

V. Educate the parents regarding the etiology and possible consequences of the disease.

   A. Counsel them regarding the risks involved with additional pregnancies.

   B. Evaluate the infant's neurological status at discharge; teach parents techniques to stimulate normal development.

   C. Teach about developmental needs, dietary guidelines, etc., as for any newborn.

Evaluation

I. Transfusion complications due to human error do not occur.

II. Transfusion complications are promptly detected and treated.

III. Phototherapy is conducted without avoidable complications.

IV. Neurologic and developmental status is evaluated and protected.

V. Nutrition and fluid-electrolyte balance are adequate.

VI. Parents understand the disease and take appropriate precautions against its recurrence in subsequent pregnancies.

HEREDITARY SPHEROCYTOSIS (CHRONIC FAMILIAL JAUNDICE)

Definition

Red cell membrane abnormalities result in hemolytic anemias, similar to hemoglobinopathies. *Hereditary spherocytosis* is a dominantly inherited hemolytic anemia. The syndrome is typified by spherocytes in the peripheral smear and the presence of fragments. The red cells assume a spherical shape because of a deficiency in membrane lipids which allows for an influx of sodium ions and water. It is difficult for the spherical cells to pass through capillary circulation. The spleen is the site primarily responsible for destruction of the red cells. The red cells are normally polished and cleaned by the spleen. Cleaning implies plucking excess membrane from the erythrocytes. The membrane loss further predisposes the spherocytic cells to hemolysis.

Most patients with hereditary spherocytosis are asymptomatic. Infection or stress, however, may stimulate further hemolysis which results in intermittent jaundice, anemia, splenomegaly, and hyperpigmented stools and urine. Supportive transfusions may be required.

Splenectomy is the preferred treatment for management of the hemolysis. Some lysis may still occur after splenectomy, but it is minimal. The child of 5 years of age or older is a candidate for splenectomy as problems with infections are decreased. With splenectomies at a later age, gallstones may occur secondary to the chronic breakdown products of red cell hemolysis. Leg ulcers, heart murmurs, and radiologic findings of thickened parietal and frontal bones may be associated with spherocytic anemia and its course.

Assessment

Data sources are the patient, the parents, the extended family, and the patient's past medical record.

I. Health history.
  A. Jaundice, yellow sclerae.
  B. Pallor.
  C. Decreased exercise tolerance.
  D. Dark urine.
  E. Dark stools.

II. Physical assessment.
  A. Eyes—yellow sclerae.
  B. Mucous membranes—pale.
  C. Skin—pallor, jaundice.
  D. Heart—flow murmurs.
  E. Abdomen—splenomegaly.
  F. Extremities—leg ulcers.
  G. Urine—dark.
  H. Feces—hyperpigmented, constipation.

Problems

I. Anemia.
II. Family's potential knowledge deficit regarding disease and treatment.

Goals of Care

I. Modify activity by degree of anemia (with stress or infection).
II. Patient/parents will understand the genetic implications of the disease, and the possibility of splenectomy.

Intervention

I. Modify activity by degree of anemia (see "Aplastic Anemia").
II. Provide patient/parents with genetic information about this dominantly inherited disease. They should realize that until splenectomy, the young child may experience several episodes of severe anemia, requiring transfusions. See also "Thrombocytopenia."

Evaluation

    I. Activity does not exceed tolerance.
    II. Preventable infections and stress are avoided.
    III. The family is well informed about the disorder and its management.

HEREDITARY ELLIPTOCYTOSIS (HEREDITARY OVALOCYTOSIS)

Definition

Hereditary elliptocytosis is an example of autosomal dominant, hemolytic anemia. It may be several months before the infant manifests elliptocytes. Jaundice may be present secondary to hemolysis with or without clinical anemia. As there is no abnormal hemoglobin in the cell, it is thought that the condition results from a deficient cell membrane. Eventually, elliptical cells may represent 50 percent of the circulating red cell population. Splenomegaly may be present early in the child's life. If rapid destruction of red blood cells occurs, splenectomy may be suggested. Transfusions, if indicated, constitute the supportive therapy.

Assessment

See "Hereditary Spherocytosis."

Problems

See "Hereditary Spherocytosis."

Goals of Care

See "Hereditary Spherocytosis."

Intervention

See "Hereditary Spherocytosis."

Evaluation

See "Hereditary Spherocytosis."

GLUCOSE 6-PHOSPHATE DEFICIENCY (G6PD)

Definition

Glucose 6-phosphate deficiency is classified as a nonspherocytic hemolytic anemia and is transmitted genetically as an X-linked recessive. The deficiency occurs in black American males (10 percent), is frequently demonstrable in Mediterranean populations, and is found in certain Oriental populations. The disease is more severe in Caucasians and Orientals. The newborn may present with prolonged jaundice. Later in childhood, the anemia of G6PD does not become apparent except in the presence of a precipitating factor, such as infection, diabetic acidosis, hepatitis, chronic renal failure, the ingestion of fava beans, or exposure to oxidizing compounds such as sulfonamides, nitrofurans, antipyretics and analgesics. Transfusions may be required.

Assessment

Data sources are the parents, the patient, the extended family, and previous medical records of patient and family.
I. Health history.
  A. Presence of similar symptoms in other male family members.
  B. Stillbirths or early childhood deaths of males.
  C. Pallor, neonatal jaundice.
  D. Weakness, fatigue.
  E. Recent infection.
  F. Recent exposure to drugs or chemicals.
II. Physical examination.
  A. Temperature—elevated.
  B. Skin and mucous membranes—pallor, jaundice.

Problems

I. Anemia.
II. Potential complications of transfusion therapy.
III. Possible family knowledge deficit regarding crisis prevention with G6PD.

Goals of Care

I. Modify activity by degree of anemia.
II. Monitor for maximum protection from complications of transfusion therapy.
III. Teach parents that drugs which precipitate hemolysis must be avoided.

Intervention

I. Modify activity by degree of anemia (see "Aplastic Anemia").
II. Monitor for maximum protection from complications of transfusion therapy (see "Hemolytic Disease of the Newborn").
III. Be certain that patient/parents understand compounds to be avoided with G6PD: sulfonamides, nitrofurans, antipyretics (except acetaminophen), analgesics, fava beans, primaquine and pamoquine, quinine, quinidine.
IV. Educate patient/parent that infection, diabetic acidosis, hepatitis and chronic renal failure may precipitate a hemolytic episode.

Evaluation

I. Activity level does not exceed tolerance.
II. Preventable transfusion complications do not occur; others are promptly recognized and treated (see "Hemolytic Disease of the Newborn").
III. Parents (and child, if old enough) are well informed about avoidance of precipitating factors.

SICKLE CELL ANEMIA (HEMOGLOBIN SS DISEASE)

Definition

Sickle cell anemia is the most common of the several sickling syndromes. All are characterized by an abnormality of the chemical makeup of the hemoglobin molecule which predisposes the red cells to assume a sickle (crescent) shape under certain circumstances. The sickled cells obstruct the microvasculature, causing decreased blood flow to the tissues. The lowered oxygen transport produces metabolic acidosis, and the decreased pH in turn precipitates sickling of more red blood cells. Severe sickling episodes are called *sickle cell crises*.

Crises in sickle cell anemia may be induced by dehydration, fever, infection, surgery, prolonged or relative anoxia such as may occur in underwater swimming or sudden exposure to high altitudes, and sometimes pregnancy. There are four types of sickle cell crisis: aplastic crisis, vasoocclusive or pain crisis, hyperhemolytic crisis, and sequestration crisis in which blood pools in the viscera with resultant shock and possibly death. Recurrent crises damage the liver, kidneys, eyes, heart, brain, and spleen. Sickle cell anemia decreases life expectancy, but childhood death is not universal and should not be considered the fate of each child with the disease. Death may result from overwhelming infection (due in part to decreased splenic function caused by repeated infarcts), infarction of vital organs, congestive heart failure caused by severe anemia, or the hypovolemia of sequestration crisis. Obviously, the care of patients with sickle cell anemia is directed at preventing crises by avoiding factors which precipitate them and at effectively treating crises which occur. Crisis treatment usually consists of controlling pain, providing adequate hydration, giving supplemental oxygen, and transfusing with whole blood or packed red cells.

Sickle hemoglobin is found primarily among blacks, but there are numerous instances of the hemoglobin abnormality in other races and in persons who are phenotypically white. Sickle cell anemia is an inherited homozygous disorder. The incidence among American blacks has been estimated at 1 in 600.

Assessment

Data sources are the patient, parents, the extended family, and the patient's past medical record.
  I. Health history.
    A. Frequent infections.
    B. Jaundice—"yellow eyes" or yellow sclerae.
    C. History of the disorder in the family, extended family, nuclear family; children who died in infancy or early childhood.
    D. Joint, abdominal, or back pain.
    E. Swollen joints.
    F. Frequent headaches.
    G. Pallor.
    H. Decreased exercise tolerance, dyspnea.
    I. Hand and foot swelling (due to vasoocclusion).
  II. Physical assessment.
    A. Height and weight.
    B. Skin—pallor (nailbeds, mucous membranes), jaundice.
    C. Cardiac exam—with anemia, presence of flow murmurs.
    D. Abdominal exam—increase or decrease in spleen size; possibly increased liver size.
    E. Extremities—joint or bone abnormalities, ulcerations, hand and foot swelling in infants.
    F. Funduscopic exam—retinal changes secondary to infarcts.
    G. Neurologic exam—use appropriate developmental tool (e.g., DDST).
    H. Delayed puberty.

Problems

    I. Parents and child need to be knowledgeable about the disease and its treatment.
    II. Sickle cell crisis.
    III. Possible altered self-concept due to limitations in activity or delayed puberty.
    IV. Increased susceptibility to infection.

Goals of Care

    I. Patient and family must understand the disease and its management.
    II. Avoidable crises will not occur.
    III. Minimize sequelae of crises.
    IV. Maximize protection against infection.

Intervention

    I. Teach family the inheritance pattern of the disease and explain the implications for other offspring in the family.
    II. Teach about the anatomic and physiological alterations that characterize the disease and the objectives and methods of treatment.
    III. Teach parents the home management of child to prevent crises and complications.
        A. Notify doctor about temperature of 101°F or higher for 4 h or more.
        B. Encourage the use of acetaminophen (not aspirin) with fever (does not alter blood pH).
        C. If child has acute back pain, abdominal pain, persistent headaches, nausea, or vomiting, notify doctor.
        D. Encourage hydration: suggest a minimum daily hydration of 1 to $1\frac{1}{2}$ times maintenance (1500 to 2200 mL/m² per 24 h). Suggest 2 times maintenance (3000 mL/m² per 24 h) during extremes in environmental conditions and stressful situations.
        E. Emphasize crisis prevention.
    IV. Inform and counsel as necessary regarding the following:
        A. Child may be smaller than peers.
        B. Child should receive appropriate immunizations.
        C. May need folic acid supplements.
        D. Should have regular dental and ophthalmologic evaluations.
        E. Observe for unusual urinary patterns (bed-wetting, an increased frequency). The disease may cause chronic kidney problems.
        F. Limit stressful activity such as football, basketball, soccer, track.
        G. Contact school system regarding sickle cell guidelines.
    V. Minimize noxious and harmful sequelae of crisis.
        A. Monitor vital signs.
        B. Maintain pain-free status (lowered stress lowers oxygen requirements).
        C. Accurate intake and output.
        D. Encourage oral fluids (if vomiting, all fluids must be parenteral).
        E. Use of humidified oxygen may be indicated, particularly in pulmonary problems. The use of oxygen in other crises is controversial.
        F. Use of antipyretics.
        G. Use of transfusions as necessary (see "Hemolytic Disease of the Newborn" for precautions).
    VI. Encourage a positive self-image (patient/parent) reinforcing activities appropriate for patient's development.
        A. Observe for feelings of guilt on part of parents or child.

     B. Observe for childhood depression or poor self-concept, and support realistic aspirations and activities.

     C. Anticipate delayed puberty.

VII. Refer to appropriate agencies for further information and support (see Table 15-1).

Evaluation

I. Blood relatives of the patient must understand the inheritance pattern of the disease. Patient's siblings are tested for the sickling trait. Appropriate genetic counseling is provided.

II. Parents (and child, at appropriate developmental level) demonstrate understanding of measures to be taken to avoid crises and of home and hospital care.

III. Crises occur infrequently and are promptly treated. Avoidable sequelae do not occur.

IV. Child's development, adjustment, and self-concept are adequate.

SICKLE CELL TRAIT (HEMOGLOBIN AS DISEASE)

Definition

Sickle cell trait is the carrier state of sickle cell anemia (hemoglobin SS disease, previously discussed). Sickle cell trait is a heterozygous condition in which some of the red cells contain sickling hemoglobin and some contain normal hemoglobin. Persons with the trait are less susceptible to problems and sickling crises than are those with the homozygous (SS) disease. Infections pose no unusual threat to persons with the trait. Children with sickle cell trait do not ordinarily demonstrate growth disturbances or delayed puberty. Any of the symptoms described under sickle cell anemia may arise, but the probability of their occurrence is markedly less. *Surgery is one of the common precipitators of crisis.* Crisis, when it does occur, is vasoocclusive (pain crisis) rather than aplastic, sequestration, or hemolytic. Approximately 8 percent of American blacks carry the sickle cell trait. One-fourth of the offspring of two carriers can be expected to have sickle cell anemia and half can be expected to have the trait, on the average. Hence, genetic counseling is highly important for persons with the sickling trait.

Keeping in mind the above distinctions between sickle cell trait and sickle cell anemia, refer to the section on sickle cell anemia for nursing care guidelines.

ADDITIONAL HEMOGLOBINOPATHIES (HEMOGLOBIN SF DISEASE, HEMOGLOBIN CC DISEASE, HEMOGLOBIN SC DISEASE)

Definition

There may be multiple abnormalities in synthesis or structure of the hemoglobin molecule. *Hemoglobin SF disease,* or sickle thalassemia, refers to the heterozygous presence of sickle hemoglobin and elevated fetal hemoglobin characteristic of β thalassemia. SF disease is one of the mildest and most common sickling hemoglobinopathies. The fetal hemoglobin retards the sickling phenomenon, largely protecting the individual from the sequelae of sickle cell trait or sickle cell disease. Minimal intervention is necessary in the management of the disease. It is important to counsel the individual and family regarding the sickle cell trait (see "Sickle Cell Trait").

Hemoglobin CC disease is a homozygous, inherited disease, which can have manifestations as serious as sickle cell anemia (see "Sickle Cell Anemia"). The sequelae of hemoglobin CC disease are very similar to hemoglobin SS disease, although the numbers of crises and problems with management may be somewhat fewer with hemoglobin CC. Preventive measures, management of crises and counseling for CC disease should follow the guidelines of sickle cell anemia.

TABLE 15-1 / INFORMATION FOR PARENTS AND PROFESSIONALS

Sickle cell:
  National Association for Sickle Cell Disease, Inc., 945 South Western Avenue, Suite 206, Los Angeles, Calif. 90006

Hemophilia:
  The National Hemophilia Foundation, 25 West 39th Street, New York, N.Y. 10018. (212) 869-9740

Leukemia:
  American Cancer Society, state divisions (for listings, see *Ca: A Cancer Journal for Clinicians*)

  Candlelighters, 123 C Street S.E., Washington, D.C. 20003. (202) 544-1696

  Leukemia Society of America, Inc., 211 East 43rd Street, New York, N.Y. 10017. (212) 986-3330

  National Cancer Institute, Office of Cancer Communications, Building 31, Room 10A17, Bethesda, Md. 20014

Hemoglobin SC disease is more often encountered than hemoglobin CC. The implications and findings of SC disease are the same as SS disease, though the crises and other manifestations of the disease are fewer, as in CC disease.

The person with sickle trait or SF disease experiences fewer side effects than in the person with SC disease or CC disease, who experiences fewer side effects than the person with SS disease. The comparison is a generality and each person possessing any of the hemoglobin abnormalities should be granted maximum benefits of counseling and intervention.

With the above considerations in mind, refer to the section "Sickle Cell Anemia" for nursing care.

β THALASSEMIA MAJOR (COOLEY'S ANEMIA, MEDITERRANEAN ANEMIA)

Definition

Thalassemia represents a series of inherited conditions in which there is a decreased production of one or more globin chains. Although thalassemia has been noted to be most common in those of Mediterranean and Oriental origin, the phenomenon occurs across ethnic delineations.

Clinical findings associated with β thalassemia include:

1. Ineffective erythropoiesis with marrow hyperactivity evidenced by "bossing" of the forehead.
2. Growth retardation, most noticeable by 9 to 10 years of age.
3. Gallstones.
4. Hyperuricemia and possibly gout.
5. Increased size of liver and spleen.
6. Increased susceptibility to infection.
7. Absence or delay of secondary sex characteristics.
8. Diabetes mellitus.
9. Congestive heart failure.

Chronic anemia is a primary causative factor in heart disease, though the condition may be accentuated by iron deposits in the myocardium. Iron accumulation (hemosiderin deposits) may be detectable in the skin (bronzed appearance) and internal organs as well as in the myocardium, as a result of frequent transfusions and breakdown of red blood cells.

Three avenues of supportive therapy are available to promote optimal activity. The first entails maintaining the hemoglobin between 7 and 8 g per 100 mL of blood by regular transfusions. The second alternative uses hypertransfusion therapy, maintaining a hemo-globin of 10 g per 100 mL or greater with concomitant deferoxamine therapy. Hypertrans-fusions have been used to help allay growth retardation. The third alternative includes splenectomy, with continued transfusion therapy. Splenectomy is indicated only when the spleen has progressively enlarged and the transfusion requirements have increased. If the child weathers preadolescence with minimal supportive therapy, the outlook is optimistic that he or she will continue to do so.

Assessment

Data sources are the patient, parents, the extended family, and the patient's past medical record.
I. Health history.
  A. Occurrence of similar findings in other family members: facies, anemia, heart problems.
  B. Mediterranean or Oriental origin of family.
  C. Jaundice.
  D. History of pallor, decreased exercise tolerance.
  E. Stillbirths, infant deaths in the family.
II. Physical assessment.
  A. Height, weight—plot on growth chart; may be below third percentile.
  B. Skin—pallor, jaundice.
  C. Face—"bossing" of forehead.
  D. Cardiac exam—murmurs.
  E. Abdominal exam—hepatosplenomegaly.
  F. Extremities—structural abnormalities.

Problems

I. Parents' and child's possible knowledge deficit regarding thalassemia, side effects, and treatment.
II. Anemia requiring frequent transfusions.
III. Altered self-concept secondary to disease and treatment.

Goals of Care

I. Facilitate patient's and parents' understanding of thalassemia and its implications.
II. Modify daily activity according to degree of anemia.
III. Encourage a positive self-image, reinforcing activities appropriate for development.

Intervention

I. Teach patient and parents:
  A. Genetic considerations.
    1. β thalassemia is a recessively inherited disorder in which the red blood cells contain decreased amounts of normal hemoglobin and anemia results.
    2. The transmission of thalassemia is 1:4 recessive.
    3. Explain the inheritance of the condition and the prospects for siblings of the homozygous carrier.
  B. Therapeutic considerations.
    1. For transfusion precautions, see "Hemolytic Disease of the Newborn."
    2. Explain and instruct about therapy. May include patient- or parent-administered deferoxamine injections.

    C. Miscellaneous considerations.
      1. Child may be smaller than peers.
      2. Child may have more infections, especially if splenectomy has been performed.
      3. Child should receive appropriate immunizations.
      4. Child may not be able to tolerate stressful sports such as football, basketball, soccer.
      5. Child may have delayed puberty.
II. Modify activity according to degree of anemia (see "Aplastic Anemia").
III. Encourage a positive self-image, reinforcing activities appropriate for development.
    A. Observe for feelings of guilt or denial on part of parents and child.
    B. Observe for childhood depression or poor self-concept. Suggest realistic aspirations and activities.
    C. Anticipate delayed puberty.
IV. Refer to appropriate agencies for further information and support (see Table 15-1).

Evaluation

I. Family members understand inheritance pattern of the disease and avail themselves of genetic counseling.
II. Avoidable complications of transfusion do not occur; others are promptly recognized and treated.
III. Parents and child demonstrate understanding of and compliance with treatment, including home care.
IV. Activity does not exceed tolerance.
V. Development, adjustment, and self-concept are adequate.

POLYCYTHEMIA OF CYANOTIC HEART DISEASE

Definition

Cyanotic heart disease induces a state of *polycythemia,* or increased numbers of red blood cells, to compensate for hypoxia of heart disease. Once the rise in hematocrit has exceeded 60 percent, the blood viscosity becomes markedly increased. To exemplify the alteration in viscosity, a hematocrit of 60 percent represents an increase in viscosity of four times the viscosity at 40 percent.

Characteristic symptoms are the result of sludging of blood and include headache, irritability and shortness of breath. Polycythemia of the newborn (with or without heart disease) presents with convulsions, hypoglycemia, hypocalcemia, priapism, decreased platelets, and renal vein thrombosis, all attributable to the increase in red cell mass.

Partial exchange transfusion is one temporary measure used in managing polycythemia. Removal of the blood must be done gradually, as a rapid loss can result in vascular collapse and cerebral insults. Optimally, the lowered hematocrit leads to a lowered peripheral resistance, producing a more efficient, larger stroke volume with an increased oxygen perfusion to tissues. With correction of the heart disease, the polycythemia resolves.

Assessment

Data sources are the patient, the patient's past medical record, and parents.
I. Health history.
    A. Congenital cyanotic heart anomaly.
    B. Shortness of breath.
    C. Irritability.

          D. Headache.

          E. Convulsions or seizures.

    II. Physical assessment.

          A. Skin—ruddy complexion in face, cyanotic extremities.

          B. Chest—pulmonary: use of accessory respiratory muscles.

          C. Cardiac exam—presence of murmurs associated with heart defect.

          D. Genitalia—priapism.

          E. Neurologic exam—neurologic deficits.

Problems

    I. Poor tissue perfusion and resultant altered activity.

    II. Potential complications from side effects of therapy.

    III. Susceptibility to bleeding.

    IV. Potential parental knowledge deficit regarding cyanotic heart disease and prevention/detection of thrombosis.

Goals of Care

    I. Optimum activity considering altered tissue perfusion.

    II. Maximum protection from complications of treatment (exchange transfusions).

    III. Prevention of bleeding.

    IV. Parental education regarding potential complications and promotion of comfort and safety for the child.

Intervention

    I. Advise parents, school personnel, and child, if old enough, that child should rest as necessary and avoid strenuous activities. (Infants, toddlers, and preschoolers usually restrict their own activity to their level of tolerance; school-age children and adolescents often do not.)

    II. For care of child having exchange transfusion, see "Hemolytic Disease of the Newborn."

    III. Teach parents, child, and teachers that good hydration is essential to reduce the risk of thrombosis (child must have free access to school drinking fountain, etc.).

    IV. For management of susceptibility to bleeding, see "Aplastic Anemia," although bleeding episodes may not be reflective of platelet counts.

    V. Evaluate for renal vein thrombosis (anuria, uremia).

    VI. Observe for signs of cerebral thrombosis (sudden vertigo, headaches, convulsions, nausea and vomiting, fainting, confusion).

    VII. Observe for signs of cardiac thrombosis (chest pain).

    VIII. See Chap. 13 for care of children with cyanotic heart disease.

Evaluation

    I. Activity does not exceed tolerance.

    II. Avoidable complications of transfusion do not occur; others are promptly detected and treated.

    III. Child is adequately hydrated.

    IV. Bleeding is avoided as possible; bleeding which does occur is properly treated.

    V. Thrombosis is detected and properly treated.

NEUTROPENIA

Definition

Neutropenia is a deficiency in circulating granulocytes. An absolute granulocyte count of less than 1500 per cubic millimeter in older children and adults and less than 1000 per cubic millimeter in infants 2 weeks to 1 year is considered neutropenia. Granulocytes (polymorphonuclear cells), particularly neutrophils, are active in phagocytosis, a major defense against infection. Therefore, the incidence of infection, particularly bacterial, increases in direct proportion to the severity of neutropenia.

Infections result when *exogenous* organisms (those which are not part of the normal flora) enter a receptive site, become established and multiply. *Endogenous* organisms (normal, harmless residents in the body) can cause severe infection when they are introduced into an area where they are not normally found, or when a change in the normal floral balance is favorable to their excessive multiplication.

The most common sites of infection are those to which organisms gain easiest entry: the skin, the respiratory tract, the mucosa, the bloodstream, and the bladder and kidneys. Frequent high spikes in temperature are usually the major sign. Due to the absence of neutrophils, *purulent exudates are not formed and the usual signs of infection may not be seen.* If meningitis develops, children may manifest the usual meningeal signs.

Many cancer chemotherapeutic agents and radiotherapy delivered to areas of the body which include large portions of functioning bone marrow have a potentially toxic effect on rapidly dividing cells of the bone marrow and can lead to profound neutropenia. The onset, degree, and duration of neutropenia varies with different agents. Often the dosage and administration of therapy will be adjusted to minimize these effects.

Drug-induced neutropenia is a syndrome of decreased production of granulocytes caused by an idiosyncratic drug reaction. The mechanism for the reaction is not clearly understood. Presumably, affected individuals have an inherent sensitivity to the agent. The drugs which most commonly cause neutropenia are the phenothiazines, aminopyrine or its derivatives (Pyralgin), chloramphenicol, sulfonamides, propylthiouracil, and phenylbutazone. The Registry on Blood Dyscrasias of the Council on Drugs of the American Medical Association maintains a list of drugs suspected of causing neutropenia.

The onset of neutropenia may be sudden, as with aminopyrine, which produces an immunologically mediated destruction of circulating neutrophils, or may occur days to weeks after the institution of drug therapy.

The disease is usually self-limiting. The duration of neutropenia is variable and death from overwhelming infection can occur.

Cyclic neutropenia is an unusual disease characterized by periodic episodes of neutropenia, fever, and infection, particularly oral ulceration. Serious infections are rare. The duration of the cycle is usually about 3 weeks (range 14 to 30 days). With each cycle there is approximately 1 week of illness followed by a period of well-being. The onset of the disease is usually early in childhood and it persists, becoming milder with age.

The most important therapeutic measure is identification and elimination of any agent that may be contributing to the neutropenia. Infections are treated with appropriate antibiotics. Early detection and prompt treatment enhance the effectiveness of therapy.

Assessment

Data sources are the patient, parents, and previous medical history.

I. Health history.
   A. Recurrent or recent infections.
   B. Exposure to drugs, chemicals, radiation.
   C. Previous drug reactions.
   D. Home environment—potential for adequate hygiene, separate sleeping facilities.

II. Physical assessment.
   A. General—elevated temperature, pulse, respiratory rate, lethargy, malaise, irritability.
   B. Skin—cutaneous ulcerations, furunculosis, absence of pus and usual signs of infection.
   C. Mucous membranes—ulceration, stomatitis, perianal abscess, pain, vaginal drainage, and redness.
   D. Lungs—cough, rhonchi, rales, tachypnea, dyspnea, decreased breath sounds.
   E. Neurological—rigidity of neck and spine, irritability.

Problems

I. Exposure to offending agent (drug-induced).
II. Increased susceptibility to infections.

Goals of Care

I. Protect patient from offending agent.
II. Protect patient from exogenous and endogenous organisms.
III. Control infections.
IV. Continuation of normal activities during periods of neutropenia.

Intervention

I. Offending agent.
   A. Identify and eliminate, if possible, offending agent.
   B. Indicate hypersensitivity in medical record.
   C. Consider Medic-Alert bracelet.
   D. Instruct patient, family, and schoolteacher on the hazards of reexposure.
II. Infectious organisms.
   A. Strict handwashing (there is little evidence that other isolation techniques such as masks, gowns, gloves, etc., provide greater protection. These measures may have an adverse effect on the patient's emotional state and may discourage needed nursing attention).
   B. Use iodine skin preparation prior to any puncture g)intravenous injection, finger puncture).
   C. Protect skin integrity: evaluate carefully the need for punctures, rotate puncture site, use paper tape rather than regular adhesive tape, maintain good hygiene, turn bedfast patient hourly, massage as needed.
   D. Limit rectal manipulation—temperature, enema, exam, suppositories, etc.
   E. Assist patient with mouth care qid.
   F. Restrict visitation to parents and family; screen visitors and staff carefully for infections.
   G. Plan staff assignments to avoid cross contamination.
   H. Provide high-calorie, high-protein diet; consider need for vitamin supplementation.
   I. Plan and implement exercise program appropriate for patient's condition.
   J. Date and change intravenous infusion tubing daily; apply antibiotic ointment and sterile dressing to insertion site daily; scalp vein needles are recommended.
   K. Keep patient's fingernails and toenails short, clean, and well manicured.
   L. Ensure that perineal care is performed for postpubescent females twice daily.
   M. Teach females proper wiping technique for bowel movement.
   N. Discuss sexual hygiene, techniques, and contraindicated practices in sexually active patients.

    O. Administer stool softeners.

    P. Avoid bladder catheterization; when necessary use smallest possible catheter, strict aseptic technique, and adequate lubrication. Maintain a *closed* sterile drainage system.

    Q. Clean and dress wounds as needed (at least bid), use strict aseptic technique.

    R. Ensure good pulmonary hygiene by coughing, deep breathing, physiotherapy.

    S. Teach patient and family to avoid exposure to pigeon droppings, people with obvious infections, particularly herpes zoster, varicella, or measles.

    T. Teach patient and family to notify physician immediately if exposure to varicella has occurred (in some cases hyperimmune gamma globulin can be administered within 72 h of *exposure* and the disease can be prevented or attenuated).

    U. Teach patient and family about the role of neutrophils in control of infection, the implications of neutropenia, and the rationale for the interventions listed above.

III. Infections.

    A. Observe closely for signs and symptoms of infection (may be masked by absence of pus).

    B. Notify physician immediately if signs and symptoms are detected.

    C. Administer antibiotic therapy as prescribed.

    D. Prevent the spread of infection with strict handwashing and hygiene (removal of drainage from wounds if present).

    E. Monitor for signs of reaction if granulocyte transfusion is administered.

    F. Teach patient and family the signs and symptoms of infection and what to do if they are detected.

IV. Activities.

    A. Evaluate the safety of return to school (based on absolute neutrophil count).

    B. If return to school is indicated, counsel teacher and school nurse.

    C. If isolation is required, arrange for homebound instruction until absolute neutrophil count increases.

Evaluation

  I. Reexposure to causative agent is avoided.

  II. Avoidable infections do not occur.

  III. Infections are controlled.

  IV. Activities appropriate for developmental stage are continued as condition permits.

DISORDERS OF PHAGOCYTOSIS

Definition

Chronic granulomatous disease (CGD) is a hereditary disorder of neutrophil bactericidal function. In the majority of cases it is transmitted in a sex-linked recessive pattern, though it can rarely be an autosomal recessive disease. Recurrent pyogenic infections are characteristic.

There are adequate numbers of neutrophils which are capable of phagocytizing but not killing bacteria. There is a defective leukocyte respiratory metabolism which prevents the cell from producing hydrogen peroxide, an integral part of the normal biochemical response to phagocytized bacteria.

The clinical manifestations of the disease are usually evident before 2 years of age. Infections are treated with appropriate antibiotics. Early detection and identification of the organism causing the infection may enhance the effectiveness of treatment. Generally, the prognosis is poor and patients succumb to infection early in childhood.

Chediak-Higashi syndrome (CHS) is an autosomal recessive hereditary disorder of leukocytes associated with an unusual group of clinical features: partial albinism, photophobia, nystagmus, hepatosplenomegaly, and cranial and peripheral neuropathies. There is an associated increased incidence of lymphoreticular malignancies. Granulocytes contain characteristic giant cytoplasmic granular inclusions.

The characteristic predisposition to severe bacterial infections is not entirely understood but is thought to be caused by the fact that the giant granules fail to release the appropriate enzymes and interfere with the bactericidal reaction.

Clinical features are usually recognized in the first months of life. Treatment is primarily management of infectious episodes with appropriate antibiotics. The use of ascorbic acid is currently under investigation. The prognosis is poor; children usually die of sepsis early in life.

Assessment

Data sources are the patient, parents, and the previous medical record.
I. Health history.
  A. Family history of similar disorder.
  B. Recurrent or recent infections.
  C. Changes in abdominal girth.
  D. Abnormalities of gait, bone pain with osteomyelitis (CGD).
  E. Changes in bowel pattern; diarrhea, pain with defecation (CGD).
  F. Abnormalities of sensorium, gait, fine or gross motor movements, sensory function (CHS).
  G. Photophobia (CHS).
II. Physical assessment.
  A. General—elevated temperature, pulse, respiratory rate, lethargy, malaise, irritability.
  B. Skin—eczematoid dermatitis, furunculosis, pus present to produce the usual signs of infection (CHS); light pigmentation.
  C. Mucous membranes—ulcerations, perianal abscesses.
  D. Lymph nodes—enlarged, suppurative.
  E. Abdomen—hepatosplenomegaly, tenderness.
  F. Skeletal—tenderness, swelling, warmth (particularly hands and feet).
  G. Lungs—rales, rhonchi, tachypnea, dyspnea, decreased breath sounds.
  H. Neurological—hyporeflexia or areflexia, ataxia, weakness, footdrop, sensory loss, seizures.
  I. Eyes—retinal albinism, horizontal nystagmus, squinting in light.
  J. Hair—gray or light brown in color.

Problems

I. Phagocytic dysfunction and consequent susceptibility to infection.
II. Cranial and peripheral neuropathies (CHS).

Goals of Care

I. Protect patient from exogenous and endogenous organisms.
II. Control infections.
III. Continuation of normal activities insofar as condition permits.
IV. Treat neurological problems and protect from related injury.

Intervention

Refer to "Neutropenia," and see Chap. 19 for intervention for neurological problems.

Evaluation

Refer to "Neutropenia," and see Chap. 19 for evaluation of care of children with neurological problems.

LEUKEMIA

Definition

Leukemia is a malignancy of unknown etiology characterized by a replacement of the normal marrow elements with abnormal accumulations of leukocytes and their precursors. The cytologic classification of the disease depends on the type of white blood cell which is predominant in the bone marrow and peripheral blood. Approximately 85 percent of the cases of childhood leukemia are classified as acute lymphocytic or lymphoblastic leukemia (ALL). The majority of the remaining cases are acute myelocytic or myeloblastic leukemia (AML). Myeloblastic leukemia is less responsive to therapy, and patients suffering from it have a poorer prognosis than do those with ALL. Erythroleukemia, also called di Guglielmo syndrome, is a variant of acute leukemia, involving primarily erythroid precursors. Promyelocytic leukemia is a variant of myeloblastic leukemia. Coagulopathy is a particular problem with this disease.

Results of recent investigations suggest that other factors, such as immunologic cell surface characteristics and clinical features, should be considered in classifying acute leukemia. It appears as though leukemias which can be identified as T or B cell in origin have a poorer prognosis than those in which the cell of origin cannot be identified (null cell).

The clinical features may be related to the disease process itself or to the therapy used. Anemia results from erythropoietic failure and from blood loss. The complications of anemia experienced by the child with leukemia are similar to those discussed under "Aplastic Anemia."

Patients with leukemia often demonstrate qualitative defects in neutrophil functions which provide inadequate resistance to infection. Profound neutropenia may result from leukemic replacement of bone marrow or drug toxicity. Overwhelming infections are the cause of death in 60 to 80 percent of children with leukemia.

Hemorrhage is usually the result of thrombocytopenia. There appears to be a synergistic relation between thrombocytopenia and infection. Occasionally a child with a low platelet count may not manifest signs of bleeding until an infection develops. In most cases thrombocytopenia alone may account for the bleeding.

Leukemic invasion of any organ system in the body can result in alteration or failure of that organ system. Disease occurring in an organ other than the bone marrow is termed extramedullary. Common sites of leukemic infiltration are the liver, spleen, lymph nodes, central nervous system, lungs, kidneys, bones, testicles, and ovaries.

When therapy is instituted and large numbers of cells are rapidly destroyed, hyperuricemia may result. If there is crystallization of the uric acid, obstruction of the renal tubules and impaired renal function may result. Hyperuricemia usually can be effectively controlled with increased fluid intake, alkalinization of the urine, and administration of allopurinol.

Untreated leukemia progresses rapidly, with death occurring within weeks to months after diagnosis. Utilization of chemotherapeutic agents enables greater than 90 percent of children with newly diagnosed cases of ALL to achieve at least one remission.

When a child is in remission, he is free of signs and symptoms attributable to leukemia. As many as 40 to 50 percent of children are being maintained in their initial remission states in excess of 5 years. Current recommendations have been to discontinue therapy after 3 years if the child has remained in continuous complete remission. Most children who reach this point will never experience a relapse.

In spite of this optimistic outlook for many children, a significant number are not able to experience long-term control of their disease. A number of clinical features have been used as prognostic factors: the age of the patient at the time of diagnosis, the initial white blood count, the degree of organomegaly and the presence of detectable extramedullary disease. Generally, a child between the ages of 2 and 10 years, with a white count of less than 10,000 per cubic millimeter and no significant extramedullary disease, has a much better prognosis.

If the child's leukemic cells become resistant to the drugs being used, the abnormal cells return and a relapse occurs. Extramedullary relapses are frequently followed by bone marrow relapses. The duration of remission is variable. There is a tendency for successive remissions to become increasingly shorter. A child may experience several remissions and recurrent relapses before he succumbs to complications of the disease.

The goal of therapy is eradication of leukemia cells and restoration of normal marrow function. Numerous drugs can be used in a variety of combinations to induce and maintain a remission. Side effects of chemotherapy are experienced by all children, but the severity of these side effects varies from one child to another.

The *induction* course of therapy is designed to reduce the leukemic cell population sufficiently to achieve a complete remission. Certain drugs are more effective in inducing a remission than others. The chemotherapy of choice in this phase is a combination of prednisone given daily and vincristine given weekly. Other agents such as daunomycin and L-asparaginase may be added to the vincristine and prednisone combination.

Generally, after 4 to 6 weeks of induction therapy, a remission is achieved. At this point, some treatment programs include a course of *consolidation* or *intensification* chemotherapy designed to further reduce the number of leukemia cells. This can be done by administering single agents such as methotrexate or L-asparaginase in intensive courses, or multiple agents in cyclic or combination therapy.

Central nervous system prophylaxis is administered early in the course of the illness. Generally, therapy consists of cranial irradiation, plus intrathecal methotrexate. Some treatment programs include initial intensive intrathecal therapy with methotrexate alone or in combination with cytosine arabinoside and hydrocortisone followed by intrathecal treatment every 2 months.

The consistent side effect of cranial irradiation is alopecia of the scalp. The severity and duration of alopecia varies from patient to patient, but generally, children lose all their hair before the completion of therapy. Hair grows back within several months, but may be of a different color and texture. Episodes of fever, irritability, lethargy, headache, nausea, and vomiting occur less commonly. Preliminary data indicate that prophylactic central nervous system radiotherapy in the treatment of acute lymphoblastic leukemia produces no clinically detectable neurologic or psychologic impairment. More investigation is needed, however.

The goals of *maintenance* or *continuation* chemotherapy are to maintain remission and to continue reducing the residual leukemic cell population toward zero. A combination of 6-mercaptopurine administered daily and methotrexate administered weekly comprises effective continuation therapy and is associated with minimal complications of drug toxicity.

In an effort to increase the duration of remission, some investigators have employed *reinduction* or *reinforcement* therapy. With this approach, prednisone or prednisone plus vincristine "pulses" are given every 3 to 4 months for 2 to 4 weeks.

When a relapse occurs, induction therapy with vincristine and prednisone may be administered. When these agents are no longer effective, L-asparaginase, cytosine arabinoside, daunomycin, Adriamycin, and other investigational agents may be used as single agents or in combination. After the remission has been reinduced, maintenance therapy will be administered. Usually, however, the occurrence of a single relapse, whether in the bone marrow or in an extramedullary site, means that permanent control of the disease will be impossible.

Unfortunately, AML is less responsive to therapy. Combinations of drugs such as vincristine, prednisone, Adriamycin, cyclophosphamide, daunomycin, cytosine arabinoside, 5-azacytidine, and 6-thioguanine are effective for remission induction in approximately 40 to 50 percent of children with AML. Some of these agents, particularly cytosine arabinoside and 6-thioguanine, are used for maintenance also, but the duration of remission is short—usually about 6 months. Long-term survival is rare in children with AML.

Two modes of therapy, bone marrow transplantation and immunotherapy, have been used. Because of a number of factors such as cost, inaccessibility of donors and treatment failure, the role of bone marrow transplantation is questionable. Numerous clinical trials of immunotherapy in acute leukemia have failed to support the promising experience reported by Mathé in 1963. Though further investigation is under way, it is doubtful that immunotherapy will become part of standard therapy.

Supportive therapy is essential during periods of bone marrow imbalance. Early recognition of infection and prompt institution of appropriate measures can be lifesaving. Antibiotics are used aggressively to combat the infectious process. Transfusion is used to counteract the complications of bone marrow suppression. Packed red blood cells are generally transfused in place of whole blood to avoid volume overload. The use of platelet concentrations has helped to control the hemorrhagic manifestations of thrombocytopenia. Granulocyte transfusions have been used for profound neutropenia. A combination of inaccessibility of leukophoresis equipment and the brief life-span of infused granulocytes has limited the benefits from this measure. Another measure used to combat complications of leukopenia is protection in a germ-free laminar airflow unit. However, such facilities are currently available in only a limited number of institutions.

The diagnosis of leukemia has a tremendous emotional impact on the child, his or her family, and the community. Cancer carries a stigma that is feared by all. Despite increasing evidence that leukemia is controllable and possibly curable, the initial reaction is to the threat of a fatal illness.

There are three possible courses of the illness: (1) treatment and no response, leading to death; (2) temporary control of the disease until recurrence and ultimate death; and (3) indefinite control of the disease. The uncertainty of the outcome is perhaps the most difficult aspect of this disease. Parents and children are encouraged to return to their normal lifestyle, but treatment regimens usually make this an impossibility.

The responsibility of administration of therapy and observation for side effects must be shared by the family. At a time of extreme stress, families are expected to assimilate a new and confusing body of knowledge.

It is well recognized that a multidisciplinary team is best able to appreciate and meet the complex psychosocial and physical needs of the leukemic child and the family. Consequently, treatment is usually coordinated through a comprehensive center.

Assessment

Data sources are the patient, parents, and schoolteacher.

I. Health history.
   A. Recurrent or recent infections.
   B. Exposure to offending agent such as benzene or radiation (rare).
   C. Anorexia, weight loss.
   D. Lethargy, fatigue, malaise.
   E. Easily bruised, bleeding from nose or gums.
   F. Pain (bone, abdominal).
   G. Home environment: potential for adequate hygiene, separate sleeping facilities (to decrease transmission of infections to the child).
   H. Family experience with chronic illness, cancer, death; coping patterns.
II. Physical assessment.
   A. General—elevated temperature, pulse, respiratory rate; lethargy, malaise, irritability.
   B. Skin—petechiae, ecchymoses, cellulitis, furunculosis, absence of pus and usual signs of infection (depending on degree of neutropenia), cutaneous nodules (rare).
   C. Lymph nodes—generalized adenopathy.
   D. Mucous membranes—bleeding from gums and nose, ulceration, stomatitis, perianal abscess, pain.
   E. Abdomen—hepatosplenomegaly.
   F. Musculoskeletal—muscle wasting, bone pain, joint pain.

      G. Lungs—cough, rhonchi, rales, tachypnea, dyspnea, decreased breath sounds.

      H. Cardiac—flow murmur.

      I. Neurological, with central nervous infiltration—nausea, vomiting, lethargy, head-ache, irritability, convulsions, cranial nerve palsies, papilledema, pain upon neck flexion, hyperphagia, blindness.

      J. Genital, with testicular infiltration—progressive painless enlargement; involved testes become nodular and firm.

Problems

    I. Replacement of normal marrow with blast cells.
      A. Anemia.
      B. Bleeding.
      C. Increased susceptibility to infections.
   II. Infiltration of tissues with blast cells.
      A. Tracheal compression due to mediastinal mass.
      B. Intestinal obstruction due to abdominal adenopathy.
      C. Increased intracranial pressure due to central nervous system infiltration.
      D. Pain.
  III. Hyperuricemia.
  IV. Toxicity of antineoplastic therapy.
      A. Nausea and vomiting.
      B. Anorexia and weight loss.
      C. Increased appetite and weight gain.
      D. Mucositis.
      E. Peripheral neuropathies.
      F. Alopecia.
      G. Sterile hemorrhagic cystitis.
      H. Local tissue irritation due to extravasation.
   V. Potentially fatal disease.

Goals of Care

      I. Modify activity by degree of anemia, and ensure maximal benefit from transfusion therapy.
     II. Prevent and/or control bleeding.
    III. Protect patient from exogenous and endogenous agents; control infections.
    IV. Decrease blast cell population.
     V. Manage tracheal compression, intestinal obstruction, and increased intracranial pressure if any of these arise.
   VI. Prevent and relieve pain.
  VII. Prevent uric acid nephropathy.
 VIII. Prevent and relieve nausea and vomiting.
   IX. Enhance intake of nutritious diet.
    X. Prevent and relieve mucositis.
   XI. Prevent constipation.
  XII. Modify activities according to degree of weakness.
 XIII. Prepare patient, family, and others for alopecia.
 XIV. Prevent hemorrhagic cystitis.
  XV. Prevent tissue necrosis due to extravasation of drugs.
 XVI. Facilitate the patient's and family's understanding of the disease and treatment.
 XVII. Encourage the patient and family to return to normal activities.
XVIII. Support the normal grieving process.
 XIX. Enhance the staff's ability to provide consistent, compassionate care.

Intervention

See the sections on anemia, "Thrombocytopenia," and "Neutropenia." Also *see* Chap. 14 regarding airway obstruction, Chap. 16 regarding intestinal obstruction, and Chap. 19 regarding increased intracranial pressure.

I. Pain.
   A. When pain is anticipated, devise a plan for controlling it involving the medical and nursing staff, the patient, and family *prior to the onset.*
   B. Explain to the patient and family that the plan is made and that comfort measures are available. Do so in positive manner conveying confidence that the pain will be controlled.
   C. Obtain a thorough assessment of the patient's pain, including the location, nature, intensity, and pattern; patient's, family's, and staff's reaction, and measures which have controlled pain in the past.
   D. Explain the nature of the pain experience to patient and family in a language that is understandable.
   E. Provide a comfortable, nonthreatening environment: remove offensive sights, sounds, and smells.
   F. Ensure patient's and family's trust and confidence by demonstrating compassion, knowledge, and competence.
   G. Assist patient to a comfortable position.
   H. Employ measures designed to relieve pain: distraction is useful (reading, records, movies, games) if appropriate; encourage the patient to imagine pleasant sensations or situations, which family can help support with stories, music, pictures, smells, etc.; decrease perception of pain with sensory and tactile stimulation (massage, vibration, heat, cold, motion, gentle scratching) based on gate-control theory.
   I. Administer analgesics as prescribed (those which do not interfere with platelet function).
   J. Evaluate each measure for effectiveness.
   K. Record a detailed description of pain experience, relief measures, and effectiveness.
II. Fluid-electrolyte balance.
   A. Ensure adequate hydration (twice maintenance) with oral or parenteral fluids.
   B. Administer allopurinol as prescribed (if mercaptopurine is administered concomitantly, adjust dose).
   C. Monitor urine pH (should be 7.0 or greater).
   D. If urine becomes acidic, administer alkalinizing agents as prescribed (sodium bicarbonate, Diamox, Scholl's solution).
III. Specific nursing concerns.
   A. Nausea and vomiting.
      1. Alert patient and family to the potential for nausea and vomiting in a positive manner, assuring them that there is a plan for managing it (avoid dwelling on the possibility, as the power of suggestion is great).
      2. Allow the patient and family to participate in making the decision about timing of administration of nauseating agents (often evening administration is preferred).
      3. Administer antiemetics, sedatives, or tranquilizers as prescribed *before* administering nauseating agent.
      4. Teach patient and parents about the potential for aspiration, and preventive measures.
      5. Eliminate offensive sights, sounds, and smells.
      6. Assist patient to a comfortable, safe position (elevated upper torso may be best).
      7. Have emesis basin within reach but out of sight.
      8. Cleanse mouth, particularly after each vomiting episode (some patients are relieved by sucking on a sourball).
      9. Employ measures to decrease anxiety and perception of nausea such as distraction and fantasy.

B. Nutrition.
1. Obtain a thorough assessment of eating patterns and food preferences.
2. Offer preferred foods—many patients will tolerate foods that their mother commonly offers during illness.
3. Encourage family to prepare foods at home or in hospital.
4. Ensure that environment is conducive to eating at mealtime—that patient is clean (hands and face washed, mouth cleansed), relaxed, rested, and free from pain and fear; offensive sights, sounds, and smells are removed.
5. Assist patient to a comfortable position.
6. Suggest that patient eat with other patients or family members.
7. Use a positive approach when discussing eating.
8. Offer small portions of food in frequent feedings.
9. Offer foods high in protein and calories.
10. Make food tray attractive and appropriate for age.
11. When appetite is increased from steroids or hypothalamic disease, limit the amount of food at each feeding rather than the frequency of feedings; offer foods low in salt.
12. Warn patient and family that fluctuations in appetite and weight may be marked and frequent—i.e., requiring a new wardrobe and middle-of-the-night snacks.

C. Mucositis.
1. Examine mouth and perianal area carefully prior to chemotherapy.
2. Instruct patient and family in the importance of immediate reporting of stomatitis.
3. Administer mouth care four times a day. Many approaches are used. A soft-bristled toothbrush should be used unless ulceration or bleeding occurs. Then a sponge or cotton-tipped applicator may be substituted. The mouth should be rinsed with 1:1 solution of hydrogen peroxide and saline. Rinsing with a Water Pik is most thorough and provides the stimulation of the gums which normally occurs with mastication. Mouthwash can be added to the rinse but should be diluted to avoid burning.
4. Notify physician immediately if lesions occur.
5. Modify chemotherapy doses as prescribed.
6. Examine area closely for signs of superinfection with opportunistic organisms.
7. If superinfection occurs, administer antibiotics as prescribed and instruct patient and family in method of administration.

D. Constipation.
1. Obtain a thorough assessment of normal bowel pattern.
2. Ensure a high fluid intake.
3. Employ natural laxatives such as prune juice, high roughage foods; exercise.
4. Administer stool softeners and cathartics as prescribed.

E. Weakness.
1. Warn patient, family, and schoolteachers of the potential for weakness.
2. Assist in the selection of activities which patient can achieve (may be able to ride a bicycle or tricycle but unable to walk long distances or climb stairs; may be able to write with larger diameter pencil, fasten zipper but not button).
3. Refer to Chap. 19 for additional guidelines.

F. Alopecia.
1. Warn patient, family, and others that alopecia will occur.
2. Make patient and family aware of alternatives such as wigs, scarfs, caps, etc.
3. Inform family of financial assistance for purchase of wigs if available.
4. During period of hair loss, change patient's clothes and bed linen frequently as hair accumulates. Patient may want to cut hair or wear a hair net to catch loose hair.
5. Prepare patient for others' reactions by encouraging expression of feelings using role play, etc.

G. Cystitis.
   1. Administer Cytoxan early in the day to allow patient to keep emptying bladder frequently while metabolites are excreted.
   2. If large bolus is given, ensure high fluid intake (twice maintenance).
   3. Ensure continuous high fluid intake with daily dose.
   4. Instruct patient and family to report immediately any sign of dysuria, frequency, urgency or hematuria; discontinue Cytoxan until further notice from physician.
   5. If bleeding occurs, continue high fluid intake.
   6. Monitor urine output (formation of clots may cause obstruction and distension).
H. Extravasation.
   1. Do not inject with the same needle used to withdraw medication from the vial.
   2. Administer drug through scalp vein needle, using largest available vein.
   3. Before injecting drug into any IV line, confirm that the line is patent and not infiltrating by infusing at least 5 mL of normal saline and observing for blood return (more may be needed if the vein is deep in subcutaneous tissue).
   4. When patency and integrity of the vein is confirmed, inject the medication slowly.
   5. Observe the site of injection continuously for signs of infiltration.
   6. Periodically confirm patency of the line with blood return.
   7. After the medication is injected, flush the line with at least 5 mL of normal saline.
   8. If infiltration occurs:
      a. Discontinue the infusion immediately. Contact with a minute amount of the drug is enough to cause severe tissue reaction, necrosis, and sloughing.
      b. Remove the IV.
      c. Apply ice packs immediately and continue intermittently for 24 h.
      d. Instruct the patient to keep the site of injection elevated.
      e. If swelling subsides, apply hot packs (again at frequent intervals) until inflammation subsides.
      f. Observe the site frequently for signs of tissue breakdown and infection.
      g. Instruct the patient to notify the physician if complications develop.
IV. Communicating with the patient and parents.
   A. Explain the nature of the disease and treatment in clear terms appropriate for developmental level and degree of stress.
      1. Repeat explanations as often as needed.
      2. Provide written information about the details of treatment and side effects.
      3. Encourage patient and family to demonstrate their knowledge with return explanations.
      4. Facilitate communication with other patients and parents.
   B. Assess the patient's ability to participate in activities.
      1. Communicate strengths and limitations clearly to patient and family.
      2. Modify activities to degree of limitation (homebound instruction, etc., if needed).
      3. Communicate with significant family members and others to clarify objectives.
      4. Provide positive reinforcement for involvement in activities.
      5. Acknowledge and allow patient's and family's anxiety.
   C. In working with the grieving process, the nurse should realize that there is not a pattern of progression through stages that is optimal. The nurse's role is to observe and assess the patient's behavior, support the patient at any phase and create an environment that will allow for progression as the patient is ready. It should be recognized that defense mechanisms are necessary and should not be denied. Possible interventions for each phase include:
      1. Denial:
         a. Establish reality of recent past. Relate to and discuss illness leading up to diagnosis.
         b. Have parent or child express what has been done during present hospitalization, establishing further reality of present.

       c. Clarify feelings of parents—"I know you must feel tired and worn out"—etc.

       d. With shock or bewilderment, encourage activities, allowing parents and child to hold on to reality, particularly those routines that have been part of the family's routine prior to diagnosis.

2. Anger:
   a. Have family and patient go over events to this point.
   b. Elicit the family's impression of those serving patient.
   c. Help family identify source of its anger.
   d. Supply consistent and truthful information.
   e. Observe for self-directed anger and/or self-inflicted punishment.
      (1) Channel anger away from individuals and redirect energies to the present, i.e., constructive participation in the child's treatment.
      (2) Reassure that the onset of disease was not anyone's "fault."
   f. Encourage verbalization of feelings.
   g. Offer family the opportunity to talk with other parents of children with cancer who have accepted disease and treatment.
   h. Give family decision-making abilities.

3. Bargaining:
   a. Acknowledge and allow feelings.
   b. Be aware of signs of guilt, "if only." (See 2e, above.)
   c. Encourage intrafamily support. Evaluate family resources, financially, emotionally.

4. Depression: (Especially with "silent" or "reflective" depression).
   a. Encourage consistency of those staying with child.
      (1) Limit visitors.
      (2) Provide scheduled times to relieve family and allow patient to rest or relax and not feel he or she has to entertain.
   b. Encourage routine self-care activities on part of family and child and permit them to feel productive and worthwhile.
   c. Offer praise for efforts expended.
   d. Slowly encourage patient to expand activities of daily living (school, play, etc.).
   e. Watch out for an abundance of relatives and other visitors which can be taxing to child and family.

5. Acceptance:
   a. Continue to provide consistent information to the parents and child, not giving them opportunity to mistrust.
   b. Ask the family to help other parents, as this can help keep the family at a level of acceptance and coping with their own child's disease.
   c. Continue with positive reinforcement and realistic hope.

V. Provide staff with opportunities for ventilation.
   A. Provide opportunities for rotation to other areas (e.g., outpatient clinic).
   B. Establish routine patient care planning sessions.

VI. Refer to appropriate agencies for further information and support (see Table 15-1).

Evaluation

I. Activity does not exceed tolerance.

II. Avoidable complications of transfusion do not occur; others are promptly detected and treated.

III. Bleeding is minimized.

IV. Infections are minimized.

V. Medication regime is followed; side effects are promptly detected and properly managed.

VI. Signs and symptoms of leukemic invasion of body tissues are recognized and treated.

VII. Renal function is maintained.
VIII. Side effects of therapy are minimized and effectively treated.
IX. Family is well informed about the course and prognosis of the disease and copes adequately.
X. Child's adjustment and development are adequate.

HEMOPHILIA

Definition

Hemophilia is an inherited coagulation disorder. The most common forms of the disease, classic hemophilia (hemophilia A, or factor VIII deficiency) and Christmas disease (hemophilia B, or factor IX deficiency), account for 95 percent of the hemophilias, with classic hemophilia accounting for 84 percent of the total.

Classic hemophilia and Christmas disease are transmitted in a sex-linked recessive manner, generally from an asymptomatic carrier mother to an affected son. The disease is due to deficient activity of the coagulation factor involved. Children with less than 1 percent of the plasma factor activity are considered severe hemophiliacs. Children with more than 1 percent of the factor activity may have a mild to moderate form of hemophilia. These children may be free of spontaneous bleeding and require replacement therapy only in the event of surgery or trauma.

The disease is characterized by recurrent episodes of hemorrhage. The bleeding may be spontaneous or caused by slight injury. The specific manifestations depend on the area involved. Prolonged hemorrhage may occur following circumcision or immunization. For the toddler who experiences frequent falls, bleeding into soft tissue and from mucous membranes is common. Injuries of the nose and mouth cause most of these bleeding episodes.

Perhaps the most debilitating complication of the disease is hemarthrosis, or bleeding into a joint. Early signs are pain, tenderness, and limitation of motion. As bleeding progresses, the joint may become swollen and warm. Muscle spasms and changes in soft tissue structure occur, resulting in the formation of flexion contractures. Recurrence of bleeding causes further degenerative changes which may lead to permanent fixation of the joint.

The goal of therapy is prevention of morbidity from bleeding episodes. When there is evidence of serious bleeding, plasma replacement therapy should be started immediately. Infusion of appropriate sources of the deficient factor will raise the plasma factor level sufficiently to allow hemostasis. Use of cryoprecipitate or commercial concentrates of factor VIII are the treatments of choice for classic hemophilia. Cryoprecipitate is easily prepared in the blood bank from fresh plasma, but must be stored in the frozen state. Several commercial concentrates are available. They are stored at 5 to 10°C and are therefore more convenient for home transfusion and travel. Hemarthroses may require continuation of replacement therapy for 3 to 4 days. Plasma from which cryoprecipitate has been removed and commercial factor IX concentrates are used to treat Christmas disease.

In some cases where the disease is severe and frequent transfusions are required to control bleeding, prophylactic infusion programs are instituted. Therapy is administered routinely two to three times a week. The goal of this approach is maintenance of adequate levels of the clotting factor and prevention of bleeding. The prophylactic approach may be used to eliminate the risk of bleeding when the patient is participating in aggressive rehabilitative physical therapy programs and must be able to engage in active exercise.

The cost and inconvenience of frequent infusions have promoted the development of home management programs. In these programs, patients and their families are taught to administer the infusions. Early institution of therapy permits earlier control of bleeding, fewer complications, and less interruption of normal activity. In some situations children as young as 5 and 6 years of age are administering their own cryoprecipitate.

ε-Aminocaproic acid (EACA or Amicar) may be administered in conjunction with factor replacement to control mouth bleeding. EACA is an inhibitor of the fibrinolytic enzyme system, which is particularly active in mucosal tissue. Suspected renal bleeding usually is a contraindication for administration of Amicar.

Approximately 10 percent of patients with classic hemophilia will develop an IgG antibody to factor VIII. This inhibitor in the patient's plasma results in the inactivation of factor VIII in normal plasma. The development of an inhibitor calls for an alteration of the plan for treatment of bleeding problems. Alternative approaches to management are currently being investigated.

The psychosocial implications of the disease are great. The genetic aspect has obvious implications. Many mothers feel responsible and guilty. This often leads to overprotection. Two behavior patterns commonly seen in hemophiliac children are probably a result of maternal overprotection: passive-dependence and risk-taking. Fathers and siblings may resent the child's limitations. The constant threat of hemorrhage interferes with many family activities and stands between the child and his peers who are able to lead active lives. The average cost of replacement therapy for one bleeding episode ranges from $50 to $350 depending on the severity of the bleeding and the weight of the patient.

The team approach to treatment of hemophilia is essential. Ideally the team should consist of the child and his family, a pediatrician, a hematologist, an orthopedist, a dentist, a physical therapist, a psychologist, a social worker, and a nurse. Coordination of the efforts of all members of the team should provide a smooth, comprehensive management of this complex disease and afford the patient the opportunity to function as a healthy, independent individual.

Assessment

Data sources are the patient, parents, the previous medical record, and the medical record of affected family members.

I. Health history.
   A. Family history of bleeding tendency.
   B. History of bleeding tendency: prolonged bleeding after circumcision, intramuscular injections, lacerations, trauma.
   C. Bleeding into joints.
   D. Bleeding into muscles.
   E. Gastrointestinal bleeding.
   F. Hematuria.
   G. Spontaneous bleeding which often occurs in phases or cycles.
   H. Maternal overprotection.
   I. Paternal rejection.
   J. Child is passive-dependent or risk-taking.
II. Physical exam (during a bleeding episode).
   A. General—agitated, in pain.
   B. Skin—bruises, soft tissue bleeding, pain, swelling.
   C. Mucous membranes—persistent oozing from lacerations, particularly the frenulum in toddlers.
   D. Muscular—pain, warmth, swelling of muscle mass.
   E. Skeletal—pain, warmth, swelling at joints, limitations of motion, contractures and ankylosis from previous episodes if therapy was not instituted early.

Problems

I. Bleeding.
II. Anemia.
III. Pain.
IV. Musculoskeletal deformities.
V. Maternal guilt and overprotection.

VI. Paternal rejection.
VII. Alteration of life-style for family.
VIII. Confusion regarding disease and treatment.

Goals of Care

I. Prevent and/or control bleeding.
II. Modify activity according to degree of anemia, and ensure maximum benefit from transfusion therapy.
III. Control pain.
IV. Prevent musculoskeletal deformities.
V. Reduce maternal guilt, and encourage mother to allow independence.
VI. Encourage paternal bonding.
VII. Facilitate family's participation in normal activity.
VIII. Teach patient and family about disease and management.

Intervention

I. Prevention of bleeding.
   A. Pad crib and playpen for infants.
   B. Remove hazards such as hard toys, sharp furniture, and throw rugs from environment for toddlers.
   C. Instruct adolescent in the use of electric razor.
   D. Avoid deep intramuscular injections; administer immunizations when replacement factor is being given for bleeding episode if possible.
   E. Apply pressure for 5 min after intramuscular or intravenous puncture.
   F. Teach patient and family to avoid drugs which interfere with platelet function (aspirin, antihistamines).
II. Control (when bleeding occurs).
   A. Reassure patient and family that bleeding will be controlled.
   B. Encourage patient to rest by removing upsetting stimuli from environment.
   C. Apply ice and pressure to affected area.
   D. Pack nose or mouth with hemostatic agents as prescribed (for mucosal bleeding).
   E. Immobilize affected area.
   F. Elevate and support joints in a slightly flexed position (for hemarthroses).
   G. Prepare for administration of replacement factor as prescribed.
III. See interventions for anemia in "Aplastic Anemia."
IV. See "Leukemia."
V. When bleeding is controlled, encourage active range of motion to the level of pain as prescribed. Encourage cautious ambulation as prescribed (may begin within 48 h).
VI. Communicating with parents.
   A. Encourage mother to verbalize feelings of guilt and reassure her that this is a normal reaction.
   B. Encourage mother to identify her strengths as a mother, and help her develop a plan for allowing child independence.
   C. Reassure her during stress of allowing independence.
   D. Facilitate communication with other parents of hemophiliac children.
   E. Encourage father to verbalize any feelings of resentment, and reassure him that resentment is a normal reaction.
   F. Encourage father to identify his strengths as a father and involve him in child's care.
   G. Facilitate communication with other parents of hemophiliac children.
   H. Encourage parents to contact supportive agencies such as the National Hemophilia Foundation.

VIII. Assess patient and family readiness for home transfusion program.
   A. Begin preparation with demonstration of techniques.
   B. Encourage patient and/or parents to gradually attempt procedure. Begin by drawing up factor, applying tourniquet, etc.
   C. Reassure patient and parents as they learn techniques.
   D. Observe patient and parents as they repeat demonstrations.
   E. Provide written and verbal instructions about indications for replacement therapy, dose calculation, procedure for administration, and procedure for contacting professional if indicated.
   F. Counsel teacher or employer as indicated.
   G. Inform family of summer camps for hemophiliacs if available.
   H. Provide written and verbal information about the nature of the disease, signs and symptoms of bleeding, measures to control bleeding, indications for replacement therapy, and procedure for obtaining medical assistance. Schedule teaching when patient is stable and relaxed.
   I. Ask patient's family to repeat information to nurse at a later time.
   J. Encourage patient to verbalize his resentment and fear; reassure him that these feelings are normal.

IX. Refer to appropriate agencies for further information and support (see Table 15-1).

Evaluation

I. Avoidable bleeding does not occur; bleeding that does take place is adequately treated.
II. Activity does not exceed tolerance or reasonable safety.
III. Avoidable complications of transfusion do not occur; others are promptly recognized and treated.
IV. Pain is well controlled.
V. Musculoskeletal deformities are minimized.
VI. Child's adjustment and development are adequate.
VII. Parents' adjustment and parenting styles are adequate.
VIII. Parents and child, as age permits, understand hemophilia and competently carry out their parts of the treatment regime.

VON WILLEBRAND'S DISEASE

Definition

Von Willebrand's disease is a hereditary coagulation disorder with an autosomal dominant pattern of inheritance. It is characterized by a prolonged bleeding time and a deficiency of factor VIII. There is reduction of both the molecular concentration and activity of factor VIII. The prolonged bleeding time is due to a deficiency of a component of the factor VIII molecule involved in platelet adhesiveness. The deficiency, therefore, produces a defect in platelet adhesion as well as plasma coagulation.

The clinical manifestations of the disease are variable among patients and occasionally in the same patient at different times. Skin and mucosal bleeding is common. Hemarthroses are rare. Menorrhagia and bleeding following dental extraction, surgery, or trauma may be severe.

Local hemostatic measures are usually effective in controlling nosebleeds. Serious bleeding is treated with transfusions of cryoprecipitate or whole fresh frozen plasma.

Assessment

Data sources are the patient, parents, previous medical records, and the medical records of affected family members.
I. Health history.
   A. Family history of bleeding tendency.
   B. History of bleeding tendency: prolonged bleeding after circumcision, intramuscular injections, lacerations, trauma.
   C. Gastrointestinal bleeding.
   D. Mucosal bleeding.
   E. Menorrhagia.
   F. Bruises easily.
II. Physical examination (during a bleeding episode).
   A. General—agitated, in pain.
   B. Skin—ecchymoses, petechiae.
   C. Mucous membranes—persistent oozing from nose or gums.

Problems

I. Bleeding.
II. Anemia.
III. Confusion regarding disease and treatment.

Goals of Care

I. Prevent and/or control bleeding.
II. Modify activity according to degree of anemia.
III. Ensure maximum benefit from transfusion therapy.
IV. Teach patient and family about disease and management.

Intervention

See "Hemophilia" and "Thrombocytopenia."

Evaluation

See "Thrombocytopenia."

THROMBOCYTOPENIA (IDIOPATHIC AND ACQUIRED)

Definition

A reduced number of circulating platelets, less than 100,000, characterizes *idiopathic thrombocytopenia* (ITP). The hematologic abnormality occurs secondary to an increased platelet destruction caused by platelet antibodies or other humeral factors. The causative agent cannot be specifically identified. The reduced platelet population exists in the presence of a relatively normal bone marrow.

Over one-half of the cases of ITP are preceded by a recent illness, and as many as 85 percent recover after 4 months of observation. A debate exists as to the efficacy of steroid therapy in ITP. Steroids are thought to increase platelet production and decrease vascular fragility. Steroids or similar drugs are chosen to minimize the possibility of a serious bleeding episode. For those who do not respond to drug therapy or who do not improve without therapy, splenectomy may be indicated. Platelet transfusions are not helpful, because the mechanism which destroys the host's platelets destroys transfused platelets as well.

Acquired thrombocytopenia (AT) is similar to ITP, but a causative agent is identifiable. Several drugs or chemicals are linked with the disorder (see history). With infection-induced thrombocytopenia, the agent may be a virus, as in Rocky Mountain spotted fever (RMSF) and Colorado tick fever (CTF), or malarial, or bacterial. With either drug-induced or infection-induced thrombocytopenia, the platelet count recovers when the offending organism is removed. In acquired platelet disorders, a health history and titers may be the most helpful data.

Assessment

Data sources are the parents, the patient, and schoolteachers.
  I. Health history.
    A. Recent bleeding, epistaxis, blood in feces, hematemesis.
    B. Recent infection.
    C. Past history of similar bleeding or bruises.
    D. Recent exposure to chemicals (AT)—insecticides, paint, kerosene, gasoline.
    E. Recent exposure to drugs (AT)—diphenylhydantoin, barbiturates, sulfonamides, antihistamines, quinidine, quinine, digitoxin, paraminosalicylic acid.
    F. Recent exposure to or contraction of Rocky Mountain spotted fever, Colorado tick fever, virax malaria, bacteremia, viral infection (AT).
  II. Physical assessment.
    A. Skin—presence of petechiae, purpura on torso, face, extremities.
    B. Mucous membranes—bleeding from orifices, epistaxis, scabs.
    C. Abdominal examination—hepatosplenomegaly feasible with infection-induced purpura; absent in drug-induced purpura.

Problems

  I. Increased susceptibility to serious bleeding.
  II. Potential complications from therapy (usually ITP only)—bone marrow stimulating agent.
  III. Anemia secondary to blood loss.
  IV. Altered self-concept secondary to disease and treatment.

Goals of Care

  I. Prevention of and observation for serious bleeding.
  II. Therapy-related:
    A. Maximum protection is given from adverse side effects of steroid/androgen therapy.
    B. Education of patient/parents regarding side effects of steroid/androgen therapy.
  III. Modify activity according to degree of anemia.
  IV. Encourage a positive self-image, reinforcing activities appropriate for development.
  V. Protect patient from reexposure to offending agent (AT).

Intervention

I. Prevention of and observation for serious bleeding (see "Aplastic Anemia").
II. Therapy-related:
  A. Maximum protection from adverse side effects of steroid/androgen therapy (see "Aplastic Anemia").
  B. Education of patient/parents regarding side effects of steroid/androgen therapy (see "Aplastic Anemia").
III. Modify activity according to degree of anemia: suggest modified levels of activity with rest periods, until hemoglobin value returns to normal.
IV. Encourage a positive self-image (patient/parents), reinforcing activities appropriate for patient's development.
  A. Observe for feelings of guilt on part of parents or child.
  B. Observe for depression or poor self-concept on part of child. Support realistic activities appropriate for growth and developmental age.
V. Protect patient from reexposure to offending agent. (See "Neutropenia.")

Evaluation

I. Avoidable serious bleeding does not occur; other bleeding is promptly detected and treated.
II. Side effects of therapy are detected early and minimized.
III. Parents and child, if old enough, are well informed about the disease and the side effects of therapy, and they cope well.
IV. Activity does not exceed tolerance.
V. Development and adjustment are adequate.
VI. Reexposure to causative agent is avoided (AT).

IMMUNE THROMBOCYTOPENIA

Definition

Immune thrombocytopenia results from maternal antibody formation to fetal platelets and subsequent destruction of platelets in the fetus and newborn. Maternal ITP at any point during pregnancy can result in platelet antibodies crossing the placental barrier and destroying the fetal platelets.

Signs of thrombocytopenia may include a purpuric rash, jaundice from the absorption of heme products from the purpuric areas, frank bleeding from any orifice, and platelet counts below 100,000. Generally no therapy is needed. With active bleeding, however, platelet transfusions are indicated. Maternal platelets are often used for the platelet transfusions. Treatment may consist of steroids, which are thought to stimulate the bone marrow's production of precursor cells, particularly platelets. The tapering-off precautions observed with chronic steroid therapy in ITP are not applicable to the short-term steroid use in immune thrombocytopenia. Therapy is supportive, as the condition only lasts for a few weeks.

Assessment

Data sources are the mother, the patient, and the mother's past medical record.
I. Health history.
  A. Maternal history of thrombocytopenia.

  B. Prolonged cord bleeding at birth.
  C. Prolonged bleeding from invasive procedures.
II. Physical assessment.
  A. Skin—purpuric lesions, jaundice.
  B. Mucous membranes—bleeding.

Problems

  I. Increased susceptibility to serious bleeding.
  II. Potential complications from therapy.
  A. Bone marrow stimulatory agent.
  B. Platelet transfusions.

Goals of Care

  I. Prevention of and observation for serious bleeding.
  II. Therapy-related:
  A. Maximum protection from adverse side effects of steroid therapy.
  B. Maximum protection from adverse side effects of platelet transfusion.

Intervention

  I. Prevention of and observation for serious bleeding.
  A. See "Aplastic Anemia."
  B. Postpone elective procedures such as circumcision.
  II. Therapy-related:
  A. Maximum protection is given for adverse side effects of steroid therapy.
    1. Observe for:
      a. Elevations in blood pressure.
      b. Gastrointestinal irritability—vomiting, hematemesis.
    2. Consider administering drugs with feedings to decrease gastrointestinal irritability.
    3. Consider contraindications if used concomitantly with diuretics or antibiotics.
    4. See "Aplastic Anemia" for a complete list of steroid effects.
  B. Maximum protection is given for adverse side effects of platelet transfusion. (See "Hemolytic Disease of the Newborn.")

Evaluation

  I. Avoidable bleeding does not occur; bleeding which does arise is detected early and treated adequately.
  II. Avoidable side effects of therapy do not occur; family is well informed about inevitable side effects and copes well.

HENOCH-SCHÖNLEIN PURPURA (ANAPHYLACTOID PURPURA)

Definition

Henoch-Schönlein purpura (HSP) is a syndrome characterized by systemic vasculitis, often precipitated by a recent illness. The basic cause is unknown.

The vasculitis is most apparent on legs, buttocks, and perineal areas with the thorax clear from obvious lesions. The lesions are urticarial at onset, later developing into hemorrhagic areas. Scattered petechiae may be present. The kidney may have lesions similar to those apparent in the skin, causing hematuria, hypertension, and sometimes long-term renal disease. There may be associated edema of the head and neck. Painful joints are common, with the pain arising from periarticular swelling. If the gastrointestinal system is affected, abdominal colic may be present with gastrointestinal bleeding. Often steroid therapy is used to increase the integrity of the endothelium, to minimize the pain associated with swollen joints and the abdominal symptoms.

Assessment

Data sources are the parents, the child, and the schoolteacher.
I. Health history.
   A. History of recent infection.
   B. Recent fever.
II. Physical assessment.
   A. Skin—diffuse, red, raised, nonblanching rash over lower torso and legs.
   B. Head and neck—possibly some edema.
   C. Extremities—some observable, palpable swelling.
   D. Gastrointestinal—hematemesis, occult blood in stools.
   E. Genitourinary—hematuria.

Problems

I. Altered renal function secondary to vascular changes of the disease.
II. Altered gastrointestinal function secondary to vascular changes of the disease.
III. Pain.
IV. Informational needs for family and patient regarding disease and treatment.

Goals of Care

I. Observe for adequate renal function.
II. Observe for adequate gastrointestinal function.
III. Encourage patient to assume activities of daily living with pain relief.
IV. Inform patient and family about disease and treatment.

Intervention

I. Observe for adequate renal function:
   A. Record intake and output, observing for altered renal function.
   B. Observe patterns of hemoglobinuria, hematuria, proteinuria; report an increase in frequency or amount.
   C. With maintenance intake (1500 to 1800 mL/m^2 per 24 h) urine output should be 400 to 1000 mL/m^2 per 24 h.
II. Observe for adequate GI function:
   A. Evaluate stool daily for occult blood.
   B. Record consistency, color, and frequency of stools.
   C. With hematemesis, suggest patient be NPO.
   D. Suggest diet modifications with blood in stool—consult dietitian for minimally irritating diet.
III. Encourage patient to assume activities of daily living when pain has been relieved.
   A. Administer steroids as ordered to minimize symptoms of HSP and associated pain.
   B. Have alternate pain medications available.

   C. Monitor and report complaints of abdominal pain, since infection and intussusception are possible.
   D. Encourage activity as tolerated.
IV. Inform patient and family about disease and treatment.
   A. Counsel patient and family regarding course of disease and precautions.
   B. Counsel regarding side effects of steroids. (See "Aplastic Anemia.")

Evaluation

I. Aberrations in renal or gastrointestinal function are prevented or detected promptly and treated.
II. Pain is controlled.
III. Family demonstrates understanding of disease and treatment.

HISTIOCYTOSIS

Definition

Histiocytosis is a disease category which includes several overlapping syndromes. *Eosinophilic granuloma* (EG) is the mildest disorder and consists of lytic lesions of the bones of the skull. Frequently there are tender, sometimes elevated areas over the radiologically well-circumscribed lesions. EG may progress to more severe syndromes or may resolve with or without treatment. There is no involvement of skin, viscera, or other soft tissues.

Hand-Schüller-Christian syndrome (HSC) is an eosinophilic granulomatous lesion of the skeleton, viscera, or skin, and carries an optimistic prognosis. *Letterer-Siwe* disease (LS) is a malignant form of eosinophilic granulomatous disease seen primarily in infants and involving skin, bones, and organs. The outset of LS is marked by systemic symptoms of fever, weight loss, and malaise with apparent skin and/or skeletal lesions. Radiologically, the skeletal lesions of HSC and LS have sharp, nonreactive borders. The liver, spleen, and lymph nodes may or may not present with evidence of disease in LS and HSC. Exophthalmos, diabetes insipidus, pulmonary infiltrates, and retarded growth and development can be observed with the more extensive involvement of eosinophilic granulomatous diseases.

Diagnosis is confirmed by surgical excision and histologic evaluation of the suspicious area. EG is treated by curettage and/or radiation therapy. With HSC and LS, cytotoxic drugs (steroids, vinblastine, nitrogen mustard, Cytoxan, methotrexate, 6-mercaptopurine, Chlorambucil) have been used, as well as curettage and radiation. Younger children are in the poorest prognostic category of histiocytosis. Disseminated disease at diagnosis also has a poor prognostic index. In all cases, response to therapy is slow.

Assessment

Data sources are the patient, the parents, and the patient's past medical record.
I. Health history.
   A. Recent fever, weight loss, malaise (HSC, LS).
   B. Polyuria, polydipsia (usually LS, though can be HSC as well).
   C. Bony lesions (EG, HSC, LS).
II. Physical assessment.
   A. Height, weight—plot on growth curve, within normal limits.
   B. Skin—presence of granulomatous lesions on skin, scalp; pallor.
   C. Eyes—exophthalmos (LS, sometimes HSC).
   D. Abdomen—increase in liver/spleen size (LS, sometimes HSC).
   E. Lymph nodes—presence of palpable, tender, immobile nodes (LS, HSC).
   F. Skeletal—bony lesions or nodules (EG, HSC, LS).

Problems

I. Potential progression of disease.
II. Potential complications from therapy (HSC, LS).
III. Potential endocrine imbalance.

Goals of Care

I. Monitor for sites of exacerbation of disease.
II. Educate patient and parents regarding disease and therapy.
III. Monitor endocrine status.

Intervention

I. Monitor for sites of exacerbation of disease:
   A. Measure and describe cutaneous lesions at regular intervals (i.e., every 2 to 3 months).
      1. It is helpful to measure the skeletal lesions on x-rays of the skull.
      2. Inspect for new lesions.
   B. Evaluate lymph nodes, spleen, and liver size at regular intervals.
   C. Evaluate chest for evidence of disease:
      1. X-rays.
      2. History of cough, congestion.
II. Educate patient and parents regarding disease and therapy:
   A. Inform patient and parents about the specifics of the diagnosed condition (i.e., EG is a mild form of histiocytosis). Include treatment in discussion.
   B. If drug therapy is used, counsel regarding side effects. Generally, side effects may include myelosuppression, increased susceptibility to infections, and mild nausea.
   C. If radiation therapy is used, counsel regarding side effects:
      1. Temporary loss of hair in radiation field.
      2. Temporarily decreased skin integrity in field of radiation; skin may be more sensitive to sun, irritants.
      3. If cranial radiation is used, may have some temporary nausea or vertigo.
      4. Long-range—hypofunction of gland or organ in radiation field, such as loss of salivary gland function when radiating mandibular area.
III. Monitor endocrine status:
   A. Evaluate urine regularly for specific gravity (to rule out diabetes insipidus).
   B. Obtain a careful history regarding fluid intake and output at regular intervals (to rule out diabetes insipidus).
   C. Monitor height and weight.

Evaluation

I. Evidence of progressive disease or complications is detected promptly.
II. Disease and therapy are well understood by family.

STORAGE DISEASES (NIEMANN-PICK DISEASE AND GAUCHER'S DISEASE)

Definition

Niemann-Pick and *Gaucher's* diseases are two examples of a condition in which lipid materials are abnormally stored in various systems. The initial sites of the deposition are generally in the reticuloendothelial system. Although both diseases have various presenting signs and symptoms, there is generally a psychomotor component, including mental retardation, indicative of storage deposits in the central nervous system; hepatosplenomegaly; and a decreased life-span. The earlier the disease presents, the earlier death may occur.

A liver biopsy is performed to confirm the diagnosis and presence of storage cells in the liver. The primary means of differentiating between the two diseases is biochemical.

The treatment is generally palliative and supportive and may include antibiotics and transfusions. The diseases have a predilection for occurring in families of Semitic origin and are transmitted as autosomal recessive disorders. An important aspect of treatment includes genetic counseling.

Assessment

Data sources are the parents, the patient, the patient's past medical record, and the extended family history.
I. Health history.
   A. Presence of similar symptoms in immediate family and/or extended family.
   B. Any known disease history from previous generations.
   C. Growth and developmental history: retardation of gross motor, fine motor, language and psychosocial skills.
II. Physical assessment.
   A. Skin—brown pigmentation.
   B. Abdomen—hepatosplenomegaly.
   C. Lymph nodes—palpable, nonmobile, sometimes tender.
   D. Neurologic evaluation—loss of gross motor function, fine motor, and speech and social interactional skills; hyporeflexia; mental retardation.

Problems

I. Disease-induced neurologic deficits.
II. Disease-induced pancytopenia.
III. Possible parental knowledge deficit regarding the storage disease, side effects, and treatment.
IV. Altered family function with diagnosis of a potentially fatal familial disease.

Goals of Care

I. Monitor neurologic status.
II. Monitor hematologic status.
III. Provide genetic counseling.
IV. Support the family in moving toward a state of psychosocial health.

Intervention

I. Monitored neurologic status:
   A. Use a standard neurological evaluation tool (i.e., DDST, Washington Developmental), to monitor progression of the disease.
   B. Encourage tasks achievable and appropriate for development of child.
   C. Discuss methods of stimulating child with parents and other care providers.
   D. Be prepared to use supportive measures, such as gavage feeding.
   E. See Chap. 19 for details of care for neurologically impaired children.

II. Monitored hematologic status: see "Aplastic Anemia."
III. Genetic counseling:
    A. Include information about the disease process.
    B. Facilitate parental understanding of the probability of having future offspring with storage diseases.
IV. Support the family in moving toward an equilibrium:
    A. Identify and include important support persons in discussions of care.
    B. Observe for guilt feelings on the part of parents and encourage openness in communication among care-givers.
    C. Reinforce decisions that incorporate appropriate growth and development needs for child and parents.

Evaluation

I. Developmental level is assessed and care is appropriate to developmental level (stimulation, protection, etc.).
II. Avoidable complications of neurologic disease (injuries or aspiration during convulsion, etc.) do not occur.
III. Avoidable complications of hematologic disorders (anemia, etc.) and treatment (drugs, transfusions, etc.) do not occur. See "Aplastic Anemia."
IV. Parents are well informed about the disease course and therapy.
V. Family members avail themselves of genetic counseling.
VI. Family receives the psychosocial supportive services needed to maximize individual coping and family function.

IMMUNOGLOBULIN DEFICIENCY

Definition

Immunoglobulin deficiency includes disorders of varying severity. Transient hypogammaglobulinemia is a frequently occurring condition in childhood, resolving over a period of months. Isolated deficiencies of IgG, IgA, IgM, IgD, and IgE have been documented as a second example. A third classification is X-linked agammaglobulinemia, which represents an absence of IgA, IgM, and IgD with an absence of lymphocytes and lowered levels of IgG. Finally, severe combined immunodeficiency is a disease incorporating an absence of B- and T-cell lymphocyte function with a deficiency of immunoglobulins.

On presentation, the child may have a history of repeated infections which have not responded to traditional antibiotic therapy. Malabsorption and failure to thrive are two other presenting sequelae.

In addition to measuring immunoglobulins to ascertain their decreased or absent function, good medical practice includes testing for the delayed hypersensitivity mechanism through skin tests, such as streptokinase-streptodornase (SKSD) or *Candida.* Titers may be obtained to evaluate the antibody response to foreign antigens produced by immunizations. It is important *never* to give a live attenuated virus or live virus of any kind, as the child can succumb to an overwhelming infection from the instilled organism.

Treatment of an immunoglobulin deficiency entails replacement with gammaglobulins, which should be given for symptomatic control in mild cases and regularly with severe deficiencies. If the child does not improve on gammaglobulin therapy, fresh frozen plasma is an alternative. The child should find a "buddy" if possible. A "buddy" is a person who can consistently offer plasma for the child. Such donor consistency minimizes complications such as hepatitis. The long-term prognosis is variable and depends on the severity of the disease. Prognosis is guarded in the severe immunodeficiencies.

Assessment

Data sources are the patient, the parents, and the patient's past medical history.

I. Health history.
  A. History of recent infection.
  B. Cough, productive or nonproductive.
  C. Skin infections.
  D. Malabsorption, diarrhea.
  E. Weight loss or poor weight gain.
II. Physical assessment.
  A. General—evaluate thoroughly for sites of infection.
  B. Height, weight.
  C. Skin—lesions or inflamed areas, pallor.
  D. Nose—rhinorrhea.
  E. Chest—rhonchi, rales; cough.
  F. Lymph nodes and tonsillar tissue are present.

Problems

I. Altered immunologic defense mechanisms with propensity for overwhelming infection.
II. Altered gastrointestinal function and malnutrition.
III. Potential alteration of homeostasis secondary to gammaglobulin therapy.
IV. Potential altered well-being secondary to disease.

Goals of Care

I. Maximum protection from overwhelming infection.
II. Optimal nutrition.
III. Observation for tolerance of gammaglobulin therapy.
IV. Maintenance of optimal self-image secondary to the side effects of disease and treatment.

Intervention

I. Maximum protection is given for complications of overwhelming infection (see "Neutropenia").
II. Optimal nutrition:
  A. Suggest a high protein, high caloric diet. Consult dietitian regarding specific dietary deficiencies.
  B. Take daily weights (if hospitalized), and weekly weight evaluations at home.
  C. Monitor character and consistency of bowel movements.
III. Observation and promotion of tolerance of gammaglobulin therapy:
  A. Rotate injection sites.
  B. Observe injection sites for signs of abscess formation.
  C. Use of warm compresses on injection area after instillation of gammaglobulin.
  D. Encourage use of muscle after injection. Counsel patient/parents regarding tenderness around injection site.

Evaluation

I. Avoidable infections do not occur.
II. Nutritional status is maximal.

III. Preventable complications of therapy do not occur.

IV. Family demonstrates understanding of disease course and therapy, and copes well.

V. Child's adjustment and development are maximal.

WISKOTT-ALDRICH SYNDROME

Definition

Wiskott-Aldrich syndrome is an X-linked recessive condition, characterized by thrombocytopenia, eczematous dermatitis, immunoglobulin deficiency of IgM and an increase in IgA, decreased lymphocytes, and a subsequent susceptibility to a variety of infectious agents. The condition may be diagnosed early in life by a family history of the disease and occurrence of thrombocytopenia in a child. The problems associated with the syndrome range from hemorrhage to infections to the possibility of developing a malignancy. Temporary joint inflammations have been observed.

Symptomatic treatment is the primary mode of intervention. Although splenectomy is used to intervene with ITP, it is not advantageous in the thrombocytopenia of Wiskott-Aldrich syndrome, since the removal of the spleen increases the risk of death by infection.

A further differentiation between ITP and Wiskott-Aldrich is that the immunoglobulins and isohemagglutinins in ITP are normal, whereas in Wiskott-Aldrich the values are not normal. A complete history can be quite helpful in combination with the lab data for confirming the compilation of symptoms characteristic of Wiskott-Aldrich syndrome.

Assessment

Data sources are the parents, the patient, the extended family, and the patient's past medical record.

I. Health history.

A. Family history, noting presence of similar symptoms in extended family.

B. Infant deaths in immediate family.

C. Recent or presenting otitis media, meningitis, pneumonia, generalized sepsis.

II. Physical assessment.

A. Temperature—increased.

B. Skin—eczema on face, arms, hands; petechial lesions, ecchymotic areas.

C. Evidence of infection.

Problems

I. Increased susceptibility to serious bleeding.

II. Decreased defense mechanisms to infection.

III. Altered skin integrity (eczema).

IV. Potential altered self-concept secondary to disease and treatment.

Goals of Care

I. Prevention of bleeding.

II. Maximum protection from infectious agents.

III. Maximum skin care.

IV. Maintenance of self-concept with an understanding of disease and treatment.

Intervention

I. Prevention of bleeding (see "Aplastic Anemia").
II. Maximum protection from infectious agents.
   A. See guidelines in "Neutropenia," with particular attention to detection of infection.
   B. Use bacteriostatic (Betadine) skin preparation before invasive procedures.
III. Maximum skin care.
   A. Keep skin clean.
   B. Keep skin well lubricated to prevent cracking.
   C. Watch for erythematous, edematous areas, as skin infections are common.
   D. Steroid creams may be used for eczema.
IV. Maintenance of self-concept with an understanding of disease and treatment.
   A. Identify strengths and weaknesses of family system, support figures.
   B. Watch for feelings of guilt on part of child or parents.
   C. Reinforce decisions that incorporate normal growth and development needs.
   D. Provide an understanding of disease and treatment and measures patient and family may take to prevent complications.

Evaluation

I. Avoidable bleeding does not occur.
II. Avoidable infections do not occur.
III. Skin integrity is maximal.
IV. Child's adjustment and development are adequate.
V. Family members avail themselves of genetic counseling.
VI. Parents demonstrate understanding of the disease course and therapy, and cope adequately.

BIBLIOGRAPHY

Beck, W. S. (ed.): *Hematology,* The Massachusetts Institute of Technology Press, Cambridge, 1973. This collection of lectures provides an abbreviated explanation and review of blood disorders. Although not as comprehensive as some other texts, it provides a quick reference.

DeAngelis, C., M. Guthneck, N. Straub, and J. Smith: "Introduction of New Foods into the Newborn and Infant Diet," *Issues in Comprehensive Pediatric Nursing,* **1**:23–33, April 1977. Although this article is not exhaustive, it presents good suggestions and guidelines for infant diets with adequate vitamins, minerals, and calories.

Feudenberg, H. H., D. P. Stites, J. L. Caldwell, and J. V. Wells: *Basic and Clinical Immunology,* Lange Medical Publications, Los Altos, Calif., 1976. This book explains basic immunology. It contains concise information about pathophysiology, diagnostic tests, and treatment. Specific immunologic phenomena are presented as they pertain to various diseases and body systems.

Greene, Trish, et al. (eds.): "Cancer in Children," *Nursing Clinics of North America,* **2**(1):1–114, 1976. These nine papers, written by practicing nurse-specialists in leading cancer treatment centers, address the following issues: therapy for acute leukemia, care of the child on immunosuppressive therapy, outpatient care, bone marrow transplantation, immunotherapy, psychosocial reactions, care of the dying child, and care by parents.

Honig, G. R.: "Sickling Syndromes in Children," *Advances in Pediatrics,* **23**:271–313, 1976. This excellent article should be required reading for those participating in the care of children with sickling syndromes. Differences are delineated among sickle cell disease, sickle trait, and sickle thalassemia. A lengthy bibliography is included.

Nathan, D. G., and F. A. Oski: *Hematology of Infancy and Childhood,* W. B. Saunders Company, Philadelphia, 1974. This fine book is both comprehensive and easy to understand. It describes hematologic pathophysiology and treatment from infancy through adolescence.

Pearson, H. A., and J. E. Robinson: "The Role of Iron in Host Resistance," *Advances in Pediatrics,* **23**:1–33, 1976. There are few discussions of iron therapy which are as understandable. The authors encourage an analytical evaluation of the use of iron as opposed to flagrant use of iron for anemias and infections.

Rudolph, A. M. (ed.): *Pediatrics,* 16th ed., Appleton Century Crofts, New York, 1977. This is the current edition of the earlier text edited by Barnett. It is one of the most comprehensive pediatric texts and presents recent statistical data.

Sutow, W. W., T. J. Vietti, and D. J. Fernbach: *Clinical Pediatric Oncology,* The C. V. Mosby Company, St. Louis, 1973. This comprehensive text includes discussions of the principles and implications of childhood cancer and its treatment. Illustrations and diagrams are used extensively.

16
The Gastrointestinal System
Elizabeth Butler Marren and Linda M. Burton

GENERAL ASSESSMENT

I. Health history.
  A. Note any presenting complaints, especially regarding elimination, pain, and feeding problems.
  B. Prenatal history: Explore possible guilt feelings the mother or father may have concerning condition of the child.
  C. Birth history: Note hypoxia, color, respiration, appearance (explore feelings of first viewing of baby with obvious defect).
  D. Neonatal history: What is the defecation, urination, and feeding pattern? Is there jaundice, any respiratory distress with feeding?
  E. Nutritional history to present time: Examine the feeding history of patient, the type and amount of formula and solids, tolerance of solids, vomiting, chewing, and weight gain or loss.
  F. Elimination: Note the defecation pattern. Is there constipation or diarrhea (type, amount, color, consistency, odor)?
  G. Developmental history: Is the child's behavior appropriate to the age, or are there delays?
  H. Are there any allergies to food, milk, or other substances?
  I. Family history: Note presence of any congenital defects, colitis, cancer, ulcers, pyloric stenosis, or colostomy in family.
  J. Socioeconomic factors: Note any pertinent information about the financial and housing situation of the family. Does the family have adequate support systems?
II. Physical assessment.
  A. Vital signs.
    1. General appearance: alert, irritable, thin, obese, presence of congenital deformities.
    2. Skin—pallor, cyanosis, jaundice, turgor, texture, hydration.
    3. Head—color of sclerae, defects of oral cavity, dentition.
    4. Chest—shape, respiration, retractions.
    5. Lungs—breath sounds, rate and quality of respirations.
    6. Abdomen—size, shape, distension, bowel sounds, palpable masses, liver, spleen size, hernias.
    7. Genital or rectal abnormalities—rectal tone, sphincter control, anal opening.
    8. Extremities—size, symmetry, muscle tone, range of motion.

OBSTRUCTIONS

Pyloric Stenosis

Definition   *Pyloric stenosis* is a progressive hypertrophy of the pyloric muscle at the outlet of the stomach. (See Fig. 16-1.) The cause is unknown. The highest incidence is in Caucasian males, and familial tendencies exist. The main symptom is vomiting, becoming projectile in the second to sixth week of life. The vomitus is not bile-stained, because the obstruction is proximal to the ampulla of Vater. There is weight loss, constipation, and excessive hunger; the infant sucks eagerly after vomiting. The medical treatment is pylorotomy.

Assessment

I. Preoperative:
  A. Feeding history: usually takes bottle eagerly after vomiting episode.
  B. Projectile vomiting.
  C. Observable peristaltic waves passing left to right during or after feeding.
  D. Palpable olive-sized mass (pylorus) in right upper quadrant.
  E. Dehydration, which may become severe as evidenced by weakness and lassitude, sunken fontanels and eyes, pale color; decrease in skin turgor; dry mucous membranes; absence of tears; decreased output of urine with a high specific gravity; rapid, shallow respirations; and rapid heart rate.
  F. Malnutrition and reduced body fat and muscle; weight loss.

II. Postoperative:
  A. Feeding: ability to retain feedings.
  B. Vomiting: type and amount.
  C. Incision: infection, redness, swelling, drainage.

Problems

I. Preoperative:
  A. Vomiting.
  B. Dehydration.
  C. Preparation of child and parents for surgery.
  D. Assess level of baby's development.

II. Postoperative:
  A. NPO initially.
  B. Reinstitution of oral feedings.
  C. Teaching parents feeding routine.
  D. Including parents in as much care and contact as possible.

Goals of Care

I. Preoperative:
  A. Prevent aspiration due to frequent vomiting episodes.
  B. Assist in restoring hydration and electrolyte balance.
  C. Prepare the child for surgery through adequate parenteral hydration, stomach decompression, chest physiotherapy.

II. Postoperative:
  A. Prevent vomiting due to pyloric edema and delayed peristalsis.
  B. Gradually increase type and amount of oral feedings to prevent vomiting.
  C. Overcome the parents' negative conditioning to baby's constant vomiting.
  D. Encourage maternal-infant bonding.

FIGURE 16-1 / (a) Normal pylorus. (b) Pyloric stenosis. Notice the hypertrophied muscle mass and narrowed lumen.

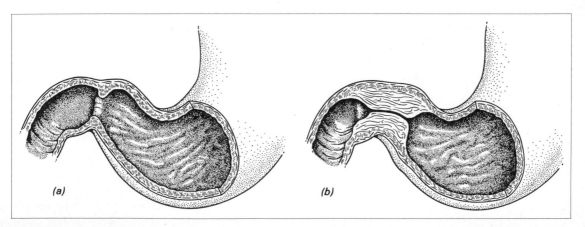

(a)   (b)

Intervention

I. Preoperative:
  A. Give and record feedings as prescribed.
  B. Keep accurate daily weight records.
  C. Observe and chart vomiting.
  D. Position baby on side or in infant seat.
  E. Give pacifier prn.
  F. Parenteral fluids.
  G. Use nasogastric tube to decompress stomach.
  H. Monitor intake and output.
  I. Prepare parents for surgery: appearance of child after surgery, where to wait, etc. Be honest in answering their questions.
II. Postoperative:
  A. NPO, usually 12 to 24 h.
  B. Administer parenteral fluids as prescribed until patient is able to tolerate oral feedings.
  C. Turning, humidity, pulmonary toilet.
  D. Monitor daily weights.
  E. Gradually increase oral feeding (half-strength glucose water to full-strength formula).
  F. Prevent aspiration due to vomiting by burping well and leaving upright for 60 min after feeding.
  G. Support parents in their effort to feed. Include them in patient's care, especially at feeding time.
  H. Involve parents in plan of care.
  I. Include visual stimuli for child, i.e., mobile, toy, colored pictures.
  J. Provide physical comfort for infant.
  K. Discharge teaching: Make sure parents understand wound care and feeding techniques. Mother and father may need help with routine newborn care. Home nurse referral.

Evaluation

I. The infant responds to parenteral therapy with adequate hydration.
II. There are no respiratory complications.
III. The patient retains oral feedings after surgery.
IV. The parents exhibit feeding skills.

Case Study

Dan B. was a 5-week-old white male admitted to a pediatric surgical unit with a 2-week history of increasingly severe vomiting after feedings. For the 4 days previous to admission he had vomited regularly 1 h after feeding. The vomitus was often projected 1 ft or more into the air. It was described as undigested food without bile. The parents had seen peristaltic waves. Dan had lost 300 g in the 5 days preceding admission.

Mr. and Mrs. B. were 20 years old, and Dan was their first baby. There was no family history of pyloric stenosis. Dan had had his first health maintenance visit to his pediatrician.

Physical examination revealed a thin, long, white male with visible peristaltic waves from the left upper quadrant to the right upper quadrant, and an olive-sized mass palpable in the right upper quadrant.

The parents expressed concern over Dan's vomiting and weight loss. The mother spoke with frustration about her "inability to feed" her child. The nurse discussed these feelings with Mr. and Mrs. B. and reassured them that nothing they did or did not do caused the vomiting.

Preoperative nursing included placing the baby NPO and inserting a nasogastric tube on low intermittent suction. The tube drained clear fluid without bile. An IV of 5% dextrose in normal saline was begun. Intake and output (urine bag) were measured. The urine specific gravity was 1.006. Abdominal girth was measured every 2 h with vital signs. Dan was positioned in a cardiac chair.

He went to surgery within 18 h for a pylorotomy. On his return from the recovery room, he was awake and alert. The nasogastric tube was disconnected after 12 h and he was put on a schedule of gradually increasing oral feedings, starting with 10 mL of glucose water.

By 24 h after surgery he tolerated 10 mL of formula every 3 h. There had been no postoperative vomiting. The IV was discontinued.

Postoperative care included wound care, measurement of intake and output with urine specific gravity, elevation in a cardiac chair, and observation and recording of Dan's tolerance of oral feedings. Mr. and Mrs. B. were included in his care and Mrs. B., who was rooming in, gave him most of his feedings. She was encouraged to express her concerns about Dan's feedings and his past history of vomiting, and her frustration lessened in the absence of postoperative vomiting. The parents demonstrated a good understanding of the disease process and the need for follow-up care. Dan was discharged 4 days after surgery.

Malrotation and Volvulus

Definition

Malrotation is an abnormality of intestinal rotation in embryologic development. Instead of the cecum and terminal ileum rotating across the peritoneal cavity to lie in the right lower quadrant, the process is arrested and they lie in the right upper quadrant. The duodenum may be compressed and become obstructed. Because the mesentery is not firmly attached to the abdominal wall, twisting of the small intestine (*volvulus*) may occur. The volvulus may wrap around the mesentery, causing bowel strangulation. Symptoms occur in the first 3 weeks of life and include vomiting, abdominal distension, and failure to pass stools. The medical treatment is the surgical correction of malposition and resection of bowel with impaired circulation.

Assessment

I. Bile-stained vomitus.
II. Absence of stool, especially in first 24 h of life.
III. Bloody mucoid drainage from rectum.
IV. Abdominal distension.

Problems

I. Preoperative:
   A. Risk of aspiration due to vomiting.
   B. Nasogastric tube to decompress stomach.
   C. Shock due to blood loss.
   D. Electrolyte imbalance due to loss of electrolytes in vomitus (containing bile, gastrointestinal fluids, pancreatic enzymes).
   E. Preparation of family for surgery.
      1. Prognosis guarded.
      2. Bonding may be impaired due to critical condition of infant.
      3. Assessment of parents' ability to cope with prognosis.
II. Postoperative: possibility of ileostomy.
   A. Intravenous fluids.
   B. NPO until peristalsis returns.
   C. Continue nasogastric suction.
   D. Wound care.
   E. Vomiting may occur.
   F. Postoperative diarrhea.
   G. Needs for:
      1. Stoma care.
      2. Normal newborn care.
      3. Outpatient follow-up.

Goals of Care

I. Preoperative:
   A. Prevent aspiration due to vomiting.
   B. Record type of vomitus.
   C. Record type or absence of stool.
   D. Prepare family for surgery.
II. Postoperative:
   A. Maintain IV fluids adequate for hydration.
   B. Maintain patency of nasogastric tube.
   C. Prevent aspiration of vomitus.
   D. Observe and chart type of stool.
   E. Provide patient with visual and tactile stimulation.
   F. Prepare parents for home care.

Evaluation

    I. Early recognition of symptoms of shock is essential.
   II. Early recognition of electrolyte imbalance is essential.
 III. Parents cope adequately with their child's surgery.
 IV. The stool assumes normal consistency and color.
  V. The child tolerates oral feedings postoperatively.
 VI. Postoperative complications are avoided.
VII. The child and the parent-child relationship develop satisfactorily.

Intussusception

Definition

Intussusception is invagination or "telescoping" of a portion of the intestine into a more distal segment (see Fig. 16-2). It is three times more common in males than females. The majority of patients are Caucasians 6 months to 2 years old. A barium enema may succeed in reducing intussusception by hydrostatic pressure. If not, surgery is performed.

Assessment

   I. Sudden onset of severe abdominal pain (draws legs to abdomen, shrill cry).
  II. Bile-stained emesis.
 III. "Currant jelly" stools (brown, bloody, mucoid).
 IV. Palpable sausagelike mass along transverse or ascending colon.

Problems

I. Preoperative:
  A. Severe abdominal pain.
  B. Vomiting.
  C. Possibility of bowel rupture and peritonitis.

FIGURE 16-2 / Intussusception. Small bowel is invaginated and passed by peristalsis into the cecum. Bowel obstruction and ischemia result.

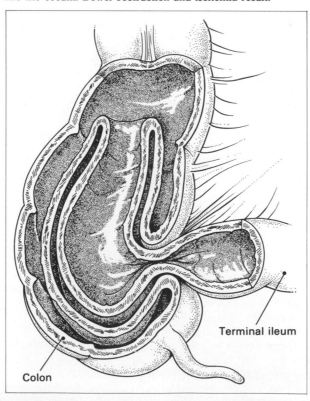

Terminal ileum

Colon

  II. After barium enema: prepare family for discharge 24 to 48 h after procedure.

  III. Postoperative:

   A. Incision care.

   B. Reestablishment of peristalsis.

   C. Parent teaching.

Goals of Care

  I. Preoperative:

   A. Control pain.

   B. Prevent aspiration of vomitus.

   C. Report any increase in the severity of symptoms indicative of shock and peritonitis: high heart rate, high respiratory rate, low blood pressure, low or high temperature, lethargy, pallor, increased abdominal distension.

   D. After barium enema: increase parents' confidence in caring for child by involving them in early care.

  II. Postoperative:

   A. Ensure adequate nasogastric tube drainage through observation of drainage, irrigation, repositioning.

   B. Ensure adequate hydration by maintenance of IV fluids.

   C. Prevent wound infection.

   D. Prepare parents for discharge through teaching about wound care, diet, necessity of outpatient follow-up.

Intervention

  I. Preoperative:

   A. Relieve pain through positioning.

   B. Record vomiting: type, amount.

   C. Record stools; type, amount.

   D. Monitor vital signs frequently.

   E. Measure intake and output.

   F. Report signs of shock.

   G. Take *axillary temperatures*, rather than rectal.

  II. After barium enema:

   A. Gradually increase feeding as prescribed.

   B. Prepare parents for discharge.

  III. Postoperative:

   A. Maintain patency of nasogastric tube.

   B. Monitor IV fluids.

   C. Measure intake and output.

   D. Take daily weight.

   E. Monitor incision care.

   F. Increase feedings as ordered.

   G. Instruct parents for discharge.

   H. Provide for as normal parent-child interaction as possible.

Evaluation

  See "Malrotation and Volvulus."

Meckel's Diverticulum

Definition

  Meckel's diverticulum is an outpouching of the terminal ileum resulting from incomplete obliteration of the yolk stalk which feeds the embryo in early gestation. The lining of the diverticulum contains aberrant acid-secreting gastric mucosa which produces symptoms that simulate peptic ulcer. Intestinal obstruction can occur (see Fig. 16-3). Medical treatment is resection of the diverticulum and anastomosis.

Assessment

  Massive, sometimes painless rectal bleeding is present, with shock secondary to blood loss or peritonitis. There is usually abdominal pain.

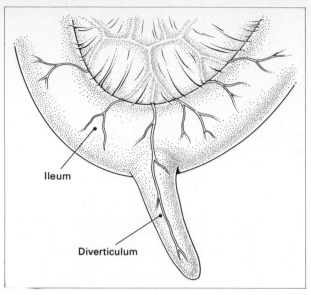

FIGURE 16-3 / Meckel's diverticulum, a blind pouch resulting from incomplete closure of an embryonic duct.

Problems

   I. Preoperative:
      A. Rectal bleeding.
      B. Shock.
      C. Possible perforation, leading to peritonitis.
  II. Postoperative: As for other gastrointestinal surgery.

Goals of Care

   I. Preoperative: early detection and prompt control of shock.
  II. Postoperative: same as for other gastrointestinal surgery.

Intervention

   I. Preoperative:
      A. Monitor vital signs.
      B. Measure intake and output:
         1. Diaper weights (1 mL urine weighs approximately 1 g).
         2. Urine specific gravity.
         3. Daily weight.
         4. Measure nasogastric tube output.
         5. Check stool for blood.
      C. Observe for rectal bleeding.
      D. Monitor intravenous fluids, which may include blood or plasma.
  II. Postoperative: same as for any gastrointestinal surgery.

Evaluation

See "Malrotation and Volvulus."

Inguinal Hernia

Definition

The testicle normally descends into the scrotum, preceded by the peritoneal sac, in the seventh month of gestation. If this sac does not close off, there is a potential opening for the intestine to descend into the inguinal canal, producing a hernia. If the intestine becomes trapped and cannot be reduced, the hernia is said to be *incarcerated*. *Strangulation* (obstruction and circulatory compromise) of intestine is common in children with hernias. The medical treatment is herniorrhaphy.

Assessment I. Palpable mass in the inguinal area, especially with straining.
II. Symptoms of partial bowel obstruction include:
  A. Fretfulness.
  B. Anorexia, vomiting.
  C. Pain and tenderness in inguinal area.
  D. Irreducible mass.
  E. Decreased bowel sounds.
III. Symptoms of complete bowel obstruction include:
  A. Shock.
  B. High temperature.
  C. Absent bowel sounds.
  D. High white blood count.
  E. Bloody stool.

Problems I. Preoperative:
  A. Straining increases risk of incarceration.
  B. Incarcerated hernia is a surgical emergency.
  C. Preparation of child and family for surgery.
II. Postoperative:
  A. Ambulation.
  B. Respiratory toilet.
  C. Resumption of feeding.
  D. Wound care.

Goals of Care I. Preoperative:
  A. Prevent incarceration through prevention of straining.
  B. Observe for obstruction.
  C. Prepare child psychologically for surgery.
  D. Inform and assist parents regarding surgery.
II. Postoperative:
  A. Stasis pneumonia can be prevented by having the patient turn, cough, and deep breathe. Blowing up a balloon with a mouthpiece is helpful.
  B. The reestablishment of peristalsis can be determined by the presence of flatus, bowel sounds, and stool.
  C. Prevent wound infection.
  D. Prepare for discharge by involving parents in care as soon as feasible.

Intervention I. Preoperative:
  A. For simple hernia, prevent straining.
    1. Decrease crying by keeping child quiet and contented.
    2. Prevent constipation through regulation of diet.
  B. If incarceration is present, *do not attempt to reduce hernia* (perforation may result).
    1. NPO.
    2. Sedation prn as prescribed.
    3. IV fluids.
    4. Nasogastric tube.
    5. Control fever using Tylenol, if prescribed, and cool baths.
    6. Monitor vital signs frequently.
    7. Use Trendelenburg's position.
    8. Preoperative teaching to relieve child's and parents' anxiety is necessary.
II. Postoperative:
  A. Observe for return of peristalsis.
  B. Respiratory care.
  C. Gradually increase diet as tolerated.
  D. Early ambulation.
  E. Wound care.

    III. Discharge teaching for the parents:
        A. The child must avoid straining.
        B. There must be no strenuous play for 1 month, including bicycling.
        C. Parents must observe wound for any signs of redness, warmth, and drainage.
        D. They must understand the importance of scheduled outpatient care.

Evaluation

    I. The child and family are adequately prepared for surgery.
    II. Parents and child understand discharge teaching as demonstrated through verbal feedback.
    III. Postoperative complications do not occur.

Umbilical Hernia

Definition

An *umbilical hernia* is a protrusion of the small intestine at the umbilicus, due to imperfect closure of the umbilical ring. Usually, spontaneous closure occurs before the fourth year. Strangulation is rare in children. The incidence of umbilical hernia is increased in blacks, premature babies, and in infants with hypothyroidism.

    Abdominal binders are contraindicated. They do not help correct the hernia and may lead to skin breakdown and umbilical infection. The "home remedy" of taping a coin over the hernia is decidedly dangerous. The medical treatment is surgery, but only if the hernia is very large and increasing in size.

    Nursing care is as for inguinal hernia, except peristalsis is delayed and the child is NPO until bowel activity returns. Gradually increase diet from clear liquids. Postoperative vomiting is not unusual. Use a pressure dressing on incision.

    The evaluation is the same as for inguinal hernia.

INFLAMMATORY DISORDERS

Necrotizing Enterocolitis (NEC)

Definition

Necrotizing enterocolitis (NEC), a condition of newborns, primarily premature babies, is characterized by ischemic necrosis of the small bowel. The cause is poorly understood, but perinatal hypoxia has been implicated. It is suspected that hypoxia causes a protective shunting of blood from the mesenteric vascular bed to the vital organs (heart, brain, kidneys). The intestinal cells are consequently damaged so that they stop secreting protective mucus, and autodigestion ensues. Symptoms occur in the first 2 or 3 weeks of life. Bowel perforation and overwhelming sepsis often result and may be fatal. Studies have linked glucose and formula feeding of hypoxic infants with NEC. Breast milk may protect against the disease through the induction of passive enteric immunity.

    Medical treatment includes GI decompression and broad-spectrum antibiotics; bowel resection with colostomy or ileostomy.

Assessment

Observe premature infant for:

    I. Jaundice.
    II. Apnea.
    III. Delayed gastric emptying.
    IV. Vomiting.
    V. Distension.
    VI. GI bleeding.
    VII. Bowel perforation.

Problems

    I. It is important to recognize the gradual onset of NEC, since successful treatment depends on early detection.
    II. Prepare family for possible surgery.
    III. Support family throughout the course of a grave illness.
    IV. Provide for needs of mother and infant for bonding.
    V. Provide for infant's needs for love, touch, and visual stimulation.
    VI. Be alert for postoperative "short bowel syndrome" due to removal of extensive portion of bowel.

Goals of Care   I. Early detection of impending NEC.
    II. Facilitation of survival and recovery.
   III. Assist family in understanding and coping with child's condition.

Intervention   I. Observe newborns, especially prematures and those with breathing difficulty, for inability to absorb glucose or formula feedings. Check food absorption by aspirating stomach contents through the nasogastric tube prior to feeding. Record amount of aspirate and stage of digestion. Return to stomach and subtract this total from present feeding.
    II. Observe and report symptoms of developing NEC:
       A. Abdominal distension.
       B. Ileus.
       C. Bloody or guiac-positive stools.
       D. Bile or bloodstained vomitus.
       E. Bradycardia.
       F. Sudden listlessness.
       G. Gray or cyanotic color, especially if baby is on a respirator.
   III. Measure abdominal girth, monitor vital signs.
   IV. Report any of the following:
       A. Abdominal girth increase of 1 cm or more.
       B. Elevated axillary temperature.
       C. Increased or decreased pulse, low blood pressure.
       D. Respiratory distress.
       E. Absent bowel sounds.
       F. Abdominal tenderness.
       G. Involuntary rigidity of abdominal wall.
    V. For infants who are diagnosed with NEC but have not yet had surgery:
       A. Adjust nasogastric tube to low intermittent suction. Maintain patency by irrigation prn.
       B. Administer antibiotics as prescribed.
       C. Culture blood, urine, and stool.
       D. Assess electrolytes, acid-base balance.
       E. Avoid abdominal trauma.
          1. Decrease activity of patient.
          2. Do not diaper; use pad under buttocks.
       F. Skin care to avoid breakdown:
          1. Expose buttocks to air and/or heat, light.
          2. Clean area meticulously after stool.
          3. Apply zinc oxide or aluminum paste to buttocks if necessary.
       G. Observe for signs of perforation.
       H. Support parents through ordeal using patience and frequent explanations. Allow them to touch their child and call and visit whenever possible.
   VI. Postoperative care of infant with colostomy or ileostomy:
       A. Insert intravenous line.
       B. Connect nasogastric tube to suction.
       C. Monitor vital signs, including axillary temperature, heart rate, respiratory rate, and blood pressure.
       D. Respiratory care should include repositioning (turning) of child and use of suction.
       E. Measure intake and output, including specific gravity of urine.
       F. Take daily weights.
       G. Stoma care:
          1. Stoma will be covered with vaseline gauze until resumption of stool.
          2. Use karaya gum sheet over abdomen.
          3. Use urine bags over stoma or collect stool on a 4- by 4-in pad secured with gauze wrapped around abdomen.
          4. Use zinc oxide or aluminum paste to protect surrounding areas of skin. If excoriated, put thickened amphogel on skin and sprinkle with karaya powder.
          5. Record amount, color, and consistency of stool.

H. Employ meticulous wound care to avoid contamination from stool.

I. Hyperalimentation.

J. Prepare parents before they visit their child by explaining what a colostomy or ileostomy is and how it functions.

K. Include parents in care of child as soon as possible to encourage bonding and familiarity with stoma care. Allow mother to supply breast milk if she desires. Encourage calls and visits.

Evaluation

I. The symptoms of impending or worsening NEC are recognized early.

II. The parents are able to express their fears about diagnosis and prognosis.

III. The skin around stoma does not become excoriated.

IV. The wound and hyperalimentation line do not become infected.

V. The baby does not exhibit signs of severe emotional withdrawal.

VI. The parents are able to cope and be involved in the child's care.

Case Study

Alex B. was a 995-g black male born at 31 weeks' gestation. Shortly after birth he experienced respiratory distress. His P_{O_2} was 38, P_{CO_2} 42, pH 7.26. He was placed on 50 percent oxygen. The chest x-ray revealed "ground glass" appearance of the lungs. He had frequent episodes of bradycardia with apnea. On the third day of life he was started on hyperalimentation and intralipids. On the fifth day he had not yet had a bowel movement without rectal stimulation, and began to have bile-colored emesis. The x-ray revealed free air in the abdomen. A diagnosis of necrotic bowel was made, and Alex was taken to surgery.

Alex's preoperative nursing included careful observation of vital signs, bowel movements, and respiratory adequacy; cutdown and hyperalimentation line care; strict intake and output; urine specific gravity; prevention of aspiration due to vomiting; measurement of abdominal girth with vital signs; care of nasogastric tube; and daily weights.

The surgical procedure was excision of the necrotic bowel and externalization of three stomas. Postoperatively Alex was on a respirator. He had a nasogastric tube to low intermittent suction. Hyperalimentation and intralipids were continued. Postoperative nursing was a real challenge, mainly because of his small size and the proximity of the stomas to his incision. A karaya sheet was applied to his abdomen wherever possible (not on the incision). Vaseline gauze was placed over the stomas, then small fluffs, and the dressings were wrapped around the abdomen with small Kling. No colostomy bags were used, and this necessitated *frequent* dressing changes. After the wound healed, small colostomy bags were used over the proximal stoma. The stomas were dilated with feeding tubes. Hyperalimentation and intralipids were continued for 5 months until the bowel was reanastomosed.

Oral feedings, begun after anastomosis, were poorly tolerated. Alex had frequent diarrhea. However, after 5 months of cutdowns and intravenous feedings, he had no more sites for a hyperalimentation line. Bile salts were added to his formula, which improved absorption and decreased the diarrhea.

Alex's parents visited him almost daily throughout his hospitalization and responded eagerly to nursing instruction about cuddling him and participating in his care. By the time of his discharge they knew how to feed him skillfully, give medicines, and recognize signs of dehydration. A community health nurse referral was made, and the hospital nurses kept in touch with the family by telephone for several days.

Appendicitis

Appendicitis with perforation can be a life-threatening problem in younger children. Although it is rare in the first 2 years of life (peak incidence is 15 to 21 years), the younger child is most seriously affected. This is because the omentum is very short; consequently, the infection is not well walled off and spreads quickly to generalized peritonitis. Early diagnosis is essential but difficult due to the nonspecificity of presenting symptoms.

Appendicitis is discussed at length in Chap. 29.

Gastroenteritis

Definition

Gastroenteritis is an inflammation of the gastrointestinal tract, either viral or bacterial in origin. The incidence and severity are highest in infancy and early childhood, when the dehydration resulting from vomiting and diarrhea can be life-threatening. Antidiarrheal medications are not usually very effective. Antiemetics may help control vomiting.

Assessment

I. Vomiting and frequent loose, watery stools.
II. Fever.
III. Dehydration.

Problems

I. Vomiting.
II. Diarrhea with possible skin breakdown.
III. Dehydration.
IV. Electrolyte imbalance.
V. Intravenous therapy.
VI. The child may be in restraints (because of IV).
VII. Acute separation of child from mother, interruption in developmental tasks.

Goals of Care

I. Administer intravenous fluids at rate and amount ordered by physician.
II. Observe child's condition carefully and report any signs of deterioration.
III. Prevent skin breakdown from frequent diarrhea.
IV. Prevent spread of infection.
V. Resume oral hydration as soon as tolerated.
VI. Meet child's developmental needs.
VII. Involve parents in care and meet their needs for support.

Intervention

I. Record response to oral feedings.
II. Observe and record vomiting type and frequency.
III. Observe and record stools: amount, frequency, color, odor.
IV. Observe and report symptoms of dehydration.
V. When NPO, give mouth care and pacifier.
VI. Administer intravenous fluids. Monitor flow rate, observe for infiltration. Child will be restrained.
VII. Care of child in restraints:
    A. Provide passive range of motion of restrained extremities during the child's bath and prn.
    B. Change position frequently.
    C. Position so that child does not aspirate vomitus.
VIII. Take daily weights (twice daily if child is severely dehydrated).
IX. Measure intake, output, and urine specific gravity. Use bag for urine or weigh diapers (1 mL urine weighs approximately 1 g).
X. Monitor vital signs, report temperature above 38.5°C, pulse above 130, respirations above 40.
XI. Assess activity and level of consciousness.
XII. Provide skin care, including frequent change of soiled diapers.
XIII. Institute isolation procedures, with careful hand-washing.
XIV. Reassure the child during procedures in understandable language. Hold child if mother is unavailable. Provide favorite toy, blanket, etc.
XV. Reinstate oral feedings, progressing as follows:
    A. Electrolyte solution.
    B. Clear liquids, bananas, rice, cereal, crackers, and toast.
    C. Half-strength formula or skimmed milk.
    D. Full-strength formula or whole milk.
XVI. Involve parents in care as much as possible.

Evaluation
I. The patient exhibits adequate hydration.
II. The buttocks do not become excoriated.
III. The intravenous line does not infiltrate.
IV. No other patients on unit develop symptoms due to poor technique.
V. Child develops well; parents cope and manage effectively.

TRAUMA

Corrosion Ingestion

Definition
The ingestion of caustic material such as lye, ammonia, acids, or bleach typically results in severe burns and inflammation of the mouth and esophagus. Esophageal scarring results in stricture. The age of peak incidence of ingestion is 18 months to 3 years.
Emergency care required at the time of ingestion is presented in Chap. 45.

Assessment
I. Child with recent injury:
   A. Burns in oral cavity.
   B. Degree of respiratory distress.
   C. Level of consciousness.
   D. Ability to swallow.
   E. Degree of pain.
II. Child with old injury and esophageal stricture:
   A. Ability to swallow.
   B. Psychological adjustment.
   C. Speech development.

Problems
I. Immediate:
   A. Edema of lips, cheeks, tongue, and pharynx.
   B. Respiratory distress due to edema and spasm of pharynx on swallowing.
   C. Possibility of tracheostomy.
   D. Parents' guilt.
   E. Child's pain and fright.
II. Long-range:
   A. Eating disturbances secondary to stricture.
   B. Psychological problems secondary to inability to eat normally, and secondary to repeated esophageal dilatation treatments.
   C. Possible speech defect secondary to oral scarring.

Goals of Care
I. Recognize and treat respiratory distress promptly.
II. Prevent strictures through medicinal regime.
III. Assist child and parents in coping.
IV. Facilitate child's psychological adjustment to long hospitalization and painful, difficult-to-understand procedures and treatments.
V. Teach parents about home safety for young children.
VI. Pave the way for parental cooperation with follow-up care which may be necessary (dilatations, speech therapy, psychological assistance).

Intervention
I. Child with recent injury:
   A. Have tracheostomy set at bedside.
   B. Monitor vital signs, observe for respiratory distress.
   C. Provide humidification.
   D. Medicate as prescribed (neutralizers of ingested substance, steroids).
II. Child with recent or old injury:
   A. Administer pain medicine as prescribed.
   B. Position for salivary drainage if unable to swallow.
   C. Restrain as necessary to protect IV and gastrostomy.
   D. Provide frequent mouth and facial skin care.

   E. Comfort measures for child:
    1. Parents should be present as much as possible.
    2. Have favorite toy from home.
    3. Explain and reassure as appropriate for age.
    4. Substitute oral activities as permitted for child who cannot eat (pacifier, blow toys).
   F. Assist parents with their feelings and the difficulties of long-term disability and treatment.
   G. Observe child for edema, bleeding, and respiratory distress following dilatations.
   H. Oral and/or gastrostomy feedings as prescribed. Observe for intolerance of feedings.

Evaluation
   I. Respiratory distress is minimized, detected promptly, and/or effectively dealt with.
   II. Skin complications are avoided (face, gastrostomy).
   III. Feedings as prescribed are well tolerated.
   IV. Parents cope well with guilt and fear.
   V. Child demonstrates good adjustment and developmental progress for age.
   VI. The child is able to cooperate during the dilatation with sedation or restraints.
   VII. The parents "child-proof" their house before discharge.
   VIII. On discharge the parents state their understanding of need for follow-up care.
   IX. On discharge the parents demonstrate proper method of feeding, either oral or gastrostomy.

CONGENITAL MALFORMATIONS

Cleft Lip and Palate

Definition
  These conditions are an abnormal development of the upper lip and palate, and may be extensive, involving premaxilla, maxilla, and tissues of the soft palate and uvula. Arrested embryonic fusion of premaxillary and maxillary processes results in a cleft lip; failure of the palatal process to fuse results in cleft palate. The two defects may occur separately or together. Genetic factors are contributory, but clefts may occur without a familial history.

  Cleft lip repair by a qualified plastic surgeon usually is done at 1 to 2 months of age with sufficient weight gain and absence of oral, respiratory, or systemic infections. Revisions are done later at 4 to 5 years. Palate surgery is postponed until a child is 12 to 18 months old, depending on the degree of deformity: if it is done too early, it may damage tooth buds; if it is done too late, the child may develop poor speech patterns. Subsequent revisions and reconstructions are delayed until adolescence, and are done when there is no infection present. Prognosis can be very good using the excellent skills of a competent plastic surgeon and with overall management for long-term care utilizing the multidisciplinary team. Parental acceptance and involvement is essential.

Assessment
   I. Deformity of upper lip.
   II. Opening in palate.

Problems
   I. Parent-child bonding.
   II. Nutrition.
   III. Prevention of infection both before and after surgery.
   IV. Coordination of cleft lip/palate team.
   V. Preoperative teaching.
   VI. Child needs to develop sense of identity and good self-image.
   VII. Parents need to accept infant with obvious defect.
   VIII. Initially, the psychological trauma to parents and other family members can be severe so it is imperative that they be allowed to ventilate feelings and be informed of prognosis.
   IX. Children with cleft palate are prone to otitis media (food enters eustachian tube) and resultant hearing loss.

     X. Child is in restraints after surgery.
    XI. Discharge planning.

Goals of Care

    I. Promote parents' relationship with obviously deformed baby.
    II. Establish adequate nutrition.
    III. Prevent infection both before and after surgery.
    IV. Coordinate efforts of cleft lip/palate team for optimum functioning.
    V. Prepare the child adequately to alleviate apprehension.
    VI. Prevent injury to suture site through use of restraints.
    VII. Prepare parents adequately for discharge care of child.

Intervention

    I. Immediately after birth and before repair:
        A. The nurse should show acceptance of infant, and support parents in immediate grief and guilt about having a deformed child.
        B. Because baby may not be able to suck due to inability to create a vacuum, consider different feeding devices:
            1. Lamb's nipple.
            2. Nipple for premature infants with holes enlarged.
            3. Asepto syringe with rubber tubing attached.
            4. Brecht feeder.
        C. Hold baby upright during feeding, feed slowly, and burp often.
        D. Decrease baby's contact with people who have colds or other infections.
        E. Team members usually include plastic surgeon, primary nurse, speech therapist, orthodontist, and ear, nose, and throat physician. The primary nurse should coordinate their efforts.
        F. Discharge teaching should include:
            1. Feeding technique.
            2. Avoidance of infection.
            3. Early recognition and prompt treatment of otitis media.
            4. Equipment to use at home.
            5. Visiting nurse referral if necessary.
    II. Following cleft lip repair:
        A. Elbow and limb restraints may be necessary.
        B. Do not allow child to lie face down or rub face on bed or pillow; position in infant seat or on side.
        C. Observe for respiratory distress.
        D. Give gentle suction of mouth and nose if ordered.
        E. Avoid stress on suture line, including that caused by crying.
        F. Care of suture line:
            1. Use of Logan bow.
            2. Cleansing with half-strength solution hydrogen peroxide on cotton swab after feeding.
            3. Application of antibiotic ointment as prescribed.
        G. Feedings should be by dropper or rubber-tipped syringe. *Do not allow baby to suck.* Generally, the child is on clear liquids until sutures are removed—3 to 14 days after surgery.
    III. Following cleft palate repair:
        A. Observe for respiratory distress.
        B. Use elbow and limb restraints.
        C. *Do not put anything into the mouth—no straws or nipples.*
        D. If packing is inserted, observe for bleeding and position on side to allow bloody mucus to drain.
        E. Humidify the environment.
        F. Feeding techniques: Give clear liquids, gradually increasing to a soft diet by cup or edge of spoon. Use a rubber-tipped syringe and rinse mouth with clear water after feedings.

G. Weigh daily.

H. Administer pain medicine as prescribed.

I. Encourage and assist parents to care for and comfort child.

J. Discharge instructions for parents should include:
1. Normal growth and development of child, emphasizing the tendency to put things in the mouth. Parent should use elbow restraints at home to prevent this.
2. Full liquid or soft diet should be continued at home.
3. Do not permit child to suck or blow.
4. Avoid infections and injury to operative site.
5. Stress the importance of close follow-up with surgeon, speech therapist, dentist, and audiologist.
6. Acquaint parents with financial aid available, as well as any parent groups or published material that may help them.
7. Support the parents and reinforce the expectation that the child can lead a normal life. Give positive reinforcement for parents' continued efforts.

Evaluation
I. The parents are able to care for the child at home by demonstrating feeding, positioning, and oral hygiene. Parents can describe the need and discuss means to prevent infection.
II. The child gains weight.
III. The temperature does not go above 38°C.
IV. Asphyxia and aspiration pneumonia do not develop.
V. There is no damage to the suture line after surgery.
VI. The child evidences a good self-concept and socialization.

Esophageal Atresia and Tracheoesophageal Fistula

Definition
Esophageal atresia is the abnormal embryonic development of the esophagus, resulting in the formation of a blind pouch or inadequately sized lumen preventing normal passage of materials (secretions and foods) from pharynx to stomach. *Tracheoesophageal fistula* is the abnormal development of a sinuslike passage between the esophagus and trachea. Several variations and combinations of the defect occur (see Fig. 16-4).

Esophageal atresia and tracheoesophageal fistula, alone or in combination, are life-threatening. Pneumonia and atelectasis or massive airway obstruction result from overflow of feedings and saliva from the blind upper esophageal pouch into the trachea and/or reflux of gastric secretions through the fistula into the respiratory tract. Surgical intervention is undertaken as soon as possible after the diagnosis is confirmed, but may be delayed if the infant is premature or critically ill, or if other major anomalies are present. Ligation of fistula is done immediately in most cases. End-to-end anastomosis of the esophagus is performed if parts are sufficiently long. Anastomosis may be deferred to allow for growth of the esophageal ends; in this event measures are taken to prevent pneumonia and provide nourishment. Construction of an esophagus by insertion of a colon segment may be done at 6 months to 2 years of age.

The prognosis for these defects depends upon early diagnosis, degree of prematurity, and coexistence of other serious defects. The survival rate for premature infants is 35 to 40 percent; that for full-term infants is 80 to 85 percent.

Assessment
I. Astute observation is imperative for early diagnosis in the newborn. Signs and symptoms of atresia/fistula appear soon after birth.
   A. Excessive mucal secretion and hypersalivation.
   1. Continuous drooling.
   2. Frothing from nose and mouth.
   B. Respiratory distress.
   1. Intermittent or circumoral cyanosis.
   2. Nasal flaring.
   3. Tachypnea.
   4. Retractions.
   5. Coarse or diminished breath sounds.
   6. Rales/rhonchi heard on auscultation.

C. Distended or scaphoid abdomen.
D. Dysphagia and inability to retain first feedings.
   1. Coughing and choking after first few swallows.
   2. Return of fluids through nose and mouth.
   3. Infant anxious and irritable.
   4. Cyanosis developing with above symptoms.
E. Fever or subnormal body temperature.
F. Inability to pass tubing through esophagus to stomach—stops in blind pouch at atretic site.

II. Evidence of esophageal stenosis in an older infant often may not appear until chopped or solid foods are started.
A. Child chokes and gags with solids.
B. Occasionally vomits undigested foods.
C. "Fussy eater."
D. Unable to pass nasogastric tube through to stomach.

Problems

I. Immediate and preoperative:
A. Danger of aspiration of excessive nasopharyngeal secretions.
B. Danger of reflux of gastric secretions into tracheobronchial tree.

FIGURE 16-4 / Esophageal atresia and tracheoesophageal fistulas. (a) Esophageal atresia with distal fistula. (b) Esophageal atresia without fistula. (c) Tracheoesophageal fistula without atresia. (d) Esophageal atresia with proximal fistula. (e) Esophageal atresia with proximal and distal fistulas. (f) Esophageal stenosis.

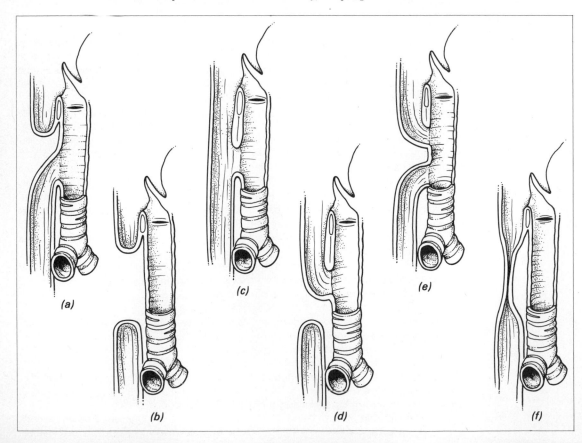

(a)   (b)   (c)   (d)   (e)   (f)

  C. Prematurity with fluctuant or subnormal body temperature.

  D. Need for fluids, electrolytes, and medications.

  E. Preparation for surgery.

 II. Postoperative:

  A. Essentially the same whether surgery is corrective or merely palliative.

  B. Continued danger of respiratory complications.

  C. Hydration and nutrition.

  D. Care of gastrostomy.

  E. Care of cervical esophagostomy.

  F. Care after esophageal reconstruction.

  G. Infant's emotional and developmental needs, and parental needs and involvement.

Goals of Care I. Immediate and preoperative:

  A. Support respirations and remove nasopharyngeal secretions, helping to prevent aspiration pneumonia.

  B. Prevent reflux of gastric juices into tracheobronchial tree, avoiding chemical pneumonia by properly positioning infant.

  C. Establish a controlled environment to maintain body temperature, provide humidity and oxygen, and help prevent infection.

  D. Administer fluids and medications as prescribed.

  E. Prepare for surgery and be prepared for emergency resuscitation and care.

 II. Postoperative:

  A. Provide intensive postoperative care, avoiding complications.

  B. Maintain a patent airway, prevent asphyxia, and prevent chemical pneumonia or pneumothorax.

  C. Monitor parenteral fluids and provide nutrition as ordered.

  D. Provide gastrostomy care and feedings effectively.

  E. Provide good care of cervical esophagostomy and promote adequate drainage of secretions.

  F. Provide care after esophageal reconstruction with care of left thoracotomy and laparotomy incisions.

  G. Provide infant with emotional stimulation.

  H. Support parents and encourage early acceptance of child and involvement to assure early bonding and attachment.

Intervention I. Immediate and preoperative:

  A. Support respirations.

   1. NPO.

   2. Begin immediate suctioning.

  B. Prevent gastric reflux by positioning infant with head and chest elevated 20 to 30°.

  C. Control environment:

   1. Place infant in incubator with monitored heat, oxygen, and humidity (may use vaporizer).

   2. Culture nasopharyngeal secretions.

   3. Monitor vital signs at regular intervals.

  D. Fluids and medications:

   1. Administer medications and fluids as prescribed.

   2. Prepare for cutdown procedure.

   3. Monitor intake and output.

  E. Prepare for surgery:

   1. Accompany for diagnostic tests and to operating room.

   2. Be prepared for possible emergency tracheostomy.

 II. Postoperative:

  A. Intensive postoperative care:

   1. Monitor vital signs every 30 to 60 min.

    a. Auscultate chest for lung sounds and apical heartbeat.

        b. Doppler blood pressure every hour.

        c. Rectal or axillary temperature every 4 h.

    2. Change position every hour and stimulate to cry every 2 h.

    3. Monitor accessory apparatus: cardiac monitor or controlled ventilation.

    4. Keep equipment for intubation nearby.

B. Airway and ventilation:

    1. NPO for 7 to 10 days.

    2. Monitor suction equipment. Change tubes every 2 to 3 days.

    3. Oxygen as necessary.

    4. Positioning as ordered—may vary:

        a. Usually head and chest elevated 20 to 30°.

        b. Flat (supine) with anastomosis.

        c. Prone in semi-Fowler's position with palliative treatment.

        d. To the left with cervical esophagostomy.

    5. Care of chest tube with water-seal drainage if left thoracotomy done.

C. Hydration and nutrition:

    1. Measure intake and output.

    2. Daily weights.

    3. Administer parenteral fluids, medications, and feedings as prescribed.

D. Gastrostomy care:

    1. Tube care:

        a. Fixation of tube to prevent displacement and continuous irritation to skin.

        b. Irrigate with 2 mL normal saline every 3 h while open to gravity drainage.

        c. Connect to intermittent low suction after first 24 h.

    2. Skin care:

        a. Keep skin clean and dry.

        b. Observe for signs of excoriation.

    3. Initiation of feedings as prescribed (withhold if vomiting or abdominal distension occur):

        a. Tube is suspended from top of isolette not more than 6 in above abdomen and attached to a 10 mL syringe.

        b. Prior to feeding, measure gastric residual and return.

        c. Maintain patency of tube by instilling 5 to 10 mL of dextrose and water every 2 h.

        d. Tube is not clamped until infant tolerates full feedings.

        e. Give pacifier at same time gastrostomy feedings are given.

        f. Begin teaching parents to administer feedings.

E. Cervical esophagostomy care:

    1. Suction at frequent, regular intervals during initial 2 to 3 days.

    2. Avoid hyperextension of neck when positioning and keep to left to promote drainage.

    3. Prevent excoriation of skin by putting a thin layer of petroleum jelly around skin edges.

    4. Soft, thick, absorbent dressings should be secured appropriately to absorb drainage.

    5. Teach parents ostomy care and how to prevent excoriation. Teach suctioning.

F. Following esophageal reconstruction:

    1. Astute monitoring of water-seal chest drainage is needed.

    2. Care for nasogastric tube, with regular, frequent suctioning for 2 to 3 days postoperatively.

    3. Continue gastrostomy feedings and care until tube is removed—usually with resumption of peristalsis.

    4. Observe for complications of anastomotic leaks, perforations or strictures:

        a. Continuous monitoring of vital signs is necessary.

        b. Notify physician at first indication of respiratory distress.

        c. Observe and note dysphagia or vomiting during months after initial repair.

  d. Instruct parents to observe for symptoms of complications and persistence of bowel odors from oral cavity.

G. Infant's emotional and developmental needs:
1. Meet needs for gratification and security.
 a. Use pacifier to meet sucking need and to coincide with gastrostomy feedings.
 b. Talk to, cuddle, and hold the child.
 c. Provide with comfortable, safe environment.
 d. Institute care plan to consistently meet and anticipate needs.
2. Developmental assessment and provision for developmental needs:
 a. Care plan should change as infant's needs change.
 b. Verbal and tactile stimulation is needed.
 c. Mobility—active/passive range of motion.
 d. Socialization associated with mealtime.

H. Parents' needs:
1. Encourage earliest possible parental involvement in care when readiness assessed.
2. Teach care of cervical esophagostomy and gastrostomy.
3. Emphasize infant's developmental needs, teaching and anticipating to avoid needless developmental delays.
4. Plan with the parents for immediate and continuing care utilizing community resources and multidisciplinary team approach—refer for community nursing service if necessary.
5. Provide parents with support:
 a. Allow ventilation of feelings.
 b. Keep in contact by phone calls immediately following discharge and refer to the visiting nurse.
 c. Demonstrate acceptance of child.

Evaluation

I. Immediate:
A. Adequate respiration.
1. Effective and easy removal of liquefied secretions is accomplished without accumulation.
2. Symptoms of respiratory distress, including choking and gagging, are avoided.
B. Prevention of gastric reflux and absence of chemical pneumonia.
C. Controlled environment:
1. Temperatire is maintained within normal range.
2. Humidified nasopharyngeal secretions are easily removed.
3. Cyanosis is minimal or absent.
4. Infections are absent.
D. Fluids and medication:
1. Adequate hydration.
2. There are no metabolic disturbances—fluid/electrolytes are in balance.
3. Medication is given as prescribed.
E. Child and parents are adequately prepared for surgery.

II. Postoperative:
A. Complications are avoided.
B. Infant's developmental needs are effectively provided for.
1. Emotional behavior in response to intervention becomes responsive, calm with minimal irritation and anxiety.
2. There are minimal developmental delays during prolonged period of care..
3. Motor development (fine and gross) attains normal limits within expected period of time.
4. Baby is responsive to parent's stimulation.
C. Parental needs are effectively provided for.
1. Parents demonstrate ability to cope with feelings toward infant, form attachment and become involved in care at earliest possible time.
2. They participate in and learn gastrostomy and cervical esophagostomy care.

3. Parents can maintain gastrostomy care and feeding, esophageal care with feeding technique, and suctioning prn at home with assistance of visiting nurse.
4. Parents demonstrate ability to understand child's developmental needs. They provide appropriate verbal, tactile, and sensory stimulation. Infant has activities and toys appropriate for age.
5. Continue close medical follow-up and be alert for a raspy cough at 6 to 24 months, eating problems, and frequent upper respiratory infections (URI).
6. Provide child with adequate nutrition as recommended by physician.

Omphalocele

Definition
Omphalocele is the protrusion or herniation of abdominal viscera into the base of the umbilical cord. The visceral mass is covered by a transparent avascular membrane which ruptures easily (sometimes in utero or at birth). The defect is centrally located on the abdomen and includes the umbilicus. Sac size depends upon visceral contents and may range from a slight enlargement at the base of the cord to a large sac containing colon, liver, and spleen. Associated anomalies may be present, including defects of intestines, heart, and great vessels; macroglossia, and gigantism.

At birth, immediate measures are taken to prevent infection and hypothermia and to avoid rupture of an intact membrane. Surgical intervention depends on the size and contents of the sac but is essentially the same as for gastroschisis with two exceptions:

1. Gastrostomy is performed. Oral feedings are not initiated until healing is extensive.
2. Large defects are treated with applications of antibiotics and coagulating agents until granulation and epithelialization occurs and the sac has receded sufficiently to allow for skin flap closure. Final closure may not be performed until infant is 10 to 12 months old or later.

Prognosis is influenced greatly by postoperative care and is good once skin closure is attained. Mortality rate is highest during the first few days of life.

Since care for the patient with an omphalocele is essentially the same as for gastroschisis, only the care during conservative therapy will be outlined here. See "Gastroschisis" for more detailed information.

Assessment
I. Respiratory distress.
II. Hypothermia.
III. Abdominal distension.
IV. High risk of infection.
    A. Septicemia.
    B. Peritonitis.
V. Possible renal and cardiac problems.

Problems
There is a prolonged high risk of infection with the large membranous sac susceptible to easy rupture.

Goals of care
I. Prevent local and systemic infection.
II. Promote epithelialization of membranous sac.

Intervention
I. Absolute incubator isolation with strict sterile technique is necessary.
II. Painting of sac with solutions (Mercurochrome, Zephiran, silver nitrate) as prescribed by physician.
    A. Observe for signs of mercury poisoning.
    B. Monitor urinalysis (mercury may appear there first).
III. Exercise extreme caution when positioning and during care to avoid rupture.
IV. Sac must contact nothing unsterile.

Evaluation   **I.** Infection is absent or controlled.
                 II. Membranous sac remains intact and epithelialization occurs.

Gastroschisis

Definition   *Gastroschisis* is a congenital full-thickness anterior abdominal wall defect with varying degrees of eviscerating bowel due to failure of the embryological tissues to mature in the abdominal layers. There is no membranous sac covering the thickened-appearing eviscerated abdominal contents. The defect is located below, to the right, and separate from the umbilicus, which is in its normal position. The herniated viscera consist mainly of small and large bowel. Associated problems may include prematurity, atresia of the small intestine, some degree of intestinal malrotation, and renal and cardiac problems.

Medical treatment includes surgery, which may be done in stages if the defect is large. The mortality rate for gastroschisis ranges from 15 to 50 percent and depends upon the degree of prematurity, the management of infections, and the seriousness of associated anomalies.

Assessment   **I.** Defect is apparent at birth, with exposed eviscerated bowel.
                II. Respiratory distress.
                III. Low body temperature.
                 A. Profound and rapid hypothermia.
                 B. Dehydration.
                IV. Abdominal distension.
                 A. Vomiting.
                 B. Gastric inflation.
                V. High risk of infection.
                VI. Possible renal and cardiac problems.

Problems   **I.** Immediate and preoperative:
                 A. Susceptibility to infection.
                 B. Rapid and profound loss of body heat.
                 C. Gastric distension and edema of extruding bowel.
                 D. Vomiting.
                 E. Dehydration.
                 F. Preparation for surgery.
                II. Postoperative:
                 A. Routine postoperative care.
                 B. Decompression of stomach.
                 C. Abdominal surgical wound care.
                 D. Prolonged nonfunctioning of GI tract.
                 E. Emotional needs of infant.
                 F. Parental needs to form attachment to infant with guarded prognosis.

Goals of Care **I.** Immediate and preoperative:
                 A. Initiate immediate infection control.
                 B. Help reestablish and maintain normal body temperature.
                 C. Decompress stomach and GI tract and help reduce edema of extruded viscera.
                 D. Prevent aspiration of vomitus and secretions.
                 E. Provide for IV administration of parenteral fluids and medications.
                 F. Maintain patient in generally stable condition.
                 G. Support parents and encourage parent-child relationship.
                II. Postoperative:
                 A. Provide for comfort and safety and minimize postoperative complications.
                 B. Prevent abdominal distension and promote removal of gastric secretions.
                 C. Provide good wound care.

    D. Prevent evisceration of wound edges and infection, and promote healing.

    E. Provide and administer parenteral fluids, medications, and nutrients.

    F. Provide infant with a sense of gratification and security.

    G. Promote parental involvement at earliest possible opportunity.

Intervention

I. Immediate and preoperative:
- **A.** Infection control:
  1. Cover exposed viscera immediately with sterile towels or sponges saturated with normal saline solution.
  2. Moisten sponges at regular intervals, never allowing them to dry.
  3. Cover moist sponges with dry sterile towels.
  4. Maintain sterile technique.
- **B.** Prevent or control hypothermia:
  1. Immediately place baby in incubator.
  2. Wrap infant in plastic or foil covered with warm, dry towels or blankets.
  3. Monitor and record vital signs at frequent, regular intervals.
  4. Handling and exposure must be minimal.
- **C.** Reduce distension and edema by inserting a nasogastric tube and monitoring function.
- **D.** Prevent aspiration by removing nasopharyngeal secretions by suction prn and at regular intervals.
- **E.** Intravenous fluids and medications:
  1. Administer and monitor IV medications and fluids as ordered.
  2. Measure intake and output.

II. Postoperative:
- **A.** Routine care:
  1. Maintain incubator care.
  2. Continue monitoring of vital signs.
- **B.** Prevent distension and promote removal of secretions.
  1. Suction nasopharyngeal area when necessary.
  2. Monitor functioning of nasogastric tube.
- **C.** Wound care:
  1. Exercise extreme caution in positioning and covering to prevent tension on sutures.
  2. Observe and record appearance of wound edges for signs of infection or necrosis.
  3. Maintain sterile technique until healing of wound occurs.
- **D.** Fluids, medications, nutrients:
  1. Record intake and output accurately.
  2. Administer parenteral fluids and medications as prescribed.
  3. Administer hyperalimentation feedings as prescribed and monitor.
  4. Oral feedings begin with returned peristaltic activity, after two to three stools.
     - *a.* Begin oral feedings with caution.
     - *b.* Initial feedings are given usually with sterile water or Pedialyte.
     - *c.* Note and record infant's tolerance of feedings.
- **E.** Infant's needs:
  1. Utilize pacifier for sucking.
  2. Frequent verbal and tactile stimulation is important.
- **F.** Parental involvement:
  1. Assess parents' reactions and methods of coping to determine their readiness and ability to become involved with the child.
  2. Encourage participation in care when appropriate.
  3. Begin and continue teaching about condition and effect of treatment, emphasizing infant's growth and development needs.
  4. Individualize care continuously—e.g., use baby's name.
  5. Evaluate needs for continuing care by involving parents in early discharge planning and ongoing care.

Evaluation

I. Immediate and preoperative:
   A. Local and systemic infections are absent.
   B. Body temperature is maintained at normal level.
   C. Absent or minimal abdominal distension with diminishing edema in extruding bowel.
   D. Nasopharyngeal secretions are removed adequately: aspiration pneumonia does not develop.
   E. Adequate hydration and nutrition are attained without complications: insertion sites are free of infection and infiltration.
   F. Infant's general condition remains stable or changes are noted with appropriate, immediate intervention.

II. Postoperative:
   A. Routine postoperative care is provided with accurate observations of complications or changes, and progress recorded.
   B. Gastric decompression is maintained and air-swallowing is prevented.
   C. There is adequate wound healing: no dehiscence of wound edges, silastic nondisplaced, no infection, no abnormal drainage.
   D. Adequate hydration and nutrition are maintained.
      1. Hyperalimentation feeding is accurate and without complications.
      2. Successful oral feedings are achieved with infant learning sucking, tolerating feedings, and gaining weight.
   E. Infant thrives.
      1. Learns sucking of pacifier.
      2. Responds to verbal and tactile stimulation.
      3. Develops normally.
   F. Parents adapt.
      1. Respond to encouragement and form attachment with infant.
      2. Take part in providing care.
      3. Visit frequently rather than avoiding.
      4. Show ability to work through feelings of guilt without blaming selves or each other for infant's condition or suffering.
      5. Demonstrate openness to teaching and plan realistically for immediate and future needs of infant.

Hirschsprung's Disease (Congenital Aganglionic Megacolon)

Definition

Hirschsprung's disease is the congenital absence of parasympathetic ganglion nerve cells in the mesenteric plexus of the descending colon, resulting in absence of peristalsis in the affected part of the colon. The aganglionic area remains persistently contracted and the proximal colon becomes distended with gas and feces. Chronic constipation and abdominal distension ensue. The distended bowel may ulcerate. Medical treatment is resection of the aganglionic portion of the bowel and anastomosis of the normal colon to the anus; sometimes a temporary colostomy is created. The prognosis depends upon the age of the child (20 to 30 percent mortality in the neonatal period) and the length of the colonic segment involved. There is a predisposition to Crohn's disease.

Assessment

I. Neonatal period:
   A. Failure to pass meconium for 24 to 48 h.
   B. Reluctance to eat.
   C. Bilious vomiting.
   D. Abdominal distension.
   E. Rapid breathing and grunting.
   F. Constipation with overflow diarrhea.
   G. Baby has worried, frowning look with thin features.
   H. Baby feeds poorly, is irritable, and fails to thrive.

    II. Early infancy:
       A. Obstinate constipation.
       B. Stools: offensive odor and ribbonlike shape.
       C. Progressive abdominal distension.
       D. Prominent veins over abdomen.
       E. Visible peristaltic activity.
       F. Palpable fecal masses and impactions.
       G. Temporary and minimal relief of constipation with enema.
       H. Failure to thrive.
       I. Hypochromic anemia and hypoproteinemia.

Problems

I. Preoperative:
  A. Constipation.
  B. Abdominal distension.
  C. Malnutrition.
  D. Possible emotional deprivation and developmental delays.
II. Postoperative:
  A. Routine postoperative care.
  B. Colostomy care.
  C. Abdominal surgical wound care.
  D. Abdominal distension.
  E. Emotional and developmental needs of child.
  F. Parents' needs.

Goals of Care

I. Preoperative:
  A. Facilitate evacuation of bowel and prepare for surgery.
  B. Observe for evidence of progressive abdominal distension and assist in decreasing distension.
  C. Help promote weight gain by providing adequate nutrition.
  D. Provide parents and child with opportunities for meeting emotional needs.
II. Postoperative:
  A. Provide good postoperative care and observe for complications.
  B. Provide good care of colostomy to assure its functioning and avoid excoriation of tissues.
  C. Prevent abdominal distension.
  D. Meet child's emotional and developmental needs during hospitalization.
  E. Help parents participate in care and understand procedures and need for good consistent follow-up care.

Intervention

I. Preoperative:
  A. Evacuation and preparation of bowel for surgery:
    1. Give enemas as prescribed (solution, frequency, medications).
      a. Observe for water intoxication.
      b. Note return and degree of distension.
      c. Siphon if no return.
    2. Constantly monitor characteristics and frequency of stool.
    3. Take *axillary temperature only*.
  B. Feedings and nutrition:
    1. Give diet as ordered—usually low-residue.
    2. Offer frequent small feedings.
    3. Have patient in upright position.
  C. Relieve distension:
    1. Observe for respiratory distress—position with head and chest elevated.
    2. Observe for abdominal tenderness and visible peristalsis.

       3. Note extent and degree of distension before and after colonic irrigation.

       4. Assure functioning of nasogastric tube.

   D. Parent-child needs:

       1. Encourage parents to visit as often as realistically possible.

       2. Hold the child frequently and give tactile and verbal stimulation during wakeful periods.

       3. Encourage age-appropriate play activities.

  II. Postoperative:

   A. Routine postoperative care—continue axillary temperature procedure.

   B. Care of temporary colostomy.

       1. Provide good skin care to surrounding area.

          a. Frequent nonabrasive cleansing.   *c.* Apply protective agents to skin.

          b. Change dressing prn or as ordered.   *d.* Expose to air periodically.

       2. Observe for signs of obstruction.

          a. Irritability, vomiting, fever.

          b. Abdominal tenderness.

          c. Decreased colostomy output.

       3. Assure proper functioning; position; record characteristics of output.

   C. Abdominal wound care:

       1. Observe for signs of infection (local, systemic).

       2. Maintain sterile technique with dressing change.

       3. Reposition at regular intervals with care not to dislodge tubing.

   D. Relieve distension:

       1. Nasogastric tube,

       2. Begin oral feedings as ordered before NG tube removal.

          a. Have child sit in upright position.   *c.* Avoid overfeeding.

          b. Bubble frequently.   *d.* Observe tolerance.

   E. Emotional and developmental needs of child:

       1. Promote parent-child interaction.

       2. Play activity as tolerated.

       3. Frequent holding with stimulation during wakeful periods.

   F. Parents' needs:

       1. Facilitate discussion of feelings toward disease, treatment, and reaction to it.

       2. Begin teaching colostomy care and encourage earliest possible participation.

       3. Teach parents growth and developmental levels and tasks child needs to attain and how to achieve.

       4. Encourage them to treat child as normally as possible.

Evaluation

  I. Preoperative:

   A. Relief of constipation is achieved, there is absence or decrease of distension, absence of water intoxication, and absence of respiratory embarrassment.

   B. Infant tolerates feedings and gains weight.

   C. Infant or child remains calm and parents demonstrate acceptance by participating in care.

  II. Postoperative:

   A. Respiratory problems are absent.

   B. Colostomy functions appropriately without excoriation of surrounding tissues.

   C. Local and systemic infections are absent.

   D. Feedings are tolerated and there is no recurrence of distension after removal of NG tube.

   E. Child's emotional reactions and development attain and remain within normal range.

   F. Parents assume responsibility for care, interact maturely with child, and provide for ongoing and comprehensive health care.

Imperforate Anus

Definition
    Imperforate anus is the congenital absence of a patent anal opening. The severity of the defect varies, as shown in Fig. 16-5. Associated fistulas are common. In the male, there may be rectovesicular, rectourethral, or rectoperineal fistulas. In the female, rectovaginal and rectoperineal fistulas may occur. Surgical intervention is essential and is determined by the type and extent of the anomaly:

1. *Stenosis* can be treated with digital dilatations continued for several months.
2. A thin *membrane* with visible meconium and no other anomaly can be treated by surgical perforation of membranous tissue.
3. For *low agenesis,* surgical correction is done through perineum.
4. For *high agenesis* and *atretic* types:
   a. Transverse colostomy is done immediately.
   b. Sacroabdominoperineal pull-through is delayed until child is 6 to 12 months old.

    The prognosis depends on the birth maturity of infant and the severity of other associated anomalies. The overall mortality rate is 20 percent but increases to 55 percent for premature infants and infants with severe associated anomalies. In less severe types 1 and 2, the prognosis is good with few functional problems. Problems with fecal continence increase with the extent of the anomaly.

Assessment
    The condition is usually apparent in the immediate neonatal period from the following:
    I. Absence of anal opening.
    II. Absence of meconium stool.

FIGURE 16-5 / Imperforate anus. (*a*) Stenosis of otherwise well-formed tract. (*b*) Membrane occludes anal opening. (*c*) Low agenesis (less than 1.5 cm). (*d*) High agenesis (greater than 1.5 cm). (*e*) Anal atresia.

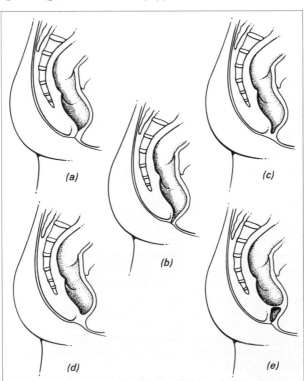

    III. Meconium-stained urine (if fistula to urinary system exists).
    IV. Inability to insert thermometer or small finger into rectum.
    V. Progressive abdominal distension.

Problems
    I. Preoperative:
       A. Need for emergency surgery.
       B. Possibility of associated anomalies.
    II. Postoperative:
       A. Routine postoperative care.
       B. Colostomy care.
       C. Care of anoplasty.
       D. Care of abdominal-perineal pull-through.
       E. Dehydration and electrolyte imbalance.
       F. Psychological needs of parents and child.

Goals of Care
    I. Preoperative:
       A. Maintain stability of general condition and prepare for emergency surgery.
       B. Continue to observe for associated anomalies or condition change.
    II. Postoperative:
       A. Provide postoperative care and avoid complications.
       B. Provide colostomy care to assure functioning and avoid excoriation of tissues.
       C. Provide care of anoplasty.
       D. Provide care of abdominal-perineal pull-through.
       E. Prevent dehydration, electrolyte imbalance, and malnutrition by providing fluids and calories.
       F. Help parents accept infant, understand diagnosis, and participate in care, providing child with physical and emotional needs.

Intervention
    I. Preoperative:
       A. Prepare for emergency surgery.
          1. NPO status maintained.
          2. Nasogastric tube insertion and care.
       B. Observe for possible associated problems.
          1. Stool from fistula.
          2. Meconium-stained urine.
          3. Symptoms of tracheoesophageal fistula (a frequently related anomaly).
    II. Postoperative:
       A. Give routine postoperative care, and intervene at first indication of complications.
       B. Colostomy care.
          1. Appropriate care and precautions are necessary.
          2. Assure parents colostomy is a temporary measure until infant has definitive surgery.
             a. Instruct mother in care.
             b. Refer to visiting nurse.
       C. Perianal anoplasty.
          1. Keep perineum exposed to air.
          2. Position infant as recommended by physician:
             a. Supine with legs extended and at 90° angle to trunk.
             b. Prone.
          3. Keep area meticulously clean.
             a. Irrigate from syringe with warm saline solution.
             b. Dry gently with absorbent cotton.
       D. Care of abdominal-perineal pull-through.
          1. NG or gastrostomy tube is connected to suction or gravity drainage as ordered.
          2. Urethral catheter care.
             a. Anchor catheter to avoid displacement.

        b. Connect to sterile collection system.

        c. Measure and record output every 8 h.

     3. Observe and report complications of respiratory distress, perineal bleeding, or abdominal distension.

     4. Teach anal dilatation to parents to prevent stricture at anastomotic site.

   E. Hydration and nutrition.

     1. Monitor parenteral fluids.

     2. Begin oral feedings as ordered.

        a. Usually begin same day.

        b. Withhold until peristalsis begins.

   F. Parent-child needs.

     1. Encourage parents to become involved in care as soon as they are able.

     2. Reinforce teaching that colostomy is a temporary measure.

     3. Provide parents with supportive professional help in home and keep in contact.

     4. Review the physical, emotional, and developmental needs of infant with parents.

     5. Listen to parents and allay anxieties.

Evaluation

 I. Preoperative:

   A. Stable condition maintained.

   B. Anomalies or complications noted and appropriately cared for.

 II. Postoperative:

   A. Complications are avoided or are promptly recognized and treated.

   B. Colostomy functions properly without excoriated tissues.

   C. There is no infection of perineal area.

   D. Urethral catheter functions adequately.

   E. Infant is well hydrated and gains weight adequately.

   F. Parents participate actively in care, and overcome their anxieties.

METABOLIC DISORDERS

Cystic Fibrosis

 See Chap. 14.

Celiac Disease (Gluten-Induced Enteropathy)

Definition

 Celiac disease is a chronic disorder with a symptom complex characterized by intestinal malabsorption resulting in malnutrition. The exact cause is unknown, but the disease is thought to result from an inborn error of metabolism exacerbated by ingestion of wheat or rye gluten. Fats and sugars are poorly absorbed from the intestine. As a result, the child passes huge, frothy, malodorous, floating stools and suffers from wasting and from fat-soluble vitamin deficiencies and their consequences, such as osteoporosis and bleeding. Symptoms appear insidiously in the first 2 years of life. Dietary restriction of glutens effectively reverses the intestinal cellular abnormalities, although response to diet therapy takes 6 to 8 weeks. Most children eventually outgrow their intolerance of glutens. Prognosis is good but depends on good management and parents' and child's cooperation with the dietary regime.

Assessment

 I. Diarrhea (chronic or recurrent).

 II. Stools: foul odor, bulky, greasy, floating.

 III. Signs of wasting and/or malnutrition.

   A. Flattened buttocks with loosely hanging skin folds.

   B. Progressive abdominal distension.

   C. Round, plump cheeks with saddened facial expression.

       D. Retarded growth (below third percentile).
       E. Developmental delays.
    IV. Notable mood changes: irritable, passive and withdrawn, temper tantrums.

Problems
    I. Erratic behavior; mood swings.
    II. Anorexia and malnutrition.
    III. Regression and passive withdrawn behavior.
    IV. Distorted parent-child relationship (hostile, overprotective).
    V. Complication of celiac crisis and susceptibility to URI.
    VI. Long-term dietary restriction may lead to child's manipulative behavior or, in adolescence, to avoidance of social situations.

Goals of Care
    I. Understand behavioral changes and mood swings in relationship to the disease and prevent precipitating situations.
    II. Follow gluten-free diet regimen exactly as prescribed to provide calories for weight gain, and help parents understand the relationship of diet in controlling the disease.
    III. Provide diversional activities appropriate for age and severity of disease.
    IV. Assist and teach parents how to interact with child during severe stages and subsequent periods; promote a healthy relationship and understanding of progressive developmental needs.
    V. Be aware of the signs and symptoms of celiac crisis and upper respiratory infections, providing care when needed and teaching parents preventive measures.

Intervention
    I. Behavioral changes.
       A. Allow child to express feelings—listen to older child and console toddler.
       B. Note and avoid situations that are emotionally disturbing or upsetting to child.
       C. Individualize care plan to assure consistency of effective behavior approaches.
       D. Make routine care a pleasant socializing time.
    II. Diet regime.
       A. NPO during initial period of severe illness or crisis.
       B. Initial diet given is high protein, low fat, and starch free. *No wheat or rye products.*
         1. Sweeten milk protein or skim milk with sucrose or banana powder.
         2. Add individual foods one at a time at 2 to 3 day intervals or as prescribed (lean meats, cottage cheese, egg white, raw ground apples).
         3. Starchy foods (bread and potatoes) added last.
         4. Vitamin supplements as prescribed.
       C. Begin with frequent feedings of small portions.
         1. Do not force-feed.
         2. Feed slowly.
         3. Socialize.
       D. Note child's reaction to and behavior changes during or after mealtime.
       E. Eliminate foods that precipitate recurrent symptoms.
       F. Take measures to prevent ambulatory child from obtaining restricted foods.
         1. Alert all staff.
         2. Older pediatric patients may assist by not taunting and tempting, and may help supervise.
         3. Enlist parents' cooperation to avoid bringing snacks.
       G. Discuss diet with parents and arrange for meeting with nutritionist or dietician.
    III. Regressive behavior.
       A. Be patient.
       B. Avoid exhaustive play for severely ill child.
       C. Play introduced should be age-appropriate.
       D. Encourage social interaction and play involving other children gradually and consistently.
       E. Accept regressive behavior in recurrent episodes or crisis.
       F. Consider play therapy.

IV. Promote a good parent-child relationship.
   A. Encourage parents to visit frequently and involve them in care and play activities.
   B. Allow parents time to discuss feelings.
   C. Provide genetic counseling (disease tends to recur in the family).
   D. Emphasize need for parents to set limits for child at home and avoid emotionally upsetting situations in child's presence.
   E. Encourage parents to keep ill child's needs in perspective in relation to their needs and needs of other family members.
   F. Refer to social worker to intervene with known social problems or anticipated difficulty with family interrelationships.
V. Infections and celiac crisis.
   A. Observe for and teach parents signs and symptoms of celiac crisis:
      1. Large, watery stools.   3. Excessive perspiration.
      2. Restless sleep.   4. Cold extremities.
   B. Treat and manage as ordered:
      1. NPO.
      2. Parenteral therapy.
      3. Observation of changes.
   C. Instruct parents to seek immediate medical care if child develops an upper respiratory infection.
   D. Urge continued regular medical follow-up.

Evaluation
I. Improved physical and psychological condition is demonstrated with weight gain, adherence to diet, improved disposition.
II. Child interacts sociably with diminished regressive behavior.
III. Parents exhibit understanding and acceptance and are able to deal effectively with child in routine daily procedures.
IV. Absence of crisis and infections, or immediate appropriate care provided.
V. Continuous follow-up management.

OTHER GASTROINTESTINAL DISORDERS

Dental Caries

Definition
Dental caries is a disease of the teeth which is characterized by a progressive destructive lesion of the calcified dental tissues eventually involving the pulp. Caries is chiefly a bacterial disease with the principal causative organisms being streptococci and *Lactobacillus acidophilus*. Organisms form and adhere to gelatinous plaque on the tooth surface. Action of the organism and substrates from foodstuffs, mainly carbohydrates (sucrose), produce acids that rapidly decalcify tooth enamel, with destruction of the tooth the end result. Untreated caries results not only in pain and tooth loss, but in consequent malocclusion, weakening of the muscles of mastication, and cosmetic defects that can be damaging to the person's self-concept. Abscesses may lead to bone destruction and bony or systemic infection. Children with congenital or rheumatic heart disease are at risk for bacterial endocarditis secondary to dental decay. Caries is the principal oral problem of children and adolescents, affecting over 90 percent.

Factors contributing to tooth decay include lack of fluoride, lack of oral hygiene, poor state of general health, and poor dietary practices. Decay of the primary (deciduous) teeth is encouraged by the practice of giving milk or other sugar-containing fluids in a nursing bottle at naps and bedtime because of the continuous flow of sugars over the teeth while the child sucks during sleep.

Assessment
I. Oral cavity.
   A. Discoloration of teeth.
   B. Decayed areas with pitting and fissures.

       C. Excessive plaque on tooth surfaces.
       D. Accumulation of food debris between teeth.
       E. Inflammation and pain of gingiva.
       F. Missing and misaligned teeth.
  II. Poor dietary practices.
       A. Excessive weight loss or gain.
       B. Excessive intake of refined sugar .
       C. Poor appetite for chewable foods and at mealtime.
  III. History of congenital cardiac disease or rheumatic heart disease.
  IV. Developmental delays and associated problems.
       A. Withdrawal and isolation secondary to dental disfigurement.
       B. Articulation and speech problems of dental origin.

Problems

  I. Untreated decay of primary or secondary teeth.
  II. Poor oral hygiene with evident lack of preventive measures.
  III. Poor dietary practices.
  IV. Speech problems.
  V. Problems with self-concept because of dental disfigurement.

Goals of Care

  I. Prevent progress of decay and infection.
  II. Teach parents the necessity for care of primary teeth (including fillings, if decay is present) to ensure health and proper alignment of secondary teeth.
  III. Teach principles of good oral hygiene and its effect on prevention of caries.
  IV. Teach the value of good nutrition in preventing caries.
  V. Encourage speech evaluation if speech problem persists after dental repair.
  VI. Assist parents in understanding appropriate management of needs for oral gratification and socialization in children and adolescents.

Intervention

  I. Provide treatment.
       A. Discuss need for immediate treatment and refer to appropriate source.
       B. Assess current oral hygiene practices, parental supervision, and dietary practices.
  II. Teach principles of good oral hygiene.
       A. Assess knowledge and current practices.
       B. Instill understanding of need for early and regular visits.
          1. Begin at 18 to 30 months for checkup and cleaning so child becomes familiar with dentist without necessarily associating pain with treatment.
          2. Adolescent should have regular visits every 3 to 6 months.
       C. Teach proper brushing and care.
          1. Toothbrush appropriate size for age of child.
          2. Up-and-down technique.
          3. Daily brushing after meals and at bedtime.
          4. Flossing between teeth regularly.
       D. Explain the effectiveness of fluoridation on strengthening calcification of tooth enamel.
       E. Seek parental assistance and guidance with younger children to assure frequent proper brushing.
       F. Individualize teaching plan.
          1. No bottles of milk at bedtime after eruption of teeth. Substitute water.
          2. Encourage early weaning, as the purpose of the teeth is mastication.
  III. Teach nutrition.
       A. Assess and evaluate current dietary habits.
       B. Teach improvement and preventive measures:
          1. Decrease between-meal snacks to improve appetite at mealtime.
          2. Substitute fresh fruits and vegetables for refined sugar snacks.
          3. No milk or milk products before bedtime without rinsing or brushing.
          4. Evaluate speech. Refer to speech therapist for continued evaluation and therapy.

5. Developmental and personality concerns.
  a. Assess in cooperation with parents initially and note if there is any change after treatment.
  b. Review needs of child during various stages of development.

Evaluation

I. Care is obtained early with appropriate treatment done and primary teeth functional until eruption of permanent teeth. No infections.

II. Parents demonstrate understanding of good oral hygiene by supervising child's habits and seeking early care if decay begins again.

III. Parents demonstrate understanding by adhering to dietary recommendations with resultant improvement in nutritional status and reduction of dental caries.

IV. Speech problems resolved.

V. No evidence of personality problems or developmental delays.

BIBLIOGRAPHY

Barlow, B., et al.: "An Experimental Study of Acute Necrotizing Enterocolitis—The Importance of Breast Milk," *Journal of Pediatric Surgery,* **9**(5):587–595, October 1974. In an experimental study of newborn rats in which hypoxia was induced it was found that breast milk prevented necrotizing enterocolitis through the induction of passive enteric immunity and control of intestinal flora. It may be inferred that breast milk may also protect the premature infant at risk.

Barnes, C. M.: "Support of a Mother in the Care of a Child with Esophageal Lye Burns," *Nursing Clinics of North America,* **4**(1):53–57, March 1969. Through the intervention of a clinical specialist the mother of a child with esophageal burns was able to manage her care, including dilatations, at home.

Bishop, W. S., and J. H. Head: "Care of the Infant With a Stoma," *Maternal Child Health Nursing,* **1:** 315–319, September–October 1976. Because of the patient's small size and delicate skin, the most important aspect of stoma care in infants is preventing wound contamination and skin breakdown. The nurse must also be aware of the impact on the family of a sick baby with a stoma.

Bliss, V. J.: "Nursing Care of Infants With Neonatal Necrotizing Enterocolitis," *Maternal Child Health Nursing,* **1:** 37–40, January–February 1976. NEC often has an insidious onset, and the nurse is in a unique position to detect and intervene in this disease. The article deals with the cause, nursing care, and treatment.

Filler, R. M.: "Total Parenteral Feeding of Infants," *Hospital Practice,* **9:** 79–86, June 1976. Review of hyperalimentation procedure and its hazards. The child with a hyperalimentation line requires scrupulous nursing observation and care.

Grant, J. N.: "Patient Care in Parenteral Hyperalimentation," *Nursing Clinics of North America,* **8**(1): 165–181, March 1973. The article reviews the nurse's responsibilities to the patient receiving hyperalimentation.

Gross, Linda: "Ostomy Care, A Letter to Parents," *American Journal of Nursing,* **74**(8):1427–1428, August 1974. In order to deal with their child's ostomy surgery and care, parents must first face their own feelings and overcome any guilt or fear. The author points out ten ways to support the child.

Williams, L. F.: "The Acute Abdomen," *American Journal of Nursing,* **71**(2):299–303, February 1971. Important observations about abdominal pain, diagnostic studies, and intervention are discussed by the author, a surgeon.

17

The Endocrine System

Diana W. Guthrie[1]

The endocrine system is diffuse and multifaceted, involving many organs and organ systems. The function of the endocrine system is to serve as a signaling device for the rest of the body. A hormone, once it is secreted into the bloodstream, goes to every cell and thus affects every other bodily function. This widespread effect is unique among body systems and makes assessment of endocrine disorders very complex. In endocrine-system assessment not only the endocrine organ itself but also every other organ of the body must be assessed, since those other organs are end organs for endocrine effects.

The first step in any good assessment is a careful health history. The astute nurse can identify the great majority of endocrine disorders by history alone. Any particular endocrine disorder may arise from any of several different causes, all of which may produce the same symptoms. Consequently, health disorders in this chapter are organized according to the organ which gives rise to them rather than by the classifications of neoplasm, inflammation, congenital defect, and so forth that are used in the other pediatric chapters. Table 17-1, however, lists endocrine disorders by etiology.

GENERAL ASSESSMENT

I. General physical examination.
- A. The child's general appearance. Endocrine dysfunctions can subtly or markedly affect shape, size, color, and maturation of the body.
- B. Height and weight. Not only should gross height and weight be assessed and compared with the norms, but height and weight should be compared:
  1. With each other.
  2. With the measurements of bodily parts (upper segment versus lower segment, head circumference, arm span, etc.).
- C. Affect. Compare to behavioral norms and expectations for age.
- D. Activity. Compare to norms for age. For example, is the child over- or underactive as a reflection of thyroid gland activity?

II. Systemic review.
- A. Ectoderm and appendages.
  1. Skin—assess color, pigmentation patterns, moistness, dryness, scaliness, etc.
  2. Hair—check amount, texture, location, distribution, and pattern (particularly of pubic hair).
  3. Nails—assess growth and texture.
  4. Teeth—note condition, repair, and mottling.
- B. Head and neck.
  1. Note head shape and size.
  2. Check patency of fontanels.
  3. Assess hair texture and distribution on head and face.
  4. Determine facial shape, symmetry, appearance, and pigmentation.
  5. Ears—check shape and size.
  6. Nose—note shape, size.
  7. Eyes—note shape, color, closeness together, protrusion (exophthalmia), movement of eyes and lids (lid lag on eye movement, etc.), presence of stare, luster, blurred vision, or diplopia.

[1] The author gratefully acknowledges the guidance and assistance of her husband Dr. Richard Guthrie, a pediatric endocrinologist.

TABLE 17-1 / CLASSIFICATION OF CHILDHOOD ENDOCRINE DISORDERS BY ETIOLOGY

Disorders of Genetic Origin

Gigantism:
    Beckwith syndrome of giantism, exophthalmos, and macroglossia
Congenital hyperpituitary function
Pituitary dwarfism
Cretinism (congenital hypothyroidism)
Congenital hypoparathyroidism
Congenital hyperparathyroidism
Diabetes mellitus
Delayed puberty and hypogonadism
Precocious puberty:
    Hypothalamic origin (constitutional)
    Due to extrapituitary disease, e.g., adrenogenital syndrome
Adrenogenital syndrome
Cushing's and Addison's diseases

Disorders of Rate of Growth
Giantism—excess growth hormone secretion Dwarfism—lack of growth hormone secretion or unresponsiveness to growth hormone Hypothyroidism—congenital or acquired Diabetes mellitus—poorly controlled diabetes may result in growth failure (also, diabetes mellitus often arises during the preadolescent growth spurt and is known as "growth onset diabetes")

Disorders of Environmental Origin
The infant of the diabetic mother The infant of the hypercalcemic mother Hyperthyroidism Hypothyroidism, acquired Ambiguous genital development secondary to maternal hormones Diabetes insipidus Hypopituitarism due to trauma or destruction of hypothalamus and/or pituitary gland Diabetes mellitus secondary to tumor, surgery, trauma, or pancreatectomy Addison's and Cushing's diseases Hypoparathyroidism with tetany secondary to surgical destruction of the parathyroid or tumor Hypogonadism due to destruction of the ovaries and testes by tumors, surgery, or chemical suppression

Disorders Caused by Infections
Thyroiditis with hypothyroidism Addison's disease Diabetes mellitus(?) Graves' disease (hyperthyroidism) (?)

      8. Neck—check thyroid size and adenopathy.
      9. Mouth—assess moistness or dryness, and tongue size.
    C. Chest and heart.
      1. Chest:
        a. Check anteroposterior diameter.
        b. Assess shape.
        c. Assess excursions and breath sounds.

   2. Heart:
      a. Assess size and position.
      b. Assess rate for tachycardia or bradycardia.
      c. Check heart sounds and murmurs.
D. Abdomen.
   1. Check for hernias or weaknesses of abdominal wall.
   2. Assess liver, spleen, and kidney size.
   3. Check for masses or tenderness.
   4. Listen to bowel sounds.
E. Extremities and spine.
   1. Extremities:
      a. Compare length with norms and with body size (upper versus lower segment measurements).
      b. Check mobility of joints.
      c. Check for limb deformities—bowlegs are a sign of rickets, for example.
      d. Assess muscle tone and irritability (carpopedal spasm and Chvostek's sign are indications of hypocalcemia in hypoparathyroidism, for example).
      e. Assess shape and size of fingers and toes.
   2. Spine:
      a. Note symmetry and flexibility.
      b. Check for scoliosis and kyphosis.
F. Nervous system (neurologic examination).
   1. Reflexes—assess for hyper- or hyporeflexia of deep tendons.
   2. Assess superficial reflexes.
   3. Check for abnormal reflexes.
   4. Assess level of consciousness.
G. Genitourinary system.
   1. External genitalia:
      a. Assess for state of maturation by comparison to the Tanner scale (1).
      b. Assess size and shape of genitalia.
         (1) Assess size of penis in males.
         (2) Assess size of clitoris in females.
         (3) Assess testicular size for age in males.
         (4) Check for ambiguity of genital formation.
   2. Internal genitalia:
      a. Assess prostate size and shape by rectal examination in the male.
      b. Assess vagina, ovaries, and uterus by vaginal and/or rectal examination in the female.

DISORDERS OF THE ANTERIOR PITUITARY GLAND

Anterior Pituitary Gland Functions

The anterior pituitary gland was once thought to be the body's "master gland," producing hormones that control the thyroid, adrenals, gonads, growth, and lactation. It is now understood that the anterior pituitary performs its functions under the influence of the *pineal gland* and *hypothalamus.*

For most pituitary hormones the hypothalamus produces a *releasing hormone* which stimulates the pituitary gland to release a specific hormone, which then stimulates hormone secretion by the target gland. The hormone from the target gland in turn suppresses the amount of releasing hormone from the hypothalamus, completing the arc. This sequence of regulatory events is called a *feedback arc* and resembles the thermostatic control mechanism of a furnace. For example, on the hypothalamic-pituitary-thyroid axis:

Step 1. The hypothalamus produces a hormone called thyrotropin-releasing hormone (TRH).

Step 2. TRH causes the pituitary to release its hormone, called thyroid-stimulating hormone (TSH).

Step 3. TSH causes the thyroid gland to release its hormone, called thyroxine (T_4).

Step 4. Thyroxine then exerts its effect on every bodily cell to stimulate metabolism. It also suppresses TRH production, which reduces the level of circulating TSH, and consequently causes the thyroid gland to decrease its own production.

Step 5. Reduced production of T_4 then allows TRH to rise, and the cycle repeats.

Certain hormones, such as growth hormone, have no target gland to produce a hormone to complete the feedback arc. In these instances the hypothalamus secretes not only the stimulating or releasing hormone but also an inhibitory hormone to prevent its oversecretion.

As far as is now known, there are six clearly defined hormones of the anterior pituitary gland:

1. *Thyroid-stimulating hormone* (TSH), which is controlled by thyroid-releasing hormone (TRH) from the hypothalamus and causes the release of thyroxine (T_4) by the thyroid gland.
2. *Follicle-stimulating hormone* (FSH) and *luteinizing hormone* (LH), which are controlled by FSH-releasing hormone (FSH-RH) from the hypothalamus and in turn control gonad functions (spermatogenesis, ovogenesis, and the production of estrogen, progesterone, and testosterone).
3. *Adrenocorticotropic hormone* (ACTH), which is controlled by an as yet undefined releasing factor from the hypothalamus (ACTH-RF) and which controls the hormonal secretions of the adrenal cortex (primarily cortisol and aldosterone, but also small amounts of estrogens, progesterone, and testosterone).
4. *Human growth hormone* (HGH), which is controlled by both a hypothalamic-stimulating hormone (HGH-RH) and an inhibiting hormone called somatostatin or HGH-RH–inhibiting hormone (HGH-RH–IH).
5. *Prolactin,* which is controlled only by an inhibiting hormone (PrIH) from the hypothalamus. Sucking at the breast initiates a neuroendocrine arc which inhibits PrIH and allows prolactin production and lactation.

Etiology of Anterior Pituitary Disorders

I. Disease states can be produced by:
  A. Increased or decreased hypothalamic hormone secretion.
  B. Increased or decreased pituitary hormone secretion.
  C. Increased or decreased hormone secretion of the target gland.

II. States of increased or decreased hormone secretion anywhere in the cycle may be caused by:
  A. Genetic inheritance.   E. Infections.
  B. Metabolic factors.   F. Drugs.
  C. Trauma.   G. Unknown (idiopathic) causes.
  D. Tumors.

III. Regardless of etiology, the end result is usually the same: the symptoms or signs are those of increased or decreased hormone secretion of the target gland hormone.

  Example Deficiency of hypothalamic TRH or anterior pituitary TSH results in the same physical problems as failure of the thyroid gland itself to produce T_4. The difference is that TRH and TSH levels will be high if the defect is in the thyroid gland, while TRH will be up but not TSH in pituitary disease, and all will be low in hypothalamic disease.

IV. Disease of the hypothalamus and/or pituitary may involve a single hormone or several.
  A. Diseases of genetic or congenital origin tend to affect a single hormone, e.g., isolated growth hormone deficiency.

B. Diseases of destruction, such as tumors, surgical ablation, trauma, etc., tend to show multiple deficiencies, e.g., panhypopituitarism, which causes deficiencies of hormones from all the target organs (thyroid, adrenals, and gonads) as well as growth hormone and prolactin.

Disorders Due to Excess Anterior Pituitary Hormone Production

Gigantism and Giantism

DEFINITION

Gigantism, also known as Beckwith's syndrome, is a congenital disorder of newborns. The etiology is unknown. The syndrome consists of exophthalmos, giantism, and macroglossia. Affected infants often also have hypoglycemia and omphalocele. Since the disease, strictly speaking, is not an endocrine disease even though the infants do have hyperinsulinemia, it will not be further discussed here.

Giantism is a disease of overproduction of human growth hormone (HGH) and is characterized by excessive growth. When the disease occurs in childhood before epiphyseal closure, very large stature of normal proportions results, and the condition is termed *giantism.* If the condition occurs after puberty and epiphyseal closure has occurred, only those areas with open epiphyses (jaw, hands, and feet) grow, and the face, hands, and feet become excessively large in proportion to the rest of the body. This condition is known as *acromegaly.* Both giantism and acromegaly may be caused by a variety of conditions of the hypothalamus or pituitary gland, but most commonly they result from an adenoma of the pituitary gland.

ASSESSMENT

I. Height rapidly increases on the growth chart in giantism.
II. Disproportionate growth of the lower jaw, hands, and feet exists in acromegaly.
III. In either condition, x-rays of the wrists and hands reveal advanced bone age; x-rays of the skull may show an enlarged sella turcica (the bony crater which houses the pituitary gland).

PROBLEMS

I. The child must be directed to medical attention so that adenoma, if present, can be treated.
II. The most outstanding nursing problem is the child's psychological development related to his or her oversized body. The acromegalic features are particularly disturbing but, especially for girls, so is the tall stature.

GOALS OF CARE

I. Direct the child and family for immediate medical diagnosis (skull x-rays, computerized tomography scan, growth hormone assay, etc.) and treatment (surgical or radiologic ablation of the tumor).
II. Prepare child and family for surgery if indicated.
III. Assist child's adjustment to altered features or tall stature.
IV. If the excessive growth is genetic (*constitutional tall stature*) rather than hormonal, prepare the child and family for the changes which will occur in sexual development if hormonal therapy (sex hormones) is used to hasten epiphyseal closure and stop growth.

INTERVENTION

I. Prepare and support patient during hospitalization and diagnostic procedures.
II. Prepare patient for surgery and the surgical outcome if surgery is planned.
III. Preparation for radiation therapy and its outcome will be necessary if radiation is indicated. Surgical removal or radiologic ablation of a pituitary tumor usually results

in destruction of the pituitary gland with subsequent hypogonadism, hypothyroidism, and hypoadrenalism, all of which must be treated with the appropriate replacement hormones to sustain life.

IV. Prepare patient for hormonal therapy to induce epiphyseal closure if no organic lesion is found.

V. Help patient with emotional adjustment to excess height, awkwardness, and incoordination.

VI. Patient may need help adjusting to derogatory remarks from others.

VII. Help patient prepare for and adjust to signs of sexual maturation when hormonal therapy is used.

EVALUATION

I. Parents and child can accurately describe what to expect if child is to be hospitalized.

II. Both are knowledgeable about the diagnostic tests that are to be performed.

III. They clearly understand the possible side effects of radiation if it is to be used.

IV. Both parents and child can adjust adequately to the child's height and/or sexual maturation.

CASE STUDY

K.C. at 12 years of age had already reached a height of 5 ft 9 in. Both her parents were of average size (father, 5 ft 11½ in; mother, 5 ft 4¼ in). K.C. was suspected of having a pituitary adenoma with resultant excessive growth hormone secretion. Neither condition was found. It was determined that K.C. had constitutional (genetic) tall stature, and she was given estrogen therapy to hasten epiphyseal closure. She had been quite shy due to derogatory and curious comments made about her height. K.C. was prepared mentally for the rapid physical changes that would take place with sex steroid treatment, but she became even more self-conscious as she matured rapidly. She also appeared more mature physically than she was mentally or socially. Preventive counseling directed at acceptance of her age role rather than a sex role beyond her years was effective, along with positive response and support from her parents. K.C. is now 16 years old, less outstanding in height and physical appearance, and, although still tall (5 ft 11 in) and of slightly below-average intelligence, apparently accepted by herself and others.

Precocious Puberty

DEFINITION

Precocious puberty is the premature maturation of the genital tissues and reproductive organs. It may be due to tumor of the hypothalamus, pituitary, or gonads, or occasionally of the adrenals.

There are a few rare syndromes which include precocious puberty. The least rare of these is the McCune-Albright syndrome, probably a genetically transmitted disorder, in which precocious puberty is associated with skin and bone lesions. By far the most common cause of precocious puberty is simply the "early alarm clock" or early onset of puberty due to unknown causes and without evidence of organic disease. This is called *constitutional precocious puberty.*

Puberty may begin at any age, even in infancy, and is called precocious if menstruation occurs before 8 years of age or if there are signs of maturation before age 10 in boys. The major danger, especially for the constitutional type of precocious puberty, is early epiphyseal closure and resultant short stature. If tumors are present, they should, of course, be removed.

ASSESSMENT

I. Parents are usually very cognizant of early sexual development and promptly seek professional attention.

II. A careful history of the sequence of appearance of sexual characteristics should be obtained, including history of vaginal bleeding in the female and spontaneous erections and ejaculation in the male.

III. Physical examination should include external and internal examination of the genital organs and an assessment of sexual maturation according to the Tanner scale (2).

PROBLEMS
I. Child must be referred to a physician to identify or rule out tumors.
II. Psychosocial adjustment of child and parents to advanced sexuality is necessary.
III. Sexual abuse must be prevented.

GOALS OF CARE
I. See that the child obtains medical diagnosis to determine the etiology of the precocious development.
II. Assist family to appropriate medical or surgical treatment when organic lesions are found (minority of cases), and provide support during treatment.
III. Counsel child and parents regarding maturation.
IV. Counsel child and parents about handling sexual feelings.
V. Prevent sexual abuse.

INTERVENTION
I. Medical referral is necessary.
II. Instruct and counsel child and parents.
III. Other persons (teacher, pastor, perhaps close friends) may need instruction and guidance. The teacher may be asked to intervene in specific instances when attention is drawn by classmates to the child's early sexual development or when difficult situations appear to be arising from the child's school contacts.
IV. Parents may need help in recognizing that early sexual development, while uncommon, is not a calamity. It does, however, have inherent problems.

EVALUATION
I. Physician's diagnosis and treatment are obtained.
II. Child, family, and involved community members cope adequately.
III. Child's psychosocial development is adequate.

CASE STUDY
M.T. was brought to the clinic when her mother noted that the 6-year-old had some pubic hair (Fig. 17-1). Laboratory studies revealed postpuberty levels of luteinizing hormone (LH) and follicle-stimulating hormone (FSH), but not the high levels expected with tumors. No tumors of the hypothalamus, pituitary, or ovaries were found. The medical diagnosis of constitutional precocious puberty was made. Menstruation occurred at age 8. With sexual counseling, M.T.'s development has been reasonably smooth, without evidence of problems relative to menstruation, sexuality, or sexual abuse. She has been told that she simply is growing up earlier than others her age and that they will catch up with her. Usual adolescent adjustment is expected.

Cushing's Disease   Cushing's disease is only rarely caused by lesions of either the hypothalamus or the pituitary. It will be discussed under diseases of the adrenal gland, with which it is more commonly associated.

Disorders Due to Deficient Anterior Pituitary Hormone Production

---

Dwarfism   **DEFINITION**
Dwarfism is the failure of growth in height to keep pace with norms. It is generally defined as a growth rate of less than 2 in per year and an attained stature more than two standard deviations below the mean. There are many causes of dwarfism, of which lack of growth hormone is only one. Insufficient nutritional intake, central nervous system damage, heart or lung disease, malabsorption disease of the gastrointestinal tract, chronic infection, inborn errors of metabolism, hypothyroidism, uncontrolled diabetes mellitus, and a host of rare congenital syndromes are some of the causes in addition to pituitary failure. Only dwarfism due to growth hormone deficiency will be discussed here, but in the assessment of a patient

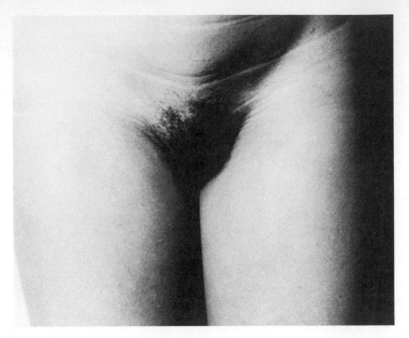

FIGURE 17-1 / Precocious puberty, age 6 years.

with short stature all the above must be looked for and ruled out before the endocrine evaluation is started.

By far the commonest cause of short stature, particularly in males, is delayed development. This condition goes by various names, including *constitutional dwarfism, constitutional delayed growth, delayed development,* and *delayed adolescence.* All these terms refer to the child who has no organic disease but simply grows slowly. These children ultimately attain their predetermined height and reach puberty, but usually 2 to 3 years later than their peers. Adolescence can be accelerated in these children, making them more like their peers in body size and appearance (pubic hair, beard, etc.), by the use of sex steroids, but with the sacrifice of 1 to 2 in of adult height because of early epiphyseal closure.

Pituitary dwarfism can be an isolated growth hormone deficiency, for which treatment is the replacement of growth hormone by every-other-day injections of human growth hormone; or it may be a part of multiple pituitary deficiencies or even panhypopituitarism, in which all pituitary function is lost. In panhypopituitarism there are multiple endocrine deficiencies affecting the gonads, adrenals, and thyroid. All must be recognized and treated.

ASSESSMENT

I. A careful health history is important, since many nonendocrine causes of dwarfism (e.g., malabsorption diarrhea) can be discovered by the history.

II. Since most short stature is genetic (constitutional), a family history of parental and family heights, growth patterns, and ages of puberty is very important, also.

III. A history of the pattern of the child's growth (height and weight at various ages plotted on a growth chart) can be very helpful because different causes of short stature produce different patterns of growth. For example, cretins grow slowly from birth, while growth hormone deficient children grow normally for the first 1 to 2 years and then begin to slow down and fall below the curve.

IV. The most important element of nursing assessment is the evaluation of the height and weight. These measurements should be carefully taken and plotted on a growth chart and properly interpreted. Standing height and sitting height should be measured in order to determine the ratio of the upper and lower segments. (Some conditions such as achondroplasia and cretinism produce fairly normal trunk length but short extremities so the upper segment exceeds the lower, while genetic dwarfs and pituitary dwarfs have proportional growth with nearly equal upper and lower segments.)

V. Head circumference and arm span should also be measured and recorded.

PROBLEMS

I. Short stature and delayed puberty are not socially as acceptable in American culture as is tall stature, so short people may develop psychologic problems related to their self-concept and social acceptability.

II. Organic problems such as tumors must be found and corrected.

GOALS OF CARE

I. Refer to physician to:
  A. Find and correct organic lesions if any.
  B. Find and correct metabolic problems if present.
  C. Identify deficiency of growth hormone if present and treat with supplemental growth hormone.
  D. Determine the value or desirability of sex hormone treatment if short stature is constitutional.

II. Facilitate proper psychosocial adjustment to short stature and/or treatment regime.

INTERVENTION

I. Refer to physician if this has not been done.

II. Counsel on good nutrition to be sure intake is adequate to achieve full potential growth.

III. Prepare child and family for treatment regimes (growth hormone is given by injection, so child or parent must be taught injection technique).

IV. Counsel as to adjustment of a short person in a tall person's world to prevent or treat psychosocial adjustment problems.

EVALUATION

I. Physician referral and follow-up care are obtained.

II. Family can complete food records and prepare diet plans.

III. Parents (or child if old enough) can give injections or oral medications.

IV. Parents can take accurate height measurements and keep records of them.

V. Parents and child can discuss their feelings about size, and cope and adjust adequately.

CASE STUDY

D.G. began to notice that he was shorter than his classmates around age 6. Since his parents were with him every day, they were not acutely aware that he was small. Their health care visits were infrequent, so assessment by growth chart records was not available. D.G. was below the 3d percentile in height and weight when he induced his parents to take him to a physician at age 8. He was hospitalized and tested and found to be deficient in growth hormone. On acceptance by the National Pituitary Agency, he began receiving growth hormone by injection at age 9. He progressed rapidly. Now as a 12-year-old with 3 to 5 years of potential growth left, he is at the 16th percentile in height and although some growth hormone treatment has been completed he will continue to grow with sex hormone treatment. He may reach the 50th percentile in growth. He has learned some pretty sharp "comebacks" to comments about his height. His confidence appeared to improve as he became aware of many famous short people who did not have the advantage of the therapy which he is receiving.

Addison's Disease

Addison's disease is a deficiency of adrenocorticosteroids from the adrenal glands. It may be due to hypothalamic or pituitary deficiency, but is usually caused by destruction of the adrenal glands themselves. The symptoms and signs are the same in any of the three situations except that the skin pigmentation characteristic of adrenal gland failure does not occur with ACTH deficiency. In adrenal gland failure, ACTH from the pituitary gland is elevated, along with melanophore-stimulating hormone (MSH), because of lack of cortisol feedback. These hormones cause increased pigmentation of the skin. In pituitary deficiency, ACTH and MSH are deficient and no pigmentation occurs. Isolated ACTH deficiency is rare in children. It usually appears along with other pituitary hormone deficiencies as a result of hypothalamic or pituitary destruction by a tumor or as a result of infarction of the pituitary gland during periods of profound hypotensive shock, and is known as Sheehan's syndrome or Simmond's disease.

Since ACTH deficiency is rare, and Addison's disease more commonly results from primary adrenal failure, care of the child with Addison's disease will be discussed in the later section on the adrenal glands.

Gonadotropin Deficiency

DEFINITION

The gonadotropins—*follicle-stimulating hormone* (FSH) and *luteinizing hormone* (LH)—are responsible for stimulation of the ovaries or testicles to produce sex hormones and reproductive cells. Deficiency of FSH and LH results in poor development of the gonads, lack of sexual development, lack of secondary sex characteristics, and infertility. Lack of sexual development may be due to failure of the gonads, in which case FSH and LH will be elevated. This condition is known as *hypogonadism* and has many causes. Deficiency of FSH and LH may be caused by hypothalamic or pituitary deficiency and is called *hypogonadotropic hypogonadism*. This condition may be genetic but more commonly is due to destruction of a portion of the hypothalamus or pituitary by trauma, infection, tumor, etc. Gonadotropin deficiency may be an isolated deficiency or may be a part of multiple pituitary or panpituitary deficiencies. The primary sign of this disease is delayed or absent puberty and infertility.

ASSESSMENT

I. Secondary sexual hair (pubic hair, axillary hair, beard) is absent.
II. Penis and testicles are small.
III. Voice deepens, however, in the male.
IV. External genitalia in the female are infantile.
V. Female's body contours remain boyish, without breast development.
VI. Pelvic examination reveals small ovaries and an infantile uterus.
VII. Menstruation is absent.
VIII. Note: Puberty is not considered delayed unless there are no signs of development by age 16 in the male and age 14 in the female.

PROBLEMS

I. Psychosocial problems may occur secondary to being "different." Discomfort is especially acute in situations that require undressing, such as the school locker room. Children compare genital development and, in girls, breast development, and the slow developer is the object of ridicule.
II. Child needs medical evaluation.
   A. If pubertal delay is caused by hypothalamic or pituitary disorder, tumors must be sought.
   B. Sex hormones may be indicated.
III. Infertility exists and may be permanent in spite of treatment.

GOALS OF CARE

I. Obtain medical diagnosis of the etiology of the problem, treatment of any existing lesions (e.g., tumor removal), and replacement therapy with sex steroids (testosterone for a male, estrogens and progesterone for a female). FSH and LH cannot be given since they are in short supply, expensive, and must be injected. Sex steroids can be given orally.
II. The patient will adjust well to both delayed puberty and the marked change that results from hormone therapy.

III. The ultimate goal is to enable the child to be psychosocially sound and sexually functional even though he or she may remain infertile.

INTERVENTION
I. Refer to physician if this has not been done.
II. Give encouragement about the normalization of physical development following treatment.
III. If no treatment is instituted or if little change in maturation is expected, intervention is directed toward self-image and self-acceptance.
IV. If the expected outcome is normal sexual function but continued infertility, child and parents should be given opportunities to express their feelings about infertility, to explore the possibilities of child adoption, etc.

EVALUATION
I. Medical evaluation and follow-up are obtained.
II. Child is psychosocially well adjusted, sexually functional, and normal in appearance.

CASE STUDY
P.J. was 16 years old and embarrassed in the locker room. His parents finally brought him to the doctor because he consistently refused to take gym and they had been called to the school office to discuss the matter. The parents had noticed that P.J.'s voice had not changed, but they thought that was just delayed. FSH and LH levels were low, as were plasma testosterone levels. Administration of chorionic gonadotropin by injection brought testosterone levels to normal. The medical diagnosis, then, was hypogonadotropic hypogonadism. Until a source of gonadotropin is available, P.J. is being treated with testosterone by mouth. He has developed normal penis size and normal secondary sex characteristics, and is sexually functional. His testicles, however, remain small and he is infertile. He no longer has trouble in the locker room and can defend himself against any ill humor. He will need continuing psychological help to adjust to his infertility.

Deficiency of Hormones Affecting Thyroid Function

Deficiencies of thyroid-releasing hormone (TRH) from the hypothalamus and/or thyroid-stimulating hormone (TSH) from the anterior pituitary do occasionally occur. The symptoms are those of hypothyroidism, discussed later under thyroid disorders.

DISORDERS OF THE POSTERIOR PITUITARY GLAND

Posterior Pituitary Gland Functions

The posterior pituitary gland is actually an extension of the neural tissue of the hypothalamus of the brain but sits in the bony depression called the sella turcica behind the anterior pituitary gland. Though it exists in anatomical proximity to the anterior pituitary gland, it is completely separate and has totally different functions.

The posterior pituitary produces several hormones:

1. The most important is *antidiuretic hormone* (ADH), which regulates water retention and loss by the kidney.
   a. *Increased ADH* results in water retention. ADH excess is usually temporary and is seen in diseases of the central nervous system and other conditions. It will not be discussed here.
   b. *ADH deficiency* results in marked water loss, a condition known as diabetes insipidus.
2. *Oxytocin,* which is important for uterine contractions.
3. An active blood pressure agent.

4. *Melanophore-stimulating hormones* (MSH), which affect pigmentation.
5. A let-down hormone important in breast-feeding.

Except for ADH, these hormones have not been linked to childhood illnesses and will not be discussed here.

Disorder Due to Deficient Posterior Pituitary Hormone Production

Diabetes
Insipidus

DEFINITION

Diabetes insipidus is a state of chronic and severe water loss resulting from a deficiency of antidiuretic hormone (ADH). The disease can result from trauma, infection, atrophy (genetic), vascular infarct, or tumor of the hypothalamic-pituitary axis. In children, diabetes insipidus is commonly associated with a tumor known as *eosinophilic granuloma*. This condition is part of the reticuloendothelial system malignancy called *histiocytosis X*. When an eosinophilic granuloma of the skull and diabetes insipidus exist together, the condition is known as *Hand-Schüller-Christian syndrome*.

Symptoms of diabetes insipidus are excessive urination (polyuria) followed by a compenstatory thirst (polydipsia). The condition is differentiated from diabetes mellitus in that, in diabetes insipidus, the urine is very dilute and does not contain sugar.

ASSESSMENT

I. Diabetes insipidus must be differentiated from diabetes mellitus (and from psychogenic water drinking, in which the drinking comes first and is followed by excessive urination).
II. A careful history of the drinking-urination sequence is necessary.
III. Test urine for sugar.
IV. Test urine for specific gravity. If it is 1.010 or greater, the child does not have diabetes insipidus.
V. Water deprivation test (ordered by physician): In this test the child is deprived of fluids for 4 to 12 h, and the specific gravity of the urine is tested against the osmolarity of the blood. In a normal child the osmolarity of the blood stays the same and urine specific gravity goes up as water is conserved. In diabetes insipidus, blood osmolarity increases and urine remains dilute as water continues to be lost. Note: During a water deprivation test, the child must be under continuous nursing observation. Since patients with this disorder cannot conserve water, they can become dehydrated and go into shock if not observed very carefully.

PROBLEMS

I. Dehydration and death if untreated.
II. Profound polyuria if untreated.
III. Regulation of medication is difficult to attain, as is acceptance of medication by daily injection or nasal insufflation.

GOALS OF CARE

I. Early diagnosis and treatment.
II. Parents (and child if old enough) are able to administer medication and regulate medication dose and water intake.

INTERVENTION

I. Assist in rapid diagnosis by urine testing and referring suspect children for medical evaluation.
II. Teach self-adjustment of medication by measuring urine output, specific gravity, and weight gain.
   A. If medication dose is too high, water will be retained, specific gravity of urine will increase, and body weight will go up.

B. If dose is too low, urine volume will increase as will water intake, specific gravity will decrease, and body weight will drop.

III. Teach parents (and child if old enough) to administer the medication. Treatment is by intramuscular injection, usually daily, of ADH in the form of vasopressin tannate in oil. An alternative form of therapy is the inhalation of a vasopressin powder into the nose for absorption through the nasal mucosa.

EVALUATION

I. Medical evaluation and follow-up are obtained.

II. Patient and/or family are skilled in injection or insufflation procedure.

III. Patient and/or family carry out proper weighing and urine-testing procedure.

IV. Parents (and child if old enough) are able to describe the course, signs, symptoms, and side effects of the disease and treatment.

V. Parents (and child if old enough) can describe the danger signals of dehydration and know when they need to call the health professional.

CASE STUDY

L.J. was 6 years old when her mother noted her frequent urination. She thought her daughter had diabetes mellitus when she took her to the physician. She had never heard of diabetes insipidus but recognized, on description, the weak, pale-looking urine her child was passing. Urinalysis revealed a low specific gravity and no sugar. A water deprivation test confirmed the medical diagnosis of diabetes insipidus. The mother, a licensed practical nurse, had little difficulty mastering the injection procedure and daily medication dose adjustments. The child's father and eventually the child herself responded well to teaching about diabetes insipidus and the child's care.

DISORDERS OF THE THYROID GLAND

Thyroid Gland Functions

The thyroid gland, located in the lower neck, can be felt by gentle palpation even in normal children. The gland is comprised of three kinds of tissue: (1) tissue for the secretion of the thyroid hormones, *thyroxine* (T_4) and *triiodothyronine* (T_3); (2) tissue for the secretion of *calcitonin*; and (3) the *parathyroid glands*. Calcitonin from the thyroid and *parathormone* from the parathyroids are involved in calcium metabolism.

The hypothalamic-pituitary-thyroid axis has already been explained (see "Anterior Pituitary Gland Functions," above). When the thyroid gland is stimulated by thyroid-stimulating hormone (TSH) from the anterior pituitary, a series of biochemical reactions for the metabolism of iodine occurs.

Inorganic iodine is trapped by the gland, converted to iodide and hooked to tyrosine to form a mono- or diiodotyrosine. The iodinated tyrosine molecules then condense into a double molecule called thyronine containing two, three, or four iodines. Diiodothyronine is not biologically active. Triiodothyronine (T_3) is the most potent of the thyroid compounds, but very little is produced by the thyroid gland. Most of the T_3 is produced peripherally in the blood by the deiodination of T_4.

T_3 or T_4, once manufactured by the gland, is stored in the thyroid follicles attached to a binding protein. When it is needed, T_4 is unbound and secreted into the bloodstream where it is again bound to a protein, *thyrobinding globulin* (TGB), and transported to the tissues. In the tissues, T_4 is converted to T_3 and inbound from TGB to have its desired effect on the cells. *The major effect of T_3 or T_4 on the tissues is to stimulate the rate of metabolism.*

Thus, in thyroid hormone *deficiency* metabolism slows down markedly, and all bodily processes are slowed. In thyroid *excess* all bodily processes are speeded up.

Deficiency of thyroid hormone can occur due to:

1. TRH (hypothalamus) or TSH (anterior pituitary) deficiency.

2. Lack of a thyroid gland (athyrotic cretinism).
3. Destruction of the gland (acute, subacute, or chronic thyroiditis).
4. Tumors.
5. Enzyme deficiencies at any of the steps in the formation of thyroxine, its storage, release, peripheral binding, T_3 formation, or peripheral release.

The signs and symptoms produced by these five defects are the same and are the direct result of the slowing of all metabolic processes.

Increased thyroid secretion (hyperthyroidism) can be caused by:

1. TRH or TSH excess.
2. Tumors ("hot" nodules) of the thyroid gland.
3. Inflammation of the thyroid.
4. Graves' disease (the most common cause).

Disorder Due to Excess Thyroid Hormone Production

Graves' Disease *Graves' disease,* the only cause of hyperthyroidism that is not rare in childhood, is nevertheless more commonly seen in adults. Because the nursing care of children with Graves' disease is like care of afflicted adults, information about this disorder is presented in Chap. 24.

Disorders Due to Deficient Thyroid Hormone Production

Cretinism **DEFINITION**
Cretinism (congenital hypothyroidism) is a congenital thyroid hormone deficiency due to lack of a thyroid gland or, rarely, lack of one or more of the enzymes needed for the manufacture or release of thyroxine. Lack of a thyroid gland or of the necessary enzymes causes slowing of all metabolic processes, including brain development. The most important consequence of cretinism is permanent mental retardation. Because some T_4 is passed from the mother to the fetus through the placenta, the infant may not show signs of hypothyroidism at birth. *Early diagnosis, however, is of critical importance in the prevention or minimization of brain damage.* For this reason many states now require T_4 screening for all newborn infants so that treatment can be started soon after birth.

ASSESSMENT
I. In the newborn period, cretinism may be discovered by T_4 screening. If not, when the infant is seen later, the history will reveal an unusually "good" baby who sleeps a great deal, feeds poorly, and has a low level of activity.
II. In spite of poor feeding there may be obesity and puffiness (myxedema).
III. Signs of slow metabolism are:
A. Dry, scaly skin.
B. Slow heart rate and low blood pressure.
C. Slow neurologic development (behind the developmental milestones).
D. Blank look and lack of playfulness.
E. Constipation.
IV. Large, thick tongue may be present.
V. Facial features are coarse.
VI. Umbilical hernia may be present.
VII. Growth is poor, especially in height.

PROBLEMS
I. Progressive permanent mental retardation will occur *unless* thyroid replacement therapy is started promptly. Maximal brain growth and development is completed by 6 months of age. For every day treatment is delayed, some intellectual capacity is irreparably lost.

II. All other problems (dry skin, bradycardia, constipation, growth, etc.) will respond to therapy and correct themselves. Growth, if long neglected, may not reach maximum genetic potential, but if treatment is started in the first year or so of life growth should ultimately be normal.

GOALS OF CARE
I. Cretinism must be recognized early (within hours or days after birth).
II. Early institution of thyroid replacement therapy is essential.
III. Even if diagnosis is delayed, thyroid replacement should begin immediately thereafter.
IV. Euthyroid state should be established and maintained throughout life.

INTERVENTION
I. Assess newborn for possibility of cretinism.
II. Establish a T_4 screening program for every institution in which babies are born.
III. Educate the child's parents about the prescribed medication and expected outcomes of treatment.
IV. Educate parents about consequences of discontinuing the medication (occurrence of hypothyroidism at any age).
V. Educate parents in recognizing signs of too much medication (hyperthyroidism).
VI. If diagnosis is delayed, evaluate child's neurologic development.
VII. If child is retarded, counsel parents about enrollment in special programs, such as early infant stimulation program.
VIII. Monitor child to maintain euthyroid state.

EVALUATION
I. Newborn's hypothyroidism is promptly recognized and treatment is begun.
II. Parents understand and cooperatively participate in the treatment regime.
III. Euthyroidism is achieved and maintained throughout life.
IV. Parents and child accept and adjust to remedial programs if they are indicated.

CASE STUDY
At birth, T.G. was noted to have rather coarse features and a large tongue. She was also somewhat hypoactive for a newborn. X-rays showed a retarded bone age, strongly suggesting that the child was a cretin. A T_4 was drawn and thyroxine therapy was begun pending the laboratory determination. Three days later the T_4 result came back showing 0.25 μg per 100 mL (normal is 4 to 12 μg per 100 mL) and confirming the presence of hypothyroidism. Medication was continued. The parents were given explanations about the medication, developmental stimulation, and expectations for growth and development. The importance of careful follow-up was explained. In 1 week the T_4 was 10 μg per 100 mL. The child was discharged and followed weekly by the physician for T_4 dosage adjustments to achieve suppression of TSH and maintenance of T_4 within the normal range. Return visits were reduced after 4 weeks to once monthly and then every 3 months. T.G. is now 3 years old and physically and developmentally normal, with T_4 of 8.6 μg per 100 mL and bone age equal to chronologic age.

Acquired Hypothyroidism

DEFINITION
Acquired hypothyroidism has many causes, such as iodine deficiency, destruction of the gland by tumor, infection, or inflammation (thyroiditis), or surgical extirpation. Iodine-deficient goiter with hypothyroidism is now rare in the United States because iodination of salt, bread, and other foods has practically eradicated iodine deficiency. Acquired hypothyroidism in children is now most commonly secondary to subacute or chronic thyroiditis (Hashimoto's disease).

Hashimoto's disease, seen most often in preadolescent girls, is thought to be an autoimmune disorder. The gland begins to fail, TSH is released in increased amounts, and the gland hypertrophies to form a goiter. The medical treatment is thyroxine replacement therapy. After 1 to 3 years of suppression the problem may remit and the patient be normal.

INTERVENTION

I. Guide patient to appropriate medical care.

II. Prepare patient for hospitalization and diagnostic tests.

III. Carefully supervise endocrine testing procedures (accurate collection of 24-h urine, properly timed blood specimen, etc.).

IV. Prepare patient for surgery.

V. Counsel patient and family for postsurgical adjustment and cooperative participation in the treatment regime, especially if bilateral adrenalectomy or pituitary ablation is required, since the child will then have a lifelong adrenal insufficiency or panhypopituitarism which requires careful and delicate medical management and patient compliance.

EVALUATION

I. Physician referral and follow-up are obtained.

II. Parents (and child if old enough) understand and cooperate with the treatment regime.

CASE STUDY

R.M., a 10-year-old boy, was seen in the endocrine clinic because of obesity of recent onset. History also revealed polydipsia and polyuria. Physical assessment findings included short stature, obesity, round moon facies, facial hair, buffalo hump, and large red striae in each flank. A presumptive diagnosis of Cushing's disease was made, and R.M. was admitted to the hospital for diagnostic studies. Cushing's disease was confirmed by findings of serum cortisol levels twice normal, ACTH absence, and abnormal glucose tolerance. Arteriograms, retroperitoneal air studies, and a renal-adrenal radioactive scan revealed a small tumor in the right adrenal cortex. A right adrenalectomy was performed with complete cure of the problem. The hospital course was uncomplicated. R.M. has regained normal appearance and has made a normal adjustment.

Cushing's Syndrome

Cushing's syndrome is a group of signs and symptoms resembling Cushing's disease (see above) but due to administration of exogenous adrenocorticosteroids rather than to their excessive production within the body. The syndrome is frequently seen when large doses of steroids are given in the treatment of such diseases as leukemia, nephrosis, and collagen diseases. Though Cushing's syndrome is reversed by discontinuation of the steroids, this treatment is often not possible because of the underlying disorder for which the steroids were given. Nursing intervention then takes the form of helping the child and family to adjust to the problems created by the drug—altered appearance and body image, susceptibility to infection, poor growth, etc., as outlined above under "Cushing's Disease."

Disorders Due to Deficient Adrenocortical Hormone Production

Addison's Disease

DEFINITION

Addison's disease is a general term for adrenal insufficiency (lack of secretion of adrenocortical hormones). Adrenal insufficiency usually involves failure of production of both cortisol (a glucocorticoid) and aldosterone (a mineralocorticoid). (See "Adrenal Gland Functions," above.) Of these deficiencies, the loss of aldosterone is the more important. The function of this hormone is to facilitate the retention of sodium by the kidney. In the absence of aldosterone there is marked loss of sodium in the urine, resulting in serum sodium reduction (hyponatremia), which causes nausea and vomiting and, with further salt loss, convulsions, vascular collapse, shock, and death. This severe state of salt depletion is known as *Addisonian crisis*.

Addison's disease may be caused by a deficiency of hypothalamic-releasing factor or of ACTH but more commonly is due to destruction of the adrenal gland by tumor, trauma, hemorrhage, or infection. In the past, the most common cause of Addison's disease was destruction of the gland by tuberculosis. Histoplasmosis is still a common etiology of gland destruction. A recently described cause of adrenal destruction is an autoimmune response similar to that of thyroiditis and indeed often occurring concurrently with it. Autoimmune adrenal and thyroid disease occurring with diabetes is called *Schmidt's disease.*

Addison's disease is less common now than formerly, since the incidence of tuberculosis has decreased, but it should be watched for in children with diabetes and/or thyroiditis since an Addisonian crisis is potentially fatal.

Nursing care of children with Addison's disease does not differ appreciably from that of afflicted adults, which is outlined in Chap. 24. The following case material is presented to demonstrate the course of the illness in a child.

CASE STUDY

A.K., 12-year-old son of a physician, had been seen by his pediatrician over a 2-year period with a history of nausea, vomiting, and vascular collapse. These episodes were usually accompanied by an infection. The pediatrician suspected Addison's disease, but the father refused to believe that this was the case, dismissing the boy's increased skin pigmentation as simply a good suntan. Eventually A.K., in acute Addisonian crisis with a serum sodium of 113 meq/L and potassium of 7.2 meq/L, was referred to a pediatric endocrinologist to prove or disprove the diagnosis of Addison's disease. Intravenous administration of a saline solution raised the serum sodium to 124 meq/L, and in a few hours the blood pressure rose from 60/30 to a normal reading of 90/60. Serum cortisol levels were repeatedly undetectable and serum ACTH was markedly elevated; the medical diagnosis of Addison's disease was confirmed. Hydrocortisone administration promptly returned the serum sodium to normal without futher intravenous fluids.

Hydrocortisone by mouth proved to be sufficient treatment to maintain the serum sodium. The father and the pediatrician monitor the serum sodium daily to adjust the hydrocortisone dose. The parents have been instructed to increase the medication during infections. A.K. has done well for 2 years without further crisis.

Adrenogenital Syndrome (AGS)

DEFINITION

There are three basic biochemical pathways of steroid synthesis:

1. *Mineralocorticoid synthesis,* the end product of which is aldosterone.
2. *Glucocorticoid synthesis,* which produces cortisol.
3. *Sex steroid synthesis,* which produces testosterone and, from it, estrogen.

Several steps are involved in the final synthesis of each compound. Each step requires an enzyme to catalyze the chemical reaction. Any one of these five or so enzymes may be congenitally lacking, resulting in a block of that step. Since some early steps are common to all three pathways, a block at a later stage in synthesis of the final compounds, especially cortisol and aldosterone, will result in shunting of synthesis into alternate pathways, particularly toward testosterone synthesis. There are some enzymes involved in early stages of steroid synthesis which block all three pathways and consequently produce feminization (from lack of testosterone) and severe salt loss (from lack of aldosterone). Unless recognized and treated within the first few hours of life, this severe form of the disease is fatal. The most common enzymatic blocks occur later in the pathway of cortisol and aldosterone synthesis and do not involve the testosterone pathway. When this happens, cortisol and aldosterone deficiencies cause failure of the normal suppression of ACTH. Under continual ACTH stimulation, the adrenal glands, in an attempt to make cortisol, hypertrophy (*adrenocortical hyperplasia*). Since cortisol and aldosterone still cannot be manufactured in spite of the glandular hypertrophy, ACTH continues to rise, which causes an increase in that synthesis which *can* occur, namely testosterone production. Increased testosterone during fetal life causes masculinization of the fetus of either sex. If the child is male, the genitalia become hypertrophied (*macrogenitalia precox*). If the condition is not treated in the male there will be continued masculinization, causing precocious puberty. In the female fetus, masculinization results in ambiguous genitalia. The external genitalia show fusion of the labia and an enlarged clitoris, and the infant may mistakenly be thought to be a male with severe hypospadias. Early differentiation is necessary both for proper gender identification and for prompt treatment of possible salt loss that could otherwise lead to Addisonian crisis.

Some of these infants have blocks only in cortisol synthesis and are not salt-losers. Especially if these children are male, the problem may not be discovered until precocious puberty results. If there is a block in aldosterone production as well as cortisol, as there often is in the common form of the disease (12-hydroxylase enzyme deficiency), then salt loss is the main problem and must be detected early to prevent death from hyponatremia and shock (Addisonian crisis).

The adrenogenital syndrome is so complex a pathogenic process that it is not feasible to correct and/or prevent salt loss and at the same time stop the masculinization of the child. Treatment includes replacement of glucocorticoids, hydrocortisone, and mineralocorticoids, which require close physician follow-up for dose adjustments. Later surgery may be necessary to correct the abnormal appearance of the female's external genitalia. The labia must be separated, the vagina opened, and the clitoris resected to decrease its size.

ASSESSMENT
I. AGS can usually be recognized at birth by genital examination.
   A. The male infant's penis is usually much larger than normal, and the testes very small.
   B. The female's genitals are masculinized and may look like those of a male with severe hypospadias, but close inspection will reveal no testicles in the labia, a vestibule rather than complete labial fusion, a perineal urethra in the vestibule, and a phallus which is really a large clitoris rather than a small penis. X-ray of the genitals will reveal a vagina and uterus.
II. Note: A careful examination of the external genitalia should always be part of the nurse's evaluation of the infant at birth, preferably in the delivery room or transitional care nursery. *Proper assessment at this time may prevent salt loss and Addisonian crisis and may be lifesaving.* Also, correct sex identification is obviously important for naming the child and orienting the parents.

PROBLEMS
I. Puberty is precocious in older children.
II. Genitalia are ambiguous in infants.
III. Danger of Addisonian crisis exists.
IV. Gender identification may be difficult.
V. Patient's and/or family's acceptance of gender assignment may be difficult, also.
VI. Salt loss and steroid management must be controlled as child grows.
VII. Plastic repair of genitalia is necessary for female.
VIII. Parent's and child's participation in and cooperation with long-term treatment regime must be obtained.

GOALS OF CARE
I. Prompt and correct gender identification is made.
II. Prompt medical diagnosis and initiation of treatment are obtained.
III. Physician follow-up for adjustment of medication is continued.
IV. Medication can be adjusted properly by parents during periods of illness.
V. Parents (and child, when old enough) understand and cooperatively participate in the treatment regime.
VI. Genitalia become normal-appearing and functional.

INTERVENTION
I. Physical examination of neonate for prompt and correct gender identification is very important.
II. *Alert the medical team for possible salt-losing syndrome.*
III. Accuracy is vital in specimen collection (24-h urines, blood samples to be drawn at specified times, etc.).

IV. Carefully observe weight, feeding, blood pressure, and urinary output in response to medications.

V. Educate parents and counsel about:
   A. Child's gender.
   B. Potential psychological problems related to abnormal genital appearance.
   C. Adjustment of medication doses by physician as the child grows.
   D. Regulation of salt intake and medication dose by parents during periods of illness or other stress.
   E. Need for long-term medical follow-up.
   F. Signs and symptoms of abnormal salt loss and impending crisis.
   G. When to call for medical or nursing help.

EVALUATION

I. Gender identification is prompt and correct.

II. Addisonian crises are avoided.

III. Parents understand, cooperate in, and cope well with the plan of care.

IV. Child adjusts well and is free of problems related to gender.

CASE STUDY: ADRENOGENITAL SYNDROME IN A FEMALE

T.D. was born in an outlying hospital. She was thought to be a boy with hypospadias and was assigned a boy's name. On the second day of life she began to vomit. By the third day of life she was retaining no feedings and so was in impending collapse. She was transferred to the medical center, where her serum sodium was found to be 110 meq/L and her serum potassium was 9 meq/L, values which in themselves are virtually diagnostic of Addisonian crisis. Twenty-four-hour urines revealed absence of 17-hydroxysteroids (the breakdown products of cortisol) and very high 17-ketosteroids (the breakdown or excretion products of testosterone). ACTH assay procedures were not yet available at that time. Normal saline was given intravenously, and the child stabilized. When the laboratory values confirmed the diagnosis of AGS, she was given hydrocortisone and fluorohydrocortisone (a mineralocorticoid) by mouth, and the dose was adjusted to maintain the proper serum values. When T.D. was 9 years old, she underwent plastic repair of her genitalia and is now a normal, functional 14-year-old girl.

Physician follow-up includes careful monitoring of growth pattern, bone age, weight gain, and blood pressure as well as serum electrolytes and drug dosage adjustments. Drug doses, particularly of hydrocortisone, are doubled during infections. With good nursing guidance T.D. and her family have adjusted well and do not evidence any uncertainty about her gender identity.

CASE STUDY: ADRENOGENITAL SYNDROME IN A MALE

M.J. was admitted at 5 years for evaluation of rapid growth and the development of pubic hair. His mother had not noticed the changes until he was arrested for breaking into a drugstore to steal a "girlie" magazine. Physical assessment revealed a child at the 90th percentile in height for a 5-year-old boy. He had acne, some facial hair, a deep voice, axillary and pubic hair, and a large penis and small testicles (Fig. 17-2). Bone age was 12 years. 17-hydroxysteroids in the urine were very low, and 17-ketosteroids were markedly elevated. Serum electrolytes were normal. The medical diagnosis, then, was non-salt-losing AGS. Glucocorticoids were prescribed and adjusted to suppress the urinary 17-ketosteroid level. Mineralocorticoids were not needed.

M.J. ceased growing and his sexual development regressed. By age 10, bone age had advanced to 14 years and he underwent spontaneous puberty without further growth. He had been a very large and tall child but ended up a short adult because of the early epiphyseal closure. M.J. is now 15 years old and sexually normal. He is fertile if he remains on steroid treatment but would become infertile if steroids were stopped, since the increased testosterone from the adrenal gland would suppress gonadotropins from the pituitary gland and prevent testicular formation of sperm.

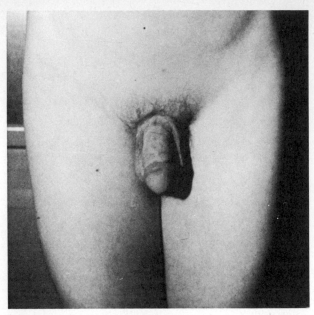

FIGURE 17-2 / Non-salt-losing adrenogenital syndrome, age 5 years.

DISORDERS OF THE PANCREAS

Pancreatic Function

Pancreatic endocrine disorders are characterized by insufficient, absent, or excessive insulin. The hormone *insulin* is responsible for keying glucose into muscle and fat cells, preventing fat mobilization, and promoting protein synthesis by increasing the permeability of cell membranes to amino acids as well as to glucose. Pancreatic diseases may be inherited or may be caused by trauma, infection, or tumor. *Congenital disorders* due to mutation or other alteration in the genes result in inadequacy of the insulin-making process, especially in the presence of stress such as viral infection, severe illness, or prolonged emotional strain. *Trauma* may lead to partial or total removal of the pancreas, causing loss of the number of cells necessary to produce adequate amounts of insulin. *Infection* of the pancreas may lead to an alteration of the insulin-making cells (the beta cells in the millions of islets of Langerhans scattered throughout the acinar tissue of the gland), setting up an antibody response which can then lead to autoimmune action against the beta cells. *Tumors* cause either increased or decreased functioning of cells.

Disorder Due to Excess Pancreatic Hormone Production

Hypoglycemia Excessive secretion of insulin occurs as a result of islet cell hyperplasia in infants (a disease known as *nesidioblastosis*) or, in older children, as a result of islet cell tumors. Both of these conditions are sufficiently rare as to warrant only minimal discussion here. Both disorders cause severe *hypoglycemia*, usually accompanied by convulsions, and are diagnosed by confirmation of the hypoglycemia by blood sugar measurement and documentation of the hyperinsulinism by measurement of serum insulin levels. Treatment of both conditions is surgical removal of the tumor or pancreas.

Disorder Due to Deficient Pancreatic Hormone Production

Diabetes
Mellitus

DEFINITION

Diabetes mellitus is a disorder resulting in an insulin-dependent or non-insulin-dependent state due to inadequate functioning of the beta cells of the islets of Langerhans. It is characterized by frequent urination, thirst, and weight loss in the insulin-dependent state (called *juvenile diabetes mellitus*), and by fatigue, slow healing of wounds and infections, obesity, and blurred vision in the non-insulin-dependent state (*maturity onset diabetes*). Of the 10 million American people with diabetes, 10 percent are dependent on insulin injections. One of 600 school children has been found to have this disease. Children may develop diabetes in infancy, early childhood, late childhood, or adolescence.

Juvenile diabetes mellitus is a disease associated with a lack of insulin production. During early treatment the diabetes may appear to go into remission in which little if any exogenous insulin is needed to maintain normal metabolism, but the beta cells evidently continue to decrease in number until most youths on insulin become totally dependent on it. Juvenile diabetes is sometimes recognized at an earlier stage in which the fasting blood sugar is normal but the 4- to 6-h glucose tolerance test results are abnormal at the times of two or more of the specimens. It is then called *chemical diabetes*.

Untreated juvenile diabetes mellitus results in nausea, vomiting, oliguria, abdominal pain, coma, and death. Besides blood glucose levels markedly elevated beyond 110 mg/dL (hyperglycemia), laboratory studies also reveal ketones in the urine (*diabetic ketosis* results from the body's effort to burn fats for energy when glucose is not available to the cells because insulin is not available), dehydration, and electrolyte imbalance (*diabetic ketoacidosis*).

ASSESSMENT

I. Family history of diabetes.
II. History of water drinking, eating, and urination patterns.
III. Test urine for sugar and acetone.
IV. Test blood for glucose.
V. Assess growth for age.
VI. If child is a known diabetic and not acutely ill, assess parent's and child's understanding of the disease and its treatment.
VII. Assess for ketoacidosis. *The child suspected of ketoacidosis requires immediate assessment and intervention to prevent rapid deterioration into convulsions and coma.*
  A. Evaluate level of consciousness and behavioral status as compared to child's usual behavior.
  B. Deep, rapid respirations (Kussmaul respirations) may be present.
  C. Note hypotension.
  D. Poor skin turgor and soft eyeballs indicative of dehydration may be present.
  E. Blood specimens must be analyzed for electrolytes.
  F. Test urine for sugar and acetone.
  G. Test blood for glucose.

PROBLEMS

I. Dehydration and death will occur if untreated.
II. If treated but managed incompletely, complications of eye, kidney, nervous system, and blood vessels can be expected. Adequate treatment prevents or delays complications.
III. Inadequate support by family and health personnel may result in child's nonacceptance of diabetes and consequent resistance to treatment and poor adjustment to lifelong disease.
IV. If parents and child have insufficient knowledge about diabetes and its management, small problems may develop into crises before help is obtained.
V. Lipodystrophy [atrophy (see Fig. 17-3) or hypertrophy] may occur 6 months to a year after insulin injections are begun.

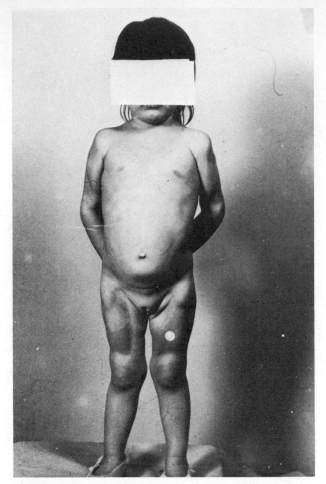

FIGURE 17-3 / Diabetes mellitus with lipoatrophy.

VI. If the diabetes is not adequately treated, the child's growth may be sporadic and he or she may be undersized (see Fig. 17-4).

GOALS OF CARE
  I. Early diagnosis and treatment adequate for child's growth and developmental stage are obtained.
 II. Adequate education is provided for the child and family to learn self-management of diabetes and to know when to call the physician or other health professional for assistance.
III. Parents (and child, if old enough) need to be able to carry out the mechanical aspects of self-care such as withdrawal and injection of insulin; mixing of insulins; rotation of injection sites; urine testing; urine and insulin record keeping; meal planning; recognition, treatment, and prevention of insulin reactions (hypoglycemia); and good health and exercise practices.

FIGURE 17-4 / Improved growth as a result of improved control of diabetes mellitus. *(Adapted from National Center for Health Statistics, NCHS Growth Charts, 1976, Monthly Vital Statistics Report, Health Resources Administration, Rockville, Md., June 1976, vol. 25, no. 3, supp. (HRA) 76–1120. Data from the National Center for Health Statistics. © 1976 Ross Laboratories.)*

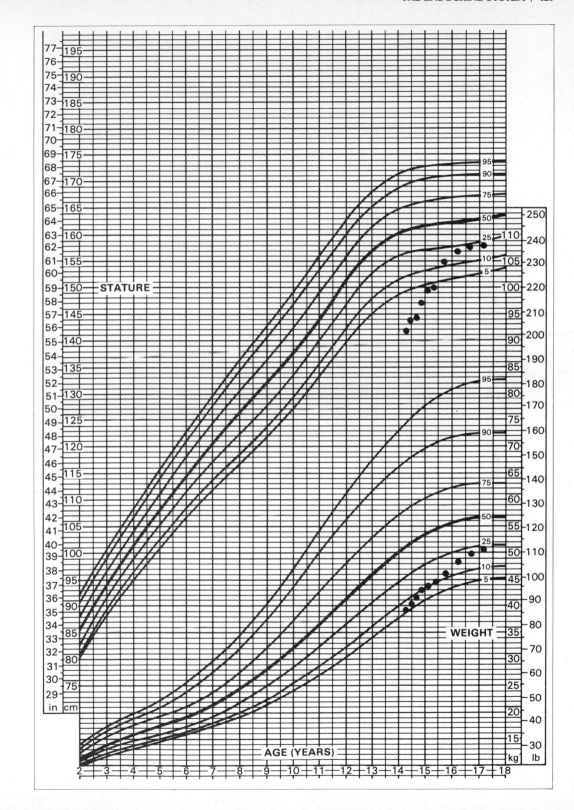

IV. Child and parents adjust to and accept the child's having a chronic disease.

V. Parents (and child if old enough) know how to alter the basic management of the disease to meet stresses of change in activity, injury, or illness.

VI. The overall objective in the nursing of a diabetic child is to enable the boy or girl to function at top capacity with the best possible control of the disease. *This goal can best be attained if diabetes management is designed to fit the child's life-style rather than the reverse.* Frequent communication and continual teaching are the best means by which this may be accomplished.

INTERVENTION

I. Identify diabetes early by adequate nursing assessment.

II. Assist child to immediate medical attention.

III. Teach parents, child, and schoolteachers or others involved to recognize and respond to hyperglycemia and hypoglycemia.

IV. Promote psychological adjustment.

V. For avoidance of long-term complications teach parents and child daily care and management of:
  A. Meal planning.
  B. Urine testing.
  C. Injection procedure with good site rotation.
  D. Hygiene of skin, hair, and teeth.
  E. Regular eye examinations for retinopathy.
  F. Prevention (as well as treatment) of hypoglycemia, which can be induced by illness or other stress.
  G. Exercise program.
  H. Regularity in daily living.

VI. Teach duration of action of the various insulins:
  A. Short-acting insulin (regular and semilente), 6 to 8 h.
  B. Intermediate-acting insulin (NPH, globin, lente), 14 to 16 h.
  C. Long-acting insulin (PZI and ultralente), 36 to 72 h.

VII. Closely monitor child during ketoacidotic episodes for vital signs, urine output, glucose and acetone in the urine, fluid intake, and level of consciousness.

EVALUATION

I. Parents (and child, if old enough) demonstrate good understanding of the disease and its course and treatment.

II. Parents (and child, if old enough) demonstrate techniques for injection of insulin and testing of urine.

III. Accurate and complete records (insulin and urine) are kept by the child or parents.

IV. Parents (and child, if old enough) keep adequate food records when requested and are able to adjust food intake to activity level.

V. Parents (and child, if old enough) are able to describe the cause, course, treatment and prevention of both hyperglycemia and hypoglycemia.

VI. Parents (and child, if old enough) know when to call the health professional:
  A. When the child's urine tests do not show the kind of control they expect.
  B. When there are ketones in the urine accompanied by elevated urine glucose (2 percent or higher) more than a few times.
  C. When glucose appears in increasing amounts in the urine.
  D. When a severe insulin reaction occurs.

VII. Child accepts the disease and is well adjusted for age.

VIII. Parents (and child, if old enough) recognize and respond correctly to his or her unique individual symptoms of hyperglycemia and hypoglycemia.

IX. Child's daily activities are adequately regulated and disciplined to promote general health as well as diabetes control.

X. Episodes of hyperglycemia and hypoglycemia are infrequent and well managed.

CASE STUDY

During one of my home visits, L.T. ran into the room saying he was having an insulin reaction. His mother, obviously very anxious, literally ran to the kitchen to get him a piece of candy. Once the candy was in the boy's hand and on the way to his mouth, he said he thought he was feeling better. The mother continued to appear anxious as she patted and talked to the child about how he was feeling. My observation of L.T. revealed no pallor, flushing (adrenaline response), overdilated pupils, or confusion. After the boy left the room, I asked the mother if this often happened. She said yes. I asked her to think back on her son's symptoms or signs that had made her believe he was having a reaction. She came to the conclusion that there were no positive indicators and that she was responding entirely to his verbal outburst. At that time, we also dealt with her panicky response. She had been talking to some other mothers and had unknowingly built up such a fear of insulin reactions that even the suggestion of one made her nervous. We continued to work with her feelings. She reviewed signs and symptoms of insulin reactions. L.T. was counseled as to his feelings and needs. He and his mother worked out a token system: When he felt like he'd "like to have" an insulin reaction and di*1* not follow through with attention-seeking behavior in this manner, he could give himself a token. Goals were set for a book, toy, outing, or similar reward. In the next few weeks, the incidence of hypoglycemic episodes was much reduced and the child began to learn to respond to honest symptoms of low blood glucose.

DISORDERS OF CHROMOSOMAL ORIGIN

Overview

Diseases of chromosomal origin usually are accompanied by a variety of abnormalities unrelated to the endocrine system. Only two chromosomal problems, in which endocrine disturbances are important, will be discussed—Turner's and Klinefelter's syndromes. The exact mechanism of chromosomal abnormalities is not known. For those diseases to be discussed here, however, the problem is thought to be one of defective *meiosis* (the cell division phase of the egg or sperm). During meiosis the chromosomes normally divide in such a way as to put one-half of the chromosomes in each daughter cell. When fertilization occurs, the normal number of chromosomes is reestablished.

Occasionally during meiosis of the egg or sperm, the chromosomes do not distribute evenly between the daughter cells, so that one cell may contain an extra chromosome and one may be deficient. If, during fertilization, a normal cell combines with a cell containing the extra chromosome, the cells of the fetus will have an extra chromosome. This condition is called *trisomy,* and many combinations of trisomy are known. Only one trisomy pattern is important from an endocrine point of view and that is the syndrome of an extra X (female) sex chromosome in a male, a condition known as Klinefelter's syndrome, to be discussed later.

Disorder Due to Chromosomal Deficiency

Turner's
Syndrome

DEFINITION

When a sex cell with a missing chromosome combines in fertilization with a normal sex cell, the cells of the fetus consequently lack a chromosome. Most of these situations are incompatible with life and the fetuses die and are aborted. One such syndrome can survive. This is Turner's syndrome, in which there is only one X chromosome and the other sex chromosome is absent. (This chromosomal configuration is often written XO.) Since persons with Turner's syndrome have no Y (male) chromosome, they are females. When only one X chromosome is present, however, sexuality is deficient in that the female has no ovaries and thus is sexually infantile even in adulthood.

It is important that Turner's syndrome be recognized prior to puberty so that estrogen replacement can begin in order to sexualize these girls. Turner's syndrome is suspected from physical examination and confirmed by chromosomal analysis. A presumptive diagnosis may be made in a phenotypic girl by means of a *buccal smear*, which is obtained by scraping the superficial cells of the mucous membrane of the cheek with a flat stick and spreading the cells on a microscope slide. The cells are stained and examined under a microscope for the absence of *Barr bodies*. Whenever two X chromosomes are present in any body cell, one of them is inactivated and deposited as a tight, dark-staining ball (called a Barr body) on the edge of the nucleus. Barr bodies may be seen in any cell containing two or more X chromosomes but are easiest to identify in white blood cells or buccal mucosal cells. In Turner's syndrome there is *no* Barr body even though the patient is female and one would be expected.

ASSESSMENT
I. Health history.
    A. Poor growth.
    B. Sometimes a hearing loss.
    C. Abnormal physical appearance.
    D. If old enough, sexual infantilism.
II. Physical examination.
    A. Short stature.
    B. Webbing of the neck.
    C. Low hairline.
    D. Wide-spaced nipples and shield-shaped chest.
    E. Cubitus valgus.
    F. If old enough, sexual infantilism.
    G. Sometimes hearing loss, mental retardation, and/or coarctation of the aorta.

> *Note* The physical findings such as short stature, webbing of the neck, and cubitus valgus are usually striking enough that girls with Turner's syndrome can be identified from the history and physical examination alone. If the child is below the age of expected puberty, the lack of gonads will not be evident. Often, however, the girl will not be brought in until adolescence, when she comes in because of amenorrhea and lack of sexual development. A buccal smear provides presumptive diagnosis and a karyotype is diagnostic. The external genitalia show a normal female configuration but are immature and childlike. Examination reveals an infantile uterus and vagina. Ovaries are absent and are replaced by a streaklike gonad that contains no hormonally functional cells and no ova, so females with Turner's syndrome will never be fertile.

PROBLEMS
I. Short stature.
II. Hearing loss.
III. Occasional mental retardation.
IV. Possible coarctation of the aorta.
V. Sexual infantilism.
VI. Infertility.
VII. Psychologic problems related to short stature and sexual infantilism.

GOALS OF CARE
I. Disorder is identified before the normal age of puberty.
II. Estrogen replacement is given to aid sexual development.
III. Patient achieves normal sexual functioning.
IV. Patient adjusts to continued short stature and infertility, which are not correctable.
V. Other defects such as coarctation or hearing loss are corrected if present.

INTERVENTION
I. Recognize probable Turner's syndrome by history and physical assessment.
II. Obtain appropriate laboratory confirmation (buccal smear and/or karyotype).

III. Obtain medical consultation for estrogen replacement if at pubescent age.
IV. Obtain medical assistance for associated medical problems (hearing loss, coarctation).
V. Assist psychologic adjustment to short stature and infertility.
VI. Assist adjustment to sexual maturation as it results from medication.

EVALUATION
I. Girl is psychologically normal.
II. Sexual function is normal.
III. Hearing and cardiac problems are corrected appropriately.

CASE STUDY
M.M. presented at 15 years of age with a complaint of poor growth and no menstruation. Physical examination was typical of Turner's syndrome. The external genitalia were normal for a 6-year-old girl. A short time later M.M. had surgery for an inflamed appendix, and examination of the internal genitalia was concurrently carried out. The uterus was infantile but well formed, as were the fallopian tubes. In place of ovaries, however, only a genital streak was found. The streak was biopsied and found to contain only strumal tissue and no functional ovarian tissue.

M.M. was begun on estrogen therapy on a daily basis for 2 years. During this time, she developed breast tissue and pubic hair. The external genitalia became more adult in appearance and the vagina became well epithelialized. Uterine bleeding began after 2 years of estrogen therapy, so cyclic hormonal therapy was begun in order to establish a normal menstrual cycle. A hearing aid was prescribed for M.M.'s hearing loss. Continuous counseling was needed for adjustment to the short stature and developing sexualization. With some difficulty, she made the adjustment and is now married and sexually functional though infertile.

Disorder Due to Chromosomal Excess

Klinefelter's Syndrome

DEFINITION
The patient with Klinefelter's syndrome is a male with an extra X chromosome. If an ovum which contains both X chromosomes as an outcome of abnormal cell division is fertilized by a normal Y sperm, the resultant fetal cells will have two X chromosomes and one Y chromosome. Since a Y is present, the child will be male with male external and internal genitalia. The extra X chromosome, however, will exert an effect and feminize the individual. The primary effect of the extra X chromosome is to suppress the testosterone production and spermatogenesis of the testicles. Feminine physical characteristics and infertility are the result. Klinefelter's syndrome is suspected by physical appearance and confirmed by buccal smear (the Barr body is present, as explained above under "Turner's Syndrome") and karyotype.

ASSESSMENT
I. Health history.
    A. Rapid linear growth with tall stature.
    B. Failure of sexual development.
II. Physical examination.
    A. Patient is tall.
    B. Patient has feminine physical characteristics.
        1. There is a female fat distribution pattern, including fat around the hips.
        2. Breasts are developed (gynecomastia).
    C. Masculinization is lacking, if patient is at pubescent age.
        1. Penis is small.
        2. Testicles are small and sometimes undescended.
        3. There is no pubic, axillary, or facial hair.
        4. Voice is high-pitched.

PROBLEMS

I. Appearance is feminine (broad hips with fat pads, breast development).
II. Masculinization is lacking (small genitalia, absent secondary sexual hair, high voice).
III. Infertility is usually but not always present.
IV. Psychologic problems exist related to feminization, lack of masculinization, and infertility.

GOALS OF CARE

I. The syndrome is recognized well before adolescence and before psychologic problems develop.
II. Testosterone is replaced.
III. Plastic correction of gynecomastia is arranged.
IV. Patient is aided with psychologic adjustment.

INTERVENTION

I. Health history and physical examination are necessary for early recognition of the syndrome.
II. Obtain appropriate laboratory confirmation (buccal smear contains inappropriate Barr body).
III. Obtain medical attention for testosterone replacement to masculinize the patient if at pubescent age.
IV. Obtain medical attention for plastic repair of gynecomastia and other inappropriate fat deposits.
V. Counsel to assist adjustment to his problem, to the changes effected by treatment, and to continued infertility.
VI. Counsel regarding sexual matters as sexual development progresses.

EVALUATION

I. There is regression of feminine appearance and increasing development of masculine features (growth of penis, appearance of body and facial hair, deepening of the voice, awakening of sexual interest).
II. Erection and ejaculation should be possible though these individuals are usually infertile (indeed they are often discovered in infertility clinics).

CASE STUDY

R.S. was 16 when he presented in the endocrine clinic for lack of sexual development. He was having severe psychological problems related to his lack of development. On one occasion, boys in his high school undressed him in the locker room, dragged him across the hall, and threw him into the girls' locker room so that the girls could make fun of him.

R.S. was quite tall with broad, feminine-appearing hips with ample fat deposition, moderate breast development, a high squeaky voice, a very small penis, small testicles, and no facial or body hair. A buccal smear revealed a Barr body. The karyotype showed an extra chromosome in the sex chromosome group, with the configuration XXY. Testosterone administration was begun on a daily basis. Linear growth increased for a few months, then ceased with epiphyseal closure. Body fat began to disappear and musculature increased remarkably. Penis size rapidly increased; pubic, axillary, and facial hair appeared; and the voice deepened. R.S. developed into a normal-appearing male except for gynecomastia, which was surgically repaired.

R.S. is now 6 ft 5 in tall and weighs 185 lb. His musculature is such that the boys no longer dare tease him or expose him to potential ridicule. He is able to achieve spontaneous erection and can ejaculate, though there are few sperm in the ejaculate. He will in all probability be sterile. Libido is now normal. Counseling for psychologic adjustment to his previous ridicule and to his awakening sexuality has been necessary.

REFERENCES

1. J. M. Tanner, *Growth at Adolescence,* 2d ed., J. B. Lippincott Company, Philadelphia, 1962.
2. Ibid.

BIBLIOGRAPHY

Chinn, P. L., and C. J. Leitch: *Child Health Maintenance,* The C. V. Mosby Company, St. Louis, 1974. A pediatric nursing text aimed at expected normal growth and development and the alterations caused by illness, injury, or stress. A useful tool accompanying this text is called *A Guide to Clinical Assessment.*

Gardner, L. (ed.): *Endocrine and Genetic Diseases of Childhood and Adolescence,* W. B. Saunders Company, Philadelphia, 1975. A medical text devoted to management of various endocrine-related diseases in children. Various authorities in the field are the authors for this text. The author for the diabetes chapter appears to have some limitations in expressing the need for close control.

Guthrie, D. W., and R. A. Guthrie (eds.): *Nursing Management of Diabetes Mellitus,* The C. V. Mosby Company, St. Louis, 1977. A composite of subjects and authors chosen to represent various areas of thought as well as information in the United States, to assist the health professional in offering the highest quality of patient care and professional education.

Jackson, R. L., and R. A. Guthrie: *The Child with Diabetes,* UpJohn Monograph, Kalamazoo, Mich., 1976. This medical monograph centers on the child with diabetes. Dr. Jackson's experience dates back to the late 1930s and his philosophy of close, regulated control is now being supported by more scientific evidence to show that control of the disease does make a difference in long-term outcome.

Kupperman, H. S.: *Human Endocrinology,* F. A. Davis Company, Philadelphia, 1973. An overview of human endocrinology and accepted patient management as of 1973.

Marlow, D. R.: *Textbook of Pediatric Nursing,* 4th ed., W. B. Saunders Company, Philadelphia, 1973. An informative pediatric nursing text dealing with various aspects of short- and long-term care of both well and ill children. Diabetes is described in the section on long-term care. There are informative charts on general care and on the comparison of insulin shock and coma.

Scipien, G. M., M. U. Barnard, M. A. Chard, J. Howe, and P. J. Phillips (eds.): *Comprehensive Pediatric Nursing,* 2d ed., McGraw-Hill Book Company, New York, 1979. Diabetes in children is presented in a compact and organized form as part of an in-depth study of children in various states of health. In this book, diabetes is described as a disorder or deviation in the chapter "The Endocrine System." Nursing management is included under each problem heading, (e.g., diabetes).

Spencer, R. T.: *Patient Care in Endocrine Problems, Monograph in Clinical Nursing,* W. B. Saunders Company, Philadelphia, 1973. An approach to endocrinology in both adults and children. This monograph emphasizes the adult, either with maturity-onset or insulin-dependent diabetes.

Tanner, J. M.: *Growth at Adolescence,* 2d ed., J. B. Lippincott Company, Philadelphia, 1962. This is the classic definitive work on physical growth of adolescents.

Villee, D. B.: *Human Endocrinology: A Developmental Approach,* W. B. Saunders Company, Philadelphia, 1975. This medical text approaches various endocrine diseases as they affect the individual throughout life.

William, R. H. (ed.): *Textbook on Endocrinology,* 5th ed., W. B. Saunders Company, Philadelphia, 1974. The classic text of medical management of endocrine diseases. This book includes a conservative approach in the care of diabetes mellitus as well as other endocrine diseases.

18

The Urinary System

Annette Crosby Frauman
and Cyrena M. Gilman

GENERAL ASSESSMENT

I. Interview with child and family.
   A. Name: Both full legal name and name used at home.
   B. Age: Also obtain birth date.
   C. Place in family: Is this child the oldest? The youngest? An only child?
   D. Number of hospitalizations: Where? Why?
   E. Chief complaint: What is the reason for seeking health care at this time?
   F. Understanding of the illness: What does the family think is wrong? How long has the condition existed? What is believed to have caused it? Does the patient's understanding vary significantly from that of the family on any of these points?
   G. Expectations about illness: What do patient and/or family think will happen (short-term and long-term expectations)?
   H. Health goals: What does family want for the patient? A cure? Control of problem with medication? Just avoidance of death? Do patient's goals correspond with family's?
   I. Residence/home environment: Address. Is there city water? Indoor plumbing? Electricity? Phone? Cooking facilities? Food storage facilities? Public transportation available from home to hospital or clinic?
   J. Family background.
      1. Cultural background: External appearances may not be accurately indicative.
      2. Socioeconomic: Income figures, housing, clothing, and transportation may be indicators.
      3. Religious: Discuss beliefs, but make no judgments. Certain religions have relevance for nursing care, e.g., Catholics may not want birth control counseling, Jehovah's Witnesses are opposed to blood transfusions.
   K. Significant data.
      1. Sleeping patterns: What were normal habits before illness or before hospitalization? Does patient nap? When? Does patient require a night light? What are usual bedtime rituals? With whom does patient sleep?
      2. Eating and drinking habits: What did the patient consume in the last 24 h? Is this a typical diet? If not, what is? What are favorite foods? What foods are particularly disliked? Can patient feed self? Does patient eat strained, junior, or table foods? Are there any medical or religious dietary restrictions? What does patient drink?
      3. Allergies: Are there any drug, food, or environmental contact allergies? Is this noted prominently on the chart? What are allergic manifestations—e.g., skin, gastrointestinal (GI), pulmonary?
      4. Elimination habits: Is child toilet-trained? What are the words child uses for urine, voiding, feces, defecating? When does child usually void and/or defecate? Can child void on demand? Is child incontinent? Does enuresis exist? Does child strain, dribble, incompletely empty bladder; experience hematuria, oliguria, polyuria, frequency, urgency, burning, or anuria?
      5. Activity levels: What were they prior to illness? What are they now? Is child hyperactive or lethargic? How long is child able to engage in vigorous activity without tiring?
      6. Recreational preferences: What kinds of activities does child prefer? Active?

Quiet? What particular toys, games, sports is child interested in or fond of? Does child participate in organized sports or play groups? What TV programs does child prefer? Does child read regularly? What types of books are preferred?

7. Communications skills/impairment: Is child verbal? Are communications skills appropriate for age? Is speech understandable to strangers? To family only? Are there speech defects? Does child speak/understand English? If not, are translations supplied by family?

8. Temperament: Is child usually calm? Excitable? Anxious?

9. Coping mechanisms: How does child deal with problems or frustrations? Does child withdraw, cry, act out, have temper tantrum, or manipulate? Is this age-appropriate?

10. Dependency/independency: Is child behaving appropriately for age? Illness often fosters dependency; to what degree has this occurred with this child?

11. Security measures: What makes the child feel comfortable or secure? What favorite toys give comfort? What rituals add to the child's security?

12. Special needs/procedures: Does the child require treatments or have drainage appliances to be cared for on a daily basis? Does child do or participate in any of these procedures? This is a good place for the interviewer to ask, "Is there anything else that I should know about the child that we haven't yet discussed?"

13. School: Does the child attend any type of school, day care center, or preschool? How does child feel about this? Does illness preclude attending regular school? What other arrangements are made for education (homebound, tutors, etc.)?

II. Observations of child-family interactions.
    A. Communication skills/impairment.
    B. Temperament.
    C. Dependency/independency: Does the family appear to encourage or discourage the child's behavior?
    D. Coping mechanisms exhibited.
    E. Child-family relationships, particularly the parent-child interactions relevant to the illness.

III. Physical assessment: Physical assessments may be made in a formal session, or informally during regular nursing procedures such as feeding, bathing, rocking, administering medication, or giving treatments.
    A. Vital signs: Many children with renal disease experience growth failure, weight gain from edema, wasting of muscle mass, decreased body temperature, and increased respiratory and pulse rates.
        1. Height: Record on growth chart for later comparison.
        2. Weight: Record on growth chart for later comparison.
        3. Head and chest measurements: Record up to the age of 2 years. Also record on growth chart for later comparison.
        4. Temperature.
        5. Pulse: May be bounding in hypertension. Rate generally increases with anemia of renal disease.
        6. Respiration: Rate and character.
        7. Blood pressure: This is very important in a child with renal disease. It should be done as consistently as possible (same cuff, same arm, same time of day). At least once a day it should be measured in three positions: lying, sitting, and standing.
    B. General appearance: Does the child appear well or ill?
        1. Sex: Do not leap to conclusions. Many children with urological problems have ambiguous genitalia.
        2. Growth and development: The use of a formal developmental assessment tool such as the Denver Developmental Screening Test is recommended. A continuing developmental assessment should be done by simply looking for age-appropriate behavior.

3. Nutritional status: Is the child obese? Are there signs of nutritional deficit? Is the child emaciated? Is the child dehydrated, well-hydrated, or overhydrated?

4. Appliances/prostheses: What are they? Where are they? Do they fit well? Are they in good condition? Do they function well?

C. Skin: Color(s)? Temperature? Turgor? Are there blemishes, infections, wounds, bruising, or petechiae?

D. Head, eye, ear, nose, and throat: Is there periorbital edema? What is the visual acuity? Are there cataracts (especially after long-term prednisone therapy)? Any unusual facies? Are the pinnae of the ears above a line extended from the inner canthus of the eye through the outer canthus and beyond? (Low-set or malformed ears are sometimes associated with urogenital anomalies.) Are there signs of ear or throat infections? Is the hair sparse, dry, or brittle? What is the state of repair of the teeth? Are they cleaned adequately? Is the breath uremic?

E. Thorax: Is there increased fat deposition (as in Cushing's syndrome)? Are there unusual breath sounds: rales, ronchi, squeaks, wheezes? Are there unusual cardiac sounds: murmurs, venous hums, or shunt bruits near the armpits, or friction rubs (as in pericarditis)? Is there pain on percussion at the costovertebral angle?

F. Abdomen: Is it scaphoid or protuberant? Is the liver down lower than is appropriate for child's age? Is there ascites? Are there pain, tenderness, or masses on palpation? Is the bladder enlarged? Are there stomas or scars from previous surgery?

G. Genitalia: Are they at all ambiguous? Are any of the following present: hypospadias, epispadias, phimosis, unusual redness, discharge, or swelling?

H. Spine and back: Is there any sign of neural tube defect? Is the spine straight? Is there any bone pain?

I. Neurological: Is there lethargy? Are there paresthesias? Are reflexes intact?

IV. Laboratory and radiographic data: While the decision to obtain these data is usually a medical one, the collection of specimens is generally a nursing function. In addition, monitoring the various values will enable the nurse to make better care plans.

A. Obtaining specimens.

1. Urine for urinalysis.

   a. If the child is not toilet-trained, bagging is necessary.

   b. Use equipment to which the child is accustomed, if possible. For example, a potty-chair may be used instead of a toilet.

   c. It may be very difficult to get a male toddler to void in a urinal in bed.

2. Clean catch.

   a. Infant: Scrub perineum well with Betadine or other antiseptic, dry with sterile sponge, and apply sterile bag. Be sure to retract foreskin when cleaning penis.

   b. Five-year-old or older: Use same method as for adult, assisting only as necessary.

   c. Toddler to 4-year-old: Need to adapt approach to the individual child. Most in this age group are uncooperative with either bagging or adult method.

3. Twenty-four-hour urine.

   a. Void at beginning of 24-h period and dispose of urine. Save all urine thereafter. Have child void as near the 24-h mark as possible, and include this specimen with total collection.

   b. It is important to impress the older child with the need to save all urine, as a toilet-trained youngster may void in the toilet without telling anyone.

   c. An infant should be bagged with a bag that can be emptied while left in place. Removal and rebagging with each voiding rapidly lead to skin breakdown.

   d. Most 24-h urine collections should be kept on ice or in preservatives. Check with the laboratory if unsure.

4. Catheterized specimen: Rarely done in children unless no alternative is available, then usually done only by a physician.

5. Suprapubic tap: Often done in infants and small children instead of catheterization to obtain a sterile specimen. Nursing responsibility in this procedure is restraint of child, maintenance of sterile technique, and comforting of child after procedure.

6. Stoma catheterization (to obtain a sterile specimen). The following method is illustrated in Fig. 18-1.

   a. Remove bag from stoma, and clean area with Betadine on sterile 4- by 4-in square of gauze.

   b. Wearing sterile gloves, gently insert the dropper end of a sterile plastic eyedropper. The bulb portion should have been cut off using sterile techniques.

   c. If the child is old enough, a deep breath, slowly exhaled, relaxes the stoma. This makes passage of the eyedropper much easier.

   d. When eyedropper is in place, gently guide a sterile No. 5 to 12 French infant feeding tube through it.

   e. Aspirate urine through the tube with a sterile syringe.

   f. Remove dropper and feeding tube from stoma simultaneously.

B. Hematology: Normal values (may vary with each laboratory).

   1. Complete blood count (CBC).

     a. Red blood cells (RBC): 4,500,000 to 5,000,000 per cubic millimeter.

     b. White blood cells (WBC): 5000 to 10,000 per cubic millimeter.

     c. Hematocrit (Hct): 43 percent.

     d. Hemoglobin (Hb): 13 g.

   2. Platelets: 200,000 to 400,000 per cubic millimeter.

C. Chemistries: Normal values.

   1. Blood urea nitrogen (BUN): 5 to 20 mg per 100 mL.

   2. Creatinine: 0.05 to 0.5 mg per 100 mL.

   3. Electrolytes.

     a. Sodium: 135 to 145 meq/L.   *c.* Carbon dioxide: 21 to 28 meq/L.

     b. Potassium: 3.2 to 6.0 meq/L.   *d.* Chloride: 94 to 106 meq/L.

FIGURE 18-1 / **Catheterization of urinary stoma. Use sterile technique. Have patient exhale slowly if possible.**

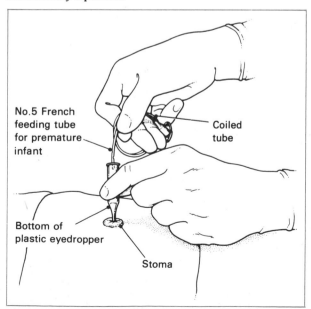

No.5 French feeding tube for premature infant

Coiled tube

Bottom of plastic eyedropper

Stoma

       4. Calcium: 9.0 to 11.5 mg per 100 mL.

       5. Phosphorus: 5 to 6 mg per 100 mL.

   D. Urinalysis: Normal values.

       1. Color: Pale straw to amber.

       2. pH: 6 (acidic).

       3. Specific gravity: 1.003 to 1.025.

       4. Sugar: Should be negative, unless recently ingested high-carbohydrate meal.

       5. Acetone: Should be negative.

       6. Protein: Should be negative, unless renal disease or dehydration is present.

       7. Blood: Should be negative.

       8. Microscopic: A few WBCs, RBCs, casts, and crystals may be normal.

   E. X-rays commonly done in the child with a renal disorder:

       1. Kidney, ureters, bladder (KUB): To check for gross anomalies or tumors.

       2. Intravenous pyelogram (IVP): To evaluate anatomy and pathological alterations.

       3. Bone age: To check for bone maturation, also used to check for calcification of bones.

       4. Voiding cystourethrogram: Evaluation for bladder anomalies, reflux, and strictures of the urethra.

   F. Nuclear medicine: A kidney scan is done (after intravenous injection of isotope) to examine blood flow through the kidney.

   G. Sonography: Ultrasound waves are used to chart kidney's outline and position in body.

V. Records.

   A. Previous medical records.

   B. School records.

VI. Other health care personnel to whom the child or family is known.

CONGENITAL MALFORMATIONS

Polycystic Disease

Definition

Polycystic disease begins in fetal life. The ureteric bud gives rise to the ureters, pelvis of the kidneys, and lower collecting ducts. The metanephrogenic cap gives rise to the glomeruli, tubules, and upper collecting ducts. If these upper and lower ducts fail to join properly in fetal life, polycystic kidneys result. The disease is divided into two types. The infantile type is autosomal recessive, and approximately 25 to 90 percent of the renal tubules are cystic. It usually presents in the neonatal period and can result in death in the first 2 months of life. In the adult type, which is autosomal dominant, symptoms may not occur until the fourth decade of life, as less than 10 percent of the tubules are affected. Approximately 10 percent of individuals with the adult form will manifest symptoms as children or adolescents. Medical treatment consists of medication for pulmonary and cardiac complications; shunting for portacaval hypertension; genetic counseling for parents; and dialysis and transplantation for end-stage renal disease.

Assessment

I. Infantile type.

   A. Large bilateral flank masses which are tense, symmetrical, and do not transilluminate.

   B. Variable urinary output; oliguria is common.

   C. Hypertension.

   D. Congestive heart failure: Tachycardia, tachypnea, gross hepatomegaly.

   E. Respiratory distress due to large kidneys, pneumothorax, or pneumomediastinum.

II. Adult type.

   A. Growth failure.

   B. Hypertension.

   C. Splenomegaly and hypersplenism.

  D. Esophageal and gastric varices and resultant hematemesis due to portacaval hypertension.

  E. Decreasing renal function, shown by elevated BUN and creatinine, leading to osteodystrophy and anemia.

Problems

  I. Infantile type.

  A. Low urinary output.

  B. Hypertension.

  C. Predisposition to congestive heart failure.

  D. Respiratory distress.

  II. Adult type.

  A. Growth failure.

  B. Hypertension.

  C. Thrombocytopenia.

  D. Hematemesis from esophogeal and gastric varices.

  E. End-stage renal disease.

Goals of Care

  I. Infantile type.

  A. Monitor urinary output.

  B. Observe for and control hypertension.

  C. Observe for and prevent congestive heart failure.

  D. Observe for and treat respiratory distress.

  II. Adult type.

  A. Foster maximum possible rate of growth and weight gain.

  B. Observe for and control hypertension.

  C. Prevent bleeding, especially when thrombocytopenia is present.

  D. Note onset of end-stage renal disease as seen in laboratory values. The earlier treatment is begun the fewer and/or less severe the complications (such as osteodystrophy or anemia) will be.

  E. Provide counseling for parents about hemodialysis and transplantation. Help child prepare for dialysis and transplantation.

Intervention

  I. Infantile type.

  A. Strict recording of intake and output. If necessary, weigh diapers to estimate urinary output (1 mL of urine weighs approximately 1 g).

  B. Frequent blood pressure readings. Nurses may certainly monitor blood pressures as often as they may deem necessary; a physician's order is not needed. Indications of headache or congestive heart failure warrant frequent blood pressure readings.

  C. Frequent vital signs and abdominal palpation for hepatomegaly if cardiac or respiratory rates are increased. Tachycardia, tachypnea, and a lower-than-normal liver margin are cardinal signs of congestive heart failure in the young child or infant.

  D. Report any signs of congestive heart failure immediately. Digitalization, antihypertensives, and low sodium feedings may be ordered; such orders are to be followed scrupulously.

  E. Observe for and immediately report any respiratory distress. Pneumothorax and pneumomediastinum are not infrequent complications. Oxygen via oxyhood, intubation, or ventilator may be required.

  II. Adult type

  A. Provide high-calorie meals within framework of any dietary restrictions of protein, sodium, and potassium.

  B. Monitor blood pressure frequently. Give antihypertensive medication as directed.

  C. Immediately report any bleeding, especially if hard to control. Hypersplenism can lead to thrombocytopenia.

  D. Monitor BUN and creatinine values. Rising values indicate onset of end-stage renal disease; this may come about quickly or slowly.

E. Provide genetic counseling for parents.

F. Provide parents an opportunity to discuss their child's defect and hemodialysis and transplantation. Provide as much information as they are ready to hear about both procedures.

G. Prepare child for hemodialysis and transplantation by visiting dialysis unit, playing with dolls who have "similar problems," telling stories, and drawing pictures. Be honest about possible discomforts.

Evaluation

I. Is intake and output strictly recorded?

II. Are blood pressures read frequently? Is blood pressure read each time child is irritable, complains of headache, or shows signs of congestive heart failure? Are antihypertensives given on schedule?

III. Are vital signs monitored frequently? If tachycardia and tachypnea are present, is liver also palpated? Is level of liver margin recorded in nursing notes?

IV. Does child show signs of respiratory distress or cyanosis? If so, is prompt action taken?

V. Is child taking in adequate number of calories for size? Is child cheating on dietary restrictions? A reasonably intelligent child will find an astounding number of ways to obtain forbidden foods, even in a hospital. Are both family and personnel aware of child's restrictions?

VI. Does spontaneous bleeding occur? Does hematemesis occur? Is bleeding hard to control? Do laboratory reports show lowered platelet counts?

VII. Are BUN and creatinine values stable or rising? If rising, are they doing so slowly or quickly?

VIII. Are parents given the opportunity for genetic counseling?

IX. Do parents understand what hemodialysis and transplantation will involve?

X. Is child prepared for hemodialysis and transplantation? Does child understand what is to happen and why? Is child given opportunities to act out anxieties verbally or in play?

Vesicoureteral Reflux

Definition

Vesicoureteral reflux is characterized by a backflow of urine from the bladder into the ureters. The backflow is due to incompetence of the distal portion of the ureter, which forms a valve as it joins the bladder wall (Fig. 18–2). The valve may be congenitally incompetent or it may be incompetent as a result of repeated infections. Continued backflow may result in dilatation and damage to the ureters and kidneys. Usual medical intervention is surgical reimplantation of the ureters into the bladder, forming a vesicoureteral valve.

Assessment

I. Careful attention to voiding habits. Dribbling, frequent small voidings, or the ability to void again immediately after the first voiding can be indicative of this condition.

II. Careful collection of a clean catch urine specimen.

Problems

I. Inadequate drainage of the urinary tract.

II. Infection due to urinary stasis.

III. Preoperative preparation and postoperative care.

Goals of Care

I. Maintain drainage of urinary tract to prevent back pressure and infection.

II. Treat existing infections.

III. Keep drainage tubing in place after surgery.

IV. Prevent residual psychological trauma from surgery.

Intervention

I. Promote drainage.

A. Keep catheters patent.

B. Prevent dependent loops in drainage tubing.

     C. Change child's position frequently (every 1 to 2 h).

     D. Careful intake and output.

     E. Empty drainage bag at least every shift.

  II. Prevent/treat infection.

     A. Careful catheter technique.

       1. Avoid irrigations.

       2. Change drainage bag and tubing every day.

     B. Administer antibiotics and/or urinary antiseptics on schedule.

     C. High fluid intake.

 III. Postoperative care: Prevent dislodging of "stints" (ureteral catheters, sometimes incorrectly called "splints") and urethral or suprapubic catheter.

     A. Restrain judiciously.

       1. Avoid using restraints as much as possible.

       2. Night restraints only as needed.

       3. Fully explain all restraints to patient and family.

       4. When restrained, provide routine respiratory toilet every 2 h or as necessary.

       5. When restrained, provide sensory stimulation and mental diversion.

     B. Tape catheters well to prevent dislodging.

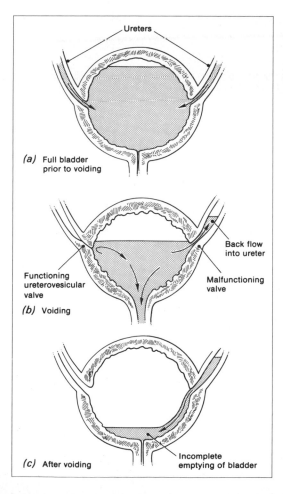

FIGURE 18-2 / **Vesicoureteral reflux.** (*a*) note the incompetent valve on the right and competent valve on the left. (*b*) during voiding, urine is refluxed into the right ureter. (*c*) after voiding, the urine returns from the right ureter to the bladder. [*From G. M. Scipien et al.* (*eds.*): *Comprehensive Pediatric Nursing, McGraw-Hill Book Company, New York, 1975.*]

IV. Prevent psychological trauma.
  A. Deal with fears of mutilation.
    1. Allow 3- to 6-year-old males to ventilate fear of penile amputation in surgery.
  B. Fully explain all tubes to child.
    1. They are not permanent.
    2. Unusual drainage sites; for example, suprapubic tubes are a necessary part of treatment at this time.

Evaluation
  I. Is urinary output consistent with intake?
  II. Did infection occur? Was existing infection controlled?
  III. Were drainage tubes kept patent? Did drainage tubes remain in place until removed by physician? Were drainage tubes removed on schedule?
  IV. Did postoperative complications, such as bronchiectasis or pneumonia occur?
  V. Did child demonstrate fearful behavior? Did child become withdrawn?

Exstrophy of the Urinary Bladder

Definition
Exstrophy of the urinary bladder actually consists of a group of congenital defects, of which the open bladder is the most obvious. The other defects include failure of the symphysis pubis to fuse and lack of urethral tubularization. There is thought to be a familial tendency for this disorder. It occurs about twice as frequently in males as in females. Surgery to repair the defect is often unsuccessful and a diversionary procedure with cystectomy is sometimes the treatment of choice.

Assessment
  I. Condition of skin and mucous membrane around and in defect.
  II. Assess stability of gait if child is walking.

Problems
  I. Drainage of urine onto skin.
  II. Cosmetic defect including possible genital deformities.
  III. Unstable gait if pelvic girdle is anomalous.
  IV. Susceptibility to infection.

Goals of Care
  I. Promote adequate drainage, with accurate recording of amounts.
  II. Acceptance of defect by child and family.
  III. Prevent injury from falls due to unstable symphysis pubis.
  IV. Prevent skin breakdown and promote healing if breakdown has occurred.
  V. Prevent infection.

Intervention
  I. Watch for possible obstruction of urine flow. Diaper should be constantly wet; if dry for a period of time, obstruction has probably occurred.
  II. If accurate intake and output is necessary, weigh diapers (1 mL urine weighs approximately 1 g).
  III. Bagging of defect should not be done as it will result in severe skin breakdown.
  IV. Assist family in accepting malformed child: Demonstrate acceptance; promote resolution of grief; as parents become ready to learn, teach care of the child.
  V. Advise parents that this child may be slower to walk and may require more practice with support. He may fall more often.
  VI. Protect from falls in hospital. Pad crib sides as necessary.
  VII. Change diapers frequently. Advise parents to wash and rinse well and sun-dry periodically to reduce ammoniacal bacteria. Use Karaya rings or powder around defect.
  VIII. Protect against fecal contamination of bladder by careful diapering, positioning infant on back (elevatd frame with canvas lying surface with hole for fecal drop-through

may be helpful), and maintaining scrupulous cleanliness. High oral fluid intake to "flush" bladder.

Evaluation
    I. Is drainage constant? Is output approximately equal to intake?
    II. Do parents hold and interact with child? Do they verbalize feelings about defect freely and realistically?
    III. Are injuries from falling avoided?
    IV. Do skin and mucous membranes remain intact?
    V. Is infection or reinfection avoided?

Posterior Urethral Valves

Definition
    Posterior urethral valves are anomalous folds of mucosal tissue in the male urethra, which act as one-way valves. Unfortunately, the valves open in toward the bladder, not out. This creates a severe obstruction which results in hydroureter, hydronephrosis, and ultimately renal failure. Because urine is produced in fetal life, this damage begins in utero. Usual medical intervention is immediate establishment of drainage, by use of urethral catheter, suprapubic catheter, ureterostomy, nephrostomy, or vesicostomy.

Assessment
    I. Bladder palpable above symphysis.
    II. Careful attention to voiding habits, especially dribbling and straining to void.

Problems
    I. Urinary drainage is imperative.   IV. Electrolyte imbalance.
    II. Infection due to urinary stasis.   V. Surgery.
    III. Overhydration.

Goals of Care
    I. Maintain drainage of urinary tract to prevent further damage to kidneys and ureters and to discourage infection.
    II. Treat existing infections.
    III. Prevent, detect early, or manage overhydration.
    IV. Prevent, detect early, or manage lectrolyte imbalance.
    V. Provide for smooth preoperative and postoperative course.
    VI. Prepare child and family to deal with drainage in the home situation.

Intervention
    I. Keep catheter patent by "milking" tubing as needed.
    II. Prevent dependent loops in drainage tubing.
    III. Change child's position every 2 h.
    IV. Careful intake and output; empty drainage bag at least every shift.
    V. Careful catheter technique.
        A. Avoid irrigations.
        B. Change tubing and drainage bag each day.
    VI. Administer antibiotics and/or urinary tract antiseptics on schedule.
    VII. Force fluids (as tolerated by renal function).
    VIII. Careful intake and output.
    IX. Monitor laboratory values.
    X. Skin care for overhydrated child.
        A. Avoid pressure.
        B. Treat any small break in skin immediately.
        C. Prevent friction in intertriginous areas by use of cornstarch, powder, or lubricants.
    XI. Provide pre- and postoperative teaching and comfort.
    XII. Observe for clinical signs and symptoms of overhydration.
    XIII. Prevent catheter or "stint" from dislodging (see interventions described for postoperative care of child with vesicoureteral reflux.)

XIV. Promote mobility in spite of drainage tubes. Use leg bag with harness (Fig. 18-3).
XV. Help parents and child become comfortable about drainage appliances and competent in their care.
    A. Cleaning and care of skin.
    B. Proper fitting and sealing of appliance.
    C. Sterile technique.

Evaluation

I. Is drainage adequate? Is urinary output consistent with intake? Is drainage tubing patent? Does child exhibit signs of urinary stasis, such as pain or fever?
II. Is infection controlled?
III. Are laboratory values for electrolytes within normal limits? Does child show clinical signs or symptoms of electrolyte imbalance, such as tetany or cardiac arrhythmias?
IV. Do parents and child demonstrate understanding of events and care associated with surgery? Are they free of unnecessary anxiety?
V. Are all drainage tubes patent and in place? Is child feverish? Are rales and ronchi present in lungs? Is child moving about in bed at least every 2 h?
VI. Is child up and about as permitted? Is child able to manage drainage appliances so they do not interfere with movement?
VII. Can family demonstrate ability for total care of drainage tubing and appliances independent of nursing assistance?

Hypospadias and Epispadias

Definition

Hypospadias is a misplaced urethral meatus at any point along the underside or ventrum of the penis. *Epispadias* is a misplaced meatus on the upper side or dorsum of the penis. Either of these congenital defects may be associated with chordee, ambiguous genitalia, or cryptorchism. Usual treatment is urethroplasty, which may be done in stages.

Assessment

Carefully inspect male neonates to locate the site of the meatus: retract the foreskin and look at the perineum. If any evidence is found of either hypospadias or epispadias, circumcision should *not* be done (the prepuce will be needed for reparative plastic surgery).

Problems

I. Parents' and child's feelings about deformed external genitalia.
II. Surgery.

Goals of Care

I. Assist parents in obtaining and understanding information about child's good prognosis for normal urological and reproductive functioning with successful surgery.
II. Good psychological development of child in spite of attention focused on his anomaly and in spite of genital surgery, which may be performed more than once.
III. Successful surgical outcome.

Intervention

I. Provide and interpret factual information.
II. Explore and help resolve parental attitudes toward anomaly.
III. Preoperative preparation of child.
    A. Cognitive-psychological preparation appropriate for age.
    B. Clear up any diaper rash or other skin breakdown in the operative area.
IV. Postoperative care.
    A. Take precautions to prevent pulling or dislodging the urethral catheter or otherwise traumatizing the surgical repair. Restrain child if necessary. (See discussion of restraining under postoperative interventions for child with vesicoureteral reflux.)
    B. Careful records of intake and output should be kept. Drainage bag should be emptied at least every 8 h. If drainage slows or stops, tube may be milked to achieve patency, but irrigation should be done only as a *last* resort.

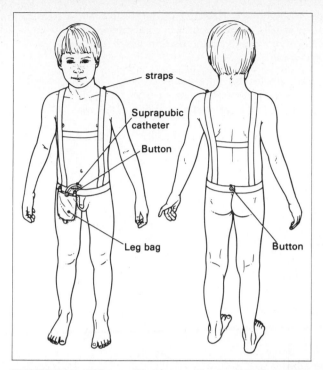

straps

Suprapubic
catheter

Button

Leg bag

Button

FIGURE 18-3 / Harness for securing "leg bag" to suprapubic catheter. Buttons for
drainage bag may be placed anywhere on the hip band. Straps are muslin. If a short
catheter is used, the catheter loop does not interfere with drainage. Harness can also be
used for child with nephrostomy tube, in which case the hip-level band pictured here
can be raised to the waist.

Evaluation

I. Is child well adjusted?
II. Are parents able to state feelings about the defect, cause, care, and prognosis openly
and accurately?
III. Does catheter remain in place until removed by physician? Do postoperative complications of infection, pneumonia, or catheter obstruction occur?

Undescended Testicles (Cryptorchism)

Definition

Cryptorchism is a condition in which one or both testes do not follow the normal
developmental progress of descent from their fetal origin on the urogenital ridge in the
upper abdomen to the lower abdomen, and down through the inguinal ring to the bottom
of the scrotum. This normal descent may not occur due to an abnormality in the testis itself,
to lack of endocrine stimulation, or to structural defects in the inguinal canal or scrotum. The
descent of the testis may be interrupted at any level, so it may be found in the inguinal canal
or in the abdomen. Spontaneous descent usually occurs in early childhood; 10 percent of
newborn males are cryptorchid, but only 0.3 percent of adult males are. This condition may
be treated medically by administration of missing hormone(s), orchiopexy, or, rarely,
orchiectomy. If surgical correction is necessary, this is usually done between the ages of 5
and 9.

Assessment

I. Scrotal sac is empty on one or both sides.
II. Testis may be palpated in inguinal canal.

III. Inguinal hernia may be palpated.
IV. Pain in testis usually indicates onset of complications.
V. Differentiate from pseudocryptorchism in which testes will descend when patient is relaxed and warm.

Problems

I. Undescended testicles are more prone to injury if fixed in one position, particularly in the inguinal canal. Traumatic orchitis may follow.
II. Structural defects that lead to undescended testes also predispose to torsion of the testes.
III. Males with undescended testes have patent inguinal canals (the canal normally closes once the testis descends), and hence are at risk for inguinal hernia.
IV. Undescended testes are 50 times more likely to develop malignancies than are normal testes.
V. The empty scrotal sac may be detrimental to the body image and self-esteem of the school-age child or adolescent.
VI. Bilateral cryptorchism will cause sterility after puberty.

Goals of Care

I. Case finding.
II. Integrated body image and good self-esteem.
III. Early detection of any complications that develop.
IV. Smooth, successful surgical course if surgery is done.

Interventions

I. Assessment for presence of testes in scrotum is part of routine assessment for all boys.
II. Any boy with undescended testes who complains of pain or shows signs of inguinal hernia or inflammation must be referred to a physician.
III. Preoperative preparation for child and family if surgery is planned. Detect and deal with castration anxiety.
IV. Prevent postoperative complications.
   A. Pulmonary toilet and moving about in bed during period of bed rest.
   B. Encourage mobility as soon as permitted.
   C. Observe for signs of ischemia in testes.
   D. Maintain traction apparatus (Fig. 18-4).

FIGURE 18-4 / Traction apparatus used following orchiopexy.

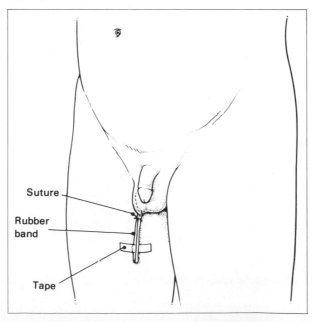

Suture

Rubber band

Tape

   E. Observe for recurrent hernia.
  V. Foster integrated body image and self-esteem. Encourage child to discuss his concerns.
  VI. Postoperatively teach child and/or parent to perform testicular examination at regular intervals.
   A. Palpate for masses or irregularities.
   B. Detect changes in size of testicle, either hypertrophy or atrophy.
   C. Seek prompt medical attention if above examinations are positive.

Evaluation
 I. Is child complaining of pain in affected groin? Is area swollen and reddened? Is child feverish? Is hernia palpable?
 II. Is child showing signs of bronchiectasis or productive cough?
 III. Does child ambulate freely as soon as permitted?
 IV. Is traction apparatus intact?
 V. Is child showing fearful or anxious behavior?
 VI. Is child and/or family able to give return demonstration of testicular exam, and to explain abnormalities being sought?

ABNORMAL CELLULAR GROWTH

Wilms' Tumor (Nephroblastoma)

Definition
Nephroblastoma is a malignant tumor arising from embryonic renal tissue. The most pronounced early symptom is an abdominal mass, often discovered by parents in bathing or dressing the child. Other symptoms include hematuria and pain. Usual age at diagnosis is birth to 3 years, though it is seen rarely in older children. Usual treatment is excision followed by chemotherapy. Using this regimen, prognosis has improved dramatically in recent years.

Assessment
 I. Abdominal mass.
 II. Hematuria.
 III. Abdominal pain.

Problems
 I. Parental anxiety regarding malignancy.
 II. Pain may be present.
 III. Surgery.
 IV. Nausea and vomiting with chemotherapy or radiation therapy.
 V. Anorexia.
 VI. Extended therapy.
 VII. Body image changes with chemotherapy.

Goals of Care
 I. Assist family to deal with feelings and fears related to malignancy, surgery, and chemotherapy.
 II. Control pain from tumor and surgery.
 III. Prevent postoperative complications such as bleeding, pneumonia.
 IV. Control nausea and vomiting.
 V. Ensure adequate nutritional and fluid intake.
 VI. Promote adjustment to change in appearance secondary to therapy.

Intervention
 I. Allow family to discuss concerns both separately and together. Provide information and assistance with grief.
 II. Preoperative preparation of child and family.
 III. Pain may be controlled by medications, position, diversion, and other comfort measures. Be alert to effective pain-relieving measures in each individual child.
 IV. Observe carefully for changes in color, breathing patterns, body language. Obtain vital signs as necessary.

V. Provide respiratory toilet. Small infant may need to be allowed to cry to aerate lungs. This needs to be carefully explained to parents. Older child should be taught to cough and splint wound before surgery; then assisted to cough, deep breathe after surgery. Other useful devices include a blow glove, blow bottle, and party favors.

VI. Provide foods liked and tolerated by child; avoid greasy foods. Small, frequent portions, attractively served are better tolerated. Carefully record intake and output to be sure adequate fluids are taken in. Distractions may help prevent nausea. Avoid noxious odors; don't keep emesis basin in sight. Room temperature should be cool. Rinse mouth after vomiting. Medication may be necessary.

VII. Carefully explain necessity for IV therapy to child at his developmental level. Explain reasons for therapy to parents. Explain how it is done, what will be done. Provide exercise for other extremities in bed. Walking may be done with IV pole on wheels.

VIII. Allow child to ventilate feelings about loss of hair, weight loss. Drawing a picture of self may be helpful, or engaging in play therapy with doll who gets chemotherapy. Carefully explain cause and time span of changes at child's developmental level. Wigs, scarves, caps may be welcome.

Evaluation

I. Does family (including child) voice realistic view of disease and prognosis? Are they able to state facts about the disease correctly?

II. How frequent are complaints of pain? Is pain relieved by the measures taken?

III. Is postoperative bleeding promptly detected and controlled? Does pneumonia or atelectasis occur?

IV. How frequently does vomiting occur?

V. Is child's nutritional intake adequate for age and weight?

VI. Do problems of immobility occur? How often does IV need to be replaced because of dislodging?

VII. Does child see self as essentially the same person despite body changes? Is he or she able to state that changes are temporary?

Benign Tumors

Benign tumors of the kidney are extremely rare in children. One type of benign tumor is associated with tuberous sclerosis, and hemangiomas of the kidney may occur rarely in infants and children. Treatment is usually surgical, and nursing care is essentially the same as for any surgery on the kidney.

INFLAMMATORY DISORDERS

Urinary Tract Infections

Definition

At one time, *urinary tract infections* were described in terms of the part of the tract exhibiting the most striking symptoms, for example, cystitis or pyelonephritis. The more accepted term at the present time is urinary tract infection. Infections are more common in males in the first year of life, due to seeding from septicemia. After the first year of life, infections are more common in girls, at least partially due to the short urethra. Therapy is directed toward identifying and treating the specific organism involved and the prevention of recurrence.

Assessment

I. Voiding patterns.

II. Clean catch specimen for urinalysis and/or culture and sensitivity.

Problems

I. Susceptibility to infection.

II. Infection.

Goals of Care	I. Prevent infection or recurrence of infection.
	II. Treat existing infection according to prescribed regimen and symptoms.

Intervention
I. Teach female children prophylaxis.
  A. Wear cotton underwear.
  B. Avoid prolonged contact with wet swim suits.
  C. Drink adequate fluids, especially in summer.
  D. Avoid dirty kiddie pools.
  E. Avoid bubble baths.
  F. Wipe front to back after elimination.
II. Administer prescribed medications accurately.
III. Reduce fever, if it occurs, by tepid sponging, prescribed medication, adequate fluids, reducing environmental temperature.

Evaluation
I. Does infection, symptomatic or asymptomatic, occur? What is the time interval of recurrence? What is the organism?
II. Do parents and child comply with the preventive regimen?

Acute Poststreptococcal Glomerulonephritis (Nephritis, Nephritic Syndrome)

Definition
Poststreptococcal glomerulonephritis is an acute condition which follows an infection with a streptococcal organism, usually group A, beta hemolytic, and is thought to be an immunologic reaction to the organism. Symptoms include hypertension, hematuria, oliguria, and periorbital edema. Treatment is largely supportive, with steroid treatment not usually indicated. The great majority of these patients recover.

Assessment
I. History of streptococcus infection in past 14 days, especially strep throat or impetigo.
II. Hematuria (brownish or red).
III. Periorbital edema.
IV. Hypertension.

Problems
I. Hypertension.
II. Dietary management.
III. Weakness, malaise.
IV. Fluid and electrolyte imbalance.

Goals of Care
I. Avoid complications of hypertension.
II. Maintain adequate nutrition and any prescribed dietary restrictions.
III. Provide adequate recreation and stimulation without overtiring the child.
IV. Prevent or control complications of fluid and electrolyte imbalance.

Intervention
I. *Closely* monitor blood pressure, being as consistent as possible (same arm, same position, same size cuff).
II. Observe for headache, restlessness, lethargy, convulsion, tachycardia, cardiac gallop.
III. Administer antihypertensives as ordered.
IV. Carefully monitor IV fluids as ordered.
V. Bed rest if indicated for elevated blood pressure.
VI. Diet should be planned after discussion with child and parents. Compliance will be more consistent if dietary plan is as near as possible to child's normal diet. Explain that restrictions are probably temporary. Sodium should not be restricted unduly, as this often results in not eating with a consequent inadequate caloric intake. Provide small, attractive, frequent meals using foods the child likes. For example, peanut butter provides protein, and popsicles provide fluid and calories. These may be well tolerated by the anorexic child.

VII. Provide activities that are interesting without being tiring. Assist child with care, having him do some parts of the care each day, as his physical condition permits.

VIII. Observe for symptoms of fluid and electrolyte imbalance. Monitor lab test results. Weigh daily.

Evaluation

I. Does hypertension occur? Does hypertensive encephalopathy or cardiac involvement occur? Are measures for reducing blood pressure effective?

II. Does child consume adequate diet?

III. Does fatigue or listlessness occur?

IV. Do fluid and electrolyte imbalances occur?

Nephrotic Syndrome (Nephrosis)

Definition

Nephrosis includes proteinuria, hypoproteinemia, edema, ascites, hyperlipidemia, and sometimes oliguria, all due to increased permeability of the glomerular membrane. The etiology is obscure. Nephrosis may follow an episode of glomerulonephritis. The course is characterized by remissions and exacerbations. Medical treatment usually consists of steroids and IV administration of salt-poor albumin.

Assessment

I. Proteinuria.

II. Edema, including ascites.

III. Decreased urinary output.

IV. Skin lesions secondary to edema.

Problems

I. Edema, which may be massive.

II. Increased need for protein intake.

III. Immobility.

IV. Body image distortion secondary to edema and steroids.

V. Fatigue.

VI. Anorexia.

VII. Marked susceptibility to infection (especially skin, respiratory).

Goals of Care

I. Prevention of skin breakdown.

II. Avoidance of complications of immobility.

III. Adjustment to changes in appearance.

IV. Adequate rest with appropriate diversion.

V. Adequate nutrition.

VI. Prevention of infection.

Intervention

I. Avoid pressure and abrasion injuries to skin (sheet burns, bedpan abrasions, tape burns, etc.). Support edematous scrotum with Bellevue bridge, shown in Fig. 18-5. Prevent friction in intertriginous areas with baby powder or cornstarch.

II. Give attractive, frequent, small feedings of preferred high-protein foods.

III. Carefully monitor IV protein infusions. Regulate rate accurately; prevent clogging of tube by rinsing with normal saline; use filter to remove crystals and sediment of protein.

IV. Promote activity as tolerated. Enjoyable activities will be met with the best cooperation.

V. Pulmonary toilet for inactive child.

VI. Explore child's body image, as through art work. Tell child the changes in his appearance are temporary. If cognitive development permits, explain edema and Cushing's stigmata in simple terms.

VII. Plan care to provide times for resting.

VIII. Do not allow contact with staff, visitors, or other patients who show signs of infection.

Evaluation

I. Any skin breakdowns?

II. Reduction in edema?

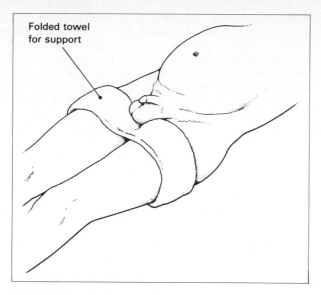

FIGURE 18-5 / Bellevue bridge for scrotal support.

III. Does child show sense of well-being?
IV. Does child accept changes in his or her appearance and know that they are temporary?
V. Is crying, cranky behavior minimal or nonexistent?
VI. Are there few or no complaints of tiredness?
VII. Do infections occur?

OBSTRUCTIONS

Neuropathic (Neurogenic) Bladder

Definition   *Neuropathic bladder* is a condition caused by impairment of the motor and/or sensory nerve supply of the bladder. Urinary incontinence and/or retention result. If uncorrected, neuropathic bladder leads to infection, reflux, and possibly renal failure. The social problems stemming from incontinence are also of great concern. The cause is most commonly a spinal defect such as meningomyelocele, but spinal cord injuries can also be responsible. Treatment is aimed at achieving continence and drainage as well as the prevention of backflow and infection.

Assessment   I. History of constipation: frequency of bowel movements, quality.
II. Malodorous urine.
III. Diaper rash, or irritation and redness of perineal area.
IV. Palpation of bladder height (retention).
V. Rectal tone.
VI. Urinary incontinence.

Problems   I. Incontinence.
II. Tendency to urinary tract infection.
III. Constipation.

Goals of Care   I. Achieve continence.
II. Prevent urinary tract infection.
III. Bowel movement at least every other day.

Intervention

I. Continence may be achieved in several acceptable ways, and the specific method selected by the physician depends on many factors such as sex, age, and the presence of reflux or renal damage. The nurse is involved in all these methods in teaching the parents and/or patient how best to perform the procedures.

   A. The Credé method may be selected for an infant with no reflux: Gentle pressure downward is applied with fingertips or the entire hand to the bladder.

   B. Self-catheterization, a clean, not sterile technique, may be selected for a patient old enough to learn it. The patient, usually female, carries with her a clean catheter, sometimes of a soft metal, and uses this as often as necessary (about every 2 h) to empty the bladder while sitting on the toilet.

   C. Most frequently, however, an ileal conduit is created surgically.

      1. The single most important aspect of conduit nursing care, because this is a permanent procedure, is teaching the parents and child how to manage the care after the child is discharged. This should be kept in mind while the nurse is performing care, and some part of teaching should be done each time.

      2. Another important part of the care of the patient with an ileal conduit is the incorporation of the stoma into the child's body image. Young males may greatly fear the loss of their penis now that it is no longer used for voiding. The nurse's acceptance of the stoma in a matter-of-fact way and a straightforward approach to teaching and answering questions go a long way toward helping the patient accept the stoma as a part of him- or herself.

      3. Clean rather than sterile technique should be used.

      4. The type of appliance most commonly used consists of a faceplate, a tag, and a belt. The faceplate is covered with an adhesive substance that creates a watertight seal with the skin around the stoma. The belt gives further support to the appliance when the container is heavy with urine. However, the appliance should be emptied frequently to avoid undue stress on the seal.

      5. Skin breakdown around the stoma, a continuing problem for most patients, can be easily cared for by substituting a special Karaya-containing seal on the faceplate. If the appliance is properly sealed, the patient may swim, shower, or take a tub bath without leakage.

II. Fluid intake must be adequate according to body size, especially in summer because of increased insensible loss. Recommend fluids liked and tolerated by the patient.

III. Bladder should be kept as empty as possible. Methods used for emptying should avoid injuring or bruising bladder walls.

IV. Diet should include fruits, fruit juices, and leafy vegetables to stimulate bowel peristalsis.

Evaluation

I. Is the child dry at all times? Is a urine odor present? Does the patient verbalize acceptance of the method and comply with the procedure? Does skin breakdown occur?

II. What is fluid intake per day? Do infections occur?

III. How often does child have bowel movement? What is size, color, consistency of stool? Does child cry or strain to pass stool?

VASCULAR DISORDERS

Renal Vein Thrombosis

Definition

Renal vein thrombosis is a condition in which thrombi form in the arcuate, interlobular, and main renal veins. Seventy percent of the affected children are less than 1 month old. Some causes are thought to be the high Hct characteristic of the neonatal period, dehydration, severe hypoxia, and/or a diabetic mother. Other predisposing problems are shock, septicemia, cyanotic heart disease, renal anomalies, pyelonephritis, and nephrotic syndrome. Medical management of the problem consists of (1) correcting underlying problems, such as electrolyte imbalance or sepsis; (2) hydration; (3) administering heparin intravenously to treat disseminated intravascular clotting; and (4) surgical excision of thrombi. The mortality rate has been as high as 60 percent, usually due to sepsis or uncorrected fluid and electrolyte imbalance. Fortunately, the prognosis has improved in recent years.

Assessment
I. Hard flank mass on affected side(s).   III. Oliguria.
II. Gross hematuria.

Problems
I. Vomiting.   III. Pain.
II. Shock.   IV. Dehydration.

Goals of Care
I. Maintain adequate nutrition.   III. Treat shock.
II. Maintain adequate hydration.   IV. Relieve pain.

Intervention
I. Maintain IV line by careful taping or splinting of site. This will provide adequate route for IV nutrition and hydration.
II. Keep strict records of intake and output. Weigh diapers if necessary to estimate urinary output (1 mL urine weighs approximately 1 g).
III. Test urine for blood and protein.
IV. Monitor skin turgor, fontanels, eyes, and temperature for signs of dehydration.
V. Take blood pressure frequently to determine if child is hyper- or hypotensive.
  A. Elevate feet and keep warm, if hypotensive.
  B. Also reassess hydration if hypotensive; suspect hypovolemia, as well as shock.
VI. Give pain medication as needed. Help child assume position of comfort. Encourage turning frequently (every 1 to 2 h) to prevent pulmonary stasis.

Evaluation
I. Is IV line patent? Has IV infiltrated?
II. Is child well nourished? Are electrolytes in balance?
III. Is child oliguric or anuric? Is there hematuria? Proteinuria?
IV. Is child dehydrated? Are fontanels and eyes sunken? Is skin turgor poor? Is temperature elevated?
V. Is child hypertensive? Hypotensive? Normotensive?
VI. Are conservative efforts sufficient to reverse shock?
VII. Does child appear to be in pain? Is child irritable or restless? Does administration of pain medication as ordered appear to give relief?

Renal Artery Thrombosis

Definition
Renal artery thrombosis is an extremely rare condition which, until recently, was usually diagnosed at autopsy. Causative factors are external trauma such as surgical manipulation; embolism from bacterial endocarditis or thrombosed ductus arteriosus; prolonged umbilical artery catheterization; or renal artery aneurysm. If medical diagnosis is made promptly, surgical embolectomy followed by heparinization can give good results. If the disease is not treated promptly, however, complete or partial nephrectomy may be necessary.

Assessment
I. Sudden flank pain.   III. Albuminuria.
II. Hematuria.   IV. Severe hypertension.

Problems
I. Pain.   III. Shock.
II. Vomiting.   IV. Severe hypertension.

Goals of Care
I. Relieve pain.
II. Maintain adequate nutrition and hydration.
III. Treat shock.
IV. Monitor blood pressure.

Intervention

I. Give pain medication as needed. Help child assume position of comfort. Encourage turning frequently (every 1 to 2 h) to prevent pulmonary stasis.

II. Maintain patent IV line by careful taping and/or splinting of site. This will provide adequate route for IV nutrition and hydration.

III. Take blood pressure frequently to determine if hypertensive, hypotensive, or normotensive.

    A. If hypotensive, treat shock by elevating feet and maintaining body heat. Assess hydration by examining eyes, fontanels, skin turgor, and temperature.

    B. If hypertensive, give antihypertensives as ordered. Elevate head to prevent headache.

IV. Keep strict records of intake and output. Weigh diapers if necessary to estimate urinary output (1 mL urine weighs approximately 1 g).

V. Test urine for blood or protein.

Evaluation

I. Is child irritable or restless? Does child appear to be in pain? Does administration of pain medication as ordered give relief?

II. Is IV patent? Has IV infiltrated? Does child appear well nourished? Are electrolytes in balance?

III. Is child dehydrated? Are fontanels and eyes sunken? Is skin turgor poor? Is temperature elevated?

IV. Are conservative efforts successful in reversing shock?

V. Is child hypo- or hypertensive? Does child appear to have a headache? Do antihypertensives lower blood pressure sufficiently?

VI. Is child oliguric or anuric? Is there hematuria? Proteinuria?

TRAUMA

Renal Injury

Definition

The kidneys are particularly susceptible to childhood injury because of the child's level of activity, lack of perirenal fat deposits, and the relatively larger size of the kidney. Most injuries are the result of blunt trauma from falls, blows, contact sports, and sledding. Degree of injury may range from contusions to cortical laceration and tearing of the collecting system to complete fragmentation and maceration of the kidney. Medical management, usually drainage and immobilization, is most commonly used for the less severe degrees of injury. Partial or total nephrectomy is performed only as a last resort to control hemorrhage or extravasion of urine. Renal injury is most frequent in males during the second decade of life.

Assessment

I. Vital signs: May be necessary to check very frequently immediately after trauma.

II. Urine dipstick for hematuria.

III. Careful record of intake and output.

IV. Daily weights.

Problems

I. Fear.
II. Shock and hemorrhage.
III. Pain.
IV. Urine output.
V. Immobility.
VI. Fever.

Goals of Care

I. Assist patient to cope with fears.

II. Control shock and hemorrhage.

III. Prevent or control pain.

IV. Maintain adequate urine output.

V. Child will choose own diversions and utilize them.

VI. Fever will remain below 37.5°C.

Intervention

I. Fears due to possible first contact with hospital and from accident which caused trauma. Explain everything that is done in terms the child can understand. This should be done even if the child seems unresponsive. Tests should be carried out in a calm, unhurried manner, and demonstrated fears dealt with in a straightforward, factual manner.

II. Monitor vital signs as necessary; may be done as frequently as every 15 min immediately after injury. Administer IV fluids at prescribed rate, use Trendelenburg's position; keep child warm.

III. Pain may be dealt with by certain positions, by changing positions, with ice to costovertebral angle (if this is helpful), and by careful monitoring of need for pain medication. In small children, pain may be evidenced only by facial expression, restlessness, and irritability.

IV. Urine output should be carefully and accurately monitored. It may be necessary to measure output as frequently as every hour immediately after trauma. Urine should be checked for hematuria, and the child should be observed for fever and hypertension, which are symptoms of urine spilling abdominally or retroperitoneally.

V. Immobilization is not well tolerated by most pediatric patients. Position carefully; ask child about positions most comfortable. Turn, cough, and deep breathe while immobile. Provide both fine and gross motor activities, as suitable for developmental level.

VI. Fever may be controlled by increasing fluids, pulmonary toilet, and fever-reducing methods such as tepid water sponging.

Evaluation

I. Is child able to verbalize or act out fear in appropriate ways?
II. Does hypovolemic shock occur, as evidenced by vital signs?
III. How often does child complain of pain? In what location? Is pain relieved by measures used? How long does relief last?
IV. Does urine output approximately equal intake? Does child complain of abdominal pain?
V. Does temperature rise above 37.5°C? Does chest remain clear? Do withdrawal and depression occur?
VI. If fever above 37.5°C occurs, how long does it persist? Does shivering occur during reduction? (If this happens, fever-reducing method should be stopped or modified, as shivering causes a physiological rise in temperature.)

DEGENERATIVE DISORDERS

Acute Renal Failure

Definition

Acute renal failure develops rapidly, over a period of days or weeks, due to compromise of the renal blood flow, injury to or disease of the kidney or its vessels, obstruction of the urinary tract, or exposure to nephrotoxic substances. It may be called acute tubular necrosis, because in many instances the cells lining the kidney tubules die and slough. Medical treatment depends on the severity of the disease, and may range from management by medication and dietary restriction to hemodialysis. The prognosis for remission is favorable if the patient's general condition is good, if the blood chemistries are not severely disordered, and if the oliguric phase does not last long. The recovery phase is usually heralded by a period of diuresis.

Assessment

I. Known previous good health.
II. Sudden onset of symptoms.
III. Edema, shortness of breath.
IV. Headache, lethargy, drowsiness.
V. Seizures or coma.
VI. Nausea and vomiting, diarrhea.
VII. Pallor.
VIII. Oliguria or anuria.
IX. Hypertension.
X. Bleeds easily, prolonged clotting time.

Problems

I. Volume overload.
II. Acidosis.
III. Electrolyte imbalance.
IV. Central nervous system (CNS) changes.

V. Hypertension.   VII. Bleeding diathesis.
VI. Anemia.   VIII. Susceptibility to infection.

Goals of Care

I. Prevent or control volume overload.
II. Decrease degree of acidosis.
III. Decrease degree of electrolyte imbalance.
IV. Detect and report any central nervous system changes as rapidly as possible.
V. Detect and control hypertension.
VI. Conserve red blood cells.
VII. Prevent infection.

Intervention

I. Keep a *strict* record of intake and output! Measure everything in *exact* milliliters. Oral fluids are usually restricted; divide allotted fluids into three 8-h portions, with amounts based on projected needs and desires for an 8-h period. Be sure to consider fluids needed to take medications as part of restriction.
II. Monitor diet carefully. Typical renal failure diet is low protein, low potassium, low to moderate sodium. Build-up of end-products of protein metabolism is one cause of acidosis. Hyperkalemia causes cardiac arrhythmias, including ventricular standstill. Forbidden high-potassium foods are bananas, nuts, oranges and other citrus fruits, potatoes, and chocolate.
III. Inform all family members and hospital personnel of child's dietary restriction. A reasonably intelligent child will find an amazing variety of food sources, even in the hospital.
IV. Monitor the child's affect, alertness, and energy levels. CNS depression may be a sign of approaching seizure activity.
V. Keep padded tongue blade in a handy place for immediate use if seizure activity begins.
VI. Monitor blood pressure frequently. If child complains of headache or visual disturbances, monitor blood pressure and notify physician. Administer ordered antihypertensives on time.
VII. Coordinate with laboratory to keep blood drawn for tests to absolute minimum. Prevent trauma as much as possible. If bleeding occurs, apply ice and direct pressure for 7 to 10 min to control bleeding.
VIII. Avoid exposure to contagious disease. Thoroughly clean any breaks in skin. Administer ordered antibiotics.

Evaluation

I. Is child in fluid balance? Are there signs of volume overload such as congestive heart failure or pulmonary edema? Are there signs of dehydration? Are intake and output charted accurately?
II. Is diet being followed carefully? Are laboratory results acceptable? Does diet need to be adjusted?
III. Are potassium levels between 4.0 and 6.0? An elevated potassium level is incompatible with good cardiac function.
IV. Are parents setting limits on dietary behavior? Is child staying within these limits?
V. Is child sleepy or hard to arouse? Has there been a change in level of consciousness?
VI. Is child hypertensive or hypotensive? Are antihypertensives taken as ordered?
VII. How severe is anemia? Is Hct falling? How fast? Is spontaneous bleeding occurring?
VIII. Has child been exposed to contagious disease? Are all wounds thoroughly cleaned? Are antibiotics being given as ordered?

Chronic Renal Failure

Definition

Chronic renal failure differs from acute renal failure in that it develops over a period of months or years. It usually passes through three stages. In the first stage, decreased renal reserve, the function of the kidney is slightly impaired, but the body's chemistry is maintained at essentially normal levels. The second stage, renal insufficiency, is usually reached when the glomerular filtration rate falls below 50 percent. Wastes are beginning to accumulate in the blood, and the body is slow in coping with electrolyte changes. The final stage, in which kidney function is minimal or nonexistent, is called uremia, azotemia, or end-stage renal disease. If left untreated, chronic renal failure ends eventually in death. The medical treatment of choice in children is dialysis, (peritoneal or hemodialysis), and eventual kidney transplant.

Assessment

I. No clear-cut history of distinct change from health to illness.
II. Fatigue, lethargy.
III. Headache.
IV. Oliguria may be present.
V. Hypertension.
VI. Poor growth.
VII. Delayed sexual maturation.
VIII. Dry skin, severe itching.
IX. Paresthesias.
X. Pallor, anemia.
XI. Tendency to bleed easily, prolonged clotting time.
XII. Nausea and vomiting.
XIII. Bone pain.

Problems

I. Acidosis.
II. Electrolyte imbalance.
III. CNS changes.
IV. Hypertension.
V. Anemia.
VI. Tendency to bleed easily and/or spontaneously.
VII. Delayed growth and sexual maturation.
VIII. Dry skin, itching.
IX. Osteodystrophy.

Goals of Care

I. Decrease degree of acidosis.
II. Decrease degree of electrolyte imbalance.
III. Detect and report any central nervous system changes as rapidly as possible.
IV. Detect and control hypertension.
V. Conserve red blood cells.
VI. Promote adjustment to disease, promote integrated body image.
VII. Moisturize skin, control itching.
VIII. Prevent or control osteodystrophy.
IX. Assist adjustment to change in life-style on dialysis.
X. Prepare for transplantation.

Intervention

I. Keep a *strict* record of intake and output! Measure everything in exact millimeters. Oral fluids are usually restricted; divide allotted fluids into three 8-h portions, allocated according to anticipated needs and desires. Be sure to consider fluids needed to take medications as part of intake.
II. Monitor diet carefully. Typical renal failure diet is low protein, low potassium, low to moderate sodium. Build-up of end-products of protein metabolism is one cause of acidosis. Hyperkalemia causes cardiac arrhythmias, including ventricular standstill. Forbidden high-potassium foods are bananas, nuts, oranges and other citrus fruits, potatoes, and chocolate.
III. Inform all family members and hospital personnel of child's dietary restriction. A reasonably intelligent child will find an amazing variety of food sources, even in the hospital.

IV. Monitor the child's affect, alertness, and energy level. CNS depression may be a sign of approaching seizure activity.

V. Keep padded tongue blade in a handy place for immediate use if seizure activity begins.

VI. Monitor blood pressure frequently. If child complains of headache or visual disturbances, monitor blood pressure and notify physician. Administer ordered antihypertensives on time and in the correct amount.

VII. Coordinate with laboratory to keep blood drawn for tests to absolute minimum. Prevent trauma as much as possible. If bleeding occurs apply ice and direct pressure for 7 to 10 min to control bleeding.

VIII. Prepare the child and family for dialysis by showing them the dialysis unit, introducing them to the staff, and having them meet children who are already on dialysis and their families. Encourage questions. Be *honest* in your answers. Allow younger children the opportunity to work through their anxieties through play or by drawing pictures. Allow older children and parents the opportunity to talk about their anxieties.

IX. Explain to family that optimal chemical environment is necessary for growth. Ensure that the child is brought for dialysis on schedule.

X. High-calorie diets are also helpful in promoting growth. High-calorie carbohydrate supplements should be taken if adequate calories are not otherwise consumed. Dietary restrictions on protein, fluids, potassium, or sodium should not be relaxed in the effort to increase calories.

XI. Encourage frequent, liberal use of hand lotion to keep skin moisturized. Use of bath oils or moisturizers should also be recommended.

XII. Ensure that calcium and aluminum hydroxide are taken as ordered to prevent or control osteodystrophy.

XIII. Never, never give a renal failure patient any medication containing magnesium. In this disease, magnesium aluminum hydroxide is not a substitute for aluminum hydroxide.

XIV. Allow the child and the parents to talk as needed about the inconvenience of being on dialysis. Transportation to the nearest dialysis center suitable for children and the large amount of time expended in dialysis and en route are common problems.

XV. Prepare the child and family for renal transplantation by talking about the operation, showing pictures of the procedure, discussing changes in postoperative life-style, and introducing them to the Intensive Care Unit (ICU) staff. Again, provide many opportunities for all involved to work through their anxieties.

Evaluation

I. Is child in fluid balance? Are there signs of volume overload such as congestive heart failure or pulmonary edema? Are there signs of dehydration? Are intake and output accurately recorded?

II. Is diet being followed carefully? Are laboratory results acceptable? Does diet need to be adjusted?

III. Are potassium levels between 4.0 and 6.0? An elevated potassium level is incompatible with good cardiac function.

IV. Are parents setting limits on dietary behavior? Is child staying within these limits?

V. Is child sleepy or hard to arouse? Has there been a change in level of consciousness?

VI. Is child hypo- or hypertensive? Are antihypertensives taken as ordered?

VII. How severe is anemia? Is Hct falling? How fast? Is spontaneous bleeding occurring?

VIII. Has child been exposed to contagious disease? Are all wounds thoroughly cleaned? Are antibiotics being given as ordered?

IX. Is child ready for dialysis? Can child give an elementary explanation of what will be happening? Is child anxious about procedure? What coping mechanisms are being used?

X. Is child dialyzed adequately? Is growth occurring?

XI. How many calories are consumed each day? Is this adequate?

XII. Is skin dry and flaking? Are moisturizers in use? Is itching a severe problem?

XIII. Is the proper medication being given? If not, why not?

XIV. Are the child and parents asking questions and talking about their anxieties? What other coping mechanisms are in effect?

XV. Is the child ready for transplantation? Can the child and family explain simply what will be happening? How are anxieties about this being coped with?

METABOLIC DISORDERS

Renal Tubular Acidosis

Definition

Renal tubular acidosis is a disease in which the kidney is unable to excrete sufficient hydrogen ion and loses too much bicarbonate ion in the urine. In addition, sodium, calcium, and potassium are lost in large amounts along with the bicarbonate ion. Generally, the loss of calcium and sodium is responsible for most symptoms. Most authors divide this disease into two types. The first, called classical or persistent primary renal tubular acidosis, is thought to be a disease of the distal convoluted tubules. It is familial (autosomal dominant), and presents mainly in 2-year-old girls. The second type, transient, or proximal renal tubular acidosis, is rare. It occurs mainly in males in the first year of life; the etiology is unknown. Medical treatment of both types of renal tubular acidosis consists of administration of alkali (sodium bicarbonate and/or sodium citrate) as well as high doses of vitamin D.

Assessment

I. General appearance of failure to thrive, including retarded growth, retarded bone age, low weight, lethargy, anorexia, vomiting, irritability.
II. Recurrent dehydration with polyuria, thirst, polydypsia, constipation.
III. Loss of calcium from bones resulting in rickets, bone pain, deformity, pathological fractures.
IV. High serum calcium which leads to nephrocalcinosis, nephrolithiasis, renal colic.
V. Loss of serum potassium with muscular hypotonia, cardiac arrhythmia.
VI. Costovertebral angle tenderness.

Problems

I. Malnutrition.
II. Dehydration.
III. Acidosis.
IV. Hypercalcemia.
V. Hypokalemia.
VI. Nephrocalcinosis/nephrolithiasis.

Goals of Care

I. Foster good nutrition.
II. Maintain adequate hydration.
III. Prevent pathological fractures.
IV. Detect cardiac arrhythmias, and treat early.
V. Detect stone formation and treat.

Intervention

I. Provide several small, light meals each day as long as anorexia and/or vomiting persist. Offer favorite foods as much as possible.
II. Offer fluids frequently; give fluids as often as requested by child. Monitor skin turgor, fontanels, eyes, and temperature for signs of dehydration.
III. Change diaper frequently to prevent skin irritation due to polyuria.
IV. Give medication as prescribed, in spite of child's dislike of taste, to combat acidosis, bone disease, and stone formation.
V. If bone disease is advanced, handle child as little as possible and discourage strenuous exercise to prevent pathological fractures. Provide for quiet diversion and sensory stimulation.
VI. If laboratory results show hypokalemia, maintain child on cardiac monitor to detect cardiac arrhythmias as quickly as possible. Notify physician immediately.
VII. Test all urine for hematuria; strain for calculi. Observe for symptoms of renal colic. Notify physician if any of these is present.

Evaluation

I. Is child well nourished? Is child growing? Gaining weight? Is child reluctant to eat, or vomiting?

II. Is child dehydrated? Is skin turgor good? Are fontanels or eyes sunken? Is temperature elevated?

III. Is child's skin intact in diaper area?

IV. Is child taking medication in sufficient amounts on schedule? Is serum acidosis corrected? Is rickets improving?

V. Are pathological fractures present? Are they healing well? Is child kept as quiet as possible to prevent other fractures? Is child suffering sensory deprivation?

VI. Do laboratory results show hypokalemia? Is child maintained on cardiac monitor?

VII. Are stones being formed? Is there hematuria? Urinary calculi? Does child have symptoms of renal colic?

BIBLIOGRAPHY

Charny, Charles W., and William Wolgin: *Cryptorchism,* Paul B. Hoeber, Inc. Harper & Brothers, New York, 1957. Although not recent, this is a comprehensive treatise covering the embryology, etiology, pathology, symptoms, complications, diagnosis, and treatment of cryptorchism. Written in a readily understandable style, it combines a review of the then-current literature with the authors' own experiences. It is referred to by many authors as a primary source.

Harrington, Joan O., and Etta R. Brener: *Patient Care in Renal Failure,* W. B. Saunders Company, Philadelphia, 1973. This is a very complete explanation of the anatomy, physiology, pathology, and treatment of renal failure, along with descriptions of treatment modules available. Nursing care is emphasized. This is a useful book for student and practitioner alike.

Kelalis, P. P., L. R. King and A. B. Belman (eds.): *Clinical Pediatric Urology,* vols. I and II, W. B. Saunders Company, Philadelphia, 1976. This comprehensive book is invaluable to the nurse who wishes to understand the surgical management and goals of care for the pediatric patient with a urological problem.

Lieberman, Ellin (ed.): *Clinical Pediatric Nephrology,* J. B. Lippincott Company, Philadelphia, 1976. A truly comprehensive work by 21 contributors that covers the workup and medical management of a wide range of nephrological conditions in the pediatric patient. Written for physicians.

Scipien, Gladys M., et al. (eds.): *Comprehensive Pediatric Nursing,* 2d ed., McGraw-Hill Book Company, New York, 1979. This outstanding textbook includes chapters on the urinary and reproductive systems in which embryology, anatomy, and physiology of the systems are discussed and nursing care for children with a wide range of health care disorders is presented. The nursing process and growth and development are given extensive treatment elsewhere in the book.

Vaughn, Victor C., R. James McKay, and Waldo E. Nelson (eds.): *Nelson Textbook of Pediatrics,* 10th ed., W. B. Saunders Company, Philadelphia, 1975. This widely used book, although written for medical students, is an invaluable reference for nurses seeking detailed information about children's diseases and their medical treatment.

Vander, Arthur J.: *Renal Physiology,* McGraw-Hill Book Company, New York, 1975. This is a well-written comprehensive text designed primarily for medical students. It is easily understood by those with some background in anatomy and physiology. Study is guided by learning objectives printed at the beginning of each chapter and test questions at the end of the book. There is also a list of suggested readings for each chapter.

19

The Nervous System

Beverly A. Bowens

GENERAL ASSESSMENT

I. Vital statistics
   A. Age.
   B. Sex.
   C. Birth date.
      1. Actual.
      2. Expected date of birth.
   D. Birth weight.
II. Data sources
   A. Patient.
   B. Family.
   C. Significant others.
   D. Available records.
      1. Child's.
      2. Mother's.
         a. Prenatal.
         b. Delivery.
III. Chief complaint.
   A. Patient and family's impressions of presenting problem.
   B. Explore time and sequence of symptom development.
      1. Diseases that develop acutely over a period of minutes to hours are usually of a vascular or traumatic nature.
      2. Diseases that peak in a day to several days are usually a result of a toxic process, an electrolyte imbalance, or an infectious process.
      3. Diseases that develop insidiously over many days, weeks, or months are usually associated with neoplastic, inborn metabolic, or degenerative processes.
   C. Attempt to determine whether symptoms are increasing, remaining the same, or improving.
IV. Family history.
   A. Age and status of siblings (alive, dead, and aborted).
   B. Parents.
   C. Grandparents.
   D. Siblings of parents.
   E. Cultural background.
   F. Socioeconomic background.
      1. Educational level and occupations of parents.
      2. Where does family live?
      3. Do other persons live in the home?
      4. Financial status.
   G. Family health history: Are there family members who have suffered from:
      1. Seizures?
      2. Mental retardation?
      3. Deafness?
      4. Blindness?
      5. Mental illness?
      6. Movement disturbances?
      7. Weakness?
      8. Cerebral palsy?
      9. Dementia?
V. Significant history.
   A. Prenatal.
      1. Dietary practices.

    2. Medications taken.

    3. Illnesses (record month of pregnancy in which illness occurred).

       a. Infections.   *d.* Surgery.

       b. Exposure to infectious diseases.   *e.* X-rays.

       c. Accidents.

B. Labor and delivery.

    1. Length of labor.

    2. Type of delivery.

       a. Breech or unusual presentation.

       b. Forceps.

    3. Type of anesthesia used.

    4. Delay in respirations or cry (Apgar score).

    5. Did baby require oxygen?

C. Postnatal.

    1. Cyanosis.

    2. Jaundice.

    3. Infections.

    4. Seizures.

    5. Anemia.

    6. Medications.

    7. Did mother and baby go home at the same time?

D. Developmental.

    1. Developmental milestones.

    2. Current status.

       a. Gross motor and fine motor skills.

       b. Socialization.

       c. Language.

    3. School performance.

E. Illnesses.

    1. Hospitalizations.

    2. Operations.

    3. Injuries.

    4. Has child ever been unconscious?

    5. Has child ever been poisoned?

    6. Has child ever had seizures?

       a. With fever?

       b. Without fever?

       c. If so, describe.

    7. Medication history.

F. Immunization record.

G. Eating and drinking patterns.

H. Sleeping patterns.

I. Elimination patterns.

J. Independency/dependency patterns.

K. Temperament.

VI. Physical assessment.

A. Vital signs.

B. Height and weight.

    1. Plot on graph for comparison to past and future measurements.

    2. Abnormalities may:

       a. Point to endocrine imbalances resulting from pituitary tumors.

       b. Be associated with genetic and congenital syndromes that include central nervous system (CNS) involvement.

C. General appearance.

D. Head.

    1. Circumference.

        a. Plot on graph for comparison to past and future measurements.

        b. A rapidly increasing head circumference or a measurement out of proportion to the chest circumference suggests increased intracranial pressure.

    2. Increased resonance that occurs on percussion of the skull (Macewen's sign or "cracked-pot" sound) is associated with increased intracranial pressure.

    3. Shape.

        a. Children with hydrocephalus often show cranial enlargement in the anteroposterior plane.

        b. Children with chronic subdural hematoma often exhibit bitemporal cranial enlargement.

        c. Irregularities in head shape may indicate premature closure of one or more cranial sutures.

        d. Asymmetry may be due to cranial trauma leading to scalp hematoma formation and/or displaced fractures.

        e. A long, narrow, receding forehead with a small cranium and flat occiput is associated with microcephaly.

    4. Size and condition of fontanels and suture lines.

        a. Tense, bulging fontanels and separated sutures indicate increased intracranial pressure.

        b. Prematurely closed sutures may be one of a variety of symptoms seen in syndromes involving the CNS.

    5. Transillumination: Useful in identifying CNS defects such as cysts and absence of brain structures.

    6. Ecchymotic areas on skull or face may indicate basilar skull fracture (Battle's sign—postauricular ecchymosis).

    7. Intracranial bruits may be heard in children who have arteriovenous malformations.

    8. Sudden, severe headaches may indicate meningeal irritation.

E. Eyes, ears, nose, mouth, and throat.

    1. Look for normal placement of eyes and ears.

    2. Note any abnormalities of nose, mouth, and throat.

    3. "Sunset" eyes are a late sign of hydrocephalus.

    4. Serosanguineous drainage from ears or nose following trauma may be cerebrospinal fluid, indicating presence of basilar skull fracture.

F. Neck: Make particular note of nuchal rigidity (neck stiffness), which is a sign of meningeal irritation.

G. Chest, heart, breasts, axillae.

H. Abdomen.

    1. An abdominal mass is often the first sign of neuroblastoma.

    2. Persistent vomiting may be seen with increased intracranial pressure and with brain tumors causing direct pressure on the emetic center.

I. Extremities and spine.

    1. Flaccid or spastic lower extremities may accompany myelomeningocele or other spinal cord lesions.

    2. Defects in spinous processes may indicate spina bifida occulta.

    3. Examine spine for curvature, dimples, tufts of hair, and sinus tracts that may indicate skeletal and/or cord irregularities.

J. Skin: Café au lait spots and subcutaneous tumors on extremities and trunk may accompany neurofibromatosis.

K. Genitourinary (GU): Constant dribbling of urine and flaccid anal sphincter indicate abnormality of the spinal cord resulting from such things as congenital malformations of the cord, spinal cord tumors, and spinal cord trauma.

VII. Neurological assessment.

A. Cerebral function: Level of consciousness, overall behavior, orientation, intellectual performance, cortical sensory interpretation, cortical motor integration, and language.

1. Developmental tests, such as the Denver Developmental Screening Test, are good measures of cerebral function.
2. Declining level of consciousness is a good indicator of increased intracranial pressure.
3. Excessive drowsiness may be caused by metabolic problem, hypothalamic disease, or brain tumor.
4. Disorientation occurring acutely may result from inflammatory, toxic, metabolic, or traumatic brain disorders.
5. Hyperactivity may be present in children with minimal brain dysfunction.

B. Cranial nerves.

1. Cranial nerve I (olfactory).
   a. Rarely affected in neurological diseases of childhood.
   b. Loss of smell (anosmia) most often due to upper respiratory infections, frontal lobe tumors, and fractures of cribriform plate.
2. Cranial nerve II (optic).
   a. May have varying patterns of visual field loss with tumors impinging on the optic chiasm.
   b. Optic nerve gliomas are not uncommon in children.
   c. Papilledema may occur with increased intracranial pressure.
3. Cranial nerves III, IV, VI (oculomotor, trochlear, abducens).
   a. Involvement of these nerves can be an invaluable clue to the location of lesions.
   b. Involvement of third nerve may indicate impending uncal herniation.
   c. Diplopia, strabismus, and nystagmus may be symptoms of brain tumor.
4. Cranial nerve V (trigeminal) may be involved in trauma, brainstem tumors, and cerebellar pontine angle tumors.
5. Cranial nerve VII (facial).
   a. Bilateral peripheral facial palsy may be congenital as with Möbius' syndrome.
   b. Brainstem and cerebral infections may lead to facial nerve palsy.
   c. Acoustic neuromas may affect facial nerve function.
6. Cranial nerve VIII (acoustic) may be affected by tumors such as neurofibromas.
7. Cranial nerves IX and X (glossopharyngeal and vagus) may be affected by tumors in the posterior fossa.
8. Cranial nerve XI (spinal accessory) involvement indicates lesion in foramen magnum.
9. Cranial nerve XII (hypoglossal) involvement may be due to vascular, neoplastic, or congenital lesions in posterior fossa.

C. Cerebellar function (balance and coordination).

1. Symptoms of cerebellar dysfunction include disturbances in balance and integrated movements; nystagmus; dysarthria; broad-based, staggering gait; intention tremor; hypotonia.
2. Causes of cerebellar dysfunction.
   a. Head trauma.
   b. Congenital abnormalities.
      (1) Hydrocephalus.
      (2) Dandy-Walker syndrome.
   c. Infections.
   d. Metabolic disorders.
   e. Neoplasms in the posterior fossa.
   f. Toxic substances.

D. Motor function (size, tone, and strength of muscles and presence of abnormal movements).

1. Symptoms include muscle weakness, generalized wasting, spasticity, flaccidity, rigidity, decreased strength, abnormal muscle movements, atrophy.
2. Causes of disturbances in motor function.

    a. Muscular dystrophy.
    b. Anterior horn cell disease.
    c. Lower motor neuron disease of spinal cord or brainstem.
    d. Cerebral palsy.
E. Reflexes.
  1. Assess superficial, deep, and pathologic reflexes.
  2. Reflex changes may be caused by:
    a. Trauma to brain or spinal cord.
    b. Neoplasms of the cord.
    c. Lesions of the pyramidal tract or motor neurons.
    d. Infections such as meningitis.
    e. Cerebral palsy.
F. Sensory.
  1. Often difficult to assess in child.
  2. Impairment may result from:
    a. Trauma to spinal cord.   *c.* Peripheral nerve injuries.
    b. Neoplasms of the cord.   *d.* Congenital abnormalities.

CONGENITAL MALFORMATIONS

Spina Bifida Occulta and Spina Bifida Cystica

Definition

Spina bifida occulta may be defined as a congenital failure of closure of the vertebral column without protrusion or displacement of intraspinal contents. This defect is found in 25 percent of hospitalized children and in 10 percent of the general pediatric population. It most frequently involves the posterior arches of the fifth lumbar and first sacral vertebrae. Spina bifida occulta is generally asymptomatic and discovered accidentally on routine spinal films. The appearance of dimples, tufts of hair, and small fatty masses along the spinal column may be indicative of this defect. Sphincter control may be difficult.

Spina bifida cystica is a more serious defect in which the inadequately closed vertebral column is accompanied by displacement of intraspinal contents into a saclike structure on the exterior surface of the spine (Fig. 19-1). The incidence is estimated to be 0.2 to 4.2 per 1000 live births. These defects are of two types—meningoceles and myelomeningoceles. The meningocele, accounting for 25 percent of the cystic type, contains spinal fluid and meninges in the saclike mass. The myelomeningocele, making up the remaining 75 percent, contains these elements plus neural tissue. These defects may be covered by a very thin membrane, by meninges, by dura, or at times, by normal skin. Approximately 80 percent of myelomeningoceles are located in the lumbar and lumbosacral region.

About three-fourths of the infants with myelomeningocele also have hydrocephalus. Early surgery to correct the spinal defect and the hydrocephalus in these infants results in a survival rate of approximately 65 percent. Ninety percent of these newborns have associated malformations and infections of the urinary tract.

The treatment of children born with myelomeningocele continues to be hotly debated in the neurosurgical community. Management protocols vary from one extreme to the other, with some physicians recommending surgical intervention for *every* child and others advocating that *none* of these children be surgically repaired. Of course, the opinions of most physicians are somewhere between these two extremes. The quality of life for the children who survive has been a large part of the debate, since many of them are left with significant mental retardation and neurological defects, including paraplegia. Many have locomotor problems due to associated musculoskeletal anomalies such as clubfoot, dislocated hips, contractures, and scoliosis. Special education is eventually required for many of these children, and personality and disciplinary problems are common. These facts provide some insight into the impact of the birth of such a child on the family, the health care system, and society as a whole.

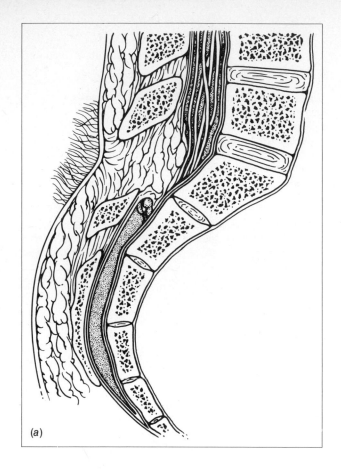

(a)

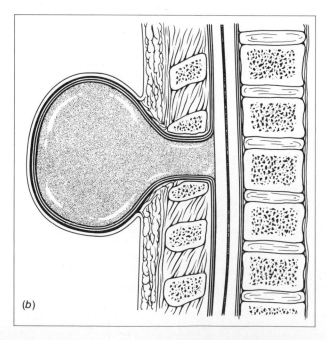

(b)

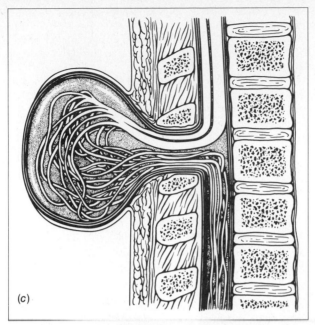

(c)

FIGURE 19-1 / Congenital malformations of the spine: (*a*) spina bifida occulta, (*b*) meningocele, (*c*) myelomeningocele.

Problems   I. Potential inability of parents to adjust to the birth of a defective child.
    A. Goals of care.
       1. Maintenance of the family's decision-making ability regarding the child and his care.
       2. Maintenance of intrafamily communication.
       3. Support of the family as they move through the grief process.
    B. Intervention.
       1. Allow the family to grieve.
       2. Provide time and quiet place for the parents to talk about the child's condition with the nurse and/or other health team members.
       3. Be as honest as possible in responding to questions.
       4. When the parents visit the child, remain nearby to answer questions and provide emotional support.
       5. Involve parents in the care to the extent that they are able—physically and emotionally—to participate.
    C. Evaluation.
       1. Parents verbalize feelings of grief.
       2. Parents exhibit mood appropriate to stage of grief process.
       3. Parents show affection toward child.
       4. Both parents visit and care for child.
   II. Parents may lack knowledge regarding the defect.
    A. Goals of care: Parents will demonstrate an understanding of the anatomy and physiology of the defect and future implications.
    B. Intervention.
       1. Assess current knowledge level and readiness to learn.
       2. Teach basic information through the use of charts, books, pictures, etc.
       3. Provide written material and pictures.
    C. Evaluation.
       1. Parents verbalize basic facts about the anatomy and physiology of myelomeningocele.

    2. Parents verbalize realistic questions and statements about the child and his condition.

III. Possible meningitis secondary to rupture and contamination of the sac.
    A. Goals of care: Protect sac from pressure and infectious agents at all times.
    B. Intervention.
        1. Position child on abdomen. Bradford frame may be used if available.
        2. Use strict aseptic technique when changing bandage.
        3. Keep perineal area scrupulously clean at all times.
        4. Do not use diapers.
        5. Plastic sheeting (such as ordinary kitchen wrap) may be used to keep urine and feces away from the bandaged area (Fig. 19-2).
    C. Evaluation.
        1. Absence of drainage from the sac.
        2. Temperature less than 38.5°C (101°F).
        3. Absence of irritability, nuchal rigidity, and lethargy.
        4. Absence of tense, bulging fontanels.
        5. Head circumference within normal limits.
        6. Negative Kernig's and Brudzinski's signs.
IV. Potential parental lack of knowledge and anxity regarding surgery.
    A. Goals of care.
        1. Decrease anxiety.
        2. The parents will demonstrate an understanding of the preoperative and postoperative routines.
    B. Intervention.
        1. Assess current knowledge level and readiness to learn.

FIGURE 19-2 / **Application of plastic wrap to protect spinal defect from contamination by urine and feces. (a) Plastic wrap (ordinary kitchen variety) is taped to skin. (b) Plastic wrap is folded back over the tape applied in (a) and secured to the thighs.**

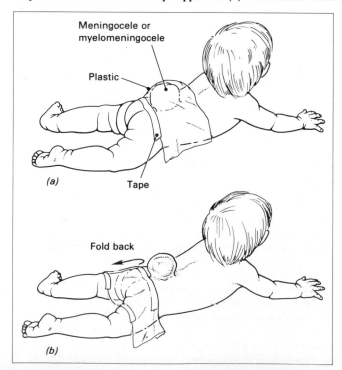

       2. Give information about hospital routines, how child will look after surgery, and the parents' role.

       3. Provide time for questions.

   C. Evaluation.

       1. Parents verbalize preoperative and postoperative routines.

       2. Parents verbalize feelings of anxiety.

       3. Absence of signs of excessive anxiety, such as constant, repetitive questions; crying, depression, and irrational behavior; withdrawal.

V. Possible postoperative infection and breakdown of suture line.

   A. Goals of care: Adequate healing of the surgical incision.

   B. Intervention.

       1. Protect bandage from urinary and fecal contamination.

       2. If bandage becomes soiled, change, using strict aseptic technique.

       3. After bandage is removed, keep suture line clean.

       4. Do not use diapers until suture line completely healed.

       5. Avoid pressure and traction on suture line.

       6. Provide diet high in protein, calories, and vitamins.

   C. Evaluation.

       1. Temperature less than 38.5°C (101°F).

       2. Absence of drainage from the incision

       3. Wound clean and dry

       4. Absence of excessive redness and warmth around incision.

VI. Possible hydrocephalus (see "Hydrocephalus" in this chapter).

VII Possible nutritional and/or metabolic problems.

   A. Goals pf care: Child will have adequate food and fluid intake and adequate metabolic balance.

   B. Intervention.

       1. Feed child slowly and allow frequent rest periods.

       2. "Bubble" baby during and after feeding.

       3. Teach parents effective methods of feeding baby.

       4. Assess electrolyte values as laboratory reports become available.

       5. Weigh daily.

   C. Evaluation.

       1. Baby retains formula and gains weight.

       2. Electrolyte values remain within normal limits.

       3. Parents feed infant adequate amounts.

       4. Parents handle infant in a comfortable manner.

       5. Parents verbalize plans for feeding—formula and solid foods.

VIII. Possible contractures and skin breakdown.

   A. Goals of care.

       1. Maintenance of an intact integumentary system.

       2. Prevention of lower extremity contractures.

   B. Intervention.

       1. Frequent skin care with particular attention to knees, toes, ankles, elbows, and ears.

       2. Apply petroleum jelly to perineal area.

       3. Change sheets under patient whenever wet or soiled.

       4. Passive range of motion exercises to lower extremities.

       5. Release restraints on upper extremities and exercise at least every shift.

   C. Evaluation.

       1. Skin free of redness, rashes, and breakdown.

       2. Joints movable through full range of motion.

IX. Urinary incontinence and potential urinary tract infection.

   A. Goals of care: Maintenance of adequate urinary tract function.

   B. Intervention.

       1. Teach parents Credé method of emptying bladder.

2. Force fluids.
3. Encourage juices that acidify the urine (cranberry, grape, apple).
4. Teach bladder training techniques when child is old enough for toilet training.
5. Teach use of external collection device for boys.
6. Teach self-catheterization when child is old enough.
7. Teach signs and symptoms of urinary tract infection.
8. Teach importance of keeping child clean and dry.

C. Evaluation.
1. Temperature less than 38.5°C (101°F).
2. Absence of flank pain.
3. Urine free of foul odor and dark color.
4. Output compatible with intake.
5. Family demonstrates Credé method.
6. Family verbalizes understanding of incontinence.
7. Family verbalizes basic points taught.

X. Fecal incontinence.
A. Goals of care: The child will have regular bowel movements and will be clean at all times.
B. Intervention.
1. Teach bowel training regime once child is old enough for toilet training.
   a. Check rectum for impaction every other day.
   b. Insert a suppository against the wall of the rectum every other day at the same time of day.
   c. Place child on toilet.
2. Give a stool softener twice a day if indicated.
3. Dietary counseling regarding bulk, avoidance of foods likely to cause diarrhea, importance of fruits and vegetables, etc.
C. Evaluation.
1. Family verbalizes understanding of fecal incontinence.
2. Regular bowel movement pattern.
3. Family verbalizes bowel training regime.

XI. Potential delayed developmental milestones.
A. Goals of care: Promotion of optimal development within limits of disability.
B. Intervention.
1. Encourage parents to cuddle, stroke, and talk to child, even during acute phase of illness.
2. Provide continuity in staff assignment to the extent possible.
3. Provide appropriate toys and bright objects for visual stimulation.
4. Include specifics of developmental stimulation in plan of care.
5. Provide written information about play and developmental stimulation.
C. Evaluation.
1. Parents verbalize importance of and understanding of developmental stimulation.
2. Parents demonstrate techniques taught.
3. Child exhibits development appropriate for age.

XII. Overwhelming financial burden to family.
A. Goals of care: Family will be able to cope with the financial demands of rearing child.
B. Intervention.
1. Provide verbal and written information about available financial assistance.
2. Refer to state crippled children's agency.
3. Refer to social worker.
C. Evaluation.
1. Parents verbalize willingness to take advantage of financial assistance.
2. Parents verbalize available financial resources.
3. Parents verbalize method of obtaining assistance.

Hydrocephalus

Definition

Hydrocephalus is characterized by an increased amount of cerebrospinal fluid and consequent increased intracranial pressure. In young children whose skull sutures have not yet fused, characteristic enlargement of the head is seen. Hydrocephalus is usually classified as either communicating or noncommunicating. In the communicating type, there is unobstructed flow of cerebrospinal fluid (CSF) through the ventricular system. The defect lies along the absorptive surfaces of the brain—the subarachnoid space. The fluid cannot be absorbed due to a thickened arachnoid, most often secondary to meningitis or intracranial hemorrhage. In the noncommunicating type, there is a block to CSF flow within the ventricles. The blockage may be a result of tumor, hematoma formation, or malformation of the ventricular system.

Problems

I. Increased intracranial pressure.
   - A. Goals of care: Maintenance of adequate neurological functioning.
   - B. Intervention.
     1. Elevate head of bed 20 to 30°.
     2. Assess vital signs and level of consciousness every 4 h or as ordered.
     3. Perform nursing activities in such a way as to avoid unnecessarily stressing child (group procedures together, allow time for rest).
     4. Monitor fluid intake carefully.
     5. Ensure patent airway.
   - C. Evaluation.
     1. Vital signs within normal limits for age.
     2. Absence of decreasing level of consciousness and increasing irritability.
     3. Equal movement and strength of extremities.
     4. Pupils equal and reactive to light.
     5. Absence of seizures.

II. Possible inadequate nutrition.
   - A. Goals of care: The child will ingest and retain adequate nutrients and fluids.
   - B. Intervention.
     1. Weigh daily.
     2. Investigate food preferences.
     3. Offer small, frequent feedings.
     4. If child vomits, allows rest period and then feed again.
     5. Dietary consultation.
   - C. Evaluation.
     1. Weight the same as or greater than on admission.
     2. Retains food.
     3. Blood values within normal limits.

III. Potential parental anxiety regarding diagnostic procedures and implications of results.
   - A. Goals of care: Decrease anxiety.
   - B. Intervention.
     1. Assess current knowledge level and readiness to learn.
     2. Provide information about tests. Use pictures, tell what to expect after test completed, when results will be available.
     3. Allow time for questions.

IV. Potential lack of knowledge and anxiety regarding preoperative and postoperative routines.
   - A. Goals of care.
     1. Parents will demonstrate an understanding of pre- and postoperative routines.
     2. Parental anxiety will be within expected, tolerable limits.
   - B. Intervention.
     1. Assess current knowledge level and readiness to learn.
     2. Give information about hospital routines, how child will look after surgery, and the parents' role.

      3. Provide time for questions.

   C. Evaluation.

      1. Parents verbalize pre- and postoperative routines accurately.

      2. Parents' anxiety is not excessive for the situation.

V. Possible postoperative infection (wound infection or meningitis).

   A. Goals of care: Prevent contamination of surgical incision.

   B. Intervention.

      1. Keep bandage clean and dry.

      2. If bandage becomes soiled, change under strict aseptic conditions.

      3. Look for signs of inflammation around incision site. If present, notify physician immediately.

      4. Avoid pressure and traction on suture line.

      5. Assess vital signs and level of consciousness every 4 h or as ordered.

      6. Assess fontanels and measure head circumference daily.

   C. Evaluation.

      1. Dressing clean, dry, and free of drainage.

      2. Temperature less than 38.5°C (101°F).

      3. Fontanels soft, not bulging.

      4. Head circumference within normal limits for that child.

      5. Absence of nuchal rigidity, restlessness, irritability, and lethargy.

      6. Absence of excessive redness and warmth around incision.

      7. Absence of drainage from suture line.

VI. Possible malfunctioning shunt.

   A. Goals of care: Maintenance of adequate neurological functioning.

   B. Intervention.

      1. Discharge teaching regarding signs and symptoms of shunt malfunction.

      2. Provision for long-term follow-up; referral to Public Health Nurse and/or Crippled Children's Service.

   C. Evaluation.

      1. Parents verbalize signs and symptoms of shunt malfunction.

      2. Parents verbalize understanding of need for long-term follow-up.

VII. Possible skin breakdown of scalp overlying pumping chamber.

   A. Goals of care.

      1. Prevention of trauma to shunt site.

      2. Maintenance of scalp skin integrity.

   B. Intervention.

      1. Turn frequently.

      2. Avoid positioning child directly on shunt site.

      3. Encourage adequate nutritional intake for healing.

      4. Discourage manipulation of pump chamber unless "pumping" ordered by physician.

   C. Evaluation.

      1. Skin over pumping chamber normal color, free of drainage, and free of signs of abrasion or breakdown.

      2. Parents verbalize understanding of positioning.

Arnold-Chiari Malformation

Definition   *Arnold-Chiari malformation* is frequently associated with obstructive hydrocephalus and spina bifida cystica of the lumbosacral region. The most common type has malformations at the base of the skull and upper cervical region with hydrocephalus which exerts a downward pressure and spina bifida cystica which tethers the cord in the lumbosacral region resulting in downward traction. The pons and medulla may be kinked and malpositioned. The only treatment for this condition is surgical. Frequently a shunting procedure is done to relieve symptoms of increased pressure. The problems and nursing care are the same as for a child with hydrocephalus.

Encephalocele

Definition   *Encephalocele* occurs when the bones of the fetal skull fail to unite properly, resulting in protrusion of brain tissue through the defect. Treatment is aimed at protection of the sac until surgical closure of the defect is accomplished. Nursing care is the same as for spina bifida cystica.

Microcephaly

Definition   *Microcephaly* is defined as a head circumference at least two standard deviations below the mean, and is secondary to a small brain. There are many causes for this abnormality— genetic, chromosomal, irradiation, infectious, or chemical. Maternal infections that have been implicated in the occurrence of microcephaly are toxoplasmosis, cytomegalovirus, and the rubella virus. Nursing care is directed toward the management of mental retardation, which is usually severe, and of seizures or other related problems.

Craniosynostosis

Definition   *Craniosynostosis* is defined as premature closure of one or more cranial sutures. This defect, often present at birth, interferes with normal skull expansion and thus results in impaired brain growth. Depending on which sutures are closed, there will be various cosmetic deformities of the skull and face. The incidence is less than 5 per 10,000 births and the exact etiology is unknown. The treatment is early surgical opening of the prematurely closed suture. Surgery carries an excellent prognosis for normal appearance and neurological and intellectual function. Nursing care is directed toward early diagnosis and care of the child and family through the surgical episode.

Arteriovenous Malformations

Definition   These abnormalities of arteries and veins of the nervous system result from a failure of capillary development during embryonic growth. This leads to abnormal veins and dilated, tortuous arteries. Arteriovenous malformations (AVM) are the most common vascular abnormalities found in children. Symptoms generally develop between the ages of 10 and 30 years, with 10 percent presenting during the first 10 years of life and 45 percent by the third decade. Most often the condition is recognized secondary to an intracranial bleed— intraventricular, subarachnoid, intracerebral, or subdural.

The prognosis varies depending on the location of the malformation. Mortality for intracranial hemorrhage in the neonatal period nears 100 percent, drops to 80 percent in infancy, and to about 50 percent in older children (1). The only definitive treatment is surgical ligation.

Nursing care is directed toward measures for the prevention of a massive intracranial hemorrhage and increased intracranial pressure. The nurse also plays the primary role in teaching and providing emotional support for the child and the family both preoperatively and postoperatively.

TRAUMA

Accidents are the leading cause of death in children between the ages of 1 and 15. CNS trauma occurs in a large percentage of fatal injuries, particularly if the injuries resulted from a motor vehicle accident. Head injuries account for about 15 percent of all admissions to pediatric wards.

Concussions, Contusions, Lacerations, Skull Fractures, and Hematomas

Definition

Concussion is a type of injury that is still not completely understood. With this injury, transient neuronal dysfunction occurs, resulting in a temporary loss of consciousness. This is generally considered to be without any permanent damage to brain tissue. There is amnesia for the accident itself and for varying periods of time preceding the injury (retrograde amnesia).

Contusions and *lacerations* are more severe types of injuries with hemorrhagic lesions and tears of brain tissue. Damage is often accompanied by cerebral edema, which worsens the condition.

Ninety percent of pediatric head injuries are of the closed type, but skull fractures *do* occur. The skull of the child is more pliable, thus accounting for the low incidence of fractures. *Linear fractures* are classified as simple fractures without displacement of bone, and are the most common type in childhood. These fractures generally do not require any special treatment or observation *unless* they cross the path of major vessels or enter the paranasal sinuses. *Basilar skull fractures* are those which extend through the base of the skull and are rare in children. Basilar fractures may be accompanied by CSF rhinorrhea or otorrhea, by bleeding from the nasopharynx or middle ear, and/or by postauricular ecchymosis (Battle's sign). *Depressed fractures* are those with displacement of the bony fragment. These may be accompanied by contusion of the brain and laceration of the dura.

An *epidural hematoma* is located between the dura and the skull, usually resulting from the tearing of an artery (Fig. 19-3). Since the bleeding is arterial, the hematoma accumulates rapidly. Characteristically, the child is unconscious only briefly, or not at all, followed by a lucid period, and then progressively deteriorating neurological functioning over a period of minutes to several days. Though this is the classic chain of events with epidural hematoma, it does not always hold true for children. Rather, they may present with headache, vomiting, irritability, unequal pupils, hemiparesis, and stupor or coma. These symptoms must be recognized early in order to prevent permanent brain damage and death.

A *subdural hematoma* is the collection of blood between the dura and the brain substance itself (Fig. 19-3). In children subdural hematomas usually result from damage to the cortical bridging veins that drain into the dural sinus. Since these hematomas are a result of venous bleeding, accumulation and subsequent symptoms develop very slowly. The symptoms, as they develop, are those of increased intracranial pressure.

Problems

I. Increased intracranial pressure secondary to cerebral edema and/or hematoma formation.
    A. Goals of care.
        1. Prevention of cerebral edema.
        2. Maintenance of adequate neurological functioning.
    B. Intervention.
        1. Keep airway clear (elevated carbon dioxide leads to increased cerebral edema which leads to increased intracranial pressure).
        2. Elevate child's head 30° to promote venous drainage.
        3. Monitor fluid intake carefully to avoid overhydration.
        4. Assess neurological functioning at least every 30 min for the first 24 h and report changes to physician immediately.
    C. Evaluation.
        1. Absence of drowsiness, irritability, and confusion.
        2. Absence of vomiting.
        3. Absence of headache.
        4. Equal and reactive pupils.
        5. Absence of bradycardia and widening pulse pressure.
        6. Equal movement and strength of extremities.
        7. Absence of seizure activity.
        8. Negative Babinski sign.

II. Possible CSF rhinorrhea or otorrhea.
   A. Goals of care.
      1. Early recognition of leaks.
      2. Avoidance of CNS infection.
   B. Intervention.
      1. Check pillow and sheets for signs of drainage.
      2. If drainage is present on bedding, note if there is a "double ring" pattern. Such a pattern would indicate two types of drainage—blood plus CSF.
      3. If possible, collect some of the drainage in a test tube to check presence or absence of glucose. A test positive for glucose would be indicative of CSF.
      4. Report the presence of drainage to physician immediately.
   C. Evaluation.
      1. Absense of fluid leakage from nose and ears.
      2. Absence of signs and symptoms of meningitis. (Refer to problem III under "Spina Bifida Cystica" in this chapter for a discussion of meningitis.)
III. Parental anxiety regarding the possibility of brain damage.
   A. Goals of care: Decrease anxiety.
   B. Intervention.
      1. Be honest in answering parents' questions about child's condition.
      2. Encourage questions.
      3. Developmental testing as soon as child's condition permits.
      4. Teaching regarding usual pattern of recovery from cerebral injury.
      5. Refer to Community Health Nurse for follow-up testing and counseling if indicated.
   C. Evaluation.
      1. Parents verbalize anxiety.
      2. Parents ask realistic questions about child's condition.
IV. Possibility of child abuse or neglect.
   A. Assessment.
      1. Is the history (explanation of how the injury occurred) consistent and logical?
      2. Are there other suspicious injuries (bruises, burns, fractures in various stages of healing)?
      3. Are there signs of neglect (severe diaper rash, malnutrition, developmental delay)?

FIGURE 19-3 / (a) Epidural and (b) subdural hematomas.

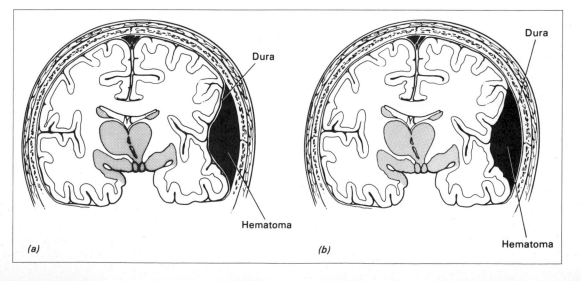

(a)   (b)

    4. Does child or siblings have a history of similar injury?

    5. Are parents intoxicated?

    6. Assess parent-child interaction.

B. Goals of care: Detect and intervene in abuse or neglect if they exist.

C. Intervention.

    1. Ensure child's immediate protection and safety.

    2. Refer to social agency if abuse or neglect is suspected.

D. Evaluation.

    1. Abuse or neglect is ruled in or ruled out.

    2. Appropriate social agency referral is instigated if abuse and neglect are not ruled out.

Spinal Cord Injury

Spinal cord injury generally results from hyperextension or hyperflexion of the neck or from vertical compression of the spine by falls on the head or buttocks. The most common sites for childhood cord injuries are vertebrae C5 to C6, T12 to L1, and C2 to C3. The most common type injury leading to cord damage is fracture dislocation.

Since trauma to the vertebral column and spinal cord is fairly uncommon in children, accounting for less than 5 percent of childhood injuries, it will not be discussed in great detail here. The interested reader is referred to a more complete discussion of this condition in Chaps. 23 and 31. Principles of nursing managemnt are essentially the same for children and adults.

ABNORMAL CELLULAR GROWTH

Intracranial Tumors: Cerebellar Astrocytoma, Medulloblastoma, Ependymoma, Brainstem Glioma, and Craniopharyngioma

Definitions   *Intracranial tumors* are the second most frequently occurring neoplasm in infants and children, preceded only by leukemia. Since 75 percent of all brain tumors in children are gliomas, the chances of finding a benign tumor at operation are quite small. In children, 50 to 60 percent of brain tumors are found below the tentorium, as opposed to 25 to 30 percent in this location in adults.

The signs and symptoms of brain tumor vary considerably, based on location, tissue type, and other factors. These symptoms are often so varied and nonspecific that they can easily be mistaken for an everyday, harmless childhood malady. The tumors generally manifest themselves as increased intracranial pressure and/or focal neurological deficit. The signs and symptoms most frequently seen are headache, impaired consciousness, cranial enlargement, vomiting, diplopia, strabismus, papilledema, nystagmus, impaired vision, cranial nerve involvement, personality changes, ataxia, seizures, and hypothalamic and endocrine dysfunction.

The discussion of terms such as benign and malignant becomes complex when related to brain tumors. Malignancy depends less on the histological assessment of the mass than on such factors as its accessibility to chemotherapy, irradiation, or surgery, the extent of its interference with brain function and CSF circulation, and the amount of increase in intracranial pressure.

Cerebellar astrocytomas, peak incidence 5 to 8 years, account for approximately 25 percent of all brain tumors in children. These tumors occur almost exclusively in childhood and early adolescence and are the most benign type. They arise from either the vermis or the cerebellar hemispheres, are almost always well circumscribed, and have a tendency toward cyst formation. The treatment of choice is surgical since these tumors are not sensitive to radiotherapy. The prognosis is good, with about 90 percent of the patients surviving from 5 years to several decades. Approximately 90 percent of these survivors have no permanent significant neurological disturbances.

Medulloblastoma, the peak incidence of which occurs during the first decade of life, is a malignant, invasive tumor accounting for 20 percent of all childhood and adolescent brain tumors. Approximately 40 percent of the posterior fossa tumors in children are of this type. It arises from the roof of the fourth ventricle, involves the vermis, and may extend to fill the fourth ventricle, thus blocking the flow of CSF. Medulloblastoma is different from other tumors in that it frequently "seeds" to other parts of the CNS via the CSF pathways.

The treatment for this tumor is often threefold—surgical excision, radiotherapy, and chemotherapy. Radiotherapy generally includes the head, as well as the total spine, to destroy the tumor cells that have "seeded" to other areas. In spite of the fact that the tumor is highly radiosensitive, the outlook for long-term survival remains poor, with only 30 percent surviving longer than 3 years.

Ependymomas arise most frequently from the floor of the fourth ventricle, fill the ventricle with tumor, and interfere with the flow of CSF, thus producing signs and symptoms of obstructive hydrocephalus. Children with this tumor may present with persistent vomiting (due to direct pressure on the emetic center) as an early manifestation of the disease. Total surgical removal is impossible since the tumor is inseparable from the floor of the fourth ventricle. Therefore, the aim of surgery is to clean out the ventricle and establish free flow of CSF. Radiotherapy may also be directed to the posterior fossa postoperatively. The survival varies from several months to 10 years or longer.

Brainstem gliomas are malignant, invasive tumors that most often arise from the pons. They account for about 10 percent of all intracranial childhood tumors and have an average age of onset of approximately 6 years. Brainstem gliomas present with cranial nerve involvement and vomiting, with increased intracranial pressure as an infrequent finding. Surgical intervention is seldom if ever indicated, since these tumors are such an integral part of vital brain structures. Even with radiotherapy, the child rarely survives longer than 12 months.

Craniopharyngiomas, comprising 5 to 13 percent of all intracranial tumors in childhood, are of congenital origin and are believed to be a remnant of embryonic squamous cells. As the tumor grows, it may compress the optic chiasm and the pituitary gland, and extend into the third ventricle, interfering with the flow of CSF. Thus, the presenting symptoms are almost classically those of increased intracranial pressure, visual distirbances, and endocrine and hypothalamic dysfunction.

The treatment of choice is surgical since these tumors are relatively resistant to radiotherapy. Response to treatment is generally good if careful consideration is given to endocrine balance before, during, and after the surgical procedure. Even with subtotal removal, the interval between surgery and recurrence is several years.

Problems

I. Persistent vomiting.
  A. Goals of care: Maintenance of adequate nutrition.
  B. Intervention.
    1. Weigh daily and record on growth chart.
    2. Careful dietary history on admission, with special attention to likes and dislikes.
    3. High protein, between-meal feedings.
    4. Provide light meal in mornings (the time vomiting most frequently occurs).
    5. If vomiting occurs, allow rest time and feed again.
    6. Careful recording of all foods eaten.
    7. Avoid performing frightening, painful procedures near mealtime.
    8. Make tray and food as attractive as possible.
    9. Provide group eating if possible.
  C. Evaluation.
    1. No weight loss.
    2. Absence of lethargy.

      3. Normal attention span for age.
      4. Adequate energy levels for activities of daily living.
      5. Hemoglobin (Hb) and blood protein levels within normal limits.

II. Headache.
  A. Goals of care: The child will be maximally comfortable an1 rsted.
  B. Intervention.
      1. Elevate head of bed 30°.
      2. Keep room dim and quiet when headache begins.
      3. Give pain medications as ordered.
  C. Evaluation.
      1. Absence of complaints of pain.
      2. Relaxed facial expression.
      3. Participation in activities of daily living.

III. Potential accidents due to vision, gait, and coordination disturbances.
  A. Goals of care: The child will be free of injury.
  B. Intervention.
      1. Keep side rails up at all times.
      2. Provide soft toys.
      3. Be sure food and liquids are a safe temperature.
      4. Keep walkways uncluttered.
      5. Do not leave child in bathtub unattended.
      6. Teach parents child's limitations and how to help child protect self.
  C. Evaluation.
      1. Absence of cuts, scrapes, bruises, and burns.
      2. Parents verbalize understanding of protective measures.
      3. Child complies with and understands protective measures.

IV. Possible frustration due to vision, gait, and coordination disturbances.
  A. Goals of care: The child will be able to cope with limitations imposed by neurological condition.
  B. Intervention.
      1. Carefully assess child's abilities and limitations.
      2. Allow child to perform those tasks of which he or she is capable.
      3. Teach parents and significant others importance of child's maintaining independence.
      4. Provide playtime to ventilate frustrations.
  C. Evaluation.
      1. Willingness to engage in activities of daily living.
      2. Absence of excessive crying and inappropriate behavior.
      3. Absence of withdrawal.

V. Parental guilt or grief.
  A. Goals of care: The family will be able to verbalize feelings and cope with guilt.
  B. Intervention.
      1. Provide quiet place and time for family to talk.
      2. Provide information that might help dispel guilt.
      3. Support in grief as appropriate to stage of grieving.
      4. Promote intrafamily communication.
      5. Refer to mental health professional or clergy as indicated.
  C. Evaluation.
      1. Absence of blame placing.
      2. Ability to make rational decisions about child's care.
      3. Absence of behavior designed to "make up" for failure, i.e., excessive gift buying, planning for elaborate trips, no limitations on behavior.
      4. Ability to carry out activities of daily living.

VI. Potential anxiety regarding diagnostic procedures.
  A. Goals of care.
      1. The child and/or family will understand the diagnostic procedures.

    2. The child will be able to cooperate during the procedures.

    3. The child will be maximally rested and comfortable following the procedures.

  B. Intervention.

    1. Provide preprocedure teaching compatible with developmental level.

    2. Use dolls, toys, and pictures as teaching media.

    3. Provide playtime and materials before and after procedures to work out anxieties.

    4. Accompany child to procedure if possible.

    5. Provide time for questions.

    6. Provide rest period following procedure.

  C. Evaluation.

    1. Ability to verbalize facts about procedure.

    2. Absence of excessive overt signs of anxiety, i.e., constant crying, short attention span, irritability.

    3. Absence of nightmares following tests.

VII. Potential anxiety regarding surgical outcome.

  A. Goals of care: The family will be able to verbalize and cope with their anxiety.

  B. Intervention.

    1. Provide quiet time and place for questions.

    2. Engage physician's aid in correcting misconceptions regarding surgical outcome.

    3. Be honest and open in discussions.

    4. Contact clergyman if family desires.

    5. Provide pre- and postoperative information to child appropriate to development. Use dolls, pictures, and hospital equipment as indicated.

    6. Provide family explicit details about postoperative course; exactly how child will look, frequent vital signs, medications, how long the surgery can be expected to take, when they can expect to talk with the physician, etc.

  C. Evaluation.

    1. Absence of excessive, repetitive questioning.

    2. Ability to correctly restate facts regarding surgical routines.

    3. Ability to make decisions regarding child's care.

VIII. Embarrassment secondary to loss of hair.

  A. Goals of care: The child will be able to cope with loss of hair.

  B. Intervention.

    1. Discuss with child rationale for cutting hair.

    2. If possible, avoid cutting hair until immediately before surgery (preferably after child is asleep in the operating room).

    3. Plan with child ways of covering head postoperatively (hats, wigs, colorful scarves, etc.).

  C. Evaluation.

    1. Absence of withdrawal.

    2. Participation in planning.

    3. Ability to verbalize concerns directly or through play activities.

IX. Potential increased intracranial pressure (postoperatively). (See "Hydrocephalus" earlier in this chapter.)

X. Possible diabetes insipidus (particularly following surgery in the area of pituitary). (Refer to Chap. 17.)

  A. Goals of care: Maintenance of adequate fluid and electrolyte balance.

  B. Intervention.

    1. Intake and output every hour or as ordered.

    2. Urine specific gravity every hour (if catheter in place), or with each voiding.

    3. Weigh every day.

    4. Review electrolyte values as available.

  C. Evaluation.

    1. Urine specific gravity within normal limits.

    2. Electrolyte values within normal limits.

        3. Urine output compatible with intake.

        4. Absence of physical signs of dehydration.

XI. Potential seizures.

  A. Goals of care.

    1. Protection of child during seizure activity.

    2. Documentation of seizure activith.

    3. Alleviation of child's and parents' anxiety if seizures occur.

  B. Intervention.

    1. Place padded tongue blade at bedside.

    2. During seizure activity

      a. Remain with child.

      b. Remove toys and other potentially injurious objects from bed.

      c. Insert padded tongue blade between teeth.

      d. Turn child or child's head to side to avoid aspiration.

      e. Do not restrain.

    3. After seizure, record:

      a. Time of onset.

      b. Location of neuromuscular activity.

      c. Length and pattern of seizures.

      d. Activity immediately preceding seizure.

      e. Incidence of incontinence.

      f. Level of consciousness.

    4. Allow child time to rest.

    5. Give explanation of seizure activity to parents (and to child if child requests it).

  C. Evaluation.

    1. Absence of injury from seizure.

    2. Recognition and documentation of seizure activity.

    3. Absence of unnecessary anxiety.

    4. Normal respiratory function (no aspiration).

XII. Possible discipline problems.

  A. Goals of care: Parents will be able to set limits on child's behavior.

  B. Intervention.

    1. Discuss with parents importance of limits in providing child with security.

    2. Support family's attempts to set limits.

    3. Assist nurses in implementing plan for limit-setting.

    4. Provide quiet time and place for parents to discuss concerns.

  C. Evaluation.

    1. Increased instances of controlling unacceptable behavior.

    2. Decreased anxiety regarding discipline.

    3. Increased participation of child in "normal" daily activities.

XIII. Potentially fatal diagnosis: A large aspect of caring for these children is dealing with the fact that many of them will die very soon. The nurse has a key role in supporting the terminally ill child and the family during this crisis. Refer to other chapters of this handbook and to references on death and dying for a complete discussion.

Extracranial Tumors: Neuroblastoma and Intraspinal Tumors

Neuroblastoma is a malignant tumor of early life. It is probably the most common solid, malignant tumor of childhood, accounting for about half of malignant tumors in the neonate. It is an embryonal tumor which arises from neural crest ectoderm. Incidence is highest during the first 5 years of life with a peak incidence before the age of 3 years.

Neuroblastoma arises most commonly from the adrenal medulla or along the sympathetic chain in the chest or abdomen. However, it may be found anywhere in the body where sympathetic nervous tissue is located. It is difficult to discover neuroblastoma in the early stages because the beginning symptoms are so nonspecific—weight loss or failure to gain, abdominal pain, feeding problems. These tumors metastasize early by vascular and lymphatic spread to a variety of body areas, typically to lymph nodes, bones, bone marrow, or liver. Consequently, most children have extensive disease by the time they come to medical attention.

The most common presenting symptom is an abdominal mass that may be discovered by the parents during bathing or by the nurse or physician during a routine physical exam. Other indications may be subcutaneous nodules, periorbital swelling due to a retro-orbital tumor, bone pain, limp, paresis of lower extremities, anemia, and irritability.

The nurse's first responsibility in neuroblastoma is for case finding and referral. Once the child is hospitalized, nursing care involves pre- and postoperative preparation and care. Due to the poor prognosis for the majority of these children, the nurse must be prepared to be helpful to both the terminally ill child and the family.

Intraspinal tumors occur approximately one-fifth as often as intracranial tumors. The most common intraspinal tumors are lipomas, dermoid and teratoid tumors, neuroblastomas, and intramedullary gliomas.

It is imperative that these tumors be diagnosed in the early stages because: (1) irreversible neurological dysfunction may occur when the diagnosis is delayed; (2) most tumors, even gliomas, may respond dramatically to surgical excision and radiation therapy; (3) intraspinal tumors may be associated, even after only partial excision, with prolonged relief of signs and symptoms. The most frequently occurring signs and symptoms are disturbances of gait and posture, pain, weakness, reflex changes, impaired bladder and bowel function, sensory impairment, and cutaneous and skeletal changes.

Treatment depends on tumor type and location, but it primarily includes surgical decompression, radiation therapy, and corticosteroid and/or other chemotherapy. Nursing care is directed primarily toward the following areas:

1. Case finding and referral.
2. Prevention of deformities and maintenance of bodily functions during hospitalization.
3. Teaching for child and family.
4. Play therapy to help child cope with anxiety.
5. Planning for rehabilitation.

ABNORMAL NEURONAL DISCHARGE: SEIZURES

"A seizure is an episodic involuntary alteration in consciousness, motor activity, behavior, sensation, or autonomic function" (2). Paroxysmal, neuronal discharge within the CNS can best be viewed as a symptom of a disease rather than the disease entity itself. Convulsions during childhood result from a variety of conditions: congenital defects, trauma, metabolic disorders, fluid and electrolyte imbalances, temperature elevations, intracranial tumors, epilepsy, invasion of the CNS by infection, drugs, or toxins.

Febrile Convulsions; Epilepsy; Grand Mal, Petit Mal, Psychomotor, and Focal Seizures; Infantile Spasms

Definitions   *Febrile convulsions* occur with a sudden rise in temperature during acute febrile diseases, primarily upper respiratory disorders such as tonsillitis, pharyngitis, and otitis. These seizures occur in approximately 8 percent of infants and children between the ages of 6 months and 3 years. They are seen rarely after the age of 7 years. Some authors feel that there are factors, such as age, degree of temperature elevation, nature of illness, genetic makeup, and rate of fever rise, which contribute to a predisposition for febrile seizures.

Epilepsy may be defined as recurrent, paroxysmal neuronal discharges leading to disturbances in consciousness or in autonomic, motor, or sensory function. It is not one specific disease, but rather a group of recurrent seizure patterns. Accurate figures on the incidence of epilepsy are not available, since this is not a reportable condition. The most common estimate is that 1 in 100 individuals in the United States suffers with epileptic seizures (about 4 million persons). Other investigators feel that the number is much higher, possibly as many as 1 in 50.

Approximately 90 percent of all epileptics develop their initial symptoms before the age of 20. Though epilepsy may first appear at any time during childhood, there are three specific periods when it is *most* likely to occur: (1) during the first 2 years of life, (2) from 5 through 7 years of age, and (3) at puberty (more often in females than males). The peak during the first 2 years of life is felt to be related to cerebral damage occurring prenatally or during the birth process. The reason for the second peak remains obscure. The peak at puberty is believed to be related to the complex chemical and physiologic changes going on in the body at that time.

The epilepsies have been classified over the years using a variety of systems, such as clinical, anatomic, electroencephalographic, and etiologic. The etiologic system that divides these patterns into two broad patterns appears frequently in writings on the subject. Children who develop seizures without any demonstrable cerebral damage are said to have *idiopathic* or *genetic* epilepsy. Epilepsy is identified as *organic* or *symptomatic* when it develops subsequent to cerebral change or damage.

A *grand mal seizure* (convulsion) is the type of epilepsy most commonly found during childhood. Classically, there is an aura followed by loss of consciousness and rolling up of the eyes. There is generalized tonic contraction of body musculature leading to the emission of a sharp cry and a period of apnea and cyanosis. During the clonic phase, the trunk and extremities alternately contract and relax. This activity may cause biting of the tongue and urinary and fecal incontinence. The seizure may last from a few seconds to a few minutes. Usually the child will sleep for a time following the seizure and, upon awakening, may continue to be drowsy and confused. There may be some transient neurologic deficit which may be helpful in pinpointing the origin of the seizures.

Petit mal seizures are often described as "staring" or "absence" episodes. These are transient losses of consciousness that may be accompanied by lipsmacking, fluttering of the eyelids, eye rolling movements, drooping of the head, or slight clonic contractions of the limb and trunk muscles. These attacks are so brief that they may not be noticed until their occurrence begins to interfere with school performance and behavior. Petit mal seizures may be precipitated by flashing light or hyperventilation.

Psychomotor seizures are periods of abnormal but apparently purposeful behavior which the patient is not able to remember after the seizure is over. Children frequently experience an aura of intense fear prior to the seizure. An aura of epigastric discomfort, smelling a bad odor, or buzzing in the ear may also precede the attack. There are a variety of motor symptoms which may appear as manifestations of the seizure. Some of the most common are jerking of the mouth and face, aphasia, tonic posturing, and repetitive coordinated but inappropriate movements (walking or running in circles, swallowing, smacking, chewing).

Focal (Jacksonian) seizures, as the name implies, involve a specific, localized part of the brain. The Jacksonian type of focal seizure originates in one area of the cortex and progresses to involve the entire motor strip. Quite often this seizure escalates to a grand mal attack.

Infantile (myoclonic) spasms are seizures peculiar to infancy. Generally, the EEG shows a characteristic pattern known as hypsarrhythmia. In approximately 50 percent of the cases, the etiology is unknown. The other 50 percent arise from a variety of causes—developmental anomalies, birth trauma, anoxia, postnatal birth trauma, meningitis, and encephalitis. Most frequently, the attacks are characterized by sudden, forceful contractions of the musculature of the trunk, the extremities, and the neck. The child is noticed to suddenly adduct and flex the limbs and drop the head. The prognosis for these children is rather bleak, since development is arrested or regresses with the onset of seizures. As the attacks continue, there is further deterioration of motor and mental abilities. Eventually, approximately 10 to 15 percent of the children die. Of those that survive, greater than 90 percent are mentally retarded.

The first step in the management of epilepsy is to document the occurrence of seizures, and obtain an accurate description of the seizure pattern. The second step is to rule out an organic cause for the seizures which would be amenable to medical or surgical intervention.

The child is generally admitted to a hospital for this phase of management. If no organic cause can be found, the child is then begun on a drug regime to bring the seizures under control. See Table 19-1 for a list of those drugs used most often.

Problems

I. Anxiety regarding the hospital environment and the diagnostic tests.
   A. Goals of care.
      1. The child and parents will be able to cope with hospitalization.
      2. The child and family will understand the diagnostic procedures.
      3. The child will be able to cooperate during the procedure.
      4. The child will be maximally rested and comfortable following the procedure.
   B. Intervention.
      1. Encourage parents to bring toys and other familiar objects from home.
      2. Provide continuity in nursing assignments to the extent possible.
      3. Assess current knowledge level and readiness to learn.
      4. Before diagnostic tests, provide explanations compatible with developmental level (use dolls, toys and pictures if indicated).
      5. Accompany child to procedure if possible.
      6. Provide playtime and materials before and after procedure to work out anxieties.
      7. Provide rest period following procedures.
   C. Evaluation.
      1. Ability to verbalize facts about procedure.
      2. Absence of signs of excessive anxiety.
      3. Child sleeps well without nightmares.
      4. Parents verbalize anxiety. Child expresses anxiety verbally or through play activities.

II. Potential embarrassment regarding seizures.
   A. Goals of care: Assist parents/child in recognizing and expressing feelings regarding epilepsy.
   B. Intervention.
      1. Provide time and a quiet place for parents to discuss concerns with nurse and/or other health team members.
      2. Provide structured play situations to help child express and work through feelings.
      3. Provide written information about epilepsy.
      4. If appropriate, put family in contact with families in the community who have a child with epilepsy.
   C. Evaluation.
      1. Verbalizes feelings.
      2. Verbalizes plans for informing others about seizures as appropriate—school, friends, family.

III. Possible injury or aspiration during seizure activity.
   A. Goals of care: Child will be free of injury and aspiration.
   B. Intervention.
      1. Padded tongue blade at bedside. Instruct family in its use.
      2. Keep bed rails up.

TABLE 19-1 / DRUGS USED IN THE CONTROL OF EPILEPTIC SEIZURES

Grand Mal	Petit Mal	Psychomotor	Myoclonic
Phenobarbital	Zarontin	Tegretol	Valium
Mysoline	Tridione	Mysoline	ACTH
Dilantin		Dilantin	Corticosteroids
			Ketogenic diet

    3. Remove toys and other potentially injurious objects from bed if seizure activity occurs.

    4. Position child on side or turn head to side during seizure activity.

    5. Remain with child during seizure.

    6. Do not restrain during seizure.

  C. Evaluation.

    1. Absence of bruises and abrasions.

    2. Normal respiratory function (no aspiration).

IV. Possible noncompliance with medication regime.

  A. Goals of care: Medication will be taken as ordered.

  B. Intervention.

    1. Teach parents and child importance of drug therapy.

    2. Provide written instructions on when to take drugs.

    3. Investigate financial resources for securing drug.

    4. Teach family importance of keeping drug out of reach of other children at home.

  C. Evaluation.

    1. Absence of seizures.

    2. Adequate blood levels of drug.

    3. Verbalizes willingness to take drug.

V. Possible toxic effects from the drug therapy.

  A. Goals of care: Prevention and recognition of toxic symptoms.

  B. Intervention.

    1. Provide written list of toxic symptoms.

    2. Give written instructions on measures to be taken if toxic symptoms occur.

    3. Caution against changing drug dosage unless instructed to do so by physician.

  C. Evaluation.

    1. Parents (and child, if old enough) can describe toxic effects.

    2. Parents (and child, if old enough) accurately describe drug regime.

INFLAMMATORY DISORDERS

Meningitis

Definition   *Meningitis* is inflammation of the meninges, the coverings of the brain and spinal cord. There are numerous organisms, both bacterial and viral, that cause meningitis. These organisms may reach the meninges through any of several routes: through the bloodstream from a focus of infection elsewhere in the body, by invasion from structures that adjoin the CNS, or through direct introduction into the CNS (e.g., traumatic injuries of the skull, birth defects such as myelomeningocele).

Bacterial meningitis occurs more frequently during childhood than at any other time in the life cycle, and is one of the most serious types of infection that a child may contract. Meningitis is particularly lethal during the first year of life because the signs of meningeal irritation may be less distinct and the sequelae more frequent when bacterial agents attack the immature brain. Although almost any bacterium is capable of causing meningitis, certain age groups seem predisposed to meningitis caused by particular organisms.

Prior to the age of 2 months, gram negative organisms and group B, beta-hemolytic streptococci are the most frequent offenders. The most common cause of meningitis between the ages of 4 months and 3 years is *Hemophilus influenzae*. Pneumococci and meningococci are the most common organisms causing meningitis in children over the age of 4 years (3).

The signs and symptoms of bacterial meningitis vary, depending upon the age of the child, the infecting organism, and the duration of illness. Those most often seen are irritability, vomiting, lethargy, anorexia, fever, signs of meningeal irritation, headache, confusion, and seizures. It is imperative that antibiotic treatment be started *immediately* in these children, since delays drastically increase mortality and sequelae.

Problems

I. Elevated temperature.
   A. Goals of care: Reduction of fever as rapidly and safely as possible.
   B. Intervention.
      1. Administer antipyretics as ordered.
      2. Keep room cool and child lightly clothed.
      3. Sponge with tepid or cool towels.
      4. Avoid overchilling since shivering will only elevate the temperature more.
   C. Evaluation: Temperature less than 38.5°C (101°F).

II. Restlessness, irritability, photophobia, nuchal rigidity.
   A. Goals of care: Keep child as comfortable as possible.
   B. Intervention.
      1. Place child in private room if possible (imperative for meningococcal meningitis).
      2. Limit visitors.
      3. Group nursing activities and treatments together to allow uninterrupted rest periods.
      4. Keep lights in room dim.
      5. Ask parents to bring a favorite toy.
      6. Avoid moving child unnecessarily during the acute phase of the illness.
   C. Evaluation.
      1. Parents verbalize understanding of restrictions.
      2. Decreasing episodes of restlessness and irritability.
      3. Increased periods of rest and sleep.

III. Potential inadequate nutrition and metabolic imbalances secondary to nausea and vomiting.
   A. Goals of care: Maintenance of adequate nutritional and metabolic status.
   B. Intervention.
      1. Offer small amounts of clear liquids frequently. Gelatin and popsicles are often well accepted.
      2. Weigh daily if child's condition permits.
      3. Monitor intake and output carefully.
      4. As child improves, try to obtain favorite foods to stimulate appetite.
   C. Evaluation.
      1. Electrolyte values within normal limits.
      2. Absence of weight loss.
      3. Moist mucous membranes.
      4. Adequate urinary output.

IV. Possible increased intracranial pressure (see "Hydrocephalus" earlier in this chapter).

V. Long-term IV antibiotic therapy.
   A. Goals of care.
      1. Maintenance of patent intravenous line.
      2. Prevention of sensory deprivation.
   B. Intervention.
      1. Restrain as necessary.
      2. Tape IV needle securely.
      3. Assess IV site every 2 h for signs of infiltration and/or irritation.
      4. Teach parents and child necessity and importance of IV antibiotics.
      5. Encourage family to talk to and touch child while awake.
      6. As condition improves, provide play activities compatible with age and within constraints of IV.
   C. Evaluation.
      1. IV fluids infuse as ordered.
      2. Absence of redness and edema around IV site.
      3. Child interested in and participates in play activities.

VI. Possible parental anxiety regarding child's future development.
   A. Goals of care: Emotional support for family.

B. Intervention.
   1. Provide time and a quiet place for parents to discuss concerns with nurse and/or other health team members.
   2. Explain difficulty in making predictions during the acute phase of the illness.
   3. Developmental assessment prior to discharge.
   4. Teach parents methods of developmental stimulation.
   5. Community health nurse referral for further evaluation in the home environment.
C. Evaluation.
   1. Parents verbalize anxieties.
   2. Parents verbalize and demonstrate developmental stimulation.
VII. Meningococcal meningitis is easily transmitted.
   A. Goals of care: Other persons will not become infected.
   B. Intervention.
      1. Family contacts and exposed staff members must be evaluated as to need for prophylactic antibiotic.
      2. Place child in respiratory isolation.
   C. Evaluation: No new cases.

Encephalitis

Encephalitis is an inflammatory process of the brain, most often of viral origin. Pathological changes are generally cellular infiltration, proliferation of microglial cells, arteritis, and/or other changes in the blood vessel walls. Encephalitis may appear in children as complications of other disease processes, such as chickenpox, mumps, measles, and herpes simplex.

Encephalitis may begin insidiously or have an abrupt, explosive onset. The signs and symptoms most often seen are changes in level of consciousness, fever, headache, vomiting, ataxia, seizures, and nuchal rigidity. The treatment and nursing care are symptomatic and supportive.

Reyes' Syndrome

Reyes' syndrome is a disorder with an obscure etiology that was first described in 1963. The incidence of this disease has been relatively unknown. However, recent epidemiological data seem to indicate that this syndrome is one of the most common neurological complications of viral infections in childhood. It is characterized by fever, seriously impaired consciousness, hypoglycemia, seizures, and impaired hepatic function. Mortality has been reported as high as 85 percent. Treatment is primarily of a supportive nature.

METABOLIC AND TOXIC DISORDERS

Lead Poisoning

Definition *Lead poisoning* may result from either ingestion or inhalation of lead. In children, it most frequently results from repeated ingestion of inorganic lead compounds. Children ages 1 to 5 years are at risk for lead poisoning, with the peak incidence being between 12 and 36 months of age. The majority of cases occur in pica-prone toddlers living in poorly maintained homes built prior to the 1940s. The child ingests lead by chewing wood coated with old paint, or by eating crumbling plaster or paint flakes. Although there are federal laws prohibiting the use of lead paint, there are no laws requiring removal of old paint containing lead from preexisting homes.

Chronic lead poisoning, with an insidious onset, is the most common in children. Ninety percent of these children present with overt signs of lead encephalopathy. The tragedy of this statistic becomes apparent when it is realized that 30 to 40 percent of the children who receive treatment after the onset of neurologic involvement suffer severe, irreversible brain damage—i.e., spasticity, quadriplegia, hemiparesis, blindness, deafness, convulsions, and mental retardation.

Although early detection is crucial, the task seems almost impossible because the initial symptoms are so nonspecific. The child may be more irritable, less active, more sleepy, may have diarrhea, constipation, nausea and vomiting, and incoordination. Such symptoms may be passed off by the family—as well as the physician—as everyday childhood illness. Lead poisoning is generally detected once the child develops seizures and symptoms of increased intracranial pressure.

Problems

I. Increased intracranial pressure.
  A. Goals of care: Maintenance of adequate neurological functioning.
  B. Intervention.
    1. Administer osmotic diuretics (urea or mannitol) as ordered immediately.
    2. Monitor intake and output carefully.
    3. Assess and record neurological status every hour. Report deterioration to physician immediately.
  C. Evaluation: Absence of deteriorating neurological status.
II. Possible intractable seizures.
  A. Goals of care: Careful observation and protection of child during seizure activity.
  B. Intervention.
    1. Administer anticonvulsants as ordered.
    2. Keep bed rails up at all times.
    3. Remove toys and other objects from bed if seizures occur.
    4. Remain with child.
    5. Position child on side or turn head to side to prevent aspiration.
    6. If seizure activity persists, notify physician immediately.
  C. Evaluation.
    1. Decreased severity and incidence of seizures.
    2. Absence of injury and aspiration.
III. Possible respiratory depression secondary to high doses of anticonvulsants.
  A. Goals of care: Maintain adequate respiratory function.
  B. Intervention.
    1. Keep an accurate record of medications given.
    2. Assess respiratory pattern and rate every hour or as ordered with vital signs.
    3. Report respiratory impairment immediately.
    4. Institute respiratory support until physician arrives.
    5. Assess blood gas values and electrolytes as reports become available.
  C. Evaluation.
    1. Respiratory rate and rhythm within normal limits.
    2. Blood gases and electrolytes within normal limits.
IV. Potential parental lack of knowledge regarding treatment regime.
  A. Goals of care: Parents will understand rationale behind therapy.
  B. Intervention.
    1. Provide information about drugs used and expected results.
    2. Notify physician of unrealistic parental expectations and misconceptions regarding treatment.
    3. Provide time and quiet place for questions.
  C. Evaluation.
    1. Parents verbalize treatment regime accurately.
    2. Parents verbalize realistic outcomes of therapy.
V. Possible family guilt regarding poisoning.
  A. Goals of care.
    1. Support of family during their feelings of guilt.
    2. Maintenance of intrafamily communication.

    B. Intervention.
        1. Provide family with facts regarding lead poisoning.
        2. Emphasize difficulty in recognizing early symptoms.
        3. Provide parents a place to discuss concerns with each other.
        4. Notify clergyman if indicated.
    C. Evaluation.
        1. Parents verbalize feelings regarding poisoning.
        2. Parents are able to involve themselves in child's care to a realistic degree.
        3. Absence of blame placing.
VI. Possible separation anxiety.
    A. Goals of care.
        1. Prevention of child's withdrawal.
        2. Promotion of adjustment to hospitalization.
    B. Intervention.
        1. Staff and parent teaching regarding separation anxiety.
        2. Encourage parents to bring familiar objects from home.
        3. Encourage parents to stay with child if feasible.
        4. Provide continuity in nursing assignment.
    C. Evaluation.
        1. Child relates to staff as appropriate for developmental level.
        2. Child maintains relationship with parents.
        3. Absence of withdrawal and apathy.
VII. Possible recurrence of poisoning following discharge.
    A. Goals of care: Prevent further poisoning.
    B. Intervention.
        1. Refer to Social Service and Public Health for assistance in identifying source.
        2. Discuss with family importance of identifying source and preventing recurrence.
    C. Evaluation.
        1. Absence of recurrence.
        2. Family verbalizes willingness to remove source of poisoning.
VIII. Potential delayed developmental milestones.
    A. Goals of care.
        1. Identification of deficit.
        2. Promotion of development.
    B. Intervention.
        1. Developmental assessment as soon as condition permits.
        2. Include specific developmental stimulation in nursing plan of care.
        3. Teach parents importance and methods of stimulation.
        4. Public Health Nurse referral for follow-up evaluation.
    C. Evaluation.
        1. Staff engages in appropriate developmental stimulation.
        2. Family verbalizes and demonstrates stimulation.

Phenylketonuria

Phenylketonuria (PKU) is an inborn error of metabolism which affects the conversion of phenylalanine to tyrosine. PKU is genetically transmitted as an autosomal recessive trait. It occurs about once in 10,000 births. Mental retardation is the primary result of the disorder and is the basis for concern about early diagnosis and treatment. Although still a source of much controversy, a low phenylalanine diet is the treatment of choice. Nurses are generally involved in case finding, in family teaching regarding dietary management, and in family support.

Maple Syrup Disease

Maple syrup disease is a familial cerebral degenerative disease caused by a defect in amino acid metabolism. The disease is characterized by the passage of urine with an odor of maple syrup. This disorder is transmitted as an autosomal recessive trait. The only known treatment is dietary restriction of specific amino acids.

Tay-Sachs Disease

Tay-Sachs disease results from a disorder in lipid metabolism involving one of the lysosomal enzymes. It is inherited as an autosomal recessive trait and occurs almost exclusively in Jews of Eastern European origin. There is no known effective treatment.

By the age of 6 months, these children generally exhibit irritability, apathy, lack of interest in the environment, lack of visual fixation, and unusual sensitivity to noise. The child has delayed developmental milestones. As the disease progresses, the child develops seizures, blindness, macular cherry-red spots, spasticity, decerebrate posturing, and dementia. Death usually occurs between the ages of 2 and 4 years of age.

DEVELOPMENTAL DISORDERS

Mental Retardation

Definition

Mental retardation is a label traditionally attached to those individuals who perform two standard deviations below the mean on a standardized psychologic test. Such a definition might prove useful in certain circumstances but serves little purpose in the planning and delivery of health care. The American Association on Mental Deficiency adopted an official definition of mental retardation in 1958. In this statement, mental deficiency refers to subaverage intellectual functioning which originates in the developmental period and is associated with impairment in adaptive behavior. In the final analysis, the primary concerns for the individual are the ability to *adapt* to the environment and to compete successfully in society.

Mental retardation is one of the most serious conditions in our society today because of the major health, social, and economic problems that it encompasses. Approximately 3 percent of the population are mentally retarded. In 1970 there were more than 6 million retarded individuals in the United States, with over one third of these being under the age of 20 years. Of those under 20, approximately 75 percent were mildly retarded, 15 percent were moderately retarded, 8 percent were severely retarded, and 2 percent were profoundly retarded (unable to care for themselves).

A discussion of etiology is somewhat unrewarding since, in a large percentage of children, the cause is not known. The most frequently used system for classification is based on causative factors. The system proposed by Baker and Barton (4) is based on the development of the child when the condition occurred. See Table 19-2 for an outline of the most common conditions in their classification system.

The IQ score has been used, rightly or wrongly, to group retarded individuals into three major categories:

1. Educable mentally retarded.
   a. IQ between 50 and 75.
   b. Can reach third- to fifth-grade level of academic achievement.
   c. Independent in activities of daily living.
   d. As adult, generally functions independently.
   e. Able to work as unskilled or semiskilled laborer.

TABLE 19-2 / CLASSIFICATION OF MENTAL RETARDATION

Prenatal Period	
Chromosome anomalies:	Maternal factors:
Down's syndrome (trisomy 21)	Rubella (German measles)
Klinefelter's syndrome	Some other viral illnesses of mother
Errors of metabolism:	Syphilis
Phenylketonuria (PKU)	Anoxia
Hypothyroidism (cretinism)	Blood type incompatibility
Hurler's disease (gargoylism)	Malnutrition
Malformation of the cranium:	Toxemia
Microcephaly	
Hydrocephaly	
Neonatal or Perinatal Period	
Anoxia	Kernicterus
Intracranial hemorrhage	Prematurity
Birth injury	
Postnatal Period	
Infections:	Physical injury:
Meningitis	Head injury
Encephalitis	Asphyxia
Poisoning:	Hyperpyrexia
Insecticides	Brain tumors
Medications	Social and cultural factors:
Lead	Deprivation
Degenerative disease:	Emotional disturbance
Tay-Sachs disease	Nutritional deficiency
Huntington's chorea	
Niemann-Pick disease	

Source: Amanda Baker and Pauline Barton, "The Mentally Retarded Child," in
G. Scipien et al. (eds.), *Comprehensive Pediatric Nursing,* McGraw-Hill Book
Company, New York, 1975.

2. Trainable mentally retarded.
   a. IQ between 25 and 50.
   b. Rarely learns to read or write.
   c. Can learn self-care activities.
   d. Can learn social skills such as acceptable behavior, table manners, acceptable means of communication.
   e. Requires assistance as adult.
   f. Can learn simple job skills and function within a sheltered workshop or the home environment.
3. Severely or profoundly retarded.
   a. IQ between 0 and 25.
   b. Acquires no academic skills.
   c. Requires assistance with essentially all activities of daily living.
   d. Can learn the tasks of infancy, i.e., to sit, to stand, to relate to others, to play with toys.
   e. As adult, requires continual care and protection.
The beginning of effective nursing is to view mentally retarded children first as children

who have the basic needs of all children. Having accomplished this, the nurse must try to assess the child and design care in terms of functional level rather than chronological age. This can be quite a task indeed when, for example, the child is a big 10-year-old functioning at a toddler level.

The nursing of children who are mentally retarded cannot be discussed in detail here. The following list of common problems is offered to alert the nurse to some important early considerations. Refer to the bibliography for additional assistance.

Problems

    I. Inability of the nurse to confront and work through his or her feelings toward defective or handicapped persons.

    II. Potential pressure upon parents by professionals and relatives to institutionalize child.

    III. Possible parental fixation in the denial stage of the grief process.

    IV. Lack of confidence in parenting abilities.

    V. Potential failure of the nurse to correctly identify the child's developmental level.

    VI. Potential knowledge deficit regarding developmental stimulation (applies to health workers as well as family).

    VII. Inadequate self-concept (child).

    VIII. Potential inability of parents to discipline child.

    IX. Possible inability of family to cope with societal rejection of child.

    X. Overwhlming financial burden.

    XI. Potential problems with siblings secondary to excessive parental involvement with retarded child.

Cerebral Palsy

Definition

"Cerebral palsy is a nonspecific, descriptive term pertaining to disordered motor function, beginning in early infancy, characterized by spasticity and/or involuntary movements of the limbs. The dysfunction is caused by brain impairment and is not episodic or progressive (5). It is estimated that cerebral palsy occurs in approximately 1 to 6 children per 1000 live births. The incidence in the population is estimated to be about 0.2 percent.

Cerebral palsy is most often classified according to neurologic signs and symptoms: (1) spastic, (2) choreoathetotic, (3) ataxic, (4) dystonic, (5) ballismic, and (6) mixed. The spastic forms account for 60 to 70 percent of the affected children. These categories may be further refined as to limb(s) involved, suspected etiology, and functional capacity. In addition to motor impairment, the child may have other associated problems, such as hearing and vision impairment, mental retardation, learning disabilities, and seizures.

There are a variety of factors occurring before, during, and shortly after birth which may lead to cerebral palsy: (1) nutritional deficiencies, trauma, infections, and radiation, which may interfere with CNS development during the prenatal period; (2) prematurity; (3) prolonged, difficult labor; (4) asphyxia and hypoxia during or immediately following birth; (5) kernicterus from neonatal hyperbilirubinemia; (6) infectious conditions (meningitis, encephalitis) following birth. Nursing is one member of the multidisciplinary team that provides services to the child and the family. Some of the problems are listed below.

Problems

    I. Inability of the parents to accept the birth of a defective child.

    II. Difficulty in maintaining effective respiratory function.

    III. Difficulty in swallowing and sucking.

    IV. Chronic fatigue secondary to nonpurposeful motor activity.

    V. Difficulties in performing activities of daily living.

    VI. Inadequate speech development.

    VII. Disturbed vision.

    VIII. Parental overprotection and other disturbances in family functioning.

    IX. Impaired self-concept.

Minimal Brain Dysfunction

Definition   *Minimal brain dysfunction* (MBD) is a descriptive term applied to

children of near average, average, or above average intellectual capacity with certain learning and/or behavioral disabilities ranging from mild to severe, which are associated with deviations of function of the central nervous system. These deviations may manifest themselves by various combinations of impairment in perception, conceptualization, language, memory, and control of attention, impulse or motor function. These aberrations may arise from genetic variations, biochemical irregularities, perinatal brain insults, or other illnesses or injuries sustained during the years critical for the development and maturation of the central nervous system . . . (6).

MBD may be the most common cause of chronic behavior problems in children (7). The incidence in the pediatric population is estimated to be between 5 and 10 percent, with males affected 4 to 5 times as often as females. Therapy is generally directed toward family education and counseling, and medication, educational management, and psychotherapy for the child (Fig. 19-4). Nurses most frequently called upon to work with these children and their families are those engaged in community settings such as schools, health departments, physicians' offices, mental health clinics, and other outpatient clinic settings. Children are rarely hospitalized with MBD as a primary diagnosis. However, children hospitalized for other reasons who display "behavior problems" may well have MBD as a coincidental difficulty.

FIGURE 19-4 / Venn diagram depicting three major target symptoms and possible symptomatic combinations in minimal brain dysfunction: (1) learning disabilities, no motor disabilities, no behavioral difficulties; (2) learning disabilities and behavioral difficulties; (3) behavioral difficulties, no motor disabilities, no learning disabilities; (4) learning disabilities and motor disabilities; (5) learning disabilities, behavioral difficulties, and motor disabilities; (6) behavioral difficulties and motor disabilities; (7) motor disabilities. [From Francis S. Wright, "General Considerations and Approach to Learning Disabilities," in Kenneth F. Swaiman and Francis S. Wright (eds.), The Practice of Pediatric Neurology, The C. V. Mosby Company, St. Louis, 1975; courtesy Dr. Kenneth F. Swaiman.]

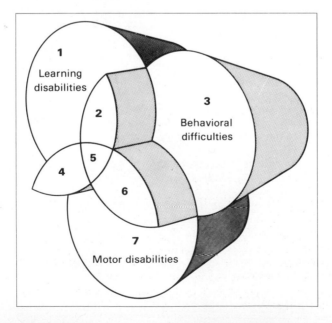

Problems
    I. Short attention span and easy distractability.
   II. Hyperactivity.
  III. Poor motor control.
  IV. Emotional lability.
   V. Poor impulse control.
  VI. Disorders in perception of space, form, movement, and time.
 VII. Delayed language development.
VIII. Parental guilt.
  IX. Parental doubt in child-rearing abilities.
   X. Inability of classroom teacher to cope with child's problems.
  XI. Poor self-concept (child).

Hearing Impairment

Definition
Profound deafness occurs about once per 1000 live births. It is estimated that approximately 25 out of 1000 newborns have a moderate to severe hearing loss. There are approximately 39,000 school age children in the United States who either were born deaf or lost their hearing before speech and language patterns were developed.

Deafness is often associated with syndromes involving other organ systems, such as kidney disease, thyroid disease, disorders of pigmentation, bone diseases, conductive defects in the heart, and eye anomalies. Listed below are some etiologic factors which are generally implicated in hearing impairment:

1. Genetics.
2. Infection.
   a. Prenatal: rubella, syphilis, toxoplasmosis, cytomegalovirus.
   b. Postnatal: meningitis, measles, mumps, chronic otitis media, tympanomastoiditis.
3. Hyperbilirubinemia.
4. Neonatal hypoxia.
5. Drug toxicity.
6. Trauma.
7. Neoplasms.

There are different methods of classifying hearing impairment based on anatomic factors, severity of hearing loss, and onset and course. Usually, the impairment is referred to as either a conductive loss or a sensorineural loss. A conductive loss is most often due to eustachian tube obstruction or dysfunction which results in serous otitis media or mucoid otitis media. This type loss may be associated with external ear and/or facial anomalies and with renal anomalies. In children, a conductive loss can usually be treated with a hearing aid. A sensorineural loss is related to cochlear pathology, damage to the acoustic nerve (cranial nerve VIII), or damage to hearing centers in the brain. This type of loss is still poorly understood.

Hearing loss is difficult to detect in very young children. However, it is imperative that these defects be identified early in order to provide the special training and support needed by such children. This disorder is frequently overlooked in children who are retarded, emotionally disturbed, or who have visual or motor handicaps. Hearing impairment should be suspected in any child who appears unresponsive to sound or who does not develop language soon after the age of 12 months. Hearing impairment should be suspected in children who exhibit the following behaviors:

1. Delayed or impaired speech development.
2. Failure to awaken from sleep when called without being touched.
3. Failure to respond to speech or to name being called.
4. Tilting head or assuming unusual postures when listening.
5. Poor school performance.

6. Poor scores on verbal intelligence testing.
7. Constantly spends time alone even in presence of other children.
8. "Self-stimulation" or other "autistic-type" behaviors.

The care and training of a hearing impaired child requires a multidisciplinary approach, especially when deafness is paired with other handicaps.

Problems
    I. Possible undetected hearing loss.
    II. Possible parental guilt.
    III. Potential knowledge deficit regarding the implications of genetic hearing loss.
    IV. Poor self-concept (child).
    V. Parental anxieties regarding child-rearing abilities for such a child.
    VI. Possible inadequate or inconsistent discipline.
    VII. Parental overprotection.

Visual Impairment

Definition
The critical period for developing acute vision is between 1 and 6 years of age. It is imperative that visual screening be done before the child reaches the age of 4 years. There are approximately 16 million children in the United States between the ages of 3 and 6 years. Of this number, only about 500,000 (3 percent) are tested annually for visual disturbances. It is estimated that 1 child in 20 has visual problems of one kind or another.

There are numerous disorders which may lead to blindness or vision loss in childhood. Among them are various genetic anomalies and degenerative disorders, congenital rubella, congenital syphilis, trauma, infection during delivery, retrolental fibroplasia, neoplasms, trachoma and other infections involving the eye postnatally, primary developmental glaucoma, and untreated strabismus (leading to loss of vision in the affected eye).

The nurse needs to be aware of signs of visual impairment in children. Blindness may be suspected in an infant who does not reach for toys or bottle, or who does not smile in response to the mother's smile. Signs that may be seen in older children are: (1) walking into furniture, (2) frequent rubbing of the eyes, (3) holding objects very close to the eyes, (4) excessive blinking, squinting, and frowning, (5) watery, inflamed eyes, (6) tearing and photophobia, (7) difficulty reading, seeing the blackboard, or doing close work.

Blind children require complex education and training from a multitude of specialists. They need special training in routine activities of daily living, as well as special opportunities for educational and social experiences.

Problems
    I. Possible undetected visual disturbances.
    II. Possible sensory deprivation.
    III. Potential lack of parental understanding in development of other sensory modalities.
    IV. Parental guilt.
    V. Overwhelming financial burden to family.
    VI. Possible inability of family to accept a defective child.
    VII. Family concern about who will care for child in later years.
    VIII. Poor self-concept.
    IX. Excessive dependency.

REFERENCES

1. Kenneth F. Swaiman and Francis S. Wright, *The Practice of Pediatric Neurology,* vols. I and II, The C. V. Mosby Company, St. Louis, 1975.
2. Ibid., p. 829.
3. Ibid., p. 543.

4. Amanda S. Baker and Pauline H. Barton, "The Mentally Retarded Child," in G. Scipien et al. (eds.), *Comprehensive Pediatric Nursing,* McGraw-Hill Book Company, New York, 1975.
5. Swaiman and Wright, op. cit.
6. Sam D. Clements, "National Project on Minimal Brain Dysfunction in Children: Terminology and Identification," Monograph no. 3, Public Health Service Publication no. 1415, U.S. Government Printing Office, Washington, D.C., 1966.
7. Paul H. Wender, "Minimal Brain Dysfunction in Children—Diagnosis and Management," *Pediatric Clinics of North America,* **20**(1):187–201, February 1973.

BIBLIOGRAPHY

Alexander, Mary M., and Marie Scott Brown: "Physical Examination, Parts 17 and 18: Neurological Examination," *Nursing 76,* **6**:38–43, June 1976; **6**:50–55, July 1976. These two articles present a method for performing a neurological assessment on a child. The first article gives a brief review of the anatomy of the nervous system and presents assessment of cerebral and cranial nerve function. The second article reviews cerebellar, motor, sensory, and reflex functions; there is a discussion of reflexes during infancy.

Barnard, Kathryn E., and Marcene L. Powell: *Teaching the Mentally Retarded Child: A Family Care Approach,* The C. V. Mosby Company, St. Louis, 1972. This book is directed to the care of handicapped infants and preschoolers who live at home. Child development concepts are presented and used as the rationale for nursing interventions in work with the mentally retarded child and the family. Specific instructions are given for designing a plan for helping the child progress. Although the book is intended for use with retarded children, the same principles are useful in stimulating development in any child.

Chard, Marilyn A., and Candace G. Woelk: "The Mentally Retarded Child and His Family," in G. Scipien et al. (eds.), *Comprehensive Pediatric Nursing,* 2d ed., McGraw-Hill Book Company, New York, 1979. The retarded child is viewed as having the same needs as ordinary children, although at a different rate and chronological age. Nursing for the child and family is discussed for home, community, institution, and general hospital settings.

Clements, Sam D: *"National Project on Minimal Brain Dysfunction in Children: Terminology and Identification,"* Monograph no. 3, Public Health Service Publication no. 1415, U.S. Government Printing Office, Washington, D.C., 1966. A compendium of the characteristics and classification of MBD.

Conway, Barbara Lang: *Pediatric Neurologic Nursing,* The C. V. Mosby Company, St. Louis, 1977. This book was designed as a supplement for nurses who already have beginning knowledge in basic neurologic nursing care. Therefore, little space is given to step-by-step descriptions of nursing management. The first two chapters deal quite extensively with embryology and physiology and provide a good foundation for the neurologic disorders discussed later in the book.

DeLa Cruz, Felix F., Bernard H. Fox, and Richard H. Roberts (eds.): "Minimal Brain Dysfunction," *Annals of the New York Academy of Sciences,* **205**:1–396, February 28, 1973. This is a collection of 35 conference papers covering the broad range of topics related to MBD. One paper focuses on the nurse's role in case finding and intervention.

Ford, Frank R.: *Diseases of the Nervous System in Infancy, Childhood, and Adolescence,* (5th ed.), Charles C Thomas, Springfield, Ill., 1966. This classic text first appeared in 1937 and presents an exhaustive study of abnormalities of the nervous system. The discussions are liberally interspersed with photographs and x-rays to illustrate the disorder under consideration. The author includes a presentation of clinical features, etiology, pathological anatomy, diagnosis, prognosis, and principles of treatment.

Passo, Sherrilyn: "Outcomes of Neurosurgical Care for the Myelomeningocele Child and His Family," *Journal of Neurosurgical Nursing,* **6**(2):122–126, December 1974. This article presents a clinical evaluation tool for the care of children with myelomeningocele and their families. The use of the tool is demonstrated with a newborn whose myelomeningocele has been surgically repaired. Nursing objectives, patient outcomes, and family outcomes are specified by the tool.

Scipien, G., and Marilyn A. Chard: "The Special Senses," in G. Scipien et al. (eds.), *Comprehensive Pediatric Nursing,* 2d ed., McGraw-Hill Book Company, New York, 1979. Embryology, anatomy, and physiology of the eye, the ear, and the sense organs of smell, taste, and touch are summarized. Assessment of children for visual and auditory acuity is presented. The bulk of the chapter is a discussion of specific nursing care for a comprehensive range of childhood eye, ear, and nose problems.

Swaiman, Kenneth F., and Wright, Francis S.: *The Practice of Pediatric Neurology,* vol. I and II, The C. V. Mosby Company, St. Louis, 1975. The book is divided into three sections. Section I places emphasis upon the historical, physical, and laboratory examinations. Section II attempts to develop differential diagnoses based on the chief complaint. This enables the reader to consult the text utilizing the child's signs and symptoms as a guide. Section III is designed to provide the reader with a detailed description of the diseases that affect the nervous system during childhood.

Wender, Paul H.: "Minimal Brain Dysfunction in Children—Diagnosis and Management," *Pediatric Clinics of North America,* **20**(1):187–201, February, 1973. Presents MBD as highly responsive to minimal treatment. Recognizable characteristics of MBD are described (motor, attentional, cognitive, learning, impulsive, interpersonal, emotional, family, and neurological phenomena; and congenital stigmata and psychological test performance). Discusses diagnosis and management. Good bibliography.

20
The Integumentary System

Patricia Harris

The functions of the skin are to give protection against injury, to maintain a barrier between the internal and external environments, to regulate heat, and to serve as a mechanism for the sensory perception of touch, pain, heat, and cold. These functions are developing but immature in the infant and child.

The severity of a dermatologic problem often depends far more on community and family reaction to the child's condition than upon its seriousness as a medical problem.

Certain situations arise with such regularity in the nursing of children with skin disorders that the following generalized approaches are introductory to the rest of the chapter.

1. To facilitate the normality of the child and preserve his or her self-esteem, listen to parents' and child's beliefs concerning the etiology of the skin problem. Supply honest, accurate information about prognosis, communicability, etc. Help the child and others keep the child's skin condition in perspective as one among a great many of his or her qualities.

2. To decrease scratching, divert the child (and teach parents diversion techniques) to age-appropriate activities that require two hands, such as finger painting, water play, block building, model construction, etc. Restrain sparingly (restraints for infants and young children are illustrated later in the chapter), allowing for comfort and thumb-sucking. Children who receive antipruritic medications need periodic evaluation for therapeutic and side effects of the drugs: Is itching under control? Is the child too sleepy to progress with schoolwork, too active to concentrate, etc.?

3. To assist the child and family to complete treatment regimes which are often time-consuming and messy and which may extend over prolonged periods of time, again divert the child's attention to pleasurable, developmentally appropriate activities during treatments. For example, read a story or arrange for the child to hear a favorite record or television show during a 20-min soak. It is very important to allow the child to have as much control over the treatment as possible; e.g., the child may be permitted to choose whether the treatment is to be done before or after mealtime and should be allowed to perform as much of the treatment as is feasible and desired, such as gathering the equipment, running the water, measuring and adding the chemical, etc. Children should be appropriately rewarded and acknowledged for their cooperation and participation, particularly after painful procedures.

GENERAL ASSESSMENT

Assessing the skin is one of the simplest and, at the same time, one of the most revealing parts of the physical assessment. An accurate description of the skin is an important part of the child's health assessment, and changes in the integument are often major clinical indexes of overall health status. Lighting must be adequate, and the child should be completely undressed. A small magnifying glass is an important aid. Palms, soles, scalp, and body folds are important assessment areas that are often overlooked.

Skin lesions are described according to color, elevation, desquamation, weeping, blistering, purulence, size, configuration, etc. Once the lesion is described, its location and distribution add more information and suggest a diagnosis. Some skin disorders, such as seborrhea, acne, and herpes zoster have characteristic patterns.

Laboratory studies often add information which is helpful in making a diagnosis or in evaluating the effectiveness of therapy.

I. Histologic study of chronic lesions is a major diagnostic aid. Skin biopsy is usually an office procedure. It is important to prepare the child for biopsy by explaining what will happen and how it will feel. Explanations should, of course, be geared to the child's developmental level.

II. Bacterial infections require culture of the exudate to determine sensitivity.

III. Suspected fungal infections can be studied in several ways:

A. By use of a potassium hydroxide (KOH) preparation, in which a skin scraping is treated with potassium hydroxide and examined under a microscope for mycelial filaments.

B. By culturing sample in a Sabouraud medium (this procedure requires incubation for 2 weeks at room temperature).

C. Use of dark-field microscopy.

D. A Wood's lamp may identify fungal infection.

IV. Skin testing for allergy may be done for children who have contact dermatitis or atopic dermatitis. Intradermal and patch tests are done using various suspected allergens. The general consensus is that skin testing is not recommended for children under 5 years of age unless symptoms are severe and there is a strong family history of allergies.

History

The history of a skin rash is important, and a detailed family history is also a basic part of the assessment. A history helps the health team sort out those skin problems which are primarily integumentary from those which are secondary to systemic illnesses. The history should list contact with allergens, past skin problems, general health, habits, family history, sports activities, hobbies, clothing, daily routines, and response to stress. Both the family and the child, if old enough, should be interviewed.

Differential Diagnosis

The skin, as a window to the overall health of the child, may reveal many secondary indications of disorders in other body systems. Discussion of such indications is beyond the scope of this chapter but they are treated under the chapter headings of the systemic illnesses. Examples of such secondary skin changes are:

1. Multiple bruising secondary to severe anemia, leukemia, or child abuse.
2. Rashes with fever secondary to common communicable diseases such as chickenpox, scarlet fever, measles, and rubella.
3. Specific skin changes which are associated with conditions such as prune-belly syndrome, Alport's syndrome, and Letterer-Siwe disease.

CONGENITAL SKIN CONDITIONS

Nevi

Nevi (singular: *nevus*) are colloquially called birthmarks, even though not all of them are present at birth. The category nevus generally includes both the vascular nevi and the pigmented nevi, including "moles," but some of the professional literature subsumes only the vascular *or* the pigmentary defects under the term (i.e., there is not uniform usage of the word *nevus*). Nevi are also categorized, particularly the vascular ones, as *involuting* (self-correcting) or *noninvoluting*. Clinical findings are frequently less clear-cut than the following discussion suggests, because two or more histologic types may be mixed in a single nevus. Etiology is unknown, but heredity evidently plays a role.

Vascular
Nevi (1, 2)

DEFINITION

I. Telangiectatic nevi (those consisting principally of capillaries).
   A. Salmon patch (also called erythema nuchae, nevus simplex, and stork bite).
      1. This is a flat, pink to red nevus found on the upper eyelids, nape, lip, or forehead of perhaps 30 to 60 percent of newborns. The color becomes redder when the infant cries, which causes concern to parents.
      2. The marks gradually fade as the child grows older and the skin becomes thicker. The majority disappear during infancy or early childhood.
   B. Spider nevus (also called nevus araneus).
      1. Named for its shape, the spider nevus consists of a tiny flat or very slightly elevated central arteriole with capillaries radiating out from it. Approximately 50 percent of children develop one or more spider nevi, usually during the school-age years and usually on the hands, neck, or face.
      2. They blanch with pressure and refill from the center outward. Many disappear spontaneously, particularly after puberty.
   C. Port-wine nevus (also called nevus flammeus).
      1. This flat, purple-red lesion is composed of a dilated, congested capillary mass under the epidermis. It is always present at birth, blanches only slightly with pressure, and becomes darker with crying.
      2. The port-wine nevus does not involute and does not become larger except to maintain its distribution as the child grows. It frequently involves the face and is sometimes associated with neurologic disorders (for example, the Sturge-Weber syndrome).

II. Angiomatous nevi (those consisting principally of blood vessels larger than capillaries).
   A. Strawberry nevus (also called nevus vasculosis, capillary hemangioma, or hemangioma simplex).
      1. This sharply circumscribed, elevated, red or purplish nevus is not present at birth. It appears, usually during the first month of life, as a red macule, grows for 6 to 8 months and then gradually recedes over a period of months or years. Most disappear entirely without treatment.
      2. The strawberry nevus blanches minimally if at all and may be present on any part of the skin.
   B. Cavernous hemangioma.
      1. This vascular tumor consists of large venous pools and channels and may include arteriovenous shunts. It may be an elevated, circumscribed red mass or, if the deeper tissues of the skin are involved, a poorly circumscribed bluish mass covered by normal skin and causing some distortion of the affected body area. Either type may become more deeply colored and larger with crying.
      2. Cavernous hemangiomas are present at birth. They are usually partially compressible but refill when pressure is removed. These lesions usually do not grow except in proportion to the baby's growth and, after a few months, decrease in size.

ASSESSMENT

I. History.
   A. Determine whether nevus was present or absent at birth.
   B. Note rate of growth or involution.
II. Inspect for:
   A. Size.
   B. Color.
   C. Elevation.
   D. Texture.
   E. Blanching.
   F. Compressibility.
   G. Location.

PROBLEMS

I. Child's appearance may decrease acceptance by family and others.
II. Bleeding, ulceration, and infection are possible with some lesions. (These "complications" accelerate spontaneous involution.)

III. Encroachment into eye orbits, nares, ear pinna, etc. can interfere with their function.

IV. Active medical or surgical intervention is, in almost all cases, to be strongly discouraged.

    A. Active treatment consists of plastic revision, systemic corticosteroids, injection of sclerosing substances, irradiation, or cryotherapy.

    B. Complications, including worsening of the cosmetic defect, are not infrequent and can be severe.

    C. An essential objective in the care of children with nevi that can be expected to involute is to avoid active treatment if at all possible, at least until the nevus has had time to correct itself as much as it will. After this time skilled surgical repair can be quite successful.

GOALS OF CARE

I. The child will be accepted by family and other persons.

II. The child will develop a good self-concept.

III. Bleeding and infection will be absent or minimal.

IV. Family will wait for nevus to achieve maximum spontaneous involution rather than subjecting child unnecessarily to the risks of active treatment.

INTERVENTION

I. Teach parents about the excellent prognosis for involution (except for port-wine mark). A family history may be quite helpful, since family incidence of vascular nevi is common and most of the relatives' nevi will have regressed or disappeared.

    A. Prepare family if nevus is expected to grow before involuting.

    B. Keep accurate measurements or photographs by which the progress of involution of the child's nevus can be gauged and demonstrated.

    C. Teach use of cosmetic covering creams if desired.

    D. Search for misconceptions about etiology which may contribute to guilt or blame.

II. Support child's self-esteem.

III. Teach skin care and protection as necessary to decrease risks of trauma and infection of the nevus.

IV. Refer to physician if indications for active treatment are present:

    A. Alarming growth—nevus doubles or triples in size in less than a month.

    B. Encroachment of organs; for example, eye orbits, nares, or pinna of ear.

    C. Lesions are atypical, with unusual growth patterns.

    D. Considerable cosmetic objections may be a problem after the end of the preschool period.

EVALUATION

I. Is child-parent relationship satisfactory?

II. Are child's social patterns normal for age?

III. Is child's self-esteem adequate?

IV. Are local skin problems (bleeding, infection, ulceration) avoided or adequately treated?

V. Is unnecessary active treatment avoided?

Pigmented Nevi

DEFINITION

Pigmentary lesions are infrequently noted in infants except for Mongolian spots, discussed below. Café au lait spots (flat, tan, or brown irregularly shaped areas in otherwise normal skin) are of no consequence unless they are cosmetically disturbing, or unless they are present in numbers of six or more, in which case they suggest the medical diagnosis of neurofibromatosis (von Recklinghausen's disease), a rare neurological disorder which is not further discussed here.

ASSESSMENT

Mongolian spots are grayish blue areas present at birth in many children, particularly blacks, Orientals, and Mediterraneans. The spots appear as flat, discolored areas resembling bruises, usually in the lumbosacral region but occasionally on the back, shoulders, and extensor surfaces of the arms and legs. They have no relationship to mongolism (Down's syndrome).

PROBLEMS
I. Spots may be mistaken for bruises indicative of nursery accident or abuse.
II. Parents may consider the child defective and somewhat unacceptable.

GOALS OF CARE
I. Teach family that the pigmented areas are of no medical significance, are common in babies, and disappear in a year or so although they may become darker in the early weeks of life.
II. Avoid confusion with bruises.

INTERVENTION
I. Teach as described in "Goals of Care."
II. Distinguish from bruises by absence of other signs of trauma (swelling, abrasion, etc.), history of presence since birth, and characteristic location.

EVALUATION
I. Family members have no misconceptions about the etiology, significance, or prognosis of the spots.
II. Mongolian spots are not mistaken for bruises.

CONTACT DERMATITIS

Diaper
Dermatitis

DEFINITION
Diaper dermatitis is composed of erythematous lesions in the diaper area. It is frequently caused or exacerbated by ammonia formation from urea. Without intervention, the rash spreads throughout the diaper area and progresses from macules and papules to eroded, moist, or crusted lesions. Secondary infection may occur (see also "Moniliasis").

ASSESSMENT
I. Inspect diaper area for presence and type of rash.
II. Obtain history of present skin care methods from parent.

PROBLEMS
I. Diaper dermatitis is not simple to treat because often it has multiple causes.
II. It can be an annoying and embarrassing problem to mothers.
III. Severe excoriation and secondary infection may result.

GOALS OF CARE
I. Prevent serious complications such as stenosis of the urinary meatus and severe secondary skin infection.
II. Teach parents the principles of keeping the area dry, well ventilated, and free of irritating substances.

INTERVENTION
I. Teach parents the following:
A. Diapers must be changed frequently and rubber pants should be avoided.
B. Area must be washed thoroughly with water or with a bland soap and water.
C. Diaper area should be exposed to air during naps.
D. Disposable diapers should not be used. Diapers should be soaked in a solution of borax, or $\frac{1}{4}$ cup vinegar can be added per diaper pail. Wash in hot water and Ivory Snow. Use a double-rinse cycle with $\frac{1}{2}$ cup vinegar in final rinse.
E. Increase fluids, especially cranberry juice.

EVALUATION
I. Can parents properly care for the perineal area and the diapers?

II. Is the baby's perineal area clean, dry, and free of lesions?

Urticaria (Hives)

DEFINITION
Hives are intensely pruritic, erythematous, confluent, raised lesions that are often accompanied by a noticeable swelling of the face. They can appear on face and total body surface, with sudden onset (see Fig. 20-1). Hives are often an allergic reaction.

ASSESSMENT
Obtain history, paying special attention to any new drugs, new foods, inhalants, or insect bites reported.

PROBLEMS
I. Intense itching is present.

II. There is a possibility of anaphylaxis with subsequent exposure to the offending allergen.

GOALS OF CARE
I. Patient will obtain relief from itching.

II. Irritant will be identified and eliminated if possible.

III. Prepare child and family to treat anaphylaxis.

INTERVENTION
I. For mild cases, an antihistamine and cool baths will help.

II. Severe cases should be treated with short-term oral steroids.

III. For severe, intense pruritis, aqueous epinephrine is given subcutaneously with one or two subseqent doses 1 to 2 h later.

IV. Lesions usually fade in 12 to 24 h.

V. For urticaria after insect stings, patient should carry insect sting kit and be referred to allergist for desensitization. Teach child and family how to use the kit.

EVALUATION
I. Itching is relieved and no complications (excoriation, secondary infection) arise.

II. All reasonable precautions are taken to avoid subsequent exposure to offending allergen.

III. Family (and child, if old enough) demonstrate skill in recognizing serious allergic manifestations and in using insect bite kit if anaphylaxis occurs.

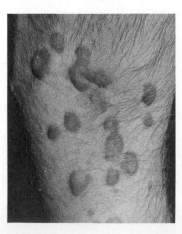

FIGURE 20-1 / Wheals, the lesions of urticaria. Welts are elevated and have pale centers with erythematous margins. Wheals are transient, lasting from a few minutes to a day or so. (*From T. B. Fitzpatrick et al., Dermatology in General Medicine, McGraw-Hill Book Company, New York, 1971.*)

Poison Ivy and Poison Oak

DEFINITION
Linear streaks of vesicles appear where plant touches the skin surface. Lesions first appear as discrete annular papules with mild erythema (see Fig. 20-2). They then become very pruritic with vesicles and weeping. The inflammation usually occurs asymmetrically on exposed body areas such as the face, arms, legs, and trunk.

ASSESSMENT
I. Note the distribution of the rash.
II. Take history, noting especially when the rash appeared and where the child had been playing.

PROBLEMS
I. Itching.
II. Rash tends to spread.
III. Risk of secondary skin infection.

GOALS OF CARE
I. Decrease itching.
II. Prevent spread of rash.
III. Control secondary infection.
IV. Prevent future exposure.

INTERVENTION
I. Teach preventive measures:
   A. Recognize and avoid plant.
   B. Wear long-sleeved shirts and long pants if playing in wooded area.
   C. Wash thoroughly with soap and water after exposure.
II. Soak the affected area for 20 min four times daily in Burow's solution or normal saline.
III. Apply calamine lotion.
IV. Oral antihistamines may be prescribed for pruritis.
V. For severe cases, short, tapered courses of corticosteroids may be needed.

EVALUATION
I. Is child following prescribed treatment?
II. Have itching and rash diminished?

NONINFECTIOUS DERMATITIS

Eczema (Atopic Dermatitis)

DEFINITION
Eczema is a generally symmetrical, reddish, slightly raised, rough-feeling inflammation, beginning as early as the first weeks of life. The lesions often develop weeping crusts. Rubbing against bedding or baby clothes exacerbates lesions (see Fig. 20-3 for characteristic distribution). The stratum corneum of the skin usually sheds, leaving patchy hypopigmentation. The skin then heals, leaving normal pigmentation without scarring. Many children outgrow infantile eczema around two years of age.

Older children have intense itching which is then rubbed or scratched, often leading to secondary infection. In persistent dermatitis, the skin takes on areas of hyperpigmentation as well as areas of paler skin. Lichenification and thickening are also common in older children.

I. Etiology. The cause is unknown. Eczema is often the earliest manifestation of an allergic tendency. The skin is more easily irritated than normal skin. This triggers the itch-scratch cycle which then causes more irritation to the skin.
II. Itch-scratch cycle. Dry, pruritic skin results in scratching, which produces excoriation, eczematization, and secondary infection. The dry skin then changes from discrete

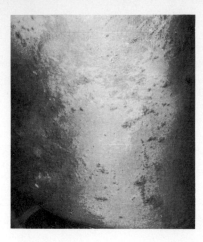

FIGURE 20-2 / Plant-induced contact dermatitis (poison ivy or poison oak). Note the vesicles in linear patches. (*From T. B. Fitzpatrick et al., Dermatology in General Medicine, McGraw-Hill Book Company, New York, 1971.*)

papules to confluent patches with thickening. This cycle presents a difficult management problem.

III. Normal course.
   A. About one person in five demonstrates some form of atopic dermatitis at some time. Eczema in many infants clears up by the age of 2 years. However, many continue to have flare-ups. Some develop asthma or hay fever as older children or adults.
   B. Atopic dermatitis often occurs in children whose parents have allergies, asthma, or atopic dermatitis themselves.

IV. Contributing factors.
   A. During cold winter months when air and skin are dry, extreme temperature changes exacerbate skin lesions and pruritis.
   B. During emotionally stressful times and during boredom, flare-ups often occur. Flare-ups also occur with excessive sweating after exercise.
   C. Eczema may be an allergic response to new foods, perfumes, or soap and drugs. Although the part that diet plays in atopic dermatitis is unclear, some children develop eczema with new foods.
   D. With systemic illnesses, especially viral infections, flare-ups may occur.

ASSESSMENT
   I. Note the distribution of the rash.
   II. Take history, paying particular attention to foods, type of clothing, and any familial history of eczema or allergy.

PROBLEMS
   I. Child is irritable and uncomfortable.
   II. Parents may have difficulty accepting child's appearance and care requirements.
   III. Secondary bacterial infections are common.

GOALS OF CARE
   I. Identify and eliminate possible allergens.
   II. Prevent scratching.
   III. Alleviate pruritis.
   IV. Promote healing.
   V. Prevent secondary infection.
   VI. Provide love, attention, and stimulation.
   VII. Assist parents in accepting and providing for child.

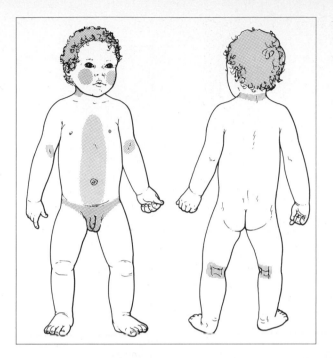

FIGURE 20-3 / Distribution of eczema. Rough, dry, erythematous lesions progress to weeping and crusting.

INTERVENTION
  I. Relief of pruritis.
    A. Antihistamines or, rarely, barbiturates may be given.
    B. Baths may be given using Aveeno or cornstarch.
    C. Elbow restraints, mittens, long pajamas, and/or occlusive dressings are sometimes necessary, especially at night, to prevent further excoriation and secondary infections (see Fig. 20-4).
    D. Trim fingernails.
 II. Topical steroids are applied after compresses during acute phase. Caution must be used due to systemic absorption of steroids, which may lead to fat atrophy, telangiectases, and possible adrenal dysfunction.
III. An elimination diet has been effective for some children. The role of milk allergy is still unclear.
IV. Avoid wool; cotton is preferable. Don't overdress babies. Humidification in the winter is important. A child's bedroom should be as dust-free as possible. Avoid excessive perspiration. Avoid extreme temperature changes. Teachers and other involved persons should be informed that the skin condition is not contagious.
 V. The skin should be cleansed with lotion. Bathing should be infrequent, no more than once a week (this protects natural skin oils when baths are taken). Tepid water should be used with mild soap. After bath, mild lotion should be applied while the skin is damp.
VI. Stress and emotion often aggravate existing atopic dermatitis. Parents often need support to set reasonable limits despite existing skin problems. Encourage parents to hold child, and give stimulation and attention.
VII. Children with atopic dermatitis and their siblings must not receive smallpox vaccination or be exposed to others with herpes infections, chickenpox, or recent smallpox vaccinations.

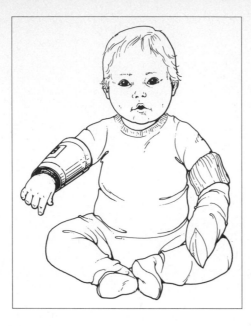

FIGURE 20-4 / A bleach bottle cut into a cylinder and applied over longsleeved pajamas is effective as an elbow restraint to prevent scratching of face, head, trunk, and upper extremities. Mittens may also be quite helpful—adult-size cotton stockings make ideal mittens (avoid wool).

EVALUATION

I. Can the family give return demonstration of care?
II. Does the child have secondary infection?
III. Is the parent-child relationship adequate?
IV. Do the parents cope well with child's condition and care regime?

CASE STUDY

In December, 2-year-old Gregory H. came to the office with his mother and grandmother for his regular checkup. Mrs. H. was very concerned, because Gregory had open, weeping lesions on the popliteal area of both knees, inner aspects of elbows, cheeks, and behind both ears. He had had eczema as a baby, but it now seemed much worse. His mother had been trying to keep the areas clean, but Gregory was constantly scratching, and was awake at night crying and scratching. Both mother and son were exhausted. Gregory had spit up as a baby and had trouble with milk formula. His skin had always been dry, and eczema on his cheeks had been a problem. But never had his skin problems been this bad.

Gregory was put on hydrocortisone cream following Aveeno bath. His mother was advised to discontinue the use of soap. She used a skin cleaning lotion and cotton balls when necessary. Even after Gregory was put on antipruritic medication, itching at night was a severe problem. Several different medications were tried. Mrs. H. trimmed Gregory's fingernails and put socks over his hands at night. She became fatigued and was disappointed with the lack of improvement. But slowly, over 3 weeks, Gregory's rash became manageable. During the day his mother rewarded him when he played with new toys which required both hands, a toy lawnmower and a large, soft beachball. (Two-hand toys decrease scratching.) Gregory continued to need antihistamines for itching, and mittens for 6 weeks, especially at night.

Flare-ups recurred in the next year, especially during the winter. Mrs. H. managed these without frequent office visits by decreased bathing and lubrication with nonperfumed lotion.

Seborrhea

DEFINITION

Seborrhea consists of oily, scaly lesions with yellowish crusts and white particles, beginning on the scalp (called cradle cap in infancy). Distribution usually extends to forehead and eyelids. Seborrhea sometimes is found in the axillae and in the diaper area (see Fig. 20-5). It usually is self-limiting.

ASSESSMENT
I. Note the distribution and appearance of the lesions.
II. Evaluate the scalp care given.

PROBLEMS
I. Seborrhea can lead to secondary bacterial infections if child scratches lesions.
II. Condition progresses without treatment and adequate hygiene.

GOALS OF CARE
I. Keep area clean, dry, and cool.
II. Prevent scratching.

INTERVENTION
I. Explain general principles of well-child hygiene and assure caretaker that bathing the scalp is beneficial.
II. For mild cases, apply baby oil to scalp, then loosen yellowish crusts and white particles with a fine-tooth comb; shampoo biweekly. Generally, once the scalp clears, the forehead and eyebrows do too.
III. More involved cases respond to a tar shampoo (Sebulex) biweekly. Ointments containing sulfur and salicylic acid may be prescribed for use following shampoo.
IV. Loose-fitting mittens may be used to prevent baby from scratching.

EVALUATION
I. Child receives proper hygiene.
II. Lesions do not spread to diaper area or axillae.

FIGURE 20-5 / **Distribution of lesions of seborrhea (intertriginous areas and scalp are primarily affected).**

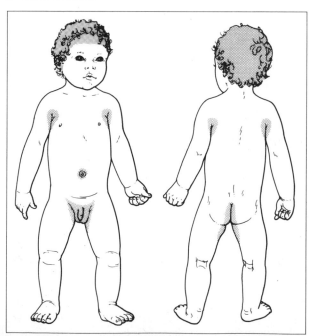

III. Secondary infection is avoided.

IV. Lesions heal.

Miliaria Rubra (Prickly Heat)

DEFINITION

Miliaria rubra is a fine, red, papular rash due to occlusion of the sweat gland pores. The torso, neck, and skin folds are most often affected. This inflammation is caused by hot weather or by being dressed too warmly.

ASSESSMENT

Inspect for characteristic rash, described above.

PROBLEMS

The major problems with prickly heat are discomfort and irritability.

GOALS OF CARE

I. Alleviate discomfort.

II. Clear up the rash.

INTERVENTION

I. Keep baby cool. Dress lightly, and give frequent, cool baths in warm weather.

II. Apply baby powder, cornstarch, or calamine lotion.

EVALUATION

Skin clears, and discomfort is alleviated.

Acne

DEFINITION

Acne is a common, chronic disorder of adolescence and young adulthood characterized by papules, pustules, comedones (blackheads and whiteheads), and in severe cases cystic lesions. Lesions are usually distributed over the face, neck, back, and chest. The precise etiology has not been pinpointed, but it is evident that the hormonal fluctuations of adolescence are one causative factor. Skin hygiene, diet, emotional stress, and a family history of acne are among other etiologic factors that have been implicated.

ASSESSMENT

I. Inspect skin for the characteristic lesions.

II. Obtain history, including possible causes of flare-ups, previous treatment efforts and their degree of success, skin care methods, cosmetic use, etc.

PROBLEMS

I. Painful skin lesions which may lead to scarring, and are considered unsightly.

II. Adjustment problems caused by flawed appearance during adolescence and young adulthood, when social development and self-esteem are extensively influenced by appearance.

GOALS OF CARE

I. Prevent or minimize scarring.

II. Decrease number of lesions.

INTERVENTION

I. Teach patient to manage the treatment plan:

   A. Clean skin with a mild soap once or twice daily (use cleaning pads for midday to accommodate daily schedule). Avoid abrasive soaps.

   B. Use peeling agents such as: benzyl peroxide or retinoic acid cream (increased pigmentation and redness often occur initially).

   C. Sunshine and/or ultraviolet light exposure may be helpful.

   D. A balanced diet, with particular attention to meeting protein and vitamin C requirements, is important.

   E. Discourage manipulation of the lesions and mannerisms such as touching the face or resting the head on the hands.

II. Additional treatment may include steroid injection of lesions (fat atrophy is a potential side effect) or incision and comedo extraction. Tetracycline may be prescribed, in which case a baseline complete blood count and urinalysis are needed and side effects must be watched for. Monilial vaginitis is a common side effect, particularly among young women who are taking birth control pills.

III. Assist the young person in dealing with stress, which often contributes to acne flare-ups. Help patient label feelings, identify alternative courses of action, set reachable goals, communicate with others, and improve peer relationships. The nurse is often instrumental in providing telephone support and overall supervision of the complicated treatment plan.

EVALUATION

I. Is the treatment plan being followed?

II. Is the treatment plan effective?

III. Is the young person coping well and adequately adjusted?

CASE STUDY

Sixteen-year-old Claudia came in for help with the rash on her face and back. She had tried many products available at the drugstore, but had been unsuccessful in clearing up her skin rash. She was discouraged. Her hair was also oily, requiring frequent shampooing. Claudia had frequent family upsets with her mother and brother, which ended in crying. At school she was an honor student. She had two close girlfriends but no boyfriends.

Physical examination revealed a well-developed postpubertal 16-year-old with cystic acne present on her nose, forehead, chin, and shoulders. The blood count and urinalysis were normal. Claudia demonstrated mild adolescent adjustment problems and poor self-esteem, probably related to her skin condition.

Treatment plan:

1. Clean face with benzyl peroxide cleansing pad during school lunch period.
2. Retin A cream was applied.
3. A peeling agent was also used.
4. Tetracycline 250 mg qid was prescribed.
5. Face and shoulders were cleansed twice daily with mild soap.

Diet was discussed. Claudia decided she could substitute a milk shake or milk for her customary carbonated drinks. She also would eat breakfast daily. Claudia agreed to come for office visits every 2 weeks for ongoing management of acne lesions. Also, at her visits she would talk about relationships with others, family functioning, and being an adolescent. Ongoing nursing care consisted of both counseling and management of the treatment plan.

After 2 months, the visits were decreased to one monthly. The tetracycline was decreased to 250 mg daily. Retin A was discontinued. Claudia was able to manage minor flare-ups with cleansing. Residual scarring was minimal.

INFECTIOUS DERMATITIS

Candidiasis (Moniliasis)

DEFINITION

The yeastlike fungus *Candida albicans* (formerly called *Monilia albicans*) is commonly present among the vaginal microorganisms of healthy women and may infect the mouths of infants during birth. Oral lesions (thrush) result and appear as white patches on the tongue, soft palate, and mucous membranes. These lesions resemble milk curds but cannot be rubbed off without revealing reddened areas. Untreated thrush is transmitted through the gastrointestinal tract to produce a severe diaper dermatitis characterized by fiery red, sharply demarcated, raw, moist lesions with peripheral islet lesions, which do not respond to usual methods of treatment for diaper rash (see Fig. 20-6). Older infants can develop *Candida* infections if the organism is transmitted to them by infected persons or if some systemic condition (diabetes mellitus, for example, or disturbance of the normal microorganism ecology following a course of antibiotics) causes overgrowth of *Candida*.

ASSESSMENT

I. Inspect for white lesions in mouth and for the perineal lesions described above.
II. Assess for indications of immunodeficiency (see immune system disorders in Chap. 15).
III. History.
  A. Has infected child or caretaker had diabetes mellitus? (Diabetics are prone to *Candida* infections which can then be transmitted.)
  B. Has patient undergone a recent course of antibiotics?
  C. Has there been known recent exposure to other children or adults with candidiasis? (Thrush is easily transmitted in newborn nurseries or other infant care group settings.)

FIGURE 20-6 / Early monilial diaper rash. Islet lesions at the periphery of the confluent, bright red rash are typical. Note the presence of the rash mainly in the body folds, which distinguishes it from a contact type of diaper dermatitis.

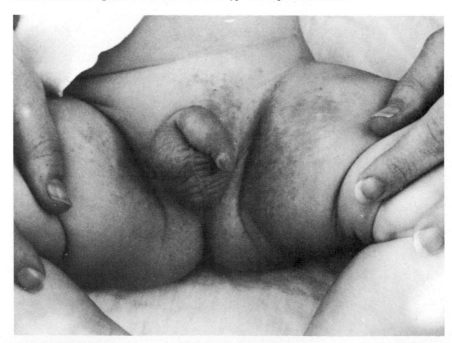

IV. Laboratory studies.
    A. Sabouraud's medium culture (of limited value due to 7- to 10-day wait for results).
    B. Potassium hydroxide preparation.
    C. Wright's stain.

PROBLEMS

I. Oral lesions can interfere with feeding and if untreated lead to further erosion of the oral tissues and very severe diaper dermatitis.
II. Monilial diaper dermatitis is severe and progressive and predisposes to bacterial infection and bacteremia.
III. Breast-feeding mothers of infants with thrush can contract monilial infection of their nipples.
IV. Infection can be transmitted to other persons.

GOALS OF CARE

I. Eliminate lesions.
II. Prevent spread of infection to other persons.

INTERVENTION

I. Nystatin oral suspension is used for oral lesions: nystatin cream or Mycolog cream for diaper area. Very mild cases of oral thrush may respond to $\frac{1}{8}$ tsp baking soda in $\frac{1}{2}$ cup water swabbed on oral lesions after each feeding.
II. Expose diaper area to air; do not use rubber pants or disposable diapers.
III. Wash nipples, pacifier, and toys thoroughly; isolate toys and bottles from other children. Insist on careful handwashing by all caretakers.
IV. The mother breast-feeding an infant with thrush should apply baking soda solution, nystatin, or Mycolog to nipples after each feeding.
V. Treat any underlying disorder such as diabetes, monilial vaginitis of mother, or immune system deficiency of child.
VI. Lesions not responding well to above-named drugs may be treated with gentian violet.

EVALUATION

I. Lesions are successfully treated and eliminated in 1 week.
II. Infection does not spread to other persons.

Impetigo

DEFINITION

Impetigo is an infectious skin disorder caused by streptococci or staphylococci and is characterized by pruritis, vesicles, and pustules which weep and develop thick, yellowish crusts. The initial lesions develop adjacent satellite lesions and spread (see Fig. 20-7). Impetigo follows some interruption in skin integrity, commonly scabies or insect bites that have been scratched. Besides being a progressive, annoying, contagious disorder that predisposes to other bacterial infection and frequently carries some degree of social stigma, impetigo is important because it places the child at risk for acute glomerulonephritis (a sequela of streptococcal infections).

ASSESSMENT

I. Inspect for characteristic lesions.
II. Obtain history, especially of insect bites at locations of lesions.

PROBLEMS

I. Streptococcus infection may lead to glomerulonephritis.
II. Without treatment, lesions spread quickly.
III. Infection spreads easily from one child to another in a classroom or play group.

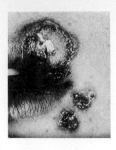

FIGURE 20-7 / Impetigo. Note crusting and developing satellite lesions spreading out from the parent lesion. (*From T. B. Fitzpatrick et al., Dermatology in General Medicine, McGraw-Hill Book Company, New York, 1971.*)

GOALS OF CARE
I. Employ hygienic methods as feasible to prevent impetigo (insect control, skin cleanliness).
II. Treat existing lesions to prevent spread.
III. Monitor for signs of glomerulonephritis (hypertension, hematuria, periorbital edema) which may follow strep infection in 7 to 14 days.

INTERVENTION
I. Culture lesions to identify organism.
II. Treat with appropriate antibiotic. Child may return to school 48 h after oral antibiotic is begun.
III. Cut child's fingernails to discourage scratching.
IV. Clean lesions thoroughly with soap and water and apply bacitracin. Instruct family so they will be able to provide this treatment at home.
V. Antihistamines may be used for itching.
VI. Identify and treat impetigo in siblings or other contacts.
VII. Instruct family to recognize and immediately report signs of glomerulonephritis if streptococcus is the infecting organism (dark urine, puffy eyes).
VIII. Help family explore feasible ways of decreasing risk of recurrence.

EVALUATION
I. Treatment regime is followed, lesions clear up.
II. Spread of infection to others is avoided or controlled.
III. Glomerulonephritis, if it occurs, is promptly recognized and treated.

CASE STUDY
Sixteen-month-old Freddie was brought in with an impetiginous lesion at the base of his nose and another, newer one on his forearm. His older brother also had several lesions on his face where he had scratched mosquito bites open.

A culture was taken. The nurse showed the boys' mother how to cleanse the lesions vigorously with soap and water and apply antibiotic ointment. The mother reported to the outpatient nurse that the lesions were spreading after 2 days. The culture revealed streptococci and staphylococci. Freddie and his brother were then put on an oral antibiotic and antihistamine for pruritis. Their mother cut their fingernails very short and put mittens on both boys at night. One week later the lesions were healing. Urinalysis and blood pressures were done to assess for glomerulonephritis. After 2 weeks, all lesions were gone and there was no scarring. Repeat urinalysis and blood pressure measurement were normal.

Herpes Simplex Type 1

DEFINITION
The herpes simplex type 1 inflammation is caused by the *Herpesvirus hominis*. The incubation period is 3 to 5 days. Vesicular lesions occur on the mucous membranes and skin (but not below the umbilicus). Acute gingivo-stomatitis usually presents with soreness of the mouth and salivation, fever, and malaise, and lasts 1 to 3 weeks. Vesicles break, then

grayish ulcerations form. The gums appear inflamed and swollen, and bleed. The submandibular lymph nodes are enlarged. Factors promoting recurrence are stress, physical trauma, sunlight, and fever. Vesicles and ulcers often recur around vermilion border of lips. Herpes is chronically recurrent throughout life.

ASSESSMENT

An inspection of the lesions reveals a group of vesicles or vesicopapules with the surrounding skin demonstrating edema, tenderness, and erythema.

PROBLEMS

I. Oral lesions and tender regional lymph nodes make child reluctant to eat.
II. It is difficult for child to drink adequate fluids.
III. Virus is transmissible from open lesion.

GOALS OF CARE

I. Assure adequate fluid intake.
II. Control temperature and alleviate discomfort.
III. Promote healing of lesions.
IV. Prevent spread of infection to other persons.

INTERVENTION

I. Relieve pain and fever with acetaminophen.
II. Apply topical anesthetics (viscous lidocaine) to lips and mouth to decrease discomfort and consequently increase fluid intake.
III. Use mouth washes with a tetracycline base to prevent secondary infections.
IV. Soak lesion to remove thick crust.
V. Apply zinc oxide ointment.
VI. Isolate from persons with burns or eczema.

EVALUATION

I. Is child's intake adequate?
II. Is child afebrile and free of pain?
III. Infection does not spread to other persons.

Herpes Zoster (Shingles)

Shingles is a painful infection of the nerve structure. It is caused by the same virus that causes chickenpox. There is vesicular eruption unilaterally along the dermatomes of the infected nerve root, which is thought to be a secondary manifestation of infection by the virus. Herpes zoster often occurs in newborns 2 or 3 weeks of age whose mothers were exposed. Children who are not immune to chickenpox may develop it after exposure to someone with herpes zoster, and adults may develop shingles after contact with a child with chickenpox. *Children receiving corticosteroids or immunosuppressive therapy, e.g., children with rheumatoid arthritis, leukemia, or nephrosis, are highly susceptible to the virus of chickenpox and herpes zoster, and the infection may be fatal for them.*

For additional discussion of herpes zoster, see Chap. 33; chickenpox is presented in Chap. 22.

Slapped Cheek Syndrome (Fifth Disease, Erythema Infectiosum)

DEFINITION

This mild, self-limiting infection is caused by a filtrable virus. The incubation period is 7 to 28 days. It is often confused with atypical measles, drug rashes, and lupus erythematosus, and is most commonly seen in 2- to 12-year-olds.

ASSESSMENT
I. History of course of illness.
   A. Child is active and apparently healthy prior to the appearance of an intensely flushed face.
   B. The infection occurs in two stages.
      1. An erythematous, coalescent maculopapular rash forms on malar prominences— "slapped cheek"—and lasts 1 to 4 days.
      2. One week later, a coalescent, then ribbonlike rash forms on buttocks, thighs, and arms, and on palms and soles. It is frequently pruritic.
II. Associated symptoms include headache, pharyngitis, coryza, and gastrointestinal upsets.

PROBLEMS
After the rash has disappeared, it may reappear days or weeks after the initial infection.

GOALS OF CARE
I. Relieve child's discomfort.   II. Teach parents about course of the infection.

INTERVENTION
I. This condition resolves spontaneously without complications.
II. Both parents and children need to understand that there is no effective method of treating this disease and it must run its course.
III. No isolation is necessary.
IV. Give antipyretics and analgesics as necessary for relief of symptoms.

EVALUATION
I. Do child and parents demonstrate understanding of the illness?
II. Is child comfortable?

Vitiligo

DEFINITION
Patches of skin depigmentation occur with borders of hyperpigmentation. The areas are often symmetrical, and are usually located on the face, chest, wrists, and hands. The cause is unknown, but one form is thought to be genetic.

ASSESSMENT
I. Obtain history of condition.   II. Inspect lesions.

PROBLEMS
I. Appearance of the skin decreases self-esteem.
II. Parents have difficulty accepting this condition, which usually cannot be cured.

GOALS OF CARE
Help child and parents to accept and live with the condition, if repigmentation cannot be achieved.

INTERVENTION
Counsel the parents and child and listen to their concerns.

EVALUATION
I. Are the child's self-esteem and peer relationships satisfactory?
II. Are parents coping adequately?

Hidradenitis Suppurativa

DEFINITION

This is a severe chronic, recurrent bacterial infection of the apocrine sweat glands in the axillae, groin, and intergluteal folds in postpubertal males and females. It is frequently misdiagnosed as furunculosis.

ASSESSMENT

Examine the lesions and obtain history of the course of the disease.

PROBLEMS

I. Occlusion of the apocrine glands results in scarring and sinus drainage.
II. Complete excision of apocrine-bearing sites, including full-thickness grafting, is often required.

GOALS OF CARE

I. Improve hygienic care.   II. Clear up bacterial infection.

INTERVENTION

I. Use antibacterial deodorants.
II. Teach proper cleansing of areas with soap and water.
III. Institute antibiotic therapy.

EVALUATION

I. Has the adolescent improved hygienic habits?   II. Have lesions decreased?

Pityriasis Rosea

DEFINITION

This acute but mild and self-limiting inflammatory disease is probably of viral origin. Involvement is limited to the skin. There are no sequelae.

ASSESSMENT

I. Examine lesions. There usually will be a scaling patch with a raised border, slightly erythematous to tan in color (*herald patch*). The center of the lesion has fine, branny scales. Lesions usually appear on the trunk, upper arms, or thighs.
II. Obtain history, as a slight sore throat or malaise sometimes may precede the lesion.

PROBLEMS

I. Pruritis.   II. Danger of secondary infections.

GOALS OF CARE

I. Reduce pruritis.   II. Prevent secondary infection.

INTERVENTION

I. An antihistamine such as Benadryl is useful to reduce itching. Discourage hot baths as they increase itching. Decreased scratching will decrease danger of secondary infection.
II. Sunlight tends to hasten resolution of the disease.

EVALUATION

I. Has scratching been eliminated?   II. Have lesions disappeared in 2 to 6 weeks?

Tinea Capitis (Ringworm of the Scalp)

DEFINITION

Ringworm of the scalp is caused by several species of fungi. Some (*Microsporum audouini* and *Trichophyton tonsurans*) are human-borne and hence can pass from child to child, and some (*Microsporum canis*) can be contracted from infected cats and dogs. Lesions consist of rounded, slightly reddened, scaly patches of alopecia and broken hair shafts. Boggy, crusted lesions (*kerions*) may also be present. Scalp ringworm is more common in boys than in girls.

ASSESSMENT

I. Inspect for characteristic lesions.

II. Wood's lamp (black light) examination shows fluorescence of infected hair shafts, except when *T. tonsurans* is the infecting agent.

PROBLEMS

I. Clipping the affected hairs and wearing a cotton stocking cap to prevent contagion cause embarrassment and may be seen as a social stigma.

II. Some schools continue to exclude infected children until lesions are completely cleared.

III. The specific medication (oral griseofulvin) has serious potential side effects including leukopenia, gastrointestinal upsets, urticaria, and headaches.

GOALS OF CARE

I. Eradicate the source of infection.

II. Prevent contagion.

III. Treat the infection.

IV. Monitor for side effects.

INTERVENTION

I. Clip hair short around the lesion.

II. Scrub scalp with nonfat synthetic soap every day.

III. Administer a topical antifungal agent as prescribed.

IV. Give oral griseofulvin as prescribed.

V. Inspect pets and treat if infected.

VI. Avoid sharing of hats, combs, brushes, wigs, etc.

VII. Provide school authorities and other involved persons with accurate information about the risk of contagion for the particular fungus involved.

EVALUATION

I. Infection responds to treatment after 3 to 4 weeks.

II. Spread of infection to other persons is avoided.

III. Side effects of drug are detected early and appropriately treated.

IV. Child's self-esteem is maintained.

Tinea Corporis (Body Ringworm, Tinea Circinata)

DEFINITION

Body ringworm is a fungal infection which is usually produced by *Microsporum canis*. It is carried by infected cats and dogs, and produces characteristic lesions, generally on the face, hands, or arms. The lesion is a raised, erythematous, scaly patch which assumes a ringlike shape as it spreads outward and clears up in the center. Mild itching is common.

ASSESSMENT

Inspect for characteristic lesion.

PROBLEMS
I. A secondary bacterial infection may develop.
II. Body ringworm is transmissible to others.
III. Topical antifungal agents may be ineffective or may produce allergy.
IV. Systemic antifungal medication (griseofulvin) may have serious side effects of headache, gastrointestinal upset, leukopenia, and urticaria.

GOALS OF CARE
I. Identify and treat source of infection (household pet, other child).
II. Prevent spread of infection.
III. Treat infection effectively without the development of serious side effects.

INTERVENTION
I. Scrub lesions with soap and water.
II. Administer topical and systemic (oral) medications as prescribed.
III. Treat pets as indicated.
IV. Avoid exchange of clothing between persons without laundering.

EVALUATION
I. Infection clears up in 2 to 3 weeks.
II. Side effects of drugs are detected promptly and adequately treated.
III. Transmission to others is avoided.
IV. Infected pets, siblings, and peers are treated.

Tinea Pedis (Athlete's Foot)

DEFINITION
This familiar fungal infection of the feet (occasionally the hands) is characterized by itching, papules, blisters, scaling, and fissures between the toes or on the soles and sides of the feet. Fungal infections of the nails may be associated. It is most commonly seen in postpubertal males.

ASSESSMENT
Inspect for the presence of the characteristic lesions.

PROBLEMS
I. Itching, discomfort, burning.
II. Transmissibility of infection.
III. Risk of secondary bacterial infection.
IV. High rate of recurrence.

GOALS OF CARE
I. Treat the infection.
II. Avoid spread to other persons.

INTERVENTION
I. Careful adherence to hygienic measures is very important.
   A. Dry thoroughly between toes after bathing or swimming, as moisture encourages fungal growth.
   B. Wear sandals or other well-aerated shoes with absorbent (cotton) socks.
II. Soak with Burow's solution, then apply antifungal agents.
III. Wear rubber or wooden sandals in public showers.

EVALUATION
I. Infection heals in 4 weeks.
II. Spread to others is prevented.

Tinea Cruris (Jock Itch)

DEFINITION
This fungal infection results in raised, annular, erythematous, pruritic lesions of the groin, and occurs almost exclusively in males past puberty. The perineal folds, scrotum, upper thighs, and buttocks (except the anal orifice) may be affected.

ASSESSMENT
Inspect lesions. Rule out intertriginous psoriasis, seborrheic dermatitis, and intertrigo.

PROBLEMS
I. Itching, risk of secondary infection.
II. Secondary atopic dermatitis, which may respond to systemic steroid therapy.
III. Contributing factors in relapses are sweating and \mechanical irritation.

GOALS OF CARE
I. Reduce inflammation.
II. Kill fungus.
III. Prevent recurrence.

INTERVENTION
I. Avoid mechanical irritation from athletic supporters, tight swimsuits, and underwear.
II. Wear absorbent underwear (cotton, not nylon).
III. Burow's solution sitz baths are followed by thorough drying, then prescribed topical antifungal and antiinflammatory agents are applied.
IV. Griseofulvin may be prescribed (see caution about side effects under tinea capitis above).

EVALUATION
I. Lesions respond to treatment in 2 to 3 weeks.
II. Clothing recommendations and careful drying are carried out on a long-term preventive basis.

DERMATITIS DUE TO ARACHNIDS AND INSECTS

Bites and stings of flying insects (mosquitoes, bees, "no-see-ums," blackflies, etc.), fleas, and various arachnids (spiders and mites) are common in childhood. Emergency treatment of venomous bites and stings and anaphylactic responses is presented in the emergency section of this book. Nonacute care of the allergic child is discussed in this chapter under "Urticaria." Other aspects of general care focus on relief of itching by use of cold compresses and calamine lotion, prevention or treatment of bacterial infection secondary to scratching, and institution of reasonable methods of protecting the child from reexposure to the offending insect or arachnid. These include wearing protective clothing; judicious use of insect repellants; avoiding wooded areas and woodpiles known to be infested by scorpions, ticks, spiders, and so forth; and defleaing household pets.

Pediculosis (Phthiriasis)

DEFINITION
Pediculosis, or infestation by lice, is readily transmissible to others by personal contact or by contact with articles that harbor the lice or their eggs (nits). Anyone may contract pediculosis (school epidemics are currently rather common), but infestation is classically associated with poor personal hygiene. Lice are bloodsuckers, and their bites are intensely pruritic. Lice are also transmitters of typhus.

There are three types of louse infestation:

1. *Pediculosis corpus (body lice)*. Nits and lice are found in the clothing, but seldom on the body. The bite produces erythematous macules most commonly seen on the upper back and areas where clothes are tight. Itching is intense and long scratch marks are usually present.
2. *Pediculosis capitis (head lice)*. These lice characteristically are found on the scalp (especially of females) but they sometimes infect beards or pubic hair. The lice themselves are highly mobile and short-lived, and hence are rarely seen.
3. *Pediculosis pubis (crabs)*. Nits and lice are located in the pubic hair and may be seen at the base of the hair shafts. Pruritis is severe. Infestation is transmitted primarily by sexual contact but also by clothing or bedding.

ASSESSMENT

I. Observe for lice or nits. Lice are oval and gray, about 2 to 4 mm long, wingless, and six-legged. Nits are white, oval, translucent, 0.5 mm long, and are firmly attached to the hair shafts near the scalp or to clothing. Nits may superficially resemble dandruff, but they cannot be easily dislodged.
II. Louse bites may produce slate-colored macules which result from the chemical action of the animal's saliva on bilirubin.

PROBLEMS

I. Lice are vectors for typhus and constitute a major public health problem.
II. Intense itching predisposes to secondary infection.

GOALS OF CARE

I. Early diagnosis is essential to control or prevent spread.
II. Prevent secondary bacterial infection.
III. Destroy and remove nits and lice.
IV. Cleanse and sooth irritated skin.

INTERVENTION

I. Have patient bathe, and wash both underclothing and outer clothing.
II. Nits must be manually removed with a fine-tooth comb.
III. Use benzyl benzoate emulsion or benzine hexachloride lotion, cream, or shampoo (Kwell).
IV. Dust personal articles and clothing with DDT after boiling.
V. Use calamine lotion for itching.
VI. All family members should be treated.

EVALUATION

I. Lice are killed, rash clears up.
II. Secondary infections are adequately treated.

Scabies

DEFINITION

Scabies is a rash caused by a tiny crab-shaped mite, *Sarcoptis scabiei*. Transmission of scabies is by direct skin contact and, rarely, by contaminated bedding and undergarments. Pruritis, which is intense, is usually worse at night. The primary lesion is a burrow, made in the skin by the impregnated female mite, in which she lays her eggs.

ASSESSMENT

I. The mite's burrow is a grayish brown, threadlike, often tortuous line or dotted line several millimeters long. It is often difficult to see with the naked eye. Inflammation results in the formation of papules, vesicles, excoriation, and crusting.

II. Lesions are distributed in the interspaces of the fingers, the flexor surfaces of the wrists, the nipples of postpubertal females, the belt line, buttocks, and male genitalia. In children the head, neck, and legs are also commonly involved.

III. Diagnosis is made by opening a burrow with a sewing needle and examining it in mineral oil under low-power magnification or with a hand lens in order to identify the mite.

PROBLEMS

I. Scabies is highly transmissible.

II. Itching is extreme.

III. Secondary infection is common (see "Impetigo").

GOALS OF CARE

I. Early diagnosis is necessary to control or prevent spread.

II. Prevent secondary bacterial infection.

III. Destroy and remove organism.

IV. Clean and sooth irritated skin.

INTERVENTION

I. Patient is bathed thoroughly with soap and water.

II. One percent γ-benzene hexachloride cream or lotion, or 25 percent benzyl benzoate lotion is applied to the entire body at prescribed intervals.

III. Triamcinolone ointment may be prescribed for pruritis.

EVALUATION

I. Lesions respond to treatment in a week or two.

II. Secondary infection is prevented or adequately treated.

III. Spread of infection to others is prevented or minimized; contacts are treated as necessary.

REFERENCES

1. Andrew M. Margileth, "Developmental Vascular Abnormalities," *Pediatric Clinics of North America,* **18**(3): 773–800, August 1971.
2. Joan E. Hodgman, Robert I. Freedman, and Norman E. Levan, "Neonatal Dermatology," *Pediatric Clinics of North America,* **18**(3): 713–756, August 1971.

BIBLIOGRAPHY

Chalker, Dan K., and J. Graham Smith: "Acne Vulgaris: Causes and Preferred Regimens," *Medical Times,* June 1977, pp. 57–62. This article includes explanations and illustrations of treatment regimes and recent bibliography.

Dupont, C. P. A.: *The Management of Skin Diseases,* London, Henry Kimptom Publishers, 1973. Short guidelines and descriptions of treatments.

Dynski-Klein, Martha: *Color Atlas of Pediatrics,* Medical Publishers, Inc., Chicago, 1975. Includes color illustrations of many skin problems.

Fitzpatrick, Thomas B., Kenneth A. Arndt, Wallace H. Clark, Jr., Arthur Z. Eisen, Eugene J. van Scott, and John H. Vaughan: *Dermatology in General Medicine,* McGraw-Hill Book Company, New York, 1971. An in-depth resource on skin disorders.

Hall-Smith, Patrick, Robert J. Cairns, and R. L. B. Beare: *Dermatology,* Grune and Stratton, New York, 1973. Presents a general description of skin problems. A detailed explanation of atopic dermatitis and psoriasis is given.

Hodgman, Joan E., Robert I. Freedman, and Norman E. Levan: "Neonatal Dermatology," *Pediatric Clinics of North America,* **18**(3):713–756, August 1971. Common and exotic skin disorders of the newborn.

Hoole, Axalle J., Robert A. Greenberg, and Glenn C. Pickard, Jr.: *Patient Care Guidelines for Family Nurse Practitioners,* Little, Brown and Company, Boston, 1976. Quick guidelines to medications and treatments of adult and pediatric skin problems. Indexed by disease. No photographs.

Margileth, Andrew M.: "Developmental Vascular Abnormalities," *Pediatric Clinics of North America,* **18**(3):773–800, August 1971. Excellent review of the vascular nevi.

Marvin, Janet A., Inez K. Teefy, and Judith M. Johnson: "The Integumentary System," in Scipien, Gladys M., et al. (eds.): *Comprehensive Pediatric Nursing,* McGraw-Hill Book Company, New York, 1975. Presents the nursing process in detail as it pertains to children with skin disorders.

Pillsbury, Donald M., Walter B. Shelley, and Albert M. Kligman: *A Manual of Cutaneous Medicine,* W. B. Saunders Company, Philadelphia, 1965. Concise, helpful reference on pediatric and adult skin problems.

21

The Musculoskeletal System

Sherrilyn S. Passo

GENERAL ASSESSMENT

I. Health history: Interview parent and child.
   A. Record vital statistics.
      1. Age.
      2. Sex.
      3. Birth date.
   B. Note chief complaint, in child's and parent's own words.
   C. Explore history of present illness.
      1. Note date of onset of symptoms and/or when alteration was recognized.
      2. Pinpoint mechanism and time of injury, and type of first aid; note transport to health care facility.
      3. Describe kind, duration, and degree of symptoms.
      4. Define chronological course of disease, including any therapy.
   D. Note past health history, including:
      1. General health status prior to illness.
      2. Perinatal health—prenatal, birth, neonatal.
      3. Developmental milestones and current status: gross motor, fine motor, social, and language skills.
      4. Diseases.
      5. Hospitalizations, injuries, or transfusions.
      6. Allergies.
      7. Immunizations.
   E. Examine family history, including:
      1. Age and health of parents and siblings.
      2. Heredity—past and present illnesses in extended family members.
      3. Cultural, religious, and socioeconomic background.
      4. Family relationships and availability of family.
      5. Family's perception of child's illness.
   F. Examine patient profile with reference to the following:
      1. Child's perception of illness and body image.
      2. Patterns of independence or dependence: self-help skills, relationships.
      3. Emotional status.
      4. Mechanisms for coping with stress.
      5. School adjustment and work history.
      6. Hobbies or special interests.
      7. Dietary habits.
      8. Sleep habits.
      9. Elimination patterns.
   G. Review systems.
      1. Joints: swelling, pain, heat, redness, stiffness, deformity.
      2. Muscles: soreness, swelling, weakness.
      3. Bones: old fractures, new fractures—deformity, heat, redness.
      4. Movement: a decrease in movement or activity level, or limitation of function (a young child's refusal to move the involved limb may be a sign of pain, which child cannot describe).
      5. Other body systems.

II. Physical examination.
  A. Record vital statistics.
    1. Note vital signs.
    2. Measure height or length, and weight.
       a. Plot on growth chart for comparison with past and future measurements and for relationship between height and weight percentiles.
       b. Note that obesity frequently complicates immobilizing disorders.
       c. A slipped upper femoral epiphysis often occurs in tall, thin teenagers or those who are obese.
  B. Examine other body systems.
  C. Developmental considerations to remember concerning the musculoskeletal system are:
    1. Ossification of the skeleton is not completed until individual is 16 to 20 years of age.
    2. Spinal curvatures normally progress from the infant's C curve to the S curve of the adult (Fig. 21-1).
    3. Normal developmental variations can be present—e.g., slight bowleggedness of the infant or slight knock-knees of the preschooler.
    4. Some abnormalities begin as minor ones in the newborn but progress to major problems if not treated early—e.g., foot and hip deformities.
  D. Conducting the examination.
    1. Begin with a general inspection while watching or playing with the child, then proceed to more specific observations and palpation.
    2. Older children may wear underpants; infants should have diapers removed.
  E. General observations of the musculoskeletal system.
    1. Symmetry of movement: walking, running, sitting, bending, jumping, skipping.

FIGURE 21-1 / Normal spinal curves of the adult (*left*) and infant (*right*). The cervical curve appears at 3 to 4 months of age when the infant begins to hold up its head. The lumbar curve appears later, when the child begins to walk at 12 to 18 months. (*From M. Alexander and M. Brown, Pediatric Physical Diagnosis for Nurses, McGraw-Hill Book Company, New York, 1974.*)

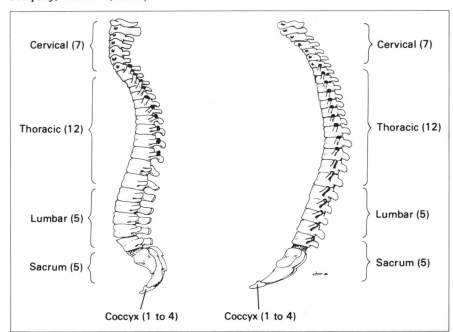

Cervical (7)
Thoracic (12)
Lumbar (5)
Sacrum (5)
Coccyx (1 to 4)

Cervical (7)
Thoracic (12)
Lumbar (5)
Sacrum (5)
Coccyx (1 to 4)

2. General alignment: position, deformities, shortenings, lengthenings, unusual postures.

    a. Growth disturbances, such as limb length discrepancies or torsional deformities, are complications of epiphyseal fractures or avascular necrosis of the epiphyseal plate.

    b. *Genu valgum* (knock-knees) is present if the medial malleoli are more than 1 in apart when the knees are touching (1). This may be normal between 2 and 3½ years of age (Fig. 21-2).

    c. *Genu varum* (bowleggedness) is present when the medial malleoli are touching and the knees are more than 1 in apart (2). This is normal in the infant who has been walking less than 1 year, or it may be caused by rickets (Fig. 21-2).

    d. *Tibial torsion* is a rotational deformity of the tibia. When the knee is facing forward, the foot is rotated inward (internal torsion) or outward (external torsion).

3. Muscles or soft tissues: symmetry, swelling, muscle wasting.

4. Skin: color (redness, cyanosis), bruises, scratches, scars.

  F. Examination of the back and spine.

    1. Alignment of spine. (Spinal curvatures are illustrated in Fig. 21-3.)

        a. *Lordosis* is an increase in the normal inward curvature in the area of the lower back, causing a hollow back deformity. It is a frequent complication of uncorrected congenital dislocated hip and muscular dystrophy.

        b. *Kyphosis* is a fixed flexion deformity of the spine which most often appears in the thoracic spine. *Scheuermann's disease,* or adolescent kyphosis, begins at puberty and progresses until vertebral growth has stopped in the late teens.

        c. *Scoliosis* is a lateral curvature. Refer to the section on scoliosis later in the chapter for observations used in routine scoliosis screening.

FIGURE 21-2 / **Genu varum and genu valgum.** (*From M. Alexander and M. Brown, Pediatric Physical Diagnosis for Nurses, McGraw-Hill Book Company, New York, 1974.*)

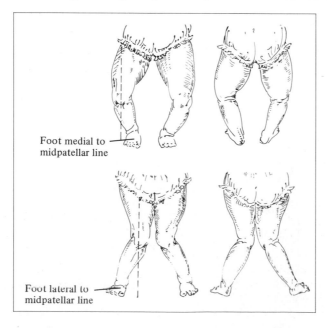

Foot medial to midpatellar line

Foot lateral to midpatellar line

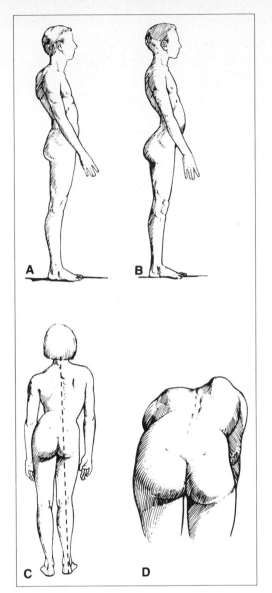

FIGURE 21-3 / Spinal deformities:
(a) kyphosis, (b) lordosis, (c) scoliosis
(standing), (d) scoliosis (bending forward).
[*From G. Scipien et al. (eds.),
Comprehensive Pediatric Nursing, 2d ed.,
McGraw-Hill Book Company, New York,
1979.*]

G. Examination of the extremities.
    1. Note the presence or absence of a part:
        a. *Congenital amputation* involves loss of the distal part of an extremity.
        b. In *dysmelia* the part may be lost proximally or axially.
        c. *Polydactyly* (extra digits) and *syndactyly* (webbing of the fingers or toes) may
            be present in varying degrees.
    2. Skin: lesions, pigmentations, lumps.
    3. Palmar or gluteal creases:
        a. A simian crease in the palm suggests Down's syndrome.
        b. Gluteal creases are often asymmetrical in congenital dislocated hip.
    4. Sensation:
        a. Signs of pressure or damage to nerves include pain, paresthesia, and paralysis.

        b. These signs may result from damage caused by fractures, a tight cast, or excessive traction.

    5. Circulation:

        a. Note pulses, color, features of nail beds (apply pressure, release, note color and circulatory filling of nail beds), temperature, edema.

        b. Signs caused by fracture or by constricting traction or casts include pulselessness, pallor, coldness, puffiness.

    6. Muscle tone and strength:

        a. Have child squeeze examiner's hands, move against resistance by examiner.

        b. Muscle weakness may be secondary to immobilization or to a disease process such as muscular dystrophy.

  H. Examination of the joints.

    1. Explore range of motion, active and passive.

        a. Describe the limits of flexion and extension by the number of degrees at the angle of the joint.

        b. Limited abduction of the hip in an infant is a sign of hip dislocation.

        c. Range of motion is frequently decreased in other conditions affecting the musculoskeletal system.

    2. Position or symmetry.

        a. Observe for foot deformities and other joint deformities.

        b. *Clubfoot* (talipes equinovarus) may be an isolated deformity or may occur secondary to paralysis.

        c. *Metatarsus adductus* is an adduction or varus deformity of the forward part of the foot.

III. Diagnostic tests (x-rays, laboratory data, etc.).

IV. Other data sources:

  A. Past records.   *B.* Referral notes.

CONGENITAL ABNORMALITIES[1]

Torticollis

Definition   *Torticollis* is an abnormality, usually congenital, in which the head is flexed and rotated by a shortening of the sternocleidomastoid muscle on one side of the neck. The etiology is uncertain; however, the defect is seen more frequently following difficult deliveries with abnormal presentations and in primiparas. At birth the degree of deformity is slight, but after a few weeks a large, firm tumor appears in the sternocleidomastoid muscle. The swelling probably results from hypertrophy of fibrous tissue in the muscle. Without treatment, the muscle remains shortened and facial asymmetry gradually develops.

Assessment

  I. Swelling of the sternocleidomastoid muscle in the neck is present.

  II. There is flexion or tilting of the head toward the affected side and rotation or twisting toward the opposite side.

  III. Facial asymmetry exists in the older child.

Problems

  I. Deformity will occur, especially if treatment is not begun early.

  II. Parents are concerned and lack knowledge about the deformity.

  III. A daily exercise program is a necessity.

  IV. The neck may be immobilized as part of the therapy.

  V. There is the possibility of damage to the thoracic duct during surgery.

  VI. There may be recurrence or progression of the deformity.

[1]The following sections are adapted from the author's work, "The Musculoskeletal System," in G. Scipien et al. (eds.), *Comprehensive Pediatric Nursing*, 2d ed., McGraw-Hill Book Company, New York, 1979.

Goals of Care

I. Detect and treat early.
II. Teach parents and older child about deformity and program of therapy.
III. Achieve complete correction or maximal correction of deformity.
IV. Prevent or detect early any recurrence of deformity.

Intervention

I. Preoperative:
  A. Detect deformity and refer for diagnosis and treatment before 1 month of age.
  B. Counsel parents and child, if old enough, about the nature of the deformity and its prognosis.
  C. Teach parents to do daily stretching exercises to correct deformity.
  D. Discuss other simple measures such as moving the child's bed so that he or she must turn away from the affected side.
  E. Prepare child and parents preoperatively when surgery is required.
II. Postoperative:
  A. Maintain cast if applied.
  B. Carry out stretching exercises from the day after surgery if a bulky dressing has been applied.
  C. Inform physician if exercises cannot be done.
  D. Observe for respiratory distress indicating damage to the thoracic duct after surgery on left side of neck.
  E. Teach parents to do postoperative exercises at home or plan for cast care at home.
  F. Arrange for long-term follow-up to check for recurrence of deformity.

Evaluation

I. Parents can maintain home therapy program and cope adequately with daily therapy.
II. Complete correction or maximal correction of deformity is achieved.
III. Recurrence of deformity is prevented or detected early.
IV. Complications and unnecessary stress associated with surgery are absent.

Clubfoot (Talipes Equinovarus)

Definition

Clubfoot is a congenital foot disorder of mixed genetic and environmental etiology. The deformity may be classified as *rigid,* in which the talus bone is abnormal at birth but no primary abnormalities of muscles, tendons, nerves, or blood vessels exist; or *flexible,* in which abnormal bony relationships are present at birth but are not severe. In either type, deformities progress, contractures worsen, and the clubfoot becomes more rigid unless treatment is instituted. Treatment should begin in the first week of life. Casts or splints correct most cases with early treatment; later diagnosis usually requires surgery.

Assessment

I. Routine screening of all newborns is essential to identify abnormal angulations or deformities of the feet.
II. Assess for equinus, adduction, and inversion of the hind part of the foot and adduction and inversion of the forward part of the foot.
III. Examine past health history and family history.

Problems

I. A foot deformity exists, leading to possible delay in weight-bearing or walking.
II. The foot may need to be immobilized in casts or splints.
III. Frequent outpatient visits for cast changes are necessary.
IV. Preoperative preparation for parents is necessary.
V. Provide postoperative care and parent teaching.
VI. The deformity may recur.

Goals of Care

I. Begin treatment before deformities become more rigid.
II. Obtain satisfactory correction of deformity.
III. Stimulate appropriate follow-up by parents.

Intervention

I. Refer for treatment within the first week of life.
II. Explain treatment program and need for follow-up to parents.
III. Discuss care of child in a Denis Browne splint—skin care, application of splint, times to be worn, and use of splint key.
IV. Preoperative preparation of parents will be necessary if surgery is performed.
V. Teach parents about postoperative care.
VI. Teach parents to care for cast at home:
  A. Check circulation, sensation, and skin condition.
  B. Soak off cast in vinegar-water solution if circulation is impaired.

Evaluation

I. Parents understand treatment program.
II. Satisfactory correction of deformity is obtained.
III. Complications of casting or splinting are avoided.
IV. Parents maintain follow-up care.

Congenital Dislocation of the Hip

Definition

Congenital dislocation of the hip is an abnormality of the joint in which the femoral head is completely outside the acetabulum. Less severe forms of congenital hip disease include the *unstable hip,* which is not dislocated but can become subluxed or dislocated upon manipulation, and the *subluxed hip,* in which the femoral head rides on the edge of the acetabulum. The etiology is unknown, but laxity of the ligaments around the hip joint, malposition in utero, and environmental factors after birth have been suspected. If the femoral head remains outside the acetabulum, bony development of the acetabulum becomes progressively abnormal and contractures develop. Therefore, the earlier treatment is begun, the better the prognosis for normal hip function.

Assessment

I. Newborn: Ortolani test.
  A. With the infant supine, the flexed hip is moved into adduction while pressing the femur downward.
  B. A click is elicited as the hip is moved into abduction and becomes located in the acetabulum.
II. Newborn to 3 months (refer to Fig. 21-4):
  A. There is limited abduction of the hip.
  B. The femur appears shortened when infant lies supine with knees and hips flexed.
  C. There are abnormal gluteal and thigh creases (more or deeper creases on the affected side).
III. After 1 year of age:
  A. A ducklike waddle or "sailor's gait" is noticeable.
  B. Trendelenburg's test is positive: When child stands on leg of affected side, pelvis drops on normal side.
IV. All ages:
  A. Past health history is taken.
  B. Family history is reviewed.
  C. Patient profile is assessed.
  D. X-rays are evaluated.

Problems

I. Newborn to 2 months:
  A. Immobilization in Frejka pillow or other abduction splint.
  B. Parents need to understand deformity and treatment.
II. After 2 months of age:
  A. Immobilization in traction or cast.
  B. Preoperative and postoperative needs of child and family.
  C. Possible recurrence, with frequent surgery and hospitalizations.
  D. Potential residual deformity, limp, or hip disease in adult life.

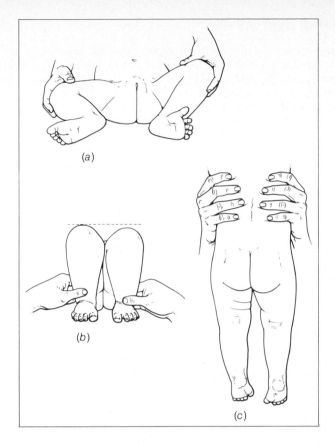

FIGURE 21-4 / **Signs of congenital dislocation of the left hip: (a) limitation of abduction of left hip, (b) apparent displacement of femoral head from the acetabulum and resultant left knee lower than right knee (both soles must be on the same level), and (c) asymmetry of gluteal and thigh folds.** [*Adapted from G. Scipien et al. (eds.), Comprehensive Pediatric Nursing, 2d ed., McGraw-Hill Book Company, New York, 1979.*]

Goals of Care
    I. Hip joint will be normal, or residual deformity will be minimal.
  II. Complications from traction, casts, and surgery will not occur.
 III. Child and family will be assisted in coping with hospitalizations and treatment.
  IV. Developmental activities of child will be maintained.

Intervention
    I. Newborn to 2 months:
      A. Teach parents to apply Frejka pillow or other abduction splint.
      B. Handle infant so that hips remain in abduction.
      C. Discuss modifications in bathing, dressing, and diaper changes with parents.
      D. Discuss appropriate activities for child in splint.
  II. After 2 months of age:
      A. Maintain traction.
        1. Bryant's traction is commonly used in the child under 2 years of age or 30 pounds.
        2. Buttocks should just clear the bed, so that a hand can pass under.
        3. Posey restraint maintains child's position in bed, and bandages encircling the legs and feet should be checked daily and rewrapped as necessary to prevent circulatory complications.

B. Explain purpose of traction and child's activity limits in traction to parents and older child.

C. Preoperative and postoperative explanations for preschooler or older child can include play in which the child applies cast to doll, as shown in Fig. 21-5.

D. Provide care for child in spica cast. Turn child *every 2 h*, check skin and circulation, and prevent cast soilage.

E. Special care is necessary for an incontinent child in a spica cast:

1. A Bradford frame allows urine and feces to drain into a bedpan below. If the child is placed directly on bed, the bed can be raised at the head to promote drainage away from the cast.

2. Petal cast as soon as dry, apply plastic wrap around edges in perineal area, fasten plastic wrap with tape, and change as necessary.

3. A folded diaper or pad is tucked under cast edges and changed frequently. Another diaper is fastened around the cast.

F. Include parents in cast care and discuss modifications for home.

G. Provide age-appropriate activities for child.

Evaluation

I. Hip joint is normal, or there is minimal residual deformity.

II. Parents maintain treatment program and provide follow-up care.

III. Complications of casting or splinting are avoided.

IV. Child is at appropriate developmental level.

FIGURE 21-5 / **Child casting doll as part of preoperative preparation.** [*From G. Scipien et al. (eds.), Comprehensive Pediatric Nursing, 2d ed., McGraw-Hill Book Company, New York, 1979.*]

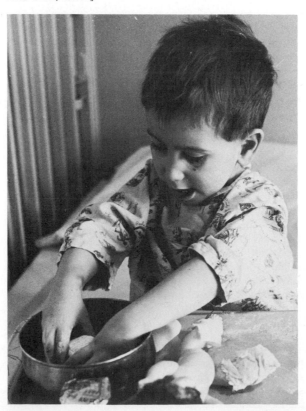

Osteogenesis Imperfecta

Definition

Osteogenesis imperfecta is an autosomal dominant hereditary disorder affecting the connective tissues, particularly the bones. Manifestations of the disease include easily breakable bones, thin skin and sclerae, poor teeth, and hypermobility of the joints. Fractures result in growth deformities including curvature or abnormal angulation of limbs, growth retardation due to injuries to the epiphyses, and kyphosis or scoliosis as a result of compression fractures of the vertebral bodies. Fractures may be associated with little pain, especially if they are incomplete. The disease is classified as the *congenital type,* in which multiple fractures are sustained in utero, or the *tarda type,* which is characterized by the occurrence of fractures later in infancy or during childhood.

Assessment

I. Fractures:
   A. Swelling.
   B. Deformity.
   C. Redness.
   D. Heat.
   E. Pain.
II. Growth deformities:
   A. Torsional deformities of limbs.
   B. Growth retardation.
   C. Kyphosis or scoliosis.
III. Evaluate x-ray results.
IV. Explore past health history and family history.

Problems

I. Frequent fractures and refracturing.
II. Growth deformities.
III. Frequent hospitalizations.
IV. Immobilization in traction or casts.
V. Child's or parents' fears of fractures.
VI. Disruption of schooling and social activities.
VII. Dental caries, breakage, loss of fillings.
VIII. Child's difficulty in becoming independent and responsible.
IX. Genetic recurrence risk.

Goals of Care

I. Prevent fractures or treat them early and completely.
II. Correct secondary growth disturbances if possible.
III. Provide a feeling of safety and security for the child and family.
IV. Maintain schooling and social activities in hospital and home.
V. Maximize child's independence according to abilities.
VI. Prevent or correct dental problems.
VII. Provide genetic counseling.

Intervention

I. Immediate:
   A. Teach patient and family the signs of fractures and early treatment measures, including splinting the fracture site before bringing child to the hospital.
   B. Handle child gently in the hospital to prevent further fractures.
   C. Monitor child's condition in traction or cast.
   D. Maintain traction or provide cast care.
   E. Teach patient and family how to care for the cast at home.
   F. Modify clothing, diapering or toileting, bathing, and feeding activities according to the child's needs.
II. Long-range:
   A. Maintain schooling and social activities while the child is hospitalized and plan with the child and parents for continuing these at home.

B. Provide long-term guidance and support for the child and family as they cope with chronic illness.

C. Discuss realistic activity allowances and limits with child and parents.

D. Plan for preventive and therapeutic dental care; teach proper dental hygiene.

E. Refer parents and older patient for genetic counseling.

Evaluation

I. Fractures from preventable trauma are avoided.

II. Present fracture is corrected satisfactorily.

III. Growth deformities are prevented or treated to achieve maximal correction.

IV. Follow-up orthopedic, pediatric, nursing, and dental care are maintained.

V. Complications of traction and casts are avoided.

VI. School and social activities are maintained to meet the child's developmental needs.

VII. Parents and child are planning realistically for the future, according to the limitations of the disease and the strengths of the child.

Case Study

Joey Sanders, 13, was admitted to the hospital with tenderness, swelling, and deformity of the right thigh. He and his family were aware that these were signs of another fracture, this one resulting from a fall from his wheelchair while roughhousing with his younger brothers. Joey had had over 100 fractures, and he was unhappy about having yet another hospitalization. He was placed in Russell's skin traction. Although school continued in the hospital and Joey met other teenagers on the unit, his behavior was a problem. He often refused meals, although he usually ate special foods when the dietitian could provide what he requested. He was very negative about bathing himself, brushing his teeth, and performing or permitting other aspects of his care and hygiene. His family seldom visited, because of transportation and financial difficulties. The nursing staff was concerned that Joey and his family might be denying the seriousness of his disease and failing to take appropriate actions to prevent fractures.

Goals formulated by the staff in a team conference included: (1) maintaining traction to promote fracture healing, (2) encouraging Joey in his school work, (3) providing opportunities for socializing with peers, (4) providing choices wherever possible in Joey's daily activities, (5) assisting family members in visiting or communicating with Joey more often, and (6) gathering more information about family members' interactions with Joey and their knowledge and attitudes about his disease.

The nursing staff drew up a plan which would provide Joey with as much control over his environment as was feasible. With one of the nurses he planned a daily schedule, including times for school work, recreation, bedmaking, and other activities. Joey was given choices wherever possible. The dietitian continued to discuss his food preferences with him. He related well to a male student nurse, who was interested in him and provided much positive feedback. At least once a day Joey's bed was moved into the recreation room for peer activities. The staff reinforced behavior which was supportive of the care plan objectives. In addition, arrangements were made for Joey to telephone home several times a week, and the social worker arranged assistance with transportation so that the family could visit.

Joey followed the schedule he had devised fairly well. He interacted well with peers and cooperated where his daily care was concerned. As a result of discussions with family members during their visits, the staff found that a pattern of behavior accompanied many of Joey's fractures: He teased his brothers until they became angry and a scuffle ensued. Mr. and Mrs. Sanders were well aware of Joey's susceptibility to fractures but they felt that their approach to the rivalries and hostilities between Joey and his brothers was inadequate. Also, they were not confident that Joey's brothers fully understood his physical problems or that Joey was coping well with his illness. The nurses continued to assess and improve Joey's understanding of and adjustment to his handicap while he remained in the hospital. The social worker worked with the parents and siblings. The outpatient clinic nurse who would continue to see Joey and his family after discharge was informed about the parents' and nurses' concerns and the family situation.

INFLAMMATORY DISORDERS

Osteomyelitis and Septic Arthritis

Definition Osteomyelitis is a bacterial infection of bone; *septic arthritis* is bacterial infection of a joint. Common causative agents are staphylococcus and streptococcus. Proteus and pseudomonas also are frequently the causes of osteomyelitis. Bacteria typically enter the body through skin infections, mucous membrane infections of the nose or throat, or open fractures or other wounds. Bacterial access to the bone or joint may be through the bloodstream or by direct extension from the focus of infection. Infection may spread from septic arthritis to neighboring bone, and vice versa. Traumatized bone seems particularly susceptible to bacteria, especially the metaphysis, which has a sluggish blood flow.

Osteomyelitis most often involves the long bones that are growing rapidly—femur, tibia, humerus, and radius, for example. (Refer to Chap. 31 for more information.) Septic arthritis most often involves the hip joint, with the knee and elbow following in frequency. More than one joint may be affected. Infants and children of 1 or 2 years have the highest incidence of septic arthritis. The inflammation begins in the synovial membrane. Pus forms in the synovial fluid, and the articular cartilage is rapidly destroyed. Osteomyelitis of the underlying bone may follow. Pathologic dislocation and necrosis of the epiphysis and epiphyseal plate can complicate the disease and produce growth disturbances in the affected limb.

Assessment
    I. There is pain in the involved joint or limb.
   II. Child is unwilling to move the limb and guards it against movement.
  III. Patient is irritable and weak.
  IV. There is soft tissue swelling, with redness and heat.
   V. Muscle spasms are present around the joint in septic arthritis.
  VI. Fever is present.
 VII. Child has poor appetite.
VIII. White blood cell count is elevated.
  IX. Wound or aspirate culture and sensitivity.
   X. X-ray (valuable after several days when destruction of bone has taken place).
  XI. Explore past health history.

Problems
  I. Immediate:
    A. Pain.
    B. Decreased mobility or immobility in affected limb.
    C. Fever.
    D. General irritability and weakness.
    E. Lack of appetite.
    F. Difficulty of diagnosis in the infant or young child who cannot describe symptoms accurately.
 II. Long-range:
    A. Restrictions of long-term intravenous therapy.
    B. Boredom, restlessness.
    C. Coping of parent and child with long-term illness and hospitalization.
    D. Potential chronic osteomyelitis.
    E. Potential growth disturbance after septic arthritis.

Goals of Care
   I. Obtain early diagnosis and treatment.
  II. Immobilize affected limb to decrease pain, prevent movement which spreads infection, and prevent contractures in soft tissues.
 III. Maintain child's comfort.
 IV. Maintain long-term intravenous therapy without complications.

V. Provide appropriate developmental stimulation.

VI. Assist parents and child in coping with illness and hospitalization.

VII. Follow up to detect chronic disease or growth disturbance.

Intervention

I. Refer child suspected of having either of these disorders to a physician for immediate diagnosis and treatment.

II. Place child on bed rest and maintain immobilization of limb or joint in traction, splint, or cast.

III. Preoperative and postoperative care following surgery for decompression of the infected bony area or exploration of the joint.

IV. Monitor and maintain system for closed infusion and drainage, if used, including accurate intake and output records.

V. Monitor and protect intravenous line.

VI. Plan for age-appropriate activities, including schooling, play, and group activities; activities can be brought to the child, or patient can be taken to them in bed or wheelchair.

VII. Provide alternative means of mobility for child, such as wheelchair or stretcher, when possible.

VIII. Involve parents in care, explaining illness and therapy program and needs of the child during long-term hospitalization.

IX. Arrange for follow-up appointments and explain importance to parents.

Evaluation

I. Infection is eradicated by early and complete treatment.

II. Child's comfort is maintained throughout course of illness.

III. Complications of therapy are prevented.

IV. Child is at appropriate developmental level.

V. Parents and child cope adequately with long-term illness.

VI. Follow-up is maintained to detect chronic disease or growth disturbance.

Juvenile Rheumatoid Arthritis

Definition

Juvenile rheumatoid arthritis is a childhood disease characterized by inflammation of one or more joints. The peak age of onset is during the preschool years. More girls than boys are affected. The etiology is unknown: Evidence suggests that the primary problem is either a hypersensitivity response in which normal immune mechanisms are exaggerated, or it is a reaction to presently unknown infectious agents.

Rheumatoid arthritis may be classified as *monoarthritis* if one joint is diseased, *oligoarthritis* if a few joints are involved, *polyarthritis* if five or more joints are affected, or *systemic* if other body systems are involved as well as the joints. Arthritis is often symmetrical, involving, for example, *both* knees, or *both* wrists, and often is "migratory"—moving from one joint to another. In an affected joint, inflammation of the synovial membrane leads to edema and cellular proliferation. Granulation tissue infiltrates the synovial membrane, causing swelling. Scar tissue replaces the granulation tissue, causing joint contractures. Secondarily, muscles are affected by inflammation and joint immobility. Other body systems and organs may be affected by inflammation. The clinical course for children with rheumatoid arthritis involves many exacerbations and remissions.

Assessment

I. Peripheral involvement:
   A. Joint swelling.
   B. Limitation of motion.
   C. Limp.
   D. Mild warmth over joint.
   E. Tenderness and pain.

II. Systemic involvement:
   A. Fever.
   B. Rheumatoid rash (salmon-pink, macular rash on chest, thighs, axillae, and upper arms).

      C. Malaise.

      D. Pallor.

      E. Subcutaneous nodules (usually on fingers, toes, wrist, elbow).

      F. Lymphadenopathy.

      G. Liver and spleen enlargement.

      H. Pericarditis.

III. Manifestations as disease progresses:

      A. *Iridocyclitis* (inflammation of the iris and ciliary body).

      B. Joint deformities (subluxation, dislocation, contractures).

      C. Growth disturbances.

IV. Diagnostic tests:

      A. Rheumatoid factor (positive in 15 percent of affected children).

      B. Enzyme and immunologic studies.

V. Explore past health history and family history.

Problems

I. Peripheral signs and symptoms:

      A. Swelling.   *C.* Limp.

      B. Stiffness.   *D.* Pain.

II. Systemic signs and symptoms:

      A. Fever.   *C.* Malaise.

      B. Rash.   *D.* Discomfort.

III. Potential complications:

      A. Iridocyclitis.

      B. Joint deformities.

      C. Growth disturbances.

IV. Parents' and child's uncertainty about the course of the disease.

V. Stress of long-term illness and therapy program.

VI. Disruption of school and social activities during exacerbations of disease.

VII. Potential complications of drugs used in therapy.

Goals of Care

I. Promote comfort.

II. Decrease stiffness and swelling of joints.

III. Control fever.

IV. Maintain adequate developmental stimulation for child during exacerbations.

V. Assist child and parent in understanding disease and treatment program.

VI. Prevent or detect in early stages complications of disease or therapy.

Intervention

I. Immediate:

      A. Be aware of side effects of prescribed drugs (refer to Table 21-1).

      B. Maintain bed rest or immobilize joints with splints during acute, painful exacerbations.

      C. Position the involved joints in extension to prevent stiffness and contractures.

      D. Provide passive range of motion if tolerated during acute, painful episodes.

      E. Reinforce active exercise program as tolerated by patient.

      F. Assist with warm baths or showers to overcome morning stiffness.

      G. Refer to occupational therapy or physical therapy.

      H. Encourage diversional activities which involve movement, when tolerated, and which are directed toward child's developmental level.

II. Long-range:

      A. Discuss disease, its course, and therapy program with child and parents.

      B. Arrange for long-term follow-up and support of child and family during course of disease.

      C. Arrange for medical follow-up of disease.

      D. Arrange for slit-lamp ophthalmologic exam every 6 to 12 months for detection of iridocyclitis.

TABLE 21-1 / DRUGS USED IN TREATMENT OF JUVENILE RHEUMATOID ARTHRITIS

Drug	Specific Action	Route of Administration	Side Effects or Toxicity
Salicylates	Antipyretic, analgesic, anti-inflammatory	PO, IV	Abdominal pain, gastric bleeding (occult blood in stool), hyperventilation in the small child, tinnitus in the older child
Gold	Unknown	IM	Skin rashes, nephritis with hematuria or albuminuria, thrombocytopenia, neurotoxicity
Steroids	Anti-inflammatory	PO, IV, IM, intra-articular	Masking of infection, peptic ulcer, vascular disorders, hypertension, increased intraocular pressure (blurry or dim vision), osteoporosis with pathologic fractures, euphoria or other mental disturbance, glycosuria, weight gain secondary to water retention, appetite stimulation

Source: G. Scipien *et al.* (eds.), *Comprehensive Pediatric Nursing,* 2d ed., McGraw-Hill Book Company, New York, 1979.

Evaluation

    I. Signs and symptoms of disease respond to treatment.
    II. Child is at appropriate developmental level.
    III. Parents and child follow treatment program and seek regular medical follow-up.
    IV. Complications of disease or therapy are prevented or controlled.

MUSCULAR DISORDERS

Duchenne's Muscular Dystrophy

Definition

    Duchenne's muscular dystrophy is a progressive muscle disorder characterized by muscle weakness. It usually becomes manifest during the preschool years but may occur in older children and young adults. The common form is found only in boys and is a sex-linked recessive trait. A second, less common form affects both boys and girls and is inherited as an autosomal recessive trait.

    Because of specific enzyme elevations, a biochemical defect in the muscle tissue is suspected to be the underlying problem. Progressive muscle wasting is accompanied by *pseudohypertrophy,* in which excessive fibrous tissue and fat cause the muscles to appear to grow larger. The disease runs a relentless course without remissions. In the commoner form, few boys survive beyond age 20. Causes of death include respiratory infection, respiratory acidosis, and cardiac complications. In the less common form, the disease progresses more slowly.

Assessment

    I. Early signs:
        A. Leg weakness.
        B. Flat feet.
        C. Stumbling and falling.
        D. Pelvic muscle weakness causing the child to "climb up his legs" with his hands to get up from the floor (*Gowers' sign*).
        E. Pseudohypertrophy of muscles.
    II. Later signs:
        A. Lordosis.
        B. Waddling gait.

      C. Walking on toes.

      D. Scoliosis.

      E. Contractures of the elbows, feet, knees, and hips.

      F. Respiratory infection.

      G. Heart failure.

  III. Diagnostic tests:

      A. Elevated enzyme levels of creatine phosphokinase (CPK).

      B. Abnormal electromyogram (EMG).

      C. Abnormal muscle biopsy.

  IV. Past health history and family history.

Problems

    I. Weakness, and gait and movement disturbances.

   II. Child's fear of falling and fear of needles used in electromyogram and other tests.

  III. Preoperative and postoperative needs of child and family in connection with muscle biopsy.

  IV. Stress of prognosis of progressive disability and death.

   V. Grieving of child and family.

  VI. Parents' needs for information on genetic transmission.

 VII. Architectural barriers in the home and community.

VIII. Need for modification of activities of daily living.

  IX. Spinal deformities (lordosis and scoliosis), and contractures of joints.

   X. Obesity due to inactivity.

  XI. Respiratory and cardiac complications.

 XII. Potential need to institutionalize child who cannot be cared for at home.

XIII. Parents' and siblings' needs for support after patient's death.

Goals of Care

    I. Meet child's safety needs.

   II. Prepare and support child and family with regard to diagnostic tests.

  III. Provide preoperative and postoperative care for child and family.

  IV. Assist child and family in understanding disease and its course.

   V. Support child and family in their grieving.

  VI. Provide information on genetic recurrence.

 VII. Help family with modifications needed in the home which encourage child's independence.

VIII. Encourage compliance with treatment program to delay or prevent complications of disease.

  IX. Support child and family in terminal stage.

Intervention

 I. Diagnostic period:

      A. Provide for child's safety needs, which will be increased due to gait and movement disturbances.

      B. Prepare child for electromyogram according to developmental age, e.g., needle play, or other dramatic play.

      C. Preoperative preparation of child and family is necessary, e.g., dramatic play of surgery, and discussion of postoperative appearance.

      D. Postoperative care around muscle biopsy will include vital signs, bed rest, and observation of wound.

      E. Explain, clarify, and reinforce parents' knowledge of nature of disease, expected course, and how parents can help their child.

      F. Support family in beginning stages of grieving.

      G. Provide information on genetic transmission and/or refer for genetic counseling.

 II. Treatment period:

      A. Refer child to physical therapy, occupational therapy, and social service.

      B. Teach child and family about special treatment measures such as drugs or bracing.

C. Discuss general care needs including activity, diet, and rest.

D. Plan for modifications needed at home to promote child's independence:

    1. Remove architectural barriers.

    2. Modify clothing.

    3. Change daily routines of bathing, dressing, feeding, urinating, and defecating.

    4. Reorganize school, social, and recreational activities, as shown in Fig. 21-6.

E. Teach proper positioning of child in wheelchair to prevent complications such as contractures.

F. Provide long-term support to help child cope with grieving and fears of death.

III. Terminal period:

  A. Support and assist parents in their grieving and decision making about care of the child in terminal stage.

  B. Provide family with an opportunity to discuss feelings and concerns after child's death.

Evaluation

  I. Parents understand nature of illness, prognosis, and genetic recurrence risks.

  II. Child and family cope effectively with diagnostic and surgical procedures.

  III. Parents plan realistically for care of child at home.

  IV. Child functions at his maximal potential throughout course of illness.

  V. Unnecessary complications are prevented.

  VI. Child deals effectively with fears and grief.

  VII. Family able to resolve their grief after child's death.

FIGURE 21-6 / **Fishing is an activity easily adapted for children in wheelchairs.** (*Courtesy of Camp Riley for Physically Handicapped Children, Bradford Woods, James Whitcomb Riley Memorial Association, Indianapolis, Indiana.*)

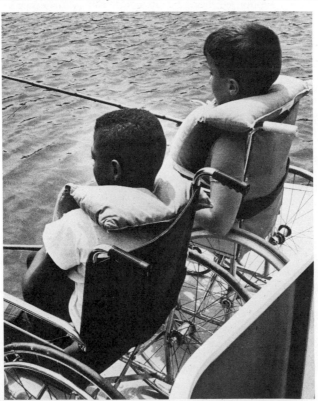

EPIPHYSEAL DISORDERS

Epiphyseal Plate Fracture

Definition The epiphyseal plate lies between the shaft of the bone and its epiphysis. The plate is the part of the bone from which new bone is produced when children grow. The epiphyseal plate can be separated from the bone shaft by trauma, with or without associated bone fracture, as shown in Fig. 21-7. Disruption of the vessels to the epiphysis causes both the epiphysis and the plate to become necrotic (*avascular necrosis*), and growth of the bone ceases.

Assessment
   I. Fracture:
      A. Swelling.
      B. Deformity.
      C. Redness, heat, and pain.
   II. Growth disturbance:
      A. Disturbance is manifested as shortness of the affected limb or an angular deformity.
      B. To measure true leg length, measure from the anterior superior iliac spine to the medial malleolus of the ankle; compare affected and normal leg lengths.
   III. Evaluate x-ray results.
   IV. Explore past health history and family history.

Problems
   I. Signs and symptoms of fracture.
   II. Preoperative and postoperative needs of child and family.
   III. Immobilization in traction or a cast.
   IV. Potential growth disturbance.

Goals of Care
   I. Satisfactorily immobilize reduced fracture.
   II. Assist child and family in coping with hospitalization, surgery, and immobilization.
   III. Detect growth disturbance, if any.

Intervention
   I. Support child and family preoperatively and postoperatively.
   II. Monitor child's condition and care for child in traction or cast.
   III. Teach parents and child about traction and/or cast.
   IV. Prepare parents for home care of child in cast.

FIGURE 21-7 / Common types of epiphyseal plate fracture: (*a*) complete separation of the epiphysis, (*b*) partial separation of the epiphysis and fracture through the metaphysis, and (*c*) fracture across the epiphyseal plate and the metaphysis.

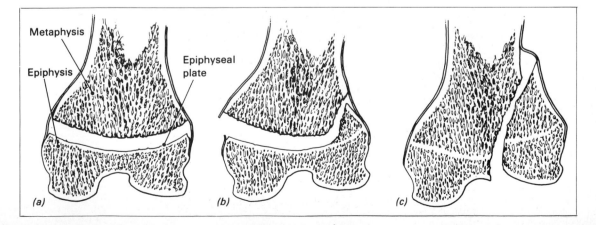

V. Discuss activity limits in hospital and at home.

VI. Reinforce the importance of follow-up appointments to detect growth disturbance.

VII. Monitor child for growth disturbance over a 1-year period or in some cases, longer.

Evaluation

I. Fracture heals adequately.

II. Parents and child are able to care for cast at home and maintain activity within set limits.

III. Follow-up is continued for detection of growth disturbance.

Legg-Perthes Disease

Definition

This is one of a group of disorders called the *osteochondroses,* which share the common pathology of idiopathic avascular necrosis of the epiphysis. The age of onset is usually between 3 and 11 years. Boys are affected four times as frequently as girls. The etiology is unknown, but physical activity or trauma may play a part.

Legg-Perthes disease progresses through four phases. In phase one, there is spontaneous interruption of the blood supply to the upper femoral epiphysis, and epiphyseal cells die. In phase two there is revascularization in the area of dead bone. Pathologic fractures occur because of bone weakness and are associated with pain and limited hip motion. In phase three, healing takes place and new bone replaces the dead bone. In the fourth phase, healing is complete. The hip joint may show residual deformity such as subluxation, flattening of the epiphysis, or limitation of motion. The disease process may be present for 2 to 8 years.

Assessment

I. There is pain in the hip or pain referred to the knee or inner thigh.

II. A protective limp is present.

III. Movement is limited in the hip joint.

IV. Muscles of the upper thigh atrophy from disuse.

V. Evaluate x-ray results.

VI. Explore past health history and family history.

Problems

I. Pain.

II. Limitation of activity.

III. Immobilization by bed rest, traction, or cast.

IV. Stress of long-term immobilization on child and family.

V. Need to modify school and social activities.

VI. Potential residual deformity.

Goals of Care

I. Immobilize joint in early phase to promote healing and prevent complications which lead to residual deformity.

II. Assist child and family in coping with immobilization.

III. Promote appropriate developmental stimulation.

Intervention

I. Refer child with suspicious symptoms for early diagnosis.

II. Maintain child on bed rest, in traction, or in cast during hospitalization.

III. Administer analgesics for relief of pain.

IV. Explain nature of disease and treatment regime to child and family.

V. Provide preoperative and postoperative care for the child and family, if surgery is performed.

VI. Plan for home care of the child in an immobilizing device.

VII. Plan for continuing school and social activities in the hospital and discuss plans for home activities with parents.

VIII. Emphasize importance of following the treatment regime over a long time period to help prevent residual deformity and promote healing.

Evaluation
    I. Appropriate treatment regime is followed by child and family.
    II. Child and family cope adequately with stress of long-term immobilization.
    III. Child is at appropriate developmental and educational level.
    IV. Contour of hip joint allows normal function after resolution of disease.

Slipped Upper Femoral Epiphysis

Definition
    This disorder is a displacement of the femoral head off the neck of the femur. It occurs most often in children aged 10 to 16. The etiology is not known, but hormonal influences and trauma are thought to play a part. Involvement may be unilateral or bilateral. The slippage of the epiphysis downward and backward is most often gradual and leads to a progressive coxa vara deformity of the femoral neck. If separation of the epiphysis from the femur is complete, the blood supply is likely to be interrupted and avascular necrosis of the femoral head is probable. After the epiphyseal plate closes by bony union, slipping can no longer take place, but residual deformity may lead to degenerative hip disease in adulthood.

Assessment
    I. This disorder most commonly occurs in very tall, thin, rapidly growing children, and in obese, inactive children with underdeveloped sexual characteristics.
    II. Early symptoms:
       A. Fatigue after walking or standing.
       B. Mild pain in the hip which may be referred to the knee.
       C. Slight limp.
    III. Later symptoms:
       A. Progressive external rotation deformity in affected limb.
       B. Restriction of movements of internal rotation, flexion, and abduction.
    IV. Evaluate x-ray results.
    V. Explore past health history and family history.

Problems
    I. Pain and fatigue.
    II. Decreased mobility, or immobility.
    III. Preoperative and postoperative needs of child and family.
    IV. Alterations in normal daily activities and schooling.
    V. Obesity and body image disturbance.
    VI. Potential residual deformity in affected limb.
    VII. Potential involvement of opposite, normal hip.

Goals of Care
    I. Immobilize affected limb to prevent further slippage.
    II. Explain nature of the disorder to child and family.
    III. Prepare child and family for surgical reduction of the slip.
    IV. Plan for alterations in home care and activities.
    V. Assist obese child with weight reduction.
    VI. Help patient deal with body image concerns.
    VII. Prevent or minimize residual deformity.
    VIII. Monitor opposite hip for bilateral involvement.

Intervention
    I. Immediate:
       A. Refer to physician at the time signs and symptoms are detected.
       B. Instruct child to avoid unnecessary weight bearing by remaining on bed rest with the affected leg in an internally rotated position.
       C. Maintain traction for further immobilization in hospital.
       D. Prepare patient and family for surgical procedures, including reduction of separation and stabilization of the epiphyseal plate or subtrochanteric osteotomy of the femur to reduce bony deformity.
       E. Care for child in cast and teach patient and family about home care.

F. Provide hospital activities and stimulation according to age-group needs.

G. Clarify child's mobility limits.

II. Long-range:

 A. Plan with child and family for changes in home routines, activities, and schooling.

 B. Begin weight reduction diet for the obese child in the hospital and plan with parents and child for diet at home.

 C. Assist child to accept body image by supportively listening to concerns, correcting misconceptions, and providing additional information about body structure and function.

 D. Arrange follow-up care to detect further slippage or deformity in the affected limb.

 E. Teach patient and parents importance of early reporting of signs and symptoms indicating bilateral involvement.

Evaluation

I. Reduction of slip is obtained and maintained.

II. Child and family are knowledgeable about disorder and treatment regime.

III. Changes are made in home and school activities which are appropriate to child's developmental needs.

IV. Successful weight reduction occurs in obese child.

V. Patient becomes more accepting of own body with a more positive body image.

VI. Residual deformity is prevented or minimized.

VII. Follow-up care is maintained to detect bilateral involvement.

Structural Scoliosis

Definition

Structural scoliosis is lateral curvature of the spine caused by structural changes of the spine. Scoliosis may develop as a result of paralysis, neurofibromatosis, or other disease entity, or it may be idiopathic. Idiopathic scoliosis tends to recur in families. The most common age of onset is early adolescence. Girls are more often affected than boys. The structural features of scoliosis include rotation of the vertebral bodies in the area of the greatest curve. The curvature increases as the child grows, causing secondary changes in the ribs and in the vertebrae, which become wedge-shaped in the middle of the curve from pressure on one side of the epiphyseal plate. In idiopathic scoliosis of adolescence, a right thoracic curve is most common. The prognosis for children with idiopathic scoliosis is best when (1) the curve is mild at the time of diagnosis and initial treatment, and (2) the curve begins at an older age and growth is near completion. Untreated scoliosis leads to degenerative joint disease of the spine in adulthood. Respiration may be compromised and pain may be progressive.

Assessment

I. Scoliosis screening program:

 A. Population—all children in grades 5 through 8 (ages 10 through 13) should be screened yearly.

 B. Setting—physical education class.

 C. Procedure—boys strip to the waist; girls may wear a bra or halter top or a bathing suit. The examiner conducts a simple, systematic examination of each child's back, as described in Table 21-2.

II. Evaluate x-ray results.

III. Explore past health history and family history.

Problems (3)

I. General:

 A. General adolescent concerns.

  1. Body image and bodily changes.

  2. Dependence-independence struggle.

  3. Sexual identity.

 B. Psychosocial needs are complicated by illness.

  1. Lack of knowledge.

TABLE 21-2 / EXAMINATION OF THE BACK: ROUTINE SCOLIOSIS SCREENING

Position of Child	Observations by the Examiner*
1. Standing erect, feet together, arms hanging straight down†	*a.* Shoulder level unequal? *b.* Hip level unequal? *c.* Waistline uneven? *d.* Spine curved? *e.* One shoulder blade more prominent than the other? *f.* Distances between arms and body unequal?
2. Bending forward at the waist, back parallel to floor, feet together, knees unbent, arms hanging freely, palms together‡	*a.* Difference in level between the two sides of the back? *b.* Hump on one side of the upper back? *c.* Compensating hump on the other side of the lower back?

*If findings are positive, there is a possibility of scoliosis.
†Examiner seated, observing child from the rear.
‡Examiner seated, observing child from front and rear.
Source: Adapted from the film, "Scoliosis Screening for Early Detection," Multi Video International, Inc., Minneapolis, 1975.

   2. Fear of pain and the unknown.
   3. Distorted perception of self.
  C. Family lacks knowledge, and suffers from guilt and apprehension.
II. Specific:
  A. Secondary problems related to associated disorders.
   1. Neurologic deficits (paralysis) may develop.
   2. Urologic problems may be present (incontinence, urinary diversion).
   3. Cardiopulmonary compromise may occur secondary to decreased vital capacity.
  B. As patient adjusts to Milwaukee brace (illustrated in Fig. 21-8), there are risks of improper fit, tissue breakdown, or noncompliance with therapy.
  C. With Cotrel traction, which is an inefficient system, the risk of tissue breakdown and fatigue is present.
  D. Discomfort and potential complications accompany the use of halo-femoral traction, another inefficient system:
   1. Skin breakdown.
   2. Footdrop.
   3. Contractures.
   4. Nerve compression causing diminished reflexes.
   5. Organ displacement.
   6. Thrombophlebitis.
   7. Respiratory compromise.
   8. Motor, sensory, and social deprivation.
  E. For patients who have Harrington rod insertion or Dwyer instrumentation and fusion:
   1. Preoperative teaching and preparation are required.
   2. Postoperative immobilization, pain, and potential complications may arise:
    a. Shock.
    b. Urinary retention.
    c. Respiratory compromise.
    d. Skin breakdown.
    e. Wound bleeding or dehiscence.
    f. Neurologic deficits.

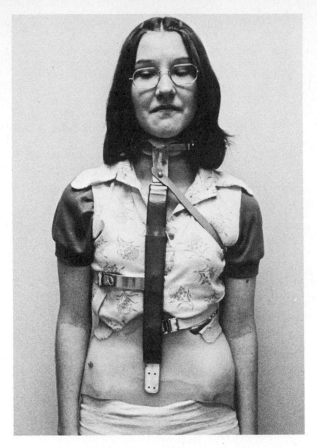

FIGURE 21-8 / Milwaukee brace. Blouse is worn under brace for purpose of photograph only. [*From G. Scipien et al. (eds.), Comprehensive Pediatric Nursing 2d ed., McGraw-Hill Book Company, New York, 1979.*]

       g. Thrombophlebitis.
       h. Superior mesenteric artery syndrome.
       i. Wound infection.
       j. Displacement of rod or hook.
       k. Constipation.
       l. Boredom.
    F. Patients with Risser jacket application experience:
       1. Immobilization.
       2. Potential complications (circulatory compromise, skin breakdown, cast deterioration).
       3. Discomfort.
    G. Alterations needed in home involve mobility, daily living activities, school, and social activities.
    H. Possible scoliosis in other family members must be considered.

Goals of Care
    I. Assist adolescent in dealing with normal age group concerns.
    II. Supply knowledge and feedback to help adolescent cope with psychosocial needs secondary to illness and therapy.
    III. Help family cope with their child's illness.
    IV. Care for secondary problems related to associated disorders.
    V. Assist adolescent in adjustment to Milwaukee brace.

VI. Maximize effectiveness of Cotrel traction.

VII. Monitor halo-femoral traction and prevent or detect complications.

VIII. Provide adequate preoperative teaching and preparation of patient and family.

IX. Provide adequate postoperative care:
- A. Meet needs for comfort, safety, and hygiene.
- B. Prevent or detect complications.
- C. Provide appropriate stimulation.

X. Assist patient in coping with Risser jacket and monitor cast for complications.

XI. Plan with patient and family for home care and follow-up care.

XII. Detect scoliosis in family members.

Intervention (4)

I. General adolescent care:
- A. Provide opportunities for expression of concerns about body image and changes.
- B. Provide privacy.
- C. Facilitate independence but recognize need for dependence.
- D. Provide health education, including sexuality.
- E. Allow for appropriate socialization.

II. Psychosocial needs complicated by illness:
- A. Provide information that supports medical plan prior to initiating plan.
- B. Involve patient in scheduling of activities.
- C. Expose patient to others who have achieved positive outcomes after similar therapy.

III. Family involvement and teaching: Include family in planning and counseling.

IV. Care of secondary problems related to associated disorders:
- A. Develop nursing care plan and interventions for each specific physical deviation.
- B. Evaluate needs for teaching and follow-through care.

V. Milwaukee brace:
- A. Monitor fit of brace; refer to orthotist for adjustments as needed.
- B. Monitor condition of skin; teach patient to remove brace at first signs of skin breakdown and gradually increase wearing time after area is healed.
- C. Assess patient's compliance with program; offer incentives to reinforce compliance.

VI. Cotrel traction:
- A. Monitor traction setup and teach patient proper use.
- B. Assess skin condition; apply lamb's wool to potential pressure areas at pelvis and mandible.
- C. Supervise activity periods in traction and rest periods out of traction.

VII. Halo-femoral traction:
- A. Monitor traction setup.
- B. Monitor patient for complications.
- C. Discuss appropriate activity and movement in traction.
- D. Teach leg exercises: dorsiflexion and plantar flexion of ankle, flexion-extension of knee, quadriceps-setting exercises.
- E. Prevent skin breakdown by preapplication of Betadine shampoo, cleansing of pin sites with hydrogen peroxide and Betadine, and frequent turning and skin care.
- F. Encourage breathing exercises and turn to prevent respiratory compromise.
- G. Provide stimulation through peer interaction, conversation, radio, television, and use of prism glasses in activities.

VIII. Harrington rod insertion or Dwyer instrumentation and fusion:
- A. Preoperatively, instruct patient and family about surgery and postoperative therapy such as logrolling, breathing exercises, and use of fracture bedpan.
- B. Postoperative care:
  1. For immobilization, logroll in bed or use Stryker frame or Circolectric bed.
  2. Keep patient as comfortable as possible and administer analgesics for pain.
  3. Observe for complications by measuring vital signs and intake and output, and by observing wound, skin at pressure points, neurologic function in lower extremities, bladder function, and bowel function.

4. Have patient perform breathing exercises: blow bottles and perhaps intermittent positive pressure breathing machine.
5. Maintain skin integrity by turning every 2 h, give skin care with each turning, and use sheepskin to pad pressure points.
6. Minimize boredom: Establish daily schedule; provide for interactions with peers; arrange activities of interest; resume schooling; and provide prism glasses, bedboard, and easels.

IX. Risser jacket application and care:
A. Prepare patient and accompany during application.
B. Maintain integrity of cast by careful handling when wet, petaling when dry.
C. Observe patient for complications by monitoring circulation, respirations, abdominal distress, and skin condition.
D. Assist patient to develop safe methods for activities and for mobility in cast, if allowed.

X. Alterations needed in home: Plan with patient and family for home care alterations in mobility, activities of daily living, school, and social activities.

XI. Recommend scoliosis screening of family members.

Evaluation

I. Therapy program is effective in preventing curve from progressing, or brings about correction of curve.
II. Patient achieves developmental tasks appropriate for age.
III. Family copes adequately with disease and therapy program.
IV. Associated problems are under control.
V. Patient is free of wound, pulmonary, circulatory, urinary tract, skin, neurologic, and musculoskeletal complications.
VI. Patient and family discuss and demonstrate knowledge and compliance with home care instructions.
VII. Home environment is adapted to patient's needs.
VIII. Follow-up care is arranged.
IX. Family members are screened for scoliosis.

Case Study

When Becky James was 13 years old, her mother noticed that the hemline on her skirts often seemed to be uneven. After a few months, it became noticeable that one shoulder blade was higher than the other. Mrs. James took Becky to her pediatrician, who stated that Becky's spine was curved and she would need to be seen by an orthopedist.

During the next few weeks, Becky's life changed significantly. On her first visit to the orthopedist, the diagnosis of curvature of the spine was confirmed. In a counseling session with the nurse, Becky and her parents were given a booklet to read about scoliosis and the treatment program. Three weeks later, Becky was measured for a Milwaukee brace. After the completed brace was checked for proper fit by the physician, an exercise program for use in and out of the brace was taught to Becky by the physical therapist. The nurse assessed Becky's and her parents' understanding of scoliosis and its treatment as well as their feelings about the changes in their lives.

The nursing plan formulated during this initial treatment period included:

1. Providing general information about scoliosis and the therapy program.
2. Reviewing the schedule for gradually increasing brace wearing time to 23 h per day.
3. Discussing changes in activities and daily living routines made necessary by the brace.
4. Teaching Becky about skin care, clothing which protects her skin, and prompt removal of the brace at the first sign of skin breakdown.
5. Providing anticipatory guidance for returning to school in the brace.
6. Helping Becky and her family recognize and cope with negative feelings toward therapy.
7. Continuing to answer questions, correct misconceptions, and assess level of understanding.
8. Reinforcing behavior which complies with the therapy program.
9. Providing continuous support so that Becky and her family can get help for problems early.

This plan was implemented during early counseling sessions and telephone conversations by the outpatient nurse. Becky and her parents demonstrated adequate knowledge about scoliosis and the program of therapy. Becky tried very hard to wear the brace as prescribed and to do daily exercises. She was motivated by her desire to prevent further curvature and disfigurement, and to please her parents and the outpatient staff. Her adaptation to wearing the brace at home was adequate, partly due to her parents' positive attitude. When a red area appeared over one rib, she removed the brace until the redness disappeared and then gradually began increasing wearing time. Returning to school presented some difficulties in adjustment. Her self-consciousness was made worse when a few classmates made ridiculing remarks. She was unhappy about sitting out of gymnastic exercises during physical education, so she planned with the nurse to spend part of her daily hour out of the brace doing gymnastics.

Becky continued to wear the Milwaukee brace day and night for the next 3 years. Her spinal curvature did not progress, despite Becky's increasing dislike for wearing the brace and refusal to wear it the total required time. The orthopedist determined that Becky could gradually decrease her wearing time, and eventually she wore the brace only at night. Becky felt fortunate to have avoided surgical correction and its resulting back stiffness. As an adult, however, she will need to be observed for progression of her curve, particularly during pregnancy and after age 40.

NEOPLASMS OF BONE

Osteogenic Sarcoma and Ewing's Sarcoma

Definition
Osteogenic sarcoma is a malignant tumor that arises from the osteoblasts (bone-forming cells) in the metaphysis of a long bone. Hence it appears at sites of active epiphyseal growth, especially the distal end of the femur and the proximal end of the tibia and humerus. Children, adolescents, and young adults compose three-fourths of all cases. Males are affected twice as frequently as females. Pain begins intermittently at the tumor site and becomes more intense and continuous. Joint function is reduced. Because this neoplasm is highly vascular, swelling over the tumor site is warm to the touch and overlying veins are dilated. Metastasis to the lungs commonly occurs early in the disease. Pathologic fractures may take place after the bony cortex is eroded. Between 75 and 95 percent of patients die within 5 years.

Ewing's sarcoma is a malignant tumor that arises in the bone marrow. Shafts of the long bones, including the femur, tibia, and humerus are common sites, as are the metatarsals and ileum. The lesion extends longitudinally in the involved bone. Rapidly growing tumor cells soon perforate the cortex of the bone to form a large, palpable, tender soft-tissue mass. Pain at the site becomes increasingly severe. As the central areas of the lesion outgrow their blood supply and degenerate, toxic products enter the bloodstream and cause fever and leukocytosis. Early metastases develop in the lungs, lymph nodes, and other bones. Ewing's sarcoma usually occurs between the ages of 10 and 20 years, but younger children are sometimes affected. The disease is twice as common in males as in females. Ninety-five percent of the children die within a few years.

Assessment
I. Clinical signs:
    A. Pain and swelling at site of tumor.
    B. Limitation of joint function.
    C. Pathologic fractures.
    D. Fever.
II. Diagnostic tests:
    A. X-ray of bone, lungs, and other sites.
    B. Surgical biopsy.
    C. Hematologic tests.
    D. Blood chemistry.
    E. Bone scan.

        F. Bone marrow test.
        G. Urine tests.
        H. Liver function studies.
    III. Assess patient's and family's understanding of possible diagnosis.
    IV. Assess coping mechanisms used by patient and family during stress.
     V. Explore past health history and family history.

Problems

      I. Pain.
     II. Mobility is decreased.
   III. Complications of illness, such as pathologic fracture or fever, may occur.
   IV. The uncertainty of a potentially fatal diagnosis causes stress.
    V. Drugs used in chemotherapy may cause complications (refer to Table 21-3).
   VI. Side effects of radiation therapy, if used, include general malaise, anorexia, skin breakdown, and decreased resistance to infection.
  VII. Amputation may be indicated in selected cases.
 VIII. Grieving process is experienced by child.
   IX. Grieving is experienced by parents and siblings before and after child's death.

Goals of Care

      I. Minimize pain.
     II. Assist child in coping with immobility.
   III. Prepare child and parents for diagnostic tests.
   IV. Detect and treat complications such as pathologic fracture.
    V. Assist child and family in dealing with uncertainty of prognosis.
   VI. Prepare child and parents for each part of therapy program.
  VII. Maintain child in therapy program.
 VIII. Minimize complications of chemotherapy, radiation therapy, or amputation.
   IX. Support child in grieving process.
    X. Support family in grieving before and after child's death.

Intervention

     I. Diagnostic period:
        A. Administer analgesics, decrease movement, and utilize other comfort measures to decrease pain.
        B. Provide alternative means of mobility such as crutches, wheelchair, or stretcher.
        C. Explain to child and parents what will be done during diagnostic tests and when and where tests will be done.
        D. Provide preoperative and postoperative care associated with surgical biopsy.
        E. Detect and treat complications of illness.
        F. Formulate a consistent approach to be used by all team members during diagnostic period.
        G. Clarify what the child and parents have been told and what terms were used.
        H. Be available to listen to misconceptions, concerns, or fears and other feelings regarding diagnosis.
        I. Clarify misconceptions and provide appropriate information about illness and therapy.
    II. Treatment period:
        A. In collaboration with team members, provide overall view of therapy program and specific preparation for chemotherapy, radiation therapy, or amputation.
        B. Chemotherapy:
            1. Monitor patient for drug side effects which are presented in Table 21-3.
            2. Provide nursing measures to control side effects.
              a. Good oral hygiene for oral ulcerations.
              b. Changes in diet for nausea and vomiting.
              c. Stool softeners for constipation.
              d. High fluid intake to prevent kidney toxicity.
              e. Reverse isolation to prevent infections.
        C. Radiation therapy:
            1. Monitor for side effects.

TABLE 21-3 / TOXIC AND SIDE EFFECTS OF DRUGS USED IN TREATMENT OF
OSTEOGENIC SARCOMA AND EWING'S SARCOMA

Drug	Toxic and Side Effects
Adriamycin (doxorubicin hydrochloride)	Myocardial toxicity; bone marrow depression; alopecia; nausea and vomiting, which may be severe; stomatitis and mouth ulcers; extravasation causes severe necrosis at injection site
Cytoxan (cyclophosphamide)	Secondary neoplasm; leukopenia; anorexia, nausea, and vomiting; hemorrhagic cystitis; alopecia
Actinomycin D (Dactinomycin, Cosmegen)	Bone marrow depression; nausea and vomiting; alopecia; injection site extravasation causes induration
Methotrexate	Bone marrow depression; liver disease; mouth, stomach, and intestinal ulceration; rashes; alopecia; nausea and vomiting; nephropathy; chills and fever
Oncovin (vincristine sulfate)	Alopecia; constipation, paralytic ileus; paresthesias; extravasation causes severe local irritation at injection site

2. Provide nursing measures to control side effects.
   a. Rest to counteract lethargy.
   b. Diet changes for anorexia.
   c. Reverse isolation to prevent infections.
D. Amputation:
   1. Give extra support to adolescent already dealing with normal concerns about body changes, body image, and sexual identity.
   2. Provide general nursing care as described in Chap. 31.
E. Provide continuity of care in hospital and outpatient department to support child in grieving process.
F. Support family members through continuity of care and counseling about child's needs.
G. Maintain long-term follow-up to detect recurrence of tumor or metastases.
III. In the period after child's death, provide support for family members to help them continue to resolve grief.

Evaluation

I. Child's comfort is maximized.
II. Child and family understand and cope adequately with diagnostic measures and diagnosis.
III. Illness and its complications are eradicated or controlled by therapy as long as possible.
IV. Child and family understand and cope adequately with therapy program and long-term illness.
V. Complications of chemotherapy, radiation therapy, or amputation are prevented or minimized.
VI. Child and family members move through grieving process adequately.

REFERENCES

1. Mary Alexander and Marie Scott Brown, *Pediatric Physical Diagnosis for Nurses,* McGraw-Hill Book Company, New York, 1974.
2. Ibid.
3. Beverly Anderson and Phyllis D'Ambra, "The Adolescent Patient with Scoliosis: A Nursing Care Standard," *Nursing Clinics of North America,* **11**:699–708, December 1976.
4. Ibid.

BIBLIOGRAPHY

Alexander, Mary, and Marie Scott Brown: *Pediatric Physical Diagnosis for Nurses,* McGraw-Hill Book Company, New York, 1974. Each chapter of this physical assessment book relates to a body system, presenting an anatomical description of the system, guides for assessment, and specific normal and abnormal findings.

Anderson, Beverly, and Phyllis D'Ambra: "The Adolescent Patient with Scoliosis: A Nursing Care Standard," *Nursing Clinics of North America,* **11:**699–708, December 1976. Intended as a guide for identifying nursing problems and establishing plans of care for the adolescent with scoliosis, this article covers the many facets of treatment.

Brewer, Earl: "Juvenile Rheumatoid Arthritis," vol. 6 in A. Schaffer (ed.), *Major Problems in Clinical Pediatrics,* W. B. Saunders Company, Philadelphia, 1970. This book presents information about diagnosis and treatment of the child with juvenile rheumatoid arthritis. Medical management, orthopedic management, and the home treatment program are discussed.

Dubowski, Frances: "Children with Osteogenesis Imperfecta," *Nursing Clinics of North America,* **11:** 709–715, December 1976. Many specific needs and problems of the child with osteogenesis imperfecta are presented, as well as nursing activities to meet those needs.

Keim, Hugo: "Scoliosis," *Clinical Symposia,* **24:**1–32, 1972. Excellent illustrations accompany an overview of the pathophysiology and treatment of scoliosis.

Salter, Robert: *Textbook of Disorders and Injuries of the Musculoskeletal System,* The Williams & Wilkins Company, Baltimore, 1970. An overview of the musculoskeletal system, this book presents pathophysiology and medical treatment of specific disease conditions and relates these to help the student understand broader concepts and relationships within the system.

Scipien, Gladys, et al. (eds.): *Comprehensive Pediatric Nursing,* 2d ed., McGraw-Hill Book Company, New York, 1979. This comprehensive textbook of pediatric nursing presents information about the nursing process; growth and development; the effects of illness; the development, function, and pathophysiology of each body system; nursing care for specific conditions of each system; and future trends in pediatric nursing.

22

Communicable Diseases

Helen L. Farrell

OVERVIEW

Immunity is the body's ability to protect itself against foreign proteins such as bacteria and allergens, and its capability to build up resistance that prevents being infected a second time by some organisms. In response to *antigens* (foreign proteins) the body's immune system produces protective proteins (*antibodies*) which are carried in the plasma and act to destroy the offending antigens. Antigen-antibody reactions include *neutralization, precipitation, agglutination,* and *opsonization,* all of which render the antigen susceptible to phagocytosis by white cells, and *lysis,* in which the antibodies cause rupture and destruction of the invading organism.

Natural immunity is an inborn, species-specific nonsusceptibility to certain infections due to the presence of naturally occurring antibodies. *Acquired immunity* is gained in either of two ways:

1. *Active immunity* results from the body's production of antibodies in response to exposure to the antigen, either by invasion by the organism or by therapeutic introduction of the organism or its antigenic by-products. Substances used to induce active immunity include killed bacteria, attenuated live bacteria, denatured toxins of bacteria, and virus vaccines. Virus vaccines are produced by passing the live virus from one animal to another until the virus is pathogenically harmless but capable of producing an immune response in humans. Dead virus may be used instead, but the reaction induced is slow.
2. *Passive immunity* results from receiving antibodies that have been produced actively by other humans or animals. The fetus's transplacental receipt of antibodies from the pregnant woman is an example of passive immunity, as is injection with immune serum. The advantage of passive immunity is that it is immediate in its response and thus can be used to increase the immunity of an exposed or infected person within minutes. The disadvantage is that passive immunity is temporary.

Infectious childhood diseases have been controlled to a considerable extent since safe and effective vaccines have been developed. However, in spite of the availability of vaccines to virtually eliminate most of the childhood infectious diseases, immunization levels in the late 1970s have dropped to an alarming low. Many, many millions of this nation's children have not been immunized against such diseases as measles, rubella, pertussis, polio, tetanus, and diphtheria, and the possibility of epidemics is ominous. Nurses are in a prime position to educate parents and children about the necessity of being immunized.

Assessment Factors in Well-Child Care

I. Infants whose mothers lack immunity to such diseases as measles, tetanus, and diphtheria are born with no immunity to those infections.
II. Socioeconomic and environmental factors may predispose to infectious diseases.
III. Travel, especially outside the country, increases the risk of some diseases in the unimmunized.

Note Many of the diseases discussed in this chapter must be reported to the state public health authority.

553

Protective Immunizations

I. See Table 22-1 for the recommended schedule of immunizations for healthy infants and children.
II. Table 22-2 presents the recommended schedule for children who for any reason were not immunized in infancy.
III. Figure 22-1 illustrates intramuscular injection sites for infants and children.

DIPHTHERIA

Definition

I. Causative agent: *Corynebacterium diphtheriae.*
II. Epidemiology.
A. Diphtheria usually is seen in late autumn, winter, and spring.
B. It is most common in children from 1 to 5 years of age.
C. The incidence is increasing in older children and adults.
D. Newborns whose mothers have diminished immunity are susceptible.
E. Unimmunized children are susceptible.

TABLE 22-1 / RECOMMENDED SCHEDULE FOR ACTIVE IMMUNIZATION OF NORMAL INFANTS AND CHILDREN

Age	Vaccine/Test
2 months	DTP,[a] TOPV[b]
4 months	DTP, TOPV
6 months	DTP[c]
1 year	Tuberculin test[d]
15 months	Measles, rubella, mumps[e]
1½ years	DTP, TOPV
4–6 years	DTP, TOPV
14–16 years	Td[f] (repeat every 10 years)

[a]DTP = diphtheria and tetanus toxoids combined with pertussis vaccine.
[b]TOPV = trivalent oral poliovirus vaccine. This recommendation is suitable for breastfed as well as bottlefed infants.
[c]A third dose of TOPV is optional but may be given in areas of high endemicity of poliomyelitis.
[d]Frequency of repeated tuberculin tests depends on risk of exposure of the child and on the prevalence of tuberculosis in the population group. For the pediatrician's office or outpatient clinic, an annual or biennial tuberculin test, unless local circumstances clearly indicate otherwise, is appropriate. The initial test should be done at the time of, or preceding, the measles immunization.
[e]May be given at 15 months as measles-rubella or measles-mumps-rubella combined vaccines.
[f]Td = combined tetanus and diphtheria toxoids (adult type) for those more than 6 years of age, in contrast to diphtheria and tetanus (DT) toxoids which contain a larger amount of diphtheria antigen. *Tetanus toxoid at time of injury:* For clean, minor wounds, no booster dose is needed by a fully immunized child unless more than 10 years have elapsed since the last dose. For contaminated wounds, a booster dose should be given if more than 5 years have elapsed since the last dose.
Note: Because the concentration of antigen varies in different products, the manufacturer's package insert should be consulted regarding the volume of individual doses of immunizing agents. Because biological products are of varying stability, the manufacturer's recommendations for optimal storage conditions (e.g., temperature, light) should be carefully followed. Failure to observe these precautions may significantly reduce the potency and effectiveness of the vaccines.
Source: Report of the Committee on Infectious Diseases, 18th ed., American Academy of Pediatrics, Chicago, 1977.

TABLE 22-2 / PRIMARY IMMUNIZATION FOR CHILDREN NOT IMMUNIZED IN EARLY INFANCY*

Under 6 Years of Age	
First visit	DTP, TOPV, tuberculin test
Interval after first visit:	
1 month	Measles,† mumps, rubella
2 months	DTP, TOPV
4 months	DTP, TOPV‡
10–16 months or preschool	DTP, TOPV
Age 14–16 years	Td§ (repeat every 10 years)
6 Years of Age and Over	
First visit	Td,§ TOPV, tuberculin test
Interval after first visit:	
1 month	Measles, mumps, rubella
2 months	Td, TOPV
8–14 months	Td, TOPV
Age 14–16 years	Td (repeat every 10 years)

*Physicians may choose to alter the sequence of these schedules if specific infections are prevalent at the time. For example, measles vaccine might be given on the first visit if an epidemic is underway in the community.
†Measles vaccine is not routinely given before 15 months of age.
‡TOPV optional.
§Td – combined tetanus and diphtheria toxoids (adult type) for those more than 6 years of age, in contrast to diphtheria and tetanus (DT) toxoids which contain a larger amount of diphtheria antigen.
Source: Report of the Committee on Infectious Diseases, 18th ed., American Academy of Pediatrics, Chicago, 1977.

    F. Diphtheria may be seen in crowded areas such as migrant farm camps and city slum areas.

    G. Major sources of infection are the asymptomatic carrier and the individual who is incubating the disease.

III. The incubation period is 2 to 4 days.

IV. Mode of transmission.

    A. Direct contact with an infected person.

    B. Indirect contact with contaminated articles.

V. Treatment.

    A. Diphtheria antitoxin. (*Caution:* Persons must be tested for sensitivity to horse serum prior to administration of antitoxin.)

    B. Antibiotics.

VI. Prognosis.

    A. Mortality is low and may be predicted by:

        1. Virulence of the organism.

        2. Severity and location of the disease.

        3. Immunization status of the client.

        4. Quality of nursing care.

Assessment

I. Manifestations: Determined by location of the disease.

    A. Nasal diphtheria:

        1. Rhinorrhea.

            a. Nasal discharge may be thick and purulent, or serosanguineous.

FIGURE 22-1 / Intramuscular injection sites for infants and children. (*a*) Midanterior muscle of thigh. Injection should be into the middle third of the anterior thigh. (*b*) Midlateral muscle of thigh. Injection should be into the middle third of the lateral thigh, anterior to the femur. (*c*) and (*d*) Two views of the deltoid muscle. Injection site is between the upper and lower portions of the muscle. (*e*) Injection site is the upper outer quadrant of the gluteal area. [*From Gladys M. Scipien et al. (eds.), Comprehensive Pediatric Nursing, McGraw-Hill Book Company, New York, 1975.*]

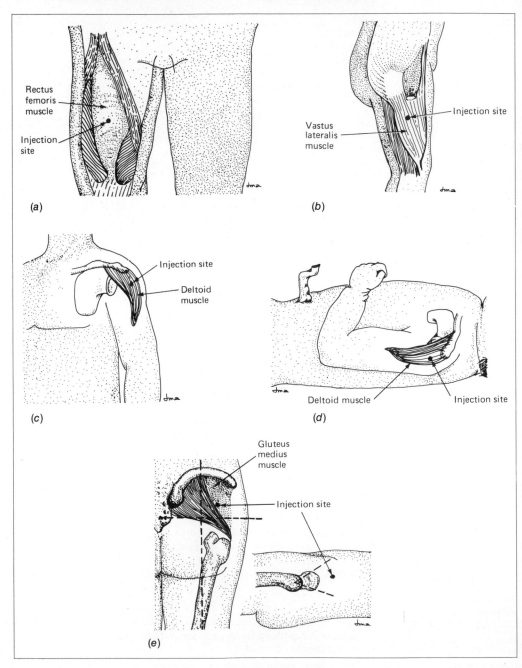

        b. There is a foul odor to discharge.

        c. Discharge may excoriate the upper lip.

    2. Nasal diphtheria accounts for a significant spread of the disease due to its mild signs and symptoms.

    3. A membrane may be present on the nasal septum.

B. Pharyngeal diphtheria:

    1. Sore throat.

    2. Headache.

    3. Malaise.

    4. Low-grade fever.

    5. Rapid pulse which is out of proportion to the fever.

    6. Foul odor to breath.

    7. A membrane forms and may extend to the nose and larynx.

    8. Cervical lymph nodes may be enlarged and tender.

    9. Edema may be present in the neck ("bull neck").

C. Laryngeal diphtheria:

    1. The laryngeal form occurs as a downward extension of pharyngeal diphtheria.

    2. Breathing is noisy and there is progressive stridor.

    3. Patient has harsh cough.

    4. Hoarseness is present.

    5. There are suprasternal and substernal retractions.

    6. Cyanosis occurs as obstruction progresses.

II. Complications.

  A. Pneumonia.

  B. Atelectasis.

  C. Cardiac failure.

  D. Circulatory failure.

  E. Nephritis.

  F. Paralysis of palate, phrenic nerve, and ocular muscles.

  G. Complications account for the greatest cause of mortality and morbidity.

Problems

    I. Communicability of the disease.

   II. Excessive secretions from nose and mouth.

  III. Respiratory distress due to airway obstruction.

  IV. Break in integrity of the skin due to excoriation of upper lip.

   V. Foul odor resulting from secretions.

  VI. Ensuring adequate nourishment and hydration.

 VII. Providing for rest while promoting normal growth and development.

VIII. Maintaining adequate hygiene.

  IX. Anticipating and recognizing complications.

Goals of Care

   I. Maintain patent airway.

  II. Prevent hemorrhage from affected mucous membranes.

 III. Protect from secondary infection.

 IV. Maintain adequate nutrition and fluid balance.

  V. Prevent or minimize complications.

Intervention

I. Place client in isolation.
   A. Teach client and all visitors proper disposal of tissues.
   B. Teach client and/or visitors principles of communicability.
II. Keep airway clear by *gentle* suctioning.
III. Provide ice collar to minimize edema of neck.
IV. Provide warm, moist air to relieve airway spasms and to aid in keeping secretions loose.
V. Apply lubricant to nose and upper lip to prevent excoriation.
VI. Ventilate room, use room deodorant, and dispose of secretions promptly to minimize odor.
VII. Oral hygiene, including the use of cleansing gargles, is necessary for cleanliness and comfort.
VIII. Offer fluids frequently.
IX. Give patient small, frequent meals of a consistency easy to swallow.
X. Maintain bed rest for acutely ill client.
XI. Observe for complications:
   A. Monitor vital signs.
   B. Monitor amount of secretions.
   C. Observe for presence of edema.
   D. Observe for regurgitation through the nose.
   E. Be alert for evidence of palatal paralysis.
XII. Notify physician immediately of signs of respiratory distress or other complications.

Evaluation

I. Respiratory distress is minimized.
II. There is no excoriation of nose or upper lip due to excessive secretion.
III. Adequate nutrition and fluid balance are maintained.

TETANUS

Definition

I. Causative agent: *Clostridium tetani*.
II. Epidemiology.
   A. Incidence is greatest in months of outdoor activity.
   B. In the United States, the incidence is higher in the Southeast and among male children.
   C. Tetanus most frequently is seen in:
      1. Unimmunized persons.
      2. Newborn infants of unimmunized mothers.
III. Incubation period.
   A. 5 to 20 days.
   B. Average of 10 days.
IV. Mode of transmission.
   A. Tetanus organism is introduced into the body during an injury.
      1. Puncture wounds, burns, and insect bites are the most frequent types of injuries by which the organism enters the body.
      2. The wound may be so slight as to go unnoticed.
   B. The organism is found in soil, water, and the intestinal tract of man and animals.

    C. For tetanus to develop there must be:
        1. Contact with the organism.
        2. Anaerobic wound conditions.
        3. A susceptible host.
V. Treatment.
    A. Administer tetanus antitoxin, but only after skin testing shows no hypersensitivity to serum.
    B. Administer antibiotics.
    C. Surgery to remove necrotic tissue may be necessary.
    D. Control muscle spasm.
    E. Tetanus immune globulin may be given.
VI. Prognosis.
    A. In the unimmunized person the fatality rate varies from 35 to 90 percent.
    B. Prognosis is related to:
        1. The age of the client (it is poorest in newborns).
        2. The number of days required for symptoms to appear (poorest with short incubation period).
        3. Extent of muscle involvement.
        4. Height of fever—prognosis is poor if fever exceeds 38.9°C (102°F).

Assessment

  I. Manifestations.
    A. Neck and jaw muscles are stiff.
    B. Spasms of masseters result in difficulty in opening the mouth and swallowing (lockjaw).
    C. Patient experiences headache and restlessness.
    D. Spasms of other muscle groups occur as the disease progresses.
    E. Opisthotonus (extension spasm of trunk and neck) develops.
    F. Abdominal rigidity is present.
    G. Patient experiences apprehension.
  II. Complications: the types of complications depend upon the quality of nursing care and the age of the client. They include:
    A. Pneumonia.
    B. Atelectasis.
    C. Pneumothorax.
    D. Mediastinal emphysema.
    E. Oral lacerations.
    F. Intramuscular hematomas.
    G. Fractures of the thoracic vertebrae.
    H. Malnutrition.
    I. Fluid and electrolyte imbalance.

Problems

    I. Severe seizures can occur.
   II. Pulmonary complications may develop.
  III. Seizures are precipitated by the slightest stimuli.
  IV. Excessive secretions may result from inability to swallow.
    V. Dehydration and malnutrition may result from an inability to take foods and fluids orally.
  VI. Skin excoriation may occur due to incontinence of urine and feces.
 VII. The client may experience extreme anxiety since sensorium is usually clear.

Goals of Care

I. Maintain airway.
II. Prevent seizures.
III. Protect client from injury.
IV. Prevent or minimize complications.

Intervention

I. Remain with the client constantly since a life-threatening seizure may develop.
II. Keep room quiet and avoid any unnecessary stimuli: vocal, tactile, or auditory.
III. Administer sedatives as prescribed to prevent seizures. If sedation is sufficient to render the client unconscious, nursing intervention is the same as for any unconscious person:

A. Turn frequently.
B. Maintain body alignment.
C. Maintain patent airway.
D. Monitor vital signs.
E. Monitor intake and output.
F. Provide meticulous skin care.
G. Perform oral hygiene measures.
H. Perform passive exercise for range of motion.
I. Provide food and fluid by gavage.

IV. Nasopharyngeal suctioning of airway is necessary.
V. Give tube feedings for those who are unable to swallow.
VI. Keep intake and output record.
VII. Monitor parenteral fluids.
VIII. Maintain a weight record if possible.
IX. Explain each procedure to client to allay apprehension.

Evaluation

I. External stimuli are reduced with resultant lessening of muscle spasm or convulsion.
II. Client does not develop muscle contractures, fractures, or intramuscular hematomas.
III. Full range of motion in all joints is maintained.
IV. Airway remains patent.
V. Patient remains hydrated and maintains normal electrolytes.
VI. There is no weight loss.
VII. Skin remains intact.
VIII. Apprehension expressed by client is minimal.

PERTUSSIS (WHOOPING COUGH)

Definition

I. Causative agent: *Bordetella pertussis.*
II. Epidemiology.

A. Pertussis is very contagious for unimmunized persons.
B. Adults are frequently susceptible since immunization during childhood does not produce lifelong immunity.
C. Infants born of mothers with a low immunity level are especially susceptible.
D. There is less seasonal variation than with other respiratory diseases.
E. There is a high incidence of the disease in developing countries.

III. The incubation period is 7 to 14 days.

IV. Mode of transmission.

    A. Direct contact with discharges from the laryngeal and bronchial mucous membrane of infected persons.

    B. May be contracted through indirect contact with contaminated articles.

V. Treatment.

    A. Antibiotics eliminate the organism but do not shorten the paroxysmal phase of the disease.

    B. Supportive nursing care is essential

    C. Complications are treated with specific forms of intervention.

VI. Prognosis: The mortality rate is as high as 40 percent for infants under 5 months of age.

Assessment

I. Manifestations: Pertussis occurs in three stages and has a combined duration of several weeks.

    A. Catarrhal stage:

        1. Low-grade fever:

        2. Rhinorrhea.

        3. Cough.

    B. Paroxysmal stage:

        1. A strangling cough develops with a characteristic whoop upon inspiration.

        2. Cough is accompanied by:

            a. Facial redness or cyanosis.

            b. Bulging eyes.

            c. Protruding tongue.

            d. Anxiety.

        3. Thick mucus is discharged from the nose and mouth.

        4. Sweating and exhaustion occur with coughing attack.

        5. Vomiting often follows coughing attack.

    C. Convalescent stage:

        1. Whooping diminishes and cough becomes less severe and occurs less often.

        2. Vomiting diminishes in relation to diminished coughing episodes.

II. Complications.

    A. Pulmonary infection.

    B. Otitis media.

    C. Atelectasis.

    D. Convulsions in infants are due to periods of anoxia during coughing episodes.

    E. Subconjunctival hemorrhage.

    F. Nutritional disturbance.

    G. Electrolyte imbalance.

Problems

I. Pertussis is highly contagious.

II. Tenacious mucus may cause excoriation of skin around nose and mouth.

III. Paroxysms of coughing may produce anoxia and convulsions.

IV. Airway may become obstructed due to excessive, thick mucus.

V. Vomiting may result in weight loss and electrolyte disturbances.

Goals of Care

I. Minimize paroxysms of coughing.

II. Maintain airway.

III. Prevent or minimize complications.
IV. Maintain adequate nutrition and fluid balance.
V. Reduce anxiety.

Intervention

I. Isolate client due to communicability of disease.
II. Provide quiet environment since sudden noise and excitement may precipitate paroxysms of coughing.
III. Maintain humidified environment to liquefy secretions.
IV. Maintain airway by suctioning as necessary.
V. Administer oxygen for cyanosis.
VI. Protect child from injury if convulsions develop.
VII. Provide small, frequent meals.
VIII. If vomiting occurs due to coughing, refeed immediately.
IX. Offer fluids frequently to keep client hydrated and to aid in liquefying secretions.
X. Observe for episodes of apnea, especially in the young infant.
XI. Remain with child to allay anxiety during coughing episodes.

Evaluation

I. Paroxysms of coughing are infrequent.
II. Secretions are easily expectorated.
III. There are no episodes of cyanosis or apnea.
IV. Client maintains normal weight and normal fluid balance.
V. A minimal degree of apprehension is expressed during paroxysms of coughing.

RUBEOLA (MEASLES)

Definition

I. Causative agent: measles virus.
II. Epidemiology.
   A. Occurrence is worldwide.
   B. Epidemics were seen about every 2 to 4 years prior to the introduction of measles vaccine.
   C. Seen most often in unimmunized children.
   D. Infants of susceptible mothers have no immunity at birth.
   E. Infants of immunized mothers acquire immunity passively from their mothers which lasts about 6 months.
III. The incubation period is about 10 days from exposure to the initial fever, or about 2 weeks until rash appears.
IV. Mode of transmission.
   A. Direct contact with droplets from an infected person.
   B. May be spread by means of contaminated articles, but this is rare.
V. Treatment.
   A. Sedatives.
   B. Antipyretics to control fever.
   C. Lotion for skin irritation.
   D. Bed rest.
   E. Humidification of room.
   F. Antibiotics for treatment of complications.
VI. Prognosis.
   A. Prognosis is affected by age (poorest in infants and older adults) and the severity of symptoms.
   B. Fatality rates have declined in the United States because of improved socioeconomic conditions and the use of antibiotics to treat complications.

Assessment

I. Manifestations: Measles is characterized by three stages:
   A. Incubation stage, which has few if any symptoms.
   B. Prodromal stage.
      1. Low-grade fever.
      2. Slight cough.
      3. Coryza and conjunctivitis.
      4. Koplik's spots.
         a. Koplik's spots appear on buccal mucosa as grayish white dots with a reddish areola.
         b. They appear during the prodromal stage and disappear within 2 days.
         c. They tend to occur opposite the lower molars and may spread irregularly over rest of buccal mucosa.
      5. Photophobia.
   C. Rash stage.
      1. A fever of 40 to 40.5°C (104 to 105°F) is common.
      2. The rash develops as faint macules on the upper lateral parts of the neck, along the hairline, and on the preauricular part of the cheeks.
      3. The rash then spreads rapidly over the face, upper arms, and chest. Finally, the rash appears on the back, abdomen, legs, and feet.
      4. The rash fades in the direction in which it appeared and begins to fade on the face as it reaches the feet.
      5. A fading rash may produce temporary brownish discoloration of the skin.
II. Complications.
   A. Otitis media.
   B. Pneumonia caused by the measles virus itself.
   C. Bronchopneumonia due to secondary bacterial infection.
   D. Encephalitis.
   E. Laryngitis, tracheitis, and bronchitis.
   F. Exacerbation of tuberculosis.
   G. Myocarditis occurs infrequently.

Problems

I. Communicability of disease.
II. Maintaining bed rest.
III. Excoriation of skin around nose due to nasal discharge.
IV. Formation of crusts around eyes due to conjunctivitis.
V. Fever may result in febrile convulsions.
VI. Itching may cause the child to scratch with resulting break in the skin producing secondary infection.
VII. Coughing may interfere with sleep.
VIII. Loss of appetite may result in weight loss.
IX. Complications must be recognized early.

Goals of Care

I. Prevent spread of disease.
II. Protect client from secondary infection.
III. Decrease possibility of febrile convulsions.
IV. Prevent or minimize complications and recognize them early.
V. Minimize general discomfort due to coughing, itching, or exposure to light.

Intervention

I. Isolate infected child from the time measles is diagnosed until 5 days after the rash appears.
II. Provide environment conducive to bed rest and keep febrile child in bed. Quiet activities such as coloring or having stories read may help to keep patient at rest.
III. Use tissues to keep nose free of secretions and dispose of them properly. A paper bag may be pinned to the bedside for this purpose and may be burned when it becomes full.
IV. Keep eyes free of crusts by bathing them with warm water.
V. Keep room dimly lighted or provide older child with dark glasses.
VI. A lubricant may be used around the nose to prevent excoriation of the skin.
VII. Monitor vital signs, including temperature, every 4 h or as otherwise indicated.
VIII. Administer antipyretics as prescribed for high fever.
IX. Keep client in a comfortably warm environment. Clothing should be of lightweight and nonirritating material, as it will facilitate heat loss and decrease itching.
X. Apply soothing lotion to the skin to reduce itching.
XI. Keep room humidified to minimize cough and to keep secretions loose.
XII. Offer small feedings served attractively to encourage eating.
XIII. Maintain hydration by offering water and other fluids such as fruit juice frequently.
XIV. Observe for signs of complications and report at once.
XV. Teach parents the importance of immunization for other unimmunized and uninfected children.

Evaluation

I. Child accepts bed rest with minimal resistance.
II. Eyes are clear of matting and crusts.
III. There is no excoriation of skin around the nose.
IV. There are no febrile convulsions.
V. No secondary infection results from scratching.
VI. Child sleeps throughout the night with minimal coughing.
VII. No weight is lost due to failure to eat.
VIII. Patient remains adequately hydrated.
IX. Preventable complications do not occur.
X. No other person in family contracts the disease.

RUBELLA (GERMAN MEASLES)

Definition

I. Causative agent: rubella virus.
II. Epidemiology.
   A. Epidemics occur approximately every 5 or 6 years.
   B. Rubella is more prevalent in winter and spring.
   C. It is seen mostly in childhood but affects more adults than rubeola. Appreciable epidemics occur at military camps and college campuses.
   D. In the United States, 80 percent of a population screened will show serologic evidence of previous infection.
   E. Transplacental immunity is effective for the first 6 months of life.
   F. Lifelong immunity is conferred with one attack.
   G. In pregnant women, the virus is transferred to the fetus during the period of viremia via the placenta.

H. The risk of congenital anomalies appears to be quite high if the mother contracts rubella during the first 8 to 12 weeks of pregnancy, but it declines as pregnancy advances and is as low as 4 percent in the second and third trimester.

III. Incubation period.
   A. From 14 to 21 days.
   B. Average is 18 days.

IV. Mode of transmission.
   A. By droplet spread or by direct contact with the patient.
   B. Indirectly by contact with article freshly soiled with discharge from the nose or mouth.
   C. Via placenta to the fetus from infected mother.

V. Treatment and prevention.
   A. Treatment is symptomatic unless complicated by bacterial infection, then treatment is directed toward specific infection.
   B. Active immunization.
      1. It is especially important that girls be immunized prior to childbearing age.
      2. Pregnant women should not come in contact with infants with congenital rubella.
      3. An intramuscular injection of immune serum globulin (ISG) may be offered the exposed susceptible person.
         a. Effectiveness of ISG is not predictable.
         b. Effectiveness depends in part upon the antibody content of the blood used.

Assessment

I. Manifestations.
   A. Mild catarrhal symptoms during prodromal phase may go unnoticed due to mildness and short duration.
   B. The characteristic sign is retroauricular, posterior cervical, and post-occipital adenopathy. Nodes are tender for the first 1 or 2 days and are palpable for several weeks.
   C. Red spots may appear on the soft palate and may coalesce into a red blush prior to the eruption of the skin rash.
   D. The rash begins on the face and rapidly spreads over the rest of the body.
      1. The maculopapular rash is conspicuous.
      2. There are large areas of flushing which spread over the entire body within 24 h after rash appears.
   E. Pharyngeal and conjuctival mucosa are slightly inflamed.
   F. Fever is slight and if present occurs when the rash is at its height. Temperature does not usually exceed 38.3°C (101°F).
   G. Polyarthritis may occur with pain, swelling, tenderness and effusion, and generally disappears without consequence.

II. Complications.
   A. Complications are relatively uncommon in childhood rubella.
   B. Neuritis and arthritis occasionally occur.
   C. Encephalitis occurs rarely.
   D. With the congenital rubella syndrome, the most common defects are:
      1. Cataracts.
      2. Cariovascular anomalies.
      3. Deafness.
      4. Mutism, secondary to deafness.
      5. Microcephaly.
      6. Mental retardation.
   E. Spontaneous abortions occur in about one-third of pregnant women who contract rubella during the first trimester.

Problems

I. Communicability.
II. Maintaining bed rest in child with fever or arthritic symptoms.
III. Persuading the child and parents that she or he should remain at home, away from others, until rash has disappeared.
IV. Teaching parents the importance of immunization for all their children.

Goals of Care

I. Prevent spread of disease by isolating patient and immunizing susceptible population after establishing susceptibility by hemagglutination inhibition (HI) test.
II. Minimize discomfort due to lymphadenopathy and pharyngeal inflammation.
III. Minimize pain and fever resulting from polyarthritis.
IV. Prevent complications.
V. Prevent exposure of pregnant women.

Intervention

I. Isolate child as soon as diagnosis is established.
II. Dispose of tissues properly.
III. Maintain bed rest for child who has arthritis or fever.
IV. Have patient use warm gargles to relieve sore throat.
V. Wash eyes with warm water if drainage is present.
VI. Administer aspirin or other analgesics as prescribed to relieve arthritic pain and reduce fever.
VII. Report any persistent fever, abnormal neurologic signs, or excessive arthritic symptoms.
VIII. The school nurse should initiate an immunization program for all susceptible children in the elementary schools.
IX. Teach parents the expected reaction to the vaccine and how to care for child.
    A. Rash develops about 10 days after immunization.
    B. Fever may develop.
    C. An antipyretic such as aspirin may be given for fever.
    D. Apply warm compresses to the injection site to relieve tenderness.

Evaluation

I. Bed rest is maintained during period of fever and arthritic symptoms.
II. Sore throat is nominal.
III. Fever does not exceed 38.3°C (101°F).
IV. There are no complications.
V. All susceptible school age children in specific exposed population are immunized.
VI. Pregnant women are not exposed.

MUMPS

Definition

I. Causative agent: mumps virus.
II. Epidemiology.
    A. Mumps is endemic in most urban populations.

B. It affects males and females equally.

C. The majority of infections occur prior to adolescence.

D. Epidemics occur at all seasons of the year but are more common in winter and spring.

III. Mode of transmission.

  A. Mumps is spread by droplets and by direct contact with an infected person.

  B. Indirectly, mumps can be spread through articles contaminated by infectious saliva and possibly urine.

  C. About 30 to 40 percent of cases are subclinical.

IV. The incubation period is from 2 to 3 weeks.

V. Treatment and prevention.

  A. Treatment is symptomatic.

  B. Diet should be easy to chew with no sour foods.

  C. Treatment for complications is specific for the particular condition.

  D. Active immunization with live attenuated virus vaccine is an effective preventive in most children.

VI. Prognosis: Recovery is usually complete in uncomplicated cases.

Assessment

I. Manifestations.

  A. Prodromal symptoms are not usually present but may include:

    1. Fever.   3. Headache.
    2. Muscular pain.   4. Malaise.

  B. Onset of disease is characterized by pain and swelling in one or both parotid glands.

    1. Swelling begins by first filling the space between the posterior border of the mandible and the mastoid.
    2. It extends downward and forward and is limited by the zygoma.
    3. The swelling may progress rapidly and reach a peak within a few hours after onset or it may develop over a few days.
    4. The earlobe is pushed upward and outward by the swollen tissue.
    5. Swelling may occur in one gland only, but is more often bilateral.
    6. Swollen area is tender and painful.
    7. Fever accompanies the parotid swelling and is usually moderate.
    8. Swelling of submandibular glands frequently accompanies or closely follows parotid swelling.

II. Complications.

  A. Meningoencephalomyelitis is the most common complication of childhood mumps.

  B. Orchitis and epididymitis are complications seen in adolescents and adults.

  C. Deafness: Mumps is considered a leading cause of unilateral nerve deafness. Deafness is permanent.

  D. Oophoritis.

  E. Pancreatitis.

  F. Nephritis.

  G. Thyroiditis.

  H. Myocarditis.

  I. Arthritis.

  J. Ocular complications.

Problems

I. Communicability of disease.

II. Pain in neck with difficulty in opening the mouth.

III. Inability to eat due to swollen parotid glands.
IV. Fever may cause dry, crusted lips.
V. Complications of a serious nature may develop.

Goals of Care

I. Prevent spread of disease to susceptible persons.
II. Minimize pain in neck.
III. Maintain adequate nutrition and hydration.
IV. Maintain bed rest during febrile period.
V. Prevent or minimize complications.

Intervention

I. Maintain isolation until all swelling has disappeared.
II. Provide ice collar to relieve pain in swollen parotid glands.
III. Provide diet that is easy to chew and avoid sour or strongly flavored foods that would cause an increased amount of pain in the parotid gland.
IV. Give frequent oral hygiene.
V. If fever is present, give tepid baths to help reduce fever.
VI. Maintain bed rest during febrile period.
VII. Monitor temperature, since a sudden fever may indicate the development of complications.
VIII. Observe for complications.
IX. Teach parents and other family members preventive measures that can be taken to protect susceptible persons from becoming ill with the disease.

Evaluation

I. Disease does not spread to susceptible persons.
II. Amount of pain due to swollen glands is minimal.
III. Fever remains below 38.8°C (102°F) during febrile period.
IV. Adequate nutrition with minimal weight loss is maintained.
V. Hydration remains adequate.
VI. Lips are free of crusts and cracks.

CHICKENPOX (VARICELLA)

Definition

I. Causative agent: *Herpesvirus varicella*.
II. Epidemiology.
   A. Chickenpox is a highly contagious disease that may occur at any age. The vast majority of children contract chickenpox before the age of 10 years with 5 to 9 years being the peak years of occurrence.
   B. Chickenpox may be seen during the neonatal period.
   C. The rate of infection of susceptible household members approaches 100 percent.
   D. The disease is seen most often from winter to early spring.
III. The incubation period is from 2 to 3 weeks, most commonly from 13 to 17 days.
IV. Mode of transmission.
   A. Direct contact.
   B. Droplet or airborne spread.

    C. Indirectly from articles freshly soiled by discharges from the skin and mucous membrane of person infected with the disease.

  V. The treatment is symptomatic:

    A. Relieve itching by use of antipruritic agents or sedation.

    B. Give antiseptic baths to reduce incidence of secondary infection.

    C. Administer antibiotic therapy for treatment of secondary infection.

    D. If varicella pneumonia develops, treatment is supportive.

  VI. Prognosis.

    A. The prognosis is usually good.

    B. Fatalities result from complications.

Assessment

  I. Manifestations.

    A. Prodromal symptoms appear at the end of the incubation period:

      1. Fever, which is slight.

      2. Malaise.

      3. Anorexia.

    B. Rash appears rapidly:

      1. Rash begins as crops of small red papules.

      2. These papules form into clear vesicles on an erythematous base.

        a. Vesicles become cloudy in about 24 h.

        b. Vesicles break easily and scabs form.

        c. Eruption of rash continues for about 3 days.

          (1) It begins on the trunk and spreads to the face and scalp.

          (2) Generally, involvement of the distal parts of extremities is minimal.

        d. Chickenpox is characterized by the simultaneous presence of papules, early and late vesicles, and crusts.

    C. Pruritus is constant.

    D. Vesicles on mucous membrane become macerated, especially those in the mouth.

    E. Generalized lymphadenopathy may be present.

  II. Complications.

    A. Secondary bacterial infection of skin lesions is the most frequent complication.

    B. Thrombocytopenia may occur with hemorrhage into the skin.

    C. Internal hemorrhage from ulceration may occur and may be fatal.

    D. Varicella pneumonia is more often seen in adult patients than children.

    E. Respiratory distress may be precipitated due to laryngeal edema if lesions are present on the larynx.

    F. Congenital malformations have occurred in infants whose mothers had the disease during the first trimester of pregnancy.

    G. Postinfectious encephalitis is the most common central nervous system complication.

    H. Chickenpox can be fatal to persons who take steroids (e.g., for leukemia or rheumatoid arthritis)—*avoid exposure.*

Problems

  I. Communicability of disease.

  II. Risk of secondary infection due to scratching of lesions.

  III. Extreme pruritis.

  IV. Risk of respiratory distress from edema of larynx.

  V. Sores in mouth due to macerated lesions may result in inadequate oral intake of food and nluids.

  VI. Pneumonia may develop.

Goals of Care

I. Minimize spread of disease to susceptible persons.
II. Prevent secondary infection.
III. Minimize discomfort due to pruritis.
IV. Prevent or minimize complications.

Intervention

I. Isolate patient as soon as diagnosis is established.
II. Maintain bed rest during febrile period.
III. Administer antipyretics as ordered for high fever.
IV. Separate from general laundry bed linen soiled with drainage from vesicles.
V. Keep child's fingernails clipped.
VI. Infants or young children may need mittens to prevent scratching.
VII. Change bed linen daily to reduce chance of secondary infection.
VIII. Bathe child in soothing baths to reduce itching and to keep skin clean.
IX. Keep child's hands scrupulously clean.
X. Apply lotions, such as calamine to help alleviate itching. Systemic antipruritic agents and sedation may be prescribed to prevent scratching.
XI. Provide loose-fitting, cotton clothing and change clothing at least daily.
XII. Observe for any sign of respiratory distress.
XIII. Avoid breaking vesicles.
XIV. Observe child for signs of complications and report immediately.
XV. Provide quiet play activity for child according to age.

Evaluation

I. Child does not develop secondary infection.
II. Scratching is minimal.
III. Child is content to remain in bed during febrile period.
IV. Complications are absent or minimal and, if they occur, are detected promptly.

POLIOMYELITIS

Definition

I. Causative agent: poliovirus types 1, 2, and 3.
II. Epidemiology.
   A. Outbreaks of clinically recognizable diseases occur most often in temperate zones.
   B. Disease outbreaks occur most frequently in warm months.
   C. Polio is characteristically a disease of children and adolescents, but all ages can be affected when immunity has not been established.
   D. The greatest period of communicability from known cases is during the latter part of the incubation period and the first week of illness.
III. The incubation period is from 1 to 2 weeks.
IV. Mode of transmission.
   A. Direct contact with pharyngeal secretions or feces of infected persons.
   B. The virus is detectable for a longer period of time in feces than in throat secretions.
V. Treatment and prevention.
   A. No antibiotics are effective against the poliovirus.
   B. Human immune globulin is not effective after the onset of illness.

    C. Give analgesics for pain.

    D. Maintain patient on bed rest until the temperature has been normal for several days.

    E. Maintain body alignment to prevent skeletal deformity.

    F. Give normal diet for age with high fluid content.

    G. Maintain airway.

    H. Control respiratory failure due to inadequate respiratory muscles.

        1. Use respirator.

        2. Tracheotomy may be necessary: be prepared.

    I. Active immunization of all susceptible persons against the three types of poliovirus will prevent the catastrophic epidemics of the past.

VI. Prognosis.

    A. Case fatalities during epidemics in the United States have been reported at 5 to 7 percent.

    B. Deaths usually occur during the first 2 weeks after the onset of the disease.

    C. After the age of puberty, there is a higher incidence of fatalities and a higher degree of deformity.

    D. The degree of recovery from poliomyelitis is related to the adequacy and promptness of treatment.

Assessment

I. Manifestations. Contact with the poliovirus may result in a variety of clinical presentations.

    A. Abortive poliomyelitis:

        1. This diagnosis is applicable during outbreaks of polio and in those persons known to have been exposed to another person with clinical evidence of disease.

        2. Symptoms are mild.

            a. Generally the fever does not exceed 39.4°C (103°F).

            b. Anorexia.

            c. Malaise.

            d. Vomiting.

            e. Headache.

            f. Sore throat.

        3. The person with the foregoing symptoms during an outbreak should be assessed several weeks after the illness for muscular involvement.

    B. Nonparalytic poliomyelitis:

        1. The clinical manifestations are similar to but more intense than those for abortive polio.

        2. Constipation is common.

        3. This type of polio presents in two phases which are referred to as minor and major illness. A short, symptom-free period is common between these two phases.

        4. Nuchal and spinal rigidity are positive diagnostic signs and occur during the major illness.

            a. Signs of nuchal and spinal rigidity may be obtained either actively or passively.

            b. The active test for rigidity consists of having the child sit up without assistance. Spinal rigidity is present if undue effort is used, the knees flex upward, and the child rocks somewhat from side to side, then must place the hands behind the body for support.

    C. Paralytic poliomyelitis:

        1. Symptoms are identical to those for nonparalytic poliomyelitis with the addition of muscle weakness in one or more muscle groups.

        2. Symptoms may disappear for a period of several days and subsequently recur.

        3. Paralysis is present when symptoms recur.

        D. Bulbar poliomyelitis with respiratory insufficiency:

           1. This form of polio presents with bulbar paralysis and coexisting involvement of the respiratory muscles.

           2. Clinical manifestations are:

               a. Inability to speak normally, or speaking in breathless sentences.

               b. Increased respiratory rate.

               c. Movement of accessory muscles of respiration.

               d. Inability to cough with full depth.

               e. Nasal speech due to palatal and pharyngeal weakness.

               f. Increased pharyngeal secretions.

               g. Nasal regurgitation of fluids due to palatal paralysis.

               h. Deviation of the palate, uvula, or tongue.

               i. Irregular rate, rhythm, and depth of respiration.

               j. Cardiovascular symptoms:

                  (1) Erratic blood pressure.

                  (2) Alternate flushing and mottling of the skin.

                  (3) Cardiac arrhythmias.

               k. Rapid changes in body temperature.

    II. Complications

        A. Erosions in the gastrointestinal tract.

        B. Gastric dilatation which leads to further respiratory difficulty.

        C. Hypertension, especially during the acute stage of illness.

        D. Hypercalcemia and nephrocalcinosis due to immobility.

        E. Transitory bladder paralysis.

        F. Urinary infection.

Problems

    I. Communicability of disease.

    II. Anxiety of child and parents.

    III. Maintaining body alignment.

    IV. Bladder paralysis.

    V. Malnutrition due to anorexia or inability to swallow.

    VI. Airway obstruction due to accumulation of secretions.

    VII. Fluid and electrolyte imbalance due to inability to take food and fluids.

    VIII. Respiratory failure due to inadequacy of respiratory muscles.

    IX. Fever may result in febrile convulsions as well as increase the need for oxygen.

    X. Pain due to muscle spasms.

Goals of Care

    I. Prevent spread of disease.

    II. Maintain good body alignment to prevent deformities due to muscle shortening.

    III. Maintain adequate nutrition and fluid balance.

    IV. Prevent fecal impaction.

    V. Prevent bladder infections.

    VI. Maintain patency of airway.

    VII. Prevent or minimize fear in child as well as in parents.

    VIII. Prevent aspiration.

Intervention

    I. Nursing care is dependent upon the clinical manifestation of the disease.

    II. Isolation precautions are taken with any type of polio. Concurrent disinfection of throat discharges and feces is necessary since polio virus is demonstrable in both throat secretions and the stool of infected persons.

III. Approach the child in a calm, reassuring manner since there may be a high degree of anxiety in the child or the parents, especially if respiratory involvement is evident.

IV. Nonparalytic type of poliomyelitis:
  A. Keep client on bed rest until fever disappears and there is no muscle pain.
  B. Observe for any sign of paralysis.
  C. Give antipyretics as prescribed for fever.
  D. Maintain fluid balance by providing oral fluid.
  E. Provide a diet adequate for age.

V. Paralytic poliomyelitis. Nursing measures in addition to above include:
  A. Maintenance of good body alignment to prevent deformities.
  B. Applying hot packs to relieve pain due to muscle spasm.
  C. Observing for distended bladder due to transitory paralysis of the bladder.
    1. Gentle manual compression of the bladder will aid in urination.
    2. Strict aseptic technique is to be observed if catheterization is necessary.
  D. Monitoring intake and output due to susceptibility to fluid and electrolyte imbalances.
  E. Promoting personal hygiene by keeping skin clean and providing oral hygiene. (Patient often perspires due to environmental temperature and application of hot packs.)
  F. Providing a diet of interest to encourage eating, as anorexia is often a problem in the early stages of polio.
  G. Promoting normal bowel function by increasing fluid intake and adjusting diet.
  H. Administering antipyretics as prescribed to control fever. Fans and tepid baths will aid in keeping fever down.
  I. Be alert for any sign of respiratory distress.

VI. Bulbar poliomyelitis with respiratory insufficiency:
  A. Provide quiet, calm environment because of increased anxiety of a client with respiratory insufficiency.
  B. Maintain patent airway by use of gentle suctioning and postural drainage.
  C. Accomplish feeding by gavage and parenteral fluids because of child's inability to swallow.
  D. Observe for signs of respiratory embarrassment which may necessitate a tracheostomy and use of artificial mechanical respirator. Respiratory difficulty may be due to involvement of the respiratory center in the brain or paralysis of the muscles of respiration.

Evaluation

  I. No skeletal deformities develop.
  II. Weight loss is negligible.
  III. Adequate fluid and electrolyte balance is maintained.
  IV. Patent airway is maintained.
  V. No urinary infection develops.
  VI. There is no fecal impaction.
  VII. Adequate ventilation is maintained.

TUBERCULOSIS

Definition

  I. Causative agent: *Mycobacterium tuberculosis.*
  II. Epidemiology.
    A. Tuberculosis occurs in all parts of the world.

    B. It is more commonly seen in underdeveloped countries.

    C. The incidence of tuberculosis increases with age and is usually higher in urban than rural areas.

    D. Epidemics have been reported where people are congregated in enclosed areas, such as classrooms.

III. The incubation period is about 1 to 3 months from the time of infection to development of a demonstrable primary lesion.

IV. Mode of transmission.

    A. Airborne droplets from sputum of infected person.

    B. Indirect contact through articles contaminated with the bacilli, though this does not occur frequently.

V. Treatment.

    A. Administer antimicrobial therapy.

    B. Keep on bed rest until there is improvement in the general condition.

    C. Diet should provide a good supply of protein, vitamins, and minerals.

VI. Prognosis.

    A. Recovery from the disease is the usual outcome of treated primary tuberculosis for most children.

    B. The disease goes unnoticed, undiagnosed, and untreated in the majority of children.

    C. During the first 2 years of life a high fatality rate is common.

    D. Otherwise, death rarely occurs except in tuberculosis meningitis or when the disease has progressed rapidly to the terminal stage before it is diagnosed.

Assessment

I. Manifestations.

    A. Tuberculosis may involve almost any tissue or organ of the body.

    B. Symptoms may simulate many other diseases.

    C. The majority of tuberculosis infections in children are intrathoracic.

        1. Intrathoracic tuberculosis:

            a. Initially, the organism enters the lung and causes a small area of inflammation.

            b. From this site, tubercle bacilli invade the regional lymph nodes.

            c. The above process constitutes the primary complex.

            d. The primary lesion may heal or progress to cause extensive damage.

        2. Progressive primary tuberculosis:

            a. The progressive stage represents invasion of the primary lesion into the surrounding lung tissue.

            b. Pulmonary lesions may be extensive without presenting symptoms. Physical findings are variable.

                (1) Percussion may be normal or abnormal.

                (2) Rales may be present or absent.

                (3) Cavitation occurs infrequently.

                (4) The tubercle bacilli are found in the sputum or in gastric washings.

            c. Fever is present.

            d. Patient has anorexia and weight loss.

        3. Infection of the hilar lymph nodes:

            a. Infection of the hilar lymph nodes is almost always seen in infants and children with pulmonary tuberculosis.

            b. It may not present symptoms.

            c. The greatly enlarged lymph nodes may compress the larger blood vessels, thus causing cyanosis, facial edema, and dilatation of the superficial veins.

        4. Acute miliary tuberculosis:

            a. Acute miliary tuberculosis is a bloodborne infection.

            b. It is seen in infants more often than in older children.

    c. All organs of the body may be involved.
- **(1)** The tubercle bacilli become lodged in the capillaries, resulting in necrosis.
- **(2)** Symptoms, e.g., fever, resemble those of any generalized infection.
- **(3)** The x-ray reveals a characteristic mottled lesion.
- **(4)** If untreated, the mortality rate is practically 100 percent.

5. Tubercular meningitis:
- *a.* Tubercular meningitis is the major cause of death from tuberculosis.
- *b.* It is always a secondary lesion; the primary lesion usually is in the lung.
- *c.* Meningeal symptoms are not present until the terminal stage of the disease.
- *d.* Clinically, the disease may be divided into three stages:
  - **(1)** Prodromal stage.
    - *(a)* Onset is gradual.
    - *(b)* A slight fever may be present.
    - *(c)* Mood changes appear.
    - *(d)* Drowsiness is frequent but sleep is often restless.
    - *(e)* Headache is present.
    - *(f)* There is anorexia.
    - *(g)* Vomiting may occur.
  - **(2)** Transitional stage.
    - *(a)* Convulsions occur in many children during this stage.
    - *(b)* Drowsiness becomes deeper.
    - *(c)* Nuchal rigidity is present.
    - *(d)* There is stiffness of the back and extremities.
    - *(e)* Bulging of the fontanels may occur.
  - **(3)** Terminal stage.
    - *(a)* Paralysis replaces evidence of meningeal irritation.
    - *(b)* A comatose state develops.
    - *(c)* Pulse and respirations are irregular.
    - *(d)* Fever is very high.
    - *(e)* Death occurs.

Problems

I. Maintaining bed rest in the acutely ill child.
II. Maintaining a long-term medication regime.
III. Poor appetite.
IV. Education of family.
V. Contact screening.

Goals of Care

I. Prevent complications.
II. Maintain or regain weight up to normal for age and sex.
III. Maintain the client on chemotherapy even in the absence of symptoms.
IV. Promote growth and development in hospitalized child.
V. Prevent spread of disease.

Intervention

I. Skin testing of all contacts may be the task of the public health nurse.
II. Initially, maintain the client on bed rest.
III. Provide client with games or play activity to stimulate interest, thus keeping the child at rest.

IV. Provide older child with opportunities to keep in touch with friends. A bedside phone may alleviate boredom and allow contact with peers.
V. Disguise taste of medication with fruit juice or fruit such as applesauce.
VI. Use flavored liquid medications when available.
VII. Provide a diet high in calories and protein. The older child may be encouraged to eat if given an opportunity to select foods from a menu.
VIII. Families may be provided with information about agencies which may be of assistance if finances become a problem.
IX. Teach family regarding:
   A. The communicability of tuberculosis.
   B. Treatment of the disease.
   C. Prevention of tuberculosis.
   D. The importance of long-term chemotherapy, even in the absence of symptoms.
   E. Importance of returning to the clinic for follow-up appointments after discharge from acute care.

Evaluation

I. Primary lesion heals with no complications.
II. All contacts are found and treatment initiated on all those infected with tuberculosis.
III. Client takes medication regularly for length of time it is prescribed.
IV. Client keeps all follow-up appointments.

GONORRHEA

Definition

I. Causative organism: *Neisseria gonorrhoeae*.
II. Epidemiology.
   A. Gonorrhea is widespread throughout the world.
   B. The infection occurs most frequently in the lower socioeconomic class.
   C. It is believed to be the most frequently unreported communicable disease.
      1. Gonorrhea affects both sexes and is becoming more frequent in teenagers and young adults.
      2. Newborns become infected during birth when they come into contact with the organism in the birth canal.
      3. Young children may be infected through intimate direct contact from infected adults or occasionally through indirect sexual contact with contaminated articles.
      4. Adolescents become infected as a result of sexual contact with an infected partner.
III. Incubation period: 3 to 5 days is the usual incubation period.
IV. Mode of transmission.
   A. Direct sexual contact accounts for the major transmission of gonorrhea.
      1. In gonococcal infection in children, sexual abuse must be considered a possibility and ruled in or out.
      2. A child infected with gonorrhea may transfer the infection to other children if they engage in sex play.
   B. Articles contaminated with infected exudate may be a source of infection in young children.
   C. Infants may become infected during birth if the mother has the disease.
V. Treatment: Penicillin is the drug of choice in the treatment of gonorrhea.
VI. Prevention.
   A. Sex education should begin no later than the seventh grade and should include information about venereal disease.

        B. Routine cultures for gonorrhea in family planning clinics and prenatal clinics will prevent the spread of the disease to newborn babies if the mother receives treatment before the infant is born.

        C. Instill prophylactic drops or salve into newborn's eyes at birth.

VII. Prognosis: With appropriate and adequate treatment with antibiotics, the prognosis is excellent.

Assessment

I. Manifestations.

    A. Gonorrhea of venereal origin:

      1. In males, a purulent discharge from the urethra appears a few days after exposure to the organism.

      2. Urethral irritation with dysuria occurs, particularly in males.

      3. Urinary meatus is red and swollen, particularly in males.

      4. If untreated, symptoms become worse.

        a. There is hematuria.

        b. Headache and malaise sometimes occur.

        c. If the client had anal sexual intercourse symptoms may include diarrhea, anal itching, and a purulent discharge adhering to the stool.

      5. Symptoms in the female may include:

        a. Vaginal discharge.

        b. Frequency of urination.

        c. Abdominal pain.

        d. Many females with gonorrhea are asymptomatic.

    B. Gonococcal vulvovaginitis:

      1. This form occurs as an inflammatory reaction in prepubescent girls.

      2. There is redness and swelling of the mucous membrane.

      3. Occasionally there is vaginal discharge.

      4. Dysuria is present.

    C. Gonococcal ophthalmia neonatorum:

      1. There is acute redness and swelling of the conjunctiva of one or both eyes.

      2. A purulent discharge from the eyes is present.

II. Complications.

    A. Bartholin's abscess.

    B. Salpingitis.

    C. Proctitis resulting from rectal infection.

    D. Urethral stricture.

    E. Prostatitis.

    F. Gonorrheal arthritis.

    G. Sterility.

    H. Blindness due to ophthalmic infection.

Problems

I. Education of young people may be a problem due to parental objection.

II. Locating contacts.

III. Failure of clients to report for follow-up care.

IV. Preventing complications.

Goals of Care

I. Educate about gonorrhea in order to prevent infection and/or reinfection.

II. Provide early and adequate treatment.

III. Prevent complications.

Intervention

I. In adolescents and adults:
  A. Educate about the cause, transmission, prevention, and treatment of the disease.
  B. Administer antibiotics as prescribed. Watch for adverse reactions to medications.
  C. Advise client to refrain from having sexual intercourse until cure is established. Reexamination should be done 3 days after treatment.
  D. Advise client not to drink alcohol for a period of 2 weeks after treatment (alcohol may interfere with blood level of penicillin).
  E. Locate, culture, and if indicated treat all sexual contacts for the 2-week period prior to the onset of symptoms.
II. Children and young adolescents for whom sexual abuse cannot be ruled out must be referred to appropriate social agency.
III. All gonococcal infections must be reported to local health authorities.

Evaluation

I. Reculture is negative after treatment.
II. Client returns to clinic at appointed time for reexamination.
III. All contacts are identified and treated.
IV. No complications develop.

SYPHILIS

Definition

I. Causative agent: *Treponema pallidum,* a spirochete.
II. Epidemiology.
  A. Syphilis is a widespread communicable disease.
  B. It is most frequently seen in adolescents and young adults.
  C. It is more prevalent in urban areas.
  D. Males are more often infected than females.
  E. Syphilis is transmitted to the fetus from the mother via the placenta.
III. The incubation period is from 2 to 10 weeks, usually 3 weeks.
IV. Mode of transmission.
  A. Sexual contact is the most common mode of transmission.
  B. Direct contact (mucous membrane, break in skin) with body fluids such as saliva, semen, blood, and vaginal discharges of an infected person can result in infection.
  C. Transmission from the infected mother to the fetus via the placenta may occur after the fourth month of pregnancy.
V. Treatment and prevention.
  A. All cases of early infectious syphilis must be reported to the local health authority.
  B. Advise client to refrain from sexual intercourse with untreated previous sexual partners.
  C. Investigate contacts for preceding 3 months for primary syphilis and for 6 months for secondary syphilis.
  D. Administration of 2.4 million units of benzathine penicillin is generally effective for primary and secondary syphilis.
  E. Congenital syphilis is treated with various doses and types of penicillin depending on the age of the child.
  F. A serologic test for syphilis should be done on all pregnant women.
  G. Education about venereal disease is essential in any effort to control syphilis.
VI. Prognosis.
  A. Recovery occurs with adequate treatment.
  B. Complications that develop prior to treatment are not reversible.

Assessment

I. Manifestations.
   A. Acquired syphilis occurs in three stages:
      1. Primary stage.
         a. A chancre appears at the site of infection.
         b. Swelling of local lymph nodes occurs a few days after the appearance of the chancre.
         c. The chancre is painless and disappears without treatment in a few weeks.
         d. The serological test may be negative up to 8 weeks after infection.
      2. Secondary stage.
         a. The patient may develop a maculopapular rash which can be so slight as to go unnoticed.
         b. Bald spots may develop on the head.
         c. Coldlike symptoms may develop.
         d. Severe headaches are not uncommon.
      3. Tertiary stage.
         a. This stage may develop soon after initial infection or as long as 25 years after infection.
         b. The disease may affect almost any system of the body during this stage.
         c. Symptoms vary according to system or systems affected.
   B. Congenital syphilis.
      1. Fever.
      2. Anemia.
      3. Failure to gain weight.
      4. Rash.
      5. Rhinitis.
      6. Unless treated, the infant may develop such signs of congenital syphilis as:
         a. Saddle nose.
         b. Rhagades.
         c. Hutchinson's incisors.
II. Complications: A few of the destructive complications of tertiary syphilis are:
   A. Deafness.
   B. Blindness.
   C. Bone destruction.
   D. Mental impairment.
   E. Aortic valve incompetence.
   F. Aortic aneurysm.

Problems

I. Education of the client about the cause, transmission, and prevention of the disease, and the consequences of untreated syphilis.
II. Early detection.
III. Prevention of spread of disease through contaminated articles.
IV. Motivating the client to return for reexamination.

Goals of Care

I. Prevent progression of disease.
II. Prevent congenital syphilis.
III. Educate the client about the disease.
IV. Prevent spread of disease through articles contaminated with moist exudate from syphilitic lesions.

Intervention

    I. Acquired syphilis:
       A. Administer prescribed medication.
       B. Observe client for any reaction to drug.
       C. Teach client how syphilis is transmitted and prophylactic measures.
       D. Ensure that articles soiled with discharges from infected lesions do not come in contact with others.
       E. Investigate contacts.
    II. Congenital syphilis:
       A. Ensure that all pregnant women have serology test for syphilis.
       B. Administer prescribed medication.
       C. Prevent excoriation of upper lip due to rhinitis by keeping secretions cleaned away. A lubricant for the lip may help.

Evaluation

    I. All contacts are found and treated.
    II. Client receives adequate treatment.
    III. Disease does not progress.
    IV. Client learns how the disease is transmitted and does not become reinfected.

CAT-SCRATCH DISEASE

Definition

    I. Causative agent: unknown. A virus has been thought to be the causative agent, although it has not been identified.
    II. Epidemiology.
       A. Cat-scratch disease is uncommon but has a worldwide distribution.
       B. It occurs during all seasons.
       C. It affects males and females equally.
       D. The infection is seen in young children more often than in adults.
    III. The incubation period is from 1 to 2 weeks from inoculation to the development of the primary lesion.
    IV. Mode of transmission.
       A. Transmission is from the domestic cat to humans by scratching, biting, or licking.
       B. Cats which transfer the disease to humans do not appear ill and do not react to the antigen when they receive it by intradermal injection.
    V. Treatment: No specific treatment is known to be helpful.
    VI. Prognosis.
       A. The prognosis is good.
       B. Within 3 months the enlarged nodes regress without treatment.

Assessment

    I. Manifestations.
       A. Generally, the client does not appear acutely ill.
       B. There is headache.
       C. Patient experiences malaise.
       D. Low-grade fever is present.
       E. There is lymphadenitis.

F. Nodes may be strikingly large.

G. Nodes may be tender.

H. Redness and swelling are present at the site of the lesion.

    1. It may resemble an insect bite.

    2. Pus obtained from the lymph nodes is bacteriologically sterile.

II. Complications: Central nervous system involvement may follow the acute stage:

    A. Encephalitis.   *C.* Myelitis.

    B. Encephalomyelitis.

Problems

I. Control of fever.

II. Control of headache.

III. Malaise may result in child's unwillingness to eat and drink adequately.

IV. Pain due to enlarged lymph nodes.

Goals of Care

I. Minimize discomfort.

II. Maintain fluid balance.

III. Maintain weight by providing interesting meals that child will eat.

IV. Maintain good hygiene.

V. Prevent or detect any early central nervous system involvement.

Intervention

I. Administer analgesics as prescribed for headache.

II. Administer antipyretics as prescribed to control fever.

III. Keep child at rest until fever and pain due to swollen lymph nodes subside. Provide child with quiet play activities appropriate for age.

IV. Serve small meals at frequent intervals to ensure an adequate intake of food.

V. Offer fluids such as fruit juice to keep child hydrated and aid in control of fever.

VI. Warm, moist compresses may alleviate the tenderness associated with the swollen nodes.

VII. Observe for and report any sign of central nervous system involvement.

Evaluation

I. Headache is relieved.

II. Child remains in bed during acute febrile period and is relatively content.

III. Patient does not lose weight.

IV. Child remains hydrated.

V. Disease is resolved without any central nervous system involvement.

ROCKY MOUNTAIN SPOTTED FEVER

Definition

I. Causative agent: *Rickettsia rickettsii.*

II. Epidemiology.

    A. Rocky Mountain spotted fever occurs throughout the United States.

    B. It is seen in the spring and summer.

    C. It is most prevalent in the southeastern states.

    D. This disease affects adult males in the Western United States more frequently than others and is most often seen in children in the East.

        1. Differences relate to the conditions of exposure to the infected tick.

        2. In the Western United States the wood tick is the common vector.

        3. In the Southern United States the dog tick is the vector.

III. The incubation period is from 3 to 10 days.

IV. Mode of transmission.

    A. Rocky Mountain spotted fever is transmitted by the bite of an infected tick.

    B. Several hours of attachment of the tick are necessary for the organism to infect the human.

    C. The disease can be contracted through contamination of the skin with a crushed tick body or tick feces.

V. Treatment.

    A. Antibiotics have greatly reduced the mortality and morbidity of rickettsial infections.

    B. Give supportive treatment.

    C. Administer parenteral fluids for those who are severely ill, as well as:

        1. Sedation.

        2. Oxygen.

VI. Prevention.

    A. Avoid tick-infested areas.

    B. Search body at least every 3 h for ticks when in a wooded area.

    C. Remove tick by exerting gentle, steady traction in order to avoid leaving the tick head embedded in the skin.

    D. Place tick-repellent collar on family dog or dip in liquid tick repellent.

    E. Vaccine containing killed *R. rickettsii* is available but is not very effective, thus is generally administered only to those at high risk, such as forest rangers.

VII. Prognosis.

    A. Recovery in uncomplicated cases generally occurs by the end of 3 weeks after onset.

    B. In the absence of treatment, the fatality rate is about 20 percent.

Assessment

I. A history of tick bite is reported in the majority of cases.

II. Manifestations.

    A. There is fever, moderate to high.

    B. Patient has poor appetite.

    C. Patient is restless.

    D. Chills occur.

    E. A maculopapular rash is observed about the third day.

        1. Rash begins on the extremities.

        2. It spreads to the palms and soles, then to the entire body.

    F. Myalgia is present.

    G. Splenomegaly is present in many cases.

    H. Severe manifestations include:

        1. Central nervous system symptoms.

        2. Edema of the face.

        3. Myocarditis.

        4. Renal involvement.

        5. Thrombocytopenia.

III. Complications: Multiple coagulation problems are being reported and may account for the highest risk of death.

Problems

I. Loss of weight and strength due to anorexia.
II. Fever may produce febrile convulsions.
III. Child is restless.

Goals of Care

I. Maintain bed rest during acute illness.
II. Relieve headache and other physical discomforts.
III. Maintain normal weight.
IV. Educate family about tick-borne disease and how to reduce risk of tick bite.

Intervention

I. Keep febrile child in bed and at rest. Provide quiet activities such as reading to encourage rest.
II. Administer medications as prescribed.
III. Monitor intake and output to ensure adequate hydration.
IV. Weigh daily to ensure that there is no drastic weight loss.
V. Provide a diet that the child is likely to eat.
   A. Small feedings spaced throughout the day may be better received than three large meals.
   B. Older children may enjoy selecting their own food.
VI. Monitor temperature and report rising fever. Be alert for febrile convulsion in child with high fever.
VII. Observe and report any sign of central nervous system disturbance.
VIII. Observe skin for signs of hemorrhage and report any such evidence.
IX. Teach family the preventive measures that should be taken to avoid tick bites.

Evaluation

I. Child is content to rest in bed during febrile period.
II. Patient remains adequately hydrated.
III. No unusual weight loss occurs.
IV. There are no complications.
V. Family takes measures to reduce tick population in home environment.

INFECTIOUS MONONUCLEOSIS

Definition

I. Causative agent: Epstein-Barr virus (EBV).
II. Epidemiology.
   A. Mononucleosis has a worldwide occurrence.
   B. It is most frequently seen in adolescents and young adults in developed countries.
   C. In developing countries the infection is most frequently seen in young children.
   D. College students are more commonly infected in this country than others in the population.
III. The incubation period is commonly 2 to 6 weeks.

    IV. Mode of transmission.

        A. Direct contact via the oral-pharyngeal route. Kissing may be the greatest cause of spread among young adults.

        B. Blood transfusions may transmit the disease, also.

    V. Treatment.

        A. Bed rest is generally prescribed at the onset and during the febrile period.

        B. Give supportive treatment.

        C. Corticosteroids may be used for those persons with severe symptoms.

    VI. Prognosis: The prognosis is good although there is generally a long convalescent period.

Assessment

    I. Manifestations: The onset is usually insidious, but it may be acute.

        A. Patient experiences malaise.

        B. Throat is sore.

        C. There is a fever that persists for several weeks.

        D. The lymph nodes are enlarged either early or late in the disease. Most commonly, the anterior and posterior cervical nodes are involved and may be enlarged and tender.

        E. The appearance of the throat may suggest streptococcal infection or diphtheria.

        F. The spleen is usually palpable but is not always tender.

        G. A rash is present in a few cases, most prominently over the trunk.

    II. Complications.

        A. Hepatitis.

        B. Rupture of the spleen.

        C. Neurologic involvement occurs occasionally, generally after the acute phase of the disease.

Problems

    I. Child may refuse food and fluids because of sore throat.

    II. Client may be unwilling to remain on bed rest due to compelling need to continue with school activities.

    III. Control of headache, fever, and sore throat.

Goals of Care

    I. Minimize discomforts associated with the disease.

    II. Maintain adequate nutrition and fluid balance.

    III. Maintain bed rest during acute febrile stage.

    IV. Minimize worry about missing school.

Intervention

    I. Give throat irrigations with warm water several times a day to soothe sore throat. This may be done prior to meals to lessen pain of swallowing.

    II. Offer foods that are soft and easy to swallow.

    III. Offer fluids that are not likely to burn or irritate the throat.

    IV. If there is any doubt that the client is receiving adequate fluids, maintain an intake and output record.

    V. Contact appropriate person to assist student in keeping up with studies while in bed.

VI. Administer medications as prescribed to alleviate headache and to minimize fever and sore throat.

VII. Observe for complications.

Evaluation

I. Patient remains on bed rest during acute phase.

II. Adequate food and fluid intake is maintained.

III. Patient keeps pace with schoolwork.

IV. Complaints of sore throat and headache are minimal.

CYTOMEGALIC INCLUSION DISEASE (CID)

Definition

I. Causative agent: A cytomegalovirus, a member of a group of viruses related to the herpesviruses.

II. Epidemiology.

A. The occurrence of cytomegalic inclusion disease is worldwide.

B. The prevalence of serum antibody varies from 40 percent in highly developed countries to 100 percent in developing countries.

C. The disease is more often seen in women than men.

D. It is seen in young infants as a congenitally acquired disease (by far the most significant form of the disease).

III. Incubation period.

A. Unknown.

B. Infections acquired during birth may be demonstrated from 3 to 12 weeks after birth.

IV. Mode of transmission.

A. Not completely known.

B. The infection may be transmitted via the placenta to the fetus.

C. Blood transfusions may be a source of transmission.

V. Treatment.

A. There is no known treatment.

B. Seizures have been controlled by use of anticonvulsant drugs.

VI. Prognosis.

A. The prognosis is poor in congenitally acquired infections; the fatality rate is high.

B. Those infants who survive may exhibit mental retardation as well as other grave conditions such as microcephaly, hearing loss, chronic liver disease, and motor disturbances.

Assessment

I. Manifestations of congenital CID.

A. Low birth weight.
D. Icterus.

B. Hepatomegaly.
E. Anemia.

C. Splenomegaly.
F. Thrombocytopenia.

II. Complications of congenital CID.

A. Mental retardation.
D. Motor disabilities.

B. Deafness.
E. Death.

C. Chronic liver disease.

Problems

    I. Low-birth-weight infant.
    II. Feeding difficulties due to illness of the infant.
    III. Grieving process of the parents due to concern for gravely ill infant.

Goals of Care

    I. Maintain general comfort of infant.
    II. Provide for safety of infant.
    III. Maintain adequate caloric intake.
    IV. Assist parents to deal with crisis of having a gravely ill child.

Intervention

    I. Isolate infant if virus is being excreted in urine or saliva.
    II. Feed infant via gavage if infant is too ill or weak to suck.
    III. Maintain adequate body temperature to prevent cold stress.
    IV. Nurse should stimulate infant by singing, talking, and holding as she would other infants. (*Caution:* Pregnant nurses or even nurses who are likely to become pregnant should not care for these infants.)
    V. Allow parents to talk about their feelings regarding their child. Refer to social agency if parents need such assistance for financial help in the prolonged hospitalization of their child.

Evaluation

    I. Infant gains weight.
    II. Complications due to secondary infection do not develop.
    III. No other cases develop among nursery population.
    IV. Parents are able to come to terms with their feelings of having a severely ill child.

ENTEROBIASIS (PINWORM DISEASE, OXYURIASIS)

Definition

    I. Causative agent: *Enterobius vermicularis.* This intestinal worm infects man only. Pinworms of animals are not transmitted to man.
    II. Epidemiology.
        A. The distribution of pinworm infestation is worldwide.
        B. Children are infected more often than adults; however, the infection is found commonly in an entire family when one member contracts the disease.
        C. It is prevalent where crowded conditions exist, such as in institutions.
    III. Incubation period: The life cycle of the worm is 3 to 6 weeks.
    IV. Mode of transmission.
        A. Eggs are transferred directly by the hand from the anus to the mouth.
        B. This mode of transmission may be the source of infection to other hosts, such as a mother who kisses the infected hands of her child.
        C. Eggs can be airborne in dust.
        D. Indirectly, the worm may be transmitted through contaminated clothing or food or any article contaminated with the egg of the worm.

1. The eggs are ingested and pass into the small intestine where they hatch.
2. The worms mature in the lower small intestine and upper colon.
3. Worms migrate to the rectum, crawl out through the anus and discharge eggs on the perianal skin.
4. The worms may migrate up the genital tract in females, causing such problems as salpingitis.

V. Treatment.
    A. Treatment should include all household members.
    B. Medications such as pyrantel, pyrvinium pamoate, or piperazine citrate are effective. Dose is calculated according to body weight.
    C. Control measures include:
        1. Daily bathing.
        2. Clean bed linen.
        3. Education about personal hygiene.
        4. Adequate hand washing facilities.

Assessment

I. Manifestations.
    A. Pruritus ani.
    B. Loss of appetite.
    C. Weight loss.
    D. Insomnia due to severe anal itching.

II. Complications.
    A. Secondary bacterial infection due to scratching.
    B. Appendicitis.
    C. Salpingitis.
    D. Reinfection occurs due to nontreatment of infected contacts.

Problems

I. Communicability of disease.
II. Education of family, if necessary, in hygienic measures to prevent reinfection.
III. Itching may produce secondary infection.

Goals of Care

I. Identify and treat all infected persons in the household.
II. Educate household members in the prevention and control of the disease.
III. Prevent secondary bacterial infection.

Intervention

I. Most persons with pinworm disease are treated at home.
II. Administer prescribed medication.
III. Identify all household members who are infected.
    A. Specimens for laboratory examinations may be obtained by "blotting" a piece of cellulose adhesive tape against the perianal area. The eggs will adhere to the tape and can be identified by microscope. This is best done in the morning before bathing or defecating.
    B. Teach family members how the infection is spread and instruct each member of the family, if necessary, in good personal hygiene, especially hand washing.

Evaluation

I. All infected persons in the household are identified and treated.
II. Family institutes improved hygienic measures as needed.
III. All family members remain free of infection after treatment.

HOOKWORM DISEASE

Definition

I. Causative agents: *Necator americanus* and *Ancylostoma duodenale*.
II. Epidemiology.
  A. Hookworm infestation occurs widely in tropical and subtropical countries.
  B. It occurs in temperate climates where disposal of human feces is inadequate.
  C. Man initiates the extrinsic phase of the worm's life cycle by discharging stool containing hookworm eggs onto the soil.
  D. Man in turn becomes infected by direct contact with the contaminated soil.
  E. Older children and adults are infected more often than infants and young children.
III. The incubation period depends upon the intensity of infection and the nutritional status of the host. It may be a few weeks or several months.
IV. Mode of transmission.
  A. Eggs in stool are deposited upon the ground, where they hatch.
  B. Larvae develop and become infective in approximately 1 week.
  C. Infection occurs when the larvae penetrate the skin, usually through the sole of the foot.
  D. The larvae enter the skin and travel to the lungs via the lymphatics or bloodstream.
  E. They migrate from the lungs to the pharynx, are swallowed, and travel to the small intestine where they attach to the wall.
V. Treatment and prevention.
  A. After an overnight fast, tetrachloroethylene is given. Dosage depends upon the weight of the child.
  B. The treatment may be repeated in 1 week.
  C. Preventive measures include prevention of soil contamination.
    1. Ensure that sanitary privies are built in areas with outdoor toilets.
    2. Educate the population about dangers of soil contamination and the need to wear shoes.
VI. Prognosis
  A. With specific treatment, the prognosis is good.
  B. Normal hemoglobin is regained by providing an adequate diet.

Assessment

I. Manifestations.
  A. Coughing may be present when the larvae are in the lung.
  B. Enteritis may be severe.
  C. There is anorexia.
  D. Malnutrition is a problem.
  E. Patient suffers from chronic fatigue.
  F. Anemia develops.

Problems

I. Reinfection occurs if sanitary disposal of feces is not carried out.
II. Identifying the infected persons in a family.

III. Educating the family concerning the sanitary disposal of feces and the need for family members to wear shoes.

IV. A very ill child may experience fatigue, anorexia, and severe anemia.

Goals of Care

I. Identify and treat all infected family members.

II. Educate family to wear shoes.

III. Teach family methods of sanitary disposal of feces.

IV. Restore normal hemoglobin in all clients with low hemoglobin.

Intervention

I. Administer prescribed medication.

II. Provide anorexic child with small, frequent meals high in iron content.

III. Observe child for symptoms of severe enteritis and report promptly if they occur.

IV. Teach family how disease is transmitted and how they can avoid becoming infected.

Evaluation

I. All family members with the disease are identified and treated.

II. Family demonstrates knowledge of sanitary disposal of feces. Rural families without indoor toilets construct sanitary privies.

III. All family members wear shoes outdoors.

IV. Those treated for the disease have a normal hemoglobin count within 1 month after treatment.

ASCARIASIS

Definition

I. Causative agent: *Ascaris lumbricoides*. This large roundworm may be up to 30 cm in length.

II. Epidemiology.
  A. Ascariasis has a worldwide distribution.
  B. It is most common in moist, warm countries.
  C. In the United States the disease occurs most often in the South.
  D. Young children under 10 years of age are most often infected.
  E. Rural areas where outdoor toilets are used favor the infection.

III. The incubation period is about 8 weeks after eggs are ingested.

IV. Mode of transmission: ingestion of the worm egg.
  A. The infective egg is deposited in the soil and taken into the mouth of the child on contaminated hands or toys.
  B. Children who eat dirt are often infected.

V. Treatment and prevention.
  A. There is no effective treatment for the larval stage in the lungs.
  B. The parasite is passed in the stool after treatment with piperazine citrate. Two doses, given 2 days apart, are usually adequate.

Assessment

I. Manifestations.
  A. Atypical pneumonia may occur as the larvae develop in the lungs.

      B. Allergic symptoms involving the following are frequently noted:
         1. Urticaria.   **3.** Elevated eosinophils.
         2. Asthma.
      C. Intestinal infection may produce no symptoms, or symptoms may include:
         1. Nausea.   **4.** Weight loss.
         2. Vomiting.   **5.** Sleep disturbance.
         3. Loss of appetite.
   II. Complications.
      A. Intestinal obstruction may result from a large population of parasites.
      B. Intussusception.
      C. Paralytic ileus.
      D. Appendicitis.

Problems

   I. Nausea and vomiting may result in dehydration.
   II. Weight loss may be marked as a result of poor appetite.
  III. Itching may produce secondary infection when urticaria is present.
  IV. Communicability of disease.
   V. Education of family in hygienic measures:
      A. Wash hands after eliminating and before handling food.
      B. Avoid eating food that has been dropped on the floor.

Goals of Care

   I. Maintain hydration.
   II. Maintain weight.
  III. Identify and treat all infected persons in the household.
  IV. Educate all members of the family in prevention of the disease.
   V. Prevent secondary bacterial infection.

Intervention

   I. Administer prescribed medication.
   II. Prevent dehydration by offering fluids frequently and using prescribed antiemetics.
  III. Maintain weight by offering small, frequent meals to the anorexic child.
  IV. Identify all household members who are infected.
   V. Teach family members how the parasite is contracted and instruct them in good personal hygiene, especially hand washing.
  VI. Reduce the chance of bacterial infection secondary to scratching by keeping finger nails trimmed.
      A. Apply a soothing antipruritic to hives, if present.
      B. Tepid baths with sodium bicarbonate added to the water may reduce itching.

Evaluation

   I. Child remains hydrated.
   II. Usual weight is maintained.
  III. No secondary bacterial infection occurs.
  IV. All infected family members are identified and treated.
   V. Family institutes improved hygienic measures, especially good hand washing.
  VI. Family members remain free of infection after treatment.

TRICHURIASIS (WHIPWORM INFESTATION)

Definition

I. Causative agent: *Trichuris trichiura.* Length of the whipworm may reach 50 mm.
II. Epidemiology.
    A. Trichuriasis is widely distributed, especially in warm, moist climates.
    B. The infestation is most common in older children.
III. The incubation period is indefinite.
IV. Mode of transmission.
    A. Ingestion of worm eggs picked up from contaminated soil.
    B. Eggs hatch and larvae migrate to the cecum and appendix, where they mature.
    C. Eggs may be present in the feces about 3 months after ingestion.
V. Treatment.
    A. Mebendazole is the drug of choice.
    B. Hexylresorcinol enemas (0.2 percent) may be given the hospitalized client.

Assessment

I. Manifestations.
    A. Many persons harbor the worm without symptoms.
    B. In heavy infections there may be chronic bowel irritation with bloody, mucous diarrhea.
II. Complication: prolapse of the rectum.

Problems

Child and family require teaching to promote good personal and environmental hygiene.

Goals of Care

I. Educate child and family about hygiene.
II. Educate child and family about proper disposal of feces.
III. Identify and treat infected family members.

Intervention

I. Administer prescribed treatment.
II. The nurse's major role is to teach the family good hygiene and proper, safe disposal of feces.

Evaluation

Family does not become reinfected.

BIBLIOGRAPHY

Benenson, Abram (ed.): *Control of Communicable Disease in Man,* The American Public Health Association, Washington, D.C., 1975. This is a current and complete reference manual on communicable disease. It considers every communicable disease known to exist. Its purpose is to provide current information for public health workers and others who are concerned with control of communicable disease. An outstanding reference manual.

Luckman, Joan, and Karen Sorensen: *Medical-Surgical Nursing: A Psychophysiological Approach,* W. B. Saunders Company, Philadelphia, 1976. An outstanding textbook for the student as well as the practicing nurse. The section dealing with immunity is an excellent in-depth treatment of the topic. At the beginning of each chapter there is a study guide which is most helpful for the reader and aids in providing an overview of what the reader can expect to gain from the particular chapter.

Remington, Jack, and Jerome Klein: *Infectious Diseases of the Fetus and Newborn Infant,* W. B. Saunders Company, Philadelphia, 1976. An excellent reference book for the reader seeking information about the pathology of certain infectious diseases.

Scipien, Gladys, Martha Barnard, Marilyn Chard, Jeanne Howe, and Patricia Phillips: *Comprehensive Pediatric Nursing,* 2d ed., McGraw-Hill Book Company, New York, 1979. This book lives up to its title. It does indeed provide comprehensive coverage. The communicable diseases are found throughout the book, and are discussed in relation to the system which is affected. Nursing management is thorough and the teaching responsibilities of the nurse are discussed.

Vaughn, Victor, III, R. James McKay, and Waldo Nelson (eds.): *Nelson Textbook of Pediatrics,* 10th ed., W. B. Saunders Company, Philadelphia, 1975. This latest edition of Nelson's *Textbook of Pediatrics* remains the leader in books of its kind. Comprehensive and complete, it is an outstanding reference book for the health professional.

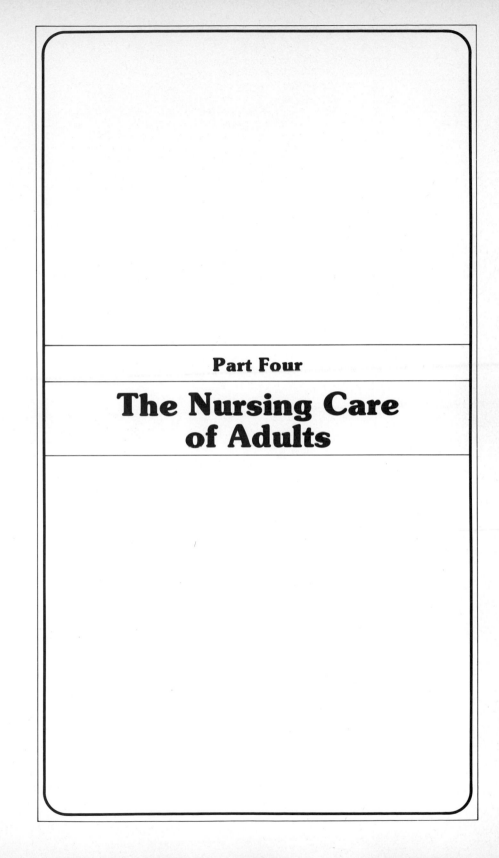

Part Four

The Nursing Care of Adults

The content of Part 4 focuses on medical-surgical problems that affect the body systems and disrupt the health of adults in a variety of settings. From Chaps. 23 to 33, a body system (nervous, endocrine, hematologic, cardiovascular, respiratory, urinary, gynecologic and andrologic, musculoskeletal, immunologic, and integumentary) is presented, and relevant disruptions are discussed within the overall framework of the nursing process.

In each chapter, content is further organized under the concepts of abnormal cellular growth, hyperactivity and hypoactivity, metabolic disorders, inflammatory disorders, trauma, obstructions, and degenerative disorders. Within this framework problems are discussed as either major or minor. *Major problems* are defined as those seen frequently in any medical-surgical setting. A definition of the problem and related pathophysiology are presented, followed by a complete implementation of the nursing process. *Minor problems* refer to those disruptions in health observed less frequently that may be either acute or nonacute. A discussion of a minor problem focuses on a brief definition, the pathophysiologic changes, and the key components of the nursing process that reflect unique differences not previously addressed.

As with other parts of this handbook, the ANA standards of nursing practice, in this case medical-surgical nursing practice, are incorporated into each discussion of a particular health problem. They are included here for reference and review.

It should be noted that nursing care, as discussed in the following chapters, has been generalized in many instances. The reader is encouraged to recognize the individual needs of each patient and to incorporate such information into the plan of care.

ANA STANDARDS OF MEDICAL-SURGICAL NURSING PRACTICE[1]

1. The collection of data about the health status of the patient is systematic and continuous. These data are communicated to appropriate persons, recorded, and stored in a retrievable and accessible system.
2. Nursing diagnosis is derived from health status data.
3. Goals for nursing care are formulated.
4. The plan for nursing care prescribes nursing actions to achieve the goals.
5. The plan for nursing care is implemented.
6. The plan for nursing care is evaluated.
7. Reassessment, reordering of priorities, new goal setting, and revision of the plan for nursing care is a continuous process.

[1] Reprinted with permission from the *American Nurses' Association Standards of Medical-Surgical Nursing Practice.* Copyright © 1974 by the American Nurses' Association.

23

The Nervous System

Gail Barlow Gall

Nursing care of the patient with a neurologic impairment must be based on an accurate assessment of the present status of the patient's nervous system combined with a knowledge of normal anatomy and physiology. This chapter will present an outline of the information needed to form a baseline assessment of the nervous system. Special nursing care for the particular diseases follow, with a brief explanation of their pathophysiology. This chapter is limited to the most frequently occurring problems, but should allow the reader to form a basis for expanding understanding and skills.

GENERAL ASSESSMENT

Assessment of the following points should be performed, presented, and recorded in an orderly format.

I. Health history.
  A. Present problem:
    1. Onset and duration.
    2. Quality of pain or impairment.
    3. Quantity of pain or impairment.
    4. Alleviating factors.
    5. Aggravating factors.
    6. Laboratory studies to date.
    7. Related problems or complaints.
  B. Past illnesses:
    1. Developmental history (birth trauma).
    2. Previous neurological problems (headache, dizziness, seizures, loss of consciousness).
    3. Significant trauma or illnesses.
  C. Family history (assess the presence of hereditary disorders, e.g., seizures).
  D. Social history:
    1. Pay particular attention to any change in behavior and patient's relationships.
    2. How does problem affect patient's day-to-day life?
II. Mental status.
  A. Level of consciousness: degree of reaction to stimuli:
    1. Alert.
    2. Confused.
    3. Delirious.
    4. Stuporous.
    5. Comatose.
  B. General behavioral-emotional status:
    1. Tense.
    2. Sad.
    3. Euphoric.
    4. Cooperative.
    5. Inappropriate.
  C. Intellectual functioning:
    1. Orientation to time, place, and person.
    2. Calculation.
    3. Recent memory (have patient recall three facts within time of examination).
    4. Remote memory (have patient recall historical data such as names of presidents).
    5. Judgment and problem-solving ability.
  D. Thought processing:
    1. Hallucinations, delusions, and/or fixed ideas.
    2. Degree of insight shown regarding problem and situation.
  E. Cortical sensory function:
    1. Ability to recognize various stimuli.
      a. Visual stimuli.
      b. Auditory stimuli.
      c. Tactile stimuli.

      2. Ability to recognize body parts and relationships.
   F. Cortical motor function: ability to carry out skilled acts in absence of motor impairment.
   G. Language:
      1. Auditory receptive: ability to recognize, retain, and understand that which is heard.
      2. Auditory expressive: ability to speak and express thought processes verbally.
      3. Visual receptive: ability to recognize, retain, and comprehend written language.
      4. Written expressive: ability to express thoughts graphically without motor impairment.
   H. Handedness:
      1. Right.   **2.** Left.
III. Cranial nerves.
   A. Olfactory: Test each nostril separately, using familiar odors such as coffee, tobacco, etc.
   B. Optic (refer to "Disorders of the Eye"):
      1. Visual acuity.
      2. Visual fields by confrontation.
      3. Fundoscopy.
         a. Condition of disk.   **b.** Condition of vasculature.
   C. Oculomotor (refer to "Disorders of the Ear"):
      1. Pupil constriction and accommodation.
      2. Symmetry and range of eye movements to upward, lateral, inward, and downward gaze.
      3. Nystagmus: oscillations of lateral gaze.
      4. Ptosis: lid droop.
   D. Trochlear (see point C, above).
   E. Trigeminal:
      1. Sensory response of:
         a. Cornea.
         b. Skin of face, anterior two-thirds of tongue, and teeth to tactile stimuli.
         c. Motor strength of muscles of mastication.
   F. Abducens (see point C, above).
   G. Facial:
      1. Sensory: response of anterior two-thirds of tongue.
      2. Motor: symmetry of face in exaggerated expressions.
   H. Acoustic (refer to "Disorders of the Ear"):
      1. Hearing.
         a. Bilateral acuity to auditory stimuli.
         b. Symmetrical response to vibrating tuning fork held midline on forehead (Rinne test).
         c. Whether air conduction of sound is better than bone is tested with a vibrating tuning fork (Webber test).
      2. Balance: vestibular function.
         a. Positional nystagmus.   **b.** Caloric testing.
   I. Glossopharyngeal:
      1. Sensory: response of posterior one-third of tongue to taste and tactile stimuli.
      2. Motor: gag reflex.
   J. Vagus: symmetry of movement of soft palate when pronouncing "ah."
   K. Accessory: muscle strength and bulk of trapezius and sternocleidomastoid muscles.
   L. Hypoglossal: midline protrusion of tongue without tremor.
IV. Motor function.
   A. Evaluate muscle groups of upper and lower extremities, left and right, for:
      1. Symmetry.   **3.** Tone.
      2. Strength.   **4.** Deep tendon reflexes.

V. Sensory function.
    A. Evaluate dermatomes (see Fig. 23-1): for response to:
        1. Pain (pinprick).
        2. Light touch (cotton).
        3. Position.
        4. Vibration (tuning fork).
        5. Temperature.
VI. Cerebellar function.
    A. Evaluate balance and coordination:
        1. Eye-hand (finger-to-nose test).
        2. Rapid alternating movement of hands and fingers.
        3. Tandem gait (heel-toe walking).
        4. Romberg test.

FIGURE 23-1 / **Cutaneous distribution of spinal nerves and dermatomes. (***From Stanley W. Jacob* **and** *Clarice Francone, Structure and Function in Man, W. B. Saunders Company, Philadelphia, 1965, p. 236.*****)**

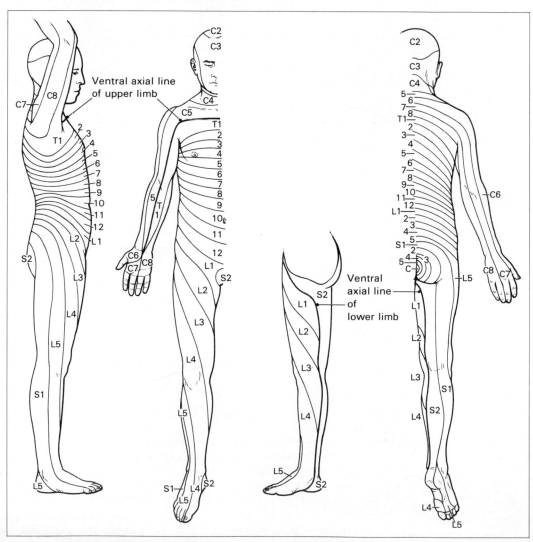

GENERAL DIAGNOSIS

  I. Alteration in comfort: discomfort secondary to pain, vertigo, gait change.
  II. Alteration in perception and coordination.
  III. Alteration in self-care activities, secondary to impaired motion.
  IV. Thought processes impaired: decreased ability to reason and make judgments.
  V. Self-concept: alteration in body image.
  VI. Alteration in nutrition: malnutrition due to loss of appetite, nausea, vomiting.
  VII. Impairment of mobility: limited range of motion, decreased muscle tone, decreased movement.
  VIII. Confusion: disorientation to person, place, time, etc.
  IX. Alteration in level of consciousness secondary to loss of consciousness.
  X. Alteration in body fluids: excess secondary to increased pulse volume, resulting in a change of mental state and/or edema.

TRAUMA

Injury to the Brain

DEFINITION
Under *trauma to the brain* are included those injuries resulting from the impact of physical force (see Fig. 23-2). *Concussion* is transient paralysis of nervous function secondary to a blow, without damage to cerebral structure. *Contusion* is bruising of the brain tissue secondary to trauma and characterized by coup and countercoup signs. *Coup* is bruising of the brain's surface at the site of injury. *Countercoup* is often more extensive and is the bruising and/or laceration on the side of the brain *opposing* the injury site. (Refer to Chap. 19 for a more detailed discussion of trauma to the brain, and refer to Chaps. 43 and 44 for a complete discussion of emergency care.)

ASSESSMENT
  I. Data sources.
     A. Patient.   *C.* Significant others.
     B. Family.   *D.* Past medical records.
  II. Health history.
     A. Stage of excitement, i.e., seeing stars.
     B. Transient decrease in mental clarity, i.e., loss of consciousness.
     C. Amnesia for impact.
  III. Physical assessment reveals:
     A. Suppression of pulse and respiration.
     B. Decreased muscle tone.
     C. Hyporeflexia.
     D. Concussion: absence of focal neurological signs. Contusion: focal neurologic signs related to area of brain damage, i.e., cranial nerve damage, hemiplegia, cerebellar disturbances, brainstem injury, convulsions.
  IV. Diagnostic tests: skull series may be needed.

DIAGNOSIS
Refer to "General Diagnosis."

GOALS OF CARE
  I. Prevent further injury to brain and spinal cord.
     A. Intervention:
        1. Maintain head and neck in fixed position, especially when transporting patient.
        2. Control any restlessness through quiet, reassurance, and sedation as ordered.

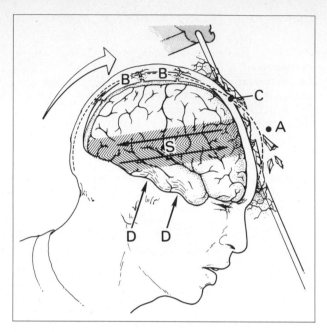

FIGURE 23-2 / Closed blunt injury of head. Skull molding occurs at site of impact. A, stippled line: preinjury contour. C, contour moments after impact with inbending at point A and outbending at vertex. B, subdural veins torn as brain rotates forward. S, shearing strains throughout brain. D, direct trauma to inferior temporal and frontal lobes over floors of middle and anterior fossa. (*From Sven G. Eliasson, Arthur L. Prensky, and William B. Hardin, Jr., Neurological Pathophysiology, Oxford University Press, New York, 1974, p. 293.*)

II. Prevent and control increased intracranial pressure (refer to Table 23-1).
    A. Assessment:
        1. Vomiting.   **5.** Decreased level of consciousness.
        2. Headache.   **6.** Increased systolic blood pressure.
        3. Papilledema.   **7.** Bradycardia.
        4. Pupillary changes.
    B. Intervention:
        1. Alert medical colleagues immediately.
        2. Administer steroids and osmotic diuretics such as mannitol and urea properly.
III. Provide adequate oxygenation of tissues.
    A. Intervention (refer to Chap. 27):
        1. Monitor respiratory function closely.
        2. Maintain airway by proper positioning; patient should be semisupine with head to one side and supported.
        3. Be prepared for tracheostomy and oxygen administration.
IV. Prevent compromise of cardiovascular system.
    A. Assessment (refer to Chap. 26):
        1. Observe skin color and temperature.
        2. Monitor pulse and ECG.
    B. Intervention:
        1. Control blood pressure.
        2. Identify and control hemorrhage from other injuries.
        3. Keep patient warm.

TABLE 23-1 / VITAL SIGNS: INCREASED INTRACRANIAL PRESSURE AND SHOCK

Vital Signs	Increased Intracranial Pressure	Shock
Blood pressure	Increased systolic, widening pulse pressure	Decreased
Pulse	Decrease in rate with initial bounding pulse	Increased
Respirations	May vary, look for trend and patterns, i.e., Cheyne-Stokes, hypoventilation, apneustic pattern (sustained contraction of inspiratory muscles), anoxia	

V. Prevent aspiration pneumonia (refer to Chap. 27).
 A. Assessment:
  1. Auscultate chest every 2 h.
  2. Monitor temperature.
  3. Observe quality of secretions for thick green-yellow mucus.
 B. Intervention:
  1. Drain secretions adequately by suction and chest therapy.
  2. Prevent accumulation of fluid by proper positioning and turning.
  3. Give proper tracheostomy care.
  4. Place nasogastric tube properly when feeding patient.
VI. Prevent pulmonary edema and emboli (refer to Chap. 26).
 A. Assessment:
  1. Auscultation and percussion of chest is necessary.
  2. Monitor respiratory rate and depth.
  3. Evaluate patient's complaints of pain to determine location, character, and radiation. Be alert for shortness of breath.
 B. Intervention:
  1. Proper positioning and turning is necessary.
  2. Adhere strictly to IV schedule.
VII. Promote normal fluid and electrolyte balance (refer to Chap. 28).
 A. Assessment:
  1. Observe relationship between intake and output carefully.
  2. The skin color and temperature indicate proper balance in hydration.
  3. The temperature, pulse, respiration, and blood pressure reflect the degree of fluid balance.
 B. Intervention:
  1. Provide nourishment for a comatose patient by intravenous and nasogastric routes.
  2. Assist a cooperative patient with food and fluid intake.
  3. Prevent urine retention by catheterization.
VIII. Optimal management of posttraumatic sequelae.
 A. Assessment:
  1. Watch for complaints of headache, giddiness, and evidence of emotional variability.
  2. Posttraumatic seizures may occur.
 B. Intervention:
  1. Control pain through adequate doses of medication.
  2. Encourage patient to express feelings and anxieties associated with injury.
  3. Provide adequate seizure control through medication.
  4. Educate patient regarding seizures.
  5. Consistently support and reassure patient during recuperation.

EVALUATION

Each goal must be measured against the baseline assessment performed and must then be reassessed at closely spaced intervals to determine success of interventions and to set new goals.

Injury to the Spinal Cord

DEFINITION

Spinal cord injury involves destruction of gray matter and hemorrhage secondary to compression of cord. It usually is caused by hyperflexion, hyperextension, abnormal rotation, or vertical compression. Areas most likely to be injured are the lower cervical spine (C4 to T1), and the thoracolumbar junction (T12 to L2).

Spinal shock involves the transient suppression of reflexes below the site of injury. Onset is usually within 30 to 60 min after trauma and gradually resolves, usually within 2 to 3 weeks, but the period may be as long as 3 years. (Refer to Chaps. 43 and 44 for a complete discussion of emergency care.)

ASSESSMENT

I. Data sources (refer to "Injury to the Brain").
II. Health history (refer to "General Assessment").
III. Physical assessment.
    A. Decreased temperature control.
    B. Decreased vasomotor tone.
    C. Decreased sweating.
    D. Urine retention.
    E. Fecal retention.
    F. Absent knee and ankle jerks.
    G. Plantar reflex variable or absent.
    H. Altered neurological responses, depending on the extent of injury.
IV. Diagnostic tests: determined by physiological changes by the extent of injury.

DIAGNOSIS

Refer to "General Diagnosis."

GOALS OF CARE

I. Immediate.
    A. Prevent further injury to spinal cord.
    B. Prevent respiratory and circulatory collapse.
        1. Assessment:
            a. Airway is patent.   *c.* Pulse is palpable.
            b. Respirations are detectable.   *d.* Note evidence of external hemorrhage.
        2. Intervention:
            a. Perform cardiopulmonary resuscitation.
            b. Control hemorrhage.
    C. Stabilization of injury. Whether medical or surgical intervention is used, nursing care will center around the subsequent immobilization of the patient.
        1. Intervention:
            a. Immobilize spinal column.
            b. Maintain position of the spinal column throughout examination, laboratory, and surgical procedures.
            c. The appropriate administration of steroids will control fluid extravasation in the spinal cord and will prevent traumatic necrosis.
    D. Maintain and support optimal respiratory function.
        1. Assessment: Level of injury will affect innervation and function of intercostal

muscles and diaphragm. A cervical injury will compromise respiratory function by interrupting diaphragmatic action. Thoracic nerves control intercostal muscles (see Fig. 23-3).

2. Intervention:
   a. Observe rate and depth of respirations.
   b. Observe symmetry of chest expansion.
   c. Assist respiration via respirator.

E. Maintain optimal drainage of secretions.
   1. Assessment: Immobility may prevent adequate drainage of secretions. Injury may interfere with normal protective mechanisms such as coughing. Pneumonia may thus complicate care.

FIGURE 23-3 / Lateral view of segments of origin of nerves supplying the limbs, diaphragm, bladder, bowel, and reproductive organs and the sympathetic outflow. A complete cord lesion above the double line causes quadriplegia; below, paraplegia. *[From J. H. Larrabee, "The Person with a Spinal Cord Injury: Physical Care during Early Recovery," American Journal of Nursing, 77(8): 1320, August 1977.]*

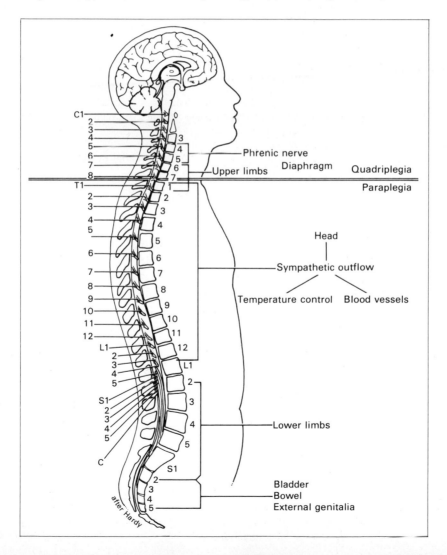

2. Intervention:
   a. Observe respirations.
   b. Observe body temperature.
   c. Regular auscultation and percussion of chest is necessary.
   d. Patient must be regularly turned within a supportive structure (e.g., Stryker frame).
   e. Ensure utilization of intermittent positive pressure breathing (IPPB) and chest therapy.
   f. Suction as necessary.
   g. Administer antibiotics appropriately.
3. Evaluation: The efficacy of acute-stage intervention should be measured against the goals of preventing further injury, stabilizing injury, and preparing for intermediate and rehabilitory stages.

II. Intermediate.
   A. Prevent complications due to metabolic disorders.
      1. Assessment: Stress of injury causes increased adrenocortical hormone production which conserves fats and glucose, utilizes protein, and causes a negative nitrogen balance. The results of anemia, decreased muscle mass and healing power, and resistance to infection leave the patient at risk for infection.
      2. Intervention:
         a. Monitor nitrogen balance through blood and urine analysis.
         b. Maintain nitrogen balance through protein supplements and protein-enriched diet.
   B. Prevent complications due to imbalance of calcium levels.
      1. Assessment: Immobilization leads to increased calcium levels in the blood, with a loss of calcium from bone. Problems which may result include pathological fractures and renal calculi.
      2. Intervention:
         a. Provide adequate hydration for optimal renal function.
         b. Regulate intake of calcium-rich foods.
         c. Promote early mobilization and weight bearing.
   C. Prevent complications due to bowel, bladder, and/or sexual dysfunction.
      1. Assessment:
         a. Interruptions of bowel and bladder function as well as sexual function are potential sources of infection, as well as barriers to the rebuilding of independence. All voluntary control over these functions is absent during the period of spinal shock.
         b. Automatic function: Reflex upper motor neuron control may return if the lesion is above the level of S2 to S4. Bowel and bladder retraining is possible, reflex sexual function may be present.
         c. Autonomic function: Lower motor neuron function is interrupted at the level of the lesion. If lesion is at the level of S2 to S4, there is no "reflex" activity, only sporadic organ response to distension. Retraining is not possible.
      2. Intervention:
         a. Straight catheterization is favored because it prevents reflux, causes less trauma to the urethral meatus, and simulates normal bladder filling and emptying, thus maintaining bladder tone.
         b. Indwelling catheters require scrupulous care to prevent infection:
            (1) A regular urine sample is collected for analysis and culture.
            (2) Utilize a closed drainage system, using gravity for collection.
            (3) The catheter must be secured appropriately to reduce meatal trauma.
            (4) Irrigate the bladder regularly.
            (5) Clamp and unclamp at regular intervals to maintain bladder tone.
         c. Promote fluid intake to improve both bowel and bladder functions.
         d. Encourage roughage in diet to improve bowel evacuation.
         e. Give stool softeners.

   f. Use suppositories, enemas, and digital evacuation to reduce fecal retention.

D. Prevent possible myocardial infarction and intracranial hemorrhage.

 1. Assessment: The patient recovering from a spinal cord injury is at risk for myocardial infarction or intracranial hemorrhage after spinal shock resolves.

  a. Autonomic dysreflexia is an abnormal response to sympathetic stimulation (usually due to bowel or bladder distension). It results in:

   (1) Disturbances of heat regulation such as flushing and sweating.

   (2) "Goose bumps."

   (3) Headache.

   (4) Postural hypotension.

   (5) Syncope.

  b. Autonomic hyperreflexia causes:

   (1) Severe, throbbing headache.

   (2) Abrupt rise in arterial blood pressure.

   (3) Bradycardia.

   (4) Flushing and sweating.

   (5) Nasal congestion.

   (6) Myocardial infarction or cerebral hemorrhage, if unchecked.

 2. Intervention:

  a. Provide adequate bowel and bladder evacuation to minimize risk of initiating the above sequence.

  b. Closely observe and report vital signs and symptoms of hyperreflexia.

  c. Protect body temperature by environmental control.

  d. Administer ganglion-blocking agents.

  e. Protect patient who has had surgical interruption of the reflex arc.

  f. Guard against syncope and postural hypotension through positioning.

  g. Provide patient and family with instruction in safeguards.

E. Prevent possible septicemia.

 1. Assessment: Immobilization, decreased sensory function, impaired circulation, and reduced healing power increase risk of septicemia secondary to skin breakdown and decubitus ulcers.

 2. Intervention:

  a. Keep skin clean and dry.

  b. Massage helps increase oxygenation.

  c. Use a positive pressure mattress.

  d. Turn patient every 2 h to avoid irreversible tissue change.

F. Prevent muscular complications.

 1. Assessment:

  a. Immobilization leads to contractures of muscle groups.

  b. After spinal shock the return of lower motor neuron activity may result in spasms.

  c. Medication may be useful in relieving spasms.

 2. Intervention:

  a. Range-of-motion exercises should be performed at regular intervals.

  b. Proper body alignment should be maintained through positioning and use of supports such as footboards.

G. Prevent psychologic complications.

 1. Assessment: The impact of the loss of body function is realized by the patient during this phase and a reaction which includes denial, anger, realization, and acceptance begins. In order to move through this process, patient and care providers must work together.

 2. Intervention:

  a. Assess patient's feelings: Allow expression of sadness, anger, and self-deprecation without recrimination.

  b. Assess personal and staff feelings through introspection, team conferences, and utilization of psychiatric consultations.

       c. Provide a trusting atmosphere through honesty and consistency. Limits should be agreed upon, set, and adhered to by all staff members.

       d. Reinforce the patient's ego by respecting his or her dignity, feelings, and privacy.

       e. Set short-term, attainable goals for emotional and physical gains.

    3. Evaluation: Progress is noted when the patient moves out of the crises of injury complications and is ready, in body and spirit, to devote energies to rehabilitation.

III. Long-term[1]: The patient will achieve maximum autonomy in setting goals and managing daily activities.

    A. Assessement:

       1. Achievement of independent bowel function restores dignity to the person and allows greater flexibility in social interaction.

       2. Physical and occupational therapy are essential in maximizing physical abilities. The role of these activities in bolstering self-esteem through realization of goals cannot be underplayed.

       3. As the patient moves toward greater physical and emotional autonomy, he or she will face more frustrations in meeting goals. As self-esteem improves, feelings may be expressed more easily. Expression of sexuality is tested.

    B. Intervention:

       1. Institute bowel retraining.

          a. Assess previous bowel habits for frequency, time of day, etc.

          b. Begin with a clean, unimpacted bowel.

          c. Provide a relaxed atmosphere.

          d. Diet should be high in roughage and fluids.

          e. If stool softeners or suppositories are to be used by the patient or family, instruction in proper use, side effects, and adverse reactions should be given.

       2. Coordinate activities of physical and occupational therapy and cooperate with the therapists in these specialties. Reinforce these activities during each shift. The nurse is the only care provider who has 24-h contact with the patient!

       3. Assess patient's feelings and allow expression without recrimination.

       4. Assess personal and staff feelings.

       5. Provide a trusting atmosphere through honesty and consistency.

       6. Incorporate family and friends into assessment of feelings and encourage their understanding and appropriate responses.

EVALUATION

I. Reassessment: close observation is essential as the patient's status may change rapidly.

II. Complications: contingent upon the level of injury (e.g., respiratory distress, renal disturbance).

ABNORMAL CELLULAR GROWTH

Brain Tumor

DEFINITION

Tumors of brain tissue vary according to the types of cells which are involved, in their predilections for areas of the brain, and in rates of growth. The brain may be the site of *either primary* or *metastatic* lesions. Tumor growth raises intracranial pressure and displaces surrounding brain tissue and vasculature. Diagnosis is made by evaluation of clinical and laboratory evidence.

ASSESSMENT

    I. Data sources (refer to "Injury to the Brain").

---

[1] The author does not attempt to condense the great range of rehabilitative nursing, but only to touch on the major points.

II. The health history usually reveals a gradual onset of symptoms.
- **A.** A decrease in mental function, or change in general behavior may be noted by the family.
- **B.** The onset of seizures in adulthood without a history of trauma is usually a symptom of tumor.

III. Signs revealed in physical assessment that heighten suspicion of a tumor include gradual changes in the neurologic assessment, particularly in mental status, and evidence of increased intracranial pressure as in papilledema.

IV. Diagnostic tests: Computerized axial tomography (CAT scan) is a noninvasive test which provides an accurate scheme of cerebral structure and density. The scan may be performed without hospitalization or involved patient preparation, and may be repeated easily to provide current information.

DIAGNOSIS
Refer to "General Diagnosis."

GOALS OF CARE
I. Symptomatic and diagnostic.
- **A.** Establish an accurate data base from which all changes may be evaluated.
    1. Assessment: Obtain a detailed history with thorough clinical information from a complete neurologic exam.
    2. Intervention: Prepare patient physically and emotionally for diagnostic procedures.
- **B.** Establish a trusting relationship between patient and care providers. A person with a suspected tumor is at the beginning of a long and often stressful relationship with the health care system.
    1. Assessment: Determine the impact of symptoms, diagnostic possibilities, and procedures on patient and family.
    2. Intervention:
        - *a.* Provide an opportunity for expression of feelings, anxieties, and fears.
        - *b.* Provide accurate information without false assurances that "everything will be okay."
        - *c.* Expedite waiting times between procedures.
- **C.** Enable patient to cope with anxiety.
    1. Assessment: Anxieties are often demonstrated by patient doubting the expertise of nurses, physicians, and technicians.
    2. Intervention:
        - *a.* Keep in mind that such doubts are based on anxieties, and also that the patient's trust must be earned, not taken for granted.
        - *b.* Patient-nurse interaction should be consistent in communications, and in the provision of physical assessment and care.
- **D.** Prevent seizures.
    1. Assessment: Seizures, either focal or generalized, are often present as the tumor growth disrupts normal neuronal function.
    2. Intervention:
        - *a.* Observe for complaints of focal seizures such as tingling, visual disturbances, temporal lobe phenomena, or olfactory hallucinations.
        - *b.* Report such symptoms to the medical team.
        - *c.* Administer medication for seizure control prophylactically, and therapeutically in the event of a generalized seizure.
        - *d.* Teach patient and family the rationale for medication as well as safeguards.
- **E.** Allow for changes in mental function and behavior.
    1. Assessment: Changes in mental function or general behavior may accompany tumor growth.
    2. Intervention:
        - *a.* Frequent, regular assessment of these factors must include information coming from patient, and often family.

   b. Protect patient from mishap. Assist in securing adequate care at home or in institution.
F. Allow for changes in sensorimotor function.
   1. Assessment:
      a. Tumor growth may impair cranial nerve function depending on the site and affect vision, hearing, vestibular function, facial sensation and pain, eye movements, swallow, and gag response.
      b. All other aspects of neuronal function, such as motor, sensory, and cerebellar modes may be affected by the tumor.
   2. Intervention:
      a. Assess the degree of impairment associated with each symptom.
      b. Protect patient against falling, choking, hitting unseen objects or tripping, and dizziness (i.e., use eye patch for double vision).
      c. Treat head and facial pain adequately.
      d. Provide physical and emotional support to alleviate symptoms and protect the patient.
      e. Report each new symptom and accompanying signs promptly and accurately.
   3. Evaluation: The observation of symptoms, the character, intensity, onset, and course, as well as accompanying signs, is measured against baseline assessment to provide data for determining tumor nature and growth. The amelioration of the symptoms becomes more likely when an accurate diagnosis can be made and therapy instituted.
II. Therapeutic stage.
   A. Alleviate and contain increased intracranial pressure. Early diagnosis and intervention of increased intracranial pressure can prevent irreversible brain damage.
      1. Assessment:
         a. Tumor growth causes increased intracranial pressure by displacing normal tissue and vasculature, and by obstructing the flow of cerebrospinal fluid (hydrocephalus.) The symptoms of brain tumor are the end products of the resultant tissue hypoxia. While the rates of onset of these symptoms may vary, the development of signs of increased intracranial pressure should alert the nurse to the need for precise monitoring of intracranial and arterial pressure.
         b. Signs: decreased level of consciousness, pupillary dilatation and loss of light reflex, paresis, increased systolic blood pressure, widened pulse pressure, slow pulse.
      2. Intervention:
         a. Monitor intracranial pressure:
            (1) Set alarm for appropriate pressure (mmHg), as prescribed.
            (2) Maintain sterility of attachment site.
            (3) Prevent excessive cerebrospinal fluid loss.
            (4) Obtain cerebrospinal fluid specimens for sugar, protein, and culture and sensitivity.
            (5) Zero balance equipment at least every 4 h.
            (6) Maintain cannula in place, and transducer in the foramen of Monroe.
            (7) Alert physician to any changes in waveform, or for signs of sudden increase in pressure.
         b. Monitor intraarterial pressure accurately.
         c. Monitor ECG.
         d. Monitor EEG.
         e. Monitor pulse, respiration, and temperature.
         f. Administer osmotic diuretics as ordered:
            (1) Catheterize to accommodate rapid diuresis, and measure urine output.
            (2) Monitor electrolytes.
         g. Assist respiration with respirator as indicated.
         h. Prevent shivering and frostbite during hypothermia therapy.

i. Administer steroids as ordered; prevent gastric irritation by using antacids.
3. Evaluation:
   a. The acute phase, or onset of increased intracranial pressure, is evaluated through the constant monitoring of the above-mentioned parameters. Ongoing assurance of accuracy should be developed and implemented for all team members.
   b. Continuing care of increased intracranial pressure requires periodic neurologic examination, with special emphasis on observation for signs of changing pressure (see "General Assessment").

B. Management of postoperative care.
1. Detect increased intracranial pressure (due to hemorrhage and/or cerebral edema) early.
   a. Assessment:
      (1) Determine level of consciousness.
      (2) Monitor pupillary signs (watch for dilatation with loss of light reflex on side of increased intracranial pressure).
      (3) Note movement and strength of extremities.
      (4) Vital signs (refer to Table 23-1).
   b. Intervention:
      (1) Report signs of increased intracranial pressure to neurosurgeon immediately.
      (2) Position patient appropriately in bed.
         (a) For infratentorial lesions, patient should be flat in bed with head stabilized.
         (b) For supratentorial lesions, place patient in a semi-forward position with head in appropriate position to maintain patent airway and adequate ventilation.
      (3) Possible steroid therapy may be accompanied by antacid medications to decrease gastric irritation.
      (4) Restrict fluids (1500 mL in first 24 h or 70 mL/h).
      (5) Mannitol may be administered (osmotic diuretic) in continuous drip or bolus for rapid diuretic effect. Measure output hourly.
2. Maintain adequate ventilation:
   a. Assessment: Observe respiratory rate and levels of blood gases.
   b. Intervention:
      (1) Maintain a position which will facilitate adequate ventilation.
      (2) Deep breathing should be encouraged frequently.
      (3) Turn patient every 2 h.
      (4) Endotracheal tube may be used, or oxygen therapy.
3. Maintain fluid and electrolyte balance.
   a. Assessment:
      (1) Daily electrolytes.
      (2) Intake and output.
      (3) Urine specific gravity.
      (4) With pituitary tumor surgery, observe for signs of diabetes insipidus.
   b. Intervention:
      (1) Replace electrolytes.
      (2) Use Foley catheter.
      (3) A vasopressor may be administered.
4. Prevent musculoskeletal complications (contractures).
   a. Assessment:
      (1) Check ability to move joints voluntarily through range-of-motion exercises.
      (2) Note skin integrity, turgor, moisture, and color.
   b. Intervention:
      (1) Perform range-of-motion exercises for all extremities at least twice daily.

        (2) Care for skin.

        (3) Turn patient every 2 h.

   5. Prevent infection.

     a. Assessment:

        (1) Observe for signs of infection at surgical site.

        (2) If a drain is used, observe for patency and nature of drainage.

        (3) Observe for increased temperature.

     b. Intervention:

        (1) Maintain sterile technique in changing dressing.

        (2) Medication specific to the type of infection present may be administered.

C. Optimize benefits of radiation therapy in arresting tumor growth.

   1. Assessment: Radiation therapy is a team process by which a patient undergoes a series of exposures to doses of radiation carefully calculated to enhance the effect of total therapy.

   2. Intervention:

     a. Have firsthand knowledge of the radiation equipment and a working rapport with the radiotherapists and technicians.

     b. Know the course of treatment and dose recommended for the patient.

     c. Assess patient's and family's feelings and understanding of the therapy and side effects.

     d. Be able to give an accurate description of the radiotherapy.

     e. Assess effects of treatment with each contact with patient, and measure physical and emotional parameters.

     f. Provide care for physical and emotional needs.

     g. Coordinate support services within the institution as well as through community agencies.

D. Optimize effects of chemotherapy while protecting patient from side effects and minimizing complications.

   1. Assessment: Chemotherapeutic cancer agents act by interfering in the reproduction of, or by destroying, rapidly proliferating cells. These include not only the malignant cells, but also red blood cells, white cells, and platelets. Due to the reduction of these normal cells the patient receiving chemotherapy is at risk for:

     a. Anemia.   *e.* Nephrotoxicity.

     b. Infection.   *f.* Cardiopulmonary toxicity.

     c. Bleeding.   *g.* Alopecia.

     d. Neurotoxicity.

   2. Intervention:

     a. Anemia:

        (1) Frequent blood counts are obtained and blood count is monitored.

        (2) Provide dietary supplements.

     b. Infection:

        (1) Know the peripheral white count. This is an indicator of the patient's resources to fight infection.

        (2) Examine skin daily for interruption of integrity and signs of inflammation.

        (3) Obtain temperature every 4 h.

        (4) Guard against infection from contamination of venipuncture technique.

     c. Bleeding. Inspect potential bleeding sites:

        (1) Skin.

        (2) Mucous membrane orifices.

        (3) Urine.

        (4) Stool; watch for occult blood.

     d. Neurotoxicity:

        (1) Assess changes in behavior and activity level.

        (2) Assess gait, coordination, bowel, and bladder function.

        (3) Report evidence of toxicity promptly.

    e. Nephrotoxicity:
       (1) Measure urine output.
       (2) Obtain analyses of urine daily.
       (3) Obtain cultures and sensitivities.
       (4) Maintain adequate hydration through oral or intravenous routes.
    f. Cardiopulmonary toxicity:
       (1) Monitor pulse and respiration closely.
       (2) Monitor neurotoxicity closely to prevent pulmonary edema.
    g. Alopecia (loss of hair): It may be beneficial to warn patient of this possibility. It is very important to provide support when it occurs.

  3. Evaluation: The triad of surgical, radiation, and chemical therapy is evaluated by the elimination of the tumor, or by reduction in its size and by its arrest. Nursing care should be evaluated along these parameters as well:
    a. There is prompt identification and management of untoward or toxic effects of therapy.
    b. The patient cooperates and complies with treatment regimen.
    c. Patient care providers work as a team.

E. Maintain ego of patient during therapeutic intervention.
  1. Assessment: The patient with a brain tumor is likely to experience valid fears regarding the diagnosis and prognosis of the disease process, and of changes in body image and possible loss of function, either resulting from the cancer or the treatment.
  2. Intervention:
    a. The nurse must be aware of his or her own feelings about this disease, and be able to express them in a supportive setting.
    b. Assist the patient in expressing anger, fear, frustration, or sadness.
    c. Provide accurate information to patient and family, and give realistic reassurance during moments of stress and doubt.
    d. Help patient utilize support services as needed, either spiritual, psychiatric, or social.
    e. Plan for continuity of care with family, utilizing occupational and community resources.
  3. Evaluation: While this area is very subjective, the key to evaluating the patient's emotional status rests in:
    a. Knowing the patient.
    b. Keeping the person progressing through emotional stresses rather than becoming trapped by each new problem.
    c. Keeping the care team appropriately involved without personalizing the patient's situation.

III. Follow-up care: Maintain an optimum level of functioning for the greatest length of time.
  A. Assessment: Frequent, thorough neurologic examinations and emotional status interviews will provide data to compare with baseline status, and degree of function present at end of the treatment regime.
  B. Intervention:
    1. Report any changes from previous assessments to medical team and appropriate specialists.
    2. Control seizures and other neurologic impairments.
    3. Reinforce emotional support as provided during previous stages.
    4. Reevaluate and enlist other resources among colleagues, patient's family, and community for occupational and physical rehabilitation.

IV. Palliative stage: Reduce physical discomfort and foster as good a mental adjustment as is possible to the loss of function and death.
  A. Assessment:
    1. Physical and emotional evaluations continue to be made.

    2. Providers agree that the patient has reached this stage.

    3. Patient and family agree that patient has reached this stage.

  B. Intervention:

    1. Provide for a safe environment where loss of function can be managed yet patient's independence can be maintained as long as possible. This might be at home, in an acute-care, or long-term care facility.

    2. Provide sufficient medication to treat pain, somatic complaints, and emotional symptoms if indicated.

    3. Maintain optimal nutrition.

    4. Help patient and family express feelings, plan care, and begin grieving process.

    5. Aid person in the utilization of spiritual and legal advice if sought.

    6. The staff must also be encouraged to express their feelings in an appropriate setting.

Spinal Cord Tumor

DEFINITION

A *spinal cord tumor* causes symptoms by compressing the cord. It may obstruct the cerebrospinal fluid. Tumors of the cord may be *intramedullary* or *extramedullary*; the latter is further categorized as either *intradural* or *extradural*. Of these, the extradural occur most frequently and are most successfully treated by surgery. Intramedullary tumors may also be treated surgically, either by laminectomy and decompression, or marsupialization. Radiation is a useful adjunct to surgical therapy and is the principal mode of treatment for intradural lesions. (Refer to Chap. 19 for further discussion.)

ASSESSMENT

  I. Data sources (refer to "Injury to the Brain").

 II. Health history.

  A. Radicular pain exists which radiates distally and is intensified by coughing, sneezing, and straining.

  B. The sensorimotor impairment is often asymmetrical, beginning with motor loss and atrophy of the muscles most distal from lesion.

III. Physical assessment.

  A. The sensory changes are distributed segmentally.

  B. Hypalgesia to pain and touch is contralateral to greatest motor loss (Brown-Sequard syndrome).

  C. There are changes in muscle strength, bulk, and in reflexes below the level of lesion.

  D. There are changes in autonomic function below level of lesion.

  E. There is local tenderness on palpation of spinal column.

IV. Diagnostic tests.

DIAGNOSIS

Refer to "General Diagnosis."

  A. Radiographic studies, including myelography.

  B. Electromyography.

GOALS OF CARE

  I. Management of problems relating to impaired function.

  A. Assessment: Initial neurologic assessment should be the baseline against which future assessments are measured.

  B. Intervention:

    1. Protect patient from cuts, burns, and secondary infection which might result from lowered appreciation of pain and temperature.

2. Assist patient with tasks which become difficult to perform secondary to motor loss:
   - a. Dressing.
   - b. Personal hygiene.
   - c. Eating.
   - d. Ambulation.
3. Assist patient and family in making adjustments in normal activities to be able to perform as many of these tasks as possible independently.
4. Provide assistance with respiration, and bowel and bladder elimination if affected by tumor (see "Injury to the Spinal Cord").
5. Provide emotional support during progressive loss of function (see "Brain Tumor").

C. Evaluation: Success of nursing intervention depends on the effect of medical, surgical, and radiation therapy. While patients should always be maintained at an optimum level of functioning, those with a favorable prognosis should demonstrate improvement and move toward rehabilitation. The patient whose tumor is not cured will have to cope with successive losses in function. In either case, function should always be measured against the baseline assessment, and the care plan revised to meet new needs.

II. Management of pain.
A. Assessment: Pain is a major problem for the patient with a spinal cord tumor and the appropriate management is largely a nursing responsibility.
1. The subjective perception of pain by the patient is influenced by culture and experience. Pain is a signal of danger to the body, and activates fears of body change and death. To the patient already racked by illness and loss of self-esteem, it may increase fears of rejection and loneliness.
2. The nursing assessment of pain will be greatly influenced by the attitude of individual care providers as well as that of the institution. Failure to effect a cure may be interpreted as total failure. Nurses need to evaluate their own feelings and know how these feelings influence care.
3. Each complaint of pain should be evaluated individually, and not assumed to be caused by the tumor.
4. Parameters by which pain is measured include:
   - a. Location.
   - b. Quality.
   - c. Severity.
   - d. Alleviating and aggravating factors.
   - e. Waxing and waning qualities.
   - f. Radiation.

B. Intervention:
1. Listening to description of pain, eliciting a history, and staying with the patient demonstrates interest, sympathy, and competence.
2. Treat each type of pain according to its character and severity.
3. Involve the patient in planning medication and setting priorities. This reinforces the patient's self-esteem, and may reduce some of the authoritarian role of the nurse in dispensing medication.
4. Once limits are established, there should be consistency in the management. Good communication among staff members is essential for this to be accomplished.
5. Prevent aggravation of pain by exercising care during treatment procedures.
6. Prevent development of new pain through maintenance of optimal function:
   - a. Body alignment.
   - b. Skin care.
   - c. Nutrition.
   - d. Elimination of body wastes.
7. Regularly assess perception of pain by the patient and act to assure continued care, understanding, and pain relief.
8. Help family understand the patient's pain, and encourage them to express their feelings.

C. Evaluation: Successful pain therapy should allow patients to maintain as much normal mental and physical function as possible while avoiding undesirable side effects. It should also allow the nursing staff and families to give care sympathetically and without guilt.

OBSTRUCTIONS

Cerebrovascular Accidents

DEFINITION
A *cerebrovascular accident* is an infarction of brain tissue which results when the cerebral blood flow is interrupted by thrombus or embolus occlusion or by hemorrhage (see Table 23-2). (Refer to Chap. 43 for discussion of emergency care, and refer to Chap. 42 for discussion of cerebrovascular accidents in relation to the aged.)

ASSESSMENT
Refer to "General Assessment."

DIAGNOSIS
Refer to "General Diagnosis."

GOALS OF CARE
I. Preserve life in the comatose patient.
  A. Assessment:
    1. Ability to react to name.
    2. Ability to withdraw from painful stimuli.
    3. Rate, rhythm, and depth of respiration.
    4. Pupillary response.
    5. Range of ocular movements.
    6. Position and posturing:
       a. Decerebrate rigidity.
       b. Decorticate rigidity.
       c. Diagonal posturing.
       d. Absence of posturing and movement.
  B. Intervention:
    1. Maintain open airway.
       a. Keep patient in a lateral position.
       b. Utilize an endotracheal tube.
       c. A respirator may be needed.
       d. Suction as necessary.
    2. Assist in regulation of body temperature.
    3. Prevent bladder distension by catheterization.
    4. Maintain fluid and electrolyte balance.
       a. Administer intravenous fluid.
       b. Feed by nasogastric tube.
    5. Prevent aspiration pneumonitis.
       a. Place patient in lateral position.
       b. Suction.
       c. Auscultate chest.
       d. Observe respiration.
    6. Prevent complications of bed rest:
       a. Observe extremities daily for signs of thrombophlebitis.
       b. Provide optimal skin care.
  C. Evaluation: Compare assessment factors against baseline continuously.
II. Assist in identifying factors that may have contributed to the stroke. This is basic to the institution of appropriate measures to halt progressive losses and restore circulation.
  A. Assessment:
    1. Health history (see Table 23-2).
    2. Physical assessment: identification of common stroke syndromes (see Table 23-3).
    3. Laboratory tests (see Table 23-4).
       a. Arteriography.
       b. Computerized axial tomography.

    B. Intervention:
        1. Provide appropriate nursing care during preparation and execution of procedures.
        2. Provide adequate and accurate information about procedure to patient and family.
        3. Assess for discomfort and side effects after arteriography and spinal tap and provide analgesics.
III. Restore circulation in the patient with a stroke due to occlusion.
    A. Assessment: Maintaining adequate blood flow to the brain is incumbent upon adequate systolic blood pressure. Positioning affects the blood pressure.
    B. Intervention:
        1. Observe and record the systolic blood pressure regularly.
        2. Horizontal bed rest for 7 to 10 days is necessary.
        3. Elevate foot of bed 14 in.
        4. Arising should be done slowly and for short periods of time at first. Patient should not be left alone.
IV. Prevent further occlusion.
    A. Assessment: Anticoagulation is useful to prevent further occlusion.
    B. Intervention:
        1. Administer heparin, Coumadin, or aspirin as directed.
        2. Observe for bleeding.
        3. Monitor prothrombin time daily.
V. Decrease need for oxygen.
    A. Assessment: Circulation is enhanced by decreasing the body's need for oxygen.
    B. Intervention: Induce hypothermia:
        1. Protect patient from frostbite.
        2. Monitor cardiac status for arrhythmias.
        3. Control shivering.

TABLE 23-2 / CEREBROVASCULAR ACCIDENTS: DEFINITIONS AND MODES OF ONSET

| | *Occlusion* | | |
	Thrombosis	*Embolism*	*Hemorrhage*
Definition	Cerebral ischemia caused by occlusion of cerebral arterial lumen		Extravasation of blood into cerebral tissue. This may be intracerebral or subarachnoid, and may be caused by hypertension, ruptured aneurysm, or ruptured arteriovenous malformation (angioma)
	Atherosclerotic thrombus which originates in cerebral vessels and is aggravated by hypertension	Thrombus carried to cerebral vessels from diseased heart.*	
Significant history	Transient ischemic attacks precede complete occlusion	Cardiac surgery, valvular disease, inadequate anticoagulation	Angiomas may produce focal seizures in late childhood or adulthood
Warning Prodrome	Transient ischemic attacks Headache not uncommon	None Headache not uncommon	None Characterized by severe headache
Time of day	Occurs during sleep or on arising	Often when getting up to void at night	Uncommon during sleep, usually with activity and exertion
Progression	Intermittent, uneven	Most rapid; several seconds to minutes	Gradual and steady, up to 24 h.

*Cardiac diseases which may generate a thrombus include valvular disease, valvoplasty, inadequate anticoagulation after cardiac surgery, endocarditis, myocardial infarction, and cardiovascular atherosclerosis.

TABLE 23-3 / CARDIOVASCULAR ACCIDENTS: COMMON SYNDROMES

Occlusion	

Internal carotid artery and branches (all of some of these deficits may be present):
    Contralateral hemiparesis
    Contralateral hemianesthesia
    Contralateral visual field
      deficit
    Homonymous hemianopsia
    Impaired language function with
      dominant side involvement
    Memory loss
	Vertebral or basilar artery (all or some of these deficits may be present):
	    Cranial nerve deficits
	      Diplopia
	      Disarthria
	      Visual field losses
	      Dysphagia
	      Hiccoughs
	    Cerebellar deficits
	      Ataxia
	    Cortical tracts
	      Contralateral motor loss
	      Contralateral sensory losses

Hemorrhage	

Intracerebral (hypertensive):
    Putamenal: eyes deviated away from lesion, hemiparesis, hemianesthesia, aphasia, altered consciousness
    Thalamic: eyes downward, pupils unreactive, hemiplegia, hemiparesis, aphasia or mutism, neck retraction
    Pontine: eyes fixed, pupils tiny and reactive, rapid coma, quadriplegia, decerebrate rigidity, death
    Cerebellar: eyes deviated laterally, no paralysis, occurs over hours, occipital headache, vertigo, vomiting, inability to walk or stand, brainstem compression evidenced by coma
	Subarachnoid (ruptured aneurysm):
	    Violent headaches, alterations in level of consciousness from alert to coma, nuchal rigidity, absence of lateralizing signs

TABLE 23-4 / CEREBROVASCULAR ACCIDENTS: CEREBROSPINAL FLUID CHARACTERISTICS

	Thrombosis	Embolism	Hemorrhage
Appearance	Clear to faint xanthochromia	Clear to slight xanthochromia	Usually bloody, deep xanthochromia*
RBC count	None	May be grossly bloody, up to 10,000 per cubic millimeter	As low as 200–400 per cubic millimeter Slight hemorrhage, but as high as 1 million per cubic millimeter
WBC count	Slight increase in leukocytes	Up to 200 per cubic millimeter if septic embolism	Leukocytosis within 24 h
Protein	Frequently raised	Elevated if septic	4 mg per 100 mL rise per 5000 RBC†

*Differentiated from traumatic tap by maintaining xanthochromia with each sample.
† M. Blount, A. B. Kinney, and K. M. Donohoe, "Analyzing Cerebrospinal Fluid," *Nursing Clinics of North America,* **9**(4):606–607, December 1974.
Source: C. Miller Fisher, Jay P. Mohr, and Raymond D. Adams, "Cerebrovascular Diseases," in M. M. Wintrobe et al. (eds.), *Harrison's Principles of Internal Medicine,* 7th ed., McGraw-Hill Book Company, New York, 1974, pp. 1743–1780.

VI. Prevent hypertension from developing.
   A. Assessment: Hypertension is the major aggravating factor in precipitating stroke due to thrombus.
   B. Intervention:
      1. Monitor blood pressure closely.
      2. Administer appropriate hypotensive therapeutic agents.
      3. Teach the patient the importance of blood pressure controls.
      4. Explore with the patient and family possible changes in life-style to enhance effect of drug therapy.
VII. Assess for underlying cardiac disease.
   A. Assessment: Underlying cardiac disease is the major factor in precipitating embolic stroke.
   B. Intervention:
      1. Identify and treat cardiovascular atheroscleroses.
      2. Maintain adequate anticoagulation therapy after cardiac surgery. Observe for bleeding.
      3. Treat subacute and chronic bacterial endocarditis (refer to Chap. 26).
      4. Identify and correct valvular disease.
      5. Teach patient about anticoagulant therapy and potential bleeding.
   C. Evaluation: Adequate management of these causative problems should reduce risk of further stroke.
      1. Establish regular evaluation of blood pressure.
      2. Regular evaluation of cardiac status, including anticoagulation as needed.
      3. Because the regulation of these problems necessitates a great deal of understanding and cooperation on the part of the patient, the nurse must serve both an educative and counseling role to evaluate and optimize compliance.
VIII. Provide physical and emotional support for the patient who is a candidate for endarterectomy or bypass grafting.
   A. Assessment: Transient ischemic attacks (TIAs) are an indication of atherosclerotic disease, and often precede complete arterial occlusion. When the site of the lesion has been identified, surgical intervention may take place to prevent a stroke.
   B. Intervention:
      1. Assist the patient throughout diagnostic examinations.
      2. Provide emotional support for patient. Patients who have undergone TIAs and cerebrovascular accidents may experience emotional outbursts that are unpredictable and uncomfortable for the patients.
      3. Maintain an accurate record of TIAs, including symptoms the patient experiences, and signs which may be found on neurologic examination.
      4. Stabilize blood pressure.
      5. Prepare patient and family for surgery.
      6. Postoperative care includes:
         a. Patent airway maintenance.
         b. Maintaining adequate circulation and prevention of hemorrhage.
         c. Fluid and electrolyte balance.
         d. Care of the surgical incision.
         e. Providing comfort and support.
         f. Assessing patient's symptoms and complaints.
   C. Evaluation:
      1. Vital signs are stabilized.
      2. There is cessation of TIAs.
      3. Patient gradually returns to normal activity.
IX. Educate patient about need to monitor blood pressure.
   A. Assessment: The prevention of further occlusion is also dependent upon the ability of the patient to control his or her blood pressure.

      B. Intervention:

        1. Determine the patient's and family's understanding of role of hypertension and diet.

        2. Develop with patient a plan for drug therapy, diet, and activity.

      C. Evaluation:

        1. Regular and frequent meetings with patient are necessary to assess blood pressure, neurologic, and emotional status.

        2. Be available for any questions or problems. Serve as a link to primary physician for prompt intervention.

X. Restore circulation in the patient with a stroke due to hemorrhage.

    A. Assessment: Controlling arterial blood pressure is essential to check hemorrhage.

    B. Intervention:

      1. Administer antihypertensive agents properly, without inducing hypotension.

      2. Maintain bed rest for 4 to 8 weeks after initial hemorrhage.

      3. Minimize occasions which increase emotional stress.

      4. Provide emotional support for patient and family.

      5. Administer sedatives and relaxants.

XI. Decrease intracranial pressure.

    A. Assessment: Intracranial pressure may be elevated.

    B. Intervention:

      1. Monitor and control intracranial pressure.

      2. Restrict activities which might increase intracranial pressure:

        a. Provide stool softeners to prevent straining with bowel movements and obviate need for enemas.

        b. Treat nausea and vomiting.

        c. Support optimal respiratory function.

      3. Promote venous drainage by elevating head of the bed 15 to 20°.

XII. Maintain fluid balance.

    A. Assessment: Adequate fluid balance must be maintained for the patient.

    B. Intervention:

      1. Administer and monitor intravenous therapy.

      2. Monitor urinary output and catheterize patient as necessary.

      3. Work with the dietician to plan meals which will be appetizing as well as nutritious.

      4. As the patient is usually fed by someone, try to provide an unhurried and pleasant atmosphere, anticipating needs and minimizing the obvious dependency.

    C. Evaluation: The greatest danger in intracranial hemorrhage due to a ruptured aneurysm is the recurrent bleeding immediately following the initial event. Of the ruptured angiomas which are not fatal, there is always a danger of subsequent bleeding. Evaluation of care following intracerebral hemorrhage is thus based on successful control of arterial blood pressure and intracranial pressure to stabilize the patient for surgical intervention.

XIII. Identify and treat ruptured angioma or aneurysm as source of seizure.

    A. Assessment:

      1. Seizures may be part of the symptoms of an angioma, or they may develop after bleeding from either a ruptured aneurysm or angioma.

      2. The patient is assessed for surgical treatment of the aneurysm by determining his or her status at the time of the initial bleeding episode; then the degree of stabilization achieved is evaluated.

        a. Factors evaluated include:

          (1) Level of consciousness.

          (2) Pupil size and reaction to light.

          (3) Arterial blood pressure.

          (4) Pulse: rate and rhythm.

(5) Respiration (deep/shallow, quiet/labored).

(6) Temperature (elevated or within normal limits).

  b. Surgical treatment.

  (1) Aneurysms:

(a) Extracranial: ligation of common carotid artery in the neck.

(b) Intracranial: resection of aneurysm, ligation of neck of aneurysm, wrapping or trapping of aneurysm.

  (2) Angiomas: block dissection if size and location permit.

B. Intervention:

1. Immediate.

   a. Administer anticonvulsive agents and evaluate effectiveness.

   b. Teach patient how to manage seizure control.

   c. Protect patient in the event of seizure.

2. Preoperative.

   a. Stabilize blood pressure and intracranial pressure as directed in previous discussion.

   b. Induce hypothermia, if ordered, protecting patient from frostbite and shivering. Monitor ECG.

   c. Prepar patient and family for surgical intervention.

3. Postoperative.

   a. Monitor vital signs and support vital functions:

   (1) Airway is open.   **(3)** Regulate temperature.

   (2) Ensure adequate ventilation.   **(4)** Arterial blood pressure is normal.

   b. Monitor and control intracranial pressure.

   c. Utilize sterile technique in wound care and observe for cerebrospinal fluid leakage.

   d. Provide safeguards for the patient with a diminished level of consciousness.

   e. Provide medication and teaching regarding seizure control.

   f. Maintain fluids and electrolytes, and monitor endocrine function for diabetes insipidus.

   g. Measure patient's neurological status and communicate changes to physician accurately.

   h. Provide counseling and support to patient and family.

   i. Assist in planning resumption of normal daily activity as well as assessing potential realistically.

   j. Discuss specific care plans with continuing care providers.

C. Evaluation: The success of surgical procedure varies, but hopefully the patient may be able to return to a normal life-style. Care should be evaluated against:

1. The neurological status as measured after hemorrhage, and after surgery.

2. The changing needs which arise over the course of convalescence and rehabilitation.

XIV. Manage patient with cranial nerve deficits.

A. Assessment: Strokes may commonly cause hemianopsia, facial nerve, and sixth nerve palsies.

B. Intervention:

1. Hemianopsia:

   a. Place objects within field of vision, especially food and utensils.

   b. Approach patient from uninvolved side.

   c. Position patient so that windows, activity, television, etc., are within his or her visual field.

2. Eating difficulties:

   a. Place food which must be chewed on uninvolved side of mouth.

   b. After patient has eaten, check to see that food is not lodged on affected side of mouth.

   c. Provide optimal oral hygiene.

        d. Assess ability to use dentures, and see that utilization is optimal. Refit if necessary.

    3. Ptosis:

        a. Prop weak eyelid open with nonallergenic tape.

        b. Instill artificial tears to protect cornea.

C. Evaluation: Measurement of cranial nerve function is outlined in the section on the neurological exam. The patient who has a stroke should have those tests of function of involved nerves repeated regularly to determine improvement or deterioration. Because language disorders often accompany these deficits, the patient cannot easily communicate discomfort or diminished ability, and one must rely on objective findings more than volunteered information.

XV. Manage patient with hemianesthesia to protect him or her from injury.

A. Assessment: Decreased sensory perception is measured by response to stimuli of pain, touch, temperature, positional changes, and vibration. Inability to recognize or respond to stimuli leaves the patient vulnerable to skin breakdown, burns, and secondary infection.

B. Intervention:

    1. Provide optimal skin care: Use massage and protective lotions.

    2. Do not allow patient to rest in linens or clothing soiled by urine or feces.

    3. Help the patient manage hot liquids.

    4. Inspect total skin surface for evidence of breakdown.

    5. Protect against pressure from infrequent changes in position.

    6. Treat pressure ulcers, burns, lacerations and irritations promptly.

C. Evaluation:

    1. Reassess sensory function at regular intervals.

    2. Skin integrity is maintained.

    3. Previously acquired pressure ulcers heal.

XVI. Manage patient with hemiparesis to obtain optimal function and prevent secondary disability or deformity.

A. Assessment: Determine muscle strength, tone, and bulk as described under "General Assessment." The patient with hemiparesis must be protected against trauma to involved limbs, contractures, pressure sores, and pneumonia secondary to immobility.

B. Intervention:

    1. Change position at regular and brief intervals.

    2. Position patient so that trunk and limbs are in good alignment.

    3. Protect involved limbs:

        a. Use sling for shoulder and arm.

        b. Sandbags will help to align hip and leg.

        c. A hand roll will keep fist unclenched.

        d. Use a footboard to prevent foot drop.

        e. An ankle brace can be used when patient is ambulatory.

        f. Supervise use of walker, cane, or other aids for ambulation.

    4. Cooperate with physical therapist to arrange therapy sessions and learn exercises.

    5. Do passive range of motion exercises with patient to point of resistance or pain.

    6. With patient and physical therapist, plan a program for gradual ambulation, and see that it is effected consistently.

C. Evaluation:

    1. Reassess muscle tone, bulk, and strength.

    2. Evaluation of overall improvements in cranial nerve, sensory, and motor areas should be integrated to determine functional capacity.

XVII. Prepare patient to perform tasks of daily living as independently as possible.

A. Assessment: The degree to which the patient can begin to assume responsibility for daily activities is based upon:

1. Functional capacity described above.
2. Mental alertness and memory.
3. Desire to achieve independence and the absence of secondary gains to remain dependent.

B. Intervention:
1. Develop a training program with patient and occupational therapy.
2. Set short-term, easily attainable goals to give patient the opportunity to feel successful.
3. Provide opportunities for patient to practice skills learned in therapy sessions.
4. Assist in obtaining special tools and equipment needed.
5. Provide support during times of frustration at not reaching goals quickly.
6. Continue to provide physical and emotional support even as patient becomes more independent. Often, as some new skill is acquired, the inability to perform a more complex task becomes apparent.
7. Assess ability of family members to allow for the slower, perhaps more awkward performance of these tasks, and reinforce the value of doing so.

C. Evaluation:
1. Continue to determine patient's ability and will to learn how to perform tasks within confines of disabilities.
2. Team assesses care plan and goal setting based on patient as a unique individual.

XVIII. Manage the patient with aphasia.
A. Definition: *Aphasia* is the impairment of the ability to produce or comprehend spoken or written communication due to a cerebral disturbance in an otherwise alert mind.
1. *Total aphasia* is the loss of nearly all function, sparing the ability to use and understand a few words; inability to read or write.
2. *Motor* or *Broca's aphasia* is verbal executive apraxia, leaving some stereotyped phrases, and sparing the ability to answer yes or no and to utter expletives.
3. *Central* or *Wernicke's aphasia* is the impairment of all language-dependent behavior. Patient cannot comprehend speech or the written word, and cannot write or communicate verbally. Hearing is diminished so patient is unaware of deficit, cannot follow directions, and talks freely.
4. *Dissociative speech disorders* include selective or mixed impairment of language-dependent behavior, which may include word deafness, mutism, or word blindness.

B. Assessment: Specific tests are executed to determine the individual's language function (see "General Assessment"). The character and extent of the aphasia may help determine the size and site of the lesion.

C. Intervention:
1. Develop means of communication with the patient, utilizing body and sign language.
2. If patient has a hearing aid, its use might enhance some language function.
3. Shouting is seldom helpful.
4. Reinforce techniques and therapy recommended by speech therapists.
5. Explore with the family other outlets for communication such as painting or drawing.
6. Continue providing audiovisual stimulation.

D. Evaluation: There is often a gradual resolution of the impairment. By utilizing the tests applicable to each patient, it should be possible to keep an accurate record describing the patient's abilities. From this, new goals might be set, or new interventions tested.

XIX. Establish healthy coping processes for patient and family. As a catastrophic event, stroke precipitates a crisis for both the patient as an individual and the family as a unit. Early and positive intervention will ease the process of responding to the stroke and will help in developing an altered life-style.

   A. Assessment:
   1. Determine how the alert patient perceives his or her situation by verbal communication, facial expression, and response to surroundings.
   2. Determine how the patient's family perceives the situation.
      a. What is the extent of the stroke and the overall prognosis?
      b. What was the role of the patient in the family?
      c. What is the experience of the patient and family with chronic disability?
      d. What are the economic, emotional, and spiritual resources of patient and family?
   B. Intervention:
   1. While it is sometimes necessary to protect the patient from an early appreciation of the extent of a stroke, the family should be aware of the threat to life.
   2. Allow the patient and family time to accept the loss of function in the patient; allow airing of feelings.
   3. Provide positive reinforcement of healthy reactions.
   4. Provide realistic reassurances.
   5. Utilize counseling resources for both patient and family; sometimes the staff will need to use a mental health consultant to deal with feelings and problems as well.
   6. Develop a way to communicate with the patient; the manner in which physical care is provided can greatly affect the way the patient perceives self.
   7. Sticking to the routine established by physical, speech, and occupational therapists reinforces the possibility of gaining improved function. These routines become *very* important to the patient.
   8. When goals are accomplished, be quick to give praise and encouragement.
   9. Do not abandon the patient as independent function returns.
   10. Allow patient and family to express concerns about a second stroke. Some common fears are:
      a. Being stricken when alone.
      b. Minor physical discomforts may be taken for signs of impending stroke.
      c. Dying without warning.
      d. Permanent disability and being a "burden."
   11. Plan for continued access to care as patient changes from hospital to rehabilitation center to home.
   C. Evaluation: The response of the patient and family to the stroke should be evaluated as an integral part of the daily care. As new problems or solutions arise, reassessment is necessary and new methods of intervention must be planned and tested.

Demyelinating Disease: Multiple Sclerosis

DEFINITION
Demyelinating disease involves the destruction of the myelin sheath of the nerve fiber, resulting in focal lesions of the brain and spinal cord (see Fig. 23-4). *Multiple sclerosis* is characterized by repeated demyelinating episodes in which the myelin is replaced by sclerotic plaques which interrupt the transmission of nerve impulses. It is difficult to determine if a person who has had one demyelinating episode, or a series of mild ones, will go on to develop a *severe* or disabling condition. For this reason it would serve very little purpose in being too prompt to label a patient undergoing a demyelinating process as having multiple sclerosis.
   As lesions may form in the brain or spinal column, varying symptom complexes arise (see

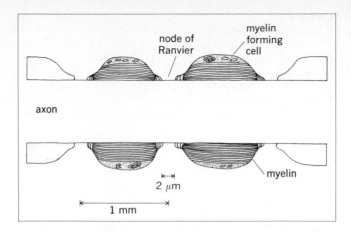

FIGURE 23-4 / The myelin sheath provides the insulation of the axon. Demyelination destroys this insulation, resulting in decreased or aberrant transmission of sensory and motor impulses. (*From Arthur J. Vander, James H. Sherman, and Dorothy S. Luciano, Human Physiology, 2d ed., McGraw-Hill Book Company, New York, 1975, p. 147.*)

Table 23-5). The onset may be fairly rapid, occurring over a few days, and there is usually some improvement within 6 to 8 weeks.

Because the cause of demyelinating disease is not fully understood, the treatment has largely been confined to providing symptomatic relief and preventing complications. Steroid therapy has been useful in reducing the severity and duration of some episodes in some cases.

TABLE 23-5 / DEFICITS CAUSED BY DEMYELINATING LESIONS

Site of Lesion	Deficits
Spinal cord	Weakness
	Ataxia
	Paralysis
	Sensory losses or disturbances
	Bowel, bladder, or sexual dysfunction
Brainstem and cerebellum	Cranial nerve disturbances:
	Diplopia
	Enlarged blind spot
	Nystagmus
	Dizziness
	Dysarthria
	Impaired facial muscle control
	Difficulty in swallowing or chewing
	Tremor
	Staggering
Cerebrum	Emotional lability
	Euphoria
	Impaired judgment and comprehension
	Difficulty with conceptualization

Source: Marci Catanzaro, "Multiple Sclerosis: Exploding the Myths That Compromise Patient Care," *R.N.*, **40**:44, December 1977.

ASSESSMENT
Refer to "General Assessment."

DIAGNOSIS
Refer to "General Diagnosis."

GOALS OF CARE

I. Identify the demyelinative process accurately in a patient with a symptom of neuronal dysfunction.

    A. Assessment:

        1. Obtain a thorough history of the present problem and past episodic dysfunction.

        2. Perform a careful neurologic examination.

        3. Record findings accurately and completely.

        4. Include evaluation of patient's emotional response to problem.

    B. Evaluation:

        1. Compare findings with medical colleagues and reach agreement on nature of deficit and the plan of treatment.

        2. Reassess neurological status regularly and compare findings with baseline assessment.

II. Protect patient from situations which might precipitate or aggravate an exacerbation.

    A. Assessment: Identify factors which have such effects:

        1. Increase in temperature, as felt by immersion in warm water, or during hot, humid weather.

        2. Injections.

        3. Fatigue.

        4. Intercurrent infections.

        5. Hormonal changes.

    B. Intervention:

        1. Recommend tepid or cool baths, and use of air conditioning.

        2. Avoid unnecessary injection therapy.

        3. Develop a regular schedule of rest and activity, increasing rest during symptomatic episodes or other illness.

        4. Identify and treat other illnesses promptly.

        5. Some patients may have increased difficulties while on oral contraceptives, or postpartum. Family planning should be thoroughly discissed.

III. Assist the patient in understanding the episodic and crisislike nature of the disease and in coping with it.

    A. Assessment: With each loss of function, there will be a question of how much return there will be. Each loss is therefore met with a grieving process in which old and new anxieties surface, and may be accompanied by depression.

    B. Intervention:

        1. Be prepared to answer questions accurately.

        2. Provide encouragement while avoiding false reassurance.

        3. Respond to patient's emotional state by a realistic appraisal of what the functional impairment might mean.

        4. Allow expression of feelings of sadness and anger by patient and family.

        5. Use other professional sources to counsel family, and to help understand one's own feelings.

        6. Be consistent in availability, amount, and quality of care.

        7. Help patient obtain support of employer or school.

        8. Assist person in obtaining help from government and social agencies to secure adequate housing, financial assistance, medical care, educational, and vocational help.

    C. Evaluation: Achieving a good nurse-patient relationship is a complicated but integral part of the care. With each new episode, the patient must develop new understanding and adjustment. Having a reliable source of care is one of the few stable factors in the patient's life. Accurate and frequent reassessment of the physical and emotional status is a must.

IV. Administer steroids safely and effectively when ordered.
  A. Assessment (see "General Assessment").
  B. Intervention:
    1. Explain the treatment regimen to the patient carefully, providing written instructions.
    2. Teach patient how to recognize side effects:
      a. Gastric gain.   c. Mood changes.
      b. Weight gain.
    3. Teach patient how to avoid side effects by means of:
      a. Antacids.   c. Reduction of demands of emotional energy.
      b. Diet.
    4. Teach patient to report any signs of viral or bacterial infection while being treated with immunosuppressive drugs.
  C. Evaluation:
    1. Reassess neurological status against baseline regularly and accurately.
    2. Side effects are absent or minimized.
    3. Demonstration of improved function while on steroids determines if their use might be helpful during other episodes.

V. Manage patient experiencing difficulties in ambulation.
  A. Assessment: Lesions of the spinal cord and cerebrum may produce motor and sensory disturbances which restrict ambulation (see Table 23-5). These deficits may be temporary, or may leave a residuum. Evaluate problem to determine nature of lesion and how it interferes with ambulation.
  B. Intervention:
    1. Provide tools for maintaining and assisting ambulation.
    2. Make sure patient can handle these tools.
    3. Develop a regimen of rest and activity to maintain muscle bulk and tone.
    4. Provide relief from spasticity through massage and medication.
    5. Physical therapy may be helpful in providing stretching exercises; it is also generally a positive experience for the patient.
    6. Plan for extended home care with continuing care providers.
    7. If the patient becomes confined to a wheelchair, the principles of caring for an immobilized patient are to be used. (See "Injury to the Spinal Cord" and "Cerebrovascular Accidents.")

VI. Manage patient experiencing difficulties with vision.
  A. Assessment: Optic neuritis is a common presenting episode, and other visual disturbances usually occur (see Table 23-5).
    1. Evaluate visual function by using examination techniques of cranial nerves II, III, IV, and VI (refer to "General Assessment").
    2. Record findings accurately.
  B. Intervention:
    1. As steroids are often used in treating optic neuritis, follow recommendations described above.
    2. Provide protection from injury secondary to visual impairment:
      a. Assess need to alter activities such as driving.
      b. An eyepatch may be helpful.
    3. Encourage utilization of aids in reading and writing.

VII. Manage bowel dysfunction.
  A. Assessment: Spinal cord lesions may interfere with normal evacuation of the bowel, causing retention of stool or incontinence. This may be aggravated by immobilization.
  B. Intervention:
    1. Institute bowel training.
    2. Provide counseling on diet and activity to help promote normal evacuation.

3. Incontinence is a humiliating experience, as is needing help with evacuation. Treat the patient with dignity and allow expression of feelings.

VIII. Maintain optimal bladder function and prevent urinary tract infections.

    A. Assessment (refer to Chap. 28):

        1. Spinal cord lesions may interfere with normal bladder drainage, either by causing incontinence or retention.

        2. Immobilization increases the risk of developing bladder or ascending urinary tract infections.

        3. Question patient about dysuria.

    B. Intervention:

        1. Work with patient to set up a schedule for voiding.

        2. To obtain a urine culture use a "clean catch" specimen or sterile straight catheter specimen.

        3. Treat an infection promptly and reculture urine after therapy.

        4. Catheterize as often as necessary to drain atonic bladder.

        5. Encourage expression of feelings (see point VII, above).

IX. Manage patient with sensory dysfunction.

    A. Assessment:

        1. Obtain a history of increased or decreased appreciation of sensory stimuli.

        2. Obtain a history of abnormal sensations such as a sunburnt feeling or tingling, electric shock with neck flexion (Lhermitte's sign), or a bandlike feeling around limb.

        3. Evaluate findings of sensory exam as described under "General Assessment."

        4. Decreased appreciation of pain and temperature make the patient susceptible to skin infections without being cognizant of their presence.

    B. Intervention:

        1. Teach the patient the importance of self-inspection and of reporting skin changes.

        2. Provide inspection of areas not accessible to patient.

        3. Protect skin by changes in position and early treatment of infection or irritation.

    C. Evaluation:

        1. Each complex of symptoms is assessed against baseline measurements.

        2. The overall ability to keep the patient at optimal function is also evaluated.

CASE STUDY

This hypothetical case is presented to illustrate problems which may arise in caring for the patient with multiple sclerosis. The case described is neither unusually mild nor dramatically severe, but represents a cross section of the physical and emotional trials of these patients. Multiple sclerosis is one of the illnesses for which the term "care of the total patient" is most aptly suited.

C.D. is a 44-year-old woman, the mother of two teenagers, who has had multiple sclerosis for about 11 years.

Her first episode was one of optic neuritis which occurred shortly after her second child was born. Her symptoms began with a sudden loss of vision. Her brief hospitalization at a medical center included consultations with ophthalmologists and neurologists, a brain scan, an electroencephalogram, and a spinal tap. Both experiencing the blindness and the "complete workup" were frightening to this young mother. She worried about her ability to raise her children, her future relationship with her husband, and her own life expectancy. Her fears were somewhat lessened by the reassurance of her physician that her vision would probably return to normal, as well as an explanation that the cause was an inflammation of the optic nerve. Improvement did begin as she began to take the prescribed corticosteroids.

C.D. was also able to talk about many of her worries to the night nurse, who would find her wide awake at 1 A.M. She expressed her doubts about her future and spoke with some ambivalence about the choice she had made to have a family rather than pursue a career. Having been taught by experience not to cut the patient off with a quick "Everything will be all right,'' the nurse listened to C.D.'s concerns, and communicated them to the primary providers who would have continuing responsibility for her care. A reduction in the dosage of the steroids allowed C.D. to sleep more easily, and avoided precipitating other side effects. Lastly, C.D. was encouraged to talk with her husband and to share her feelings.

This incident was almost forgotten when, 5 years later, during an August heat wave, C.D. had an episode of double vision. She was evaluated by the same medical team, and her exam revealed an intranuclear ophthalmoplegia, with the remainder of the physical assessment normal. The mode of onset of her symptoms and the site of the lesion as well as the history of the previous episode made the diagnosis of a demyelinating process fairly certain at this time. Without further studies, C.D. was again placed on a tapering dose of steroids and her vision gradually improved.

Emotionally, C.D. responded to her situation much differently than she had to the previous episode. She was confident that her vision would return to normal and was almost nonchalant. This was partly due to the complete resolution of her earlier symptoms, but also resulted from a more stable situation at home: her children were both in school, her husband was enjoying success, and she had begun graduate studies.

Problems arose no more than 2 months later when a demyelinating lesion of the spinal column caused difficulty with walking. The symptoms developed over 3 days and resulted in an evaluation at the health center. The examination revealed abnormally brisk knee and ankle reflexes, unilateral extensor plantar response on the left side, with a decreased appreciation of vibration and position on one leg and contralateral weakness. Within a few days, her mobility was more severely impaired, and her inability to void necessitated admission to the hospital. She was again placed on steroids and was catheterized intermittently to maintain normal bladder tone. (Sterile technique was used, and cultures were obtained regularly.)

During one catheterization procedure, C.D. began to cry, and became quite angry with the nurse. The catheterization brought out her frustration at being helpless and resurrected the fears she had experienced 5 years earlier. Several factors triggered C.D.'s outburst: the physical dependence, the depersonalization of the procedure, the crisis of the hospitalization and interruption of normal family life, the medication, and the emotional lability which may result from demyelinating lesions. Being cognizant of these factors, the nurse allowed C.D. to express her feelings without taking her anger personally. She was able to sympathize with her about the physical limitations and, having formed this alliance, helped dissolve the anger. Together, they explored some of C.D.'s feelings of frustration and anger at the illness in relation to her own expectations for herself.

As the emotional tempest abated, C.D. began to feel better. Over the next few days she began physical therapy and felt more confident with each demonstration of improved strength. Her bladder control improved, and she was taught how to regulate her liquid intake and schedule times for voiding. With these indicators of a return to normal function, she began to focus on coping with the illness.

This hospitalization was the major crisis of C.D.'s experience with multiple sclerosis. As the episode resolved and she returned to her activities at home and school, she and her husband were able to speak with the primary nurse and physician and to identify realistic goals as well as those precautions she should take. She decided to continue graduate school on a part-time basis and received some financial assistance from the state rehabilitation commission as well as vocational planning advice. After completing her studies, she was hired as a counselor in a community program for the elderly. Characterized as a cheerful member of the staff, she enjoys her work and feels that her salary contributes to the cost of hiring a person to do household work. Subsequent episodes have interrupted her work, but she has responded well to rest and has avoided drug therapy or hospitalization.

When C.D. is disabled by a demyelinating episode, the family responds as a unit and rallies to her support. However, now that the children are adolescents, the issue of autonomy can sometimes become entwined with their mother's physical limitations. Because all the family members receive their care at the same health facility, the primary nurses can coordinate their efforts to meet each individual's needs. At one point a conference of C.D.'s primary nurse, the pediatric nurse, and family social worker resulted in a referral of C.D.

and her daughter to the social worker and the development of a care plan which could be implemented consistently by all the providers involved.

It can be seen from this case presentation that the ongoing care of the patient with multiple sclerosis is far from static. The nurse must not only respond to the physical and emotional crises, but must also anticipate their emergence and intervene promptly. Accurate assessment of the patient's status as well as communication between nurse and physician is necessary to provide good care. Other professionals must also be included to broaden the base of support to the patient and family so that care is not dependent on one provider's skill or philosophy.

Neuromuscular Junction Transmission Defects: Myasthenia Gravis

DEFINITION
Myasthenia gravis is a disease of neuromuscular transmission characterized by episodic weakness and fatigability. Attacks may be acute or chronic and the condition is aggravated by various factors.

ASSESSMENT
I. Data sources (refer to "Injury to the Brain").
II. There is a health history of a deficit caused by weakness of a group of muscles (see Table 23-6).
III. Physical assessment reveals signs of weakness on sustained or repetitive performance of a task.
    A. Improved functions demonstrated after intravenous injection of Tensilon.
    B. Evaluation of the patient for underlying thyroid disease, or for presence of thymoma is also done at this time.
IV. Diagnostic tests

DIAGNOSIS
Refer to "General Diagnosis."

GOALS OF CARE
I. Protect patient from factors which may aggravate weakness.
    A. Assessment: Identify factors leading to weakness:
        1. Upper respiratory infections.
        2. Excitement or increased activity.
        3. Sleep deprivation.
        4. Menses, and possibly pregnancy.
        5. Increased carbohydrate and alcohol intake.
    B. Intervention:
        1. Identify and treat upper respiratory infections promptly.
        2. Help patient plan regular activity and rest.
        3. Help patient obtain adequate rest, nutrition, and care during pregnancy.
        4. Encourage a moderate approach to diet and alcohol, as tolerated by the patient.
    C. Evaluation: Compliance is based on the patient's ability to understand the risk in precipitating or aggravating symptoms.
II. Manage patient with common symptoms during an acute attack.
    A. Assessment:
        1. During an acute attack the aspiration of food or fluids is a danger.
        2. Respiratory function is compromised and hypostatic pneumonia is possible.
        3. Bowel and bladder incontinence may occur as a result of skeletal muscle involvement.
    B. Intervention:
        1. Provide nourishment by liquids, and intravenous or tube feedings.
        2. Enhance respiratory function by use of ventilator. Use proper technique for suction.

TABLE 23-6 / MUSCLE GROUPS COMMONLY AFFECTED BY MYASTHENIA GRAVIS

Muscle Group	Result
Ocular	Ptosis
	Paresis of eye movement: diplopia
Facial	Unequal, smooth facies
Pharyngeal and laryngeal	Husky, nasal speech
	Choking or aspiration of foods
	Regurgitation of fluids
Respiratory	Decreased respiratory exchange
Other skeletal	Neck weakness
	Stress incontinence
	Weakness of anal sphincter
	Sometimes wasting

3. Respond to changes in vital signs and breath sounds promptly.
4. Administer antibiotics and medication accurately. Treatment includes:
    a. Drug therapy with neostigmine.
    b. Low-dose steroids.
    c. Radiation of thymoma.
    d. Thymectomy (may be selected).
5. Treat side effects of neostigmine. Gastric and uterine cramps may occur and will respond to atropine.
6. Instruct in bowel and bladder care.
7. Allow patient to express fears and anxieties.
C. Evaluation: Respiratory function, alimentation, and a healthy emotional state is successfully maintained through the crisis.

DEGENERATIVE DISORDERS

Dementia

DEFINITION
Dementia is a chronic, progressive decrease in intellectual function with memory loss due to diffuse cerebral atrophy. It is usually seen in old age (*senile dementia*; refer to Chaps. 40 and 42), but may occur earlier (*Alzheimer's dementia*).

ASSESSMENT
I. Data sources (refer to "Injury to the Brain").
II. Health history and physical assessment should rule out treatable pathology:
    D. Neoplasm.
    E. Trauma.
    F. Vascular lesions.
III. Diagnostic tests.
    A. Computerized axial tomography.
    B. Other radiologic and laboratory procedures as indicated by symptoms.

DIAGNOSIS
Refer to "General Diagnosis."

GOALS OF CARE
I. Accurately assess mental capacity.
    A. Assessment:
        1. Perform tests of mental status (see "General Assessment").
        2. Record findings accurately.

    B. Evaluation:

        Adequate baseline examination and recording of findings are essential to proper management and planning for care.

II. Provide safe environment for patient.

    A. Assessment: As the loss of mental function becomes more extensive, the patient will experience increasing difficulties with anxiety, disorientation, belligerence, and nocturnal wandering. Memory loss will make such habits as smoking dangerous, and complicate simple tasks such as boiling water.

        1. Evaluate patient's living situation and resources.

        2. Evaluate family's response to problem and ability to provide adequate protection.

    B. Intervention:

        1. Work with family to achieve understanding of the illness and to help them cope with emotional factors. While some loss of function might be expected in extreme old age, it is a greater shock when it occurs in late middle age.

            a. Help family grieve the loss.

            b. Assist in obtaining financial help and in locating caretakers.

            c. If the patient must be placed in a home, help with the transition.

        2. Teach family the importance of:

            a. Maintaining patient in an adequate nutritional state.

            b. Protecting patient from injury.

            c. Continuing care of other illnesses.

    C. Evaluation:

        1. Reexamine and compare with baseline neurological status.

        2. Maintain optimum health and nutrition.

        3. Family is able to make adjustments within the family unit.

Parkinson's Disease

DEFINITION

Parkinson's disease is an extrapyramidal disorder of posture and movement. Pathophysiology is related to the absence of dopamine usually present in the basal ganglia. The disease may affect an individual in a symmetric or asymmetric pattern.

ASSESSMENT

  I. Data sources (refer to "Injury to the Brain").

  II. Health history (refer to "General Assessment").

  III. Physical assessment.

    A. Involuntary tremor.

    B. Impairment of voluntary movement.

    C. Autonomic dysfunction.

    D. Depression.

    E. Intellect and sensory and reflex functions are spared.

  IV. Diagnostic tests.

DIAGNOSIS

Refer to "General Diagnosis."

GOALS OF CARE

  I. Optimal management of symptoms is achieved through chemical and supportive therapy.

    A. Assessment:

        1. As symptoms develop, the patient should be evaluated clinically, with accurate recording of findings.

        2. The patient's emotional response should also be evaluated; the "stony-faced" expression is an effect of muscular rigidity, not a reflection of feeling.

B. Intervention:
1. Appropriate drug therapy can alleviate or minimize many of the following symptoms:
   a. Tremor.
   c. Slowness.
   b. Rigidity.
   d. Autonomic dysfunction.
2. Drug choice will depend on accurate assessment of the neurological status. Available treatment includes:
   a. L-Dopa.
   c. Anticholinergic agents.
   b. L-Dopa and carbidopa in combination.
   d. Antihistamines.
3. Take a careful history to determine contraindications to drugs including factors such as:
   a. Age.
   b. Underlying medical problems.
   c. Other medications.
4. Follow closely to evaluate side effects:
   a. Gastrointestinal distress.
   b. Kinetic disorders and other neurologic complaints.
   c. Cardiac, vascular, or respiratory changes.
   d. Psychotropic changes.
5. Teach patient how to prevent and manage mild side effects:
   a. Eat crackers at night, and take drugs containing L-dopa with meals.
   b. Change position slowly to decrease dizziness and orthostatic hypotension.
   c. Control alcohol intake.
   d. Do not operate heavy machinery if drowsy.
   e. Use hard candy to activate salivation.
6. Encourage patient to maintain a normal level of activity and social interaction to reduce rigidity and prevent muscle contractures.
7. Special facial exercises and routines for walking and changing position should be practiced daily.
8. The family should be involved in understanding the importance of keeping patient active and assisting with planning activities.
9. Counseling will help patient express sadness about the limitations of the illness.
10. Specific autonomic dysfunctions need to be treated carefully:
   a. Dysphagia: Prepare easily chewed food.
   b. Incontinence: Provide good bladder care to prevent infection and protect skin.
11. Immobilization will necessitate:
   a. Monitoring fluid and electrolytes.
   b. Prevention of skin breakdown.
   c. Prevention or control of urinary and respiratory infections.
   d. Physical therapy.
   e. Planning for ongoing care at home or in an institution.

C. Evaluation:
1. Response to medication.
   a. Over time the effect may decrease.
   b. Carbidopa potentiates L-dopa and side effects should be monitored.
2. Compare physical and emotional status with baseline data to revise care.

HYPERACTIVITY AND HYPOACTIVITY

Convulsive Disorders

DEFINITION
A *convulsion* is a complex of symptoms evoked by the abnormally excessive and disorderly discharge of nerve impulses in the cerebral cortex. Specific foci or changes in the cerebral medulla induced by metabolic or ionic changes may produce seizures.

Focal seizures are caused by identifiable lesions resulting from trauma, tumor, arteriovenous malformation, infection, or hemorrhage. Focal seizures produce symptoms related to the area of the cortex where the lesion is situated: (1) focal motor seizures, (2) focal sensory seizures, (3) psychomotor seizures (see Table 23-7).

In *generalized seizures* the lesion which causes the abnormal discharge is not readily identifiable, perhaps having occurred in utero or during childhood without providing symptoms. Generalized seizures may also be produced by metabolic and ionic changes: (1) grand mal, (2) petit mal, (3) myoclonic or akinetic seizure.

Refer to Chap. 19 for further discussion.

ASSESSMENT

I. Data sources (refer to "Injury to the Brain").
II. Health history.
    A. Onset, presence of aura.
    B. Sensory or motor dysfunction observed by patient.
    C. Observations made by onlookers:
        1. Movements of eyes and limbs.   3. Automatisms.
        2. Changes in consciousness.   4. Postictal state.
    D. Personal and family history.
    E. Possibility of new focus or changes in cerebral medulla.
III. Physical assessment.
    A. Asymmetry in body parts from right to left.
    B. Asymmetry in reflexes or gait.
    C. Automatisms or absence spells during examination.
IV. Diagnostic tests.
    A. EEG.
    B. Skull x-ray and computerized scan in adult-onset seizures.
    C. Cerebrospinal fluid evaluation for inflammatory disorders.

DIAGNOSIS
Refer to "General Diagnosis."

GOALS OF CARE
I. Manage patient in the convulsive state (grand mal).

TABLE 23-7 / CAUSES OF RECURRENT CONVULSIONS IN DIFFERENT AGE GROUPS

Age of Onset, Years	Probable Cause
Infancy, under 2	Congenital maldevelopment, birth injury, metabolic disorders (hypocalcemia, hypoglycemia), vitamin B$_6$ deficiency, phenylketonuria
Childhood, 2–10	Birth injury, trauma, infections, thrombosis of cerebral arteries or veins, beginning of idiopathic epilepsy
Adolescence, 10–18	Idiopathic epilepsy, trauma, congenital defects
Early adulthood, 18–35	Trauma, neoplasm, idiopathic epilepsy, alcoholism, drug addiction
Middle age, 35–60	Neoplasm, trauma, vascular disease, alcoholism, drug addiction
Late life, over 60	Vascular disease, degeneration, tumor

Source: Raymond D. Adams, "The Convulsive State and Idiopathic Epilepsy," in George W. Thorn et al. (eds.), *Harrison's Principles of Internal Medicine*, 8th ed., McGraw-Hill Book Company, New York, 1977, p. 132, Table 24-1.

A. Assessment:
1. Aura (possible).
2. Sudden loss of consciousness.
3. Epileptic "cry" as air is forced out of lungs.
4. Fall to ground.
5. Tonic or clonic contraction of muscles of tongue and limbs.
6. Clenching of jaw.
7. Incontinence.
8. Transient coma.
9. Confusion and drowsiness (postictal state).
10. Headache.

B. Intervention:
1. Protection from injury.
    a. Get patient to floor.
    b. If time allows, place soft, firm object between teeth to prevent tongue biting.
    c. *Never* try to force object between already clenched teeth.
2. Maintain open airway by placing in a lateral position.
3. Consciousness should return within 2 to 5 min. If seizure is repeated or continues without interruption (*status epilepticus*), anticonvulsants will be administered intravenously.
4. Reorient patient on recovery.
5. Provide emotional support.
6. Determine and treat precipitating factor, i.e., forgetting medication, infection, etc.

C. Evaluation:
1. In the case of a new onset of seizures, the patient should be brought under medical supervision and receive a diagnostic workup.
2. Prevention of any other seizures is the measure by which care should be judged.

II. Optimal nursing management for prevention and control of seizures is achieved.
A. Assessment: As the primary provider, the nurse is readily available to the patient and has the knowledge and ability to assess changes in the patient's status and recommend and effect changes in the care plan.
B. Intervention:
1. Diagnostic:
    a. Accurate observation, history, and physical exam are performed.
    b. EEG and other procedures are planned.
    c. Diagnostic procedures are explained and patient is prepared.
2. Therapeutic:
    a. Monitor effectiveness of anticonvulsants through blood values and control of seizures.
    b. Monitor side effects.
3. Provide counseling and education to the patient, family, and community.

III. Help the patient understand the nature of the seizure disorder and his or her role in its management.
A. Assessment:
1. Most patients will have to take anticonvulsants for years, if not their entire lifetime.
2. Both the risk of seizure and the constraints of therapy will place some restrictions on activity.
3. For the adolescent, the onset of seizures and the treatment regimen will be a complicated process, in which the issues of independence and control are entwined.
4. Each seizure is a crisis; the lack of control and loss of consciousness is frightening.
5. The ignorance of society in labeling patients with seizures as a special group creates a prejudice which may be very difficult to overcome.

B. Intervention:

1. Teach patient how to manage drugs.
   a. Anticonvulsants work by reaching and maintaining adequate levels in the bloodstream. Sporadic use will nullify the protection.
   b. Infection and other physical stresses (e.g., menses) may call for extra protection.
   c. Recognize and control side effects (e.g., gum hypertrophy with Dilantin).
   d. Caution patient against using other drugs—either prescription, over-the-counter, or "street"—without consulting neurology team.
   e. The reason for not drinking alcohol is that seizure threshold is lowered in alcohol withdrawal.
2. Explain rationale behind any restrictions: swimming, driving, and operating heavy machinery would be life-threatening should a seizure occur. These activities are proscribed until seizure control is adequate.
3. Adolescents do better if they are:
   a. Given an adequate description of the pathology and EEG.
   b. Allowed to feel responsible for taking the medications and making appointments.
   c. Able to identify with peers with similar problems, either in structured groups or normal social activities.
4. When a seizure occurs, the patient may feel guilty, humiliated, depressed, and have increased anxiety about being "in control."
   a. Allow expression of feelings.
   b. Assist family, friends, and peers in understanding patient's feelings.
   c. Take steps to improve seizure control.
5. Promote understanding of seizures within the professional community, and for schools and industry.
6. Utilize resources of national organization and regional facilities.

C. Evaluation:

1. Accurate diagnosis and treatment (if possible) of underlying disorder is carried out.
2. Physician, nurse, and patient are able to prevent seizures.

METABOLIC, NUTRITIONAL, AND TOXIC DISORDERS

Metabolic Disorders

DEFINITION

Metabolic disorders are related to a demonstrable fault in the general metabolism or to abnormalities of the nervous system itself. This term is also used to describe those disorders in which no vascular or structural lesion may be identified.

ASSESSMENT

I. Acute hypoxic encephalopathy.
   A. Data sources (refer to "Injury to the Brain").
   B. Health history.
      1. Strangulation.
      2. Carbon monoxide poisoning.
      3. Cardiac or respiratory arrest.
      4. Shock.
      5. Paralysis of respiratory muscles.
   C. Physical assessment.
      1. Symptoms:
         a. Mild (transient):
            (1) Decreased attention.
            (2) Poor judgment.
            (3) Incoordination.

      b. Severe
         (1) Coma.
            (a) Reversible if less than 3 to 5 min.
            (b) Irreversible if greater than 5 to 6 min.
         (2) Convulsions.
         (3) Circulatory collapse.
         (4) Death.
   2. Sequelae: seizures.
   3. Complications:

      a. Dementia.   **d.** Parkinsonism.
      b. Visual agnosia.   **e.** Cerebellar ataxia.
      c. Choreoathetosis.   **f.** Intention or action myoclonus.

D. Diagnostic tests.

II. Hypercapnia: respiratory acidosis which occurs with emphysema. Treatment includes intermittent positive pressure breathing (IPPB) and treatment of concomitant heart failure. Symptoms include:

A. Data sources (refer to "Injury to the Brain").

B. Health history (refer to "General Assessment").

C. Physical assessment.

   1. Headache.   **5.** Drowsiness.
   2. Papilledema.   **6.** Confusion.
   3. Asterixis.   **7.** Coma.
   4. Mental dullness.

D. Diagnostic tests.

III. Hypoglycemic encephalopathy: irreversible damage to neurons caused by the metabolism of lipids and proteins in the brain in the absence of sugar. It is treated by administering intravenous glucose.

A. Data sources (refer to "Injury to the Brain").

B. Health history.

   1. Insulin overdose.
   2. Pancreatic tumor.
   3. Acute alcoholic intoxication.

C. Physical assessment.

   1. First stage (recovery complete):
      a. Confusion.
      b. Drowsiness.
      c. Excitement.
   2. Second stage (recovery complete):

      a. Suckling.   **d.** Spasms.
      b. Grasping.   **e.** Decerebrate rigidity.
      c. Motor restlessness.

   3. Third stage (recovery delayed or incomplete):

      a. Deepening coma.   **c.** Slow pulse.
      b. Shallow respiration. **d.** Hypertonicity of limbs.

D. Diagnostic tests.

DIAGNOSIS
Refer to "General Diagnosis."

GOALS OF CARE
I. Preserve life; maintain life supports, if used.

A. Assessment: Absence of pulse and respirations.

B. Intervention:

   1. Perform cardiopulmonary resuscitation.
   2. Maintain an open airway.
   3. Oxygen may be administered.
   4. Hypothermia may be induced to reduce the brain's need for oxygen.

    C. Evaluation: If there is no spontaneous ability to maintain respirations, the use of a ventilator may be necessary.

  II. Manage effects of hypoxia.

    A. Assessment: Cerebral edema and convulsions may be present in the posthypoxic state.

    B. Intervention:

      1. Administration of steroids should be monitored closely.

      2. Convulsions should be watched for, and anticonvulsants given.

  III. Management of complications will depend on the presenting symptoms, and intervention should be geared to same.

EVALUATION

  I. Continuous reassessment is necessary.

  II. It is essential that each problem or complication be promptly assessed and treated in order to avoid irreversiole damage.

Nutritional Disorders

Niacin Deficiency (Pellagra) and Thiamine Deficiency (Wernicke's Disease)

DEFINITION

Deficiencies of the vitamins niacin and thiamine have the most marked effects in the nervous system. Both vitamins are present in sufficient quantities in normal diets but are deficient in starvation and alcoholic states. Not only does alcohol dependence interfere with obtaining sufficient amounts of food, but it also interferes with the body's ability to absorb these vitamins.

ASSESSMENT

  I. Data sources (refer to "Injury to the Brain").

  II. Health history (refer to "General Assessment").

  III. Physical assessment.

    A. Niacin deficiency.

      1. Acute confusional psychosis.

      2. Symmetrical posterior column peripheral neuritis.

    B. Thiamine deficiency.

      1. Bilateral ocular paralysis.   4. Poor insight.

      2. Ataxia.   5. Symptoms of Korsakov's psychosis.

      3. Disorientation.

  IV. Diagnostic tests.

DIAGNOSIS

Refer to "General Diagnosis."

GOALS OF CARE

  I. Identify and manage nutritional disorders.

    A. Assessment:

      1. History of poor diet and a progressive onset of symptoms.

      2. Changes in mental status.

      3. Symmetrical peripheral neuropathy.

      4. Presence of bilateral ocular paralysis in thiamine deficiency.

    B. Intervention:

      1. Bring patient under adequate medical care.

      2. Administer replacement therapy. Treatment for each includes:

        a. Niacin:

          (1) Oral administration of niacinamide.

(2) Maintenance of fluid and electrolyte balance.
(3) Riboflavin and thiamine.
(4) High-calorie, high-protein diet.
    b. Thiamine:
      (1) Rapid replacement of thiamine via intravenous and intramuscular routes.
      (2) Oral supplement of B vitamins. (Add B vitamins to all parenteral glucose administered.)
      (3) Normal diet.
      (4) Treat cardiac failure if present.
  3. If motivation exists, help patient seek treatment for alcohol dependence.
  4. Assess resources of family and friends for ongoing care, particularly if Korsakov's psychosis continues.
C. Evaluation: The replacement of depleted vitamins may be effective in reversing the neurologic deficits, but treating the underlying malnutrition must be the primary source of prevention.

Toxic Disorders: Environmental Pollutants

Lead Poisoning

DEFINITION

Lead is present in paints, in water from lead pipes, and in illicit whisky. Since lead poisoning is more prevalent and more dangerous in children, it is discussed in more detail in the chapter on pediatric neurology (Chap. 19).

ASSESSMENT
  I. Data sources (refer to "Injury to the Brain").
  II. Health history (refer to "General Assessment").
  III. Physical assessment.
    A. Colic.
    B. Encephalopathy (mostly in children).
    C. Peripheral neuritis.
    D. Mild anemia.
  IV. Diagnostic test: urinalysis

DIAGNOSIS
Refer to "General Diagnosis."
Diagnostic test: urinalysis.

GOALS OF CARE
  I. Identify the patient with neurotoxic disorder.
    A. Assessment:
      1. A history of acute or chronic exposure to toxic materials should be sought for as part of the normal examination.
      2. Be alert for symptom complexes which correspond to toxicity.
    B. Intervention:
      1. Assist in diagnostic procedures.
      2. Execute maneuvers to protect life and administer appropriate medications:
        a. Dimercaprol
        b. Calcium disodium versenate.
        c. Oral peincillamine.
      3. Assist in planning for removal of patient from future exposure.
    C. Evaluation: The progression of symptoms is halted and reverses are effected where possible.

Carbon Monoxide Poisoning

DEFINITION

Carbon monoxide is present in exhaust from internal combustion engines. Refer to Chap. 45 for a complete discussion of emergency care.

ASSESSMENT
I. Data sources (refer to "Injury to the Brain").
II. Health history (refer to "General Assessment").
III. Physical assessment.
   A. Symptoms are related to those of tissue hypoxia:
      1. Headache.
      2. Confusion.
      3. Fainting on exertion.
      4. Coma.
      5. Convulsions.
   B. Cherry red color of skin and mucous membranes is the noteworthy sign.
IV. Diagnostic tests.

DIAGNOSIS
Refer to "General Diagnosis."

GOALS OF CARE
See "Lead Poisoning."

INTERVENTION
I. Oxygenate tissue through natural or artificial respiration.
II. Decrease demands for oxygen by hypothermia and rest.
III. Administer pure oxygen.

Pesticide Poisonings

DEFINITION AND ASSESSMENT
See Table 23-8.

DIAGNOSIS
Refer to "General Diagnosis."

GOALS OF CARE
See "Lead Poisoning."

INTERVENTION
See Table 23-8.

INFLAMMATORY DISORDERS

Bacterial Disorders

Meningitis

DEFINITION
Meningitis is an inflammation of the pia arachnoid and the fluid which it encloses, as well as the fluid of the ventricles and always cerebrospinal fluid. (Refer to Chap. 19 for further discussion.)

ASSESSMENT
I. Data sources (refer to "Injury to the Brain").
II. Health history (refer to "General Assessment").
III. Physical assessment.
   A. Acute symptoms:
      1. Severe headache.
      2. Focal cerebral deficits.
      3. Disorders of consciousness.
      4. Stiffness of neck and back.
   B. Chronic and subacute symptoms:
      1. Hydrocephalus.
      2. Subdural effusion.
      3. Vomiting, anorexia.
      4. Confusion.
      5. Blood vessel infarction.

C. Late symptoms and sequelae:
1. Optic atrophy.
2. Fibrosis around cord roots.
3. Cerebral damage: dementia.
4. Paralysis.
IV. Diagnostic tests: Analysis of cerebrospinal fluid reveals:
A. Increased leukocytes.
B. Increased pressure.
C. Increased protein.
D. Decreased sugar.
E. Infectious agent is identified by Gram's stain and culture.

DIAGNOSIS
Refer to "General Diagnosis."

GOALS OF CARE
I. Manage patient during diagnostic process:
A. Assessment: A careful history, observation, and examination should be performed and recorded.
B. Intervention:
1. Assist patient through diagnostic procedures, particularly the spinal tap.
2. Provide analgesia such as aspirin.
II. Prevent spread of infection and terminate existing infection.
A. Assessment: Proper and adequate administration of antimicrobials is necessary to eliminate infectious organism.
B. Intervention:
1. Administer antibiotics in correct dosage through intravenous route.
2. Observe patient's responses to therapy. These should be communicated to primary physician and recorded accurately.
3. Place patient under respiratory isolation.
III. Manage patient with focal symptoms and general cerebral deficits.
A. Assessment: Each presenting problem should be managed to prevent progressive losses.
B. Intervention:
1. Control fever.
2. Maintain adequate fluid and electrolyte balance.
3. Monitor and control intracranial pressure.
4. Observe for, and control convulsions.
5. Protect hemiparetic patient from complications of immobility.
6. Ensure that the confused patient has adequate supervision of activities and is gradually reoriented.

Brain Abscess

DEFINITION
A *brain abscess* is a localized bacterial infection in the brain.

ASSESSMENT
I. Data sources (refer to "Injury to the Brain").
II. Health history (refer to "General Assessment").
III. Physical assessment.
A. Acute phase:
1. Fever (until abscess is encapsulated).
2. Headache.
3. Vomiting.
4. Seizures and focal signs.
5. Decreasing consciousness.
B. Slow onset.
1. Headache.
2. Transient focal signs.
3. Stiff neck.
4. Signs of increased intracranial pressure.

TABLE 23-8 / PESTICIDES AS NEUROTOXINS

Type	Toxicology	Prominent Neurologic Symptoms	Confirmation of Diagnosis	Treatment
Solid organochlorides	Interferes with axionic transmission of nerve impulses	Apprehension, disorientation, headache, paresthesia, twitching, and tremor convulsions	History of exposure, blood and urine tests	Open airways; treat convulsions; induce vomiting or lavage stomach; give cathartic if no evacuation in 4 h; clean skin and hair; no epinephrine or adrenergic amines; provide adequate protein, carbohydrate, and vitamins
Organophosphate: cholinesterase-inhibiting	Causes high acetylcholine concentrations at neuro-effector junctions and at skeletal muscle myoneural junctions and autonomic ganglia; impairs CNS function	During exposure or within 12 h: headache, dizziness, extreme weakness, ataxia, small pupils, twitching, tremor, blurred or darkened vision; sometimes convulsions, confusion, incontinence, unconsciousness	Lowered plasma and/or RBC cholinesterase activity; metabolites appear in urine 12–48 h after absorption	Open airways; atropine; pralidoxime for twitching; observe vital signs every 24 h; prepare for respiratory distress; if ingested, induce vomiting or lavage stomach; do not give respiratory depressants; avoid contamination from vomitus; treat convulsions
Carbamates: Cholinesterase-inhibiting	Same as organophosphate cholinesterase inhibitors	Same as organophosphate cholinesterase inhibitors	Blood tests not reliable; enzyme activities commonly revert to normal	Open airways; administer atropine; observe for pulmonary edema; bathe and shampoo; if ingested, empty stomach; follow emesis with activated charcoal; no morphine, aminophylline, phenothiazines, or reserpine

| Arsenical pesticides | Binds critical sulfhydryl-containing enzymes in tissue; produces toxic injury to brain and other organs; toxic encephalopathy manifested as speech and behavioral disturbances; peripheral neuropathy in acute and chronic cases | Acute: dizziness, muscle spasms, delirium, sometimes convulsions, headache Subacute: chronic headache Chronic: peripheral symmetrical neuropathy (paresthesia, pain, anesthesia, paresis, ataxia) | 24-h urinalysis, blood tests | Flush contaminated area; if reinated area; if reinated area; if recent ingestion, empty stomach; maintain hydration and fluid and electrolyte balance; administer dimercaprol intramuscularly. For gaseous poisoning: remove to fresh air; maintain respiration and circulation; administer intravenous fluids and dimercaprol. |
| Halocarbon and sulfuryl fumigants | Acts as CNS depressant; methyl bromide also exhibits neurotoxicity to basal ganglia | Headache, dizziness, drowsiness, tremor, ataxia, diplopia, twitching, weakness, Jacksonian seizures; regional myoclonic movements may lead to coma and death; methyl bromide poisonings may result from low-level, chronic exposures resulting in convulsions, bizarre behavior, and speech and gait impairment | Bromide levels | Remove from exposure; control convulsions; remove ingested fumigant liquids via lavage; observe for adequate pulmonary functions; provide sedation if necessary for protracted manifestations |

Source: Donald P. Morgan, *Recognition and Management of Pesticide Poisonings*, 2d ed., Environmental Protection Agency, Office of Pesticide Programs, Washington, D.C., August 1977.

IV. Diagnostic tests
- **A.** Electroencephalogram (EEG) abnormalities over site of abscess.
- **B.** Positive scan.
- **C.** X-rays of possible sites of primary infection, i.e., sinuses, lungs.
- **D.** To differentiate from tumor, where history does not suggest abscess, surgical exploration may be done.

DIAGNOSIS
Refer to "General Diagnosis."

GOALS OF CARE
- I. Manage patient during diagnostic procedures and medical treatment. Diagnostic and medical management (see "Meningitis").
- II. Manage the patient with a craniotomy.
  - **A.** Assessment:
    1. Vital signs.
    2. Intracranial pressure.
    3. Neurological status:
       - *a.* Focal signs.
       - *b.* Level of consciousness.
    4. Signs of cerebrospinal fluid drainage and hemorrhage.
  - **B.** Intervention:
    1. Administer antimicrobials as prescribed.
    2. The abscess may need to be excised (or aspirated).
    3. Provide adequate oxygenation of tissues.
    4. Monitor and control intracranial pressure.
    5. Report changes in neurological status and act upon revisions in care plan.
    6. Check for cerebrospinal fluid drainage from nasal passages, ears, and mouth.
    7. Keep dressing sterile.
    8. Protect eyes and cornea if edema is present (refer to "Disorders of the Eye").
  - **C.** Evaluation: The prognosis for recovery is good if the abscess is identified, and adequate levels of antibiotics are maintained.
- III. Control seizures (see "Convulsive Disorders").

Viral Disorders

Encephalitis

DEFINITION
Encephalitis is an acute febrile illness with meningeal involvement. It can be caused by an arbovirus, herpes simplex, and other viral or postviral allergic reactions. Refer to Chap. 19 for further discussion.

ASSESSMENT
- I. Data sources (refer to "Injury to the Brain").
- II. Health history (refer to "General Assessment").
  - **A.** Arboviruses.
  - **B.** Herpes simplex.
  - **C.** Other viral and postviral allergic reactions.
- III. Physical assessment.
  - **A.** Impaired level of consciousness.
  - **B.** Convulsions.
  - **C.** Aphasia.
  - **D.** Hemiparesis with asymmetric reflexes and Babinski response.
  - **E.** Involuntary movements.
  - **F.** Cranial nerve palsies.
  - **G.** Fever, headache, and vomiting.

IV. Diagnostic tests.
 A. Aseptic cerebrospinal fluid.
 B. EEG: abnormalities in herpes.
 C. Identification of antibodies in cerebrospinal fluid.

DIAGNOSIS
Refer to "General Diagnosis."

GOALS OF CARE
 I. Manage patient during diagnostic procedures.
 II. Manage patient with focal symptoms and general cerebral deficits (see "Meningitis").
 III. Prevent sequelae.
  A. Assessment:
   1. Amnesia and a liability to have seizures.
   2. Reactive depression and anxiety.
  B. Intervention:
   1. The anticonvulsant regime should be explained to patient.
   2. Allow patient to express feelings.

Aseptic Meningitis

DEFINITION
Aseptic meningitis is characterized by a symptom complex resulting from invasion of an infective agent which is usually viral. Coxsackie virus, echo virus, and mumps are the most common causes. Refer to Chap. 19 for further discussion.

ASSESSMENT
 I. Data sources (refer to "Injury to the Brain").
 II. Health history (refer to "General Assessment").
 III. Physical assessment.
  A. Headache.   **C.** Stiffness of neck and back.
  B. Fever.   **D.** Variable changes in consciousness.
 IV. Diagnostic tests: Analysis of cerebrospinal fluid reveals:
  A. Pleocytosis of mononuclear cells.
  B. Small increase in protein (may vary).
  C. Normal sugar.
  D. Viral isolation as opposed to positive culture and Gram's stain (follow procedure recommended by your agency).

DIAGNOSIS
Refer to "General Diagnosis."

GOALS OF CARE
 I. Manage patient during diagnostic procedures.
 II. Manage patient with focal symptoms and general cerebral deficits (see "Meningitis").
 III. Provide the patient with emotional support.
 IV. Relieve symptoms.

Guillain-Barré Syndrome

DEFINITION
Guillain-Barré syndrome is an acute, idiopathic polyneuropathy which usually follows an upper respiratory or gastrointestinal infection or the administration of flu vaccine. It is characterized by an ascending paralysis which is usually reversible.

ASSESSMENT
Refer to "General Assessment."

DIAGNOSIS
Refer to "General Diagnosis."

GOALS OF CARE

I. Manage the patient during stage of ascending paralysis.
  A. Assessment:
    1. Obtain history and perform baseline neurologic examination.
    2. Ability to maintain adequate respiratory function.
    3. Cardiac function.
    4. Urine output.
  B. Intervention:
    1. Provide adequate ventilation by use of respirator and tracheostomy.
    2. Use sterile technique to prevent respiratory infection.
    3. Maintain blood pressure.
    4. Monitor intake and output; catheterize if necessary.
    5. If steroids are given, monitor effects and side effects.
    6. Assist with management of specific symptoms:
      a. Eating is impaired due to cranial nerve palsies.
      b. Ocular palsies may exist.
      c. Immobilization due to paresis requires:
        (1) Skin care and positioning.
        (2) Range-of-motion exercises.
        (3) Diet management.
      d. Maintain adequate bowel function with regular evacuation.
  C. Evaluation: Speed of reversal of the paralysis varies. Continue assessment and compare with baseline data.
II. Manage ongoing care of patient.
  A. Assessment:
    1. Continue evaluating neurological status.
    2. Evaluate resources available to patient at home and in the community.
  B. Intervention:
    1. Provide assistance in obtaining and using crutches or cane.
    2. Arrange for physical therapy and evaluate muscle improvement.
    3. Provide management of steroid therapy, including prevention of side effects.
    4. Assess patient's emotional response to the illness and provide support.
    5. Assist in identifying social and government agencies which might help with vocational counseling and rehabilitation.
  C. Evaluation: There is a gradual return to independent function.

DISORDERS OF THE EAR

Problems of the ear will be presented as they commonly occur in the outer, middle, and inner ear, respectively. Please refer to Fig. 23-5 for the location of parts of the ear involved with the various problems which are described.

The External Ear

Otitis Externa

DEFINITION

Otitis externa ("swimmer's ear") is an infection often accompanied by inflammation with a bacterial or fungal source and is often caused by swimming in contaminated water or extensively chlorinated swimming pools. A trauma to the ear canal can also precipitate the occurrence of this problem.

ASSESSMENT

I. Data sources (refer to "Injury to the Brain").
II. Health history (refer to "General Assessment").
III. Physical assessment.
  A. Usually moderate but occasionally severe pain.

B. Occasionally, fever.

C. Edema.

D. Because of severe pain and swelling it may be very difficult to insert the otoscope for assessment.

E. Signs of injury, inflammation, lesions, infection, discharge, or bleeding.

IV. Diagnostic tests.

DIAGNOSIS

I. Alteration in comfort: discomfort secondary to pain, discharge.

II. Alteration in body temperature: increase secondary to inflammatory process.

GOALS OF CARE

I. Relieve pain.

II. Reduce infection and edema.

III. Prevent permanent tissue damage.

IV. Prevent recurrence of contact with source of infection.

INTERVENTION

I. Antibiotic therapy may be necessary.

II. Bed rest may be advisable.

III. Increase fluid intake to prevent dehydration.

IV. Analgesics or codeine may be used to relieve pain.

FIGURE 23-5 / The anatomy of the ear. (From Eldra P. Solomon and P. William Davis, *Understanding Human Anatomy and Physiology*, McGraw-Hill Book Company, New York, 1978, p. 306.)

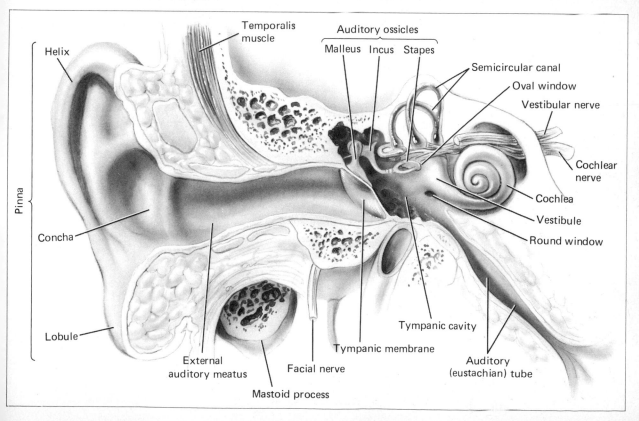

V. Wet or dry heat applications will help to soothe discomfort and increase blood supply to the area. Proper instructions for self-application of heating pad, wet compresses, or hot water bottle should be provided to the patient.

VI. Discharge and debris may be removed by medicated ear drops or instillation of Burow's solution.

VII. Antibiotic ear drops or particular steroid preparations may be applied to aid in treating inflammation.

VIII. If ear canal is not patent, a cotton airwick saturated with antibiotic solution can be inserted into the auditory canal down to the eardrum.

IX. Patient should be instructed to avoid swimming, showering, or any other source of infection until the condition is eliminated.

EVALUATION

I. Pain is relieved and signs of inflammation are eliminated.

II. Check for recurrence of problem.

External Canal Blockage

DEFINITION

The external ear canal may be blocked by a collection of cerumen (wax), foreign bodies, or insects. This may result in reduced hearing, direct tissue damage, or perforation of the eardrum.

ASSESSMENT

I. History of occurrence with identification of possible cause of the blockage.

II. Increased sensitivity and/or pain.

III. Decrease in hearing acuity.

IV. Objects are visible in ear canal.

DIAGNOSIS

Alteration in sensory perception (hearing), secondary to obstruction in ear canal.

GOALS OF CARE

I. Remove cause of blockage without damage to the external ear canal or eardrum.

II. Prevent infection.

III. Restore hearing.

INTERVENTION

I. Only skilled and experienced personnel should attempt removal of blockage.

II. In the case of insect blockage, oil drops may be instilled into the external canal with the insect hopefully floating out of the canal in the oil.

III. Foreign bodies and other objects:
   A. Remove by instrument.
   B. Gentle irrigation.
      (Caution: swelling of some objects may occur with absorption of irrigation solution, rendering removal even more difficult.) Proper technique for irrigation includes:
      1. Gentle flow.
      2. Solution at 95 to 105°F (35 to 40.6°C).
      3. Proper positioning of irrigation device (see Fig. 23-6).

IV. If irrigation is not helpful, glycerine drops or a saturated solution of sodium bicarbonate may be used 2 to 3 times daily for several days.

V. A gentle anesthetic may be required for children or excitable patients.

VI. Instruct patient and/or family regarding safety precautions to prevent further occurrence.

EVALUATION

I. Symptoms are relieved.

II. Pain is eliminated.

III. Auditory acuity is restored.

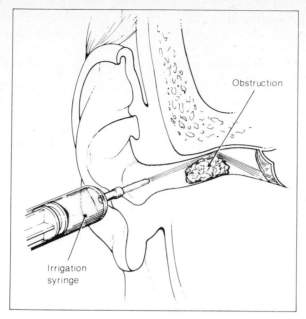

FIGURE 23-6 / Irrigation of the external auditory canal. Note that the solution is directed toward the upper wall of the canal. To gain access to the canal, pull ear in (a) superior and posterior direction in adult, (b) posterior and inferior direction in child. [*From Dorothy A. Jones, Claire F. Dunbar, and Mary M. Jirovec (eds.), Medical-Surgical Nursing: A Conceptual Approach, McGraw-Hill Book Company, New York, 1978, p. 1283.*]

Furunculosis

DEFINITION
Furunculosis or boils in the ear canal are usually caused by the entry of staphylococcus via a small crack or a fissure in the skin.

ASSESSMENT
I. Pain often felt along the jaw as well as in the external canal.
II. Diminished hearing.
III. Feeling of fullness in the ear.
IV. External ear canal swollen or totally blocked.

GOALS OF CARE
I. Relieve pain.
II. Eliminate staphylococcus contamination.
III. Prevent recurrence.

INTERVENTION
I. Insert cotton pledget saturated with Burow's solution. This should be changed every 2 to 3 h.
II. Give aspirin for relief of pain.
III. Keep ear dry.
IV. Administer antibiotic medication, especially penicillin.
V. Instruct patient to avoid scratching ear or use of any object in the ear such as bobby pins, etc.

EVALUATION
I. Observe for elimination of signs and symptoms and restored hearing.
II. Check for recurrence of problem.

The Middle Ear

Perforation of the Eardrum

DEFINITION

Perforation of the eardrum may be considered a middle or outer ear problem. The eardrum may be perforated as a result of:

1. Chronic infection, such as acute and/or chronic otitis media.
2. Trauma.
    a. Insertion of toothpicks and bobby pins, or careless use of Q-Tips.
    b. Direct blows to the side of the head, or a slap with an open palm.
    c. Burns.
    d. High-pressure flow of fluids, such as water.
    e. Blast injury.
3. Postsurgical effects.

ASSESSMENT

I. Excruciating pain at time of rupture.
II. Diminished hearing.
III. Dizziness, nausea, and vomiting.
IV. Hollow reverberating sound in the head.
V. Appearance of blood in ear canal.

DIAGNOSIS

I. Infection (potential).
II. Alteration in comfort: pain.
III. Disturbance of perception and coordination, secondary to altered balance.

GOALS OF CARE

I. Immediate.
    A. Remove cause of perforation.
    B. Restore continuity of eardrum.
    C. Prevent infection.
    D. Restore hearing.
    E. Relieve pain.
II. Postoperative.
    A. Prevent infection.
    B. Prevent recurrence.
    C. Prevent falling due to disturbance of balance.

INTERVENTION

I. Immediate.
    A. Small perforations will heal spontaneously.
    B. Give analgesic for relief of pain.
    C. Apply trichloroacetic acid frequently.
    D. Surgical procedures to close perforation may be necessary.
        1. Myringoplasty.
        2. Graft (fashion from temporal muscle, vein graft occasionally).
II. Postoperative.
    A. Give antibiotic medication for several days; it may be accompanied with application of antibiotic powder to ear canal (Neosporin).
    B. Maintain intact dressing. External dressing may be reinforced.
    C. Surgical packing is usually removed 1 week postoperatively.
    D. Do not suction or probe canal. Gentle suction may be used after 2 weeks to remove debris.
    E. Ear drops should not be used because of possibility of dislocating graft.
    F. Assist with early ambulation attempts; patient may become dizzy.
    G. Medication may be used for nausea, vomiting, or dizziness.
    H. Instruct patient to:
        1. Avoid immersing head in water, swimming, especially diving.
        2. Avoid skydiving or flying in unpressurized planes.

3. Avoid shampooing or any other contact with water as instructed by physician.
4. Continue antibiotic treatment.
5. Continue antihistamine medication for approximately 1 month if prescribed.
6. Avoid blowing nose with force.

EVALUATION
I. Signs and symptoms, especially pain and signs of infection, diminish.
II. Hearing is restored.
III. There is no recurrence of infection.

Eustachian Salpingitis

DEFINITION
Eustachian salpingitis is blockage of the eustachian tube, which connects the postnasal air channel (nasal pharynx) to the middle ear and serves as a safety outlet for secretions from the middle ear as well as an equalizer of air pressure on both sides of the eardrum. Blockage of the tube may be caused by:

1. Violent blowing of the nose without the mouth open, thereby forcing infected material into the eustachian tube.
2. Enlarged adenoids.
3. Cold or allergy attacks.
4. Enlarging tumor mass.
5. Sudden descent in poorly pressurized aircraft.

ASSESSMENT
I. History of recurrence from common causes.
II. Impaired hearing.
III. Fullness in the ear.
IV. Crackling or other noises during swallowing.

V. Sensation of fluid in the ear.
VI. Tinnitus.
VII. Dizziness.

GOALS OF CARE
I. Remove cause of blockage.
II. Prevent infection of middle ear.

INTERVENTION
I. Short course of steroid treatment is given.
II. Fluid is withdrawn by needle placed through anesthetized eardrum. (Children need to be hospitalized and placed under general anesthesia for this procedure.)
III. Fluids may be drained from middle ear by small suction tube via eardrum incision (drainage tube may be left in place for several weeks if drainage is thick).
IV. If condition is accompanied by adenoiditis or tonsillitis, removal of adenoids or tonsils may be appropriate.

EVALUATION
I. Reduction of signs and symptoms.
II. Restoration of hearing.
III. Check for recurrence or for signs and symptoms indicative of acute otitis media.

Acute Otitis Media

DEFINITION
Acute otitis media is a middle ear inflammation caused by a pathological organism which gains entry via the external auditory canal through a perforated eardrum, or through the eustachian tube.

ASSESSMENT
I. Severe, painful earache which may be of a stabbing nature and may radiate over involved side of head.
II. Sensation of fullness in the ear which may change with position alteration.

   III. Tinnitis.

   IV. Tenderness over mastoid bone.

    V. High fever [up to 105°F (40.6°C)].

   VI. Diminution of hearing.

  VII. Headache.

 VIII. Abnormal noises in head and ear.

   IX. Vertigo, nausea, and vomiting.

    X. Anorexia.

   XI. Decreased pulse.

DIAGNOSIS

    I. Alteration in balance, secondary to inflammation.

   II. Alteration in comfort: pain, tinnitus, and headache.

  III. Alteration in nutrition, secondary to nausea, anorexia.

GOALS OF CARE

    I. Reduce infection and prevent spread to mastoid and brain.

   II. Relieve pain.

  III. Restore hearing loss and prevent permanent loss of hearing.

  IV. Prevent recurrence.

INTERVENTION

    I. Antibiotic therapy appropriate for specific pathological organism is administered (penicillin and erythromycin are frequently used).

   II. Surgical intervention can include myringotomy, an incision through posterior aspect of eardrum and drainage. Rapid healing usually occurs and does not affect hearing.

  III. Instruct patient to watch for signs and symptoms of continuation of conditions.

EVALUATION

    I. Signs and symptoms are reduced.

       A. Pain is diminished.   C. Hearing is restored.

       B. Tenderness is decreased.   D. Appetite is restored.

   II. Check for recurrent signs and symptoms indicative of chronic otitis media.

Chronic Otitis Media and Mastoiditis

DEFINITION

Chronic otitis media may result from recurrence of acute otitis media and sustained entry of pathological organisms (that may continue over a period of years) caused by (1) inadequate treatment of acute otitis media or (2) organisms resistant to antibiotic therapy. Conditions may extend to mastoids, brain, larynx, and facial nerves.

ASSESSMENT

    I. Mild hearing loss.

   II. Discharge with foul odor.

  III. Signs and symptoms of perforated eardrum.

  IV. Identification of collection of soft ball of skin with invasion of eardrum.

   V. Identification of mastoid involvement via x-rays.

  VI. Signs and symptoms of meningitis.

 VII. Signs indicative of facial nerve involvement include:

       A. Facial paralysis.   D. Inability to drink fluid without dripping.

       B. Inability to close eyes.   E. Inability to whistle.

       C. Drooping mouth.

 VIII. Signs and symptoms of inflammation.

  IX. Vertigo.

DIAGNOSIS

Refer to "Acute Otitis Media."

GOALS OF CARE

I. Immediate.
  A. Reduce and eliminate source of infection.
  B. Restore hearing.
  C. Prevent complications.
II. Postoperative.
  A. Reduce postoperative pain. **C.** Prevent contamination of operative area.
  B. Prevent complications. **D.** Prevent recurrence of condition.

INTERVENTION

I. Immediate.
  A. Antibiotic therapy.
  B. Surgical intervention.
    1. Simple mastoidectomy is performed to remove involved mastoid cells.
    2. Radical mastoidectomy is performed to remove all involved tissues in mastoid and middle ear.
    3. Posteroanterior mastoidectomy (simple mastoidectomy plus tympanoplasty) is done to repair damaged eardrum and middle ear.
II. Postoperative.
  A. Give medication (aspirin, codeine sulfate, sedatives) and use an ice cap for reduction of postoperative pain.
  B. Observe for complications of facial paralysis, infection, and meningitis.
  C. Maintain good sterile technique in changing dressings. Packing may be removed third to fourth day postoperatively.
  D. Instruct patient and family regarding:
    1. Dressing and packing.
    2. Expected restoration of hearing.
  E. If stapes and cochlea are uninvolved, expect return of hearing.
  F. If cochlea or stapes are damaged, patient may require hearing aid.

EVALUATION

I. Signs and ymptoms are reduced.
  A. Infection cleared. **D.** No residual paralysis.
  B. No discharge from ear. **E.** No vertigo.
  C. Hearing restored.
II. Follow up progress of rehabilitation.

The Inner Ear

Otosclerosis

DEFINITION

Otosclerosis consists of ossification of stapes with a diminution of sound transmission through the ossicles to the inner ear. Loss of hearing with this condition is associated with development of new spongy bone in the labyrinth. The cause is unknown, with a higher rate of occurrence in females and a higher rate of recurrence in blacks. A hereditary basis may be relevant to this condition.

ASSESSMENT

I. Slow diminution of hearing without middle ear infection.
II. Abnormal bilateral buzzing and ringing noises.
III. Bone conduction is better than air conduction of sound.

GOALS OF CARE

I. Prevent infection. **IV.** Prevent falling due to balance disturbance.
II. Promote comfort. **V.** Provide information regarding prognosis.
III. Promote graft stability.

INTERVENTION

I. Immediate.
   A. Surgery.
   B. Stapedectomy is performed for removal of otosclerotic lesions and implantation of prosthesis for restoration of sound conduction.

II. Postoperative.
   A. Observe for signs and symptoms of infection (fever, vertigo, headache, eye pain).
   B. Position patient according to physician's preference.
      1. Upright (ear up) for maximum graft stability.
      2. Side of operation down to promote drainage.
      3. Patient's preferred position for maximum comfort.
   C. Administer antibiotics, sedative, and pain medication for vertigo, nausea, pain, and nystagmus.
   D. Assist in early ambulation; patient may feel dizzy for several days postoperatively.
   E. Instruct patient in the following:
      1. Avoid blowing nose for minimum of 1 week.
      2. Follow instructions for head position.
      3. Replace soiled cotton padding as necessary.
      4. It may be several weeks before full effects of surgery are known (due to tissue edema and surgical pack).
      5. Avoid smoking.
      6. Protect ears when outdoors.
      7. Avoid crowds and exposure to colds.

EVALUATION

I. Symptoms are reduced.
II. Hearing is restored.
III. Check for symptoms of recurrence.

Ménière's
Syndrome

DEFINITION

Ménière's syndrome is a dysfunction of the labyrinth that is accompanied by two characteristic effects: variable remissions and loss of equilibrium. This condition may be caused by tumors, infections, leukemia, allergies, arterio- or atherosclerosis, medical toxicity, physical or emotional stress, or genetic factors.

ASSESSMENT

I. History of common causes.

II. Attacks are characterized by:
   A. Dizziness.
   B. Tinnitus.
   C. Diminution of hearing on involved side.
   D. Headaches.
   E. Nausea and vomiting (especially with sudden head motion).
   F. Irritability.
   G. Depression or withdrawn behavior.
   H. Diminution of appetite.
   I. Vertigo.
   J. Feeling of fullness in the ear.
   K. Past pointing (inability to place finger on indicated point such as nose, elbow, etc., with the eyes closed).

III. Attacks are intermittent, often with abrupt onset, lasting from minutes to hours. Period between attacks may last months or even years.

IV. Caloric test: Insert fluid below or above body temperature with observation after insertion.
   A. Dizziness indicates normal functioning of labyrinth.
   B. No response indicates presence of acoustic neuroma.
   C. Severe attack indicates Ménière's syndrome.

DIAGNOSIS
Refer to "Acute Otitis Media."

GOALS OF CARE
I. Prevent attacks.
II. Reduce postoperative causes of discomfort.
III. Prevent injury from falling.
IV. Prevent complications.

INTERVENTION
I. Immediate.
   A. There is no universally accepted medical or surgical treatment.
   B. Administer diuretic drugs and low-sodium diet for reduction of inner ear fluid.
   C. Tranquilizers and/or antimotion medication may help.
   D. Administer antihistamines and vasodilators.
   E. Psychiatric referral may be appropriate.
   F. Surgical procedures:
      1. Destruction of part or all of inner ear (labyrinthectomy), is used only with severe or total deafness for the relief of symptoms.
      2. Ultrasonic vibrations can be applied to labyrinth.
      3. Cryosurgery (utilized infrequently).
II. Postoperative.
   A. Provide encouragement and understanding.
   B. Instruct patient to slow body movements, jerking, etc., which may precipitate an attack.
   C. Encourage bed rest for a few days postoperatively.
   D. Instruct patients regarding possibility of dizziness for 4 to 6 weeks after surgery; it will resolve itself.
   E. Observe for Bell's palsy (pain near jaw angle or behind ear).

EVALUATION
Refer to "Otosclerosis."

Motion Sickness **DEFINITION**
Motion sickness is caused by a disturbance in the nerve receptors of the inner ear resulting from shifting fluid (endolymph) within the semicircular canals. This condition may be caused by any type of transportation such as planes, buses, automobiles, trains, and boats. Individuals with a chronic infection of the eustachian tube, sinus, or the ears are quite prone to this condition. If prolonged, motion sickness may lead to dehydration, acidosis, and profound mental depression.

ASSESSMENT
I. Nausea and vomiting.
II. Dizziness.
III. Greenish pallor.
IV. Cold sweat.
V. Difficulty in breathing.

GOALS OF CARE
I. Prevent recurrence.
II. Prevent complications of prolonged course.

INTERVENTION
I. Prevention: Administer Dramamine and Bonine (long-lasting but may cause drowsiness), or Marezine (brief duration with no dizziness).
II. Patient should remain in a reclining position with head still.
III. Avoid reading, looking at scenery, or watching the horizon.
IV. Avoid alcoholic drinks.
V. Suck ice.
VI. Inhale oxygen.

DISORDERS OF THE EYE

See Fig. 23-7 to locate structures involved in various disorders.

General Assessment of the Eye

    I. Visual acuity: determined using Snellen chart.
        A. Individual stands 20 ft from chart.
        B. Each eye is tested separately with and without glasses.
        C. The large E at top of chart is scaled for normal vision at 200 ft from chart.

FIGURE 23-7 / **The anatomy of the eye. (*From Eldra P. Solomon and P. William Davis, Understanding Human Anatomy and Physiology, McGraw-Hill Book Company, New York, 1978, p. 287.*)**

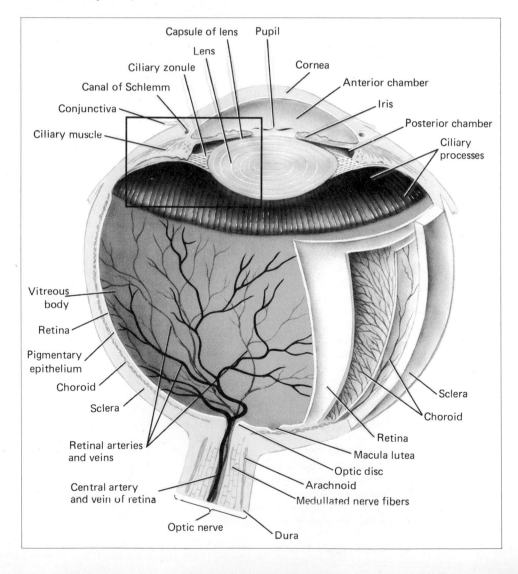

    D. The rows of letters that follow are scaled to sizes to be read at various distances (20, 40, and 100 ft).

    E. Visual acuity is expressed as the ratio of the distance in feet of the lowest line of letters which can be read to the distance in feet from the chart. Example, individual reads letters of size 40 at 20 ft from chart, visual acuity equals 40/20 vision.

  II. Refraction: Determining refractive error and prescribing correction.

    A. Examination is initiated with instillation of cycloplegic drug (i.e., atropine) into conjunctival sac. This paralyzes ciliary muscle, thus impeding accommodation process.

    B. Determination of the refractive error is accomplished with sets of trial lenses in an instrument (usually retinoscope) projecting beam of light into eye.

    C. Refractive error is identified with observation of light reflex in individual's pupil. (See Table 23-9 for common refractive errors, description, common signs, and corrections.)

 III. Visual fields: Examining peripheral and side vision.

    A. Eye is fixed at central point; field is checked with perimeter instrument.

    B. Target screen method or confrontation method may also be used.

 IV. Color vision: An individual is asked to identify colors in a color plate booklet.

  V. Extraocular muscle function: Have individual hold head in one position and follow moving object with eyes.

    A. Check six cardial positions of gaze.

    B. Observe muscle movement, coordination, and alignment.

 VI. Examination of external and internal eye structures: vessels, iris, cornea, optic disk, macula, red reflex, scleras, conjunctiva, pupils (reflexes), iris, and chambers.

    A. Direct ophthalmoscope examination: A beam of light is directed through pupil, permitting visualization of fundus.

    B. Indirect ophthalmoscope: Stereoscopic picture of larger area of retina is obtained by use of a binocular, hand-held convex lens permitting examination of extreme retinal periphery. A mydriatic agent is used to dilate pupils before examination.

 VII. Tonometry: Eyeball tension is measured with use of tonometer. Normal tension equals 11 to 22 mmHg. A local anesthetic is instilled into eye before examination.

VIII. Gonioscopy: The anterior chamber angle (iris-cornea juncture) is examined with a contact glass, illuminator, and hand microscope.

Conjunctivitis

DEFINITION

Conjunctivitis is an inflammation of the conjunctiva often caused by bacteria, viruses, allergies, or exposure to irritating chemicals.

ASSESSMENT

  I. Data sources (refer to "Injury to the Brain").

 II. Health history (refer to "General Assessment").

III. Physical assessment.

    A. Tearing and reddened eye.

    B. Purulent discharge.

    C. Itching and burning sensation.

    D. Swollen eyelids.

    E. Blurred vision, feeling that something is in the eyes.

IV. Diagnostic tests.

GOALS OF CARE

  I. Reduce inflammation.

 II. Prevent spread of contamination to other eye or to other people.

TABLE 23-9 / ERRORS OF REFRACTION

Error	Description	Symptoms	Corrective Lens
Myopia (nearsightedness)	Parallel rays of light focus in *front* of the retina	Blurred distant vision Squinting	Concave (minus) lens
Hyperopia (farsightedness)	Parallel rays of light focus *behind* the retina	Headache Burning sensation of the eye Pulling sensation in the eye	Convex (plus) lens
Astigmatism	Light rays are not refracted equally in all meridians owing to irregular curvature of cornea	Squinting Tilting head to one side	Cylinder lens
Presbyopia	Decrease in accommodative power of the crystalline lens due to aging process	Inability to see comfortably at close range, "arm's length" reading	"Reading glasses": convex lens for near vision; bifocal lenses for near and distant vision

Source: Irene C. Cullin and Nancy L. Holland, in Dorothy A. Jones, Claire F. Dunbar, and Mary M. Jirovec (eds.), *Medical-Surgical Nursing: A Conceptual Approach,* McGraw-Hill Book Company, New York, 1978, p. 1266, Table 38-2.

INTERVENTION
I. Administer antibiotic drops.
II. Sulfonamides or steroid drops may be prescribed also.
III. Hygienic measures include:
   A. Frequent handwashing.
   B. Separate toweling for infected eye.

Blepharitis

DEFINITION
Blepharitis is an inflammation of eyelid margins, usually bilateral, normally caused by staphylococcus.

ASSESSMENT
I. Irritation of eyelid margins.
II. Crusting with scale formation.
III. Ulcers on lid margins causing loss of eyelashes.
IV. Burning and itching of eyes.
V. Tearing.
VI. Thickened and inflamed eyelids.
VII. Feeling of something in the eye.

GOALS OF CARE
I. Reduce inflammation.
II. Promote comfort.
III. Prevent recurrence.
IV. Prevent spread to other individuals.

INTERVENTION
I. Use warm compresses to soften and remove crust.
II. An antibiotic or sulfonamide ophthalmic ointment is applied directly to eyelid margins after crust removal.
III. Antibiotic and steroid drops ward off secondary infections.
IV. Limit use of towels, washcloths, and cosmetics to involved individual.

Hordeolum

DEFINITION
Hordeolum (*sty*) is one of the most common inflammations of the lid margin, involving hair follicles, and usually is caused by a staphylococcal infection.

ASSESSMENT
I. Localized redness and swelling.
II. Tenderness at site of infection.
III. Burning, smarting feeling of eye.
IV. Feeling of something in the eye.
V. Tearing.
VI. Redness, pain, and swelling with appearance of small, hard, red boil at base of eyelash.

GOALS OF CARE
I. Reduce pain.
II. Promote rupture of sty and resolution of process.

INTERVENTION
I. Use warm, moist compresses for 15 min, 3 to 4 times a day.
II. An antibiotic ointment may be appropriate.

Chalazion

DEFINITION
Chalazion is an inflammation inside the eyelid involving the meibomian gland and the sebaceous eyelid gland (often occurring during pregnancy).

ASSESSMENT
I. In the acute stage, the assessment is similar to the assessment of a sty.
II. In the later stages, there is a hard, painless lump or cyst on the inner aspect of the eyelid.

GOALS OF CARE
Refer to "Hordeolum."

INTERVENTION
I. In the early stage, warm, moist compresses and antibiotic ointments are given.
II. In the later stages, excision by an ophthalmologist may be necessary.

Keratitis

DEFINITION
Keratitis is an inflammation of the cornea. *Superficial keratitis* is caused by infection from the external environment. *Deep keratitis* is caused by the spread of an etiological agent through the circulatory system or from neighboring eye structures. It is often caused by viral and/or bacterial infections and is less frequently associated with tuberculosis, syphilis, and other systemic infections.

ASSESSMENT
I. Dilatation of blood vessels around cornea.
II. A cloudy appearance of cornea.
III. Photophobia.
IV. Tearing.
V. Impaired vision.
VI. Increased sensitivity to light.

GOALS OF CARE
I. The immediate goal is treatment of condition.
II. Reduce inflammation.

INTERVENTION
I. Immediate use of antibiotics, occasionally cortisone, is necessary.
II. Treat underlying cause.

Dacryocystitis

DEFINITION
Dacryocystitis is an infection of the lacrimal sac usually caused by an obstruction of one of the tear canals that leads into the nose.

ASSESSMENT
I. Pain below eyeball.
II. Redness and flowing below the eye, may extend to the eyelids.
III. Profuse tearing.
IV. Purulent discharge.

GOALS OF CARE
I. Reduce inflammation and infection.
II. Prevent spread to cornea.

INTERVENTION
I. Apply hot compresses frequently.
II. Antibiotics may be prescibed.
III. Surgery may be necessary to open a new channel into the nose.

Uveitis

DEFINITION
Uveitis is an inflammatory condition of the uveal tract (pigmented vascular layer of the eye including iris, ciliary body, and choroid). If the iris and ciliary body only are involved, the condition is called *iridocyclitis*. When the choroid is involved, the retina will be involved also because of the close proximity of the two structures. This condition is called *chorioretinitis*. Uveitis is a unilateral disease affecting young and middle-aged people. It may be caused by the spread of infection from other structures of the eyes, parasitic invasion, systemic disease, focal infection, or allergic response.

ASSESSMENT
I. Iris:
    A. Pain (may radiate to temple).   D. Irregularly shaped pupil.
    B. Photophobia.   E. Blurred vision.
    C. Sluggish iris movement.   F. Light intolerance.
II. Choroid:
    A. Yellowish white lesions on retina.
    B. Visual loss in peripheral fields corresponding to lesion locations.
    C. Possible decrease in central acuity.
III. Skin tests to rule out tuberculosis, histoplasmosis, and toxoplasmosis.
IV. Rule out conjunctivitis and glaucoma.

GOALS OF CARE
I. Rule out conditions with similar symptoms.   IV. Prevent progression to glaucoma.
II. Reduce inflammation.   V. Relieve pain.
III. Prevent loss of sight.

INTERVENTION
I. Use warm compresses, coating, and/or aspirin.
II. Dark glasses should be worn.
III. Corticosteroids are prescribed.
IV. Reassure patient and family regarding slow progress and fear of loss of sight.

Optic Neuritis

DEFINITION
Optic neuritis is an inflammation of the optic nerve resulting from syphilis, acute infectious diseases, multiple sclerosis, internal poisonings and, rarely, meningitis or encephalitis.

ASSESSMENT
I. Sudden loss of vision, including blind spots and narrowing of visual field.
II. Pain with eyeball movement.
III. Swollen retina.
IV. Bleeding from the retina.

GOALS OF CARE
I. Relieve signs and symptoms. III. Treat underlying cause.
II. Prevent recurrence. IV. Prevent permanent loss of sight.

INTERVENTION
Immediate steroid therapy is necessary.

Malignant Melanoma

DEFINITION
Malignant melanoma is the most common malignant intraocular tumor developing in the uveal tract, usually in the choroid, which affects individuals in middle age. It is usually unilateral. (Refer to Chap. 31 for a more complete discussion.)

ASSESSMENT
I. Iris: altered color of iris and size of pupil.
II. Choroid: retinal detachment and sudden or gradual loss of vision.
III. Pain if tumor is large and causing increased intraocular pressure (glaucoma).
IV. Macular: blurring of central vision.

GOALS OF CARE
I. Preoperative and postoperative care according to intervention chosen.
II. Support patient and family through progression of diagnosis and treatment.

INTERVENTION
I. Enucleation of eyes.
II. Iridectomy when tumor is limited to small portion of iris.

Corneal Ulcer

DEFINITION
A *corneal ulcer* arises from loss of corneal epithelium resulting from extension of conjunctivitis to cornea, corneal inflammation, or direct corneal trauma. The pathological organisms involved are usually bacterial, viral, or fungal.

ASSESSMENT

I. Pain.
II. Photophobia.
III. Tearing.
IV. Bloodshot appearance to eye.
V. Involvement of iris: purulent discharge and white or yellow deposits behind cornea.
VI. Perforated corneal ulcer: prolapse of iris through cornea.

DIAGNOSIS

Alteration in comfort: pain, secondary to corneal inflammation or trauma.

GOALS OF CARE

I. Immediate.
  A. Remove positive agent or accompanying condition.
  B. Promote comfort.
  C. Relieve infection/inflammation.
II. Preoperative.
  A. Allay anxiety during waiting period for donor.
  B. Avoid increase of pressure and strain on the eye.
III. Postoperative.
  A. Promote healing.
  B. Reduce anxieties while awaiting results of surgery.

INTERVENTION

I. Immediate.
  A. Remove foreign bodies.
  B. Dark glasses should be worn.
  C. Mydriatics are administered.
  D. Examination of eye is followed by medication for relief of pain.
  E. Antibiotics are given for specific types of infection.
  F. Warm compresses are applied.
  G. Systemic antibiotics are given if appropriate.
  H. Steroid therapy may be prescribed for secondary fungal infections if present.
  I. Corneal transplantation involves a split-thickness (lamellar keratoplasty) or full-thickness (penetrating keratoplasty) transplant with fresh donor tissue to replace damaged cornea.
II. Postoperative.
  A. Cover both eyes to ensure total rest.
  B. Prepare patient for possible failure (88 percent of cases are successful).
  C. Instruct patient to wear protective shield over eye for a minimum of 6 weeks after discharge.
  D. Instruct patient regarding activities to ensure protection of eyes during healing period.

Cataracts

DEFINITION

Cataracts result from the slowly growing opaqueness of the eye lens usually accompanying the aging process, diabetes, eye infection or, rarely, exposure to chemical or physical poisons. (Refer to Chap. 42 for a discussion of cataracts in relation to the aged.)

ASSESSMENT

I. Gradual or painless loss of sight.
II. Increased opaqueness of lens.
III. Distorted or blurred vision.

IV. Irritation from glaring or bright lights.

V. In the later stage, gray or milky white appearance to pupil.

GOALS OF CARE

I. Immediate.

   A. Identify appropriate time for treatment.

   B. Reassure patient and provide information concerning progression and required surgery.

II. Preoperative.

   A. Promote comfort.

   B. Reduce any infection present.

   C. Prepar for surgery.

III. Postoperative.

   A. Prevent increased intraocular pressure.

   B. Promote comfort.

   C. Prevent complications.

   D. Support rehabilitation activities.

INTERVENTION

I. Surgical removal will be performed at appropriate stage of condition, determined by maturation of cataract, occupation, and patient's general health.

II. Preoperative.

   A. Provide safety precautions due to reduced vision of patient.

   B. Instruct patient and family regarding surgery.

   C. Administer antibiotics and take conjunctival cultures as prescribed.

   D. Instruct patient not to touch eyes.

   E. Mydriatics may be prescribed before surgery.

III. Postoperative.

   A. Avoid coughing or sneezing.

   B. Avoid rapid movements.

   C. Avoid bending from the waist.

   D. Give analgesics for relief of pain.

   E. Provide quiet and safe environment.

   F. Notify physician if sudden pain occurs (may be indicative of hemorrhage or ruptured suture).

   G. Treat nausea and vomiting immediately.

   H. Assist patient in early ambulatory activities.

   I. Instruct patient and family on administration of eyedrops, use of dark glasses, and fitting for corrective lenses.

Glaucoma

Glaucoma is caused by increased intraocular pressure due to increased production of aqueous humor and/or decreased outflow of aqueous humor, occurring in approximately 2 percent of the population over 40 years of age (refer to Chap. 42 for a discussion of glaucoma in relation to the aged.) There are two types of glaucoma in the adult: chronic simple glaucoma (wide-angle), and acute or chronic congestive glaucoma (narrow-angle). See Fig. 23-8 for the route of normal flow of aqueous humor.

Acute
(Narrow-angle)
Glaucoma

DEFINITION

In *acute (narrow-angle) glaucoma,* the dilated iris prevents drainage of aqueous humor into the canal of Schlemm (see Fig. 23-9).

ASSESSMENT

I. Severe pain.

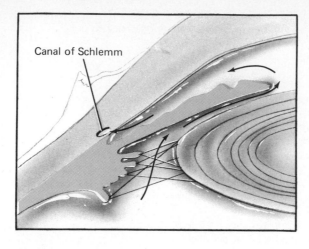

FIGURE 23-8 / Normal circulation of aqueous humor. (*From Eldra P. Solomon and P. William Davis, Understanding Human Anatomy and Physiology, McGraw-Hill Book Company, New York, 1978, p. 296.*)

II. Cloudy and blurred vision.
III. Progressive (may be rapid) diminution of vision.
IV. Dilated pupils.
V. Nausea and vomiting.
VI. Artificial lights around objects.

GOALS OF CARE
I. Prevent and or reduce progression of condition.
II. Reduce pain.
III. Prevent permanent blindness.

INTERVENTION
I. Parasympathomimetic drugs are prescribed for miotic action (to draw iris away from cornea for facilitation of aqueous humor drainage).
II. Eyedrops should not be used as they may increase severity of condition.
III. Treatment needs to be done immediately to prevent permanent blindness.
IV. Surgical intervention may be necessary to restore proper drainage (see Fig. 23-10).

Chronic (Wide-angle) Glaucoma

DEFINITION
In *chronic (wide-angle) glaucoma* the intraocular pressure increases over a prolonged period of time.

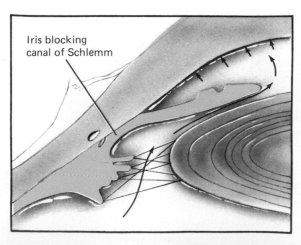

FIGURE 23-9 / Blockage of aqueous humor drainage in closed-angle glaucoma. (*From Eldra P. Solomon and P. William Davis, Understanding Human Anatomy and Physiology, McGraw-Hill Book Company, New York, 1978, p. 296.*)

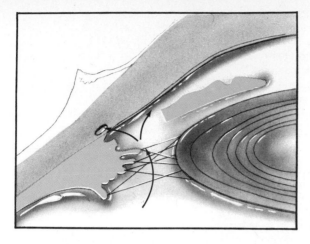

FIGURE 23-10 / Surgical intervention to restore normal drainage of aqueous humor. *(From Eldra P. Solomon and P. William Davis, Understanding Human Anatomy and Physiology, McGraw-Hill Book Company, New York, 1978, p. 296.)*

ASSESSMENT
I. Early phase: no symptoms.
II. Tired feeling in the eyes.
III. Halos or rainbows around electric lights.
IV. Hard eyeball.
V. Blind spots, slow diminution of peripheral vision.
VI. Poor night vision.

GOALS OF CARE
I. Identify condition early for prevention of permanent loss of vision.
II. Promote compliance with medication.

INTERVENTION
I. Miotic eyedrops are prescribed.
II. Close observation is necessary to determine if disease is controlled, with periodic eye examinations and visual field testing performed.
III. Surgical intervention may be necessary for proper drainage of aqueous humor.
IV. Avoid conditions which will increase intraocular pressure such as:
    A. Emotional stress.
    B. Wearing of tight clothing around waist or neck.
    C. Heavy exertion.
    D. Upper respiratory infections.

Detached Retina

DEFINITION
A *detached retina* is the separation of the retina from the choroid. It may be partial at first, but may then progress to a complete separation if it is not treated properly. Detachment of the retina is usually due to a break in the retina through which aqueous humor flows into the space between the retina and choroid, producing the separation.

ASSESSMENT
I. Flashes of light, occasionally followed by a sensation of a curtain drawn across the visual field.
II. Blurred vision.
III. Sensation of particles in visual field.
IV. Blind spots.
V. Progressive loss of vision.

GOALS OF CARE
I. Preoperative.
  A. Prevent permanent vision loss.
  B. Allay anxiety.
  C. Promote comfort.
  D. Supportive management is given through surgical intervention.
II. Postoperative.
  A. Maintain retinal reattachment.   C. Promote comfort.
  B. Prevent permanent visual loss.   D. Reduce anxiety.

INTERVENTION
I. Preoperative.
  A. Patient must stay in bed with eyes bandaged.
  B. Maintain appropriate head position for area of detachment according to physician's preference.
  C. Give support, sedation, and/or tranquilizers for comfort and to allay anxiety.
II. Surgical intervention involves repairing the separation between retina and choroid via:
  A. Diathermy.   C. Scleral buckling.
  B. Cryosurgery.   D. Photocoagulation.
III. Postoperative.
  A. Patient must stay in bed with eyes bandaged for a minimum of several days.
  B. Safety precautions must be observed in patient's environment to avoid bumping head or sudden movements.
  C. Diversional activities may help.
  D. Assist patient as ambulation progresses.
  E. Support patient through waiting period to determine effect of surgery.

Eye Disorders Resulting from Usage of Tobacco and Alcohol

DEFINITION
Excessive and/or combined use of alcohol and tobacco may cause vision changes or loss of vision.

ASSESSMENT
I. Blind spots in central vision.
II. Disturbances of color (especially red and green).
III. Eye muscle palsies.
IV. Optic nerve involvement.

GOALS OF CARE
I. Decrease or eliminate causative agent.
II. Prevent permanent loss of vision.

INTERVENTION
I. Provide information regarding cause and the effects to the patient.
II. Encourage a decrease or elimination of tobacco and alcohol.
III. Encourage balanced diet.

Eye Disorders Resulting from Usage of Common Drugs

DEFINITION
Side effects of common drugs may include vision changes or loss of vision.

ASSESSMENT
I. Digitalis:
   A. Seeing snowflakes or rainbows in visual fields.
   B. Yellow vision.
II. Cortisone:
   A. Symptoms of cataracts.
   B. Symptoms of glaucoma.
III. Tranquilizers:
   A. Blurred or double vision.
   B. Other symptoms of glaucoma.
IV. Aspirin: Retinal hemorrhages.
V. Medications occasionally used for diarrhea, gall bladder disturbances, Parkinson's disease, motion sickness, gout, and hypertension may also cause eye reactions.
   A. Symptoms of glaucoma.
   B. Blurred vision.

GOALS OF CARE
I. Identify positive agent.
II. Decrease or eliminate intake of appropriate medication.

INTERVENTION
Alleviate the observed symptoms.

Eye Disorders Secondary to Systemic Diseases

Hypertensive and Renal Retinopathy

DEFINITION
See Chaps. 26 and 28 for a discussion of hypertension and renal pathology.

ASSESSMENT
I. Narrowing of retinal arterioles.
II. Increase in capillary permeability with resultant retinal edema, exudates, hemorrhage, and papilledema.

GOALS OF CARE
I. Reduce effect of underlying disease.
II. Prevent permanent loss of vision.

INTERVENTION
I. There is no known ophthalmic treatment for hypertensive retinopathy.
II. Treatment has to be directed toward hypertension and chronic glomerulonephritis.

Rheumatoid Arthritis

DEFINITION
See Chap. 32 for a discussion of rheumatoid arthritis.

ASSESSMENT
I. Iritis and iridocyclitis.
II. Relapses of symptoms accompanying exacerbation of arthritis.

GOALS OF CARE
Provide supportive measures for patient.

INTERVENTION
There is no known satisfactory ophthalmic treatment.

Lupus
Erythematosus

DEFINITION
See Chap. 32 for a discussion of lupus erythematosus.

ASSESSMENT
I. Retinopathy with exudates and hemorrhage.
II. Nystagmus.
III. Occlusion of central retinal artery.
IV. Loss of vision.

GOALS OF CARE
Supportive management is given for complications of underlying disease.

INTERVENTION
There is no known specific ophthalmological treatment.

Anemia

DEFINITION
See Chap. 25 for a discussion of anemia.

ASSESSMENT
I. Retinal hemorrhage.
II. A decrease in red blood cell count (to less than 50 percent of normal).
III. Visual loss if hemorrhage involves maculum.

GOALS OF CARE
I. Prevent permanent vision loss.
II. Treat underlying disease process.

INTERVENTION
Treat anemic process.

Diabetic
Retinopathy

DEFINITION
See Chap. 24 for a discussion of diabetes mellitus.

ASSESSMENT
I. Microaneurysms in the venous end of capillaries in the inner nuclear retina near the optic disk and/or macula.
II. White or yellowish waxy exudate.
III. Punctate hemorrhages.
IV. Possible retinal detachment with total visual loss.

GOALS OF CARE
I. Retard progression of disease.
II. Support patient.

INTERVENTION
The most successful intervention is maximum management of the patient's diabetes.

BIBLIOGRAPHY

Eliasson, S. G., A. L. Prensky, and W. B. Hardin, Jr. (eds.): *Neurological Pathophysiology,* Oxford University Press, New York, 1974. Designed for medical students and generalists, this text presents pathophysiology of neurologic problems clearly and simply.

Fowkes, W. C., Jr., and V. K. Hunn: *Clinical Assessment for the Nurse Practitioner,* The C. V. Mosby Company, St. Louis, 1973. Concise presentation of the neurologic examination as part of the complete assessment.

Jones, D., C. Dunbar, and M. Jirovec (eds.): *Medical-Surgical Nursing: A Conceptual Approach,* McGraw-Hill Book Company, New York, 1978. The section on perception and coordination offers the reader an in-depth look at neurological disorders, and Chap. 31 presents a good neurological assessment.

Mayo Clinic and Mayo Foundation: *Clinical Examinations in Neurology,* W. B. Saunders, Philadelphia, 1971. Excellent source for evaluating problems of the nervous system. Examination techniques and interpretation of results are presented.

Melasanos, L., V. Barkauskas, M. Moss, and K. Allen: *Health Assessment,* The C. V. Mosby Company, St. Louis, 1977. A good resource for examination of the eyes, ears, and nervous system.

Thorn, G. W., et al. (eds.): *Harrison's Principles of Internal Medicine,* 8th ed., McGraw-Hill Book Company, New York, 1977. Excellent source for the generalist in identifying and managing specific disease processes.

24

The Endocrine System

Jacqueline Sicard Baran

ABNORMAL CELLULAR GROWTH

Adrenal Medullary Tumors

Definition

The main function of the adrenal medulla is to produce and secrete catecholamines (epinephrine and norepinephrine) into the circulation. The adrenal medulla is not essential to life because its function can be carried out by the sympathetic nervous system. The only abnormal clinical entities associated with the adrenal medulla are medullary tumors which hypersecrete catecholamines. These tumors are classified into pheochromocytoma, neuroblastoma, and ganglioneuroma.

Pheochromocytoma, the most common pathological condition associated with sporadic hypersecretion of catecholamines, is thought to occur as a familial autosomal trait. Although 98 percent of pheochromocytomas can be located within the abdomen (especially in the adrenal medulla), they can occur anywhere along the course of the sympathetic nerve chain, i.e., carotid body, urinary bladder. There is a 5 to 10 percent incidence of malignancy among pheochromocytomas (1). Other factors which stimulate the release of catecholamines are responses to stressful situations which can be physical or psychologic, i.e., hypotension, anoxia, altered emotional state. The reaction to such stress is often termed the flight or fight phenomenon. *Neuroblastomas* are usually large, highly malignant tumors. They occur most often in children under 5 years of age and rarely in the adult. The most common clinical features are diarrhea, weakness, malaise, and abdominal pain and are often the result of spread of the tumor (2). *Ganglioneuromas* are rare tumors which can develop during youth but occur more frequently in adulthood. They can be benign or malignant (3). In the subsequent outline, the most prominent tumor, pheochromocytoma, will serve as a model for application of the nursing process.

Assessment

I. Nursing health history.[1]
  A. Source and reliability.
    1. Patient.
    2. Family.
    3. Significant other.
  B. General survey.
    1. Age.   5. Weight.
    2. Sex.   6. Facial expression.
    3. Skin color. 7. Grooming.
    4. Height.   8. Posture.
  C. Response to interview.
    1. Attention span.   3. Ability to understand ideas.
    2. Vocabulary level.   a. Slow to grasp meaning.
     a. Simple, nontechnical terms.   b. Quick to gain meaning.
     b. Complex, technical terms.   4. Ability to recall recent and past events.
  D. History of present illness.
    1. Chief complaint(s).   b. Aggravating and alleviating factor.
    2. Reason for hospitalization. c. Setting.
    3. Description of symptoms. d. Previous treatment and response, if any.
     a. Chronology.

---

[1]Same for all endocrine disorders. Will not be repeated in subsequent sections.

668

    E. Current status and attitude.
       1. Insight into health problem(s).
       2. Expectations.
       3. Effect of illness on family and social roles.
       4. Adjustment in life-style.
          a. Work.
          b. Diet.
          c. Activity.
          d. Social habits.
       5. Previous experience with hospitalization.
          a. Positive.
          b. Negative.
    F. Emotional status.
       1. Presence of absence of anxiety.
       2. Previous experience with stress.
          a. Pain.
          b. Physical trauma.
          c. Emotional trauma: loss of job, significant other.
       3. Past reaction to stress and coping mechanisms.
       4. Past psychiatric care.
       5. Medication to relax.
       6. Effect of illness on self-concept.
       7. Adaptation of self-concept to reality.
       8. Ability to relate to others.
          a. Family.
          b. Friends.
          c. Health-team members.
    G. History of health status.
       1. Knowledge of health status.   **3.** Allergies.
       2. Knowledge of medication(s).   **4.** Compliance with medical supervision.
    H. Personal and social history.
       1. Current life situation.   **3.** Habits.
          a. Family construction.   *a.* Diet.
          b. Significant other(s).   *b.* Smoking.
          c. Employment.   *c.* Alcoholic beverages.
          d. Insurance coverage.   *d.* Elimination.
          e. "Typical day."   *e.* Sleep.
       2. Past development.   *f.* Activity.
          a. Education.
          b. Religion.
          c. Employment.
II. Physical and behavioral assessment: nonspecific.
    A. Nervous.
       1. Sensory.
          a. Heat intolerance.
          b. Headache.
       2. Motor: syncope.
    B. Integumentary.
       1. Excessive sweating.
       2. Blanched or flushed skin.
    C. Cardiovascular.
       1. Palpitations.   **3.** Tachycardia.
       2. Heart failure.   **4.** Hypertension.
    D. Gastrointestinal.
       1. Nausea, vomiting.
       2. Weight loss.

        E. Mental status.
          1. Anxiety.
          2. Nervousness.
        F. Other.
          1. Glycosuria.
          2. Hyperglycemia.
  III. Other relevant sources.
        A. Medical history.
          1. Family history.
          2. History of multiple endocrine neoplasia (MEA), type 2 medullary carcinoma of the thyroid gland, hyperparathyroidism, and pheochromocytoma.
        B. Interview with family and/or significant other.
        C. Old records.
        D. Referral note.
        E. Diagnostic tests.
          1. Urinary vanillylmandelic acid (VMA).   **4.** Intravenous urograms.
          2. Urinary metanephrine.   **5.** Suprarenal laminograms.
          3. Urinary epinephrine and norepinephrine.   **6.** Plasma catecholamines (limited).

Problems

  I. Physical.
        A. Altered nutritional status.   *D.* Stress.
        B. Pain.   *E.* Safety.
        C. Fatigability.   *F.* Body hygiene.
  II. Psychosocial.
        A. Mental fatigue.   *C.* Anxiety.
        B. Stress.   *D.* Nervousness.

Diagnosis

  I. Complains of headache, dizziness, palpitations, nausea, visual disturbances associated with elevation in blood pressure.
  II. Has abnormal glucose tolerance test (GTT) and/or fasting blood sugar.
  III. Complains of abdominal or precordial pain.
  IV. Has history of weight loss despite adequate dietary intake.
  V. Unable to tolerate heat and/or control diaphoresis.
  VI. Expresses concern about impending diagnostic test and surgery.
  VII. Sleeps in short naps only; unable to rest or "relax."
  VIII. Family expresses concern over patient's "change in personality."

Goals of Care

  I. Immediate.
        A. Minimize internal and environmental stressors.
        B. Reduce pain.
        C. Provide diet compatible with regulation of hyperglycemia and weight gain.
        D. Promote physical and emotional rest.
        E. Prepare physically, psychologically, and emotionally for diagnostic test and surgery.
        F. Provide supportive and protective care.
  II. Long-range.
        A. Promote patient and family independence in managing self at home.
        B. Return to preillness state, physically, psychologically and emotionally, if appropriate.

Intervention

  I. General.
        A. Allow patient to plan daily schedule, if possible, and anticipate changes, i.e., diagnostic test.
        B. Note and record activities and/or circumstances associated with hypertensive attacks, and try to eliminate from environment.
        C. Orient patient to room and hospital routine.
        D. Encourage frequent bathing.

    E. Administer medication(s) and record response(s).
       1. Analgesics for pain.
       2. Sedatives and tranquilizers for rest and relaxation.
       3. Antihypertensives for control of blood pressure (alpha and beta blockers).
       4. Hypoglycemic agents for control of elevated blood sugar.
    F. Allow time to verbalize fears about surgery and "tumors."
    G. Preoperative teaching (see postoperative care of laparotomy in Chap. 29).
    H. Ascertain significant other, and involve in patient care and teaching.
    I. Attend when ambulating, if indicated.
    J. Eliminate unnecessary equipment and material from room.
    K. Provide therapeutic diet compatible with regulation of hyperglycemia and weight gain and based on preferences.
    L. Monitor responses to treatment.
       1. Weigh daily: increased.
       2. Appetite improved.
       3. Urine sugar and acetone normal or improved.
       4. Blood pressure and pulse decreased.
       5. Sleep and rest improved.
       6. Mental status: able to express feeling, interested in participating in care, positive outlook.
    M. Patient and family teaching.
       1. Anatomy and physiology of illness.
       2. Expected responses from treatment.
          a. Unilateral adrenalectomy.
             (1) Curative.
             (2) No medication.
          b. Bilateral adrenalectomy: See "Adrenocortical Hypofunction."
       3. Diet.
       4. Rest and activity.
       5. Avoidance of physical and emotional stress.
    N. Behavioral counseling, if indicated.
  II. Hypertensive crisis.
    A. Nursing assessment.
       1. Rapidly rising blood pressure.
       2. Visual disturbances.
       3. Altered sensorium: confused, coma.
       4. Convulsions.
       5. Congestive heart failure.
          a. Increased pulse rate.
          b. Labored respirations.
          c. Abnormal breath sounds.
    B. Nursing intervention.
       1. Start intravenous.
       2. Place on cardiac monitor.
       3. Strict intake and output.
       4. Administer medication and fluids as ordered.
       5. Assess response to treatment measures.
          a. Blood pressure, pulse, respiration every 15 min, or as needed.
          b. Neurological signs every ½ h, or as needed.
          c. Chest sounds every ½ h, or as needed.
       6. Do not leave unattended.
 III. Postoperative.
    A. See adrenalectomy under "Adrenocortical Hyperfunction: Hypercortisolism."
    B. See point I, above.
    C. Be wary of hypotension.

Evaluation
   I. Verbally describes pathophysiology of disease.
  II. States expected response(s) from treatment and possible complications.
    A. Bilateral adrenalectomy: see "Adrenocortical Hypofunction."
    B. Unilateral adrenalectomy: curative; no hormone replacement therapy.

III. Is able to return to work and maintain family and social roles.
IV. Shows improvement in:
   A. Pulse: normal rate and rhythm; decreased palpitations.
   B. Blood pressure decreased.
   C. Mental status: decreased anxiety, nervousness.
   D. Appetite increased; weight gain.
   E. Skin: improved color; decreased sweating.
   F. Urine sugar and acetone normal.
V. Keeps medical appointment. If unable, calls and schedules another appointment.

Follow-up

I. Clinic.
II. Periodic telephone calls.

Insulinoma

Definition

Insulinomas, or functioning beta cell tumors of the pancreas, are characterized by hyperinsulinism with hypoglycemia. The consistent chemical abnormality is relative hyperinsulinism and inappropriately high serum insulin levels for the simultaneously determined plasma glucose concentration. The latter demonstrates a failure of the abnormal beta cell tissue to turn off insulin secretion normally. Insulinomas are multiple in less than 8 percent and malignant in approximately 10 percent of cases reported. Single adenomata occur in the head, body, and tail of the pancreas. Ectopic sites of the tumors are rare and usually occur along the gastrointestinal tract. Although insulinomas are composed entirely of islet tissue and amyloid deposits, beta granules are occasionally found, suggesting abnormalities in storage and release of insulin (4).

Assessment

I. Nursing health history.
II. Physical and behavioral assessment.
   A. Nervous.
      1. Sensory.   2. Motor.
         a. Visual disturbances.   a. Weakness.
         b. Lightheadedness.   b. Fatigue.
   B. Integumentary. Excessive sweating.
   C. Central nervous system.
      1. Drowsiness.   4. Loss of consciousness.
      2. Stupor.   5. Deep coma.
      3. Confusion.
   D. Mental status.
      1. Amnesia.
      2. Noisy behavior.
      3. Personality change.
III. Other relevant sources.
   A. Interview with family.
   B. Past medical records.
   C. Medical history.
      1. Other medical and endocrine problems, especially peptic ulcer associated with tumors or hyperplasia of the parathyroids, pituitary and pancreatic islets: multiple endocrine adenomatosis (MEA) type I.
      2. Family history, especially endocrine disorders.
   D. Diagnostic tests.
      1. Fasting blood sugar and insulin levels.
      2. Fasting (48 to 72 h) blood sugar and insulin.
      3. Glucose tolerance test: limited value.
      4. Provocative tests: play secondary role to prolonged fast.
         a. Intravenous tolbutamide.
         b. Intravenous glucagon.

Problems

I. General.
    A. Physical.
        1. Weakness.   **4.** Body hygiene.
        2. Fatigability.   **5.** Altered sensorium.
        3. Safety.
    B. Psychosocial.
        1. Irritability.   **3.** Anxiety.
        2. Restlessness.   **4.** Noisy behavior.
II. Subtotal or total pancreatectomy.
    A. Infection.
    B. Hormone imbalance.
    C. Other (see postoperative care after abdominal surgery in Chap. 29).

Diagnosis

I. Complains of symptoms of hypoglycemia, such as weakness, lightheadedness, loss of consciousness and visceral disturbances, usually before breakfast and relieved shortly after eating.
II. Aberrant behavior patterns and disturbances in consciousness noted to be more pronounced after prolonged fasting or vigorous physical exercise.
III. Between hypoglycemic attacks, no abnormal physical or behavioral findings may be found.
IV. May present in deep coma and respond readily to glucose infusion.

Goals of Care

I. General.
    A. Immediate.
        1. Provide optimum diet to meet nutritional needs.
        2. Promote a safe, therapeutic environment.
        3. Promote physical and emotional rest.
        4. Reduce physical and psychological stresses aggravating or contributing to illness.
        5. Prevent and/or control complications.
        6. Evaluate response(s) to treatment measures.
        7. Prepare physically and emotionally for surgery.
    B. Long-range.
        1. Prevent reoccurrence.
        2. Promote patient and family independence in managing self at home.
        3. Return to preillness state, physically, emotionally, and psychologically, if appropriate.
        4. Establish need for follow-up.
II. Subtotal or total pancreatectomy.
    A. Immediate.
        1. Relieve pain and discomfort.
        2. Assist in controlling and/or preventing complications.
        3. Assist in restoring normal fluid and hormone balance.
        4. See care of the patient having abdominal surgery in Chap. 29.
    B. Long-range: same as general long-range goals.

Intervention

I. General.
    A. Explain all diagnostic procedures and expected responses.
    B. Prevent and/or control reoccurrence of signs and symptoms.
        1. Teach signs and symptoms of hypoglycemia.
        2. Develop with medical team "plan of care" for hypoglycemic attacks.
            a. Drugs: glucagon.
            b. Intravenous solution.
            c. Laboratory work.
        3. Keep record of diet intake.
        4. Document environmental stressors contributing to attacks, and if possible:
            a. Limit visitors.

         b. Avoid room change.

         c. Avoid activity.

         d. Encourage balanced diet.

    5. Anticipate changes in normal routine.

    6. Monitor vital signs, behavior, and level of consciousness.

  C. Administer medication for sleep and rest.

  D. Involve in planning care, stressing importance of rest, diet, and moderate activity.

  E. Patient and family teaching.

    1. Anatomy and physiology of illness.

    2. Methods of treatment and expected response(s).

      a. Surgery.

        (1) Subtotal pancreatectomy.

          (a) Transient diabetes (6 to 8 weeks).

          (b) Permanent diabetes.

        (2) Total pancreatectomy: often necessary for permanent diabetes.

      b. Drugs and diet.

    3. Medication(s).

      a. Type.   **c.** Dose.

      b. Action.   **d.** Side effects.

    4. Signs and symptoms of hypoglycemia and hyperglycemia and appropriate action.

    5. Avoidance of physical and emotional stressors.

    6. Diet.

    7. Activity and rest.

    8. Safety precautions for activities such as driving or cooking.

  F. See "Diabetes Mellitus."

  G. Behavioral counseling, if indicated.

II. Subtotal or total pancreatectomy.

  A. Routine care for abdominal surgery.

  B. Observe for hypoglycemia.

  C. Monitor body temperature frequently for high elevation.

  D. Patient and family teaching: see point I, above.

Evaluation

I. Verbally describes pathophysiology of disease.

II. States medication receiving, dose, time, action, and side effects.

III. States expected response(s) from treatment and possible complications.

IV. Verbally recalls signs and symptoms of hypoglycemia and hyperglycemia and appropriate response(s).

V. Demonstrates skills taught, such as insulin administration, urine testing.

VI. Is able to return to work and resume family and social roles.

VII. Keeps medical appointments. If unable, calls and reschedules appointment.

VIII. See "Diabetes Mellitus," if applicable.

Follow-up

I. Clinic.

II. Periodic telephone calls.

III. Visiting Nurse Association.

Pituitary Tumors

Definition   *Pituitary tumors* result from the abnormal cellular growth of one or more of the secretory cells of the pituitary gland, namely, chromophobe cells, acidophilic cells, and basophilic cells. Pituitary tumors account for 10 percent of all intracranial tumors (5), and only a very small percentage are malignant (6).

Depending upon the size, location, and function of the tumor, three syndromes may occur: (1) hypersecretion of one or more pituitary hormones, (see Table 24-1), most commonly, somatotropin (GH), prolactin (PRL), corticotropin (ACTH), melanocyte-stimulating hormone (MSH), and rarely, thyrotropin (TSH) and gonadotropins (LH, FSH); (2) hyposecretion of one or more pituitary tumors due to tissue compression by the tumor, or (3) alteration of surrounding structures, such as the optic chiasm and hypothalmus (7). Figure 24-1 illustrates portions of the pituitary discussed above and the relative locations of the pituitary, hypothalmus, and optic chiasm.

The etiology of pituitary tumors is unknown. Although most tumors appear to occur spontaneously, recent evidence suggests a relationship between tumor development after induction of a hypersecretory state, i.e., adrenalectomy for Cushing's syndrome predisposes to the development of ACTH-secreting tumors (Nelson's syndrome). Pituitary tumors may arise from the anterior lobe, posterior lobe, or remnants of Rathke's pouch (8). Tumors of the posterior lobe are rarely encountered. *Anterior lobe tumors* are classified according to the character of their secretory granules: chromophobe, acidophil, or basophil; however, more than one cell type may occur in a particular tumor.

Chromophobe tumors account for 85 percent of pituitary tumors. Although considered nonsecretory, evidence of secretion of one or more pituitary hormones can be found in many cases, namely, growth hormone and prolactin. Some of these tumors may become very large and locally invasive, but distant metastases are rare (9).

Acidophilic tumors contain the same secretory granules possessed by the normal lactotropic cells (prolactin) and somatotropic cells (growth hormone). Acidophilic tumors are thought to be the cause of acromegaly, a chronic disease characterized by excessive levels of growth hormone. Acidophilic tumors grow more slowly than chromophobe tumors, and distant metastases are practically never seen (10).

Basophilic tumors are rarely of significant size to produce clinical manifestations. They occur in about 10 percent of patients with *Cushing's syndrome,* a chronic disease characterized by excessive circulating levels of ACTH (11).

TABLE 24-1 / HORMONES OF THE HYPOTHALMUS AND PITUITARY GLAND

Hypothalmus	*Anterior Pituitary*	*Posterior Pituitary*
Thyrotropin-releasing factor (TRF)	Growth hormone (GH)	Stores and releases ADH, oxytocin
Corticotropin-releasing factor (CRF)	Thyroid-stimulating hormone (TSH)	
Prolactin-inhibiting factor (PIF)	Adrenocorticotropic hormone (ACTH)	
Luteinizing hormone-releasing factor (LHRF)	Follicle-stimulating hormone (FSH)	
Oxytocin	Luteinizing hormone (LH)	
Antidiuretic hormone (ADH)	Prolactin (PRL)	
Growth hormone-releasing factor (GRF)	Melanocyte-stimulating hormone (MSH)	
Melanocyte-inhibiting factor (MIF)		
?Melanocyte-releasing factor (MRF)		
?Growth hormone-inhibiting factor (GIF)		

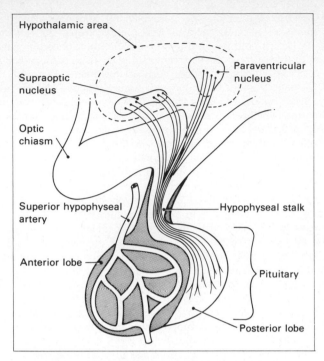

FIGURE 24-1 / Hypothalamic-pituitary relationship.

Craniopharyngiomas are believed to arise from remnants of Rathke's pouch. These nonpituitary tumors are more commonly suprasellar rather than intrasellar in location, but the clinical problems presented by these tumors resemble those of chromophobe tumors (12).

Assessment

I. Nursing health history.
II. Physical and behavioral assessment (see Fig. 24-2 for physical indications of acromegaly).
   A. Excess growth hormone: acromegaly.
      1. Sensory.
         a. Headache.
         b. Visual impairment.
         c. Deepened, husky voice.
      2. Musculoskeletal (see Fig. 24-3).
         a. Muscle weakness, atrophy.
         b. Acral bone growth (extremities).
         c. Broad face.
         d. Overgrowth of head, lips, nose, tongue, and jaw (prognathism).
      3. Integumentary.
         a. Thick, tough skin (especially hands and feet).
         b. Excessive diaphoresis.
         c. Increased facial hair.
      4. Gastrointestinal: weight gain.
      5. Mental status.
         a. Hypoactive.
         b. Emotional instability.
         c. Mental deterioration.
         d. Irritability.
         e. Anxiety.

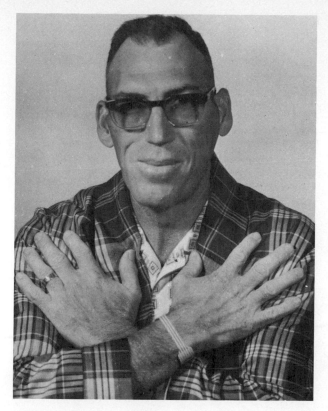

FIGURE 24-2 / Acromegaly. [*From David M. Hume and Timothy S. Harrison, in Seymour I. Schwartz et al. (eds.), Principles of Surgery, 2d ed., McGraw-Hill Book Company, New York, 1974.*]

    B. Excess prolactin.
        1. Headache.
        2. Visual disturbances.
        3. Intermittent lactation.
        4. Amenorrhea.
        5. Mild hirsutism.
        6. Anxiety.
    C. Excess corticotropin (ACTH); see "Adrenocortical Hyperfunction: Hypercortisolism."
    D. Excess melanocyte (MSH): abnormal skin and mucocutaneous pigmentation.
III. Other relevant sources.
    A. Family photographs (acromegaly).
    B. Medical history.
    C. Referral note.
    D. Interview with family.
    E. Diagnostic tests.
        1. Serum GH, PRL, T_4 (thyroxine), TSH, ACTH.
        2. Plasma cortisol (8 A.M.).
        3. Metapyrone test.
        4. Serum LH and testosterone (male).
        5. Serum LH, FSH, and estradiol (female).
        6. Urine osmolality.
        7. Skull films.

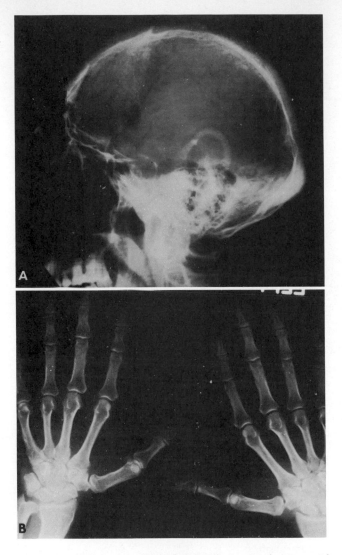

FIGURE 24-3 / **X-rays of lateral skull plus hands of patient with acromegaly.** [*From David M. Hume and Timothy S. Harrison, in Seymour I. Schwartz et al. (eds.), Principles of Surgery, 2d ed., McGraw-Hill Book Company, New York, 1974.*]

    8. Tomograms of sella tursica.
    9. Pneumoencephalogram.
  10. Cerebral arteriogram.
  11. Formal visual field test.

Problems
    I. Acromegaly.
      A. Physical.
        1. Muscle weakness.
        2. Pain (osteoporosis, arthritis, headache).
        3. Nutrition.
        4. Body hygiene.
        5. Safety.

   B. Psychosocial.
      1. Body image.   **4.** Mental fatigue.
      2. Communication.   **5.** Emotional stress.
      3. Altered sexual drive.   **6.** Anxiety.
  II. Excess prolactin.
   A. Physical.
      1. Pain.
      2. Safety.
   B. Psychosocial.
      1. Body image.
      2. Altered sexual function.
      3. Emotional stress.
 III. Excess corticotropin (see "Adrenocortical Hyperfunction: Hypercortisolism").

Diagnosis

   I. Acromegaly.
   A. Frequently complains of headache and joint pain.
   B. Has abnormal glucose tolerance test and/or fasting blood sugar.
   C. Complains of fatigue after minor activity.
   D. Complains of feeling hungry shortly after meals.
   E. May express need for assistance in activities of daily living.
   F. May have difficulty communicating with others.
   G. Has difficulty keeping skin and hair dry and clean.
   H. Often speaks of "past self" in positive terms, while present self-image is negative.
   I. Often has decreased peripheral vision.
   J. Expresses concern about diagnostic test and treatment.
   K. May voice concern about possibility of sterility and decreased libido.
  II. Excess prolactin.
   A. Frequently complains of headache.
   B. Often has impaired vision.
   C. May voice concern about possibility of sterility.
   D. Expresses concern about diagnostic test and treatment.
   E. Expresses concern about family role.

Goals of Care:
Acromegaly

   I. Immediate.
   A. Relieve pain.
   B. Maintain muscle tone.
   C. Promote a safe and therapeutic environment.
   D. Promote communication with family, significant others, and medical staff.
   E. Promote physical and emotional rest.
   F. Assist in preventing and/or controlling complications.
   G. Prepare physically, emotionally, and psychologically for diagnostic test and treatment.
   H. Evaluate response to treatment measures.
   I. Provide optimum diet to meet calorie needs and control diabetes.
  II. Long-range.
   A. Promote patient and family independence in managing self at home.
   B. Return to family and social roles.
   C. Return to preillness state physically, emotionally, and psychologically.
   D. Establish need for follow-up.

Intervention

   I. Acromegaly.
   A. Administer analgesics for pain.
   B. Orient to hospital.
   C. Prevent and/or control complications.
      1. Assess motor and sensory deficit(s).
      2. Ambulate with assistance, if necessary.

3. Assist with activities of daily living, if necessary.
4. Avoid extraneous equipment in room.
5. Maintain muscle tone.
   a. Range-of-motion (ROM) exercise.
   b. Good body alignment.
   c. Physical therapy.
   d. Encourage activity as tolerated.
6. Weigh daily.
7. Assess response to hypoglycemic agents.
   a. Urine sugar and acetone.
   b. Signs and symptoms of hypoglycemia, hyperglycemia.
8. Monitor vital signs.

D. Encourage discussion of feelings.
1. Physical changes.
2. Alterations in sexual function.
3. Family and social roles.
4. Diagnostic test and treatment.

E. Reassure that some of the physical and behavioral changes are amenable to change.

F. Involve in planning care, stressing importance of good skin care, rest, and activity.

G. Insure proper administration of diagnostic test.
1. Inservice.
2. Explain procedure(s) to patient.
3. Enlist support of patient for collecting specimens.

H. Patient and family teaching.
1. Anatomy and physiology of illness.
2. Treatment.
   a. Hypophysectomy: craniotomy, transsphenoidal; expected response(s):
      (1) Rapid decrease in growth hormone.
      (2) Pituitary hormone deficiencies: ACTH, TSH, LH, FSH.
      (3) Improved glucose tolerance.
      (4) Improved physical features.
   b. Irradiation; expected response(s):
      (1) Gradual decrease in growth hormone (months to years).
      (2) Pituitary hormond deficiencies: ACTH, TSH, LH, FSH.
      (3) Gradual improvement in glucose tolerance.
      (4) Gradual improvement of physical features.
3. Medication(s).
   a. Type:
      (1) Thyroid hormone.
      (2) Adrenocortical hormone.
      (3) Hypoglycemic agent.
   b. Action.
   c. Dose.
   d. Side effects.
4. Importance of follow-up.
   a. Complication(s) from treatment: hormone deficiencies.
   b. Regulation of medication:
      (1) Thyroid hormone.
      (2) Cortisone.
      (3) Insulin.
5. Signs and symptoms of hormone deficiencies:
   a. Hypothyroidism.
   b. Hypoadrenalism.
6. Signs and symptoms of hypoglycemia.
7. Appropriate responses to complications, infection, hormonal deficiency.

       8. Avoidance of physical and emotional stress.
       9. Activity, rest.
    10. Diet.
    11. Medic-Alert identification.
I. Specific observations after treatment.
  1. Craniotomy (see Chap. 23).
    a. Anterior pituitary hormone deficiencies.
    b. Transient diatetes insipidus.
  2. Transsphenoidal hypophysectomy.
    a. Cerebrospinal fluid rhinorrhea.
    b. Infection.
    c. Loss of smell.
    d. Transient personality change.
  3. Irradiation: outpatient.
    a. Gradual onset of hormone deficiencies.
    b. Thyroid hormone.
    c. Adrenocortical hormone.
    d. Gonadotropins.
    e. Pituitary apoplexy (spontaneous hemorrhage into pituitary tumor).
      (1) Assessment:

(a) Severe headache.	*(d)* Pyrexia.
(b) Blindness.	*(e)* Mental confusion.
(c) Shock.	*(f)* Irritability.

      (2) Treatment: immediate craniotomy.
J. Behavioral counseling, if indicated.
II. Excess prolactin.
  A. Administer medication for pain.
  B. Assess extent of visual defect, and promote safety measures.
  C. Explain all diagnostic tests and expected responses.
  D. Patient and family teaching.
    1. Anatomy and physiology of illness.
    2. Treatment.
      a. Surgery; see above.
      b. Irradiation; see above.
      c. Drugs.
        (1) L-Dopa.
        (2) Bromergocryptine: not available in United States.
    3. Medication(s).
    4. Importance of follow-up.
    5. Signs and symptoms of hormone deficiencies.
    6. Appropriate response(s) to complications.
    7. Stress.
    8. Activity, rest.
    9. Diet.
    10. Medic-Alert identification.

Evaluation

    I. Verbally describes pathophysiology of illness.
   II. States medication receiving, dose, time, action, and side effects.
  III. States expected response(s) from treatment and possible complications.
  IV. Verbally recalls signs and symptoms of hormonal deficiencies taught and appropriate response.
   V. Is able to resume previous family and social roles.
  VI. Demonstrates skills taught: insulin administration, urine sugar and acetone.
 VII. Wears Medic-Alert identification.
VIII. Keeps medical appointments. If unable, calls and reschedules appointment.

Follow-up

I. Clinic.
II. Periodic telephone calls.
III. Visiting Nurse Association.

Thyroid Tumors

Definition

Tumors of the thyroid gland can be benign or malignant. Benign tumors are termed *adenomas*. Adenomas are well-encapsulated, noninvading tumors which display autonomy of growth and function. The chief importance of thyroid adenomas lies in the need to differentiate them from malignant tumors, and in their ability in some cases to produce sufficient hormone to suppress the remaining normal thyroid tissue. The pathogenesis of adenomas is poorly understood. There is, however, some evidence that overproduction of TSH (thyroid-stimulating hormone) by the pituitary gland may be responsible for some cases of adenomas. Fortunately, malignant tumors of the thyroid gland are uncommon and rarely fatal. The prognosis is determined by many factors, namely, the histologic features and stage of the tumor and the ag and sex of the patient (13). Depending upon the cell composition, tumors can be classified as papillary, follicular, mixed, medullary, or anaplastic. *Papillary, follicular, and mixed papillary-follicular tumors* are responsible for approximately 80 percent of malignant tumors. They consist of well-differentiated cells and tend to grow and metastasize slowly. If detected at an early age and stage of development, prognosis is favorable. There are impressive data linking the occurrence of tumors to previous radiation exposure of the thyroid gland and to prolonged hyperplasia of the thyroid induced by continuous exposure to TSH. Also, these tumors are at least four times as frequent in women as in men but carry a less favorable prognosis with the latter sex group. *Medullary tumors* are the most distinctive type of thyroid tumors. They are frequently familial and are most commonly inherited as an autosomal dominant characteristic. They secrete calcitonin and are often associated with other endocrine disorders, such as pheochromocytoma, hyperparathyroidism, and Cushing's disease. Medullary tumors readily invade intraglandular lymphatics and also spread via the bloodstream to distant sites such as lung, bone, and liver. *Anaplastic tumors* are highly malignant, rapidly invading lesions composed of undifferentiated cells. These tumors metastasize throughout the body. The prognosis is very poor, regardless of early diagnosis, treatment, and/or age of the patient (14).

Assessment

I. Nursing health history.
II. Physical and behavioral assessment.
    A. Physical: thyroid nodule(s).
    B. Behavioral: none specific to disorder.
III. Other relevant sources.
    A. Medical history.
    B. Referral note.
    C. Old records: history of radiation treatment to neck, head, chest.
    D. Interview with family.
    E. Diagnostic test.
        1. Thyroid scan.
        2. Serum T_4.

Problems

I. Benign and noninvasive tumors: anxiety about impending surgery.
II. Invasive tumors: medullary, anaplastic (rarely seen).
    A. Physical.
        1. Pain.
        2. Nutrition: dysphagia.
        3. Altered respiratory status.
        4. Communication.
        5. Diarrhea.
    B. Psychosocial.
        1. Stress.
        2. Anxiety.

Diagnosis

I. Benign and noninvasive tumors: complains of feeling lump or "bump" in neck.
II. Invasive tumors: medullary, anaplastic.
    A. Complains of painful, hard mass in neck.
    B. Complains of difficulty in swallowing food.
    C. Has noted increased shortness of breath.
    D. Complains of frequent, watery stools (medullary carcinoma, increased calcitonin).

Goals of Care

I. Benign and noninvasive tumors.
    A. Immediate. Prepare emotionally and psychologically for surgery (subtotal thyroidectomy).
    B. Long-range.
        1. Return to physical, emotional, and psychological state prior to illness.
        2. Establish need for follow-up.
II. Invasive tumors.
    A. Immediate.
        1. Relieve pain.
        2. Promote physical and emotional rest.
        3. Provide physical and emotional support.
        4. Provide optimum diet to meet nutritional needs.
        5. Prepare emotionally and psychologically for surgery (thyroidectomy).
    B. Long-range.
        1. Promote patient and family independence in managing self at home.
        2. Return to family and social roles, if possible.

Intervention

I. Benign and noninvasive tumors.
    A. Preoperative teaching (see general surgery of the neck in Chap. 25).
    B. Patient and family teaching.
        1. Pathophysiology of illness.
        2. Treatment and expected response(s).
            a. Subtotal thyroidectomy. Removal of tumor *without* residual hormone deficiency.
            b. Medication. Suppress tumor with thyroxine (adenoma).
        3. See subtotal thyroidectomy (Chap. 25).
        4. Medication: type, action, dose, side effects.
II. Invasive tumors.
    A. Medicate for pain.
    B. Medicate for frequent bowel movements.
    C. Administer medication for rest and sleep.
    D. Provide high-caloric, high-protein fluids based on preferences.
    E. Assess respiratory function and institute appropriate measures.
        1. Oxygen therapy.
        2. Adequate rest between activities.
    F. Patient and family teaching.
        1. Anatomy and physiology of illness.
        2. Treatment and expected responses.
            a. Total thyroidectomy.
            b. Radical neck surgery.
            c. Irradiation.
        3. Medication.
            a. Type.   c. Dose.
            b. Action.   d. Side effects.
        4. Signs and symptoms of hypothyroidism.
        5. Importance of follow-up.
            a. Hormone replacement.
            b. Irradiation.
        6. Diet.
    G. Behavioral counseling, if indicated.

Evaluation
I. Benign, noninvasive tumors.
   A. Verbally describes pathophysiology of illness.
   B. States medication receiving, dose, time, action, and side effects.
   C. Is able to return to work and/or resume family and social roles.
   D. Keeps medical appointment. If unable, calls and reschedules appointment.
II. Invasive tumors.
   A. Verbally describes pathophysiology of disease.
   B. States medication receiving, dose, action, time, and side effects.
   C. Verbally recalls signs and symptoms of hypothyroidism.
   D. Shows improvement in:
      1. Decreased dysphagia: improved appetite, weight gain.
      2. Decreased pain.
      3. Decreased difficulty in breathing.
      4. Decreased bowel movements.
   E. Keeps medical appointment. If unable, calls and reschedules appointment.

Follow-up
I. Clinic.
II. Periodic telephone calls.
III. Visiting Nurse Association.

HYPERACTIVITY AND HYPOACTIVITY

Diabetes Mellitus

Definition

Diabetes mellitus is a chronic, complex disease characterized by alterations of carbohydrate, protein, and fat metabolism and the development of microvascular complications (thickening of the capillary basement membranes), neuropathy (peripheral sensorimotor defects, segmental demyelination), and macrovascular complications (large vessel disease) (15). Although diabetes mellitus is a common disease, affecting 1 to 5 percent of the total population, no distinct pathogenesis, etiology, invariable set of clinical findings, specific laboratory tests, and/or curative therapy exist (16).

Etiologic factors associated with diabetes include heredity, viruses, obesity, membrane receptor defects, insulin antibodies, and drugs. Although there is not sufficient evidence that stress per se can produce a permanent diabetic state in genetically normal individuals, a variety of severe stress states (psychological and physical) have been associated with glucose intolerance, i.e., pregnancy, physical and emotional trauma, and acute illnesses. For the population at risk for developing diabetes, stress may be the factor responsible for the overt expression of the disease and may subsequently hinder the individual's response to treatment.

Various terms are used to identify the kinds of diabetes, but two major types are generally considered, juvenile and adult. *Juvenile or early onset diabetes* often has a rapid onset before the age of 15 and is often characterized by acute symptoms. Because lack of insulin in this group is critical and can lead to ketosis, the term "ketosis-prone" is used to describe this form. *Adult or maturity-onset diabetes* is the more common and milder form. It frequently develops in overweight individuals during the 40- to 60-year age range. Unlike its counterpart, this group rarely develops ketosis, and is sometimes referred to as "non-ketosis-prone" (17).

Diabetes has also been classified into stages. The prediabetic stage covers the interval between conception and diagnosis and is suspected in individuals with high genetic risk. The subclinical or latent stage is characterized by normal fasting blood sugar and glucose tolerance test. Diabetes is suspected because of decreased glucose tolerance during stressful states, pregnancy, surgery, and other illnesses, or after certain drug therapy. The chemical stage overlaps the former stage, is asymptomatic, and shows normal fasting blood sugar, but the glucose tolerance test is abnormal. Overt diabetes represents the symptomatic stage (18). The fasting blood sugar is always elevated.

Another term used in reference to diabetes is brittle. The term refers to an unstable, labile diabetic state that is difficult to control. The individual fluctuates between ketosis and hypoglycemia with minor changes in insulin dose.

Assessment:
Adult Onset
Diabetes

    I. Nursing health history.
   II. Physical and behavioral assessment.
       A. Cardiovascular.
          1. Hypotension.
          2. Tachycardia, other cardiac arrythmias.
          3. Hypovolemia, dehydration.
       B. Respiratory.
          1. Abnormal breath sounds.
          2. Rate, rhythm: usually hyperpnea.
          3. Absence or presence of dyspnea.
       C. Infection. Skin lesions.
          1. Appearance, odor of urine.   **3.** Recent viral or bacterial infection.
          2. Discomfort with urination.   **4.** Breath sounds.
       D. Kidney.
          1. Urinary output.
             a. Polyuria.
             b. Anuria.
          2. Urine sugar, acetone. Specific gravity.
       E. Central nervous system.
          1. Headache.   **3.** Stupor.
          2. Drowsiness.   **4.** Coma.[2]
       F. Sensorimotor.
          1. Muscle tone depressed.   **3.** Blurred vision.
          2. Reflexes depressed.   **4.** Response to stimuli.
       G. Mental status.
          1. Nervousness.
          2. Depression.
          3. Anxiety.
  III. Other relevant sources.
       A. Medical history.
          1. Family history of diabetes or other endocrine disorders.
          2. Recent physical or emotional stress, infection, trauma, divorce, death of significant person.
          3. History of drug ingestion: glucocorticoids, birth control pills.
       B. Interview with family.
       C. Old records.
       D. Diagnostic tests.
          1. Elevated fasting plasma glucose.
          2. Abnormal glucose tolerance test, either oral or intravenous.
          3. Urine glucose and acetone.
          4. Arterial blood gases.
          5. Serum acetone.

Problems

    I. Acute stage.
       A. Physical.
          1. Hypotension.
          2. Fluid and electrolyte imbalance.
             a. Dehydration.
             b. K^+ loss.

[2]More commonly observed in the younger diabetic than in the adult patient.

3. Discomfort.
    a. Pain.   *c.* Malaise.
    b. Weakness.   *d.* Nausea, vomiting.
4. Complications.
    a. Cardiac arrythmias.   *d.* Hypoglycemia.
    b. Anuria, osmotic diuresis.   *e.* Infection.
    c. Cerebral anoxia, edema.
B. Psychosocial.
  1. Stress.
  2. Fear.
  3. Anxiety.

II. Subacute stage.
  A. Physical.
    1. Nutrition.
    2. Activity.
    3. Rest.
    4. Complications.
      a. Hyperglycemia.
      b. Hypoglycemia.
      c. Metabolic imbalance.
  B. Psychosocial.
    1. Adjustment to diabetes.
      a. Change in lifestyle.   *c.* Activity.
      b. Dietary patterns.   *d.* Occupation.
    2. Body image.
    3. Anxiety, fear.
      a. Complications.
        (1) Heart and renal disease.
        (2) Blindness.
        (3) Loss of limb.
      b. Sexual dysfunction.
      c. Loss of family, social roles.

III. Discharge stag.
  A. Promotion of self-care management.
  B. Patient and family support and education.

Diagnosis

I. Acute stage.
  A. If able, complains of polyuria and polydipsia in particular; anuria may be present.
  B. Has experienced weight loss, gain over past few weeks.
  C. Hyperpnea (Kussmal's), hypotension, tachycardia, and other cardiac arrhythmias may be present but variable in severity.
  D. Complains of anorexia, nausea, vomiting along with weakness, malaise, and muscle aches.
  E. Exhibits some degree of central nervous system depression: headache, drowsiness, stupor, and coma.
  F. Exhibits signs of dehydration.
    1. Skin dry and inelastic.
    2. Oral and nasopharyngeal membranes dry.
    3. Eyeballs sunken and softer.
  G. Is anxious and irritable about prognosis and frequent laboratory tests.

II. Subacute stage.
  A. May or may not experience episodes of hyperglycemia, hypoglycemia during regulation period.
  B. Verbally or nonverbally expresses anxiety and fears regarding complications.
    1. Loss of family and social roles.

    2. Financial status.

    3. Sexual function.

  C. May fear inability to return to previous "normal life."

  D. Expresses negative feelings about testing urine and/or giving self-injections.

III. Discharge stage.

  A. Expresses confidence in self to manage medical regime at home.

  B. Asks many questions regarding care at home, diet, insulin dose, urine testing, etc., despite teaching.

Goals of Care

I. Acute stage.

  A. Immediate.

    1. Provide physical and emotional support.

    2. Recognize and report complications.

      a. Hypoglycemia.   *d.* Cerebral anoxia.

      b. Infection.   *e.* Congestive heart failure.

      c. Cardiac arrhythmia.   *f.* Anuria.

    3. Reduce pain and discomfort.

  B. Long-range.

    1. Prevent occurrence of iatrogenic complications.

      a. Skin breakdown.

      b. Infections.

      c. Phlebitis.

    2. Establish a relationship of trust, concern, and confidence with patient and family.

II. Subacute stage.

  A. Immediate.

    1. Assist in controlling diabetes.

      a. Diet.

      b. Physical, emotional, and psychological rest.

      c. Reduce internal and external stresses.

      d. Activity.

    2. Assist in preventing and controlling immediate complications.

      a. Hypoglycemia.

      b. Hyperglycemia.

      c. Fluid imbalance.

  B. Long-range. Promote patient independence in managing case.

III. Discharge stage.

  A. Immediate. Evaluate patient and family's knowledge and skill to manage medical regime at home.

  B. Long-range.

    1. Reach and maintain ideal weight.

    2. Maintain proper nutrition.

    3. Assist in preventing and controlling immediate and long-range complications.

Intervention[3]

I. Acute stage.

  A. Define with medical team critical nursing actions to be instituted to support patient physically.

    1. Hypoglycemia.

    2. Cardiac arrhythmia.

    3. Congestive heart failure.

    4. Respiratory distress.

  B. Evaluate response(s) to treatment measures (flow sheet).

    1. Blood glucose.   **3.** Arterial blood gases.

    2. Serum acetone.   **4.** Urine sugar and acetone.

[3]Modifications based upon activity of illness and ability of patient.

      5. Serum potassium.   **9.** Temperature.
      6. Fluid balance.   **10.** Adequacy of airway.
      7. Neurological signs.   **11.** Breath sounds.
      8. Vital signs.

   C. Levine tube and/or medication for abdominal discomfort.
   D. Group nursing and treatment activities to promote rest.
   E. Provide safe and comfortable environment.
      1. Air mattress.
      2. Foot cradle.
      3. ROM exercises.
      4. Body alignment.
      5. Frequent change in position.
      6. Skin and oral care.
      7. Aseptic technique in inserting and maintaining intravenous lines and Foley catheters.
   F. Explain purpose of treatment measures to patient and family.
   G. Arrange conference time for family with physician.

 II. Subacute stage.
   A. Assist in establishing immediate and long-range goals: diet, life-style, medication, urine testing.
   B. Involve in planning daily care, stressing importance of rest, diet, and activity.[4]
   C. Monitor responses to treatment measures.
      1. Adequacy of diet.
      2. Appetite.
      3. Blood sugar.
      4. Urine sugar and acetone.
      5. Fluid balances.
      6. General emotional and physical well-being.
   D. Explain all diagnostic procedures and expected responses.
   E. Insure proper collection of specimens.
      1. Inservice: nursing staff and appropriate others.
      2. Explain procedure to patient.
      3. Enlist patient support in collecting specimens.
   F. Patient and family teaching.
      1. What is diabetes?
      2. Treatment.
         a. Oral agents: mechanism of action, duration, risks, side effects, drug incompatibilities, when not to take.
         b. Insulin: action, peak, duration, storage and care, dose adjustment, local reaction, administration.
         c. Diet.
         d. Weight control.
         e. Exercise.
         f. Stress.
      3. Urine testing: frequency, when to test for ketones, reportable results, second voided specimens, drugs affecting results.
      4. Signs and symptoms of hypoglycemia, hyperglycemia, and appropriate responses.
      5. Foot and skin care.
      6. Complications.
      7. Medic-Alert identification.
   G. Behavioral counseling, if indicated.
   H. Social service consultation, if needed.

[4]An organized diabetic activity program should be available. If not, health providers should consider establishing such a program.

III. Discharge phase evaluation.
   A. Have patient and/or family demonstrate skills taught.
      1. Urine testing.
      2. Insulin administration.
   B. Have patient state:
      1. Signs and symptoms of hypoglycemia and hyperglycemia, and appropriate responses.
      2. Difference between immediate and long-range illnesses and appropriate responses.
      3. Medication receiving, dose, frequency, action, side effects.
      4. Date of next medical appointment.
      5. Diet.
   C. Have patient describe:
      1. Relationship between diet, exercise, stress, and medication on blood glucose.
      2. Measures to control and/or prevent complications.

Follow-up
   I. Visiting Nurse Association.
   II. Clinic.
   III. Periodic telephone calls.

Adrenocortical Hyperfunction: Hypercortisolism

Definition
Hyperfunction of the adrenal cortex can produce syndromes of *hypercortisolism* (excess plasma cortisol), *mineralocorticoid* excess (aldosterone excess), viralism, or feminization. The most frequently encountered abnormalities usually result from hypersecretion of the glucocorticoids. However, mixed syndromes may occur. Figure 24-4 shows normal cortisol regulation, the detailed sequence of events leading to hypercortisolism (19).

Cushing's syndrome is the term used to describe the variety of clinical and chemical abnormalities resulting from a chronic excess of glucocorticoids, namely, cortisone and hydrocortisone. The term *Cushing's disease* refers to those cases of Cushing's syndrome in which hypercortisolism is secondary to excess secretion of ACTH (adrenocorticotropic hormone) by the pituitary gland. Cushing's syndrome can result from exogenous or endogenous factors. Cushing's syndrome is most often due to the administration of exogenous glucocorticoids (steroids) in the therapy of nonendocrine diseases. There are three major varieties of endogenous Cushing's syndrome: (1) autonomous function by an adrenocortical tumor (primary hypercortisolism: adenoma, carcinoma), (2) excessive stimulation of the adrenals by pituitary ACTH, and (3) excessive secretion of ACTH by a nonpituitary tumor (ectopic ACTH syndrome) (20).

Assessment
   I. Nursing health history.
   II. Physical and behavioral assessment (see Fig. 24-5).
      A. Motor.
         1. Decreased muscle mass, especially limbs.
         2. Poor coordination.
         3. Generalized osteoporosis.
            a. Pathological fractures.
            b. Compression fractures of the spine.
            c. Kyphosis.
      B. Skin.
         1. Fragile and thin.
         2. Facial plethora (abnormal dilatation of blood vessels).
         3. Excessive bruising on arms, legs.
         4. Purple striae on arms, breasts, thighs, abdomen.
         5. Petechial hemorrhage.
         6. Hirsutism.

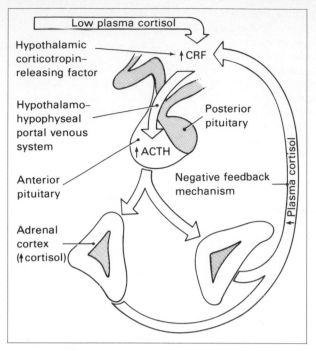

FIGURE 24-4 / **Normal mechanism for plasma cortisol regulation. Low plasma cortisol → hypothalamus ↑ CRF → anterior pituitary ↑ ACTH → adrenal cortex ↑ cortisol → ↑ plasma cortisol → hypothalamus.**

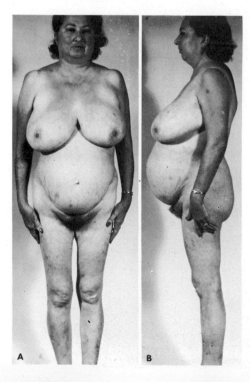

FIGURE 24-5 / Cushing's syndrome. [*From David M. Hume and Timothy S. Harrison, in Seymour I. Schwartz et al. (eds.), Principles of Surgery, 2d ed., McGraw-Hill Book Company, New York, 1974.*]

    C. Cardiovascular.
        1. Hypertension (main cause of death).
        2. Increased susceptibility to congestive heart failure, thrombosis, cardiac enlargement.
    D. Gastrointestinal.
        1. Ulcer.
        2. Obesity—proximal distribution (see Figs. 24-6 and 24-7 for comparison of the distribution with Cushing's syndrome and simple obesity).
            a. Face: moon face (marked rounding) (see Fig. 24-8).
            b. Supraclavicular.
            c. Area over seventh cervical vertebra: buffalo hump.
            d. Abdomen: truncal obesity.
    E. Mental status.
        1. Irritability.   **3.** Depression.
        2. Emotional lability.   **4.** Psychoses.
    F. Other.
        1. Hyperglycemia, glycosuria.
        2. Menses.
            a. Amenorrhea.
            b. Oligomenorrhea.
        3. Infertility.
        4. Gynecomastia.
III. Other relevant sources.
    A. Medical history.
        1. Drug use.

FIGURE 24-6 / Patient with Cushing's syndrome. Note proximal distribution of fat and striae over abdomen and thigh. (*Courtesy of Dr. Louis Avioli.*)

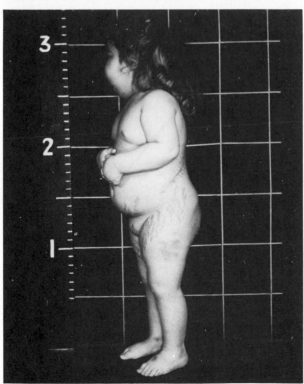

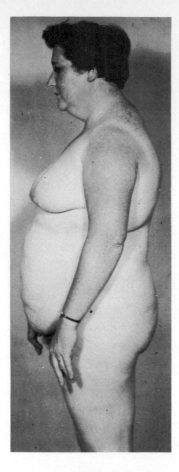

FIGURE 24-7 / Simple obesity, in contrast to Cushing's syndrome. [*From David M. Hume and Timothy S. Harrison, in Seymour I. Schwartz et al. (eds.), Principles of Surgery, 2d ed., McGraw-Hill Book Company, New York, 1974.*]

    2. Physical and emotional stress.
    3. Other medical problems: cardiac, gastrointestinal, diabetes, bone disease.
  B. Interview with family.
  C. Old records.
  D. Referral note.
  E. Consultation note.
  F. Diagnostic tests.
    1. Low-dose dexamethasome suppressive test.
    2. Plasma ACTH.
    3. Plasma cortisol (8 A.M. and 4 P.M.).
    4. 24-h urinary cortisol (free cortisol).
    5. High-dose formal dexamethasome suppression test.
    6. Glucose tolerance test.
    7. Skull films: cone views of sella tursica.
    8. Chest x-ray (ectopic ACTH).

***Problems*[5]**

I. General problems.[6]
  A. Physical.
    1. Fluid and electrolyte imbalance (sodium and water retention).
    2. Hypercalciuria.

[5]Depends upon the cause, severity, and proposed mode of treatment of Cushing's syndrome, i.e., pituitary tumor, adrenal hyperplasia, chronic use of steroids.
[6]Most commonly encountered problems regardless of cause.

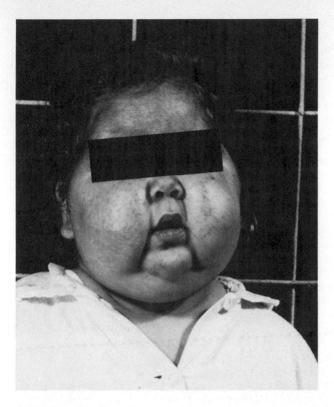

FIGURE 24-8 / Moon face of Cushing's syndrome. (*Courtesy of Dr. Louis Avioli.*)

    3. Nutrition.
    4. Weakness.
    5. Fatigability.
    6. Safety.
    7. Pain.
    8. Stress (physical and emotional).
    9. Infection.
   10. Hyperglycemia, glycosuria.
  B. Psychosocial.
    1. Body image.   4. Anxiety.
    2. Emotional lability.   5. Psychoses.
    3. Depression.
II. Adrenalectomy: adrenal adenoma(s).
  A. Preoperative (see preoperative care of laparotomy in Chap. 29).
  B. Postoperative.
    1. Hypertension.[7]
    2. Shock: more likely.
    3. Pain.
    4. Nausea, vomiting.
    5. Hormone replacement (glucocorticoid plus mineralocorticoid).
    6. Nutrition.
    7. Rest.
    8. Activity.

[7]Can occur due to manipulation of the adrenal gland(s).

III. Pituitary irradiation.[8] Cushing's disease.
  A. Hormone replacement.   D. Activity.
  B. Nutrition.   E. Stress reduction.
  C. Rest.

Diagnosis

I. General.
  A. Has experienced marked weight gain over the past few months.
  B. Has noted accumulation of adipose tissue in the facial, nuchal, truncal, and girdle areas.
  C. Complains of marked weakness and fatigability, often is unable to rise from a deep knee bend without assistance.
  D. Has noted tendency to bruise easily.
  E. Has noted denudation of skin following trivial injury, i.e., removal of Band-Aid.
  F. May complain of back pain, loss of height, and/or frequent bone fractures.[9]
  G. Complains of superficial skin infections which heal slowly.
  H. Exhibits some degree of glucose intolerance (frank diabetes rare, usually abnormal glucose tolerance test).
  I. Has high blood pressure.
  J. Has noted changes in menses: oligomenorrhea, amenorrhea.
  K. Exhibits abnormal behavior: irritability, depression, psychoses, emotional lability.
  L. May complain of pain and tenderness in kidney area.[10]
  M. May complain of midepigastric pain.
  N. May complain of feeling nauseated followed by periods of vomiting usually several hours after eating.

II. Postoperative.
  A. Complains of incisional pain.
  B. Complains of nausea and may be followed by vomiting.
  C. May experience fall in blood pressure, tachycardia, elevated temperature, restlessness.
  D. May experience critical elevations in blood pressure during early postoperative period.
  E. May have impaired wound healing.

III. Pituitary irradiation.
  A. May complain and/or exhibit signs and symptoms of pituitary hypofunction.[11]
  B. Same as noted under "Problems."

Goals of Care

I. General.
  A. Immediate.
    1. Promote physical and emotional rest.
    2. Minimize internal and external stresses.
    3. Provide optimum nutrition.
    4. Reduce pain and prevent reoccurrence, if possible.
    5. Assist in preventing and/or controlling complications, infection, ulcer, hypertension, glucose intolerance.
    6. Promote positive image of self.
    7. Promote independence.
    8. Provide a safe and supportive environment.
    9. Minimize errors in administering and/or collecting specimens for diagnostic test.

[8]Approximately one-third of patients treated with irradiation up to 5000 R have corrected hypercortisolism without producing endocrinologic deficiencies. Alternative choices: hypophysectomy via craniotomy or transsphenoidal approach.

[9]Depends upon presence and severity of osteoporotic process.

[10]May excrete 150 to 300 mg calcium per day in urine with resultant renal stone.

[11]Improvements in clinical status can take several months. As noted, two-thirds of these patients may experience concomitant hormonal deficiency thyroid, gonadotropins, ACTH. See appropriate sections for nursing diagnosis.

     B. Long-range. Prepare for proposed treatment intervention, surgery, irradiation.

  II. Postoperative (see also postoperative care of laparotomy in Chap. 29).

     A. Immediate.

       1. Reduce pain and discomfort.

       2. Assist in preventing and/or controlling complications, hypotension, infection, thrombosis.

       3. Promote wound healing.

       4. Provide optimum nutrition.

     B. Long-range.

       1. Provide knowledge regarding illness.

       2. Return to preillness state, physically, psychologically, and emotionally.

  III. Irradiation.[12]

     A. Immediate. Provide continuity of care with radiation department.

     B. Long-range.

       1. Assist patient, family in managing self at home.

       2. Assist in controlling hormonal deficiencies.

Intervention

   I. General.

     A. Orient to physical environment and hospital procedures.

     B. Explain all procedures and expected responses.

     C. Administer medication to promote rest and sleep.

     D. Medicate for pain.

     E. Group nursing and treatment activities to promote rest.

     F. Remove extraneous equipment from room.

     G. Assist with ambulation, if indicated.

     H. Prevent and/or control infections.

       1. Separate geographically from individuals with infectious diseases.

       2. Assess for sites of infection.

         a. Skin lesions, productive cough, abnormal breath.

         b. Sounds, pain, and burning upon urination, etc.

       3. Medical asepsis: catheterization, intravenous lines.

       4. Immediate attention to infectious areas.

     I. Encourage verbalization of fears and anxiety.

       1. Explain problems have a physical basis amenable to treatment.

       2. Reassure that most physical changes are reversible.

     J. Monitor response(s) to treatment measures.

       1. Weigh daily.   **4.** Medication(s).

       2. Urine sugar and acetone.   **5.** Appetite.

       3. Vital signs and temperature.   **6.** Stools for occult blood.

     K. Evaluate adjustment to illness.

       1. Patient goals: diet, medication, follow-up.

       2. Willingness to participate in care.

       3. Relationship with staff, family, and others.

       4. Expectations.

     L. Insure proper administration of diagnostic test.

       1. Inservice: nursing staff and others.

       2. Explain procedure to patient.

       3. Enlist support of patient for collecting specimens.

     M. Explain treatment measure and expected outcome(s).

       1. Preoperative teaching.

       2. Schedule and procedure for radiation therapy.

     N. Behavioral counseling, if indicated.

   II. Postoperative.

     A. Medicate for pain.

[12]Usually done in outpatient department.

B. Observe for complications.
  1. Adrenal crisis (*see* "Adrenocortical Hypofunction").
  2. Shock.
  3. Hemorrhage.
  4. Infection.
  5. Paralytic ileus.
  6. Congestive heart failure.
C. Prevent and/or control complications.
  1. Check operative site every hour.
      a. Redness.   *c.* Drainage.
      b. Swelling.   *d.* Abnormal bleeding.
  2. Aseptic wound care.
  3. Assess gastrointestinal function.
      a. Distention: patency, function of nasogastric tube.
      b. Peristalsis: type of bowel sounds, fluid tolerance.
      c. Nausea, vomiting, medication.
  4. Auscultate chest sounds every hour.
      a. Deep breathing and coughing.
      b. Position change.
      c. Intermittent positive pressure breathing (IPPB) treatments.
  5. Monitor vital signs as needed.
      a. Vasopressor drugs: every 15 min or more frequently.
      b. Every hour until stable.
  6. Strict intake and output.
  7. Monitor vital signs as needed.
D. Patient and family teaching.
  1. Anatomy and physiology of disease.
  2. Expected results from surgery.
  3. Action of corticosteroids on body organs.
      a. Signs and symptoms of adrenal crisis.[13]
      b. Signs and symptoms of Cushing's syndrome.
      c. Effect of stress, emotional and physical.
          (1) Withdrawal.
          (2) Preventing gastric ulcers.
          (3) Medic-Alert bracelet.
  4. Correction of glucose intolerance and appropriate responses.
      a. Monitor urine sugar and acetone.
      b. Signs and symptoms of hypoglycemia.
  5. Diet.[14]
      a. High protein.   *c.* Restricted calories.
      b. Adequate potassium.   *d.* Low sodium, low carbohydrate.
III. Irradiation.
  A. Send nursing care plan and nursing history to radiation department.
  B. Team conference with nursing staff from radiation therapy department.
  C. Assess need for transportation to and from hospital.
  D. Patient and family teaching.
      1. Explanation of illness.
      2. Expected responses from therapy.
          a. Physical changes.
          b. Possibility of pituitary hormone deficiencies.
              (1) Signs and symptoms of adrenal crisis.
              (2) Signs and symptoms of thyroid deficiency.
              (3) Signs and symptoms of gonadotropin deficiency.

---

[13]See "Adrenocortical Hypofunction."
[14]Depends upon residual problems involving diabetes, heart disease, and/or other medical problems.

      c. Signs and symptoms suggesting improved glucose tolerance.

      d. Appropriate action to be taken if hormonal deficiencies occur.

3. Medication(s): dose, frequency, action, side effects.
4. Medic-Alert bracelet.
5. Rest, activity.
6. Diet.[15]

a. Maintain normal body weight.	*c.* Low carbohydrate, low calcium.
b. High protein, adequate potassium.	*d.* Salt restriction.

7. Behavioral counseling, if indicated.
8. Nutritional counseling.
9. Social service consultation.
10. Importance of follow-up.

Evaluation

I. Verbally describes pathophysiology of illness.
II. Wears Medic-Alert identification bracelet
III. States medication receiving, dose, frequency, time, action, side effects.
IV. Verbally recalls signs and symptoms of hormonal deficiencies taught.
V. States appropriate action to be taken if complications occur.
VI. Maintains ideal body weight.
VII. Demonstrates skills taught for urine testing.
VIII. Demonstrates adequate nutrition: diary of food intake.
IX. Keeps medical appointments. If unable, calls and schedules another appointment.

Follow-up

I. Clinic.
II. Periodic telephone calls.
III. Visiting Nurse Association.

Adrenocortical Hypofunction

Definition

Adrenocortical insufficiency or hypofunction can be primary or secondary. *Primary adrenal insufficiency* or *Addison's disease* is the result of destruction of the adrenal cortex which impairs the capacity of the gland to secrete cortisol and aldosterone. Most often the cause of primary insufficiency is idiopathic, probably an autoimmune response. Other known causes include adrenalectomy, infection (tuberculosis, histoplasmosis), adrenal hemorrhage (trauma), amyloidosis, and metastatic disease. The clinical picture presented by patients with Addison's disease is one of deficiency in both glucocorticoids and mineralocorticoids, i.e., volume contraction, hypokalemia, impaired tolerance to stress, and diminished mental vigor.

    The destruction of the adrenal gland is a gradual process associated with compensatory increases in ACTH (adrenocorticotropic hormone) and renin. This compensatory process for a time allows the adrenal to secrete enough cortisol and aldosterone to meet the physiologic needs of the body in the absence of some physiologic or psychological stress, infection, trauma, loss of job, or loss of significant other. When more than 90 percent of the adrenal cortex is destroyed, internal homeostasis is lost, and the clinical picture of Addison's disease is evident (21).

    Cortisol deficiency occurring as a consequence of pituitary ACTH deficiency is termed *secondary adrenal insufficiency.* ACTH deficiency may be due to pituitary or hypothalamic disease. Unlike primary adrenal insufficiency, secondary insufficiency is seldom associated with a deficiency in aldosterone secretion and/or increase in MSH (melanocyte-stimulating hormone) secretion. Some of the more commonly encountered causes for ACTH deficiency are pituitary tumor or cyst and chronic suppression of ACTH by cortisol from an adrenal neoplasm or by exogenous glucocorticoids (22).

---

[15]Depends upon severity of illness and other medical problems.

Assessment

I. Nursing health history.
II. Physical and behavioral assessment.[16]
  A. Primary adrenal insufficiency.
    1. Motor.
      a. Poor coordination.
      b. Generalized weakness.
    2. Skin
      a. Wasting of fat deposits.
      b. Hyperpigmentation of skin and mucocutaneous membranes (excess MSH; tan, bronze appearance).
      c. Vitiligo: areas lacking pigmentation and surrounded by hyperpigmented borders.
      d. Dry skin
      e. Loss of skin tone.
      f. Loss of body hair.
    3. Cardiovascular.
      a. Hypotension.
      b. Syncope.
      c. Abnormal rate, rhythm, and quality of pulse.
    4. Gastrointestinal.
      a. Weight loss.   d. Vomiting.
      b. Anorexia   e. Abdominal pain.
      c. Nausea.
    5. Mental status.
      a. Apathy.   d. Confusion.
      b. Lethargy.   e. Diminished vigor.
      c. Irritability.   f. Psychosis.
    6. Others.
      a. Fasting hypoglycemia.
      b. Loss of libido, impotence.
        (1) Infertility.
        (2) Irregular menses.
  B. Secondary adrenal insufficiency. Same as primary insufficiency except for skin pigmentation.
III. Other relevant sources. Medical history.
  A. Drug use, especially steroids.
  B. Other medical problems, namely, infections, (tuberculosis, histoplasmosis) and other endocrine, disorders (hypothyroidism, diabetes mellitus, hypoparathyroidism).
  C. Interview with significant other(s).
  D. Old records.
  E. Diagnostic tests.
    1. 8 A.M. plasma cortisol ($< 3\ \mu$g per 100 mL).
    2. Cotrosyn (synthetic 1–34 ACTH) stimulation test.
    3. Plasma ACTH.
    4. Serum electrolytes.
    5. 24-h urine 17-hydroxycorticosteroids and 17-ketosteroids.

Problems

I. Physical.
  A. Shock.[17]
  B. Stress.
  C. Altered nutritional status.

[16]Physical findings depend upon duration and severity of adrenal insufficiency.
[17]When present indicates critical adrenal insufficiency (Addisonian crisis). Other signs and symptoms include anorexia, vomiting, abdominal pain, apathy, confusion, and extreme weakness. If untreated, death results.

    D. Altered fluid and electrolyte balance (sodium and water loss, potassium retention).

    E. Pain.

    F. Weakness.

    G. Fatigability.

    H. Safety.

II. Psychosocial.

    A. Confusion.

    B. Apathy.

    C. Depression.

    D. Irritability.

Diagnosis

I. General.

    A. Has experienced weight loss.

    B. Has noted progressing fatigability and weakness.

    C. Complains of anorexia, nausea, and vomiting.

    D. May complain of hunger, headache, weakness, trembling, and emotional lability in the late morning hours or 2 to 3 h after eating a high-carbohydrate meal (fasting hypoglycemia).

    E. Has noted changes in skin color (bronze, tan, and/or white patches with hyperpigmented borders.

    F. Complains of dizziness in upright position.

    G. May complain of abdominal pain.

    H. Has craved salt and/or salty foods.

    I. Displays abnormal behavior to surroundings: irritability, depression, apathy.

    J. Expresses anxiety and fear regarding self, family, and future.

II. Addisonian crisis.

    A. Presents with signs and symptoms of severe shock: hypotension, weak, thready pulse, restlessness, etc.

    B. If able, complains of profound weakness.

    C. Exhibits evidence of gastrointestinal distress: abdominal pain, anorexia, nausea, vomiting, and diarrhea.

    D. Has impaired CNS function: confused, stuporous, comatose.

    E. If able, may complain of severe headache and pain in abdomen, lower back, or legs.

    F. May have cardiac arrhythmia.

Goals of Care

I. General.

    A. Immediate.

        1. Promote physical and emotional rest.

        2. Minimize internal and external stresses.

        3. Assist in obtaining diagnostic tests.

        4. Provide optimum nutrition and fluid balance.

        5. Prevent and/or control complications.

        6. Provide a safe and therapeutic environment.

        7. Relieve pain and discomfort.

        8. Evaluate response to treatment measures, medications, diet, fluid balance.

        9. Provide emotional support.

        10. Encourage gradual activity.

    B. Long-range.

        1. Prepare patient and family to manage self.

        2. Return to preillness state, physically, emotionally, and psychologically.

II. Addisonian crisis.

    A. Assist in preventing and/or controlling complications.

    B. Assist in restoring normal hormonal balance.

    C. Assist in restoring normal fluid and electrolyte balance.

    D. Provide emotional support to the patient and family.

Intervention

I. General.
 A. Assist with activities of daily living until less fatigued.
 B. Encourage activity as tolerated.
 C. Active and passive exercises, if on bed rest.
 D. Ambulate with assistance, if necessary.
 E. Group nursing and treatment activities to promote rest.
 F. Administer medication to:
  1. Promote rest and sleep.
  2. Relieve pain.
  3. Relieve nausea, vomiting, and anorexia.
 G. If able, eliminate environmental factors contributing to physical and psychological stress.
 H. Explain all procedures and treatment measures and expected responses.
 I. Monitor responses to treatment measures.
  1. Intake and output.
  2. Blood pressure.
  3. Pulse, temperature.
  4. Weight.
  5. Mental status.
  6. Appetite.
 J. Prevent and/or control infections.
  1. Separate geographically from individual with infectious diseases.
  2. Discuss ability to return to preillness state, physically, psychologically, and emotionally.
 K. Insure proper administration of diagnostic test.
  1. Inservice: nursing staff, others.
  2. Explain procedure to patient.
  3. Enlist support of patient for collecting specimens.
 L. Patient and family teaching.
  1. Anatomy and physiology of disease.
  2. Effect of corticosteroids on body organs.
  3. Increase requirements of corticosteroids during severe physical and emotional stress, grief, infection, surgery.
  4. Medications.
   a. Type.   d. Dose.
   b. Action.   e. Side effects.
   c. Specific regimen.
  5. Signs and symptoms of adrenal insufficiency.
   a. Progressive fatigability.   e. Postural hypotension.
   b. Weakness.   f. Emotional irritability.
   c. Anorexia, nausea, vomiting. g. Headache.
   d. Restlessness.
  6. Signs and symptoms of Cushing's syndrome (see "Adrenal Hyperfunction: Hypercortisolism").
  7. Medic-Alert bracelet.
  8. Importance of follow-up.
  9. Diet.
 M. Behavioral counseling, if indicated.
II. Addisonian crisis.
 A. Start intravenous line. If unable, prepare for cutdown.
 B. Place on cardiac monitor.
 C. Monitor blood pressure, pulse, and respiration every 15 min until stable, and temperature every ½ to 1 h.
 D. Measure intake and output every hour. Report output less than 30 mL for two consecutive hours.
 E. Insert nasogastric tube.

    F. Administer parenteral fluids as ordered, usually 5% dextrose in saline solution.

    G. Administer medication as ordered.

        1. Adrenocorticosteroids.

        2. Vasopressors.

        3. Antibiotics.

        4. Antiemetics.

    H. Do not leave patient.

    I. Assign other nursing personnel to interview the family.

Evaluation

    I. Verbally describes pathophysiology of disease.

    II. Wears Medic-Alert identification.

    III. States appropriate action to be taken under special conditions:

        A. Infection.

        B. Psychological trauma.

        C. Surgery and/or extensive dental work requiring general anesthesia.

        D. Inability to take medication by mouth.

    IV. States medication(s) receiving, dose, time, action, side effects.

    V. Verbally recalls signs and symptoms of hormonal deficiencies taught.

    VI. Maintains ideal body weight.

    VII. Keeps medical appointment. If unable, calls and schedules another appointment.

Follow-up

    I. Clinic.

    II. Periodic telephone calls.

    III. Visiting Nurse Association.

Hyperthyroidism

The terms *thyrotoxicosis* and *hyperthyroidism* are used interchangeably to describe diseases associated with excess thyroid hormone. Figure 24-9 reviews the normal mechanisms for plasma thyroid hormone regulation.

Overactivity of the thyroid gland itself is the most common cause of hyperthyroidism. An increase in serum thyroxine (T_4) is the mark of hyperthyroidism and is usually accompanied by an increase in triiodothyronine (T_3). *Graves' disease* is the most common form of hyperthyroidism and consists of an enlarged and uniformly affected thyroid gland (diffuse goiter). Other forms include Plummer's disease (multinodular goiter) and toxic adenoma (uninodular goiter). Hyperthyroidism can also be caused by excessive pituitary TSH (thyroid-stimulating hormone secretion or by the ectopic production of TSH-like material by neoplasms. The latter situations occur rarely. Pregnancy and excessive ingestion of thyroid hormones are also associated with an increase in circulating thyroid hormones (23, 24).

Graves' disease is a multisystemic disorder characterized by the syndrome of diffuse goiter, infiltrative ophthalmopathy, and myxedema. The exact pathogenesis is uncertain. However, the overt clinical expression of Graves' disease and the subsequent course are modified by such constitutional factors as heredity, sex, and perhaps emotions. The tendency of Graves' disease to occur in several members of the same family is well documented, but the precise mode of its transmission is uncertain. The hereditary factor appears to involve an autoimmune response, as suggested by the increased family incidence of other autoimmune disorders, such as pernicious anemia and Hashimoto's disease. The female sex is more affected than the male sex in a ratio of approximately 7:1. Often, Graves' disease becomes evident after a severe emotional stress, such as the loss of a significant person or after an acute fright, such as an automobile accident (25).

Toxic multinodular goiter is a disorder in which hyperthyroidism arises from a nontoxic multinodular goiter of long standing. The reason that the nontoxic goiter loses its normal homeostatic regulation is unknown. The clinical manifestations of the disease are relatively mild in comparison to Graves' disease, and it is almost never accompanied by infiltrative ophthalmopathy (26).

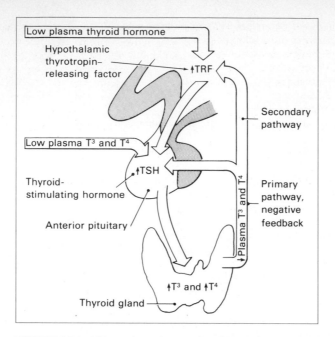

FIGURE 24-9 / Normal mechanism for plasma thyroid hormone(s) regulation. Low plasma T_3 (triiodothyronine) and T_4 (thyroxine) → anterior pituitary ↑ gland T_3 and T_4↑→↑ plasma T_3 and T_4→ feedback to anterior pituitary, pituitary, and hypothalamus. More research is needed to clarify the exact role of the hypothalamus in regulating thyroid hormone synthesis. Present evidence suggests a secondary role in which the hypothalamus determines the set point of the feedback threshold. For example, when T_3 and T_4 levels become very elevated, TRF levels drop, producing a fall in TSH levels.

Graves' Disease

Definition

Graves' disease (hyperthyroidism) is a disease of thyroid hormone excess usually caused by an immune mechanism. The excessive stimulation of the thyroid gland in Graves' disease is thought to be due to the production of a substance, long-acting thyroid stimulator (LATS), which is produced by the reticuloendothelial system and which resembles TSH.

LATS is a gamma globulin of immune system origin and like TSH stimulates the thyroid gland, except over a longer period of time. In addition, LATS or a similar substance from the reticuloendothelial system stimulates the production of retrobulbar fat causing a protrusion of the eyeballs (exophthalmos). The stimulation of the gland produces an enlargement of the gland (goiter) and an excess of thyroxine with an increase in all metabolic processes. The process can regress spontaneously but usually requires control with medication and/or surgery. Hyperthyroidism can be so severe as to be life-threatening, especially from strain on the cardiovascular system.

Control of the thyroid secretion by medication or surgery does not cure Graves' disease. Since the real disease is in the reticuloendothelial system with LATS production, all we hope to do is control the symptoms by blocking thyroxine output until spontaneous remission occurs. If, however, spontaneous remission does not occur in 3 to 5 years of treatment with thyroid-blocking drugs, or if the gland is quite large and needs removal for cosmetic reasons (very large glands rarely regress), then surgical removal of enough of the gland is carried out to ensure a euthyroid state. Radioactive iodine is never given to children who will go through the reproductive age. If medication alone is used, it is given to ensure a euthyroid state. Medication is continued for 1 to 3 years and then discontinued to see if spontaneous remission has occurred. If not, medication is restarted. If surgery is contemplated, the same medications are given to get the patient to a euthyroid state. Iodine is added for 2 weeks, then surgery is performed. Ideally, enough gland is removed to ensure against a recurrence of the hyperthyroid state, but enough is left to ensure a euthyroid state. In practice, either is very difficult. Hypothyroidism is a common complication of surgery but is easily treated.

Assessment

I. History. There is usually a history of hyperactivity, intolerance to heat, nervousness, and even on occasion psychotic behavior and weight loss in spite of voracious appetite and diarrhea.
II. Assess signs of weight loss.
III. Assess signs of hyperactivity.
    A. Smooth, sweaty skin.   *C.* Increased heart rate and blood pressure.
    B. Silky hair.   *D.* Increased reflexes with quick return.
IV. Assess thyroid size (presence of goiter).
V. Assess eye signs.
    A. Exophthalmos.
    B. Lid lag.
    C. Fixed stare.

Problems

I. Hyperactive behavior which may appear psychotic at times.
II. Exophthalmos with damage to the eyes because lids cannot be closed. Proptosis (bulging eyeball) may also stretch the optic nerve, resulting in degeneration and blindness.
III. Gland size may be painful, is unsightly, and may compress the trachea, interfering with respiration.
IV. Stimulation of the cardiovascular system may result in cardiac strain, fatigue, and high cardiac output—heart failure.

Goals of Care

I. Immediate control of cardiac decompensation.
II. Early control of thyroxine output with a return to a euthyroid state.
III. Continuation of a euthyroid state by spontaneous remission, medication, or surgery.

Intervention

I. If the patient is quite hyperthyroid and agitated, nursing attention is required to calm the patient.
II. Frequent assessment of thyroid status is required to adjust medication dose.
III. Frequent assessment of medication side effects is needed (skin rash, granulocytopenia, and liver enlargement are frequent).
IV. Frequent assessment of eye signs and gland size is needed.
V. Education as to signs of medication toxicity or allergy is needed.
VI. Education as to long-range goals, duration of therapy, and consequences should be carried out.
VII. Counseling as to the desirable method of treatment (medication, surgery, etc.) should be given.
VIII. If surgery is chosen, the patient must be prepared psychologically.
IX. The complications of surgery must be explained (hyperthyroidism with the need to take medication for life, hypocalcemia with the need to take calcium, and recurrent laryngeal nerve injury with hoarseness).
X. Follow-up for hypothyroidism after surgery and education to ensure medication compliance.

Evaluation

I. Evaluation of the success of therapy by return to a euthyroid state.
II. Evaluation of preparation for surgery by assessment of patient's psychologic state prior to surgery.
III. Evaluation of postsurgical problems by compliance with follow-up and presence of a euthyroid state.

Toxic Adenoma

Definition *Toxic adenoma* is a disorder characterized by one or more "autonomous" adenomas of the thyroid gland. The pathogenesis is unknown. The natural course of the disorder is one of slow, progressive growth and increasing function over a span of years (27).

Assessment I. Nursing health history.
II. Physical and behavioral assessment (see Fig. 24-10 for appearance of diffuse goiter of hyperthyroidism).
  A. Nervous.
    1. Sensory.
      a. Heat intolerance.   *d.* Failure of convergence.
      b. Fixed stare.   *e.* Exophthalmos.[18]
      c. Lid lag.
    2. Motor.
      a. Skeletal muscle weakness and atrophy.   *c.* Fine hand tremors.
      b. Exaggerated tendon reflexes.   *d.* Clumsiness.
  B. Integumentary.
    1. Excessive sweating.   5. Increased body temperature.
    2. Fine hair and skin.   6. Telangiectasia.
    3. Friable nails.   7. Palmar erythema.
    4. Decreased scalp and axillary hair.
  C. Neck.
    1. Enlarged thyroid.
    2. Thyroid bruit and/or thrill.
  D. Cardiovascular.
    1. Hypertension.   4. Palpitations.
    2. Wide pulse pressure.   5. Systolic flow murmur.
    3. Arrhythmias: tachycardia, atrial fibrillation.   6. Edema in lower extremities.
  E. Respiratory.
    1. Increased rate and depth.
    2. Exertional dyspnea.
  F. Gastrointestinal.
    1. Weight loss.   3. Nausea.
    2. Diarrhea.   4. Increased peristalsis.
  G. Mental status.
    1. Inability to concentrate.   3. Agitation.
    2. Nervousness.   4. Irritability.
  H. Other.
    1. Oligomenorrhea.
    2. Decreased libido and fertility.
III. Other relevant sources.
  A. Medical history.
  B. Interview with family.
  C. Old records.
  D. Referral note.
  E. Diagnostic tests.
    1. Serum T_3, T_4.   4. Serum TSH.
    2. Free T_4.   5. LATS level.
    3. Plasma TBG (thyroid-binding globulin).   6. Thyroid uptake and scan.

---

[18]Exophthalmos is common to Graves' disease. It is the result of accumulation of large quantities of mucopolysaccharides and fluid behind the eyeballs and in the external muscles of the eye, forcing the eyeballs to protrude.

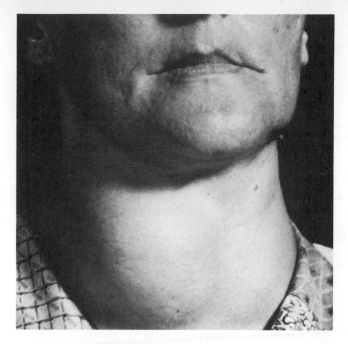

FIGURE 24-10 / **Diffuse goiter of hyperthyroidism.** (*Courtesy of Dr. Louis Avioli.*)

Problems

I. General.
  A. Physical.
    1. Muscular weakness.
    2. Fatigability.
    3. Altered nutritional status.
    4. Stress.
    5. Safety.
    6. Eye trauma.
    7. Hypertension.
    8. Dyspnea.
    9. Arrhythmias.
    10. Heat intolerance.
  B. Psychosocial.
    1. Mental fatigue.
    2. Irritability.
    3. Anxiety.
    4. Inability to concentrate.
    5. Body image.

II. Thyroid crisis or storm.[19]
  A. Shock.
  B. Fluid imbalance.
  C. Hyperthermia.
  D. Arrhythmias: often atrial fibrillation.
  E. Nausea, vomiting.
  F. Heart failure.
  G. Extreme restlessness.
  H. Abdominal pain.
  I. Tachypnea.

III. Subtotal thyroidectomy,[20] postoperative period.
  A. Hemorrhage.
  B. Respiratory obstruction.
  C. Communication.

[19]Thyroid storm is a life-threatening clinical syndrome characterized by hypermetabolism, with hyperthermia up to 106°F (41°C), vascular collapse, severe tachycardia, heart failure, and gastrointestinal and CNS dysfunction. If untreated, death results. The causes of this complication include stress, such as physical and emotional trauma, infection, and surgery.
[20]The choice of treatment depends upon the severity of illness, gland size, age, ability of the patient to follow a regimen, and the presence of complicating diseases. Treatment measures include surgery, iodine treatment, antithyroid drugs, and radioiodine.

D. Infection.

E. Pain.

F. Stress on suture line.

G. Hormone imbalance.
1. Thyroid storm.[21]
2. Tetany.
3. See postoperative care of patients with neck surgery (Chap. 25).

Diagnosis

I. General.

A. Has noted increased feelings of apprehension and inability to concentrate.

B. Has noted difficulty in interpersonal relationships and inappropriate spells of crying or euphoria.

C. Complains of fatigue with routine activities of daily living.

D. Has noted tremors of the hands.

E. May experience breathlessness with minor activity.

F. May experience difficulty sleeping despite feeling mentally and physically fatigued.

G. May have noted a feeling of fullness in the neck.

H. May complain of eye irritation and/or gravellike feeling of eyes (Graves' disease).

I. May complain of excessive fineness of the hair and inability to keep a "set."

J. May complain of continuous or episodic palpitations and/or "racing heart."

K. May have bright-eyed, staring appearance.

L. Complains of weight loss.

M. Unable to tolerate normal environmental temperatures: sets thermostat lower than average temperature, prefers winter to summer months.

II. Thyroid crisis or storm.

A. Has history of hyperthyroidism treated either incompletely or not at all.

B. Signs and symptoms usually occur abruptly and following some stressful experience, such as infection, surgery, and physical or emotional trauma.

C. Is restless and tremulous.

D. Electrocardiogram (ECG) shows tachycardia (usually atrial fibrillation) and may be accompanied by congestive heart failure.

E. Complains of nausea, vomiting, and abdominal pain.

F. Has elevation in body temperature with profuse sweating.

G. May exhibit apathy, stupor, or coma.

H. May become hypotensive.

III. Subtotal thyroidectomy.

A. May experience abnormal bleeding from operative site associated with difficulty in breathing.

B. May develop severe restlessness and difficulty breathing a few hours after surgery (bilateral laryngeal nerve damage).

C. May have difficulty speaking and/or hoarseness (unilateral laryngeal nerve damage).

D. May experience anxiety and mental depression followed by complaints of paresthesia and heightened neuromuscular excitability 1 to 7 days postoperatively (hypoparathyroidism).

E. May exhibit signs and symptoms of thyroid storm.

F. Complains of pain at operative site, especially when positioned.

Goals of Care

I. General.

A. Immediate.
1. Provide optimum diet to meet caloric and nutritional needs.
2. Promote physical and emotional rest.
3. Prevent and/or control complications.
4. Evaluate response(s) to treatment measures.
5. Provide emotional support.

[21]Can occur following surgery due to manipulation of thyroid and release of large quantities of thyroid hormone. More commonly seen in patients poorly prepared for surgery.

    B. Long-range.

        1. Promote patient and family independence in managing self at home.

        2. Return to physical, emotional, and psychological state prior to illness, if appropriate.

        3. Establish need for follow-up.

II. Thyroid storm.

    A. Immediate.

        1. Assist in preventing and/or controlling complications.

        2. Assist in restoring normal fluid and hormone balance.

        3. Provide physical and emotional rest.

        4. Relieve pain and/or discomfort.

        5. Provide emotional support to the patient and family.

    B. Long-range. Same as point I B above.

III. Subtotal thyroidectomy.

    A. Immediate.

        1. Relieve pain and discomfort.

        2. Assist in controlling and/or preventing complications.

        3. Assist in restoring normal fluid and hormone balance.

        4. Provide adequate means of communication.

        5. Provide emotional support to the patient and family.

        6. See postoperative care of patients with neck surgery (Chap. 25).

    B. Long-range. Same as point I B above.

Intervention

I. General.

    A. Orient to hospital routine.

    B. Explain all procedures and treatments and expected responses.

    C. Avoid long teaching sessions and complex medical terms.

    D. Select room and roommate to provide a quiet, relaxing environment.

    E. Restrict visitors, if necessary.

    F. Provide medication for sleep and rest.

    G. Encourage participation in planning daily care, stressing adequate rest between activities.

    H. Assist with activities of daily living, if indicated; tremors, muscle weakness.

    I. Regulate environmental temperature to provide comfort.

    J. Provide diet adequate in calories and vitamins, avoiding coffee, tea, colas, and highly seasoned, bulky foods.

    K. Prevent eye trauma.

        1. Dark glasses during the day.   **3.** Eye medication.

        2. Patch eyes as ordered, such as at bedtime.   **4.** Elevate head at bedtime.

    L. Monitor responses to treatment measures.

        1. Weigh daily.

        2. Blood pressure, pulse, respirations, temperature.

        3. Mental status.

        4. Appetite.

        5. Neuromuscular reflexes.

    M. Observe for side effects of medication, and report immediately: depends on type, dose, and duration.

        1. Rash.   **6.** Swelling of buccal mucosa.

        2. Conjunctivitis.   **7.** Excessive salivation.

        3. Pruritus.   **8.** Coryza.

        4. Sore throat.   **9.** Swollen neck veins.

        5. Fever.

    N. Reassure that most physical and behavioral changes are amenable to treatment.

    O. Patient and family teaching.

        1. Anatomy and physiology of illness.

      2. Medication(s).
        a. Type: antithyroid (Tapazole, propylthiouracil); iodine; radioiodine.
        b. Action.
        c. Dose.
        d. Side effects.
        e. Expected responses to medication.
      3. Signs and symptoms of hyperthyroidism.
      4. Signs and symptoms of hypothyroidism.
      5. Importance of follow-up.
        a. Incidence of hypothyroidism with medication and surgery.
        b. Incidence of recurrent hyperthyroidism with medication and surgery.
      6. Diet.
      7. Activity and rest.
  P. Behavioral counseling, if indicated.
II. Thyroid crisis or storm.
  A. Maintain patent intravenous line.
  B. Place on cardiac monitor.
  C. Keep accurate flow sheet of responses to treatment.
      1. Blood pressure, pulse, respirations, and temperature, every 30 min or as needed.
      2. Mental status.
      3. Intake and output: estimate diaphoretic loss.
      4. Neuromuscular reflexes.
      5. Chest sounds.
  D. Medicate for abdominal pain, nausea, anorexia, and vomiting.
  E. Insert nasogastric tube for nausea, vomiting, and/or administration of medication.
  F. Institute cooling measures.
      1. Hypothermia blanket.
      2. Tepid to cool water or alcohol sponges.
      3. Avoid chilling and skin burns.
      4. Drugs.
  G. Administer medications as ordered and observe for effectiveness and side effects.
      1. Antithyroid preparations.
      2. Iodine preparation.
      3. Beta blocking agents.
      4. Digitalis.
      5. Sedatives.
      6. Tranquilizers.
      7. Diuretics.
  H. Administer fluids as ordered.
III. Subtotal thyroidectomy.
  A. Check operative site (at least once an hour).
      1. Redness.
      2. Pain.
      3. Swelling.
      4. Drainage.
      5. Bleeding: side of and behind neck.
  B. Report complaints of neck fullness, heaviness, and/or tight dressing.
  C. Observe for respiratory obstruction, dyspnea, swelling, tight dressing, stridor, cyanosis.
  D. Keep suction equipment and tracheostomy set at bedside.
  E. Place in semi-Fowler's position on back.
  F. Immobilize head.
      1. Firm pillows, sandbags.
      2. Prevent flexion or extension.
      3. Move head with body when turning.
  G. Apply ice bag to incision.

    H. Observe for tetany once an hour.
       1. Anxiety, mental depression.
       2. Paresthesia.
       3. Twitching.
       4. Positive Chvostok's and Trousseau's signs.
    I. Check quality of voice once *every* 1 to 2 h.
       1. Tone, pitch.
       2. Hoarseness.
       3. Limit talking.
       4. Provide alternate means of communication.
    J. Observe for hypothyroidism, hyperthyroidism.
    K. ROM exercises to neck, when able.
    L. Topical cream to incision when suture is removed.
    M. Patient and family teaching (*see* point I above).

Evaluation

    I. Verbally describes pathophysiology of disease.
    II. States medication receiving, dose, time, action, and side effects.
    III. States expected response(s) from treatment and possible complications.
    IV. Verbally recalls signs and symptoms of hyperthyroidism and hypothyroidism.
    V. Maintains ideal body weight.
    VI. Is able to return to work and resume family and social roles.
    VII. Shows improvement in:
       A. Pulse: normal rhythm and rate; decreased palpitations.
       B. Temperature normal.
       C. Respirations: tolerates activity without dyspnea.
       D. Reflexes: decreased excitability; decreased tremors.
       E. Appetite increased; weight gain.
       F. Mental status: decreased nervousness, irritability, etc.
    VIII. Keeps medical appointments. If unable, calls and reschedules appointment.

Follow-up

    I. Clinic.
    II. Periodic telephone calls.

Hypothyroidism

Definition

Hypothyroidism is the term used to describe clinical disorders resulting from insufficient production of thyroid hormones, thyroxine (T_4) and triiodothyronine (T_3). Severe hypothyroidism beginning in infancy is termed *cretinism,* whereas in the adult patient, marked thyroid hormone deficiency is termed *myxedema* (28).

Hypothyroidism is classified as primary or secondary depending upon the cause for hormone deficiency. *Primary hypothyroidism* refers to thyroid hormone deficiency caused by intrinsic thyroid disease. Some of these causes include destruction of the gland (thyroidectomy, radioactive iodine, local irradiation, or idiopathic disease) or defects in thyroid hormone synthesis (chronic thyroiditis, genetic enzyme defects, therapy with antithyroid drugs, or iodine deficiency). *Secondary hypothyroidism* refers to thyroid hormone deficiency in the presence of a normal thyroid gland. This disorder is caused by disease of the anterior pituitary gland or hypothalamus resulting in deficient TSH (thyroid-stimulating hormone) or TRH (thyroid-releasing hormone) secretion. Regardless of the cause for the hypothyroidism, all organ systems are affected. The severity of clinical manifestations is closely related to the degree of hormone deficiency (29).

The term *myxedema coma* is used to describe the clinical complication of profound hypothyroidism. It is characterized by myxedema (an accumulation of mucopolysaccharides in tissues that hold body water) and *severe* central nervous system depression with hypoventilation, hypothermia, and stupor proceeding to coma. The pathogenesis of this disorder is unknown, but several factors predispose to its development, namely, exposure to cold, infection, physical and emotional trauma, and central nervous system depressants. It is associated with a very high mortality rate (30).

Assessment

I. Nursing health history.
II. Physical and behavioral assessment.
  A. Nervous.
    1. Sensory.
      a. Cold intolerance.
      b. Numbness and tingling of fingers.
      c. Deafness (occasionally observed).
      d. Periorbital puffiness (see Fig. 24-11).
      e. Thick tongue.
    2. Motor.
      a. Muscle weakness and atrophy.
      b. Slow gait.
      c. Depressed tendon reflexes.
  B. Integumentary.
    1. Dry, scaly skin.   4. Decreased sweating.
    2. Hair loss.   5. Skin pallor.
    3. Brittle nails.   6. Nonpitting edema of lower extremities.
  C. Cardiovascular. Blood pressure, pulse: low or low normal range.
  D. Respiratory.
    1. Decreased rate and depth.
    2. Exertional dyspnea.
  E. Gastrointestinal.
    1. Weight gain (moderate).
    2. Anorexia.
    3. Constipation.
  F. Mental status.
    1. Lethargy.
    2. Memory impairment.
    3. Drowsiness.
  G. Other.
    1. Loss of libido.
    2. Menstrual disturbances (menorrhagia).
III. Other relevant sources.
  A. Medical history.
  B. Interview with family and/or significant other.
  C. Old records.

FIGURE 24-11 / Periorbital puffiness of hypothyroidism. (*Courtesy of Dr. Louis Avioli.*)

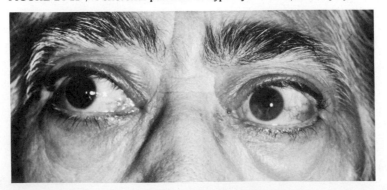

    D. Referral note.

    E. Diagnostic test.

       1. Primary hypothyroidism.

          a. Serum T_3, T_4.

          b. Serum TSH.

       2. Secondary hypothyroidism.

          a. Serum T_3, T_4.

          b. Serum TSH.

          c. TRH stimulation test.

          d. Plasma ACTH.

          e. FSH, LH, especially in postmenopausal women.

          f. Formal visual fields.

          g. Skull films with cone view of sella tursica.

Problems

I. General.

    A. Physical.

       1. Weakness.   **5.** Activity.

       2. Altered nutritional status.   **6.** Communication.

       3. Stress.   **7.** Skin breakdown.

       4. Edema.

    B. Psychosocial.

       1. Body image.   **3.** Mental fatique.

       2. Apathy.   **4.** Decreased interpersonal relationships.

II. Myxedema coma.

    A. Shock.   *D.* Respiratory embarrassment.

    B. Heat loss.   *E.* Altered nutrition.

    C. Fluid imbalance.   *F.* Altered mental status.

Diagnosis

I. General.

    A. Has noted difficulty in performing a full day's work.

    B. Family and/or associates may have noted loss of interest in work and environment.

    C. Complains of constipation.

    D. Complains of hair loss, brittle nails, and dry skin (especially women).

    E. Has noticed moderate weight gain despite decreased appetite.

    F. Has preference for warm weather, uses more blankets, sets thermostat higher than normal.

    G. May have noted periorbital puffiness and/or swelling of extremities.

    H. May have enlarged tongue accompanied by husky voice.

    I. May have slow speech and difficulty remembering events.

II. Myxedema coma.

    A. May have history of hypothyroidism.

    B. Signs and symptoms usually occur in the winter and usually follow exposure to cold, an infection, physical and emotional trauma, and CNS depressants.

    C. Clinically resembles brainstem infarction, subnormal temperature, severe hypotension, bradycardia, respiratory depression, absent tendon reflexes, and at times, seizures.

    D. Has nonpitting edema of extremities and periorbital puffiness.

Goals of Care

I. General.

    A. Immediate.

       1. Promote physical and emotional rest.

       2. Evaluate responses to treatment measures.

       3. Prevent and/or control complications.

       4. Promote a balanced diet.

       5. Promote adequate bowel elimination.

       6. Provide emotional support.

      B. Long-range.
        1. Provide patient and family independence in managing self at home.
        2. Return to physical, emotional, and psychological state prior to illness, if appropriate.
        3. Establish need for follow-up.[22]
  II. Myxedema coma.
      A. Immediate.
        1. Provide physical support.
        2. Provide emotional support to the family.
        3. Assist in preventing and/or controlling complications.
        4. Assist in restoring normal fluid and hormone balance.
      B. Long-range (same as point I B above).

Intervention

  I. General.
      A. Orient to hospital routine.
      B. Explain all procedures and treatments and expected responses.
      C. Provide a balanced diet restricted in calories and salt but within preference.
      D. Promote adequate bowel function.
        1. Encourage fluid intake.
        2. Encourage bulky foods.
        3. Encourage activity as tolerated.
        4. Administer stool softeners and laxatives.
      E. Encourage participation in planning daily care.
      F. Regulate environmental temperature.
      G. Select room and roommate to provide a quiet, relaxing environment.
      H. Provide emotional support for patient and family.
        1. Promote communication with family to enable them to understand physical and emotional changes.
        2. Encourage expression of feelings.
        3. Reassure that most of the physical and behavioral changes are amenable to treatment.
        4. Allow time for expressing self (slow speech, difficulty concentrating).
      I. Prevent skin breakdown if on bed rest.
        1. Implement active (ROM) exercises.
        2. Frequent positioning.
        3. Air mattress.
        4. Mild soaps and lotions.
      J. Monitor responses to treatment measures.
        1. Weigh daily: decreased.
        2. Intake and output.
          a. Diuresis, early clinical response.
          b. Decreased edema.
          c. Decreased periorbital edema.
        3. Appetite improved.
        4. Mental status.
          a. Improved feeling of well-being.
          b. More alert and active.
          c. Awareness of surroundings.
        5. Hoarseness gradually abates.
        6. Pulse, respirations increased.
        7. Temperature increased within 24 h.
        8. Reflexes: delay disappears.
        9. Constipation may disappear.
        10. Hair, skin improved over a period of months.

---

[22]For unknown reasons, patients with hypothyroidism have a high incidence of discontinuing their medication when they feel better or medication runs out.

K. Observe for side effects of medication(s), especially cardiac patients.

   1. Palpitations.   **4.** Hyperthermia.

   2. Angina.   **5.** Heart failure.

   3. Headache.   **6.** Tachycardia.

L. Use lower than normal doses for sedatives and narcotics, and check frequently.

M. Patient and family teaching.

   1. Anatomy and physiology of illness.

   2. Expected responses from treatment (see above).

   3. Medication(s).

      a. Type

         (1) Thyroid extract (USP thyroid): vary in biologic potency.

         (2) Synthetic thyroid hormone: more predictable effects.

      b. Action.

      c. Dose.

      d. Side effects.

   4. Signs and symptoms of hypothyroidism and hyperthyroidism.

   5. Importance of follow-up: side effects, complications.

   6. Diet.

   7. Activity, rest.

   8. Avoidance of physical and emotional stress.

N. Behavioral counseling, if indicated.

II. Myxedema coma.

A. Place on cardiac monitor.

B. Maintain patent intravenous line.[23]

C. Administer medications as ordered.

   1. Thyroid hormone.

   2. Hydrocortisone.

D. Administer fluids as ordered.

E. Support respirations (see care of the patient receiving assisted ventilation in Chap. 27).

F. Avoid external warming, but promote adequate measures to decrease further heat loss and unnecessary body exposure, drafts.[24]

G. Evaluate for infection if temperature is normal.

H. Monitor responses to treatment measures.

   1. Temperature increased within 24 h.

   2. Pulse, respiration, blood pressure increased.

   3. Intake and output: diuresis, early clinical response.

   4. Reflexes: delay improved.

   5. Regression of edema and periorbital puffiness.

   6. Mental status improved.

I. Assign other nursing personnel to interview family.

J. Other: see care of the comatose patient in Chap. 23.

Evaluation

I. Verbally describes pathophysiology of disease.

II. States medication receiving, dose, time, action, side effects, and importance.

III. States expected responses from treatment.

IV. Verbally recalls signs and symptoms of hypothyroidism and hyperthyroidism.

V. Maintains ideal body weight.

VI. States significance of rest, activity, and avoidance of physical and emotional stress.

VII. Is able to return to family and social roles.

VIII. Keeps medical appointments. If unable, calls and schedules another appointment.

---

[23]Because of the sluggish circulation and severe hypometabolism, absorption of medication from the stomach or from subcutaneous and intramuscular sites is unpredictable.

[24]Could lead to vascular collapse.

Follow-up	**I.** Clinic.
	II. Periodic telephone calls.
	III. Visiting Nurse Association, if indicated.

Hyperaldosteronism

Definition

Hyperaldosteronism, excess secretion of aldosterone by the adrenal cortex, can be primary or secondary depending upon the cause of the hypersecretion. The term *primary hyperaldosteronism* (Conn's disease), implies that the disturbance causing hypersecretion is within the adrenal cortex itself. The most common cause of excess aldosterone is an autonomously functioning adenoma. Normally, aldosterone acts on epithelial cells of the renal tubule, sweat glands, salivary glands, and gastrointestinal tract to promote sodium and chloride retention and potassium (K^+) excretion. In states of increased aldosterone, its known effects on electrolyte balance are exaggerated, leading to K^+ wasting and sodium retention (mild edema, increased blood pressure). *Secondary hyperaldosteronism* occurs as a result of the adrenal-stimulating action of angiotensin II. There are numerous situations which increase the activity of the renin-angiotensin system and secondarily increase aldosterone secretion, e.g., dehydration, upright position, sodium depletion, renal artery stenosis, cardiac failure. Unlike primary aldosteronism, secondary aldosteronism is not a specific disorder but rather a response to the pathophysiology of one or more clinical disorders (31, 32).

Assessment

I. Nursing health history.
II. Physical and behavioral assessment.
    A. Musculoskeletal weakness.
    B. Headache.
    C. Paresthesia.
    D. Muscle cramps.
    E. Excessive thirst.
    F. Frequent voiding.
    G. Mild edema (if present at all).
    H. Mild to moderate hypertension.
    I. Lethargy.
III. Other relevant sources.
    A. Medical history.
    B. Interview with family and/or significant other.
    C. Referral note.
    D. Diagnostic tests.
        1. Plasma aldosterone (supine and upright) after K^+ replacement.
        2. Urinary aldosterone, 24-h.
        3. Peripheral plasma renin levels.
        4. Serum electrolytes: Na, K^+.
        5. Urinary K^+, 24-h.
        6. Intravenous pyelogram (IVP).
        7. Renal arteriograms secondary to IVP.
        8. Adrenal vein catheterization with renin levels.
        9. Plasma renin activity (PRA).
            a. After salt-restriction diet (3 days): furosemide (Lasix) and activity.
            b. After salt-loading diet (6 g per day for 5 to 7 days).

Problems

I. Physical.
    A. Pain.
    B. Weakness.
    C. Safety.
    D. Altered fluid and electrolyte balance.
    E. Elevated blood pressure.
II. Psychosocial.
    A. Stress.
    B. Anxiety.
    C. Lethargy.

Diagnosis

I. May complain of headaches.
II. Complains of fatigue, leg cramp, and paresthesia.

III. Has lost interest in physical activity and/or projects requiring mental effort.
IV. Complains of excessive thirst and frequent voidings.
V. Expresses concern about impending diagnostic test (IVP, arteriogram) and treatment.

Goals of Care

I. Immediate.
  A. Relieve pain.
  B. Promote physical, emotional, and psychological rest.
  C. Prevent and/or control complications.
  D. Prepare psychologically for diagnostic test and surgery.
II. Long-range.
  A. Evaluate responses to therapeutic measures.
  B. Promote patient and family independence in managing self at home.
  C. Return to physical, emotional, and psychological state prior to illness, if appropriate.

Intervention

  I. Administer analgesics for pain.
 II. Administer tranquilizers and sedatives for rest and sleep.
III. Administer K^+ replacement and assess response.
IV. Group nursing and medical activities to promote rest.
 V. Allow adequate rest between activities.
VI. Assess motor and sensory deficits, and institute appropriate measures.
  A. Assist with ambulation.
  B. Remove extraneous equipment from room.
  C. Avoid hot beverages.
VII. Observe and record.
  A. Blood pressure.
  B. Intake and output.
  C. Response to provocative tests.
    1. Arteriograms.
    2. Plasma renin activity test.
  D. Electrolyte balance.
    1. Edema.
    2. Signs and symptoms of hypokalemia.
VIII. Patient and family teaching.
  A. Anatomy and physiology of illness.
  B. Treatment measures and expected responses.
    1. Primary aldosteronism.
      a. Removal of adrenal adenoma preferred treatment.
      b. Adrenalectomy (left adrenal plus 50 percent right adrenal if tumor not found).
      c. Drugs: spironolactone (aldactone).
        (1) Poor surgical risk.
        (2) Recurrent aldosteronism following surgery.
    2. Secondary aldosteronism. Treat underlying disease(s).
  C. Medication.
  D. Signs and symptoms of hypokalemia.
  E. Signs and symptoms of adrenal insufficiency. Precautionary: must be over 90 percent destruction of adrenal glands before deficiency occurs.
  F. Diet.
  G. Rest and activity.
  H. See Chap. 23 for care of the patient with metastatic carcinoma receiving radiation therapy.
IX. Behavioral counseling, if indicated.

Evaluation

  I. Verbally describes pathophysiology of disease.
 II. States medication receiving, dose, action, time, and side effects.
III. States expected response(s) from treatment.

IV. Is able to return to family and social roles.

V. Shows improvement in the following after treatment of primary aldosteronism.
  A. Decreased blood pressure: 80 percent normotensive after a few months.
  B. Decreased muscle weakness first few weeks after surgery.
  C. Decreased thirst and polyuria first few weeks after surgery.
  D. Decreased headache first few weeks after surgery.
  E. Maintains normal plasma potassium level.
  F. Decreased anxiety and lethargy.

Follow-up

I. Clinic.

II. Periodic telephone calls.

Diabetes Insipidus

Definition

The term *diabetes insipidus* refers to a deficiency of antidiuretic hormone (ADH or vasopressin). ADH exerts control on urinary water excretion, thereby controlling the concentration of body fluids. A deficiency of ADH results in the excretion of excessive amounts of dilute urine and secondary polydipsia. Figure 24-12 shows the normal mechanisms of antidiuretic hormone regulation.

The stimulus for release of ADH by the posterior pituitary (stores ADH) is believed to be regulated by osmoreceptors in the hypothalamus, namely, paraventricular and supraoptic nuclei. Changes in the plasma osmolar concentration (amount of solute in body water) are detected by the osmoreceptors, and ADH secretion is either enhanced or decreased. Pressoreceptors (carotid body) in the vascular system also control ADH secretion by sending impulses to the hypothalamus in response to pressure changes in the blood vessels. After being released into the circulation, ADH exerts its water-conserving effect by altering the permeability of the distal convoluted tubules and collecting ducts of the kidneys. Stimulators

FIGURE 24-12 / ADH regulation. Stimuli → hypothalamic receptors →↑ ADH by hypothalamus → plus, neural message sent to posterior pituitary to ↑ ADH release →↑ plasma ADH → altered membrane permeability of the distal convoluted tubules →↑ water reabsorption by ECF →↓ plasma concentration, and urine output.

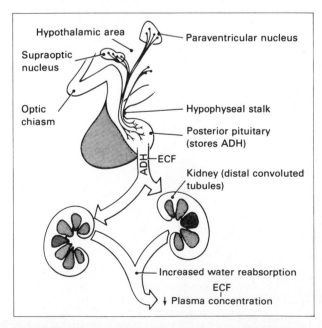

of ADH secretion include circulatory shock, hemorrhage, pain, anxiety, trauma, nicotine, morphine, acetylcholine, tranquilizers, and some anesthetics (33).

Diabetes insipidus can be permanent or transient. *Permanent* diabetes insipidus results from structural damage to the supraoptic and paraventricular nuclei of the hypothalamus, division of the supraopticohypophysial tract above the median eminence. or damage to the kidneys causing renal unresponsiveness to ADH (*nephrogenic diabetes insipidus*). Causes of diabetes insipidus can be idiopathic or familial, or can result from head trauma (accidental or neurosurgical), neoplasm, and infections (34).

Assessment

I. Nursing health history.
II. Physical and behavioral assessment.
    A. Dry skin and mucous membranes.
    B. Excessive thirst.
    C. Polyuria.
    D. Fatigue.
    E. Weakness.
    F. Hypotension.
    G. Dizziness.
    H. Nervousness.
III. Other relevant sources.
    A. Medical history.
    B. Interview with family.
    C. Diagnostic tests.
        1. Skull x-ray with view of sella tursica.
        2. Urine, 24-h: volumes of 5 to 10 L or more.
        3. Urine osmolalities: 50 to 200 mosmol/L.
        4. Plasma osmolality: > 300 mosmol.
        5. Specific gravities: 1.000 to 1.005.
        6. Water deprivation test (8 h):
            a. Urine volume remains greater than 30 mL/min.
            b. Urine concentration, less than 200 mosmol/L (280 to 300 mosmol—normal).
            c. Urine specific gravity, 1.001 to 1.005 (1.020 or above normal).

Problems

I. Physical.
    A. Dehydration.
    B. Polyuria, polydipsia.
    C. Weakness.
    D. Malaise.
    E. Safety.
II. Psychosocial.
    A. Anxiety.
    B. Nervousness.

Diagnosis

I. Complains of excessive thirst (18 to 24 L per day) and frequent urination (frequently *only* complaint).
II. Has preference for ice-cold water.
III. May complain of constipation.
IV. May complain of weakness, malaise, and dizziness.
V. Shows signs of dehydration, weight loss, dry skin and mucous membranes.

Goals of Care

I. Immediate.
    A. Prevent and/or control complications.
    B. Promote a safe environment.
    C. Promote physical, emotional, and psychological rest.
II. Long-range. Promote patient and family independence in managing self at home.

Intervention

I. Check for regularity of stools, and administer stool softeners or laxatives as needed.
II. Observe and record (especially important when no *thirst* mechanism):
    A. Intake and output.
    B. Urine specific gravity.
    C. Weight.
    D. Blood pressure, pulse (orthostatic changes), and temperature.
    E. Skin condition.

III. Explain all diagnostic tests and expected responses.
IV. Carefully observe during water restriction test:
    A. Weight before start of test and frequent weight checks during test. Loss of *3 to 5 percent* of body weight warrants immediate reporting.
    B. Intake and output.
    C. Urine specific gravity.
    D. Mental status.
V. Patient and family teaching.
    A. Anatomy and physiology of illness.
    B. Treatment and expected responses. Medication.
        1. Short-acting, aqueous Pitressin, 2 to 6 h nasal spray.
        2. Vasopressin tannate in oil, long-acting, 24 to 72 h subcutaneous or intramuscular injection (must be mixed well).
        3. Diet: low protein, low salt.[25]
        4. Diuretics, especially thiazides.
        5. Chlorpropamide: oral hypoglycemic agent.
    C. Expected responses from treatment (hormone replacement). Decreased:
        1. Thirst and urination.
        2. Feeling of malaise and weakness.
        3. Constipation.
        4. Nervousness.
    D. Use of nasal spray.
    E. Technique for intramuscular or subcutaneous administration of medication.
    F. Signs and symptoms of vasopressin deficiency.

Evaluation

I. Verbally describes pathophysiology of illness.
II. States medication receiving, dose, time, action, and side effects.
III. States expected response(s) from treatment.
IV. Demonstrates skills taught: nasal spray or intramuscular or subcutaneous injection.
V. Shows improvement in following:
    C. Weight increased.
    D. Mental status improved.

Follow-up

I. Clinic.
II. Periodic telephone calls.
III. Visiting Nurse Association.

Inappropriate Antidiuretic Hormone

Definition

The syndrome of *inapppropriate ADH secretion* (SIADH) or excess secretion of ADH results in excretion of concentrated urine with water retention and low plasma tonicity and the risk of severe water intoxication (35). The syndrome may occur from ectopic vasopressin secretion (most commonly from brochogenic carcinoma) or from inappropriate neurohypophysial vasopressin secretion (see "Diabetes Insipidus"). The latter can occur in a variety of clinical disorders of the central nervous system (trauma, neurosurgery on the midbrain, infection, cerebral hemorrhage), lungs (tuberculosis, pneumonia), or after the use of certain drugs (chlorpropamide, narcotics, barbiturates, diuretics, vincristine). In some patients, no underlying disorder can be found (36).

Assessment

I. Nursing health history.
II. Physical and behavioral assessment.
    A. Edema.   D. Muscle cramps.
    B. Nausea.   E. Mental confusion.
    C. Vomiting.   F. Coma.

[25]Dietary restrictions and diuretics only treatment measures for nephrogenic diabetes insipidus.

III. Other relevant sources.
    A. Medical history.
    B. Diagnostic tests.
       1. Electrolytes: hyponatremia.
       2. Serum urea nitrogen: low.
       3. Urine osmolality.
       4. Plasma osmolality: < 280 mosmol.
       5. Urinary sodium excretion: < 30 meq/L.

Problems

I. Physical.
    A. Altered nutritional status.
    B. Altered fluid balance.
II. Psychosocial. Altered mental status.

Diagnosis

I. Gains weight despite poor appetite and normal fluid intake.
II. Has elevated urine specific gravity.
III. Urinary output low in comparison to intake of fluids.
IV. Often is confused but may be in coma.

Goals of Care

I. Immediate. Prevent and/or control complications.
II. Long-range. Promote patient and family independence in managing self at home.

Intervention

I. Observe and record:
    A. Intake and output (strict).
    B. Blood pressure, pulse, and temperature.
    C. Weight.
    D. Urine specific gravity.
    E. Edema.
    F. Mental status.
II. Strict adherence to prescribed fluid restriction.
III. Patient and family teaching.
    A. Pathophysiology of illness.
    B. Importance of fluid restriction.

Evaluation

I. Adheres to fluid restriction, keeps accurate account of fluid intake, does not "sneak" fluids.
II. Describes pathophysiology of illness and signs and symptoms.
III. Shows improvement in:
    A. Weight, decreased.
    B. Urine output, increased.
    C. Mental status, improved.

Follow-up

I. Clinic.
II. Periodic telephone calls.

Hypergonadotropic Syndromes

Definition

The secretion of testosterone, estrogen, and progesterone (androgens) by the testes and ovaries is necessary for normal sexual development and reproduction. Synthesis of these hormones by the gonads is regulated by the anterior pituitary gonadotropins (luteinizing hormone, LH, and follicle-stimulating hormone, FSH). The hypothalamus in turn controls the secretion of pituitary gonadotropins.

    Several disorders affecting normal sexual development and reproduction can occur. The most common disorders of abnormal sexual development and function fall into the category *hypergonadotropic hypogonadal syndromes.* These syndromes are characterized by elevated LH and FSH in conjunction with testicular or ovarian failure.

Klinefelter's syndrome represents the most common example of male hypergonadism (elevated LH, FSH, and testicular failure). The primary etiologic factor is an extra X chromosome (47, XXY sex chromosomal complement). The presence of extra X chromosomes in testicular tissue is the factor responsible for the seminiferous tubule (site of spermatogenesis) and Leydig cell (site of testosterone production) failure. Variant forms of Klinefelter's syndrome occur infrequently. The clinical features of these variant forms are determined by the number of X chromosomes (37).

Turner's syndrome (ovarian dysgenesis) represents the most common clinical entity of female hypergonadotropic hypogonadism (elevated LH and FSH and ovarian failure). The majority of these patients have a 45, XO sex chromosome constitution. Some isolated cases of male Turner's syndrome have been identified (38).

Assessment	I. Nursing health history.
	II. Physical and behavioral assessment.
	A. Klinefelter's syndrome: puberty.
	1. Decreased or absent secondary sexual characteristics.
	2. Small, firm testes.
	3. Decreased libido.
	4. Gynecomastia (breast enlargement).
	5. Excessive long bone growth (extremities).
	6. May have subnormal intelligence: IQ of less than 80.
	7. Personality disorders.
	B. Turner's syndrome.
	1. Short, webbed neck.
	2. Shieldlike chest.
	3. Low-set or deformed ears.
	4. Puffiness over dorsum of the fingers.
	5. Cubitus valgus (deviation of extended forearm).
	6. Decreased breast development.
	7. Sparse pubic hair.
	8. Widely separated nipples.
	9. Amenorrhea.
	III. Other relevant sources.
	A. Medical history.
	B. Interview with family.
	C. Diagnostic tests.
	1. Kleinfelter's syndrome.
	a. Serum FSH, LH.
	b. Serum testosterone.
	c. Buccal smear (Barr body present).
	d. Testicular biopsy: selected few.
	e. Sperm count.
	f. Skull films.
	2. Turner's syndrome.
	a. Serum FSH, LH, PRL.
	b. Serum estradiol.
	c. Buccal smear (Barr body absent).
Problems	Psychosocial: body image; socialization; dependence.
Diagnosis	I. Complains of peer ridicule.
	II. Feels inferior as friends develop sexually.
	III. Has few friends.

IV. Seldom takes part in school and/or other social activities.

V. May attend special school for handicapped children.

Goals of Care

I. Immediate.

    A. Encourage communication with patient and family.

    B. Provide physical, emotional, and psychological support.

II. Long-range. Promote patient and family independence in managing self at home.

Interventions

I. Interview family regarding:

    A. Adjustment to disorder.

    B. Patient's habits: friends; social activities; hobbies.

    C. Patient's adjustment to disorder.

II. Patient and/or family teaching.

    A. Anatomy and physiology of illness.

    B. Treatment and expected responses.

    C. Medication: testosterone, estrogen (will restore secondary sexual characteristics but not fertility).

III. Behavioral counseling, if indicated.

Evaluation

I. Verbally describes pathophysiology of illness.

II. States medication receiving, dose, action, side effects.

III. Shows improvement in secondary sex characteristics.

Follow-up

I. Clinic.

II. Periodic telephone calls.

METABOLIC DISORDERS

Hyperparathyroidism

Definition

Hyperparathyroidism is a disorder of mineral metabolism characterized by excess secretion of parathyroid hormone (PTH) resulting in hypercalcemia. It is the most common disorder involving the parathyroid gland. See Fig. 24-13 for review of parathyroid hormone functions.

PTH is responsible for regulating calcium and phosphate metabolism. PTH exerts its effect on three primary sites, bone, kidney, and gastrointestinal tract, stimulating resorption of calcium and phosphate from bone; calcium reabsorption, phosphate excretion, and vitamin D metabolism by the kidneys; and directly and indirectly, absorption of calcium and phosphate from the gastrointestinal tract (presence of vitamin D in the gastrointestinal tract primarily responsible for calcium absorption). PTH activity is regulated by serum calcium levels. A fall in serum calcium stimulates PTH secretion and a rise suppresses PTH secretion (negative feedback mechanism). The effects of PTH are opposed by calcitonin, a hormone produced by the thyroid gland, which acts to lower serum calcium levels (39).

Hyperparathyroidism can be primary or secondary. *Primary hyperparathyroidism* is the result of a defect in the normal feedback control of PTH secretion. The exact etiology is unknown. However, the most common findings are an autonomously functioning adenoma of the parathyroid gland or hyperplasia of the gland. *Secondary hyperparathyroidism* is characterized by a disruption of mineral homeostasis, producing a compensatory increase in PTH secretion such as occurs due to the hypocalcemia of chronic renal failure, rickets, VDRR (vitamin D-resistant rickets), or malnutrition (40).

The possibility of a multiple endocrine neoplasia syndrome (MEA) should be considered when hyperparathyroidism is present. Two types of MEA exist. *MEA type I* includes (1) pituitary tumors which hypersecrete growth hormone, prolactin, or both, (2) primary hyperparathyroidism, and (3) islet cell tumors of the pancreas, which often secrete gastrin or insulin. *MEA type II* includes (1) medullary carcinoma of the thyroid with hypersecretion of calcitonin, (2) primary hyperparathyroidism, and (3) pheochromocytoma (41).

Assessment

   I. Nursing health history.

  II. Physical and behavioral assessment.
- **A.** Moderate hypercalcemia.
  1. Renal.
     - **a.** Back pain, hematuria: calculi.
     - **b.** Polyuria.
     - **c.** Urinary tract infection.
  2. Skeletal. Vague pain, can be severe.
  3. Gastrointestinal.
     - **a.** Pain.
     - **b.** Anorexia.
     - **c.** Nausea, vomiting.
     - **d.** Constipation.
     - **e.** Weight loss.
  4. Neuromuscular.
     - **a.** Muscular weakness.
     - **b.** Cardiac irregularities.
     - **c.** Lethargy.
     - **d.** Decreased muscle tone.
- **B.** Severe hypercalcemia.
  1. Confusion.
  2. Delusions.
  3. Stupor, coma.
  4. Any of the above (under moderate hypercalcemia).

III. Other relevant sources.
- **A.** Medical history.
- **B.** Interview with family.
- **C.** Old records.

FIGURE 24-13 / Major actions of parathyroid hormone (PTH).

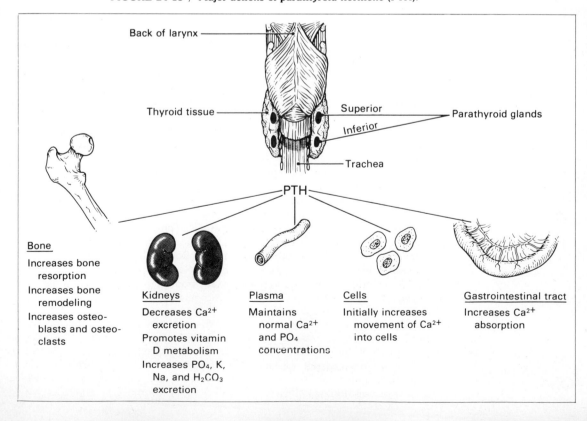

    D. Diagnostic tests.
       1. Serum calcium, phosphorus, magnesium.
       2. Ionized serum calcium.
       3. Serum PTH.
       4. Alkaline phosphatase.
       5. Tubular reabsorption of phosphorus (TRP).

Problems

I. Physical.
  A. Pain.   *C.* Anorexia, nausea, vomiting.
  B. Weakness.   *D.* Dehydration.
II. Psychosocial.
  A. Irritability.   *D.* Personality changes.
  B. Confusion.   *E.* Stupor, coma.
  C. Depression.

Diagnosis

   I. Complains of long history of vague skeletal pain.
  II. May complain of back pain associated with hematuria, burning, and frequency.
 III. Complains of anorexia, nausea, and vomiting associated with vague abdominal pain.
 IV. Complains of constipation.
  V. Frequently complains of severe polyuria and polydipsia.
 VI. Family relates history of personality or behavioral changes.
VII. Complains of weakness and lethargy.
VIII. May present in coma.

Goals of Care

I. Immediate.
  A. Relieve pain and discomfort.
  B. Promote physical, emotional, and psychological rest.
  C. Prevent and/or control complications.
II. Long-range.
  A. Promote patient and family independence in managing self at home.
  B. Return to preillness state physically, emotionally, and psychologically, if appropriate.

Intervention

   I. Administer medication for:
    A. Pain.
    B. Nausea, vomiting, anorexia.
    C. Rest and sleep.
  II. Group nursing and medical activities to promote rest.
 III. Prevent and/or control complications.
    A. Encourage fluid intake up to 3000 mL per day.
    B. Assess for dehydration.
      1. Skin.
      2. Mucous membranes.
      3. Intake and output.
    C. Encourage ambulation as tolerated.
    D. Strain all urine, if indicated, and observe for hematuria.
    E. Check stools for blood (can develop peptic ulcer).
    F. Assist with care, if indicated.
    G. Evaluate regularity of stools, and use stool softeners as needed.
 IV. Patient and family teaching.
    A. Anatomy and physiology of illness.
    B. Treatment and expected responses.
      1. Surgery: preferred and primary mode of treatment.
      2. Drugs and diet.
        a. Oral phosphate.
        b. Estrogens.
        c. Low-calcium diet.

      C. Preoperative teaching.

      D. Need for follow-up.

      E. Postoperative (see postoperative care of patient with neck surgery in Chap. 25). Assess for:

        1. Hemorrhage.   **3.** Laryngeal nerve damage.

        2. Respiratory obstruction.   **4.** Tetany.

  V. Behavioral counseling, if indicated.

Evaluation

  I. Verbally describes pathophysiology of illness.

  II. States medication receiving, dose, action, side effects.

  III. Maintains normal serum calcium level.

  IV. Shows improvement in signs and symptoms of hypercalcemia.

      A. Weight gain.   *C.* Decreased polyuria.

      B. Decreased pain.   *D.* Improved mental status.

  V. Keeps medical appointments. If unable, calls and reschedules appointment.

Follow-up

  I. Clinic.

  II. Periodic telephone calls.

  III. Visiting Nurse Association.

Hypoparathyroidism

Definition

Hypoparathyroidism is a disorder characterized by decreased secretion of parathyroid hormone (PTH). The most common cause of hypoparathyroidism is iatrogenic (postoperative hypoparathyroidism). However, with improved surgical skills and the decreased necessity for thyroid surgery, the incidence of hypoparathyroidism has declined significantly. Other causes of hypoparathyroidism include idiopathic lack of function and damage to the four parathyroid glands following hemorrhage, infection, or thyroid gland irradiation. All are very rare.

Assessment

  I. Nursing health history.

  II. Physical and behavioral assessment.

      A. Tetany.

        1. Numbness and tingling of the extremities.

        2. Feeling of stiffness in hands, feet, and lips.

        3. Cramps of the extremities.

        4. Carpopedal spasm.

        5. Laryngeal spasm: mistaken for bronchial asthma.

        6. Emotional lability.

        7. Irritability.

        8. Anxiety.

        9. Depression.

        10. Psychoses.

        11. Mental retardation: chronic untreated hypoparathyroidism.

      B. Others.

        1. Weakness.   **4.** Diarrhea.

        2. Nausea, vomiting.   **5.** Fatigue.

        3. Constipation.

  III. Other relevant sources.

      A. Medical history.

      B. Diagnostic tests.

        1. Serum calcium, phosphorus, magnesium.

        2. Serum PTH.

        3. Serum albumin.

Problems I. Physical.
     A. Weakness.
     B. Fatigue.
     C. Safety.
     D. Nausea, vomiting.
II. Psychosocial.
     A. Depression.
     B. Anxiety.
     C. Irritability.

Diagnosis I. Complains of numbness and tingling of the extremities and stiffness in the hands, feet, and lips.
II. Complains of nausea, vomiting, and constipation or diarrhea.
III. May have positive Chvostek's and Trousseau's signs.
IV. Has changes in moods and is often irritable.
V. Family or significant other has noted personality changes, depression, delusions, or other psychoses.
VI. May develop respiratory difficulty which appears to be an asthma attack.

Goals of Care I. Immediate.
     A. Prevent and/or control complications.
     B. Promote physical, emotional, and psychological rest.
II. Long-range.
     A. Promote patient and family independence in managing self at home.
     B. Return to physical, emotional, and psychological state prior to illness, if appropriate.

Intervention I. Regulate activities to allow for period of rest.
II. Administer medication for rest and sleep.
III. Evaluate response to treatment measures.
     A. Chvostek's sign.
     B. Trousseau's sign.
     C. Appetite.
     D. Somatic complaints.
          1. Numbness.
          2. Tingling.
          3. Weakness.
     E. Mental status.
IV. Keep tracheostomy set and drugs such as calcium gluconate at bedside.
V. Patient and family teaching.
     A. Pathophysiology of illness.
     B. Treatment and expected responses.
          1. Drugs: action, dose, side effects.
               a. Vitamin D (25,000 to 100,000 U daily).
               b. Oral calcium (1 to 2 g daily).
          2. Diet.
     C. Signs and symptoms of hypocalcemia.
     D. Importance of follow-up.
VI. Behavioral counseling, if indicated.

Evaluation I. Describes anatomy and physiology of illness.
II. States medication receiving, dose, action, side effects.
III. Maintains normal calcium level.
IV. Shows improvement in signs and symptoms of tetany.
V. Keeps medical appointments. If unable, calls and reschedules appointment.

Follow-up I. Clinic.
II. Periodic telephone calls.

INFLAMMATORY DISORDERS

Thyroiditis

Definition Inflammatory reactions of the thyroid gland are termed *thyroiditis*. Depending upon the stage of infection, hypothyroid or hyperthyroid states may occur, although the latter is uncommon. *Acute thyroiditis* is very rare. Subacute and chronic (Hashimoto's) thyroiditis are the most common inflammatory diseases of the thyroid gland.

Subacute (*granulomatous or de Quervain's*) *thyroiditis* is believed to be caused by a viral infection. It often follows an upper respiratory infection, mumps, or some other viral infection such as influenza or Coxsackie virus. The disease usually subsides within a few months, leaving no deficiency in thyroid function. However, repeated infections over many months can produce hypothyroidism (42).

Hashimoto's thyroiditis is thought to be caused by an autoimmune response which interferes with the normal biosynthesis of thyroid hormones, such as organic binding of thyroid iodide. There is often a family history of Hashimoto's disease, goiter, primary hypothyroidism, or Graves' disease. About 20 percent of the patients are hypothyroid when first examined. If seen during the early phase of the disease, symptoms of mild hyperthyroidism may be present. Clinical hypothyroidism commonly develops in patients who are euthyroid (normal thyroid function) when first seen. The progression to hypothyroidism develops over several years (43).

Riedel's thyroiditis is a rare disorder with no known cause. The thyroid gland is enlarged, with marked fibrosis. Clinical symptoms are related to compression of adjacent structures, namely, the trachea, esophagus, and recurrent laryngeal nerves. Hypothyroidism occurs occasionally (44).

Assessment I. Nursing health history.
II. Physical and behavioral assessment.
  A. Subacute thyroiditis.
    1. Gradual or sudden pain in thyroid region.
    2. Hoarseness.
    3. Dysphagia.
    4. Palpitations.
    5. Lassitude.
    6. Nervousness.
    7. Thyroid gland.
      a. Enlarged, firm.
      b. Tender to touch.
  B. Hashimoto's disease. Thyroid gland: goiter outstanding clinical feature.
    1. Moderately enlarged.
    2. Firm, nodular surface.
    3. Nontender.
    4. Rarely causes compression of adjacent structures.
III. Other relevant sources.
  A. Medical history.
  B. Family interview.
  C. Diagnostic tests.
    1. Thyroid hormone antibodies elevated in Hashimoto's.
    2. TSH elevated in Hashimoto's.
    3. ^{131}I uptake higher at 6 h than at 24 h in Hashimoto's; low in subacute thyroiditis.
    4. T_4 variable.
    5. Sedimentation rate elevated in subacute thyroiditis.

Diagnosis I. Subacute thyroiditis.
  A. Complains of gradual or sudden pain in area of thyroid gland lhich might be accompanied by fever.
  B. Pain is aggravated by turning head or swallowing, and radiates to the ear, jaw, or occiput.

C. Hoarseness or dysphagia may be present.

D. Complains of nervousness and lassitude.

II. Hashimoto's disease. Usually has no complaint. Goiter usually found during examination for some other complaint.

Goals of Care

I. Immediate.

    A. Relieve pain.

    B. Promote physical, emotional, and psychological rest.

II. Long-range. Promote patient and family independence in managing self at home.

Intervention

I. Administer medication such as aspirin for pain.

II. Patient and family teaching.

    A. Anatomy and physiology of illness.

    B. Treatment and expected responses.

        1. Hashimoto's disease, usually none. Thyroid hormone: alleviate goiter or hypothyroidism.

        2. Subacute thyroiditis.

            a. Thyroid hormone: suppressive doses.

            b. Glucocorticoids: severe cases.

III. Signs and symptoms of hypothyroidism.

IV. Importance of follow-up.

Evaluation

I. Verbally describes pathophysiology of illness.

II. States medication receiving, dose, action, and side effects.

III. Verbally describes signs and symptoms of hypothyroidism.

IV. Keeps medical appointments. If unable, calls and reschedules appointment.

Follow-up

I. Clinic.

II. Periodic telephone calls.

REFERENCES

1. Philip E. Cryer, *Diagnostic Endocrinology,* Oxford University Press, Inc., New York, 1976, p. 129
2. Judith A. Krueger and Janis C. Ray, *Endocrine Problems In Nursing,* The C. V. Mosby Company, St. Louis, 1976, p. 72.
3. Ibid.
4. Robert Williams, *Textbook of Endocrinology,* W. B. Saunders Company, Philadelphia, 1974, p. 650.
5. Ibid., p. 64.
6. Ibid., p. 64.
7. Krueger and Ray, op. cit., p. 17.
8. Williams, op. cit., p. 64.
9. Ibid.
10. Ibid., p. 68.
11. Ibid., p. 64.
12. Ibid., p. 64.
13. K. O. Franssila, "Prognosis in Thyroid Carcinoma," *Cancer,* **36:**1138–1146, September, 1975.
14. George O. Bell, "Cancer of the Thyroid," *Medical Clinics of North America,* **59:**459–470, March 1975.
15. Patricia Chaney, *Managing Diabetics Properly,* Intermed Communications, Inc., Horsham, Pa., 1977, p. 14.
16. George W. Thorn, Raymond D. Adams, Eugene Braunwald, Kurt J. Isselbacher, and Robert G. Petersdorf, *Harrison's Principles of Internal Medicine,* 8th ed., McGraw-Hill Book Company, New York, 1977, p. 564.
17. Ibid., p. 565.
18. Ibid.
19. Ibid., p. 532.

20. Cryer, op. cit., pp. 67, 73.
21. Williams, op. cit., pp. 270–271.
22. Ibid., pp. 274–275.
23. Thorn et al., op. cit., p. 511.
24. Cryer, op. cit., pp. 42–43.
25. Williams, op. cit., pp. 163–166.
26. Ibid., p. 185.
27. Ibid., p. 187.
28. Ibid., pp. 197–198.
29. Cryer, op. cit., pp. 45–47.
30. Ibid., p. 48.
31. Will G. Ryan, *Endocrine Disorders: A Pathophysiologic Approach,* Year Book Medical Publishers, Inc., Chicago, 1975, pp. 41–42.
32. Williams, op. cit., pp. 265–288.
33. Krueger and Ray, op. cit., p. 27.
34. Williams, op. cit., p. 87.
35. Krueger and Ray, op. cit., p. 29.
36. Cryer, op. cit., pp. 27, 28.
37. Williams, op. cit., p. 337.
38. Ibid., p. 456.
39. Krueger and Ray, op. cit., p. 121.
40. Williams, op. cit., p. 732.
41. Cryer, op. cit., p. 141.
42. Thorn et al, op. cit., p. 519.
43. Ibid.
44. Williams, op. cit., p. 227.

BIBLIOGRAPHY

Beland, Irene L., and Joyce V. PVASSOS: *Clinical Nursing,* Macmillan Publishing Co., Inc., New York, 1975; Collier Macmillan Publishers, London, 1975. This is a comprehensive source regarding the pathophysiology and management of diabetes.

Bell, George O.: "Cancer of the Thyroid," *Medical Clinics of North America,* **59:**459–470, March 1975. This reference presents a clear review of the classification and treatment of thyroid carcinoma.

Chaney, Patricia. *Managing Diabetics Properly,* Intermed Communications Inc., Horsham, Pa., 1977. The physiological and psychosocial aspects of the clinical management of diabetes are discussed in this publication.

Cryer, Philip E.: *Diagnostic Endocrinology,* Oxford University Press, New York, 1976. This book provides a basic understanding of endocrine diagnostic tests which can be utilized in planning patient teaching.

Franssila, Kaarle O.: "Prognosis in Thyroid Carcinoma," *Cancer,* **36:**1138–1146, September 1975. This reference correlates survival rates of various histological and clinical features in 227 cases of thyroid cancer.

Krueger, Judith A., and Janis C. Ray: *Endocrine Problems in Nursing,* The C. V. Mosby Company, St. Louis, 1976. This book provides a comprehensive summary of the nursing problems frequently encountered in the care of patients with endocrine disorders.

McCloskey, Joanne C.: "How to Make the Most of Body Image in Nursing Practice," *Nursing,* **766:**68–72, May 1976. This reference gives a useful discussion of the overt and covert manifestations of illness which attests body image, which is useful in the assessment of patients' reaction to illness.

McConnell, Edwina: "Meeting the Special Needs of Diabetics Facing Surgery," *Nursing,* **766:**30–37, June 1976. A general review of the physiological and psychosocial needs of diabetic patients useful in understanding the body's reaction to stress and associated insulin needs is provided in this article. The reader is encouraged to utilize a supplemental source for drug management.

Newton, David, Arlene O. Nichols, and Marian Newton: "You Can Minimize the Hazards of Corticosteroids," *Nursing,* **777:**26–33, June 1977. This article provides a current discussion of the classification of steroids including use, action, and side effects.

Read, Sharon P.: "Clinical Care in Hypophysectomy," *Nursing Clinics of North America,* **9:**617–654, December 1974. This reference gives a comprehensive review of metabolic and endocrine problems associated with a hypophysectomy for pituitary tumor. Preoperative and follow-up nursing implications are summarized.

Ryan, Will G.: *Endocrine Disorders: A Pathophysiologic Approach,* Year Book Medical Publishers, Inc., Chicago, 1975. This is a very general but easily understandable review of endocrine disorders, especially when used with other resources.

Spencer, Roberta: *Patient Care in Endocrine Problems,* W. B. Saunders Company, Philadelphia, 1973. This reference provides a useful list of patient problems and nursing interventions relevant to endocrine disorders.

Thorn, George W., Raymond D. Adams, Eugene Braunwald, Kurt J. Isselbacher, and Robert G. Petersdorf: *Harrison's Principles of Internal Medicine,* 8th ed., McGraw-Hill Book Company., New York, 1977. This reference gives a clear review of endocrine disorders, manifestations, treatment, and complications.

Tucker, Susan: *Patient Care Standards,* The C. V. Mosby Company, St. Louis, 1975. The author presents a comprehensive review of nursing implications.

Williams, Robert: *Textbook of Endocrinology,* W. B. Saunders Company, Philadelphia, 1974. This is an in-depth reference for understanding the physiological and psychosocial manifestations of endocrine disorders.

25

The Hematologic System

Mary Bigelow Huntoon

Blood is a substance composed of many cells (e.g., erythrocytes, leukocytes, etc.). It continuously circulates throughout the body, transporting oxygen and nutrients, removing carbon dioxide and body wastes, protecting the body from infection, transporting hormones, and helping to regulate body temperature. When disruption in blood formation or blood composition occurs, it can result in a multiplicity of physical and emotional changes. Gastrointestinal problems, decreased resistance to infection, enlargement of body structures, e.g., the liver and spleen, and bone pain are but a few of the changes observed. This chapter will discuss alterations that occur as a result of blood formation, coagulation, disturbances, blood cell destruction, and abnormal cellular growth. The end result of these disruptions will affect not only circulation but the entire process of oxygenation.

ABNORMAL CELLULAR GROWTH

Leukemia

Definition

Leukemia is a neoplastic disease which involves the blood-forming tissues in the lymph nodes, spleen, and bone marrow. Several types of leukemia are recognized, but all are characterized by abnormal and uncontrolled growth of immature leukocytes present in the tissue producing that cell and in the blood. The most common white cells involved are the granulocytes, lymphocytes, and monocytes.

Leukemia is also classified by the course and duration of the disease. *Acute leukemia* (more common in children and young adults) is more serious, has a rapid onset, and progresses quickly into the blood-forming organs with immature leukocytes. *Chronic leukemia* (more common in adults) has a gradual onset and a slower course, as the leukocytes are more mature and better able to defend the body against infection (refer to Table 25-1). The incidence of leukemia is on the increase, with a 50 percent rise in mortality noted over the last quarter of a century. Leukemia accounts for approximately 5 percent of all cancer and is one of the leading causes of death in children.

The exact etiology of leukemia is unknown. Several factors are associated with the disease and may contribute to its development. Viruses have caused leukemia in laboratory animals, and thus it is possible they may also cause leukemia in humans. Exposure to radiation in certain doses is linked with development of leukemia. Studies have also shown that absorption of certain chemicals and genetic disorders may be influential.

The major effects of leukemia are (1) proliferation of abnormal immature leukocytes, (2) infiltration of the cells into the blood-forming tissue, and (3) the eventual infiltration into all the body tissue. The end result is death due to primary and secondary causes.

Of all leukemias, both acute and chronic, 90 percent are lymphocytic (characterized by hyperplasia of the lymphoid tissues) while only 10 percent are monocytic and myelocytic (characterized by hyperplasia of the spleen and bone marrow). Acute granulocytic, chronic granulocytic, and chronic lymphocytic leukemia will be discussed here. (Refer to Chap. 15 for a discussion of acute lymphocytic leukemia.)

Assessment

I. Acute granulocytic leukemia (AGL): A subcategory of acute myelogenous leukemia, AGL is a malignant disease of the stem cells of the bone marrow. It represents over 80 percent of acute leukemias in adulthood and increases in incidence from middle age onward. It is more common in males, but there seems to be no difference in frequency among races.

TABLE 25-1 / CLASSIFICATION OF COMMON TYPES OF ACUTE AND CHRONIC LEUKEMIA

Major Category	Subcategory	Synonyms	Characteristic Cells and Clinical Manifestations
Acute			
Myclogenous	Granulocytic	Myelocytic, AML, AGL (includes congenital leuke- mia)	Myeloblasts Most common in adults, and infants Response to therapy 50%; me- dian prognosis 10–12 months
	Myelomonocytic	Naegli, AMML	Myeloblasts with some mono- cytic characteristics Prognosis 1–2 years
	Erythroleukemia	DiGuglielmo, EL	Proerythroblasts
	Promyelocytic	Progranulocytic, AProL	Promyelocytes Usually in adults Risk of disseminated intravas- cular coagulation (DIC)
	Oligoblastic	Smoldering, pre- leukemia	Slow progression Poor response to therapy
Monocytic	Monocytic, acute	Monoblastic, Schilling, AMonoL	Immature monocytes Usually in children or young adults Response to drugs; prognosis 6 weeks to 3 months Risk of DIC Inflamed gums common sign
Lymphocytic	Lymphocytic, acute	Lymphocytic, ALL	Immature lymphoblast Common in 95% of children; rare in adults Response to therapy; median prognosis 2.5 years Lymphadenopathy
	Undifferentiated	Stem cell, acute, AUL	Stem cell Prognosis very poor
Chronic			
Myelogenous	Granulocytic	Myelocytic, CML, CGL	Abnormal proliferation of gran- ulocytes Most common in adolescents and young adults Splenomegaly Median prognosis 3 years
Monocytic	Monocytic, chronic		Immature monocytes
Lymphocytic	Lymphocytic, chronic	CLL	Abnormal proliferation of lymphoblasts Most common in older adults Enlarged lymph nodes and spleen Median prognosis 5 years

Source: Adapted from W. J. Williams et al., *Hematology,* 2d ed., McGraw-Hill Book Company, New York, 1977, pp. 810, 820.

    A. Data sources.
       1. Patient.
       2. Family.
       3. Significant others.
       4. The patient's record (if there is one available).
    B. Health history.
       1. Patient complains of fatigue or malaise, usually of several months' duration. Exercise intolerance may be noted, along with dizziness or light-headedness.
       2. Fever may be present with or without a documented infection.
       3. Patients may also complain of easy bruising, nosebleeds, bleeding gums or petechiae; menstrual periods may increase in length and in volume.
       4. Documentation regarding previous treatment of any similar symptoms or a family history of leukemia is necessary, along with any known exposure to chemicals or radiation.
       5. Transformation of a chronic myelocytic leukemia into acute leukemia is possible. The change is accompanied by weight loss and progressive anemia.
       6. Chronic infections of the skin and respiratory tract are often noted.
    C. Physical assessment.
       1. A complete assessment of all systems and a full evaluation of general health is necessary for all patients.
       2. Marked pallor of the skin and mucous membranes is usually noted, with petechial hemorrhages and variously sized ecchymoses present. Careful documentation of bruised sites should be noted and evaluated.
       3. Tachycardia and cardiac murmurs may be heard.
       4. Splenomegaly, hepatomegaly, and lymphadenopathy may be present.
       5. Sternal tenderness is often demonstrated in these patients. When firm pressure is applied from the top to the bottom of the sternum, a small area, most commonly in the midportion, is found to be quite tender upon pressure. The patient will complain of pain at the pressure point but will have been previously unaware of its existence.
       6. Malaise and diaphoresis may be present.
    D. Diagnostic tests.
       1. Blood findings reveal a marked increase in the immature leukocytes in the peripheral blood, associated with anemia and thrombocytopenia.
       2. White blood counts may be elevated, with abnormal and immature cells.
       3. Serum uric acid levels are elevated in approximately half the patients.
       4. Bone marrow biopsy may be done (refer to Fig 25-1). It is unnecessary if numerous blasts are found in the blood.
          a. The biopsy is usually done using the sternum as the site, although the iliac crest may be used.
          b. For a sternal puncture, the patient is placed on his or her back with a pillow under the thoracic spine.
          c. The site is prepared and anesthetized.
          d. A sternal needle is inserted, and a small amount of marrow is aspirated.
          e. The patient may feel a slight pain at this time.
          f. Following the removal of the needle, the puncture site is covered with a sterile dressing.
          g. A slight soreness may be present for several days.
II. Chronic granulocytic leukemia (CGL): The first type of leukemia to be discovered, CGL is characterized by abnormal, immature granulocytes in the bone marrow. It is most common from the age of 25 through 40 and is seen more often in men. Of all cases of leukemia, 20 percent are accounted for by CGL.
    A. Date sources (refer to point I A, above).
    B. Health history.
       1. The complaints of the patient are similar to those in patients with acute granulocytic leukemia.

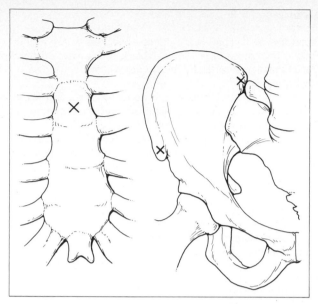

FIGURE 25-1 / The two most commonly used sites for bone marrow aspirations are the sternum and the anterior or posterior iliac crests (*Adapted from S. O. Schwartz, W. H. Hartz, Jr., and J. H. Robbins, Hematology in Practice, McGraw-Hill Book Company, New York, 1961.*)

      2. The onset is usually gradual and insidious.

      3. Complaints of aching in the long bones and of discomfort in the upper left abdomen are common.

      4. Headaches and confusion or other central nervous system symptoms may be present.

  C. Physical assessment.

      1. Findings coincide with acute granulocytic leukemia.

      2. Sternal tenderness is usually present.

      3. Hepatomegaly and splenomegaly are present, but the lymph nodes are usually not palpable.

  D. Diagnostic tests.

      1. The leukocyte count is high, revealing granulocytes in all stages of development. They appear mostly normal, with the most mature elements present in the greatest number.

      2. Mild anemia is usually present.

      3. The platelet count is high, as opposed to low, as it is in acute granulocytic leukemia.

      4. A genetic defect, the Philadelphia chromosome, is present in the white cells of 70 to 90 percent of all patients.

      5. The leukocyte alkaline phosphatase determination is low.

      6. Uric acid is usually elevated, as is the serum vitamin B_{12}.

      7. X-ray may reveal osseous lesions in the skeleton.

III. Chronic lymphocytic leukemia (CLL): The most common type of leukemia seen, CLL affects older patients (it is unusual in persons younger than 30), and it increases in frequency with age. It is, again, more common in males. CLL has few symptoms and a long duration. It is usually the easiest leukemia to diagnose and treat. It is characterized by proliferative abnormality of the lymphoid tissues, mainly affecting the small lymphocytes. Inherited or acquired immunologic defects may be significant in this disease.

A. Data sources (refer to point I A, above).
B. Health history.
    1. Similarities to the previously discussed leukemias are found.
    2. Fatigue or a sense of lack of well-being is the most outstanding complaint.
    3. Documentation of a family history of leukemia is necessary.
C. Physical assessment.
    1. Enlargement of superficial lymph nodes is noted. The cervical nodes are most often involved, as may be the axillary and mesenteric nodes. (See Fig. 25-2.)
    2. Splenomegaly is usually present.
    3. Skin lesions may be apparent. These lesions, the result of actual infiltration of the skin by leukemic cells, are generalized, discrete, and bright red or purple in color.
D. Diagnostic tests.
    1. Blood lymphocytes are elevated and are abnormal and immature.
    2. Mild anemia is usually present.
    3. Bone marrow biopsy or aspiration is of little merit in diagnosis.
    4. Uric acid levels are usually normal.
    5. Immunoglobulin levels are decreased.

Problems

  I. Predisposition to bleeding.
 II. Predisposition to infection.
III. Fatigue.
IV. Psychological adjustment to diagnosis.
 V. Complications of the disease process.

Diagnosis

   I. Vulnerability to hemorrhage, due to the thrombocytopenia.
  II. Vulnerability to infection due to the leukocytes, which are present in large numbers but are immature or abnormal and are unable to fight microorganisms.
 III. Alterations in comfort, manifested by pain and discomfort. This may be due to fatigue, as a result of anemia, to pain and pressure from enlarged organs on adjacent structures, and to tachycardia.
 IV. Alteration in nutrition, due to anorexia and fever, which may be a result of chemotherapy.
  V. Depletion of body fluids, due to fever, and anorexia, which could result in an impairment in urinary elimination and in fluid and electrolyte imbalance.
 VI. Alteration in body image and self-concept, due to the disease process and prognosis.

FIGURE 25-2 / **Axillary and cervical lymph node enlargements in a patient with chronic lymphocytic leukemia (CLL).** (*From W. J. Williams et al., Hematology, 2d ed., McGraw-Hill Book Company, New York, 1977.*)

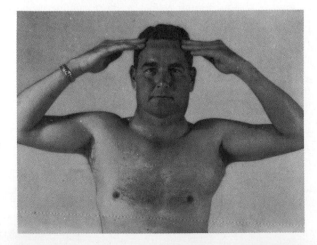

Goals of Care

  I. Immediate.
    A. Halt proliferation of leukocytes and induce a remission, if possible.
    B. Prevent bleeding and internal hemorrhage due to the altered blood values.
    C. Promote adequate food and fluid intake in order to meet bodily needs.
    D. Provide psychological support needed to adjust to the disease.
  II. Long-range.
    A. Prevent infection by providing care which optimizes health.
    B. Promote optimal functioning in activities of daily living.
    C. Treat complications of the disease process.
    D. Promote family involvement during the patient's adjustment to the disease process and changes in life-style.

Intervention[1]

  I. Constant observation for signs of bleeding or hemorrhage is necessary. Urine, feces, and vomitus must be checked for blood, along with frequent checks of the skin surfaces.
  II. The patient should be protected from falls and handled gently to prevent trauma.
  III. Anemia (or hemoglobin levels less than 8 g per 100 mL) is treated with transfusions of whole blood.
    A. Blood work should be checked frequently to assess anemic state.
    B. Thrombocytopenia may be managed with platelet transfusions.
  IV. Pressure must be applied to injection sites or any cuts for several minutes to decrease hematoma formation.
  V. Stool softeners to prevent constipation and rectal trauma may be necessary.
  VI. Adequate rest is required to prevent fatigue and an increased susceptibility to infection.
    A. Eight hours of sleep at night and short naps during the day are encouraged.
    B. Sedatives at night to aid sleeping may be necessary due to increased bone pain and resulting discomfort.
  VII. Many types of pain or discomfort accompany leukemia. Bone pain, discomfort due to the enlarged organs and lymph nodes, nerve pain, and throat pain because of ulcerations, are common.
    A. Repositioning, cooling baths, and mouth care, in addition to medication, are useful.
    B. Aspirin or Darvon with sedatives (if needed) are used.
    C. Stronger analgesics, such as codeine or Demerol, in conjunction with Phenergan and Thorazine, can be administered with more severe pain.
    D. Oral medications are preferred if thrombocytopenia is present.
  VIII. The comfort of the patient can be increased by controlling the fever and administering frequent mouth care.
    A. Antipyretic drugs such as aspirin may decrease the temperature and control pain.
    B. If bleeding is a problem, Tylenol may be just as effective.
    C. Cooling sponge baths in tepid water can help reduce the fever and increase the comfort of the patient.
  IX. Painful ulcerations in the mouth and throat make mouth care before meals and at least every 2 to 3 h very important. Viscous Xylocaine will anesthetize the throat and increase comfort. Care must be taken to be sure the gag reflex is intact before offering the patient food or liquids.
  X. If the patient has any gastrointestinal bleeding, old blood may accumulate, making the patient nauseous.
    A. Diluted hydrogen peroxide or lemon and glycerin cleanse the mouth, remove crusted blood, and decrease halitosis.
    B. Soft-bristled toothbrushes or cotton applicators should be used to remove excess debris from the teeth and gums.

[1]Although there are several varieties of leukemia, most of the principles of care are similar.

XI. Cracking and crust formation around the lips can be prevented by lubricating with petroleum jelly.

XII. Prednisone may decrease lymph node enlargement and increase the patient's level of comfort. (For a complete discussion of steroids refer to Chap. 32.)

XIII. Anorexia is often present due to painful mouth ulcerations, discomfort resulting from enlarged organs (especially the spleen and liver), and possibly from chemotherapy or radiation.

    A. Antiemetics given $\frac{1}{2}$ h before meals may help control nausea.

    B. If severe vomiting is a problem, blood electrolytes should be checked.

XIV. Small servings of soft, bland food may decrease throat irritation. Anesthetic gargles may also help, along with cold or frozen foods such as ice cream, sherbet, milk shakes, and high-protein fruit drinks.

    A. Allow the patient to choose foods that are most appealing, and consult the dietitian if necessary.

    B. Diets high in protein, vitamins, and calories are the most effective nutrition sources for leukemic patients.

XV. Patients with leukemia need an intake of 3 to 4 L of fluid a day to prevent dehydration and to dilute the high levels of uric acid that result from the abnormal leukocyte destruction by the antileukemic drugs.

    A. Alkalinization of the urine may be achieved by giving sodium bicarbonate every 6 h.

    B. Allopurinol (100 mg, 3 to 4 times per day) may also be given to inhibit uric acid crystal formation.

    C. If patients are unable to eat and drink, intravenous therapy or hyperalimentation may be required (see Chap. 29 for discussion on hyperalimentation).

XVI. Prevention of infection is a major nursing problem, as immature white cells and the effects of anticancer drugs limit a patient's resistance to infection.

    A. The patient should be monitored continuously for sore throats, temperature elevations, and chills. If infection is suspected, treatment with antibiotics, based on blood culture and sensitivity tests, must be started immediately.

    B. Blood studies should be checked frequently. If there is evidence of pancytopenia (a reduction in all the cellular blood components), the patient should be placed in a single room for protection. Reverse isolation precautions may be used.

    C. Platelet and white blood cell transfusions can be given to increase resistance and to decrease bleeding. (Donor matching increases the success rate.)

    D. Recurrent infections due to low immunoglobulin levels are treated with prophylactic doses of gamma globulin.

XVII. Management and care of the patient with leukemia should be structured to allow the patient to pursue as many activities and as full a life as long as possible.

    A. When feasible, the patient should live at home, continue work or school, and participate in social activities.

    B. It is important for the patient to have the support of significant others to help in carrying out the activities of daily living.

    C. The family, close friends, and employers will need information about leukemia, including the symptoms, treatment, complications, and prognosis.

XVIII. Despair and depression are common when patients deal with the problem of a chronic, life-threatening illness and the eventual body image changes that may result. Hope for remission may be crucial to the patient and family. However, realistic assessment and evaluation of the type of leukemia and its response to therapy are necessary in order to provide support for patients and their families.

XIX. Medical intervention in leukemia usually consists of chemotherapy alone or in conjunction with radiation or x-ray therapy.

    A. In *acute granulocytic leukemia,* chemotherapy agents may be used alone, sequentially, or in combination. The two most commonly used are 6-mercaptopurine (6-MP, Purinethol), a purine antimetabolic given in doses of 2.5 mg/kg per day orally, or a folic acid antimetabolite, methotrexate (Amethopterin), 2.5 to 5.0 mg per day orally.

B. In *chronic granulocytic leukemia,* the drug of choice is busulfan (Myleran), an alkylating agent. The dose is usually 2 mg, 2 to 4 times daily.

    1. Once the white blood cell count falls to normal limits, the drug is given intermittently.

    2. Platelet counts should be checked daily, as the major toxic effect of busulfan is irreversible thrombocytopenia, a decrease in the number of blasts and promyelocytes in the peripheral blood to below normal.

    3. Chlorambucil or 6-MP may also be used.

C. Irradiation of the spleen and administration of radioactive phosphorus may also be used in treating chronic granulocytic leukemia.

D. The chemotherapeutic agent most often selected in chronic lymphocytic leukemia is chlorambucil (Leukeran), 0.01 to 0.2 mg/kg daily in dividing doses. This is usually given after meals to decrease gastric irritation. Triethylenemelamine (TEM), 2.5 to 5 mg daily, is also used with sodium bicarbonate before meals.

E. Bone marrow transplants in suitable patients with matched donors are now being performed. The results vary.

Evaluation

I. Reassessment.

    A. Reassessment of the patient's response to therapy is continual.

        1. With effective therapy, remissions can be achieved and the length of survival extended.

        2. Chronic lymphocytic leukemia has the best prognosis of the three types of leukemia.

    B. Monthly chemotherapy and physical reevaluations are needed. The patient and family need to be taught the side effects of therapy and the need for compliance.

    C. Sensitive support to help the patient deal with body image changes and alterations in daily living patterns are important.

        1. Family members or counselors, such as marital or sexual counselors, along with the nurse, can provide this help.

        2. A decrease in libido, sterility, impotence, and menopausal symptoms are common side effects of chemotherapy. The patient should be informed of these potential changes.

    D. The patient's psychological response must be evaluated.

        1. Social workers can help the patient and family deal with the financial problems.

        2. Information about the Visiting Nurse Association regarding long-term care can be obtained from the American Cancer Society. They have information regarding special equipment that might be needed and available in-home nursing and housekeeping care.

    E. Measures to involve a minister or priest, psychiatrist, or occupational or physical therapist may be appropriate to provide the physical and/or emotional support or activities needed to help the patient handle the illness. The fear of death is always present and should be discussed, as appropriate.

II. Complications.

    A. Iatrogenic disorders result from radiation and chemotherapy.

        1. Radiation sicknesses such as nausea, platelet depression, and alopecia (baldness) may be seen. These symptoms will have to be treated as they appear.

        2. Patients should be allowed to express their feelings regarding therapy and the subsequent problems resulting from therapy.

        3. Reevaluation of the choice of therapy is often necessary.

    B. The most common complications in leukemia and usually the eventual causes of death are infections, hemorrhage, and renal failure (refer to Chap. 28).

Multiple Myeloma (Plasma Cell Myeloma)

Definition   *Multiple myeloma* is produced by malignant proliferation of plasma cells which may result in diffuse invasion and overgrowth of the bone marrow and the formation of single or multiple plasma cell tumors at various sites. This results in bone destruction throughout the body, overproduction of myeloma proteins, and later involvement of the lymph nodes, liver, spleen, and kidneys. Usually by the time of diagnosis the disease is widely spread. The condition occurs most commonly in the 50 to 60 age range and is seen twice as often in men as in women. The prognosis is generally poor, with the median survival rate less than 2 years. The incidence of multiple myeloma has increased over recent years (see brief discussion in Chap. 31).

Assessment
I. Data sources (refer to "Leukemia").
II. Health history.
   A. The onset of multiple myeloma is slow, and patients may have a long period without symptoms. However, during this period they may suffer from recurring attacks of fever, cough, and bacterial infections, especially pneumonia. Once symptoms appear, they are varied.
   B. The patient's most common complaint is usually pain. This is progressive back or rib pain which is usually increased with movements and varies in intensity.
   C. The patient may have noted a weight loss and may feel tired.
   D. Tingling and numbness may be present in the lower extremities.
   E. Changes associated with hypercalcemia may be observed, e.g., renal nocturia, anorexia, and confusion.
III. Physical assessment.
   A. Pressure or gentle palpation over osteolytic or "punched-out" lesions of the skeleton may elicit tenderness or pain (see Fig. 25-3). Pathological fractures may be present due to osteoporosis.
   B. The patient may demonstrate deformities or asymmetry in the skeleton. A change in height is often detected.
   C. Neurological disorders may be manifest due to spinal cord involvement and compression fractures of the vertebrae.
   D. The liver and lymph nodes may be enlarged.
   E. Anemia is usually present, corresponding with the loss of weight and general pallor. The patient's overall appearance must be considered, but may only be indicative that something is wrong.
   F. Complaints of blurred vision and dizziness may be present.
IV. Diagnostic tests.
   A. X-ray studies reveal osteoporosis, multiple lesions of the bone, and demineralization.
   B. The bone marrow contains large numbers of atypical or immature plasma cells.
   C. Blood studies reveal an increased concentration of serum globulin, particularly an abnormal M-type globulin.
   D. Renal function tests, e.g., calcium level tests, uric acid level tests, protein tests, will give data concerning renal function (refer to Chap. 28 for a discussion of tests).
   E. The final and most definitive sign of multiple myeloma is the appearance of an abnormal globulin, Bence Jones protein, in the urine.

Problems[2]
I. Pain.
II. Infection.
III. Difficulty ambulating.
IV. Difficulty with urination.
V. Anxiety and fear.

---

[2] Nursing problems may vary, depending upon the duration and the extent of the disease. Frequently, patients with multiple myeloma will experience one or more of the problems listed.

VI. Anemia.

VII. Hemorrhage.

Diagnosis

I. Alterations in comfort manifested by pain which may be experienced in the area of skeletal lesions or nerve compression. The pain will increase due to increased involvement.

II. Disturbances in antibody formation may result in increased susceptibility to infection.

III. Alterations in mobility are present due to pain, pathologic fractures, ossification, loss of calcium from the bones, and fear.

IV. Potential impairment of urinary elimination due to hypercalcemia, renal stones, and inadequate hydration may result in fatal renal damage.

V. Mild to severe anxiety due to the prognosis, the overall effects of the disease, and/or concern regarding the pain and the effects of the illness on family and work responsibilities may result.

VI. Anemia, secondary to marrow failure, may be manifested.

VII. Vulnerability to hemorrhage and bleeding may result from circulatory and hemorrhagic disturbances due to increased blood viscosity.

FIGURE 25-3 / **X-ray of a patient with multiple myeloma.** (*a*) **Small punched-out lesions in the skull.** (*b*) **Severe demineralization of the lumbar spine with partial collapse of the vertebral bodies.** (***From W. J. Williams et al., Hematology, 2d ed., McGraw-Hill Book Company, New York, 1977.***)

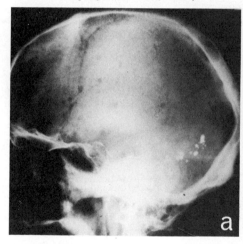

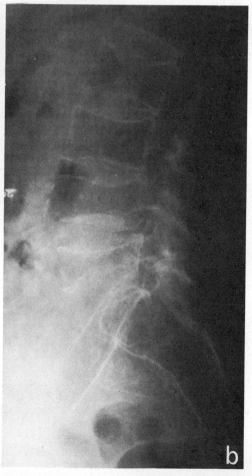

Goals of Care

I. Immediate.
   A. Control pain to enable the patient to continue as normal a life-style as possible.
   B. Promote ambulation to increase the effects of chemotherapy and to decrease the complications of immobility.
   C. Control infection to prevent a further decrease in resistance.
   D. Promote hydration to maintain renal function.
   E. Involve family members and foster supportive roles.
   F. Reduce bone tumor size and growth.

II. Long-range.
   A. Prevent further infection and the complications of infection.
   B. Slow tumor growth.
   C. Promote patient and family adjustment to illness.
   D. Treat complications of the disease as they develop.

Intervention

I. Pain can generally be controlled with medication.
   A. Aspirin and codeine may obtain relief in the earlier stages.
   B. Stronger analgesics such as Demerol may be necessary later.

II. Ambulation and maintenance of mobility are necessary to sustain a patient to allow remission through chemotherapy.
   A. Osteoporosis and calcium loss increase with immobility.
   B. Pain or fear of falling may be a major obstacle.

III. Fractures of the long bones may be pinned surgically.
   A. Supports should be used only for a short time due to atrophy and immobilization and are usually only required until pain is decreased or relieved by radiotherapy or chemotherapy.
   B. Because these patients are vulnerable to falls and accidents, they should always be accompanied when walking.
   C. Orthopedic supports or braces for the spine, ribs, or extremities may be used to stabilize the patient and to prevent further damage, such as fractures and spasms.

IV. In order to promote bone remineralization, activity, physical therapy, steroids, and vitamin D may be used.

V. If bacterial infection is present, antibiotics are administered.
   A. Isolation of the patient from sources of infection is a necessity and will involve teaching the patient and family members about adequate rest, good nutrition, and avoidance of persons with colds or sore throats.
   B. All infections must be cultured and treated promptly.

VI. Patients with multiple myeloma require between 3000 and 4000 mL of fluid per day to counteract the calcium overload and to prevent protein precipitation in the renal tubules.
   A. Hyperuricemia may be present and can be counteracted by allopurinol.
   B. Saline infusions, thiazides, and steroids may be used in treatment, if they are not contraindicated.

VII. Nausea and vomiting are often seen in these patients; therefore, along with forcing fluids, antiemetics may be administered.

VIII. Patients with multiple myeloma have a grave prognosis. Much support and encouragement is necessary to promote patient mobility and to receive chemotherapy.

IX. The patient should be given an opportunity to express fears and ask questions.
   A. Family members should be supported and encouraged to participate in care and to interact with the patient.
   B. Questions should be answered honestly and realistically.
   C. Additional support systems should be involved, including referrals to counselors, social workers, and other significant persons the patient and family may want to involve.

X. Adjustments in life-style will have to be made, and fear, anger, and grieving are reactions that will often be seen.

XI. The most common medical treatment for multiple myeloma is chemotherapy.

Alkylating agents such as phenylalanine mustard (PAM, melphalan) and cyclophosphamide (Cytoxan) are used with an approximately 35 percent chance of survival for 2 years.

XII. Prednisone has also been combined with intermittent doses of PAM or other agents; this is believed to enhance the effects of the alkylating agent and to increase the remission rate to greater than 60 percent. The choice of chemotherapy, agents, and dose schedule varies greatly and depends on many factors such as age, degree of debility, state of disease, and hematological status.

XIII. Radiotherapy may prove effective for localized bone lesions.

Evaluation

I. Reassessment: Evaluate long-term compliance. Revise care plans as necessary.

II. Complications.
   A. Neurological complications may cause spinal cord compression. If they do, a surgical laminectomy is indicated. Paraplegia may result (refer to Chap. 23).
   B. Anemia is treated with androgens and transfusions of whole blood or red blood cell concentrations.
   C. Hemorrhagic complications may be responsive to fresh blood or platelet transfusions. If they are due to hyperviscosity, plasmapheresis is necessary to remove enough plasma, containing the monoclonal protein, to reduce plasma volume. Prednisone or steroids may aggravate these symptoms.
   D. Complications of chemotherapy may be many and are varied depending on the agent used.

III. Reevaluation.
   A. Continual reassessment of the patient's health status and evaluation of complications must be made.
   B. The patient's adjustment to physical changes and level of mobility should be determined.
   C. The patient and family's psychological adjustment to the illness and prognosis must be evaluated. Revision in teaching or instituting counseling may be necessary based on assessment of adjustments.
   D. Continual follow-up care is necessary.
      1. Progress is evaluated, and serum and/or urine protein concentrations are measured.
      2. Remissions can occur, with a median duration of 21 months.
      3. However, the disease progresses and eventually becomes resistant to therapy. Some patients develop acute leukemia.
      4. The most common cause of death, accounting for 50 percent of cases, is nonhypertensive renal failure.
   E. Hyperviscosity syndrome.
      1. Indicates increased intravascular resistance.
      2. It is accompanied by heart failure, visual disturbances, and renal failure.
      3. Excess plasma load must be reduced, or death will ensue.

Polycythemia Vera (Primary Polycythemia)

Definition

Polycythemia vera is a disease of unknown etiology. It is classified as a myeloproliferative disorder caused by neoplastic overproduction of one or more of the bone marrow cells because of differentiation of the stem cell. The problem is characterized by a marked increase in erythrocytes, reflected by an elevated hematocrit and usually an increase in the leukocytes and thrombocytes. This results in an increase in blood viscosity resulting in a slowing of blood flow, an increase in the total blood volume (as much as 2 to 3 times normal), and a severe congestion of all tissues and organs with blood. Physical changes with polycythemia vera are attributed largely to the blood volume and viscosity. As these changes intensify, symptoms related to pump failure and portal congestion may occur. Prompt treatment will help reverse the more acute changes.

Assessment

I. Data sources (refer to "Leukemia").
II. Health history: The patient may state the complaints have been present for a while.
   A. Headaches, dizziness, and tinnitus, or dyspnea, visual disturbances, and weakness are often noted.
   B.• The classic symptom is the dusky red and ruddy skin color.
   C. The face, ears, nose, lips, and distal part of the extremities are usually involved.
   D. Patients are usually 50 to 60 years of age or older.
   E. The problem is commonly observed in white males of Jewish extraction.
   F. Family history rarely noted.
   G. Gastrointestinal complaints of nausea, vomiting, and abdominal pain may be present.
III. Physical assessment.
   A. On physical examination, the skin and mucous membranes may have ecchymotic areas. The conjunctiva will also be red.
   B. A ruddy complexion (plethora) will be observed.
   C. The spleen is usually enlarged and palpable, with the patient expressing upper left quadrant discomfort.
   D. If pump failure (early) is present, tachycardia and lung congestion will be present.
   E. A common complaint is pruritus, especially after a hot bath.
   F. Painful joints may be observed and swelling may be noted.
   G. Spontaneous nose bleeds and gingival bleeding may be reported.
   H. Hypertension is often noted. Examination of the extremities for signs of phlebitis is essential.
IV. Diagnostic tests.
   A. Blood tests demonstrate an increase in red cell mass.
   B. Leukocytosis and microcythemia are present in approximately 50 percent of patients.
   C. Examination of the bone marrow shows hyperplasia.
   D. The uric acid will probably be increased.

Intervention

I. The cause of polycythemia vera is unknown, so treatment and interventions are symptomatic. The most common medical treatments are:
   A. Phlebotomy (refer to Chap. 26).
      1. Often the treatment of choice, it can be used as a sole means of treatment for a period of time in approximately two-thirds of the patients.
      2. Following this intervention the hematocrit is reduced to 40 to 45. The number of 500-mL phlebotomies needed to accomplish this may vary from individual to individual.
      3. If frequent treatments are necessary or if complications such as iron deficiency anemia develop, other treatments should be tried.
      4. Foods high in iron (liver, legumes) should be avoided.
   B. Irradiation. Administration of a myelosuppressant agent such as radioactive phosphorus is used. This concentrates in proliferating cells and may cause remissions up to several years.
   C. The use of alkylating agents and chemotherapy is often preferred over irradiation. These are usually administered intravenously.
II. Nursing interventions are focused on promoting patient comfort, preventing complications, and promoting the patient's independence.
   A. Increased bleeding can lead to a high incidence of peptic ulcers and hemorrhagic gastritis.
      1. The patient should be cautioned to protect against injury.
      2. Any noted bleeding or bruising should be examined for causes and treated.
      3. Careful oral hygiene is necessary; a soft-bristled brush should be used.
   B. Anticoagulants should not be taken.
      1. Any surgical or dental procedure should be performed only if necessary and followed with caution. Any postoperative bleeding should be treated.
      2. Heparin and vitamin K antagonists have been used safely and successfully.

C. Hyperuricemia may lead to gouty arthritis and renal calculi. A large fluid intake is encouraged and may also cause a decrease in blood viscosity.

D. Dietary modifications in purine intake, such as avoidance of liver, kidney, and meat extracts, may be needed.

  1. Uricosuric agents may be given, such as allopurinol, 100 mg, 3 times a day.
  2. Acute gouty arthritis, seen in polycythemia vera, is treated in a similar manner as primary gout (refer to Chap. 31).
  3. Patients should be taught to test their own urine (alkalinity).

E. Fatigue may be due to therapy and/or treatments.

  1. Rest periods without disturbing activities and noise should be encouraged, and activities should be planned to conserve the patient's strength.
  2. Adequate nutrition should be maintained.

F. Fatigue may also be the result of anemia caused by internal bleeding and phlebotomies. Internal bleeding should be investigated and iron-deficiency anemia treated with iron supplements.

G. Pruritus may be disabling in some patients. It is believed to be due to an increase in histamine.

  1. Some relief may be obtained by myelosuppressive therapy.
  2. Sometimes antihistamines (e.g. Benadryl) may be helpful.
  3. The patient may apply pressure to the itching areas but must be encouraged to keep nails short to avoid breaking the skin integrity.
  4. Medicated baths or antipruritic lotions may decrease the itching.

H. Alteration in mobility and maintenance of activities of daily living may be a problem. Patients should be encouraged to ambulate, or if bedridden, turned frequently with range-of-motion exercises, in order to prevent stasis of the urine and development of thrombi.

I. Patients should be encouraged to perform as many activities of normal living as possible without harming themselves. Patients and families should be taught about the disease process and potential problems, and they should be given support as necessary.

Evaluation

I. Reassessment: Management of the patient with polycythemia vera varies.

  A. Interventions should allow the patient to spend time at work and with the family, with the least harm and expense as possible.
  B. The survival rate is approximately 13 years, with many patients developing leukemia-like symptoms and eventually dying.

II. Complications (refer to Chap. 26 for discussion of changes to be assessed e.g., congestive heart failure).

  A. Decreased blood flow and venous stasis.
  B. Venous thrombosis.
  C. Congestive heart failure.
  D. Infection usually occurs secondary to the disease or therapy chosen. Interventions are based upon symptomatology.

III. Revision in plan of care must be made in light of changes in the patient's health status.

HYPERACTIVITY AND HYPOACTIVITY

Aplastic Anemia

Definition

Aplastic ("having deficient or arrested development") *anemia* is a disorder associated with hypoproliferation of the precursor red blood cells in the bone marrow, resulting in a decrease in circulating erythrocytes. It is characterized by erythrocyte cellular depletion and fatty replacement of the bone marrow. It is accompanied by leukopenia and thrombocytopenia (pancytopenia or a reduction in all the cellular blood components), and it affects all age groups and both sexes. The etiology of approximately 50 percent of the cases of aplastic anemia seen is unknown; however, the source of the injury to the stem cells, which causes their decreased proliferation, is theorized to be acquired by environmental (such as exposure to pollutants) or idiopathic constitutional factors not yet identified.

The most common *known* causes of aplastic anemia are chemical and physical agents such as drugs (chloramphenicol is most often identified), radiation, and infections, both viral (hepatitis) and bacterial (tuberculosis).

Assessment

I. Data sources (refer to "Leukemia").
II. Health history.
    A. The patient usually complains of a slow onset of fatigue and weakness in conjunction with nosebleeds, fever, or infection.
    B. A careful documentation of recent infections is needed (e.g., in granulocytopenia there is a decreased resistance to disease).
    C. A suspected history of drug ingestion or exposure to other toxic substances should be noted. Occupation may be a source of toxin, e.g., carbon tetrachloride or DDT.
    D. Bleeding episodes should be clearly explained and documented.
III. Physical assessment.
    A. The examination may show nothing remarkable except for a slight pallor.
    B. Small petechiae might be seen with a skin inspection, especially around the shoulders and ankles, along with hemorrhages in the mucous membranes around the gums (thrombocytopenia).
    C. Upon eye examination, retinal hemorrhages are usually noted.
    D. Enlargement of the spleen may be noted.
IV. Diagnostic tests.
    A. Blood studies reveal red blood cell, white blood cell, and platelet counts all below normal.
    B. Bone marrow aspiration will reveal thin, bloody material showing a decrease in bone marrow elements and an increase in fatty deposits.

Problems

I. Infection.
II. Hemorrhage.

Diagnosis

I. Potential risk of infection due to decreased white blood cell count.
II. Potential risk of hemorrhage due to decreased platelet blood cell count.
III. Alterations in activities of daily living due to fatigue and anemia.
IV. Mild to moderate anxiety due to disease process and diagnosis.

Goals of Care

I. Immediate.
    A. Withdrawal of offending agent or drug to prevent further damage.
    B. Provide supportive management to keep the patient as comfortable as possible and yet "buy time" until a remission occurs.
II. Long-range.
    A. Obtain a spontaneous remission.
    B. Aid the patient and family in adjusting to the disease process.

Intervention

I. The chemical or infectious agent must be identified and removed or treated.
II. Restrictions and safeguards for the patient are needed in order to protect and support the patient.
    A. These are best managed after the patient and family have received frank and realistic information about the seriousness of the disease and the goals of intervention.
    B. Resource persons such as a psychologist may be necessary to allow the patient to ventilate fears and anxieties and to provide information needed to make adjustments in life-style.

III. Anemia may be treated with blood transfusions of platelets, whole blood, or granulocytes. The transfusions are stopped when bone marrow function resumes.
IV. To stimulate bone marrow function, the following medical courses of action may be considered:
  A. Corticosteroids and androgens (testosterone) may be given in small doses and over short periods of time. The results are usually poor in adults.
  B. Bone marrow transplants have been made, but compatible donors are hard to find and results have been varied.
  C. A splenectomy to increase the effective life span of available circulating blood cells is possible, but not necessarily common, due to the risks and variable results.
V. Infections are common and are also the usual cause of death. However, unless absolutely necessary, the patient is encouraged to continue the accustomed life-style:
  A. Reverse isolation may be necessary. This usually includes reduction of exposure to numbers of people, handwashing with an antiseptic before contact, and wearing a mask.
  B. Close observation for signs and symptoms of infection is necessary.
  C. Skin infection may be reduced with antiseptic soap.
  D. Antibiotics are used to treat known infections.
VI. Excessive bleeding is also a common problem. The patient is taught to take care in preventing injury.
  A. Stress the importance of avoiding skin injuries.
    1. Intramuscular injections should be avoided.
    2. Suggest that an electric razor be used.
  B. Stress the need of care in oral hygiene. Instruct in proper technique, if necessary.
  C. Suggest the use of a stool softener to avoid straining at defecation.
  D. Excessive menstrual flow is treated with suppressive hormonal therapy.
  E. Corticosteroids may decrease capillary bleeding.
VII. Splenectomy may be performed if the organ is enlarged and/or interfering with the development of normal cells.

Evaluation

I. Reassessment.
  A. Reassessment is continuous. Blood studies are followed closely.
  B. Supportive therapy continues, and complications are treated symptomatically in anticipation of remission.
II. Complications.
  A. The most common complications are infection and hemorrhage. Patients with a history of recent exposure to bone marrow toxins seem to do the best. Prevention of infection is critical. Early diagnosis and treatment are essential.
  B. Remissions are rare, but approximately one-third of the remissions seen are cured. If severe pancytopenia is present, death may occur from hemorrhage or overwhelming infection.
  C. Death usually occurs within a few months. The overall mortality in adults is 70 percent, with a mean survival rate of 3 months.

Agranulocytosis

Definition

Agranulocytosis is manifested by a decrease in granulocytes which leads to lowered resistance and possible bacterial invasion. This is caused by a suppression of bone marrow activity with a resulting decrease in production. It can occur at any age but is seen most often in adult women. The exact cause is not known, but it appears to be an immunologic or leukocytic antibody reaction (to drug administration) by an inherently sensitive individual. This idiosyncratic drug reaction is most often seen with phenothiazines, Thorazine, sulfonamides, and penicillin but may also be seen after large doses of antimetabolite drugs and therapy continued over a long period of time.

Assessment
    I. Data sources (refer to "Leukemia").
   II. Health history.
      A. A thorough health history of recent exposure to drugs or chemical agents is needed.
      B. Any family history of increased drug or chemical sensitivity should be noted.
  III. Physical assessment.
      A. Early symptoms assessed include fatigue, weakness, headache, and restlessness.
      B. The majority of individuals complain of a sore throat, which progresses rapidly into chills, high fever, and dysphagia.
      C. Necrotic areas are often seen in the oral mucous membranes.
  IV. Diagnostic tests.
      A. The white blood cell count is less than 5000 per cubic millimeter.
      B. The bone marrow examination reveals hypoplasia.

Intervention
    I. Treatment involves removal of the offending drug and informing the patient to avoid any further contact with drugs, chemicals, or physical agents that may affect bone marrow.
   II. General supportive care of the patient is important, with adequate rest periods, increased fluid intake, and prevention of future infections. Reverse isolation may be necessary.
  III. Good oral hygiene and adequate nutrition with a diet high in protein, vitamins, and calories should be maintained with avoidance of irritating foods and beverages.
  IV. Antipyretics and tepid baths will reduce the fever.
   V. Hot saline gargles, an ice collar, and analgesics may provide necessary comfort to the mouth and throat.
  VI. Recovery results vary depending on the promptness of treatment, the granulocyte count, bone marrow production, and whether the disease is acute or chronic; however, the recovery is usually fairly rapid if infection is prevented or treated with antibiotics in order to prevent sepsis.
 VII. In chronic agranulocytosis, leukocyte transfusion or splenectomy may eventually be necessary and prove helpful.

Evaluation
    I. Reassessment and evaluation of the patient's response to treatment should be planned at frequent intervals.
   II. Response to treatment should be reviewed and adjustments in the care plan should be made accordingly.

METABOLIC DISORDERS

Pernicious Anemia

Definition
    Pernicious anemia, the most common manifestation of vitamin B_{12} deficiency, is a chronic, progressive, megaloblastic anemia characterized by a deficiency of the intrinsic factor. Vitamin B_{12} is necessary for normal red blood cell maturation and for normal nervous system functioning. Vitamin B_{12} is obtained from foods (or the extrinsic factor) and cannot be absorbed in the small intestine unless the intrinsic factor, believed to be a glycoprotein secretion of the gastric mucosa, is present. Vitamin B_{12} deficiency, thought to be an autoimmune disorder, impedes the deoxyribonucleic acid (DNA) precursors, resulting in the appearance of megaloblasts (large, primitive erythrocytes) in the blood and bone marrow and also resulting in thrombocytopenia and leukopenia.

    Pernicious anemia affects approximately 0.1 percent of the population. The highest incidence is found mainly in men and women over age 50. It is seen fairly often in fair Scandinavians and may be due to a genetic defect in that nationality.

    Other vitamin B_{12} deficiencies that may be seen are due to inadequate dietary intake, increased vitamin B_{12} requirements such as in hyperthroidism, defective absorption caused by a total gastrectomy, and failure of absorption in the small intestine. The most common causes of lack of small intestine absorption are malabsorption syndromes such as celiac disease, blind loop, and tapeworm infestation (refer to Table 25-2). Vitamin B_{12} deficiency can result in degeneration of the lateral and dorsal columns of the spinal cord, peripheral nerve damage and parasthesia, and altered food digestion.

Assessment

I. Data sources (refer to "Leukemia").
II. Health history.
   A. The dietary history may indicate a poor dietary intake, such as a "strict vegetarian" diet or alcoholism. This is not often seen.
   B. The patient usually complains of a slow, steady onset of weakness, anorexia, indigestion, and numbness and tingling in the extremities.
   C. A weight loss may have been noted. Diarrhea is commonly seen.
   D. In older patients, shortness of breath, dizziness, palpitations, and the development of angina after exertion may be the most common complaints.
   E. Early graying of the hair may have been noted.
   F. This problem may develop slowly because the bodily requirement of vitamin B_{12} is low; therefore, symptoms may appear gradually.
   G. Irritability and mood swings may be noted.
   H. Complaints of tinnitus may be described if auditory nerve involvement is present.
III. Physical assessment.
   A. The patient appears pale, wasted.
   B. A pale yellow or lemon yellow tinge to the skin or sclera may be noted.

TABLE 25-2 / ETIOLOGIC MECHANISMS OF MEGALOBLASTIC ANEMIAS

Vitamin B_{12} Deficiency	Folic Acid Deficiency
Decreased intake:	Decreased intake:
Poor diet	Poor diet
Impaired absorption	Alcoholism
Intrinsic factor (IF) deficiency	Infancy
Pernicious anemia	Hemodialysis
Gastrectomy (total and partial)	Impaired absorption
Destruction of gastric mucosa by ingested caustics	Intestinal absorption
Anti-IF antibody in gastric juice	Steatorrhea
Abnormal intrinsic factor molecule	Sprue, celiac disease
Intrinsic intestinal disease	Intrinsic intestinal disease
Familial selective malabsorption (Imerslund syndrome)	Anticonvulsants, oral contraceptives
Illeal resection, ileitis	Increased requirement:
Sprue, celiac disease	Pregnancy
Infiltrative intestinal disease (lymphoma, scleroderma, etc.)	Infancy
Drug-induced malabsorption	Hyperactive hemopoiesis
Competitive parasites	Neoplastic disease
Fish tapeworm infestation	Skin disease
Bacteria in diverticula of bowel	Blocked activation by folic acid antagonists
Bacteria in blind loops and pouches	
Chronic pancreatic disease	
Increased requirement:	
Pregnancy	
Neoplastic disease	
Hyperthyroidism	

Source: W. J. Williams et al., *Hematology,* 2d ed., McGraw-Hill Book Company, New York, 1977, p. 304.

      C. The mucous membranes may be inflamed, and the tongue is smooth and beefy red.

      D. Bleeding of the gingivae may be noted.

      E. The spleen is usually enlarged and palpable.

      F. The most significant findings are with the neurologic examination. Signs of posterior and lateral column disease may be symmetrical paresthesias in the feet and fingers. Incoordination, impairment of position (a pragnosia) and vibratory sense, and an absence of reflexes may be noted. Alteration in balance and proprioception may be noted.

      G. Bowel sounds may be increased if diarrhea is present.

      H. Dyspnea may be present, increasing upon changes in position. Slowed capillary refill will also be noted.

      I. Tachycardia and premature ventricular beats may be heard. In advanced stages signs of pump failure may be noted.

IV. Diagnostic tests.

      A. Blood studies will show a decrease in erythrocyte count and a decreased serum vitamin B_{12} level.

      B. Bone marrow biopsy reveals an increased number of megaloblasts.

      C. A definitive test for pernicious anemia is the Schilling test, which consists of a measurement of the absorption of radioactive vitamin B_{12} both before and after parenteral administration of the intrinsic factor.

      D. Gastric juice analysis for the presence of free hydrochloric acid is another important test. A low-volume, high-pH gastric juice with no free hydrochloric acid is seen in pernicious anemia.

Problems

I. Noncompliance with therapy.

II. Gastrointestinal disturbances (gastrectomy).

III. Inadequate nutrition.

IV. Fatigue.

V. Inadequate protection from neurological and mental disturbances.

Diagnosis

I. Noncompliance with vitamin B_{12} therapy may be manifested by neurological involvement. It may be due to lack of understanding regarding medical treatment.

II. Vulnerability to gastrointestinal disturbances are a result of the decrease in hydrochloric acid which affects chemical digestion of food.

III. Potential alterations in nutrition, resulting in inadequate intake.

IV. Alteration in ability to perform activities of daily living due to fatigue may be seen as a result of the iron deficiency anemia that often develops in conjunction with pernicious anemia.

V. Inadequate protection from bodily harm may result from the paresthesia, mental confusion, and ataxia which are the results of vitamin B_{12} deficiency.

Goals of Care

I. Immediate.

      A. Vitamin B_{12} therapy to alleviate symptoms.

      B. Control gastrointestinal symptoms in order to increase comfort and nutrition.

      C. Promote nutrition with an adequate dietary intake.

      D. Provide rest in order to promote maximum function.

      E. Protection from bodily harm as a result of neurological symptoms.

II. Long-range.

      A. Patient education regarding disease process.

      B. Maintenance Vitamin B_{12} therapy for the patient's lifetime.

      C. Family involvement as a support system.

Intervention

I. Nursing interventions are in conjunction with medical therapy. Immediate vitamin B_{12} therapy is initiated with administration of cyanocobalamin, 100 μg IM, 3 times per week for 10 doses. The patient response is rapid, demonstrated by an improved appetite, normal blood studies, decreased physical symptoms, and a sense of well-being.

II. Gastrointestinal symptoms must be treated when observed.

    A. Mouth care must be done carefully in patients with severe glossitis. Frequent oral hygiene before and after meals will ease discomfort and cleanse the mouth.

    B. The patient should be instructed to avoid highly seasoned, coarse, or irritating foods, and also foods that may be difficult to digest.

III. If dysphagia is present, hydrochloric acid can be administered after meals. Hydrochloric acid stains the teeth, so it must be well diluted in water and administered through a straw.

IV. Constipation and diarrhea may be treated with medication.

V. A nutritious diet should be emphasized to patients with pernicious anemia. They should be encouraged to eat foods high in iron, protein, and vitamins such as vitamin B_{12}. This includes meat, liver, fish, eggs, and milk.

VI. Folic acid is sometimes given in conjunction with vitamin B_{12} in patients with a poor nutritional history. Caution should be used with folic acid administration, as neurological symptoms may be intensified.

VII. In the presence of peripheral edema, diuretics and decreased sodium intake will be prescribed.

VIII. Bed rest is usually necessary if severe anemia is present. Exercise should progress as tolerated. Unless contraindicated, bathroom privileges and short periods out of bed in a chair may be permitted.

IX. If the patient is bedridden, frequent turning, range-of-motion exercises, and physical therapy are necessary.

X. Iron supplements of ferrous sulfate or ferrous gluconate, 0.3 g, 3 times a day after meals, may be given. In extreme cases, blood transfusions may be needed.

XI. If the patient suffers from neurological disturbances, protection from harm is necessary.

    A. Side rails and restraints can be used.

    B. If ambulating, protect the patient from falls, especially if a gait disturbance has been noted.

    C. Accompany the patient at night, as perception disturbances cause great difficulty in maneuvering in the dark.

    D. Reduced sensations to heat and pain are often present; therefore, heating pads and hot compresses must be used with care. Check for skin reddening and do not leave a hot pad on a patient for long periods of time.

    E. Extra blankets may provide comfort to a patient, as increased sensation to cold is also a problem.

    F. Foot cradles can take the undue pressure of blankets off the feet.

    G. Bladder and rectal sphincter involvement, due to advanced disease process, may complicate nursing care.

    H. Providing a quiet environment will decrease stress of loud noises.

XII. Vitamin B_{12} therapy must be continued the rest of the patient's life.

    A. Injections of cyanocobalamin, 100 μg, may be given twice monthly or oral vitamin B_{12} may be given in daily 500- to 1000-μg doses.

    B. The patient and family *must* be taught the importance of continued medical observation and treatment.

    C. The risks of interrupted therapy *must* be stressed without causing unnecessary anxiety.

    D. If the patient and family are well informed regarding pernicious anemia and have a basic grasp of the need for continued medication, the prognosis is usually excellent.

XIII. Behavioral changes that accompany this problem may necessitate the use of restraints, mild sedation, and counseling.

Evaluation

I. Reassessment.
   A. The patient must continue taking a vitamin B_{12} preparation and should be followed periodically.
   B. If without neurological involvement, the patient should be restored to a previous level of health.
II. Complications.
   A. Follow-up is necessary, as relapses may indicate infection, renal insufficiency (Chap. 28), gastric carcinoma, benign polyps, or gastrointestinal bleeding (Chap. 29).
   B. With neurological complications, the prognosis is related to the extent and duration of involvement. Vigorous therapy and treatment can reverse some of the neurological problems.

Folic Acid Anemia

Definition

Folic acid anemia is relatively common. The causes of this condition vary and are very similar to the causes of vitamin B_{12} deficiency (refer to Table 25-2). Folic acid is necessary for normal red blood cell maturation, and its deficiency affects the synthesis of DNA. This megaloblastic anemia, like vitamin B_{12} deficiency, is characterized by the appearance of megaloblasts in the blood and bone marrow.

The incidence of folic acid anemia is higher in countries with poor nutritional sources. Although in the United States dietary intake of folic acid is high, the bodily reserves are low, and the symptoms of folic acid anemia can appear rapidly with depletion of the total body stores in 12 to 16 weeks.

Assessment

I. Data sources (refer to "Leukemia").
II. Health history.
   A. The patient's complaints are very similar to those of pernicious anemia or vitamin B_{12} deficiency.
   B. Fatigue and shortness of breath may be the major complaints.
   C. An extensive dietary history is very important. A poor intake of green vegetables or fresh fruits along with excessive cooking of food may result in folic acid anemia.
   D. Chronic alcoholics are especially susceptible, partially due to diet, but also due to increased alcohol levels which block bone marrow response to folic acid.
   E. A history of liver disease or gastrointestinal malabsorption, such as sprue (intolerance of wheat, protein, or gluten ingestion) or regional enteritis may be found.
   F. A history of any previous anemia should be noted, along with any treatment given.
   G. Drug ingestion of certain anticonvulsants (Dilantin, phenobarbital), oral contraceptives, and antimetabolites (such as methotrexate, a folic acid antagonist) must be determined.
   H. Folic acid requirements are increased during growth, pregnancy (especially during the last trimester), and in certain disease states, such as cancer and leukemia.
   I. Care must be taken to be sure the patient has folic acid anemia and not vitamin B_{12} deficiency.
   J. It commonly occurs in adults.
III. Physical assessment.
   A. The appearance of the patient is similar to that in pernicious anemia.
   B. The patient is pale and emaciated.
   C. Glossitis is usually present.
   D. The neurological changes present in pernicious anemia are *not* seen in folic acid anemia, unless they are linked to chronic alcoholism.
   E. Other disorders, such as protein and iron deficiency and electrolyte imbalances, may be seen in conjunction with folic acid anemia.
IV. Diagnostic tests.
   A. A decrease is seen in the serum and red cell folate level.

B. The Schilling test and serum vitamin B_{12} level are normal, and hydrochloric acid is present in the gastric juice.

C. Bone marrow examination reveals an increased number of megaloblasts.

D. A favorable response to a therapeutic trial of folic acid, 50 to 100 μg IM daily for 10 days, is indicative of folic acid anemia.

Problems/
Diagnosis

I. Noncompliance due to inability to alter dietary habits or lack of understanding of disease.

II. Nutritional alteration due to an intake of less than minimal daily requirements.

III. Alterations in comfort due to irritations of the oral mucosa.

Goals of Care

I. Immediate.

    A. Folic acid therapy to alleviate symptoms and disease process.

    B. Promote adequate nutrition to supplement and increase folic acid intake.

    C. Provide comfort measures to decrease glossitis.

II. Long-range: Patient education to prevent future folic acid deficiency.

Intervention

I. Oral doses of folic acid, 0.1 to 5 mg daily, are given until the blood studies improve or the cause of intestinal malabsorption is corrected. If malabsorption is a problem, parenteral doses are given initially.

II. Vitamin C is sometimes also prescribed, in addition, because it augments folic acid in promoting erythropoiesis.

III. Dietary habits and food intake must be considered.

    A. A dietitian working closely with the patient may be able to suggest foods high in folic acid and plan meals that are attainable to the patient.

    B. Consideration to cost and availability must be given.

    C. Fruits and green vegetables, including such choices as lemons, bananas, melons, spinach, broccoli, lettuce, and lima beans, are necessary to provide adequate folic acid intake.

IV. Refer to "Pernicious Anemia" for care of the mouth and neurological considerations.

Evaluation

I. Reassessment.

    A. Periodic blood determinations should be made to determine the patient's response to the drug therapy.

    B. The patient and family's understanding regarding compliance with therapy must be evaluated.

    C. If folic acid anemia is misdiagnosed and is in reality vitamin B_{12} anemia, neurological symptoms will develop.

Iron-Deficiency Anemia

Definition

Iron-deficiency anemia is one of the most common anemias, and it affects 10 to 30 percent of the world population. It is characterized by decreased or absent iron stores in the bone marrow, spleen, and liver, a low serum iron and a low hemoglobin level, and by microcytic, hypochromic (small and devoid of pigment) red blood cells. It is caused by inadequate intake or absorption of dietary iron to compensate for iron requirements or by increased loss of iron due to bleeding, whether it is physiologic or pathologic. The distribution of this anemia is related to geographic location, economic and social class, age, and sex. Iron deficiency is common in underdeveloped areas where nutrition is poor and in tropical areas where parasites such as hookworm are prevalent. Menstruating and pregnant women and young children are the most common victims. If pathological bleeding is involved, the chronic blood loss is usually from the gastrointestinal tract. Symptoms will increase and intensify unless replacement therapy begins.

Assessment

I. Data sources (refer to "Leukemia").

   A. Fatigue, irritability, and headaches are common complaints.

   B. In severe anemia, shortness of breath upon exertion and tachycardia may be noted.

   C. A complete dietary history should be obtained. If a small amount of animal protein is eaten or if clay (pica) and starch are ingested, these may be the source of the deficiency.

   D. Any history of previous anemias should be checked in both the patient and the family members.

   E. Menstrual histories are important. Recent pregnancies and any difficulties with pregnancies should be noted.

   F. Chronic bleeding or gastric surgery should be investigated as any recent trauma may also be a cause of this anemia.

   G. Patients may have a history of a recent infection or nonbacterial inflammation such as rheumatoid arthritis.

   H. Regular blood donation can result in iron loss.

   I. Iron-deficiency anemia may be observed more frequently in young adults and teenagers due to poor dietary intake.

III. Physical assessment.

   A. The patient will appear pale.

   B. The mucous membranes and conjunctiva are pale, and the normal redness in the palms of the hands is missing.

   C. The skin is dry.

   D. Flattening or concavity of the nails may be noted, along with brittleness of the hair and nails (see Fig. 25-4).

   E. Inflammation of the mucosa of the mouth (stomatitis), cracks in the corner of the mouth, and glossitis (atrophy of the papillae of the tongue) are often seen.

   F. There may be a slight enlargement of the liver noted upon palpation.

   G. Since another health problem (e.g., carcinoma, vascular occlusions, rectal bleeding) may be the primary cause of the anemia, a complete physical is essential.

IV. Diagnostic tests.

   A. The red blood cells are microcytic and hypochromic.

   B. The blood hemoglobin is reduced.

   C. A decrease in the serum iron level may be found.

   D. On bone marrow examination, hemosiderin (an insoluble form of storage iron) is absent.

Problems

I. Gastrointestinal disturbances.

II. Noncompliance to therapy.

FIGURE 25-4 / **Spoonlike concavity of the fingernails seen in iron-deficiency anemia.** (*From W. J. Williams et al., Hematology, 2d ed., McGraw-Hill Book Company, New York, 1977.*)

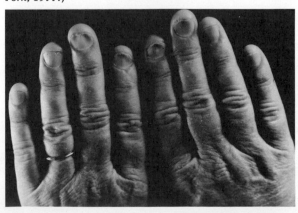

Diagnosis

I. Potential alterations in comfort due to glossitis and possible gastrointestinal disturbances due to iron therapy.
II. Promotion of understanding in patient regarding the need to find the source of the deficiency.
III. Alterations in nutrition due to inadequate intake of foods high in iron.

Goals of Care

I. Immediate.
 A. Determine and correct the underlying cause of the anemia.
 B. Correct the iron deficiency by iron preparations and a diet high in food iron.
 C. Provide care for the throat and mucous membranes in order to increase comfort.
II. Long-range.
 A. Prevent reoccurrence of the anemia.
 B. Evaluate response to therapy.

Intervention

I. The source or cause of the anemia must be determined. If gastrointestinal bleeding is suspected, numerous diagnostic tests must be performed. X-Rays of the gastrointestinal tract, stool examinations for occult blood, and gastroscopy and sigmoidoscopy examinations may be done. It is important that the patient understand the need for these studies to facilitate cooperation. (Refer to Chap. 29 for discussion.)
II. The role of the nurse involves teaching the patient about the procedures and providing support and comfort during and after the tests. The patient and family must be encouraged to ask any questions they might have regarding the tests or the disorder.
III. Iron may be given orally or parenterally.
 A. Oral medications, such as ferrous sulfate, 0.2 g, or ferrous gluconate, 0.3 g, 3 times a day after meals, are preferred.
 B. Iron salts are gastric irritants, so they must be given following food. Some dyspepsia may result anyway. However, salts should not be taken with milk, as absorption will not take place.
 C. Liquid iron preparations must be diluted and administered through a straw because they stain the teeth.
 D. The patient must be informed that iron will make stools appear tarry or dark green and that this is a harmless side effect.
 E. Ascorbic acid will help to promote iron absorption; vitamin C or orange juice can be given with the iron preparations.
 F. Diet teaching regarding foods high in iron should be done. These foods include red meat, eggs, leafy green vegetables like spinach, and iron-fortified cereals.
IV. Parenteral iron therapy is chosen only when it is necessary because of oral intolerance or continual blood loss. Imferon may be given in doses of 100 to 250 mg daily or every other day on demand.
 A. Care must be taken to prevent the medication from leaking into the tissues.
 B. The Z-tract injection technique is usually used.
  1. Do not massage the site following injection.
  2. Movement increases absorption. Excessive exercise or constricting garments should be avoided by the patient.
  3. Previous sites should be checked by the nurse for complications (e.g., hemorrhage) throughout the course of therapy.
V. Iron therapy is necessary 2 to 3 months after the hemoglobin returns to normal because the iron stores replenish at a slower rate.
VI. Refer to the other anemias for further interventions.

Evaluation

I. Reasssessment.
 A. The patient will be followed for several months. The hemoglobin level will be checked to evaluate response to therapy.
 B. If the hemoglobin level remains low, the patient will be reevaluated for the cause of the anemia.
II. Complications: rare; however, reoccurrence of anemia is often seen in cases where the iron deficiency was treated, but the underlying cause was not.

Hypoprothrombinemia

Definition *Hypoprothrombinemia* is a disorder with a deficient amount of circulating prothrombin. Prothrombin is produced in the liver, and the presence of vitamin K is necessary for prothrombin synthesis to take place. If a person is vitamin K deficient, it may be due to improper diet, gastrointestinal tract disorders which interfere with vitamin K absorption, extensive liver damage, or antibiotic therapy which sterilizes the bowel, preventing vitamin K production. Dicumarol, an anticoagulant, can cause hypoprothrombinemia in toxic doses by interfering with the conversion of vitamin K to prothrombin.

Assessment
I. Data sources (refer to "Leukemia").
II. Health history: The health history may be vague, with the patient complaining of minor bleeding episodes or ecchymosis following minimal trauma.
III. Physical assessment.
    A. Ecchymosis may be present.
    B. Hematuria and gastrointestinal bleeding may be overt symptoms.
IV. Diagnostic tests: Blood studies show an elevated prothrombin time.

Intervention
I. Vitamin K supplement is administered. Synkayvite, 5 mg IM, or Mephyton, 5 mg orally, are drugs of choice for minor bleeding.
II. If more severe bleeding is present, 10 to 15 mg of Aqua-Mephyton can be given intravenously.
III. Prothrombin can be replaced directly by transfusion.

INFLAMMATORY DISORDERS

Infectious Mononucleosis

Definition *Infectious mononucleosis* (also known as glandular fever) is a common, benign condition seen most often in young adults from 17 to 25 years of age. It is very prevalent among college students. The cause is believed to be a herpeslike virus, known as the Epstein-Barr virus, and transmission is probably due to oral contact with saliva exchange. Although infectious mononucleosis is a self-limiting disease, its symptoms are varied and its effects are seen throughout the body. The incubation period is approximately 30 to 50 days, and the onset of symptoms may be gradual.

Assessment
I. Data source (refer to "Leukemia").
II. Health history.
    A. The early complaints include chills, headache, and malaise.
    B. History of contact with an individual having similar symptoms is not uncommon.
    C. Nausea and a distaste for cigarettes are often early indicators. Patient may have decreased appetite.
    D. The patient may then have a fever, sore throat, and swollen lymph nodes. This triad is seen in 80 percent of reported cases.
    E. Complaints of increasing fatigue are not uncommon.
    F. Often effects young adults.
    G. History of decreased rest, poor eating habits, fatigue, and exposure are common.
III. Physical assessment.
    A. The diagnosis of infectious mononucleosis is based on both the clinical picture and the blood test results.
    B. On physical examination, the pharynx usually reveals reddened, infected mucous membranes near the tonsils. Exudate, petechiae, and white patches on the palates may also be noted.
    C. The cervical lymph nodes are palpable and noticeably enlarged. This is usually bilateral and may be seen in conjunction with axillary and inguinal node enlargement.

D. The liver and spleen are palpable in more severe cases.

IV. Diagnostic tests: The characteristic findings of the blood, most often seen within 10 days, are:

    A. Leukocytosis, with a white blood cell count of 12,000 to 18,000 per cubic millimeter, of which 60 percent are large, atypical lymphocytes (Downey cells).

    B. A positive heterophil agglutination test.

Intervention

I. All nursing interventions should focus on relieving the problems and preventing complications. The prognosis for infectious mononucleosis is usually excellent. However, no specific interventions hasten the process. Therefore, providing comfort and symptomatic intervention are of primary concern, as convalescence varies.

II. Bed rest is strongly encouraged until the fever, headache, and fatigue decrease. The patient should not engage in any strenuous activity, as this may result in a decrease in resistance to infection or may cause a splenic rupture. Blows to the abdomen, lifting, and straining should be avoided.

III. By decreasing the fever and discomfort of the sore throat and swollen glands, the patient's appetite and dysphagia should improve. Aspirin or other analgesics and warm saline gargles, along with cool sponge baths and a large fluid intake, will help.

IV. Nutritious foods with a high-protein and high-vitamin content should be encouraged. These foods should be nonirritating to the throat and might include soup, milkshakes, fruit juices, and soft cheeses. Steroid treatment, such as prednisone, and intravenous therapy may be indicated if the throat swelling is severe.

V. The patient should be isolated from possible sources of infection. A secondary streptococcal infection of the throat is not uncommon. Any increase in throat pain or fever should be noted so that antibiotic therapy may be started.

Evaluation

I. Reassessment: continuous. Response to therapy is good.

II. Complications.

    A. Splenic rupture is always of concern in the acute phase of infectious mononucleosis. The two major indicators are abdominal pain and shock. The pain may be left-sided and radiate. Tachycardia is often present. If this occurs, an emergency splenectomy is necessary.

    B. Acute airway obstruction can occur with extreme hyperplasia of the pharyngeal tissue.

    C. Neurological manifestations with central nervous system involvement can be seen.

    D. Hematologic complications are noted through frequent blood work.

    E. Liver damage and hepatitis can be seen.

    F. Revision in plan of care must be made in view of these complications.

OBSTRUCTIONS

Purpura (Vascular purpura)

Definition

Purpura is the name given to a group of disorders characterized by the appearance of ecchymoses or small hemorrhages (petechiae) in various places on the body or mucous membranes. The etiologies are unknown or poorly understood. Often the platelet count and function are normal, so the hemorrhages are believed to be associated with the inability of the blood vessels, usually capillaries, to maintain integrity. Thus, the blood is permitted to seep into the subcutaneous tissue. This postulated abnormality in the vascular factors involved in hemostasis may be in conjunction with increases in fragility and permeability. The causes are varied: an autoimmune reaction, due to allergy or specific drugs (iodine, belladonna); bacterial or viral infection (subacute bacterial endocarditis, Rocky Mountain spotted fever); hereditary or acquired structural disorders (Cushing's disease, scurvy); or a result of various disease processes, such as certain skin or chronic diseases (refer to Table 25-3).

TABLE 25-3 / PURPURAS

I. Vascular
    A. Nonthrombocytopenic purpura
        1. Purpura simplex
        2. Mechanical purpura
        3. Orthostatic purpura
        4. Senile purpura
        5. Adrenocortical hyperfunction
        6. Hereditary disorders of connective tissue
        7. Scurvy
        8. Purpura associated with dysproteinemia
        9. Purpura associated with infections
    B. Autoerythrocyte sensitivity
    C. DNA sensitivity
    D. Allergic purpura
II. Hereditary hemorrhagic telangiectasia
III. Thrombocytopenic purpura:
    A. Idiopathic thrombocytopenic purpura
    B. Secondary thrombocytopenic purpura

Source: Adapted from W. J. Williams et al., *Hematology*, 2d ed., McGraw-Hill Book Company, New York, 1977, p. 1313.

Assessment

I. Data sources (refer to "Leukemia").
II. Health history: Diagnosis is usually made by exclusion.
III. Physical assessment: The hemorrhages may be localized to the extremities, site of trauma, the face, or groin area.
    A. Bruising or spontaneous bleeding into the tissues may be the major complaint.
    B. Many other associated findings may be present, such as pain and gastrointestinal bleeding. The incidence varies widely depending on the process involved.
    C. A family history of bleeding may be present.
IV. Diagnostic tests: Blood studies usually are not definitive.

Intervention

I. Observe the patient continually for signs of bleeding. The patient and family should be taught to:
    A. Examine the skin and mucous membranes for petechiae or ecchymoses.
    B. Check urine and stool for frank or occult blood.
    C. Note and treat immediately nosebleeds and cuts.
    D. Watch for signs of internal hemorrhage, including weakness, faintness, dizziness, tachycardia, abdominal pain, hypotension, and confusion.
II. Prevent trauma.
    A. Teach the patient to avoid straining or lifting of heavy objects, to exercise care when walking, and to request assistance if necessary.
    B. Meticulous skin care, using oils and lotions to keep the skin soft, is needed.
    C. If the patient is bedridden, frequent turning is imperative.
    D. Only electric razors and soft-bristled toothbrushes should be used.
    E. The patient must avoid cuts. If cut, pressure must be applied for several minutes, a pressure dressing should be applied, and the site should be checked often.
    F. Stools should be kept soft to prevent trauma to the rectal mucosa. Laxatives and stool softeners can be used.
    G. Diet may need modification to prevent irritation to the mucous membranes and the gastrointestinal lining, but it should provide adequate nutrition.
    H. Extreme heat and dehydration should be avoided.

III. The family can provide excellent support and assistance if they are taught about purpura, its complications, and how they can help the patient maintain as normal a lifestyle as possible. The nurse should be available to answer any questions and to provide the resources needed.

Idiopathic Thrombocytopenic Purpura

Definition

The platelet count in *idiopathic thrombocytopenic purpura* (ITP) is below 200,000 per cubic millimeter due to premature platelet destruction. The etiology of ITP is unknown, but the major theory is that autoantibodies sensitize platelets, making them vulnerable to destruction by the spleen, or that the autoantibodies interfere with the production of platelets. Chronic ITP affects all ages and more women than men; acute ITP is most common in children (refer to Chap. 15).

Assessment

I. Data sources (refer to "Leukemia").
II. Health history.
    A. The health history is usually not indicative of any obvious sources.
    B. The most common complaint and physical manifestation are those of petechiae and minor bleeding episodes. The bleeding may have been noted for years, e.g., nosebleeds or gingival bleeding.
III. Physical assessment.
    A. Close physical examination of the skin reveals the presence of petechiae or ecchymosis.
    B. The liver and spleen may be palpable but not enlarged.
    C. In more advanced cases, dyspnea, decreased joint movement, and pain are added complaints.
    D. Fatigue may accompany the problem.
IV. Diagnostic tests.
    A. The platelet count is decreased.
    B. A prolonged bleeding time is noted (clot retraction).
    C. Increased capillary fragility is found.
    D. Prothrombin time is usually normal.

Intervention

I. Steroids such as prednisone, 10 to 20 mg, 4 times a day, increase the platelet count, thus reducing the bleeding tendency. Platelet transfusions have been used. (See Chap. 32 for care of the patient who is receiving steroids.)
II. If steroids are not effective or if large doses are necessary, a splenectomy is done. After a splenectomy, 80 percent of the patients improve or go into a remission.
Postoperative care should include prevention of hemorrhage.
IV. Immunosuppression has been used with some success in patients who did not respond well to the splenectomy.

Evaluation

I. Reassessment: continuous observation of the patient is essential throughout the postoperative period.
II. Complications: hemorrhages, especially cerebral hemorrhages. Rest and prevention of undue stress through excess activity, sneezing, or straining are necessary.

Disseminated Intravascular Coagulation

Definition

Disseminated intravascular coagulation (DIC) is an acute disorder which is characterized by widespread fibrin deposits in capillaries and arterioles and by hemolysis of platelets, thrombin, and other clotting factors, which results in bleeding. The excessive clotting activates the fibrinolytic mechanism to produce fibrin-split end products, which further inhibits platelet clotting and ultimately leads to more bleeding. The result is decreased blood flow and increased tissue damage. The etiology of DIC is not understood, but it is related to thromboplastic substances which are released into the blood. This may be due to certain chronic disease states, obstetric complications (e.q., abruptio placenta), surgical trauma, gram-negative sepsis, or shock, or may be seen after rapid transfusion of a large amount of blood. DIC may last for several hours or days. Unless this process can be reversed, death will ensue due to severe renal problems and/or hemorrhage.

Assessment
I. Data sources (refer to "Leukemia").
II. Health history.
   A. The health history may not be available or indicative of the onset of disseminated intravascular coagulation.
   B. Bleeding should be carefully assessed, if noted, as to the type, severity, location, and mode of onset.
   C. Specific predisposing factors, e.g., infections, malignant diseases, heat stroke, burns, and obstetrical complications, should be included in the history.
III. Physical assessment.
   A. Physical assessment will reveal petechiae or ecchymotic areas on the skin and mucous membranes.
   B. Hemorrhaging may be overt.
   C. Signs of shock, including oliguria, may be noted.
   D. Seizures may also occur.
IV. Diagnostic tests.
   A. A prolonged prothrombin time.
   B. A low platelet count.
   C. The lack of blood coagulation.

Intervention
I. Treatment of the underlying condition that initiated DIC is done immediately.
II. Heparin is administered to block coagulation.
III. Bleeding and shock, if present, are treated.
IV. The consumed clotting components are replaced after the heparin is started. Platelet concentrates and fresh or fresh frozen plasma are used.

Evaluation
I. Reassessment: continuous.
II. Complications: DIC can result in organ injury, and the complications of those injuries are often seen.

DEGENERATIVE DISORDERS

Hemophilia

Definition
The hemophilias are relatively rare disorders and are characterized by a defective mechanism in the coagulation process. The most common is *hemophilia A* or *classic hemophilia,* which is a factor VIII deficiency. This represents approximately 80 percent of the inherited coagulation disorders. The other type of hemophilia seen is *hemophilia B,* which is a factor IX or Christmas factor deficiency. Hemophilia is a sex-linked recessive trait seen almost exclusively in males, although females are carriers. The severity of the clotting defect can vary from mild to severe and is manifested by prolonged bleeding from trauma to the tissues and joints. Hemophilias are classified as childhood disorders, but because of new developments in treatment, this disease now extends into adulthood (refer to Chap. 15).

Assessment
I. Data sources (refer to "Leukemia").
II. Health history.
   A. A thorough health history is extremely important in patients with suspected hemophilia.

B. A detailed description of all past operations (dental extractions or surgery) and traumas and the duration of bleeding in relation to the above are significant.

C. Hematuria, epistaxis, hematemesis, and melena may be present.

D. A strong family history of "bleeders" is indicative of hemophilia, as the genetic defect is hereditary.

E. Any association of bleeding episodes with other illnesses, procedures, drugs, and diet should be noted, along with the age of onset.

III. Physical assessment.

A. The patient may exhibit a variety of signs and symptoms, as this disorder varies in severity from family to family.

B. The physical assessment usually confirms the health history, with the patient exhibiting signs of current or past hemorrhage.

C. Characteristics of chronic joint deformities, contractures, or muscle atrophy may be present.

D. Hemarthrosis, or bleeding into the joints, is seen in severe hemophiliacs.

E. Severe abdominal pain and bruising are common.

IV. Diagnostic tests.

A. A screening test for coagulation factors is usually done.

B. Blood studies show a prolonged partial thromboplastin (PTT) and prothrombin time (PT).

C. Specific assays to distinguish between factor VIII and factor IX deficiency are done.

Intervention

I. Replacement of the missing factor by transfusions of fresh or fresh-frozen whole blood or plasma is possible.

A. Antihemophilic factor (AHF) levels can be raised by administration of commercial AHF concentrates such as cryoprecipitate and Hemophil.

B. Prophylactic treatment of the missing factors are administered prior to surgery or dental extractions.

II. Topical bleeding can be controlled by pressure, using Gelfoam or hemostatics such as thrombin.

A. Continual observation for signs of internal bleeding is necessary.

B. Trauma must be avoided and the patient educated to prevent bleeding episodes.

C. Bleeding can be delayed for periods of time in hemophilia, and the manifestations of that bleeding are not seen until much later.

D. Patients must identify the fact that they have hemophilia to doctors, teachers, dentists, and employers.

III. Hemarthrosis is treated with AHF or whole blood administration, rest, protection (sometimes in a cast), and ice. Steroids may reduce joint inflammation.

Evaluation

I. Reassessment: continuous. Response to interventions and compliance with preventive teaching should be noted.

II. Complications.

A. Hemorrhage and shock.

B. The major complication associated with hemophilia is that repeated transfusion and AHF therapy will cause the patient to become sensitized to AHF and to develop autoimmune anticoagulants (anti-AHF factor). This patient will not respond to further therapy and consequently dies as a result of hemorrhaging.

C. Refer to "Hemophilia" in Chap. 15 for additional information.

Hemolytic Anemias

Definition

Hemolytic anemia is a broad descriptive name given to numerous diseases characterized by a shortened erythrocyte life span. This is due to increased destruction by the reticuloendothelial elements and failure of the bone marrow to produce sufficient erythrocytes to compensate for the vast numbers of red cells destroyed. Much about these diseases is yet unknown; however, they are most often classified as hereditary or intracorpuscular defects and acquired or extracorpuscular.

An *intracorpuscular defect* takes place within the erythrocyte. The genetic result is usually due to (1) defects in the red cell membrane, (2) defects of the glycolysis and related metabolic systems enzymes, and (3) defects of the hemoglobin molecule and its synthesis. Factors or mechanisms external to the erythrocyte that cause hemolytic anemia may be drugs, plasma components, infections, or chemical or physical agents (refer to Table 25-4 for clarification).

Hemolytic anemias are found in all age groups and both sexes. The anemia may be acute or chronic, mild or severe, depending on the rate of hemolysis. Racial and geographic incidences are noted in many of the diseases.

In adults, *hereditary spherocytosis* or congenital hemolytic jaundice is one type of hemolytic anemia seen, characterized by spherocytes (spherically shaped erythrocytes) in the blood smear and increased osmotic fragility. *Glucose 6-phosphate dehydrogenase* (G6PD) deficiency is rare and appears to be an enzymatic defect that is manifested in blacks and persons of Mediterranean extraction in response to certain drugs. *Thalassemia,* also common in those of Mediterranean heritage, is a biochemical defect in hemoglobin synthesis. Thalassemia major is seen in childhood, as is sickle cell anemia or hemoglobin S disease. *Autoimmune hemolytic anemia* is an acquired defect, the exact mechanism of which is not known. It is theorized to result from an alteration in the red cell antigen, to be a cross-reaction of that antigen, or to be induced by the lymphoid cells which produce antibodies against normal red cells.

Assessment

I. Data sources (refer to "Leukemia").
II. Health history.
    A. The major complaints of patients with hemolytic anemia will be those common to most anemias: weakness and fatigue. Dypsnea may also be noticed.
    B. If the patient is in hemolytic crisis (which may be precipitated by an acute infection), malaise, chills, fever, aches, and pains in the back and abdomen may accompany the complaint of fatigue.
    C. A strong family history of certain kinds of hemolytic anemias or signs and symptoms in other family members may be noted, including a history of jaundice, gallstones, or anemia. Some hemolytic anemias are genetic and sex-linked.
    D. Any bleeding episodes should be noted.
III. Physical assessment.
    A. Pallor may be noted, along with jaundice. A slight scleral icterus may be the only observable sign.
    B. Splenomegaly is present in congenital hemolytic anemias, except for sickle cell anemia.
    C. Cholelithiasis is common, especially in hereditary spherocytosis.
    D. Leg ulcers may be noted, especially around the ankles. They are usually bilateral and are often seen in hereditary spherocytosis and sickle cell anemia.
    E. Skeletal abnormalities of the skull and of the frontal and parietal bones are often observed in severe thalassemia major.
    F. Acquired hemolytic anemia patients may only exhibit pallor and a slight jaundice.
IV. Diagnostic tests.
    A. Blood studies reveal normocytic anemia; increased reticulocytes, due to the efforts of the bone marrow to compensate for excessive erythrocyte destruction; increased red cell fragility; and shortened erythrocyte life span.
    B. Hemoglobinuria results from the excretion of hemoglobin into the urine. The urine appears pink to red to almost black. This can be distinguished from hematuria microscopically. Intravascular hemolysis is the major cause of hemoglobinuria.
    C. Fecal and urine urobilinogen reflect the increased catabolism of urine.
    D. Serum lactate dehydrogenase (LDH) is often increased.
    E. Hyperplasia in the bone marrow is found upon examination.

TABLE 25-4 / CLASSIFICATION OF COMMON HEMOLYTIC DISEASES

I. Hereditary or intracorpuscular hemolytic disorders
   A. Erythrocyte membrane defects
      1. Hereditary spherocytosis
      2. Hereditary elliptocytosis
      3. Stomatocytosis
   B. Enzyme deficiencies in the metabolic pathways
      1. Glucose 6-phosphate dehydrogenase (G6PD)
      2. Pyruvate kinase
   C. Defects in globin structure and synthesis
      1. Sickle cell anemia
      2. Thalassemia major
II. Acquired or extracorpuscular hemolytic disorders
   A. Immunohemolytic anemias
      1. Transfusion of incompatible blood
      2. Erythroblastosis fetalis
      3. Autoimmune hemolytic anemia due to warm-reactive antibodies
         a. Idiopathic
         b. "Secondary"
            (1) Virus and mycoplasma infections
            (2) Lymphosarcoma, chronic lymphocytic leukemia
            (3) Other malignant diseases
            (4) Systemic lupus erythematosis
         c. Drug-induced
            (1) Quinidine
            (2) Penicillin
            (3) Methyldopa
      4. Autoimmune hemolytic anemia due to cold-reactive antibodies
   B. Traumatic and microangiopathic hemolytic anemias
      1. Prosthetic valve replacement and cardiac abnormalities
      2. Thrombotic thrombocytopenic purpura
      3. Disseminated intravascular coagulation
   C. Infections
      1. Malaria
      2. Bacteria
      3. Virus
   D. Chemicals, drugs, and venoms
      1. Antimalarials
      2. Sulfonamides
      3. Antipyretics and analgesics
      4. Mothballs
      5. Fava Beans
      6. Certain snake and spider venoms
      7. Mushrooms
      8. Lead poisoning
   E. Physical agents
      1. Thermal injury
      2. Ionizing irradiation (questionable)
   F. Hypersplenism

Source: Adapted from M. W. Wintrobe et al., *Clinical Hematology,* 7th ed.,
Lea & Febiger, Philadelphia, 1975, p. 721.

Problems	I. Maintenance of adequate fluid intake and renal function. II. Adequate treatment of the signs and symptoms of anemia (e.g., fatigue, weakness, etc.).
Diagnosis	I. Potential alteration in urinary elimination, due to severe hemolysis, resulting in renal failure. II. Prevent alteration in activities of daily living, due to sickle cell crisis and anemia. III. Decrease alterations in comfort secondary to the disease process and complications.

Goals of Care	I. Immediate.
	   A. Eliminate any causative factors that may precipitate hemolysis, such as certain drugs and infections.
	   B. Maintain renal function by preventing neurosis of the renal tubules.
	   C. Treat anemia by administering blood transfusions.
	II. Long-range: Educate patient regarding causative factors leading to the disease process.

Intervention	I. As a variety of disorders are found in the hemolytic anemias, further diagnostic tests and exhaustive health histories must be obtained to diagnose causative factors. Once the diagnosis is made, elimination of the factor and patient education as to the source are necessary.
	II. Renal function can be impaired as a result of severe hemolysis.
	   A. The patient must take in large amounts of water to dilute the effects of the red cells.
	   B. Input and output must be watched, and electrolytes should be checked as renal tubule absorption may be impaired.
	   C. Intravenous therapy may be necessary.
	   D. Infusions of sodium bicarbonate or sodium lactate can alkalize the urine.
	III. Anemia is treated with blood transfusions. Caution must be used, as the transfused cells will rapidly be destroyed in patients with an autoimmune hemolytic disease. Prednisolone or another corticosteroid is then administered in 10- to 20-mg doses 4 times a day until normal hemoglobin levels are reached.
	IV. Hemolytic "crisis" is often characterized by fever, abdominal discomfort, nausea, and vomiting. Comfort measures are referred to under the other anemias.
	V. Other care for anemia is discussed under the other anemias.
	VI. A splenectomy is often the treatment of choice in hemolytic anemias.

Evaluation	I. Reassessment.
	   A. Continual follow-up is necessary to prevent reoccurrence.
	   B. Patient and family education regarding the disorder diagnosed is important to prevent future episodes.
	   C. The prognosis of the disease varies, but in certain disorders such as thalassamia minor and hereditary spherocytosis the prognosis is very good.

BIBLIOGRAPHY

Coleman, Robert, John Minna, and Stanley J. Robby: "Disseminated Intravascular Coagulation: A Problem in Critical Care Nursing," *Heart and Lung,* **3**:789–796, September–October 1974. A clinical, laboratory, and pathological approach to the DIC syndrome.

Desotell, Susan: "A Brighter Future for Leukemia Patients," *Nursing 77,* **7**(1):18–23, January 1977. An update of combined drug therapy used in treating leukemia.

Eisenhower, Laurel A.: "Drug-Induced Blood Dyscrasias," *Nursing Clinics of North America,* **7**(4): 799–808, December 1972. A discussion of drug-induced anemias, agranulocytosis, and the effects of drugs on blood clotting.

Foster, Sue: "Sickle Cell Anemia: Pathophysiologic Aspects," *Heart and Lung,* **3**:955–961, November–December 1974. A clear and concise discussion of the pathophysiology of sickle cell anemia.

Rickel, Linda: "Emotional Support for the Multiple Myeloma Patient," *Nursing 76,* **6**:76–80, April 1976. An excellent article on the psychological management of the acutely ill patient.

Rossman, Maureen, Rosemary Slavin, and Edward G. Taft: "Pheresis Therapy: Patient Care," *American Journal of Nursing,* **77**(7):1135–1141, July 1977. An excellent explanation of the nursing care during leukapheresis.

Scarlato, Michael: "Blood Transfusing Today: What You Should Know and Do," *Nursing 78,* **8**(2):68–72, February 1978. This article clarifies component transfusions and provides an overview of care.

Schulman, Delores, and Phyllis Patterson: "The Adult with Acute Leukemia," *Nursing Clinics of North America,* **7**(4):743–762, December 1972. A good article on nursing care of leukemia patients.

——— and ———: "Multiple Myeloma," *American Journal of Nursing,* **75**:81–98, January 1975. A good discussion of multiple myeloma and common interventions.

Vaz, Delores D. S.: "The Common Anemias: Nursing Approaches," *Nursing Clinics of North America,* **7**(4):711–726, December 1972. A general discussion of common nursing care in various anemias.

Williams, William J., Ernest Beutler, Allan J. Ersler, and Rundles R. Wayne: *Hematology,* 2d ed., McGraw-Hill Book Company, New York, 1977. An excellent and thorough presentation of all hematologic disorders.

Wood, Camilla: "Iron Deficiency Anemia," *Nurse Practitioner,* **2**:24–25, May–June 1977. A good review of assessment and physiology of iron deficiency anemia.

———: "Macrocytic Megaloblastic Anemias," *Nurse Practitioner,* **2**:24, 25, 29, July 1977. A concise summary of the physiology of vitamin B_{12} and folic acid anemia.

26
The Cardiovascular System

Rose Pinneo

Cardiovascular nursing is the care of individuals with an alteration in cardiovascular physiologic functioning. It encompasses both the cardiac and peripheral circulatory disturbances. In caring for individuals with these disturbances, the nurse needs an understanding of the pathophysiology of related conditions as a basis for collecting meaningful data, identifying nursing problems, establishing goals for care, planning interventions, and evaluating outcomes. In performing these various aspects of the nursing process, the nurse works collaboratively with the physician and other members of the health team so that high-quality care is delivered to the patient.

This chapter provides the practicing nurse with a handy, quick reference relating to the care of patients with selected cardiovascular disorders. Because the scope of content is broad, it is not possible to provide in-depth information about each disorder. Therefore, the reader is referred to the bibliography and other sources for further information. Hopefully, the information provided in this chapter will motivate the nurse to seek other resources to increase his or her knowledge.

ABNORMAL CELLULAR GROWTH

Congenital Heart Disease: Coarctation of the Aorta

DEFINITION
Coarctation of the aorta is a constriction of the aorta, usually occurring distal to the left subclavian artery. This constriction obstructs arterial blood flow to the lower extremities and abdominal organs, thus causing blood pressure in the upper extremities to exceed that in the lower extremities.

ASSESSMENT
I. Data sources.
   A. Patient.
   B. Family.
   C. Previous hospital or medical records.
II. Health history.
   A. Age.
   B. Sex.
   C. Occupation.
III. Physical assessment.
   A. The blood pressure in the arms is higher than in the legs.
   B. Pulses in the lower extremities are diminished or absent.
   C. Patient complains of epistaxis, headaches, and leg pain with exercise.
   D. There are forceful arterial pulsations in the suprasternal notch.
   E. There may be extensive development of arm and shoulder muscles.
   F. A grade II ejection systolic murmur is present in left sternal border.
IV. Diagnostic tests.
   A. Electrocardiogram. In about 50 percent of cases, there is left ventricular hypertrophy.
   B. Chest x-rays show a dilated left subclavian artery high on the left mediastinal border. There is rib notching, secondary to intercostal artery dilation, and also left ventricular enlargement.
   C. Cardiac catheterization is helpful in ruling out other cardiac anomalies (patent ductus arteriosus, ventricular septal defect, and others). There is an abnormal pressure gradient across the coarctation.

PROBLEMS

I. Patient experiences severe headaches from the hypertension in upper extremities.

II. Patient suffers from anxiety over the increasing symptoms associated with this condition and its prognosis.

III. Coarctation of the aorta becomes progressively worse as an individual grows older. Because of the obstruction to the blood flow, increased pressure builds up proximal to the constriction. This is reflected in cerebral arteries and could cause cerebrovascular accidents and retinal hemorrhages. Because of the increased afterload which the pressure causes on the heart, it could also cause heart failure.

GOALS OF CARE

I. Restore normal circulation to prevent complications from increased blood pressure.

II. Reduce anxiety.

III. Reduce headaches.

INTERVENTION

I. Medical treatment: for heart failure, if present.

II. Surgical treatment: resection of the coarctation with an end-to-end anastomosis or with the use of a Dacron graft if the coarctate segment is long. Bacterial endocarditis is vented by prophylactic antibiotic therapy both pre- and postoperatively (see Fig. 26-1 showing coarctation of the aorta and its repair with a graft).

EVALUATION

I. Observe for postoperative complications in patients having surgery, such as hemothorax from bleeding from an artery, or abdominal pain from an increased blood flow to thin-walled mesenteric arterioles.

FIGURE 26-1 / (a) Coarctation of the aorta. (b) Repair of coarctation of the aorta.

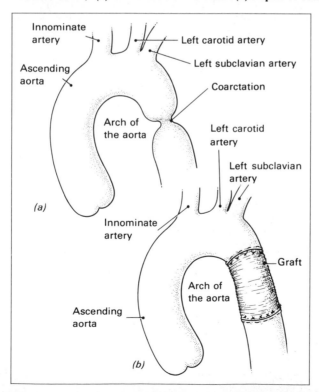

II. Observe for improvement in patients on medical therapy for heart failure.

III. Provide emotional support to the patient and family before and after surgery.

IV. Assess needs of family members and find resources to meet them.

Rheumatic Heart Disease and Heart Sounds

DEFINITION

Rheumatic heart disease is a cardiac disease which occurs as a sequel to an earlier episode of acute rheumatic fever. As a result of the streptococcal infection accompanying acute rheumatic fever, the acute inflammatory reaction may involve (1) the endocardium, including the valves, resulting in scarring, distortion, and stenosis; (2) the myocardium, where small areas of necrosis develop and heal, leaving scars; and (3) the pericardium, where there may be adhesions to surrounding tissues. The development of rheumatic heart disease in later life depends upon the severity of the damage.

ASSESSMENT

Data sources.

A. Patient's history of rheumatic fever (although there are some cases without this history).

B. Family.

C. Medical records showing previous episodes of rheumatic fever.

II. Physical assessment.

A. Symptoms of congestive heart failure include dyspnea, cough, and inappropriate tachypnea.

B. There is evidence of heart murmurs. In order to identify heart murmurs, one must have a basic knowledge of normal heart sounds:

    1. The first heart sound, S_1, corresponds with the closure of the mitral and tricuspid valves.

    2. The second heart sound, S_2, corresponds with the closure of the aortic and pulmonic valves. These two are the ones normally heard and sound like "lubb dup."

    3. Additional sounds which might be heard are:

        a. S_3, which corresponds with rapid ventricular filling in the first third of diastole.

        b. S_4, corresponds with ventricular filling in response to atrial contraction, in the last third of diastole.

C. When listening for sounds it is important first of all to identify S_1 and S_2. Systole occurs between them and diastole occurs between S_2 and the next S_1. Murmurs occurring during these periods are called either systolic or diastolic murmurs. These murmurs are related to valvular disorders and will be described under valvular heart disease. (See Fig. 26-2 for the relationship of the four heart sounds to the systole and diastole of one cardiac cycle.)

D. Locations on the chest where heart sounds are best heard are:

    1. Aortic area: second interspace, right of the sternum.

FIGURE 26-2 / Relationship of the four heart sounds to systole and diastole of one cardiac cycle. AVC, atrioventricular valvular closure (mitral and tricuspid valve); SVC, semilunar valvular closure (aortic and pulmonic valves); VF, ventricular filling; AC, atrial contraction, causing further ventricular filling.

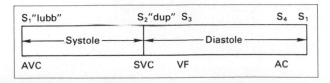

    2. Pulmonic area: second interspace, left of the sternum.

    3. Tricuspid area: fifth interspace, left of the sternum.

    4. Mitral area: fifth interspace, left midclavicular line.

    5. See Fig. 26-3 for these four locations where heart sounds are best heard.

III. Diagnostic tests.

    A. X-ray shows left atrial enlargement.

    B. Cardiac catheterization.

        1. Under local anesthesia and with fluoroscopic control, catheters are inserted in arteries and veins and passed through the great vessels into the heart chambers.

        2. Blood samples are then taken for evaluation and pressures are recorded.

        3. Following the catheterization, the patient must be observed for bleeding at the site of the catheter insertion.

        4. Blood pressures are not recorded from the extremity used for catheterization, and usually the patient is kept on bed rest for 24 h following the procedure.

        5. Pulses in the extremities are palpated frequently to assess for the presence of thrombi.

PROBLEMS

I. Valvular heart diseases are the main problems. Details about them are given below.

II. Congestive heart failure may occur as a result of valvular problems.

GOALS OF CARE

I. Avoid subsequent streptococcal infections and treat any that should occur with antibiotics.

II. Help the patient live within the limits imposed by the carditis.

III. Repair the valvular disorder by replacement, if possible.

FIGURE 26-3 / Locations on the chest wall where heart sounds are heard: aortic area, second interspace right of the sternum; pulmonic area, second interspace left of the sternum; tricuspid area, fifth interspace left of the sternum; mitral area, fifth interspace left of the midclavicular line.

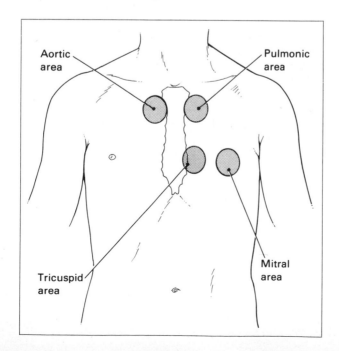

INTERVENTION

I. Medical treatment: Give therapy for congestive failure, if present.
II. Surgical treatment: Replace or repair the defective valve.
   A. Dissection of a constricted mitral valve by mitral commissurotomy.
   B. Valve replacement.

Valvular Heart Diseases

DEFINITION

Valvular diseases of the heart may develop from infections such as acute rheumatic fever, bacterial endocarditis, or syphilis, or from congenital malformation of the valves and rupture of the chordae tendineae. The damage may be perforation of the valve leaflets, stenosis, or insufficiency of the valves. These changes result in disturbances of blood flow. If stenosis is present, blood requires increased pressure to go through the valve; if insufficiency develops, blood goes in a reverse direction from normal flow. The heart valves most often affected are those in the left heart (mitral and aortic) because of the great pressure load as compared with the right heart.

ASSESSMENT

I. Data sources.
   A. Patient's past history of heart disease or an inflammatory process such as rheumatic fever.
   B. Family history of childhood diseases.
   C. Previous medical and hospital records giving information on previous infections, especially streptococcal infections.
II. Physical assessment and pathology related to the various valvular disorders.
   A. Mitral stenosis. The mitral valve thickens and leaflets fuse together. The opening narrows. The pressure increases in the left atrium and is reflected in the pulmonary vessels and the right ventricle. This may lead to right heart failure. Symptoms are:
      1. Excessive fatigue.
      2. Dyspnea, orthopnea, and paroxysmal nocturnal dyspnea.
      3. Cough and bronchitis.
      4. Peripheral edema from the right heart failure.
      5. On auscultation at the mitral area, a diastolic murmur is heard and a loud snapping first heart sound.
      6. Hemoptysis from the long-standing pulmonary hypertension.
      7. Atrial fibrillation develops in 50 to 80 percent of patients because of the left atrial enlargement. Thrombi may form, predisposing the patient to stroke if thrombi move as emboli through the arteries to the brain.
   B. Mitral insufficiency. There is scarring, thickening, shortening, and deformity of the cusps of the mitral valve with retraction of the free margins. As a result, there is incomplete closure of the mitral valve, allowing regurgitation of blood into the left atrium. Symptoms are:
      1. Fatigue.
      2. Dyspnea on exertion and orthopnea.
      3. Palpitations.
      4. Systolic thrill over the mitral area.
      5. An apical pansystolic murmur radiating into the axilla is heard. In addition, a third heart sound is heard over the mitral area.
      6. Atrial fibrillation may occur.
      7. Hemoptysis occurs less frequently than in mitral stenosis.
   C. Aortic stenosis. Valve cusps become stiff and calcified, causing a narrowed opening. Symptoms are:
      1. Fatigue may be the first symptom.
      2. Angina pectoris on exertion.
      3. Dyspnea on exertion.

    4. Syncope may occur after exertion or change of position because of inadequate blood to the brain.

    5. There is a harsh, rough midsystolic murmur over the aortic area with radiation to the carotid arteries.

    6. The pulse is slow and small in volume.

    7. Systolic blood pressure is normal, but the diastolic blood pressure is high (decreased pulse pressure).

    8. There is peripheral edema if right heart failure occurs.

    9. If left heart failure occurs, the prognosis is poor.

D. Aortic insufficiency. This condition results from scarring, retraction, and stiffening of the free borders of the leaflets. If the valve is very deformed and rigid, varying degrees of stenosis may be present also. The heart may become very large. This, in turn, can lead to mitral insufficiency.

    1. There is palpitation or throbbing of the chest, particularly when lying on the left side.

    2. Patient experiences dizziness, especially with abrupt changes of position.

    3. Dyspnea on exertion is a common symptom. It becomes progressively worse. There may be orthopnea, paroxysmal nocturnal dyspnea, and pulmonary edema.

    4. Fatigue.

    5. Angina pectoris may be related to the low diastolic pressure.

    6. A soft, blowing diastolic murmur may be heard, starting with the second heart sound (S_2). It is heard best over the aortic area and at the third interspace, to the left of the sternum.

    7. Bounding pulse (rapidly rising and collapsing), called "water-hammer" pulse.

    8. The blood pressure is high during systole and low during diastole (increased pulse pressure).

E. Tricuspid stenosis. The pathology is similar to that of mitral stenosis.

    1. Right-sided heart failure occurs, leading to hepatomegaly, dependent edema, ascites, extreme fatigue, jaundice, and cyanosis.

    2. There is a rumbling diastolic murmur, intensified with inspiration.

    3. A presystolic pulsation is present in the liver.

    4. Venae cavae may be markedly dilated. Jugular venous pressure is elevated.

F. Tricuspid insufficiency. Thickening, curling, and retraction of valve leaflets. It is more common than tricuspid stenosis. Symptoms are:

    1. Hepatomegaly.

    2. Distended jugular veins.

    3. Peripheral edema and jaundice.

    4. Holosystolic murmur, maximal at the left lower sternal border (tricuspid), and loudest during inspiration.

III. Diagnostic tests.

A. The chest x-ray shows an enlarged heart in most cases. If heart failure is also present, pulmonary congestion is also seen.

B. An echocardiogram (ultrasound) shows abnormal valve function.

C. Cardiac catheterization demonstrates abnormalities in pressures and direction of blood flow.

D. The electrocardiogram may be normal in mild cases. In severe cases, it shows hypertrophy of heart chambers, depending on which valve is involved.

E. The angiocardiogram involves the intravenous injection of a radiopaque solution to determine the circulation of blood. It is often done when cardiac catheterization is done. This technique demonstrates the location of the stenosis or insufficiency.

PROBLEMS

I. Increasing symptoms of cardiac problems result in eventual incapacitation.

II. Patient suffers from psychologic depression due to increasing symptoms.

III. Patient fears the possibility of cardiac surgery.

GOALS OF CARE

I. Prevent further valvular damage and/or replace defective valves.

II. Help patient live within the limitations imposed by the valvular damage.

III. Prevent and/or treat congestive heart failure which results from valvular diseases.

IV. Prevent further infections by giving prophylactic antibiotic therapy.

INTERVENTION

I. Medical treatment:

A. Administer antibiotic treatment to prevent recurrences of infections.

B. Treat the congestive heart failure, if present, with digitalis, sodium restriction, diuretics, and limitation of activity.

C. Provide psychological support.

D. Teach reasons for the therapy.

II. Surgical treatment: With the use of the heart-lung machine, surgery on the valves is possible. Through this means, the circulation of blood is diverted from the heart and lungs and gas exchange functions for the body are performed. Meanwhile, defective valves are replaced by artificial valves, and sewn in place.

A. Preoperative care:

1. Psychological preparation should include the following in an educational program: what the surgery entails, an orientation to the recovery room and the intensive care unit, and the equipment used following surgery. Encourage patient's discussion of fears.

2. Demonstrate and have patient practice deep breathing, range of motion, and coughing exercises.

3. Laboratory tests should include urine, blood electrolyte and enzyme studies, electrocardiogram, x-ray, echocardiogram, and cardiac catheterization.

4. Medications before surgery may include digitalis, diuretics, and antiarrhythmia drugs.

5. Patient is maintained on low-sodium diet.

6. Weigh patient daily for baseline measurements.

7. Monitor vital signs, including the apical-radial pulse.

B. Postoperative care:

1. Vital signs are checked frequently for any changes:

a. Blood pressure changes are monitored by the use of catheters threaded into arteries and veins and connected to monitors via energy tranducers.

b. Pulse rate and quality need careful, frequent, direct assessment by the nurse.

2. A cardiac monitor is used continuously to identify arrhythmias.

3. Level of consciousness is checked.

4. Pupils are examined for reaction to light or for their being unequal in size.

5. Patient must be observed for signs of cyanosis, which indicate severe hyponemia. Positive signs require immediate intervention.

6. Surgical dressings need to be checked for excessive drainage and bleeding, especially posteriorly.

7. The patient is elevated to a semi-Fowler's position to help chest drainage and lung reexpansion.

8. Oxygen is administered by ventilatory equipment, usually attached to a cuffed tracheotomy tube, so that respiration can be controlled.

9. Chest tubes and their connection to water seal drainage or Pleurevac equipment need to be cared for by milking or stripping to prevent the formation of clots. The amount of drainag in the collecting bottle needs to be measured carefully and recorded to observe for excess volume.

10. Urinary output is carefully recorded and monitored.

11. Help patient with deep breathing and coughing by splinting the chest.

12. Report any elevated temperatures over 101°F.

13. Parenteral fluids and blood transfusions are given carefully to avoid overloading the patient.

14. Laboratory studies are done frequently: These will include electrolytes, blood gases, hematocrit, hemoglobin, prothrombin time, and serum fibrinogen.
15. Daily weighing of the patient is done to assess fluid loss or retention.
16. Pain medication is given in small doses. This prevents overmedicating, and thus does not hinder the cough reflex.
17. Change the patient's position frequently, supporting dependent parts. Give passive range-of-motion exercises.
18. After the initial critical period is over, patient begins to ambulate in increasing amounts.
19. Provide psychological support to the patient and family.
20. Anticoagulant therapy is begun after insertion of prosthetic valves to lessen the possibility of thromboembolism.
21. Antibiotic therapy is used to prevent endocarditis or infected cardiotomy.

Hypertrophic Obstructive Cardiomyopathy (HOCM)

DEFINITION

This syndrome is characterized by hypertrophy of the left ventricle, involving the interventricular septum and the left ventricular outflow tract. During systole, the hypertrophied muscle in the outflow tract often narrows this region sufficiently to produce obstruction to left ventricular ejection. This condition is called various names: hypertrophic obstructive cardiomyopathy (HOCM), idiopathic hypertrophic subaortic stenosis (IHSS), and muscular subaortic stenosis (MSS). It differs from all forms of fixed obstruction in that it does not become manifest until after the early systolic ejection is underway. The severity of obstruction often varies from one beat to the next and from one phase of respiration to another.

ASSESSMENT

I. Data sources.
  A. Family history.
  B. Patient's history, including:
    1. Age when symptoms started.
    2. Discovery of a heart murmur.
    3. Abnormal electrocardiogram.
    4. Abnormal echocardiogram.
  C. Previous medical records showing diagnostic evidence of the disease.
II. Physical assessment.
  A. A jerky arterial pulse with sharp upstroke is typical. A bifid pulse may be felt, especially in the carotid artery. The initial peak results from an early unobstructed rapid ejection, and the later peak, from relief of dynamic outflow obstruction.
  B. A systolic murmur of variable intensity is present along the left sternal border and apex. The second heart sound is clearly audible.
  C. The patient's symptoms include:
    1. Exertional dyspnea.
    2. Angina pectoris.
    3. Dizziness and syncope.
    4. Fluid accumulation.
    5. Palpitations.
III. Diagnostic tests.
  A. The electrocardiogram shows signs of left ventricular hypertrophy and conduction defects such as Wolff-Parkinson-White syndrome, left anterior hemiblock and bundle branch block, and atrial and ventricular arrhythmias.
  B. A chest x-ray may not be helpful, and may be normal. Evidence of left ventricular enlargement may be subtle, since the cavity size is not increased.
  C. The echocardiogram is an important diagnostic tool. It will show the thickness of the interventricular septum and left ventricular posterior wall, and their movements during systole. It also helps in analyzing systolic motion of the mitral valve. Abnormal systolic anterior motion of the anterior mitral leaflet with its opposition against the septum localizes the outflow obstruction of HOCM.

D. Cardiac catheterization with angiocardiography: With obstruction, there is a systolic pressure difference between the lower ventricle and the chamber in the upper ventricle. This increased gradient between these pressures can be demonstrated by exercise, having patient perform the Valsalva maneuver, or by giving certain drugs (isoproterenol).

PROBLEMS
I. Disabling angina.
II. Fear of syncope.
III. Discomfort and concern over palpitations.
IV. Inability to participate in physical activity (more of a problem the younger the patient is).

GOALS OF CARE
I. Slow the heart rate to lessen obstruction and augment myocardial oxygen needs.
II. Prevent cardiac decompensation.
III. Use surgical intervention if palliative intervention is unsuccessful in relieving symptoms.
IV. Prevent bacterial endocarditis.

INTERVENTION[1]
I. Medical therapy:
  A. Give propranolol to slow the heart rate. It should be gradually increased and carefully monitored.
  B. Avoid giving digitalis, except for rapid atrial fibrillation when other drugs are unsuccessful.
  C. Nitrites are contraindicated.
  D. Use diuretics carefully so they do not cause hypovolemia.
  E. Administer anticoagulants if atrial fibrillation is present to prevent thrombi.
II. Surgical therapy involves incision of the muscular ridge obstructing the left ventricular outflow tract.
III. Prevent bacterial endocarditis, since the thickened septum or mitral valve may serve as a locus of infection.

EVALUATION
I. Evaluate the individual patient's response to propranolol. Is it slowing the heart rate without also causing decreased cardiac output?
II. Evaluate the effect of changes of body position on obstruction and the consequent symptoms.
III. Use surgery if treatment is unsuccessful.
IV. Evaluate the quality of pulse and the presence of abnormal heart sounds.

Congenital Conduction Defects

DEFINITION
Congenital conduction defect, in its strictest sense, refers to atrioventricular (AV) heart block which is present at birth. But, in a practical sense, it also refers to any AV heart block which is associated with congenital malformations of the heart in the absence of a history of other causative diseases, such as rheumatic fever or diphtheria. The conduction defect, if it occurs in several members of the family, suggests a genetic basis.

In congenital conduction defect there is disruption to the normal pathway by which impulses originate in the sinoatrial node and are transmitted through the heart. The most usual cause is related to the atrioventricular node and the bundle of His, in which impulses are hindered in being conducted or there are accessory pathways which bypass the atrioventricular node.

[1] Since the etiology of this syndrome is not fully understood, intervention is palliative.

ASSESSMENT

I. Data sources.
   A. Patient and patient's history.
   B. Family.
   C. Previous hospital and medical records showing evidence of conduction defects earlier in life.
II. Physical assessment: The conduction defects and associated arrhythmias may include:
   A. Bundle branch block.
   B. Complete heart block.
   C. Wolff-Parkinson-White syndrome (preexcitation syndrome).
   D. Atrial fibrillation.
   E. Junctional rhythm.
   F. Multifocal premature ventricular contractions.
III. Diagnostic tests.
   A. The electrocardiogram shows conduction defects and other arrhythmias stated above.
   B. Bundle of His recordings are obtained by threading a catheter into the large veins and inserting it into the right heart. As its tip is at the tricuspid valve, and a recording is done from the end of the catheter, the impulse transmission through the bundle of His can be determined.

PROBLEMS

I. Danger of fast-rate arrhythmias when accessory pathways are present.
II. Danger of slow-rate arrhythmias and/or sudden death when impulses fail to reach the ventricular myocardium.

GOALS OF CARE

I. Prevent and/or treat complications of conduction defects:
   A. Fast-rate arrhythmias.
   B. Slow-rate arrhythmias which might cause sudden death.

INTERVENTION

I. Antiarrhythmia drugs.
II. Inserting a permanent cardiac pacemaker for slow-rate arrhythmias in order to increase and control the heart rate.

EVALUATION

I. Evaluate the effect of drugs on the incidence and control of fast-rate arrhythmias.
II. Evaluate the effect of the permanent pacemaker on the heart rate and cardiac output.

Tumors of the Heart

DEFINITION

Cardiac tumors may arise from any tissue of the heart; 75 percent of these tumors are benign (1). Most of the malignant tumors are sarcomas. Primary tumors of the heart may occur at any age, but are rare in the young age group. Secondary tumors of the heart are more common than primary ones, but they infrequently cause clinical heart disease. The highest spread of metastases to the heart occurs from malignant melanoma, leukemia, and malignant lymphoma (2).

ASSESSMENT

I. Data sources.
   A. Family history of heart tumors.
   B. Patient and medical records:
      1. Evidence of malignant tumors elsewhere that might have metastasized.
      2. Symptoms of cardiac disease or diseases of other organs.

II. Physical assessment.
  A. Any tumor may cause signs and symptoms of endocarditis such as weight loss, fatigue, arthralgia, syncope, and fever.
  B. Assessment depends upon the location of the tumor in the heart.
    1. If the tumor is in the right atrium, it may obstruct the tricuspid valve, causing a delay in the closure of this valve. This delay in closure causes a wide splitting of the first heart sound (S_1) because the two components of S_1 do not close at the same time.
      a. Because of the reduced ventricular flow, there would be early pulmonic valvular closing. This would eliminate the normal physiologic splitting of S_2 on inspiration. In addition, there would be systolic or presystolic murmurs.
      b. The electrocardiogram may show a P-wave enlargement, right bundle branch block, or right ventricular hypertrophy.
      c. The chest x-ray will show a large right atrium and small right ventricle.
      d. Cardiac catheterization will show an increased right-sided pressure.
    2. If the tumor is in the left atrium, it may obstruct the mitral valve, causing mitral stenosis. There can be delay in the closure of the mitral valve due to the increase in right atrial volume and the obstructed outflow tract. There will be an accentuated apical first sound, as in mitral stenosis. The ventricular systole shortens because of decreased ventricular filling. This causes a premature closing of the aortic valve and a widely split second sound.
      a. A presystolic murmur is often heard due to atrial outflow obstruction.
      b. The electrocardiogram shows prominent P waves due to atrial enlargement, and the ventricular axis may be shifted to the right. All types of arrhythmias may be seen (3).
  C. Clinical features related to the location of the tumor.
    1. In right-sided tumor:
      a. Exertional dyspnea.
      b. Easy fatigability.
      c. Dusky skin.
      d. Osteoarthropathy.
      e. There will also be signs of right-sided failure:
        (1) Hepatomegaly.
        (2) Peripheral edema.
        (3) Distended jugular veins.
    2. In left-sided tumor:
      a. Progressive dyspnea.
      b. Orthopnea.
      c. Substernal discomfort.
      d. Palpitations.
      e. Intermittent edema.
      f. Hemoptysis.
      g. Evidence of peripheral emboli.
III. Diagnostic tests.
  A. Angiocardiography is the most accurate and precise diagnostic test to determine presence of tumor, although it has limitations in differentiating tumors from large thrombi.
  B. Echocardiography (ultrasound) is helpful in diagnosing tumors in valvular orifices.
  C. Cardiac catheterization is of limited use, other than for the purpose of angiography. It has the risk of dislodging tumor material.
  D. Phonocardiography. This procedure shows marked changes in the character or intensity of either systolic or diastolic murmurs with shifts in body position.

PROBLEMS
  I. Anxiety of patient and family over the implications of the diagnosis of a tumor.
  II. Need of early diagnosis so treatment can be provided.
  III. Constitutional disturbances which accompany tumors:
    A. Anorexia.
    B. Fever.
    C. Malaise.
    D. Cachexia.

GOALS OF CARE
I. Prevent consequences of a heart tumor:
   A. Pericardial tamponade or constriction.   D. Emboli.
   B. Obstruction of a heart chamber or valve.   E. Arrhythmias.
   C. Congestive heart failure.
II. Diagnose the tumor precisely since open-heart surgery may be needed.

INTERVENTION
I. Give x-ray therapy for cardiac metastases.
II. Cytotoxic drugs help to effect temporary regression of lesions.
III. Pericardiocentesis may be performed if tumor is in the pericardium.
IV. Open-heart surgery with cardiopulmonary bypass may be performed.

EVALUATION
I. Evaluate the efficacy of supportive therapy in diminishing symptoms.
II. Evaluate the effects of cardiac surgery on the patient.

HYPERACTIVITY AND HYPOACTIVITY

Papillary Muscle Dysfunction

DEFINITION
When the papillary muscle does not function correctly, especially on the left side of the heart, mitral insufficiency results. Normally, the papillary muscle contracts during systole to hold the mitral valve and the tricuspid valve in a closed position to prevent regurgitation of blood into the atria. When the muscle is ischemic or if the chordae tendineae attached between the muscle and the valve rupture, papillary muscle dysfunction results. When this occurs, prognosis is poor because circulation of blood is greatly altered each time the heart beats.

ASSESSMENT
I. Data sources: health history from patient and family.
II. Physical assessment.
   A. There is sudden onset of exertional dyspnea.
   B. There is sudden onset of a loud and harsh pansystolic murmur.
   C. Possibly, an S_3 and S_4 gallop may be present.
   D. Possibly, there may be no symptoms with an isolated chorda tendinea rupture.
III. Diagnostic tests.
   A. The electrocardiogram shows ST depression and T-wave changes.
   B. The x-ray shows systolic expansion of the left atrium.
   C. Left ventricular angiography shows reflux of the dye into pulmonary veins, indicating regurgitation of blood.
   D. Echocardiography shows mitral valve dysfunction.

PROBLEMS
I. There is sudden onset of symptoms of hemodynamic malfunctioning with deterioration of the clinical status.
II. The psychologic effects of the changing clinical status on the patient and family must be dealt with.
III. Careful observation of changing vital signs is essential because of deterioration of the clinical status.

GOALS OF CARE
I. An immediate goal is to prevent further deterioration, if possible. Surgery may be anticipated to accomplish this.
II. Correct the hemodynamic abnormalities through valve replacement.

INTERVENTION
Surgical replacement of the valve will be performed if the situation is acute. This, of course, requires open-heart surgery with the use of the cardiopulmonary bypass machine.

EVALUATION
I. Evaluate the postoperative course and revise plan according to the clinical status.
II. As soon as feasible, provide rehabilitation so the patient can resume normal activities.

Congestive Heart Failure

DEFINITION
Congestive heart failure is that condition in which the heart is unable to pump an adequate supply of blood to meet the oxygen and nutritional needs of the body. It may be due to:

1. Damage to heart muscle from myocardial infarction, trauma, or collagen diseases.
2. Inflow abnormalities such as fluid loss from dehydration or hemorrhage, or fluid overload from excessive IV fluids, or sodium and water retention.
3. Outflow of blood from the heart is hindered because of damaged valves.
4. Disturbances of rate, rhythm, and conduction.

The extent of the cardiac disability is directly related to the cardiac reserve the patient has. The cardiac reserve is the ability of the heart to adjust to increased demands placed upon it. When this ability is lost, symptoms of heart failure develop.

There are three main mechanisms by which the heart is able to compensate for the loss of cardiac reserve, as follows:

1. Ventricular dilatation refers to the lengthening of muscle fibers of the heart, thus increasing the volume of the heart chambers. According to Starling's law of the heart, the greater the stretch, the greater the contraction. This mechanism has its limitation, however. Beyond a certain point, added stretch no longer increases contractility.
2. Ventricular hypertrophy is the thickening of the muscle walls from the increasing diameter of muscle fibers. For a time, this compensatory mechanism increases cardiac output, but it, too, has its limitations.
3. Tachycardia, the increase in heart rate, is the least effective mechanism of the three. When the rate becomes excessively rapid, this mechanism defeats its purpose, for the filling time between contractions is greatly shortened and this in itself decreases cardiac output.

Compensation exists when these mechanisms are adequate to maintain a cardiac output and there are no symptoms of failure. When, however, the heart is unable to maintain an adequate cardiac output and symptoms develop, decompensation is said to exist.

Forms of heart failure   The heart consists of two separate but related pumping systems: the right heart, which is the pump for the pulmonary circulation; and the left heart, which is the pump for the systemic circulation. Heart failure may involve the left heart, the right heart, or both.

Left-sided heart failure   This situation almost always results from damage to the myocardium of the left ventricle. This damage causes a decrease in the pumping ability of the left ventricle, which results in its failure to eject its full quota of blood when the heart contracts. As more blood enters the left ventricle, it meets resistance from this remaining blood. This causes the left atrium to increase its pressure to overcome this resistance. In turn, this increased pressure is reflected in the pulmonary veins and capillaries. These congested pulmonary vessels impede the exchange of oxygen and carbon dioxide across the walls of the alveoli of the lungs and the capillaries. As the situation continues, fluid from the capillaries is forced by the increased pressure into the alveoli of the lungs.

Right-sided heart failure This is often a sequel to left-sided heart failure, for the increased pressure in the pulmonary vascular system causes the right ventricle to dilate and hypertrophy to meet the increased work load. Right-sided heart failure may also occur when pulmonary diseases are present which put an added burden on the right ventricle. When the right ventricle fails, it no longer ejects its normal quota of blood volume and some remains after contraction. The residual volume now impedes blood flow from the right atrium, which has to increase its pressure to exceed the pressure in the right ventricle in order to empty blood into it. This then creates a backward pressure throughout the entire peripheral venous system.

ASSESSMENT
I. Data sources.
   A. Health history.
      1. Determine the patient's usual physical activities.
      2. Note patient's health habits—types of food eaten, medications taken, sleep pattern, ingestion of alcohol, coffee, etc.
      3. Pay especial attention to the history of previous illnesses or concurrent illnesses, such as hypertension, diabetes, myocardial infarction, or valvular disease.
   B. Determine what kind of support family members give patient and what the family understands about patient's condition.
   C. Previous medical and hospital records will give data about illnesses and therapy for them.
II. Physical assessment.
   A. Left-sided heart failure. The following symptoms develop because of congestion in the lungs from the back pressure from the left side of the heart.
      1. Dyspnea (shortness of breath) may be the earliest symptom of left-sided failure. At first, it may occur only on exertion. Later, it becomes more apparent.
      2. Orthopnea. If dyspnea occurs when the patient is recumbent and is relieved when the patient sits upright, this condition is called orthopnea.
      3. Paroxysmal nocturnal dyspnea. Sudden dyspnea occurs when the patient is asleep. Patient awakens, feels suffocated, and is usually coughing and wheezing. He or she often is relieved on sitting upright in bed or opening the window.
      4. Acute pulmonary edema. This is the most extreme form of left-sided heart failure. Massive accumulation of fluid occurs in the alveoli of the lungs which greatly interferes with gaseous exchange and results in hypoxia. Unless it is corrected immediately, this leads to death from severe hypoxia and arrhythmias.
      5. As cardiac output from the left ventricle falls, arterial pressure in the kidneys decreases. The body compensates for what it senses as low blood volume by increasing enzymes which retain sodium and water. This serves to increase venous return to the heart, and increases the work load of the heart.
      6. Cerebral anoxia. When the left ventricle fails and cardiac output is decreased, the amount of oxygen going to the brain is decreased. This causes irritability and confusion. For some reason, this seems to happen at night more than during the daytime. The nurse needs to consider congestive heart failure when this symptom is noted.
      7. Fatigue and muscular weakness. Another effect of a low cardiac output is profound exhaustion. Oxygen to the tissues is diminished and removal of metabolic wastes is delayed.
      8. Physical signs to watch for are:
         a. Rales. On auscultation of the bases of the lungs, one can detect abnormal breath sounds which reflect the presence of fluid in the alveoli. As the situation worsens, rales are heard higher in the lung fields. Therefore, the height of where rales are heard in the chest is indicative of the extent of heart failure.
         b. Gallop rhythm. By auscultation of heart sounds, a triple rhythm can be heard which consists of S_1, S_2, and S_3. The third heart sound is abnormal in the

adult and indicates dilatation of the left ventricle with an increase of fluid volume entering it.

B. Right-sided heart failure. When the right side of the heart fails, the symptoms relate to the retention of sodium and water within the body which causes edema and venous congestion within the organs.

1. Distended neck veins are due to increased venous pressure. Normally, neck veins do not remain distended when a patient is sitting at an angle of 45°. In the right-sided heart failure patient, however, the neck veins remain distended at this angle because of the increased back pressure from the right atrium. This may be one of the earliest signs of right-sided heart failure.

2. Peripheral edema is caused by the increased pressure in the venous circulation which forces fluid from the capillaries into interstitial spaces. The nurse needs to look for edema in dependent parts of the body, such as the ankles if the patient is sitting in a chair, or in the sacrum if the patient remains in bed. If edema is generalized and found throughout the body, the term *anasarca* is used.

3. Weight gain corresponds to the fluid retention mentioned above. Weighing the patient is a far more precise measurement of fluid retention than observing for edema, for a person can accumulate up to 10 lb of fluid before it is obvious as edema.

4. Liver enlargement and abdominal pain. As the liver becomes congested with fluid, it enlarges and stretches the capsule surrounding it. This causes tenderness in the abdomen and is often accompanied by anorexia and nausea. When pressure is applied over an engorged liver, neck veins distend. This phenomenon is called *hepatojugular reflux*.

5. Coolness of the extremities is due to the reduction of peripheral blood flow.

6. Anxiety and fear. Patients realize that their heart is diseased and know the significance of this. They may have nightmares, become very depressed, or withdraw from reality and use denial as their coping mechanism.

III. Diagnostic tests.

A. The electrocardiogram shows an enlarged heart and tachycardia.

B. The chest x-ray shows an enlarged heart and pulmonary involvement if there is pulmonary edema.

C. There is an S_3 gallop on auscultation.

D. Rales are present at the lung bases.

E. Venous pressure is elevated.

F. *Pulsus alternans.* The strength of the heartbeat varies from beat to beat, depending on the stroke volume for each beat.

G. Arm-to-tongue circulation time is prolonged. A substance injected in the arm is timed until it is tasted by the patient. This is not a sensitive test and is not used often.

H. Albuminuria is present.

I. Blood urea nitrogen (BUN) level is elevated.

PROBLEMS

I. Patient experiences severe anxiety because of fear and difficulty in breathing.

II. There is an imbalance between oxygen needs and the oxygen supply.

III. Overloading of the circulation puts a burden on a diseased heart which cannot pump adequately.

IV. Lowered perfusion of the tissues and organs causes confusion and irritability because of cerebral ischemia and fatigue, and muscular weakness from lack of circulation to skeletal muscles.

V. Exchange of gases through alveoli walls is impeded, causing low oxygen in the circulating blood.

GOALS OF CARE

I. Immediate.

A. Obtain the cooperation of the patient and family in following a plan of care.

B. Improve the contractility of the heart to meet the demands of the body.

C. Decrease the work of the heart.

D. Supply oxygen and improve nutrition to the heart muscle and body tissues.

E. Identify and alleviate untoward effects of therapy.

II. Long-range.

A. Encourage the patient and family to adopt a life-style that will be within the limits of the heart condition.

B. Rehabilitate the patient to as full a life as is possible.

C. Teach the patient about the caloric expenditures of activities and their relationship with emotions.

D. Instruct the patient in the reasons for medications and diet.

E. Make certain the patient knows the symptoms which need to be reported to the physician and understands the necessity of regular checkups.

INTERVENTION

I. General intervention for congestive heart failure.

A. To improve contractility of the heart by use of digitalis preparations.

1. Positive effects of digitalis preparations:

   a. They increase cardiac output by enhancing the force of myocardial contraction.

   b. They slow the heart by vagal stimulation.

   c. They decrease the size of the heart because of improved contractility.

2. Toxic effects of digitalis preparations:

   a. Cardiovascular system.

   (1) Arrhythmias: bigeminy, paroxysmal atrial tachycardia with block, and atrioventricular block.

   (2) Watch for any change in heart rate, particularly rates below 60 per minute.

   b. Gastrointestinal system.

   (1) Anorexia, nausea, vomiting, diarrhea.

   (2) Depletion of potassium, especially when the patient is also on diuretics.

   c. Central nervous system.

   (1) Visual disturbances.

   (2) Headache, lethargy, confusion, neuralgia.

   d. If there are symptoms of digitalis toxicity, report them to the physician before giving further digitalis.

3. Digitalis preparations (4):

	Digitalizing Dose	*Maintenance Dose*
Digoxin	2–4 mg	0.25–0.75 mg
Digitoxin	1.0–1.5 mg	0.50–0.2 mg
Digitalis leaf	1.5 g	100–200 mg

B. To increase the work of the heart through reducing blood volume returning to the heart by use of the following drugs:

1. Morphine. Helps to relieve anxiety, especially when dyspnea is present in left-sided failure. It also causes some peripheral venous dilatation, thus relieving the heart of some fluid load. Be sure that the patient's pulse rate and respiratory rate are not slow when giving morphine. Do not give this drug if these conditions exist, for morphine will further decrease them.

2. Diuretics.

   a. Interfere with the reabsorption of sodium by the kidneys, thus aiding them in excreting fluid from the body.

      b. Electrolyte and kidney function may be disturbed when diuretics are used; therefore patient must be observed for abnormalities in the laboratory reports of electrolytes, pH, and BUN.

      c. Diuretics include the following:

        (1) Thiazide diuretics:

          (a) Chlorothiazide (Diuril).

          (b) Hydrochlorothiazide (HydroDiuril).

        (2) Furosemide (Lasix). Rapid-acting when given intravenously. May also be given orally.

        (3) Ethacrynic acid (Edecrin). Rapid-acting when given intravenously. May also be given orally.

        (4) Aldosterone antagonists: spironolactone (Aldactone).

        (5) Triamterene (Dyrenium).

   3. Record the weight daily to determine the effectiveness of the diuretic therapy in excreting fluid. The body weight should decrease as the fluid is excreted.

   4. Sodium-restricted diet.

      a. This diet is used primarily for the prevention, control, and elimination of edema. To make this goal more effective, fluid restriction should also be observed.

      b. The nurse can help make low-sodium diets more palatable by suggesting various seasonings, such as lemon juice, lime juice, mint, dill, and onion.

      c. Salt substitutes are also available if the physician agrees.

      d. If sodium becomes extremely low, the patient may develop low-salt syndrome as manifested by the following symptoms: weakness, nausea, and vomiting.

C. To decrease the work of the heart through rest. Rest is one of the most effective means of diminishing the cardiac work load. Therefore, limiting physical activity by bed rest or chair rest is basic to the intervention. Complete bed rest is undesirable, however, because of the hazards associated with immobility. Patients ar therefore urged to use a bedside commode, feed themselves, and participate to some extent in bathing themselves. As the patient improves in clinical status, activities gradually increase.

D. To improve oxygenation of body tissues, use oxygen therapy. As a result, dyspnea is greatly relieved. Oxygen may be given by means of nasal cannulas or masks.

E. To rehabilitate the patient and family to achieve the long-term goals:

   1. Assist the patient and family to make changes in their life-style. This will require their full cooperation in the plan of care.

   2. Be sure the patient has adequate knowledge concerning the disease.

   3. Motivate and encourage the patient who seems discouraged and hopeless about the future.

   4. Assist patients with little financial resources to learn how to prepare low-sodium diets without spending excessive amounts of money for food.

II. Intervention for acute pulmonary edema. Acute pulmonary edema is an extreme form of left-sided heart failure. Fluid seeps from the pulmonary capillaries across the interstitial spaces into the alveoli of the lungs. Severe dyspnea, tachycardia, pallor, frothy red-tinged sputum, wheezing, sweating, bubbling respirations, and cyanosis make up the picture. Treatment for this emergency situation includes:

A. Place the patient in a high Fowler's position to improve respirations by lowering the diaphragm and allowing lungs to expand.

B. Give morphine, 10 to 15 mg, either intramuscularly or intravenously for urgent situations.

C. Give oxygen by intermittent positive pressure equipment with a tight-fitting mask and with humidification. An antifoaming agent such as 30 percent alcohol for humidification helps to reduce pulmonary secretions.

D. Digitalization with rapid-acting digitalis drugs is needed to increase contractility of the left ventricle. These drugs are given intravenously. (See Table 26-1 for rapid-acting digitalis preparations, their dosage, and time of action.)

TABLE 26-1 / RAPID-ACTING DIGITALIS PREPARATIONS

	Initial Dose, mg IV	Average Onset of Action, min	Subsequent Doses
Digoxin	0.5	15	0.25 mg every 2–4 h until a total dose no greater than 1.5 mg is reached
Lanatoside C (Cedilanid)	0.8	10	0.4 mg every 2–4 h until a total dose no greater than 2.0 mg is reached
Ouabain	0.20	5	0.1 mg every hour until a total dose no greater than 1.0 mg is reached

Source: L. Meltzer, R. Pinneo, and J. Kitchell, Intensive Coronary Care: A Manual for Nurses, 3d ed., Charles Press, Brady Co., Bowie, Md., 1977, p. 82. Used by permission of the publisher.

E. Diuresis by rapid-acting diuretics helps to relieve the fluid overload, which is excreted via the kidneys. The most frequently used are:
1. Furosemide (Lasix) 40 to 80 mg IV push.
2. Ethacrynic acid (Edcrin) 50 mg IV push.
3. When giving these drugs, watch for potassium depletion. Potassium replacement is usually needed (5).

F. Aminophylline will relieve the bronchospasm which interferes with ventilation. It is given in a dosage of 250 to 500 mg diluted in 50 mL IV fluid over a 15-min period. If it is given rapidly, it can cause hypotension and arrhythmias. Aminophylline can also be given by rectal suppositories in dosages of 500 mg.

G. Reduction of blood volume can be accomplished by:
1. Rotating tourniquets. These trap blood in extremities, thereby reducing venous return to the heart. Rotating tourniquets are not used frequently today because rapid-acting drug therapy is usually effective.
   a. If they are to be used, apply tourniquets or blood pressure cuffs on four extremities (except for those attached to IV fluids), and tighten three of the four only enough to occlude venous return and not occlude arterial blood flow. Take the pulse distal to the tourniquet to make sure of this.
   b. Prepare a diagram so that the clockwise rotation of tourniquets will continue every 15 min.
   c. Loosen and tighten a tourniquet on an extremity, making sure of a distal pulse each time, and note on the diagram which tourniquets you worked with.
   d. When terminating, loosen only one tourniquet at a time to prevent sudden increases of circulating blood to the heart. (See Fig. 26-4 for the rotation of tourniquets.)
2. Phlebotomy. By removing 500 to 700 mL of blood, circulating blood volume can also be reduced. This method is reserved only for those cases in which other measures have failed and is seldom used. It has the danger of causing hypotension and shock.

EVALUATION
I. Observe the vital signs frequently to assess changes.
II. Monitor the heart for arrhythmias and give antiarrhythmia therapy if needed.
III. Examine the patient frequently to detect improvement of signs or symptoms of heart failure. Weighing the patient the same time each day is a valuable index of response to therapy.

IV. Watch for signs of side effects of drug therapy or low-salt syndrome.
V. Observe the results of laboratory data.
VI. Help the patient understand the reasons for the treatment program.
VII. As the patient improves, the level of activities needs to be evaluated. In 1964, the New York Heart Association developed a functional and therapeutic classification of patients with heart disease. However, these classifications have been replaced by a new classification of the patient's overall cardiac status which is based on the improved precision of modern diagnostic techniques and therapies, and on the symptoms presented by the patient (6).

Pulmonary Heart Disease

DEFINITION
Hypertrophy of the right ventricle results from certain diseases affecting the function and or structure of the lungs. The common factor preceding right ventricular hypertrophy is pulmonary hypertension. There are four factors which increase the work of the heart or affect the myocardium: (1) alveolar hypoventilation, (2) reduction in the pulmonary vascular bed, (3) intrapulmonary vascular shunts, and (4) myocardial factors (7).

ASSESSMENT
I. Data sources.
   A. Patient complains of increasing dyspnea, gradually restricted activities, and has a history of repeated respiratory infections.
   B. Family.

FIGURE 26-4 / Rotation of tourniquets (*Adapted from Joan Luckmann and Karen Sorenson, Medical-Surgical Nursing: A Psychophysiologic Approach, W. B. Saunders Company, Philadelphia, 1974, p. 642.*)

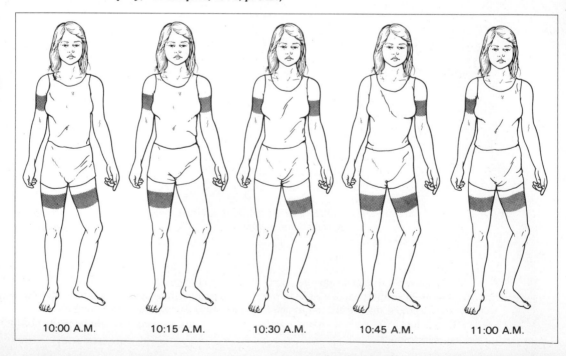

| 10:00 A.M. | 10:15 A.M. | 10:30 A.M. | 10:45 A.M. | 11:00 A.M. |

II. Physical assessment.
  A. Dyspnea is slowly progressive.
  B. Activities are gradually restricted.
  C. Ankle edema is present.
  D. There are frequent respiratory infections.
  E. Patient assumes an upright position with arms braced on supports, a position which aids breathing.
  F. Patient has a chronic productive cough.
  G. Patient has a thin, cyanotic appearance and a barrel chest. Other symptoms may be an immobile diaphragm, increased chest resonance, prolonged expiratory phase, expiratory rales, and rhonchi.
  H. Heart sounds are faint.
  I. Tachycardia of 90 to 110 heart rate per min is present.
III. Diagnostic tests.
  A. Hematocrit is elevated.
  B. Chest x-ray shows contour changes of the pulmonary artery and vascular changes in the lung fields with severe pulmonary hypertension.
  C. Cardiac catheterization helps to differentiate pulmonary heart disease from other conditions such as pulmonary emboli.
  D. The electrocardiogram shows right ventricular hypertrophy.

PROBLEMS
  I. Increasing dyspnea.
  II. Limitation of activities.
  III. Repeated respiratory infections.
  IV. Right-sided heart failure with peripheral edema.
  V. Emotional depression from increasing disability.

GOALS OF CARE
  I. Immediate.
    A. For the acute respiratory stage, improve ventilation so that dyspnea is relieved.
    B. Increase myocardial contractility to relieve the symptoms of right-sided heart failure.
  II. Long-range.
    A. Teach the patient how to live within the limitations of the disease.
    B. Teach patient the purposes of therapy.

INTERVENTION
  I. Promote rest and relaxation.
  II. Give carefully controlled low concentrations (25 percent) of oxygen for acute care (some patients need respirator assistance).
  III. Give oral bronchodilators (ephedrine and aminophylline) for acute shortness of breath.
  IV. Administer antibiotics for respiratory infections (tetracycline).
  V. Individualize exercise programs to maintain muscle strength according to the level of oxygen saturation.
  VI. If peripheral edema is present, use diuretics to promote fluid excretion and decrease the load on the heart.
  VII. Education should have as its goal to teach the patient how to control the disease.

EVALUATION
  I. Evaluate the patient's level of activities. If no symptoms occur, increase activities slowly. If symptoms do occur, decrease intensity of activities and increase their frequency, allowing for rest periods between.
  II. Evaluate drug therapy. Are antibiotics controlling infections? Are diuretics controlling peripheral edema? Change plans of intervention according to these evaluations.
  III. Evaluate the patient's emotional responses to the disease and provide psychological support.

Cardiogenic Shock

DEFINITION
The damaged heart is unable to function adequately as a pump and deliver sufficient oxygen and nutrients to the tissues of the body. Unless adequate perfusion is restored, the body cells deteriorate and die. Once the vital organs are destroyed, the situation is irreversible and treatment is of no avail. Mortality rate is 80 percent. (See Table 26-2 to follow the sequence of steps in the mechanism of cardiogenic shock. The arrows indicate the effect of one factor on another.)

ASSESSMENT
I. Data sources.
   A. Patient.
   B. Family.
   C. Medical records.
II. Physical assessment.
   A. Hypotension.
      1. The systolic blood pressure falls below 90 mmHg. This alone does not warrant calling the situation cardiogenic shock, however.
      2. The systolic blood pressure falls before diastolic pressure falls.
   B. Mental apathy and lethargy reflect lack of cerebral perfusion.
   C. Skin is cold and moist because of peripheral vasoconstriction.
   D. There is oliguria from diminished renal blood flow. Usually, urinary output is at least 1 mL/min; in cardiogenic shock, the urinary output falls below 20 mL/h, or it may cease completely (anuria).
   E. Pallor or cyanosis is present.
   F. Pulse is feeble and rapid.
III. Diagnostic tests.
   A. Arterial blood gases: There will be a low P_{O_2} and low pH (because of acidosis).
   B. Chest x-ray.
   C. An electrocardiogram will indicate if an acute myocardial infarction might have occurred and also indicate the presence of arrhythmias.

TABLE 26-2 / MECHANISM OF CARDIOGENIC SHOCK

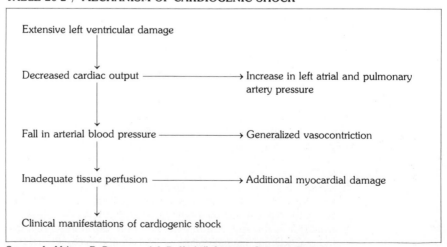

Source: L. Meltzer, R. Pinneo, and J. R. Kitchell, Intensive Coronary Care: A Manual for Nurses, 3d ed., Charles Press, Brady Co., Bowie, Md., 1977, p. 91. Used by permission of the publisher.

    D. Pulmonary artery pressures: These will show whether the left ventricular end diastolic pressure is elevated above 12 mmHg. If so, there is diminished left ventricular function.

PROBLEMS

   I. Low cardiac output and low tissue perfusion require continuous assessment of changes in vital signs and in the sensorium of the patient.

  II. An acutely ill patient needs help to compensate for the pump failure. If treatment is not successful, irreversible shock will occur.

GOALS OF CARE

Improve cardiac output without causing an extra burden on the heart so that there will be an improvement in tissue perfusion throughout the body.

INTERVENTION

   I. Supportive treatment:

    A. Give oxygen therapy by tight-fitting mask or with the use of assisted respiratory devices.

    B. Relieve chest pain from reduced coronary blood flow with small doses of morphine.

    C. Correct the metabolic acidosis with the use of sodium bicarbonate.

  II. Specific treatment:

    A. Give intravenous fluids to expand the plasma volume. Solutions, such as albumin, whole blood, or low-molecular-weight dextran improve the blood pressure and urinary output.

    B. Give inotropic drugs to improve myocardial contractility, even though these may cause oxygen deprivation. Drugs to be used are: Levophed, dopamine, Isuprel, glucagon, and digitalis. These drugs need to be tried and evaluated for each individual patient. Watch for infiltration of Levophed, for tissue necrosis can result.

    C. Vasodilator drugs may be used to combat the vasoconstriction. Because these drugs tend to lower the blood pressure, they should only be used for systolic blood pressures above 100 mmHg. Two drugs used for this purpose are sodium nitroprusside and phentolamine.

    D. Regulation of the heart rate. Giving therapy for heart rates either too slow or too fast will help achieve a more adequate cardiac output.

  III. Mechanical assistance of the circulation:

    A. By using an intraaortic balloon pump, the heart can be assisted.

    B. During diastole, the balloon is inflated, which increases pressure in the coronary arteries.

    C. During systole, the balloon is deflated so that the left ventricle does not have to pump against a pressure load. (See Fig. 26-5 for a diagram of the placement of the aortic balloon catheter in the femoral artery and the threading of it to the descending aorta. There the balloon is inflated in synchrony with the cardiac cycle as explained above.)

EVALUATION

   I. Basic physiologic measurements need to be evaluated in order to continue or alter a treatment program. These measurements include:

    A. Arterial blood pressure as determined by means of an intraarterial catheter. This is far more accurate than blood pressures determined externally.

    B. Arterial blood gases need to be determined frequently. Therefore, if an intraarterial catheter is in place, blood samples can be collected and blood studied for P_{O_2} and pH; otherwise, an arterial puncture must be done each time.

    C. Urinary output must be carefully measured every 30 min to 1 h in order to assess kidney function in excreting urine. An indwelling catheter is needed for this purpose.

    D. Monitoring the patient with the use of a pulmonary artery catheter (Swan-Ganz). This is an effective means of evaluating the performance of the left ventricle.

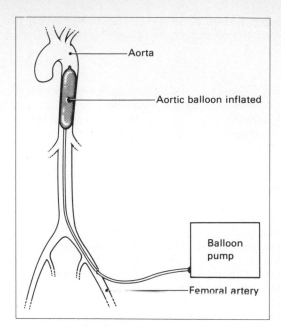

FIGURE 26-5 / Aortic balloon.

1. A double lumen tube is threaded through the large veins into the right side of the heart.
2. A balloon on the outside of the tube is inflated to help its passage to the pulmonary artery.
3. Pressure (called wedge pressure) is determined and then the balloon is deflated.
4. The catheter is left in place for further monitoring.
5. When the pulmonary catheter wedge pressure increases, it reflects reduced left ventricular emptying. Normal pressure is considered to be 5 to 12 mmHg. (See Fig. 26-6 for a diagram of the insertion of a Swan-Ganz catheter into the pulmonary artery.)

II. Evaluate the quality of pulses at the radius, carotid, and femoral arteries. In addition, listen for abnormal heart sounds at the apex and compare the apical heart rate with the peripheral pulse rate.

III. Evaluate the sensorium. It is expected that as the patient improves, mental status improves also.

Emotional Stress and Cardiovascular Diseases

DEFINITION
The relation between emotions and cardiovascular function has led to studies which have demonstrated (1) a specific type of personality frequently associated with a specific disease, (2) a correlation between emotional stress or events in the past and the onset or aggravation of a specific disease, (3) a different physiological or biochemical reaction in persons with a specific disease to experimental emotional stress, and (4) the development of a specific disorder in animals in response to experimental stress (8).

ASSESSMENT
I. Data sources.
   A. Health history: Identify the relationship of past stress to disease.
   B. Family history of diseases associated with emotional stress (gastric ulcers, hypertension, myocardial infarction, etc.).

II. Physical and behavioral assessment.
  A. Palpitations, blushing, pallor, and fainting are related to stimulation of the sympathetic nervous system.
  B. Increased blood pressure, pulse rate, or circulatory collapse with a decrease in heart rate and profound fall in blood pressure (called vasovagal response).
III. Diagnostic tests.
  A. Increased blood pressure during stress (closely correlated with increased blood pressure in sustained hypertension).
  B. Identify type A personality and recognize it as a risk factor. Characteristics of type A personality are:
    1. Aggressiveness.   **4.** Work-oriented attitude.
    2. Ambitiousness.   **5.** Chronic impatience.
    3. Competitiveness.   **6.** Preoccupation with deadlines.
  C. Increased serum cholesterol levels at the time of emotional stress.
  D. Attacks of angina during stress.
  E. Palpitations and tachycardia are effects of emotional stress.
  F. Left ventricular failure of pulmonary edema may be precipitated by emotions.
  G. Electrocardiographic changes occur during stress: inversion of T waves.

PROBLEMS
  I. Increased sympathetic stimulation with symptoms stated above occurs.
  II. Circulatory collapse and fainting result from fall in cardiac output.
  III. Congestive heart failure is often precipitated by acute emotional stress, especially in patients already having some form of heart disease.

GOALS OF CARE
  I. Immediate: Relieve the stress through medication and nursing care so that the cardiovascular disease does not progress further.
  II. Long-range: Teach patients how to cope with stressful situations, and how to avoid unnecessary stress, especially if they already have cardiac diseases.

FIGURE 26-6 / Insertion of a Swan-Ganz catheter through the right side of the heart to the pulmonary artery.

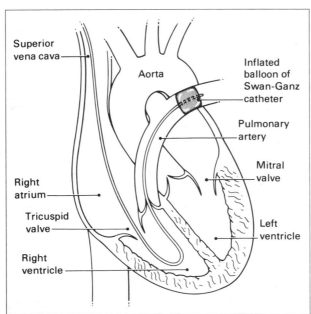

INTERVENTION

I. Reassure the patient.

II. Make an attempt to identify factors which produce stress in the patient's life; then suggest alterations which can make them more bearable. This may mean a vacation, change of scene, or regular program of physical activity, etc.

III. Drugs such as sedatives and tranquilizers may be helpful in relieving anxiety associated with stress.

IV. Teach patients how to cope with stress and how to avoid unnecessary stress.

EVALUATION

I. Evaluate the approach best suited to the individual patient.

II. Change plan of care according to the evaluation. Then, reevaluate.

Hyperkinetic Heart Syndrome (High Cardiac Output State)

DEFINITION

Hyperkinetic heart syndrome is an increased rate of ejection of blood with each heartbeat.

ASSESSMENT

I. Data sources.
   A. Age of patient: this syndrome usually occurs in young persons.
   B. Patient's statements about symptoms and their relation to factors such as exercise or rest.
   C. Patient's family.

II. Physical assessment.
   A. Peripheral arterial pulsations rise quickly, fall in volume, and collapse.
   B. Apical rate is fast.
   C. Blood pressure is elevated.
   D. Precordium is overactive with ventricular lifts and a loud first heart sound.
   E. A harsh systolic murmur is heard in the third or fourth interspaces and over the carotid arteries (9).
   F. Palpitations are present.

III. Diagnostic tests.
   A. Phonocardiogram (intracardiac): The murmur is seen to originate in both the outflow tracts but is loudest in the outflow tract of the left ventricle.
   B. The chest x-ray will show left ventricular hypertrophy in 50 percent of patients.
   C. Electrocardiogram shows evidence of left ventricular enlargement in many cases.

PROBLEMS

I. Possibility of congestive heart failure if condition continues.

II. Discomfort from cardiac palpitations and awareness of the heart beat.

III. Anxiety.

GOALS OF CARE

I. Reduce frequency of symptoms.

II. Provide psychological support to reduce anxiety.

III. Prevent the condition from worsening to congestive heart failure.

INTERVENTION

I. Propranolol can be beneficial because of its beta-adrenergic blocking action

II. Guanethidine is helpful, for it interferes with the actions of the adrenergic nervous system by depleting postganglionic stores of catecholamine (10).

EVALUATION
I. Compare frequency of symptoms before and after intervention.
II. Evaluate beginning signs and symptoms of congestive heart failure.
III. Evaluate presence of anxiety.
IV. Evaluate presence of abnormal heart sounds.

Pregnancy and Heart Disease

DEFINITION
The heart rate in pregnancy begins to rise between the eighth and tenth weeks. This totals 14,000 more beats per day. Oxygen consumption rises about the second month. Cardiac output in pregnancy increases 30 to 50 percent above the nonpregnant level. Blood volume increases during pregnancy. The electrocardiogram shows left axis deviation because the heart is displacd upward, forward, and laterally.

It is easy to see that the increase in cardiac output during pregnancy can cause problems in a woman with heart disease. The most usual form of heart disease in women of childbearing age is of rheumatic origin, causing mitral stenosis.

ASSESSMENT
I. Data sources.
   A. Patient and husband.
   B. Medical records showing history of heart disease.
   C. Family.
II. Physical assessment.
   A. A diastolic murmur may be present.
   B. X-ray may show cardiac enlargement.
   C. A systolic murmur of grade III or greater is present.
   D. The presence of a severe arrhythmia or conduction defect, atrial fibrillation, atrial flutter, or complete heart block are indicative of heart disease.
III. Diagnostic tests.
   A. Phonocardiogram to determine the presence of systolic and diastolic murmurs.
   B. X-ray to show cardiac enlargement.
   C. Electrocardiogram to show arrhythmias, cardiac enlargement, and axis deviation.

PROBLEMS
I. As pregnancy continues, the burden on the heart increases. With heart disease already present, complications such as congestive heart failure may occur.
II. Anxiety of patient and family over the patient and baby.

GOALS OF CARE
I. Assist the patient to go to term without increasing heart problems.
II. Provide psychological support to patient and family throughout pregnancy.
III. Reduce cardiac demands to levels of tolerance within the patient's cardiac capacity.

INTERVENTION
I. Most patients can go to term. Therapeutic abortions can lead to guilt and may affect later life more than the continuation of the pregnancy.
II. Medications:
   A. Digitalis.
   B. Diuretics.
   C. Sedatives.
III. Low-sodium diet.

IV. General:
  A. Patients should get extra bed rest for 2 to 3 h in the afternoon and at least 8 h sleep at night.
  B. Those in class 3 or 4 in the hospital should be on complete bed rest.
  C. All patients with a history of cardiac decompensation should be hospitalized at first and then kept on complete bed rest at home.
  D. Restrict physical activity according to individual needs.
  E. Avoid crowds and chilling to decrease the possibility of infections.

EVALUATION

I. Evaluate side effects of diuretic and digitalis therapy. The hazards of potassium depletion are real.
II. Evaluate program for activity and rest on an individual basis.
III. Evaluate presence of infections with a "clean catch" urine specimen, for example, so that infections such as cystitis can be diagnosed and treated at their onset.
IV. Evaluate presence of arrhythmias and use antiarrhythmia drugs as indicated.
V. Evaluate electrolytes, especially when digitalis and diuretics are used simultaneously.

METABOLIC, NUTRITIONAL, AND TOXIC DISORDERS

Hypertension

DEFINITION

Hypertension is a persistent elevation of the systolic blood pressure above 140 mmHg and of the diastolic pressure above 90 mmHg. A sustained elevation of blood pressure is clinically significant because it can lead to such conditions as hypertensive heart disease, arteriolar nephrosclerosis, and retinal abnormalities. Hypertension is classified as follows:

1. Primary hypertension, also known as essential hypertension, constitutes 90 percent of all cases. Types include:
  a. Benign hypertension. Gradual onset and prolonged course.
  b. Malignant hypertension. Abrupt onset and a short, dramatic course which is rapidly fatal unless treatment is successful.
2. Secondary hypertension. This type develops as a result of other primary diseases of the cardiovascular system, renal system, adrenal glands, or neurologic system (11).

ASSESSMENT

I. Data sources.
  A. Patient and health history: Identify factors in patient's life-style which might be related to hypertension. In doing a history, determine at what age the patient's blood pressure first became elevated, if there was any renal or cardiovascular disease in the past, whether patient has suddenly lost weight (sign of pheochromocytoma) or gained weight (edema), or any severe headaches, nocturia, dyspnea, fatigue, or angina.
  B. Family: Since hypertension can have a familial tendency, determine its frequency in the family history.
II. Physical assessment.
  A. The blood pressure consistently is above 140 mmHg systolic and 90 mmHg diastolic. (This is due to constricted arterioles, causing resistance to blood flow.)
  B. Eye signs: Retinal blood vessels become tortuous, thin, shiny, and may hemorrhage. These signs can be determined by an ophthalmoscopic exam. Blurrring of vision may be experienced.
  C. Severe headaches associated with nausea and vomiting are present, especially in the morning hours.
  D. Patient experiences dyspnea if there is some heart failure.

    E. Peripheral edema is present if there is right-sided heart failure.

    F. There is polyuria and nocturia. The kidneys have less ability to concentrate the urine, so there is increased volume excreted. The urine may contain protein because of kidney problems.

    G. Patient complains of palpitations.

    H. Epistaxis (nosebleeds) may occur from the increased pressure in the circulatory system.

    I. Patient is forgetful and irritable.

III. Diagnostic tests.

    A. Take blood pressure readings on both arms while the patient is supine, and then erect. For accuracy, readings are taken repeatedly over a period of 1 to 2 h.

    B. Ophthalmoscopic examination will demonstrate vascular changes in the retina. If hemorrhages, exudate, and papilledema are present, there is definite vascular damage.

    C. The electrocardiogram shows evidence of cardiac hypertrophy or other cardiac abnormalities.

    D. X-ray helps to determine cardiac size.

    E. Urinalysis will show proteinuria, bacteria (from pyelonephritis), pus cells, and red blood cells, indicating kidney disease.

    F. An intravenous pyelogram is helpful in revealing parenchymal disease of the kidney.

    G. Blood urea nitrogen and serum creatinine indicate kidney function level.

    H. Determine serum sodium, potassium, chloride, and carbon dioxide levels.

    I. Specific laboratory tests will be done to determine if the hypertension is secondary to pheochromocytoma (Regitine test), primary aldosteronism, or Cushing's syndrome.

PROBLEMS

I. Headaches.

II. Anxiety.

III. Confusion and forgetfulness.

IV. Fatigue.

V. Difficulty in breathing, especially if heart failure is occurring.

GOALS OF CARE

I. To lower the blood pressure to a level compatible with optimal functioning.

II. To lower the blood pressure to prevent complications.

III. To help the patient understand the importance of drug therapy and frequent checkups.

INTERVENTION

I. General measures:

    A. Weight reduction is necessary if the patient is obese.

    B. Patient is put on a sodium-restricted diet (to about 2 g sodium a day).

    C. Patient begins regular physical exercise.

    D. Give sedatives or tranquilizers for patients who are apprehensive.

    E. Provide a quiet environment.

    F. Listen to what the patient is saying and offer reassurance when appropriate.

    G. When giving medications, watch for side effects.

II. Drug therapy: This is the most specific form of intervention for a hypertensive patient. Since no two patients are alike in their reactions to drug therapy, they must be closely observed for expected and side effects; then alterations in drug therapy may be indicated. Those with mild hypertension may only need a diuretic; those with more severe forms of hypertension are usually given a combination of a diuretic and a vasodilator.

    A. Diuretics:

        1. Thiazides: chlorothiazide (Diuril); hydrochlorothiazide (HydroDiuril).

            a. Block tubular reabsorption of sodium and potassium.

        b. Potassium may need replacement through food or medication if thiazides and digitalis are used together.
    2. Spironolactone (Aldactone).
        a. Antagonizes the action of aldosterone, thus inhibiting reabsorption of sodium and promoting diuresis.
        b. It reduces excretion of potassium.
        c. Should not be used if patient has renal insufficiency.
  B. Vasodilators:
    1. Reserpine (Serpasil).
        a. Depletes stores of norepinephrine in brain and peripheral tissues, thus causing vasodilation.
        b. Can cause emotional depression, so watch for despondency.
        c. Also, causes nasal stuffiness.
    2. Guanethidine (Ismelin).
        a. Produces postganglionic blockade of norepinephrine.
        b. Can cause orthostatic hypotension (low blood pressure with change of body position), so warn patients not to change positions quickly.
        c. Also, diarrhea and inability to ejaculate, causing impotence.
    3. Hydralazine (Apresoline).
        a. Has direct action on blood vessels.
        b. Dilates peripheral blood vessels; increases cardiac output and renal blood flow.
        c. Can cause tachycardia, angina pectoris.
    4. α-Methyldopa (Aldomet).
        a. Acts by displacing norepinephrine in the sympathetic nerve endings with α-norepinephrine, called a "false transmitter."
        b. Dilates peripheral arterioles, usually increases glomerular filtration and cardiac output.
        c. May cause drowsiness and dryness of mouth.
        d. Postural hypotension.
        e. Toxic effects: hepatitis and hemolytic anemia.

III. Sympathectomy: This procedure results in the blockage of stimuli from the sympathetic nerve fibers to the blood vessels. This surgery is done on those few patients who cannot tolerate drug therapy. This used to be the method of choice, but it has its side effects, especially orthostatic hypotension, neuritis, loss of ejaculation in the male, and loss of perspiration in areas innervated by the sympathetic nerves.

IV. Teaching and rehabilitation:
  A. Education is lifelong. The nurse needs to teach the patient this. Hypertension is controllable, not curable.
  B. Rehabilitation should be adjusted to the particular needs of individual patients so that there will be maximum compliance to the regimen.
  C. The following should be included in the teaching plan:
    1. Patients need to be taught how to take their own blood pressures so they can continue this at home.
    2. Continue with the medications as ordered. Patients should be told to take the drugs on time, not to skip doses, not to take more than ordered, and to report side effects to the physician.
    3. Dietary restrictions. Avoid large, heavy meals. Teach the reasons for the sodium-restricted diet and what foods can be included or excluded. Teach patients not to drink large amounts of fluid, since increased fluid will increase blood volume, which in turn causes increased blood pressure.
    4. Emphasize a planned, moderate exercise program, including activities such as daily walks, gardening, and golf. Avoid strenuous exercise.
    5. Encourage the patient to develop interesting hobbies.

EVALUATION

I. Careful assessment of the effects of drug therapy is needed. Often, a combination of drugs is given when one drug alone is not effective. Watch for electrolyte imbalance, especially in regard to potassium depletion with diuretic therapy. Potassium supplements may be needed.

II. Evaluate the patient's understanding of diet therapy, drug therapy, and the alteration of life-style. Reinforce and teach areas not clearly understood.

Anemia and Heart Disease

DEFINITION

Anemia is a condition that occurs when the oxygen transport capacity of the blood is below normal due to decreased circulating red blood cells or to decreased hemoglobin. Anemia may result from (1) inadequate production of erythrocytes because of abnormal function of the bone marrow, (2) insufficient quantity of erythrocytes because of blood loss, (3) inadequate maturation of erythrocytes because of absence of an essential factor (as in pernicious anemia), and (4) increased destruction of erythrocytes resulting from acquired or hereditary factors (12). Compensation for anemia includes tachycardia and an increased stroke volume which cause an increased cardiac output. If this compensation is ineffective in increasing the cardiac output, myocardial ischemia may develop, causing angina-type chest pain.

ASSESSMENT

I. Data sources.
  A. Obtain health history from the patient as to eating habits and evidence of loss of blood. Also, determine what types of activity cause fatigue.
  B. Take family history. What is the frequency of anemia in family members?
  C. Obtain medical and health records of previous hospitalizations or clinic visits.

II. Physical assessment.
  A. Fatigue. Patients will be just as fatigued in the morning when they wake up as when they retire.
  B. Tachycardia and bounding pulse are present.
  C. Skin and mucous membranes are pale.
  D. Tongue and mouth are sore.
  E. Patient is sensitive to cold.
  F. There is loss of skin elasticity and tone. Hair thins.
  G. There are systolic bruits over both carotid arteries.
  H. There is a pulmonary ejection systolic murmur.
  I. Neurological symptoms include tinnitus, headache, spots before the eyes, fainting, drowsiness, irritability, and difficulty in concentrating.
  J. Dyspnea and some peripheral edema may be present.

III. Diagnostic tests.
  A. Blood studies will determine cell counts and amount of hemoglobin.
  B. Sickle cell preparation will identify the typical sickle cell erythrocyte.
  C. Bone marrow examination.
  D. Icterus index will determine the amount of bilirubin.
  E. Analysis of iron in the serum will diagnose iron-deficiency anemia.

PROBLEMS

I. Physical problems: weakness and fatigue.
II. Psychological problems: depression.

GOALS OF CARE

I. To improve the blood condition so the patient can live a more normal life.

Identification of arrhythmias A logical approach to arrhythmia identification is to classify them as to disturbances in impulse initiation or to disturbances in impulse transmission. Space prohibits a complete description of each arrhythmia and its significance. Threfore, the reader is referred to other texts for an in-depth discussion of this subject.

Normal sinus rhythm is said to exist when the heart rate is between 60 and 100 beats per minute, the rhythm is regular, a P wave precedes the QRS complex at a constant interval, and the QRS complex width is within normal limits (see Table 26-3). An arrhythmia exists when the above criteria are not all met. Table 26-4 provides a framework for the reader as a summary of the most frequent arryhthmias, their abnormal characteristics, and a representative rhythm strip of each.

ASSESSMENT
I. Data sources.
   A. Patient's history.
   B. Family.
   C. Medical records showing previous occurrences or showing drug therapy which might be causing the arrhythmia.
II. Physical assessment.
   A. Take the apical-radial pulse to determine if a pulse deficit is present. This occurs with arrhythmias in which there is variation in the strength of the heartbeat and the stroke volume varies in response to it.
   B. Venous distension and pulsation of great veins in the neck might indicate an atrial arrhythmia.
   C. Patient may complain of palpitations caused by an arrhythmia.
   D. Use a cardiac monitor or electrocardiogram to document what the arrhythmia is.
III. Diagnostic tests.
   A. Electrocardiogram.
   B. Cardiac monitor.
   C. Avionics tape recorder.
   D. Bundle of His recordings with the use of an electrode-tipped catheter placed near the tricuspid valve. This requires cardiac catheterization, so is done only selectively.

PROBLEMS
I. When identifying an arrhythmia, assess the patient directly for the effect the arrhythmia has on cardiac output. The blood pressure will decrease if the cardiac output decreases.
II. Identify associated symptoms such as syncope, dyspnea, and palpitations.
III. Anxiety is usually present and should be identified both as a cause and a result of an arrhythmia.
IV. Identify systemic causes of arrhythmias, such as fever, hormonal imbalance, or exercise.
V. Identify relaton of arrhythmia to drug therapy or to electrolyte disturbances attributable to drug therapy.

GOALS OF CARE
I. If there is an arrhythmia having an effect on the cardiac output, it should be treated and corrected if at all possible.
II. Treat arrhythmias so that the heart can function more normally and the patient can live a more normal life.
III. If the cause for an arrhythmia (drug therapy, infections, or electrolyte disturbances) is identified, eliminate it if possible.

INTERVENTION
The management of arrhythmias can be generalized. If the rate is slow, the objective is to increase it to improve cardiac output; if the rate is fast or there are signs of irritability, the objective is to slow it or depress the irritable focus so that cardiac output will be improved.

TABLE 26-3 / NORMAL SINUS RHYTHM AND ITS CHARACTERISTICS

Characteristics	*Representative Rhythm Strip*
Heart rate: 80 beats per minute. Rhythm: regular. P waves before each QRS complex. PR interval: normal. QRS complex: normal.	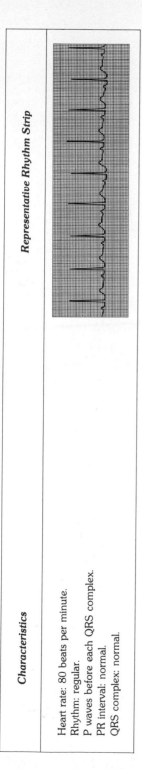

TABLE 26-4 / ARRHYTHMIAS AND THEIR ABNORMAL CHARACTERISTICS

Arrhythmias and Characteristics	*Representative Rhythm Strip*
Arrythmias Due to Disturbances in Impulse Formation	

I. Sinoatrial (SA) node arrhythmias: impulses originate in the SA node.
  A. *Sinus tachycardia.* Heart rate: 100–150 beats per minute.
 	
  B. *Sinus bradycardia.* Heart rate: 40–60 beats per minute.
	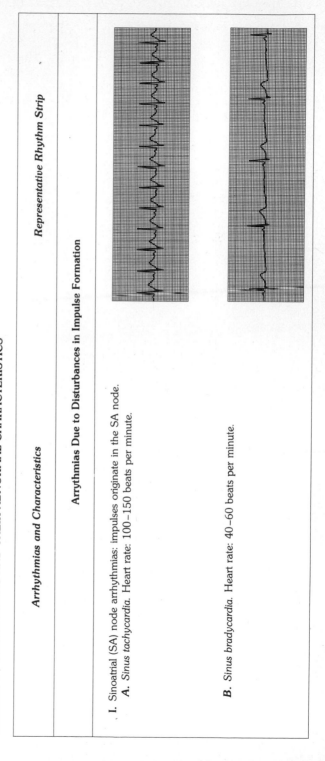

TABLE 26-4 / ARRHYTHMIAS AND THEIR ABNORMAL CHARACTERISTICS *(Continued)*

Arrhythmias and Characteristics	*Representative Rhythm Strip*
Arrythmias Due to Disturbances in Impulse Formation	
C. *Sinus arrhythmia.* Irregular rhythm of QRS complex: fast rate alternating with slow rate. Increased rate is related to respiratory inspiration; decreased rate is related to respiratory expiration.	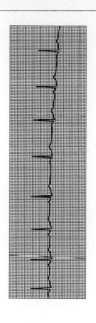
II. Atrial arrhythmias: impulses originate in the atria. **A.** *Premature atrial complexes.* A premature beat preceded by an abnormally shaped P wave.	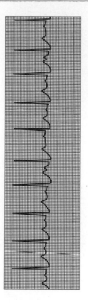
B. *Paroxysmal atrial tachycardia.* Heart rate: 150–250 beats per minute. P waves, if seen, are abnormal in shape and may be combined with T waves.	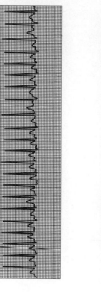
C. *Atrial flutter.* Sawtooth-appearing flutter waves instead of P waves. There is usually a ratio of these flutter waves to QRS complexes, since only a proportion are conducted to the ventricles. Ratio is expressed as 2:1, 3:1, or 4:1 atrial flutter.	

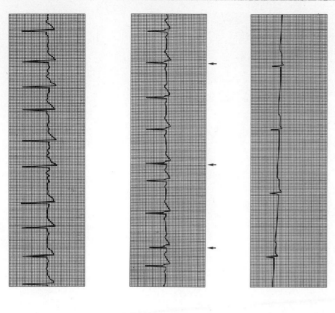

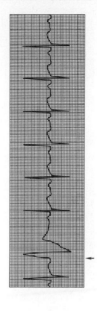

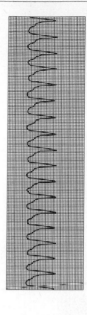

D. *Atrial fibrillation.* Irregular ventricular rhythm. P waves not present; instead there are small irregular fibrillation waves, irregular QRS complex.

III. Junctional arrhythmias: impulses originate in the atrioventricular (AV) node.

   A. *Premature junctional complex.* Shape and position of P waves may vary. They may be inverted preceding or following QRS complexes or may be hidden in the QRS complexes. The cardiac cycle comes earlier than expected.

   B. *Junctional rhythm.* Slow rate: 40-60 beats per minute. P waves have the same characteristics as in premature junctional complex above. All the beats have the characteristics stated above. (There are no identifiable P waves in the rhythm strip to the right.)

IV. Ventricular arrhythmias: impulses originate in the ventricles.

   A. *Premature ventricular complex (PVC).* Premature beat having no P wave. Widened, distorted QRS complexes. T wave oppositely directed from the QRS complex. Full pause follows the premature beat. Various patterns include ventricular bigeminy, multifocal PVC, frequent PVCs, R-on-T pattern.

   B. *Ventricular tachycardia.* Heart rate: 140-220 beats per minute. Slightly irregular rhythm. No identifiable P waves. Widened, distorted QRS complexes. T wave oppositely directed from QRS complexes.

TABLE 26-4 / ARRHYTHMIAS AND THEIR ABNORMAL CHARACTERISTICS (*Continued*)

Arrhythmias and Characteristics	*Representative Rhythm Strip*
Arrhythmias Due to Disturbances in Impulse Formation	
C. Ventricular fibrillation. Chaotic waves of varying height and width. No pattern. Patient soon becomes unconscious because of no cardiac output. Death results unless the arrhythmia is treated immediately.	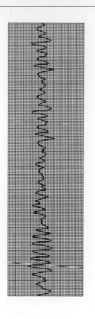
Arrhythmias Due to Disturbances in Impulse Transmission	
I. Atrioventricular node heart blocks. *A. First-degree AV heart block.* PR interval prolonged beyond 0.20 s (five small squares on ECG paper).	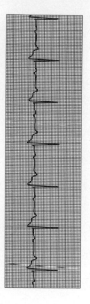
B. Second-degree AV heart block. *1. Wenckebach type.* Progressive lengthening of PR interval from beat to beat until a P wave is not followed by a QRS complex (arrows); then the sequence is repeated.	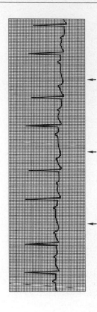

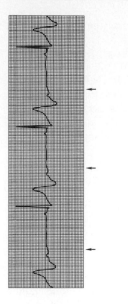

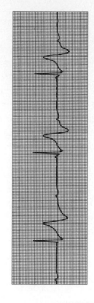

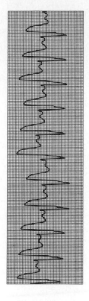

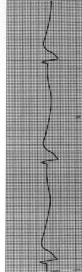

2. *2:1 AV heart block.* A ratio of P waves to QRS complexes of 2:1 (as in rhythm strip on right), 3:1, or 4:1. Beats are dropped in this ratio (arrows indicate where P waves are not conducted).

C. *Third-degree AV heart block (complete).* Slow ventricular rate: 30–40 beats per minute. P waves independent of QRS complexes.

II. Intraventricular blocks.

A. *Bundle branch block.* P waves precede wide, distorted QRS complexes. QRS complexes exceed 0.12 s (three small squares on ECG paper).

III. *Ventricular standstill.* P waves may be seen with sudden cessation of QRS complexes, or P waves are absent and QRS complexes are very slow in rate, 10–25 beats per minute, and are widened. They may be absent and only a straight line is seen. Patient is unconscious. Death results unless resuscitation is immediate.

The modes of therapy are as follows:

I. For slow rate arrhythmias (bradyarrhythmias).

  A. Drug therapy.

    1. Atropine, 0.6 to 1 mg. Atropine blocks vagal stimulation of the heart, resulting in an increase in rate.

    2. Isoproterenol (Isuprel), 2 to 4 mg in 1000 mL IV fluids. Isoproterenol stimulates conduction and contraction, thus increases the rate.

  B. Cardiac pacemaker. An artificial cardiac pacemaker is an electrical device that is used to initiate the heartbeat when the patient's rate is slow from a variety of causes, such as AV heart block and bundle branch blocks. The pacemaker consists of a battery pack which may be placed outside the body (external) or embedded under the skin (internal). The battery pack is attached to electrodes through which the electrical stimulation reaches the tissues of the heart.

    1. The methods of pacing are:

      a. Fixed rate, which stimulates at a preset rate, regardless of the patient's heart rate. This type is not used frequently because of the danger of competition. However, it may be used if the patient's heart rhythm is regular.

      b. Demand pacing, which stimulates when the patient's heart rate falls below the rate set on the pacemaker.

    2. Types of pacemakers:

      a. A temporary pacemaker is used for temporary heart block as in myocardial infarction. A pacemaker catheter with electrodes near its tip is threaded through the great veins into the right side of the heart until it is touching the endocardium. The pacemaker battery is outside the body and is attached to the distal end of the catheter.

      b. Permanent pacemakers.

        (1) Epicardial pacemaker electrodes are inserted on the epicardium (outside layer) of the heart by doing a surgical incision through the chest wall. The pacemaker is embedded under the skin.

        (2) Transvenous endocardial pacemaker electrodes are at the tips of the pacemaker catheter which is threaded into the right side of the heart until it touches the endocardium. It is attached at its distal end to a pacemaker which is embedded under the skin of the chest wall.

    3. Nursing role in cardiac pacing (for permanent pacing).

      a. Preoperative care.

        (1) Prepare the patient and family for the procedure and for what to expect following it, such as bulging of the pacemaker embedded under the chest wall, soreness and discoloration of the area where it is embedded, and a sense of heaviness from the weight of the pacemaker.

        (2) Provide psychological support.

        (3) Assess the patient's understanding of the pacemaker and how it will help the heartbeat.

        (4) Ask the patient to do range of motion exercises which will be done postoperatively to prevent a "frozen shoulder" from developing.

      b. Postoperative care.

        (1) Prevent infection by using sterile dressings over the operative site and giving antibiotics for several days (if ordered).

        (2) Monitor the cardiac rhythm. Verify the correct functioning of the pacemaker. When the pulse rate of the patient drops below the rate set on the pacemaker (if it is a demand model), there should be a pacemaker spike seen on the electrocardiogram. Following this pacemaker spike, a QRS complex should occur if the pacemaker is capturing the heartbeat. If there are pacemaker spikes not followed by QRS complexes, or if the patient's heart rate falls very low and there are no pacemaker spikes, the pacemaker is not functioning correctly and the physician should be so

notified. (*See* Table 26-5 to observe pacemaker spikes on the electrocardiogram and the QRS complexes which follow them.)

    (3) Assist the patient in moving his or her shoulder by passive range of
motion exercises to prevent the development of a "frozen shoulder."

    (4) Provide psychological support by allowing the patient to express feelings
about having a pacemaker. Help patient deal with any fears and anxieties.

  c. Rehabilitation and long-term care.

    (1) The patient's instruction should start with assessing the patient's under-
standing of the pacemaker and its purpose.

    (2) Included should be: normal function of the heart, the pacemaker function,
how to take one's pulse, the importance of follow-up visits to the clinic
or physician's office, how to recognize symptoms of malfunctioning of
the pacemaker (dizziness, syncope) and warning about being near
electrical equipment with high-frequency signals (microwave ovens).

    (3) Emphasis should be on the positive aspects following a pacemaker
insertion and stressing that normal activities can be pursued.

 C. Cardiopulmonary resuscitation for ventricular standstill (see Chap. 45).

II. For fast rate arrhythmias (tachyarrhythmias).

 A. Drug therapy.

  1. Digoxin may be used for atrial fibrillation with a rapid ventricular rate or to
terminate other fast rate arrhythmias originating above the ventricles. Its action
is on the vagus nerve to slow impulses going through the AV node, thus reducing
the number of impulses conducted to the ventricles.

  2. Quinidine is usually given orally to depress ectopic foci in the atria. Therefore,
it is helpful in controlling the atrial arrhythmias.

  3. Procainamide (Pronestyl) is used to depress ventricular ectopic foci primarily,
but also has been used for atrial arrhythmias. When given intravenously, it has
a tendency to cause hypotension.

  4. Lidocaine is used to suppress ventricular ectopic activity and, therefore, is
effective for premature ventricular complexes and ventricular tachycardia. It has
an advantage over procainamide in not causing hypotension.

  5. Propronolol (Inderal) reduces sympathetic stimulation of the heart by blocking
beta receptor cells of the heart. It decreases the strength of ventricular contraction
and the cardiac output and, therefore, should not be used if heart failure is
present.

 B. Electrical countershock. By delivering a high voltage of electric current of brief
duration through the heart, depolarization of the entire heart is accomplished. This
allows the SA node to regain its pacemaking function. Its use is:

  1. For ventricular fibrillation. The machine is set at its highest voltage and the

TABLE 26-5 / PACEMAKER-INDUCED RHYTHM AND ITS CHARACTERISTICS

Characteristics	*Representative Rhythm Strip*
Pacemaker spikes precede all QRS complexes except one: the complex designated by an arrow is initiated by the heart instead of the pacemaker.	

synchronizer switch is turned off. The current will flow through the heart as soon as the button for the electric discharge is pushed. This is called defibrillation.

2. For tachyarrhythmias (other than ventricular fibrillation). The machine is set at low voltage levels (depending on the physician's preference) and the synchronizer switch is turned on. The current will flow through the heart when the machine senses an R wave. This procedure is called elective cardioversion.

C. Carotid sinus pressure. This is vagal stimulation applied by using slight pressure over the carotid sinus in a carotid artery where baroreceptors are located. It is most effective for paroxysmal atrial tachycardia and is used by the physician. Be sure the patient is lying down, for this maneuver can cause a very slow heart rate and possibly syncope.

EVALUATION

I. If an arrhythmia causes decreased cardiac output, evaluate the patient's clinical status through direct assessment of vital signs, particularly the blood pressure. Therapy should be given and the effect reevaluated.

II. Evaluate whether symptoms such as syncope, dyspnea, or palpitations occurred simultaneously with an arrhythmia. If this is so, the arrhythmia may be the causative factor, and therapy for the arrhythmia is indicated.

III. Assess the patient for evidence of anxiety which might be the cause of fast-rate arrhythmias. Assist the patient in working through the anxiety or, in some cases, give an ordered sedative.

IV. If the patient is attached to any monitoring device, be constantly observant of the electrocardiogram, recognize significant arrhythmias, and work with other members of the health team in treating them.

Scleroderma (Systemic Sclerosis)

DEFINITION

Scleroderma is a chronic disease of unknown etiology characterized by sclerosis of the skin and subcutaneous tissues, as well as of the internal organs. The heart is involved in a large percentage of patients. Although all three layers of the heart are affected in these patients, the myocardium is affected more than the others. Cardiac muscle is replaced by connective tissue in various degrees: (1) patchy scarred areas, (2) overgrowth of vascular connective tissue which separates muscle bundles, and (3) massive replacement of cardiac muscle with nonvascular connective tissue.

ASSESSMENT

I. Data sources.
  A. Patient's health history.
  B. Family.
  C. Medical records.
II. Physical assessment.
  A. Dyspnea occurs on exertion or at rest, due to the accompanying heart failure.
  B. Chest pain simulating that of coronary heart disease is present.
  C. If tamponade has occurred, there will be pulsus paradoxus.
  D. There is fixed splitting of S_2 (second heart sound) in the absence of bundle branch block.
  E. Systemic symptoms:
    1. Swelling and stiffness of fingers (Raynaud's phenomenon), which is associated with ischemia.
    2. Weight loss, fatigue, and musculoskeletal weakness and aching.
    3. Symmetrical skin changes of shiny, edematous skin, progressing from the distal to the central portions of the extremities. Facial involvement results in a fixed expression and inability to move facial muscles.

      4. Kidney, respiratory, and gastrointestinal systems are also involved.

III. Diagnostic tests.
    A. Chest x-ray shows an enlarged heart.
    B. The electrocardiogram may be normal for cardiac disease, but shows many arrhythmias.
    C. Cardiac catheterization shows cardiac enlargement.
    D. Sedimentation rate is elevated.

PROBLEMS

I. A nonspecific disease, the symptoms of which are like other diseases.

II. Anxiety and depression of the patient who realizes nothing will alter the course of the disease.

III. Supportive measures offer the only relief from the symptoms.

GOALS OF CARE

I. Assist the patient to work through psychological reactions to the disease.

II. Provide supportive care so that the patient can live optimally within the limitations set by the disease.

INTERVENTION

I. No therapy alters the course of the disease.

II. Supportive measures are:
    A. Avoidance of exposure to cold.
    B. Physical therapy to maintain muscle strength.
    C. Treatment for congestive heart failure, if it occurs.
    D. Corticosteroids help skin lesions and any inflammatory process such as pericarditis, but they do not slow the process.

EVALUATION

I. Evaluate the effectiveness of drug therapy in preventing or relieving congestive heart failure.

II. Evaluate the patient's knowledge of the disease and compliance with a change in lifestyle.

III. Evaluate the therapy in relation to the symptoms. When it is ineffective, the therapy may need to be changed.

Periarteritis Nodosa

DEFINITION

Periarteritis nodosa is a disease of unknown etiology characterized by necrosis of blood vessel walls and aneurysm formation. The disease starts with degeneration of the media, then spreads by inflammation to the whole circumference of the vessel.

ASSESSMENT

I. Data sources.
    A. Patient's health history.
    B. Family.
    C. Medical records.

II. Physical assessment.
    A. There is fever and multisystem involvement.
    B. Tachycardia is common.
    C. Friction rub from pericarditis is present.
    D. Hypertension exists.
    E. There are symptoms of congestive heart failure.
    F. A systolic murmur is present.

III. Diagnostic tests.
  A. The electrocardiogram shows T-wave changes which are related to fibrosis. Bundle branch block may occur.
  B. Chest x-ray shows left ventricular enlargement or generalized cardiomyopathy.
  C. Biopsy of areas of active inflammation shows tissue changes resulting from circulatory disturbances.

PROBLEMS
I. The disease affects all ages.
II. Symptoms simulate those of myocardial infarction because of coronary artery involvement.
III. Therapy may prevent its spread to other arteries, but it may not prevent infarction from occlusion.
IV. Disease may be controlled, but long-term prognosis may not change.

GOALS OF CARE
I. Provide comfort to the patient by controlling the pain.
II. Watch for side effects of massive dosages of steroids.
III. Prevent congestive heart failure.
IV. Provide psychological support to patients, who may or may not respond to therapy.

INTERVENTION
The mainstay of treatment is corticosteroids to reduce pain, control symptoms, and prevent the progress of the disease. Some patients fail to respond to them, however, and the disease progresses.

Lupus Erythematosus

DEFINITION
Lupus erythematosus is a disease of unknown etiology characterized by inflammatory lesions involving many body systems: the skin, joints, kidneys, respiratory, cardiac, gastrointestinal, neurologic, and renal. In about one-half of the patients the heart is involved. When it is, the endocardium, myocardium, and pericardium are affected either singly or in combination. The lesions in the endocardium are Libman-Sacks lesions, which are wartlike in appearance and are commonly found under the mitral valve leaflets. The heart is enlarged. There may be pericarditis with effusion. In the myocardium, fibrin is deposited in the vessels and septa. (See Chap. 32 for further discussion.)

ASSESSMENT
I. Data sources.
  A. Patient's health history.
  B. Family.
  C. Medical records.
II. Physical assessment.
  A. There is hypertension due to kidney involvement.
  B. There is pain from pericarditis without pericardial friction rub.
  C. Both systolic and diastolic murmurs are heard over the mitral area.
  D. Tachycardia.
  E. Fever (may be spiking or sustained).
  F. Arrhythmias: atrial flutter, atrial fibrillation, and conduction defects.
  G. Malaise.
  H. Weight loss.
  I. Butterfly erythema over the bridge of the nose.
  J. Arthritis.

III. Diagnostic tests.
   A. Lupus erythematosus cell test.
   B. Electrocardiogram shows ST- and T-wave changes plus arrhythmias mentioned above.

PROBLEMS
I. The disease involves many systems.
II. Treatment with corticosteroids may prolong life by healing lesions, but it may also cause valvular deformity, requiring valve replacement.

GOALS OF CARE
I. Provide comfort by relieving symptoms of the disease.
II. Control hypertension.
III. Prevent and control congestive heart failure.
IV. Prevent infections.

INTERVENTION
I. Give salicylates for joint pain.
II. Give corticosteroids to suppress inflammation.
III. Avoid infections.

EVALUATION
I. Evaluate the effect of comfort measures in relieving symptoms.
II. Evaluate therapy in controlling hypertension.
III. Evaluate the presence of arrhythmias, friction rub, and heart murmurs in consequence of therapy.
IV. Evaluate side effects of drug therapy (corticosteroids).

INFLAMMATORY DISORDERS

Bacterial Endocarditis

DEFINITION
Bacterial endocarditis is a severe bacterial infection of the endocardium. The basic lesion is a friable vegetation on the heart valves, the endocardial lining of a heart chamber, or the endothelium of a blood vessel. The vegetation is made up of platelets, fibrin, white blood cells, red blood cells, some bacteria, and varying amounts of necrosis. As healing takes place, the exposed area of the vegetation becomes covered with fibrous tissue and phagocytosis of the bacteria occurs. Previous rheumatic endocarditis is the most common cause of bacterial endocarditis. The mitral valve is the site most often involved. Because of the location of these vegetations and their friable characteristic, peripheral arterial embolism is common in this disease. As the result of the embolization to other parts of the body, septic infarction and abcess formation occur, most commonly in the kidney, brain, and spleen.
   There are two forms of bacterial endocarditis:

1. Acute bacterial endocarditis. This is a severe infection, characterized by high fever, heart murmurs, embolic phenomena, and an enlarged spleen. It follows a rapid course. The endocardium is damaged early in the disease.
2. Subacute bacterial endocarditis. This is a less severe infection, characterized by a continuous fever, weight loss, fatigue, joint pains, and an enlarged spleen. Its onset is insidious and the course is prolonged. With adequate therapy, there is little or no damage to the endocardium.

Where does the infection originate?

1. Preexisting disease or injury of the heart valves predisposes the endocardium to infection.
2. Acute infection elsewhere in the body (tonsils, teeth, kidneys) is likely to cause bacterial endocarditis.
3. Heart surgery can predispose a patient to endocarditis when poor technique is used.
4. Contaminated needles and careless technique in parenteral administration of drugs or IV therapy can produce bacterial endocarditis. (Drug addicts are prone to develop it.)

ASSESSMENT
I. Data sources.
  A. Patient's health history. Look for any history of rheumatic fever, infections of other organs, dental work, etc.
  B. Family. Family records can provide information on childhood infectious diseases.
  C. Medical records can provide data on previous hospitalizations or previous diseases which might be related to bacterial endocarditis.
II. Physical assessment.
  A. Symptoms related to the infection are:
    1. Fever which is not continuous but remittent in some patients.
    2. Chills.
    3. Night sweats.
    4. Fatigue.
    5. Anorexia.
    6. Joint pains from endothelial swelling.
    7. Weight loss.
  B. Symptoms related to cardiac involvement include:
    1. Tachycardia.
    2. Enlarged spleen.
    3. Petechiae of the skin and mouth.
    4. Clubbing of fingers and toes.
    5. Pallor.
    6. Heart murmurs occur late in the disease.
  C. Symptoms related to emboli:
    1. The spleen is the most common organ involved with emboli. Symptoms of splenic infarction are tenderness and enlargement of the spleen, and pain in the upper left abdomen.
    2. Renal involvement would be evidenced by flank pain and hematuria.
    3. Brain involvement would show sudden visual problems, an inability to speak, and paralysis of one side of the body.
    4. Extremities would show circulatory problems such as gangrene.
    5. Pulmonary embolism is characterized by severe dyspnea, hemoptysis, cough, and pleuritic pain.
III. Diagnostic tests.
  A. The major diagnostic tool is a blood culture. This is repeated over several days and is usually positive by the third day.
  B. Sedimentation rate is elevated.
  C. Hematocrit is low, showing anemia.
  D. White cell count is increased (leukocytosis).
  E. Urine examination shows hematuria, proteinuria, and casts.

PROBLEMS
I. A very ill patient with high fever, if disorder is acute bacterial endocarditis.
II. A need for early diagnosis so antibiotic therapy can be instituted to combat the infection.
III. A need for comfort measures because of the high fever and chills.

GOALS OF CARE (13)

I. Identify the infectious organism.
II. Destroy the organism in order to prevent vegetations on the heart valves.
III. Protect the heart from permanent damage.
IV. Prevent relapses and recurrent fevers.
V. Surgically correct reparable valvular deformities.
VI. Provide comfort measures.

INTERVENTION

I. Supportive measures:
   A. Put patient on bed rest for signs of heart failure or fever.
   B. Administer aspirin, provide cooling measures, and force fluids for fever.
II. Drug therapy.
   A. Antibiotic therapy:
      1. It must be bactericidal rather than bacteriostatic.
      2. It must be specific for the organism, identified by blood cultures.
      3. It must be continued for at least 4 to 6 weeks.
      4. It is given by slow, continuous IV drip. Heparin added to the IV infusion prevents thrombophlebitis.
      5. Penicillin is the backbone of therapy. It is able to penetrate the fibrin of the vegetation and reach the bacteria.
      6. If the patient is allergic to penicillin, Benadryl is added to the IV drip. For such a patient, equipment for providing an airway should be on hand when the IV drip is started, in case of reactions to the penicillin. Prednisone may be used to control reactions.
   B. Surgery of the involved valve may be needed if other therapy is unsuccessful and heart failure continues.

EVALUATION

I. Effective control of bacterial endocarditis can be determined by the following criteria:
   A. Fever, sweats, and tachycardia disappear in a few days.
   B. Weight gain and improvement in the blood condition occur by the second week of therapy.
   C. Urinary function improves over the period of illness.
II. If the above improvements do not take place, therapy may need to be changed.
III. Watch for complications of bacterial endocarditis:
   A. Congestive heart failure.
   B. Embolization to other organs.

Myocarditis

DEFINITION

Myocarditis is an inflammatory process of the heart, caused by bacterial, viral, rickettsial, and parasitic diseases. Frequently, it develops secondary to endocarditis and pericarditis. The heart reacts to the infectious process by dilatation and congestive heart failure.

ASSESSMENT

I. Data sources.
   A. Patient's health history of previous infections, such as rheumatic fever, diphtheria, etc.
   B. Family history of infections.
   C. Medical records showing other infectious diseases, especially bacterial endocarditis, for myocarditis is a common complication of it.

II. Physical assessment.
  A. The disease begins like influenza and is followed by clinical features associated with cardiac enlargement and failure.
  B. There is persistent fever with tachycardia disproportionate to the degree of fever.
  C. Fatigue.
  D. Dyspnea.
  E. Palpitations.
  F. Pericardial friction rub.
  G. Gallop rhythm.
  H. Pulsus alternans.
  I. Arrhythmias: atrial and ventricular arrhythmias, heart block, and cardiac arrest.
  J. Nausea, vomiting, and anorexia.
III. Diagnostic tests.
  A. Chest x-ray reveals an enlarged ventricle.
  B. Serial electrocardiograms are nonspecific, but do show ST-T wave abnormalities.
  C. According to patient's symptoms, especially if heart failure is present that developed suddenly and without apparent cause.
  D. Leukocytosis.

PROBLEMS
I. Gastrointestinal problems of nausea, vomiting, and anorexia.
II. Persistent fever.
III. Palpitations.
IV. Arrhythmias.

GOALS OF CARE
I. Provide rest for the heart so that it can heal and overcome the infection.
II. Prevent complications by treating heart failure and arrhythmias.
III. If myocarditis is due to systemic infections, treat these infections.

INTERVENTION
I. Give supportive care for heart failure. Provide bed rest until symptoms of infection and inflammation lessen and disappear. Overexertion during the critical period can cause death.
II. Administer digitalis for heart failure.
III. Treat complications, such as arrhythmias.

EVALUATION
I. Effective control over myocarditis can be determined by:
  A. Relief of symptoms related to heart failure.
  B. Temperature returning to normal range.
  C. Decrease in the cardiac symptoms (gallop rhythm, arrhythmias, palpitations, and pulsus alternans).
  D. Decrease in size of heart as shown on x-ray.
II. Increase in the patient's sense of well-being because of decrease of fatigue, nausea, vomiting, and anorexia.

Pericarditis

DEFINITION
Acute pericarditis is an inflammatory process involving the pericardium. It may occur as a primary process, but is usually secondary to other diseases. Pericarditis may occur with or without an exudate. When there is an exudate it accumulates between the two layers of

pericardium (parietal and visceral) and impairs the heart function because of its constrictive action. Occasionally, the acute process heals with fibrosis which constricts the heart action, also. Pericarditis is classified as *acute* or *chronic*.

1. Acute pericarditis may be *fibrinous* or *exudative*.
    a. Acute fibrinous. Delicate adhesions form around the pericardial sac. There is a pericardial friction rub, described as soft and scratchy.
    b. Acute exudative. As fluid accumulates in the pericardial sac, it prevents the heart from filling during diastole. If it occurs rapidly, tamponade results.
2. Chronic constrictive pericarditis. The pericardium becomes a thick, fibrous, calcified band of tissue around the heart. It eventually causes cardiac failure.

ASSESSMENT
I. Data sources.
   A. The patient's health history may reveal other infectious or inflammatory diseases, such as rheumatic fever, collagen diseases, tuberculosis, or myocardial infarction.
   B. Family.
   C. Medical records may reveal background data.
II. Physical assessment.
   A. A pericardial friction rub occurs as the heart moves. It occurs during systole and diastole and is a scratchy, grating sound. It decreases in pericardial effusion.
   B. Dyspnea.
   C. Chest pain may be mild or severe, occurring over the precordial or substernal area. It radiates to the shoulder and neck and down the left arm. It is aggravated by swallowing, coughing, lying down, and by deep breathing.
   D. Tachycardia.
   E. Fever.
   F. The patient appears very ill, and is pale, anxious, and restless.
   G. Pulsus paradoxus (paradoxical pulse) is due to the compression of the heart by the pericardial fluid or fibrosis. This phenomenon can be elicited in the following way:
      1. Inflate a blood pressure cuff around the patient's arm to a level greater than the systolic pressure. Have the patient increase his or her depth of respiration.
      2. As the blood pressure cuff is deflated, sounds are heard while the patient exhales.
      3. The pressure difference (>10 mmHg) between the first sound (on exhalation) and the pressure level where sounds are audible during all phases of respiration gives a quantitative estimate of the degree of arterial paradox. This finding is suggestive of acute cardiac tamponade.
   H. Atrial arrhythmias, which may be transient.
III. Diagnostic tests.
   A. Electrocardiogram: There is elevation of the ST segment the first few days; the T wave inverts as the subacute phase starts. Pericarditis is differentiated from myocardial infarction in that pathologic Q waves do not occur in pericarditis. Atrial arrhythmias are demonstrated.
   B. The chest x-ray may be normal. If several hundred milliliters of fluid are in the pericardial sac, the x-ray will show an increase in heart size.
   C. An angiocardiogram, carried out with patient sitting, is helpful in detecting pericardial effusion or thickening, and differentiating pericardial effusion from cardiac dilatation.
   D. There is an increase in white blood cell count to 10,000 to 20,000 per cubic millimeter.
   E. Echocardiography, using ultrasonic techniques, helps to detect abnormal movements of the heart wall and a widened space when pericardial effusion is present.

PROBLEMS
I. Chest pain.
II. Fever.

III. The patient is very anxious.

IV. Arrhythmias may be present.

GOALS OF CARE

I. Relieve symptoms.

II. Treat underlying systemic illness.

III. Provide emergency treatment if tamponade occurs.

INTERVENTION

I. Give supportive care, bed rest, reassurance, and aspirin for pain.

II. Steroids are helpful if aspirin is ineffective in relieving the pain when the diagnosis is clearly not tuberculosis.

III. If the cause is tuberculosis, isoniazid and p-aminosalicylic acid are used and continued for at least 2 years. Streptomycin may be used in place of p-aminosalicylic acid if the patient cannot tolerate the latter.

IV. Pericardial paracentesis (aspiration of fluid from the pericardial sac) for cardiac tamponade will relieve the pressure on the heart and allow for improved cardiac functioning.

V. Give digitalis, diuretics, and a low-sodium diet for congestive heart failure.

VI. Pericardiectomy (excision of the fibrinous pericardium) for constrictive pericarditis is performed for chronic cases.

EVALUATION

I. Evaluate whether cardiac tamponade has occurred by watching for the following symptoms: dyspnea, orthopnea, tachycardia, elevated venous pressure, decreased systolic blood pressure with narrow pulse pressure, pulsus paradoxus, liver engorgement, gallop rhythm. If this is confirmed through radiologic studies, pericardial paracentesis is done. The fluid obtained should then be studied to determine the cause. Anticoagulants are discontinued (if patient was receiving them). Specific antibiotics are then given for the bacterial cause. Following this, the patient's blood pressure and venous pressure should be monitored closely.

II. Evaluate whether the therapy is relieving the symptoms. Change in therapy may be indicated if patient is not improving.

III. Evaluate whether congestive heart failure is occurring. If so, give therapy for this complication, administering digitalis, diuretics, and putting patient on a low-sodium diet.

Thrombophlebitis and Phlebothrombosis

DEFINITION

Thrombophlebitis is inflammation of the inner lining of the veins with clot formation. *Phlebothrombosis* is clot formation in the vein without inflammation or followed secondarily by inflammation (14).

Stasis Thrombi form in veins when there are areas of stagnation from slow blood flow. They consist of red blood cells enmeshed in a fibrin network. They have a "tail" that can easily become detached and travel to other sites, such as the lungs, causing embolism there. After a few days the "tail" undergoes changes and becomes more adherent to the vessel wall. As thrombi become larger, they obstruct the lumen of the veins, and because of the inflammatory process, the valves in the veins become destroyed. Conditions likely to cause stasis of blood in the veins are:

1. Prolonged bed rest.
2. Surgery.
3. Varicose veins.
4. Congestive heart failure.
5. Obesity.
6. Pregnancy.

Hypercoagulability   Hypercoagulability may be associated with malignant disease, blood dyscrasias, and oral contraceptive drugs.

Endothelial injury   Endothelial injury may be caused by IV injections, thromboangiitis obliterans (Buerger's disease), fractures, and chemical injury from sclerosing agents and opaque media for x-rays (15).

ASSESSMENT
I. Data sources.
   A. Nursing health history from the patient.
      1. Injuries to extremities.
      2. Oral contraceptive medications.
      3. Amount of ambulation.
      4. Subjective symptoms.
   B. Family.
   C. Other relevant sources.
      1. Medical history.
      2. Medical records.
II. Physical assessment.
   A. Superficial thrombophlebitis.
      1. Veins are tender and palpable.
      2. Area is tender, reddened, and warm.
      3. Fever is minimal.
      4. There is no systemic reaction.
   B. Deep thrombophlebitis confined to small venous channels.
      1. Lesion is not visible or palpable.
      2. Mild pain in the calf of the leg may be the only symptom.
      3. There is no systemic reaction.
   C. Deep thrombophlebitis in major venous trunks.
      1. Extremity is swollen.
      2. Skin is warm.
      3. Fever goes up to 101°F.
      4. When the inferior vena cava is involved, both lower extremities are swollen and cyanotic.
      5. When the superior vena cava is involved, both upper extremities as well as the neck and back become swollen and cyanotic.
III. Behavioral assessment.
   A. Patient is anxious.
   B. Patient is irritable because of calf pain and restrictions in mobility.
IV. Diagnostic tests.
   A. Phlebography is done by injecting a radiopaque media and taking x-rays. This determines how well the vein fills with blood and the location of the thrombi.
   B. Venous pressure measurements: In the affected leg, the venous pressure is higher than in the other. This is due to back pressure of blood. When collateral circulation is established, venous pressure in the involved leg may no longer be elevated.
   C. Radioactive isotopes, such as fibrinogen labeled with radioactive iodine, are injected into the involved vein. A counter determines how concentrated the isotopes are in the areas of thrombi.
   D. An ultrasonic flow detector is used as a diagnostic tool to study blood flow.

PROBLEMS
I. Painful leg with swelling and warmth.
II. Danger of complications if thrombi become emboli.
III. Anxiety.

GOALS OF CARE
I. Prevent thrombi from forming by early ambulation after surgery, leg exercises, and the use of elastic stockings. Prophylactic anticoagulant therapy is provided for patients predisposed to the development of thrombophlebitis or for those who have a history of it.
II. Prevent thrombi already formed from becoming emboli.

INTERVENTION

I. Bed rest with elevation of the involved extremity is necessary.

II. Apply hot, moist packs to alleviate pain and hasten resolution of the inflammation.

III. Give analgesics (codeine) for pain.

IV. Give anticoagulants for deep vein thrombophlebitis to prevent further clots.

V. Elastic stockings, properly applied, should be worn when the patient becomes ambulatory. They compress superficial veins and prevent venostasis.

VI. Administer fibrinolytic drugs such as streptokinase and urokinase to dissolve thrombi. These are not as effective as anticoagulants, however.

VII. Surgery may be needed if other therapies are ineffective and there is a danger of gangrene.
   A. Thrombectomy can be done to remove thrombi.
   B. Vein ligation traps the thrombi in the veins distal to the incision.
   C. Plication of the inferior vena cava is done to trap emboli.
   D. An umbrellalike prosthesis is placed in the lumen of the inferior vena cava.

EVALUATION

I. Evaluate anticoagulant therapy and watch for bleeding. If there should be bleeding, use the antidotes. Protamine sulfate is the antidote for heparin; vitamin K is the antidote for coumarin drugs.

II. Evaluate the psychological reactions of patients. Many apprehensive patients are fearful that their clots will move to their hearts and cause sudden death, so clarify any misconceptions to avoid this.

III. Evaluate the knowledge the patient has regarding future care and reinforce areas in need of it.
   A. Avoid tight garters and girdles.
   B. Avoid taking contraceptive drugs.
   C. Avoid any pressure under the knee, such as pillows. Elevate the foot of the bed, and have patient avoid crossing the legs.

TRAUMA

Traumatic Heart Disease

DEFINITION

There are two categories for injuries to the heart and great vessels: injuries due to external forces, and injuries due to diagnostic medical or therapeutic procedures.

I. Injuries due to external forces (16).
   A. Cardiac tamponade. This is usually caused by gunshot and stab wounds. Tamponade is the result of as little as 50 to 100 mL of blood in the pericardium. Wounds of the atria are likely to heal spontaneously because of the low pressure; wounds of the ventricles, however, will bleed and result in death unless treatment abates the process.
   B. Shunts. These are abnormal communications between parts, caused by trauma, such as ventricular septal defect, fistula between the left ventricle and the coronary sinus, and a fistula between the aorta and the right ventricle. Congestive heart failure occurs if the shunt is large.
   C. Valvular insufficiency. This condition results from injury to the valves of the heart. Usually, the injury is a blunt injury, such as a sharp blow to the chest wall.
   D. Myocardial dysfunction. Myocardial dysfunction follows blunt trauma. Hemorrhage occurs in the contused area and is followed by infarction. Tachycardia and arrhythmias occur frequently. The contused area can rupture.
   E. Coronary arterial insufficiency. Coronary arterial injury is rare as a result of blunt trauma. Usually, if the coronary artery is injured, the injury has caused additional serious injuries to other areas of the heart. The result of coronary arterial injury is hemopericardium.

    F. Rupture or aneurysm, or both, of the aorta. Penetrating trauma of the aorta usually has fatal results. Patients will be in severe shock or near death by the time they reach the emergency department.

    G. Arterial involvement. Major arterial injuries may result from either penetrating trauma or from blunt trauma. Either a complete or partial laceration of the artery may take place. By the time the patient is seen there may be a pulsating hematoma and formation of a false aneurysm.

    H. Embolization. A penetrating object can cause clot formation on its surface. Such clots are likely to move as emboli to other parts of the body.

II. Injuries due to medical or therapeutic procedures (17).

    A. Cardiac surgery. Various accidental events can happen following surgery, such as a prosthetic aorta valve impinging on the right coronary ostium, embolization of calcified matrial following the removal of a calcified valve, and creation of a dissecting aneurysm.

    B. Cardiac catheterization. There may be laceration of the left ventricle, hemorrhage into a ventricular wall following injection of contrast material during angiocardiography and perforation of the right atrium by a catheter which had migrated there after prolonged intravenous therapy.

ASSESSMENT

I. Data sources.

    A. Patient and history of the trauma.

    B. Interview person accompanying patient for more data about trauma.

II. Physical assessment.

    A. There is severe pain at the site of the wound.

    B. There is an open wound with hemorrhaging, if wound was caused by a penetrating object.

    C. Internal hemorrhage will occur with blunt injuries.

    D. Watch for changes in vital signs. They change quickly and must be observed carefully in order to determine the clinical status.

    E. Check for changes in the sensorium. As shock is imminent, cardiac output decreases, and this decreases cerebral perfusion.

    F. Patient experiences great difficulty in breathing if the penetrating wound was through the chest wall, causing the loss of negative pressure in the pleural cavity.

Diagnostic tests.

    A. There is usually no time for lab tests. Diagnosis is based on symptoms.

    B. For patients not acutely ill, cardiac catheterization, blood gas studies, and other lab tests may be done, depending on the type of injury.

PROBLEMS

I. The patient is actuely ill and in need of emergency therapy. If the aorta is wounded, prognosis is grave.

II. Patient may have severe respiratory difficulties.

III. The clinical status depends on the extent of the injury as well as its location.

GOALS OF CARE

I. Identify what tissues and organs are injured.

II. Determine amount of blood loss.

III. Restore the respiratory and cardiac systems to as normal functioning as possible.

IV. Prevent further hemorrhage.

V. Prevent shock or treat shock if it has already occurred.

INTERVENTION

I. Perform pericardial paracentesis for cardiac tamponade.

II. Open-heart surgery with bypass may be needed for injuries causing bleeding or shunts in the heart.

III. Insert chest tubes for drainage when there is a penetrating chest wound.
IV. Restore blood volume by blood transfusions and IV fluids.
V. Treat for shock.
VI. Do a thoracotomy if necessary.
VII. Monitor arterial pressures internally, if possible. Patient should be in an intensive care unit.
VIII. Search for the entrance and exit of bullet if wound is from gunshot.
IX. If the patient is admitted to an emergency department and there may be criminal involvement, report the case to the appropriate judicial authorities.

EVALUATION

The plan of care will need to be changed almost every minute because of the changing clinical status of patients with traumatic heart disease.

OBSTRUCTIONS

Coronary Artery Disease

Coronary artery disease is the result of the process of atherosclerosis in which (1) there are internal thickening and plaque formation within the coronary arteries due to the deposition of fatty substances along the intima; (2) there are resultant fibrosis, calcification, and narrowing of the coronary arteries; and (3) there is constriction of the blood supply to the myocardium which finally can give rise to symptoms relatd to the ischemic process. Two forms of coronary artery disease are angina pectoris and myocardial infarction.

Angina Pectoris **DEFINITION**

Angina pectoris results from temporary ischemia without myocardial tissue damage.

ASSESSMENT

I. Data sources.
   A. Patient.
      1. The patient describes some precipitating cause, such as exertion or overeating.
      2. The patient also states that the pain disappeared when the precipitating cause was removed or nitroglycerin was taken sublingually.
   B. Family. If a family member was with the patient when the pain started, the relative's account will be similar to the patient's.
   C. Previous records.
      1. Medical records help to provide information on previous attacks and their pattern.
      2. The electrocardiogram will not be of diagnostic value to determine previous episodes of angina pectoris.
II. Health history.
   A. Age.
   B. Sex.
   C. Occupation. (Stress and emotional factors in occupation can affect anginal attacks.)
III. Physical assessment.
   A. The patient experiences squeezing, burning, pressing, choking, and aching feelings under the sternum. This pain usually radiates to the arms (mostly the left).
   B. The pain is of short duration. With rest or taking of nitroglycerin, the pain usually disappears.
IV. Diagnostic tests.
   A. The electrocardiogram is normal unless it is taken during an anginal attack; it may then show ischemic changes (ST-segment and T-wave changes). Or it may show these changes after exercise testing.
   B. Coronary angiocardiogram will show the status of the coronary arteries and indicate which ones are occluded.

V. Other relevant assessments.
   A. What risk factors does the patient have? Smoking?
   B. Is there a family history of heart disease? Hypertension? Cholesterol?

PROBLEMS
Severe chest pain which causes anxiety.

GOALS OF CARE
I. To assist the patient to control personal and environmental factors which bring on anginal attacks.
II. To prevent further attacks which could become attacks of myocardial infarction.
III. To teach the patient to control risk factors.
IV. To teach the patient the proper use of nitroglycerin.

INTERVENTION
I. For relief of attacks:
   A. Have patient stop all activity and remain quiet until the pain subsides.
   B. Have patient take nitroglycerin sublingually when the pain begins. Repeat every 5 or 10 min if needed. A headache may follow the drug administration.
II. To prevent attacks:
   A. Anxious persons are referred to psychiatrists for help.
   B. If patient is obese, she or he must lose weight.
   C. A regular program of exercise should be set up.
   D. Administer long-acting nitrites such as Peritrate, Isordil.
   E. Propranolol (Inderal) reduces oxygen requirements of the myocardium.
   F. Sedatives, tranquilizers, and antidepressants help to lessen the frequency and severity of attacks.
   G. Surgery.
      1. Coronary bypass procedure is performed, using part of the saphenous vein as a bypass graft around the obstruction of the coronary artery. A coronary angiocardiogram indicates the location of the obstruction.
      2. For preoperative and postoperative care, see "Intervention" under "Valvular Heart Diseases," above.
      3. See Fig. 26-9 for a diagram of the attachment of a saphenous vein bypass graft to the aorta and anterior descending artery.

EVALUATION
I. Evaluate frequency of anginal attacks. As they become more frequent and medication is ineffective, surgery as described above may be needed.
II. Evaluate how well the patient is controlling personal and environmental factors which may cause attacks.

Myocardial
Infarction

DEFINITION
Myocardial infarction results from so much obstruction in the coronary artery that there is tissue damage to the myocardium. This obstruction can be from a narrowed lumen due to atherosclerotic plaques or from thrombosis.

ASSESSMENT
I. Data sources.
   A. The patient.
      1. The patient describes that the pain occurred following some precipitating cause, or pain may be unrelated and occur at rest.
      2. The patient also states that change of position or taking medications did not relieve the pain nor did rest have an effect on it.
   B. Family. The family member states the facts as the patient did if he or she was with the patient when the pain occurred.

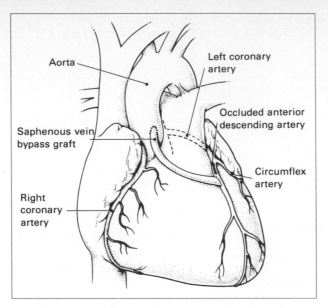

FIGURE 26-9 / Saphenous vein graft for occlusion of a coronary artery.

    C. Previous records.
        1. Medical records help to provide some diagnostic information if previous my-ocardial infarctions occurred.
        2. The electrocardiogram will show evidence of a previous myocardial infarction. Large Q waves will be seen.
  II. Health history.
    A. Age.
    B. Sex. (Males are afflicted more often than females until about 50 years of age.)
    C. Occupation. (Those working in stressful situations are more prone than others.)
 III. Physical assessments.
    A. Crushing, severe, prolonged pain is felt over the sternum that radiates to the shoulder, down the left arm, and sometimes to the right arm.
    B. Patient experiences nausea, vomiting, extreme weakness, anxiety and fear, and a feeling of impending doom.
    C. Dyspnea is present.
    D. There is tachycardia. Blood pressure is elevated at first, then it may drop.
    E. Diaphoresis.
 IV. Diagnostic tests.
    A. Electrocardiograms will show large Q waves (after 24 h) and ischemic changes (ST-segment and T-wave changes). These changes are shown in those leads nearest to the injured myocardium.
    B. Enzyme studies indicate injury to cells, but are not specific for myocardial cells, except for myocardial band (MB), an isoenzyme of creatine phosphokinase.
    C. Creatine phosphokinase (CPK) level becomes elevated 2 to 6 h after the attack.
    D. Serum glutamic oxaloacetic transaminase (SGOT) level becomes elevated after 8 h of the attack.
    E. Lactic dehydrogenase (LDH) becomes elevated on the second or third day after the attack.
  V. Other relevant assessments.
    A. What risk factors does the patient have? Smoking?
    B. Is there a family history of heart disease? Hypertension? Obesity? Diabetes? Cholesterol?

PROBLEMS

I. Severe chest pain which does not abate. With it are other symptoms of myocardial infarction.
II. Anxiety and fear are present.
III. The main nursing problem is to prevent the complications of myocardial infarction, such as arrhythmias, congestive heart failure, and shock.

GOALS OF CARE

I. To restore the patient to as normal a functioning level as possible.
II. To help in the healing of the infarction (should take about 6 weeks).
III. To prevent complications.
IV. To educate the patient about medications, activities, and diet.
V. To teach the patient the need to control risk factors (smoking, medications for hypertension, diet for obesity).

INTERVENTION

I. Acute care in a coronary unit.
  A. Relieve the chest pain with morphine or Demerol.
  B. Relieve anxiety and provide support for the patient and family.
  C. Give oxygen therapy.
  D. Attach patient to a cardiac monitor and observe for arrhythmias.
  E. Provide bed rest, but use passive exercises to prevent embolic complications.
  F. Use a stool softener to prevent the patient from straining for a bowel movement.
  G. Give a liquid diet at first.
  H. Prop patient in an upright position.
  I. Start some aspects of rehabilitation.
II. Subacute care.
  A. Gradually increase activity (for uncomplicated cases).
  B. Prevent overfatigue.
  C. Relieve anxiety.
  D. Rehabilitate and educate the patient and family as to diet, activity, drugs, avoidance of risk factors, and the meaning of a heart attack.
III. Convalescent care.
  A. Continue rehabilitation and education of the patient and family.
  B. Increase activities according to the patient's exercise tolerance, but not competitively or when fatigued.
  C. Teach patient symptoms to watch for—dyspnea, palpitations, and dizziness—that are contraindications to exercise.

EVALUATION

I. Evaluate heart sounds for presence of S_3, an indication of possible congestive failure.
II. Commend the patient for even small progress.
III. Determine how well goals are being achieved.
IV. Be alert for complications such as congestive heart failure by observing for dyspnea in various degrees and peripheral edema. Watch for cardiogenic shock by observing decreased blood pressure with cold, clammy skin and mental changes. Revise plan of care according to evaluation.

Peripheral Arterial Diseases

Atherosclerosis and Arteriosclerosis

DEFINITION

Arteriosclerosis is the loss of elasticity and the hardening of the media (middle layer) of the blood vessel wall by the deposition of calcium. *Atherosclerosis* is a type of arteriosclerosis in which there is the development of plaques containing cholesterol, fatty acids, and other substances along the intima (inner layer) of the vessel wall. It produces narrowing of the lumen and may critically reduce blood flow. There is a positive relationship between atherosclerosis and factors such as smoking, hormones, obesity, physical inactivity, emotional stress, and a high-cholesterol diet.

ASSESSMENT
I. Data sources.
   A. Patient's health history. Note especially history of smoking, patient's eating habits, obesity, physical activity, age, or any associated diseases, such as diabetes.
   B. Determine if there is a family history of cardiovascular disease.
   C. Medical records will indicate any associated diseases and history of cardiovascular diseases.
II. Physical assessment.
   A. There is pain in the lower limbs brought on by exercise that terminates when exercise ceases (intermittent claudication).
   B. Coldness or numbness of an extremity may be present.
   C. Absence of a normally palpable pulse is the most reliable sign of occlusive arterial disease.
III. Diagnostic tests.
   A. Oscillometry. A measurement of pressures in the extremity to pinpoint at what level the obstruction is.
   B. Skin temperature studies. Compare warm and cold temperatures on the extremity.
   C. Arteriography. By injecting contrast media and taking x-rays of the part, abnormalities of blood flow can be detected.
   D. Exercise tests for intermittent claudication. The patient performs some form of exercise and a record is made of the time from the onset of exercise to the onset of pain.
   E. Lumbar sympathetic block is done by blocking the sympathetic vasomotor nerve fibers supplying the ischemic extremity. A positive response means that a sympathectomy may improve circulation.

PROBLEMS
I. Pain in the extremity is brought on by exercise and relieved by rest.
II. Symptoms of ischemia in leg are coldness, numbness, and color change.
III. Patient experiences anxiety over the increasing severity of symptoms.

GOALS OF CARE
I. To preserve the extremity from the effects of ischemia.
II. To relieve the intermittent claudication.
III. To dilate the arteries to improve circulation to the extremity.

INTERVENTION
I. Reassure the patient that she or he is in no immediate danger.
II. Assist the patient to change her or his life-style (stop smoking, avoid cold temperatures, etc.).
III. Encourage an exercise program of graduated walking.
IV. Teach the patient to give the feet meticulous care.
V. Administer vasodilating drugs to increase circulation by dilating blood vessels.
VI. If the above measures fail to improve circulation, surgery may be necessary.
   A. Endarderectomy. This procedure is the removal of the intima and part of the media of the involved artery. An arteriotomy is made over the artery and by blunt and sharp dissection, the occluding material and part of the arterial wall are removed.
   B. Bypass grafting. When significant atherosclerosis is present, bypass grafting is done. A knitted Dacron graft or a part of the saphenous vein is used.
      1. If a saphenous graft is used, the vein is removed and reversed to permit the flow of blood to correspond with the direction of the venous valves and then attached by end-to-end anastomosis.

2. Another technique in using a saphenous vein graft is not to remove it but to disrupt its valves by passing a mechanical instrument along the course of the vein and then attaching it to the diseased artery by an end-to-side anastomosis.
3. Postoperative care includes:
   a. Administration of antibiotics to prevent infection developing around the graft.
   b. Peripheral pulses need to be palpated frequently. Sudden disappearance of the pulse usually indicates thrombosis of the graft or an embolus, both of which need immediate reoperation.
C. Amputation. If the above surgeries are not feasible for a patient, amputation of the involved extremity may be necessary.
D. Sympathectomy. This is an adjunct to reconstructive operations and is indicated if significant occlusive distal disease is present. Its effect is to relieve the slow circulation in the ischemic extremity by vasodilatation.

EVALUATION
I. Observe for improvement of the following symptoms: pain, pallor, cold temperature of the skin, and intermittent claudication.
II. Evaluate the patient's compliance in taking care of the extremities and in changing her or his life-style (especially stopping smoking).

Acute Arterial Occlusion by Arterial Embolism

DEFINITION
Arterial embolism is frequently the cause of acute arterial occlusion. It occurs as a sudden catastrophic event appearing without warning and threatening the loss of a limb or a life. In most of the cases, arterial emboli originate in the heart and therefore should be regarded primarily as a symptom of serious underlying heart disease. The three main causes are mitral stenosis, atrial fibrillation, and myocardial infarction. Most of the emboli originating in the heart lodge in the arteries of the extremities. They tend to lodge at the bifurcation of a major artery, such as the site where the abdominal aorta divides into the two iliac arteries to the legs. When this happens, the tissues perfused by such arteries are deprived of oxygen.

One of the greatest threats from an embolus is that it may lodge in the cerebral circulation, resulting in stroke. Most often, these affected vessels are intracranial and cannot be reached by surgery for the removal of the emboli.

The physiologic consequences of an arterial embolus are the immediate onset of ischemia with resulting anoxia of tissues distal to the occlusion. Within a few hours after the lodging of an embolus, thrombi form in the artery distal to it where the flow of blood has become stagnant. Necrosis develops in the ischemic tissues several hours after the embolus has obstructed the artery. The rate of necrosis varies according to the collateral circulation.

ASSESSMENT
I. Data sources.
   A. Obtain patient's health history, paying particular attention to whether the patient has had an acute myocardial infarction, atrial fibrillation, or mitral stenosis which might explain the origin of the embolus. Or has there been any injury to the extremity which might give a clue to the development of thrombi?
   B. Determine family history.
   C. Medical records and previous hospital records may reveal cardiovascular diseases in which emboli are likely to occur.
II. Physical assessment.
   A. There are five Ps of acute arterial occlusion (18):
      1. *Pain* in the involved extremity is the most distinctive symptom. It is described as burning, throbbing, sharp, and shooting.
      2. *Paresthesia* (tingling sensations) is due to ischemia of the peripheral nerves.
      3. *Pallor* represents varhing degrees of decreased circulation. Associated with visible pallor may be the sensation of coldness.
      4. *Pulselessness* confirms the diagnosis and localizes the site of occlusion. This is the significant physical finding.

    5. *Paralysis* is a late symptom. It indicates a severe ischemic insult and probable tissue necrosis.

    B. Muscle turgor of the involved extremity is an index of the degree of ischemia present. If the muscle is very stiff, prognosis is poor.

    C. Included in the physical assessment is the cardiac examination for underlying heart disease.

    D. If a cerebral artery is occluded, neurological symptoms such as transient ischemic attacks or a stroke develop.

III. Diagnostic tests.

    A. An arteriography may be done if there is uncertainty about the site or location of an embolus. However, if doing it delays an embolectomy, an arteriogram should not be done.

    B. Lack of pulsations in the extremities indicates peripheral embolism, and in the carotid indicates carotid occlusion.

    C. An electrocardiogram will rule out previous myocardial infarctions or indicate the presence of atrial fibrillation and ventricular hypertrophy from mitral stenosis.

    D. Obtain chest x-ray.

    E. Oscillometry may be of value in recording pulsations or absent pulsations in the involved extremity. However, physical examination is usually sufficient to determine this.

GOALS OF CARE

I. To restore normal blood flow.

II. To prevent further tissue damage from occlusion.

INTERVENTION

Immediate action is needed within a few hours.

I. Protect the extremity from pressure and other trauma. Keep it at room temperature and at a slight elevation.

II. Prompt administration of intravenous heparin is the most important therapeutic measure.

III. Surgery:

    A. Embolectomy. An incision is made over the involved artery (arteriotomy). A balloon catheter (Fogarty) is inserted beyond the embolus. The balloon is then inflated and is withdrawn in its inflated state to remove the embolus.

    B. Postoperative care includes careful observation of the distal pulses, skin color, and presence of pain; and administering heparin to prevent clot formation. Antibiotic therapy is given and continued for a few days.

EVALUATION

I. Reestablishment of palpable pulses distal to embolectomy indicates blood flow.

II. Pain disappears.

III. Motor and sensory functions return.

IV. Color and warmth return to the skin.

Thromboangiitis Obliterans (Buerger's Disease)

DEFINITION

Thromboangiitis obliterans is a disease characterized by inflammation of the arteries and veins of the lower extremities. Thrombosis often occurs with it and may lead to gangrene. It primarily affects males of less than 40 years of age.

ASSESSMENT

I. Data sources.

    A. Patient's health history. The patient is a heavy cigarette smoker, age less than 40. There is a typical history of pain in the lower extremities.

    B. Family. Is there any family member with the same disease?

C. Medical records may give helpful data on other cardiovascular diseases or history of thrombophlebitis.

II. Physical assessment.

A. Intermittent claudication. Pain in legs after exercise is relieved after resting. This is frequently the first symptom.

B. There are coldness, numbness, tingling, and burning sensations in the extremities.

C. Extremities are pale when elevated above the heart level and red when dependent.

D. Arterial pulses in the involved extremities diminish as the disease progresses.

E. Symptoms are aggravated by smoking, chilling, and emotional disturbances.

F. Ulceration and gangrene are frequent complications.

III. Diagnostic tests.

A. Arteriography.
B. Skin temperature tests.
C. Oscillometry.
D. Blood studies.
E. X-ray examinations.

PROBLEMS

I. There is pain on exercise.

II. The life-style must be changed in order to avoid further ischemia in the extremities. Patient should stop smoking and take care of the extremities.

III. The condition may progress to ulceration and gangrene.

GOALS OF CARE

I. To improve circulation in the extremities.

II. To encourage good health habits to prevent progression of the disease.

III. To protect the extremities from trauma and infection.

INTERVENTION

I. Buerger exercises alternately to fill and empty blood vessels:

A. Patient lies flat.

B. Legs are then raised above level of the heart for 2 min until blanching occurs.

C. Legs are then lowered below level of the heart and feet are exercised for 3 min until skin color is pink.

D. Patient lies flat for 5 min.

E. Patient repeats 5 times, and should do entire set 3 times a day.

II. Patient should stop all smoking in any form, as smoking constricts the blood vessels.

III. Patient must take proper care of feet by having properly fitting shoes, avoiding cold or overheating from appliances, and avoiding constricting garters.

IV. Administer vasodilator drugs.

V. Surgery:

A. Sympathetic block or lumbar sympathectomy will produce vasodilation.

B. Amputation may be necessary if gangrene occurs.

EVALUATION

I. Evaluate compliance with changes in life-style. Reinforce educational program.

II. Observe for desired effects from intervention, especially improved symptoms of circulation to the extremities. If improvement has not occurred, other interventions will need to be tried.

Raynaud's Disease

DEFINITION

Raynaud's disease is a peripheral vascular disorder of the hands in which there is paroxysmal contraction of the arteries. It is related to emotional stress and exposure to cold temperatires. There is an abnormality of the peripheral sympathetic nervous system in which there is sympathetic overactivity leading to toxic contraction of arterioles. Vasospasms in the arterial wall lead to occlusion, atrophy, and possibly gangrene.

ASSESSMENT
I. Data sources.
   A. The patient's health history usually reveals symptoms which are related to factors such as cold temperatures or emotional episodes. Does patient smoke?
   B. Raynaud's disease affects women more frequently than men.
   C. Are there family members with the same diagnosis?
   D. Medical records may contain data to help with the diagnosis.
II. Physical assessment.
   A. There is gradual onset with pallor of a few fingers on exposure to cold temperatures; then all the fingers become involved.
   B. There is bilateral involvement (both hands).
   C. Radial and ulnar pulses are palpable and normal.
   D. Skin of the hands appears white, smooth, taut, shiny; nail deformity and loss of hair may eventually occur. Later in the course of the disease scars from healed ulcerations are noted along with absence of radial or ulnar pulse.
   E. Repeated attacks of vagospasm may progress to ulceration and gangrene.
III. Diagnostic tests.
   A. A careful history is necessary to rule out the possibility of other diseases.
   B. The vasoconstrictor response to cold will be demonstrated by both hands having the characteristic pallor-cyanosis-rubor sequence following exposure to cold.

PROBLEMS
There will be severe reactions of the hands in response to cold temperatures or emotional upsets.

GOALS OF CARE
I. Teach the patient to live within the limitations of the disease.
II. Increase the circulation of blood to both upper extremities.

INTERVENTION
I. Have patient avoid exposure to cold and learn to control emotions which bring on vasoconstriction.
II. Some patients ar advised to move to warmer climates to avoid cold temperatures.
III. Patient should avoid tobacco in any form.
IV. Vasodilator drugs have been helpful for some patients.
V. Surgery: A cervicodorsal sympathectomy (removal of first, second, and third thoracic ganglia) may be performed. This is done for those patients who have progressed to trophic changes in the fingers.

EVALUATION
I. Evaluate the patient's compliance with change in life-style.
II. Evaluate symptoms. If they are not relieved, other therapies may be needed.

DEGENERATIVE DISORDERS

Varicose Veins

DEFINITION
Varicose veins are dilated, tortuous, elongated branches of the greater and lesser saphenous veins. The condition is due to incompetent valves. Because of this incompetency, there is incomplete emptying of the saphenous veins due to backward pressure on these veins from the pull of gravity. As the blood becomes stagnant in these veins, thrombosis occurs. With this increase in back pressure, there may be an increase in the permeability of the capillary walls, resulting in extravasation of red blood cells into surrounding tissues. When these red

blood cells disintegrate, they produce a characteristic brown color in the skin. Chronic edema of the subcutaneous tissue leads to inflammation, fibrosis, and atrophy. Finally, the cells die and ulceration of the skin occurs.

ASSESSMENT
   I. Data sources.
      A. Obtain patient's health history. Is there obesity? How much standing does the patient do? Pregnancy? Any history of thrombophlebitis?
      B. Do any family members have similar complaints?
      C. From patient's medical records, determine conditions which might be the cause of varicose veins, such as pregnancy, overweight, thrombophlebitis, or arteriovenous fistulas.
   II. Physical assessment.
      A. Some patients have no complaints except for the appearance of tortuous veins; others complain of aching discomfort in the legs. This aching usually occurs after a period of relatively inactive standing and is relieved by elevation of the legs.
      B. Edema of the lower leg appears during the course of the day and becomes aggravated by prolonged standing. It disappears or decreases during the night when the patient is sleeping. Because of this edema, the patient complains of heaviness due to increased fluid accumulation.
      C. Night cramps in the calves of the legs and the feet are due to contractions of muscles in the leg.
      D. There is brownish discoloration of the lower leg.
      E. Dryness and scaling with some pruritis may be observed over prominent varices, particularly at the ankle.
      F. Skin infections may occur.
      G. Ulcerations may be found with long-standing varicose ulcers. They are usually shallow, but may possibly erode veins or even arteries.
   III. Diagnostic tests.
      A. Venous pressure changes during walking. Normally, there is a marked decrease in the saphenous vein pressure with exercise, for muscular action has increased the flow of blood. Those patients with varicose veins have less of a decrease in venous pressure during exercise because of the reflux of blood down the veins.
      B. Trendelenburg's test will demonstrate the backward flow of blood through the incompetent valves into the saphenous veins. The patient lies down and elevates the involved leg until the superficial veins collapse. Then a tourniquet is applied high on the leg to occlude the superficial veins. The patient then stands and the tourniquet is taken off. If the valves are incompetent, the veins distend quickly because of the backflow of blood.
      C. Phlebography. Angiographic contrast media is injected into the saphenous veins followed by x-rays before and after the patient stands. This visualizes the valves.

PROBLEMS
   I. Patients, particularly women, are embarrassed because of the appearance of their varicose veins.
   II. Discomfort from edema, weight, and night cramps disturbs patients.
   III. Danger exists of condition progressing to ulcerations which are difficult to heal, some requiring plastic surgery.
   IV. Patients find it difficult to stand for any length of time.

GOALS OF CARE
   I. Improve circulation of blood through the saphenous veins so that thrombophlebitis or other complications are avoided.
   II. Teach the patient the proper care of the lower extremities.
   III. Promote the use of elastic support.

INTERVENTION

I. Educate the patient about elastic support for legs, the avoidance of tight constrictions on legs, and proper care of legs and feet.
II. Antigravity measures to increase blood flow from the legs to the heart include:
   A. Elevation of the legs above the level of the heart, and sleeping with the foot of the bed elevated.
   B. Avoidance of prolonged standing.
   C. Avoidance of constrictions on the legs, such as garters and tight girdles.
   D. Using elastic support on the legs to decrease venous pooling in the veins. The support hose should be individually prescribed so that it fits properly.
III. Walking helps to promote muscular contraction on the veins lith improved circulation.
IV. Surgery includes vein ligation and stripping. The greater saphenous vein is ligated at the groin and stripped from groin to ankle. This is done by threading a wire into the vein and pulling the wire with the vein. Following the operation, elastic support hose are applied and the foot of the bed is elevated above the level of the heart.
V. Treatment of the varicose ulcers:
   A. Patient is on bed rest and feet are elevated above level of the heart.
   B. Continuous warm, moist compresses are applied to eliminate infection and relieve discomfort.
   C. After the ulcer is free of infection, skin grafting may be needed.

EVALUATION

I. Evaluate compliance with instructions as to elevation of legs, the use of support hose, and proper care of the legs.
II. Evaluate the relief of symptoms of varicose veins or the aggravation of symptoms.
III. Watch for signs of ulcerations.

Aneurysms

DEFINITION

An *aneurysm* is a dilatation of an artery. The most common cause is arteriosclerosis. Other causes are degenerative connective tissue disease of the media, syphilis, and trauma. The main problem is weakness of the arterial wall. The various types of aneurysms and their most common locations are:

1. Fusiform (spindle-shaped dilatation of a segment). This type is found most often in the aorta, especially in the abdominal aorta and in the iliac arteries.
2. Saccular (outpouching from an artery due to thinning of the media). Saccular aneurysms are found most often in the abdominal aorta and popliteal arteries.
3. Dissecting (splitting the arterial wall by blood that is forced between the layers because of a tear in the intima). This type is found most often in the thoracic aorta with other arteries being involved by its extension into their walls. As dissection progresses, branch vessels are obliterated.

ASSESSMENT

I. Data sources.
   A. Patient's health history of diseases such as syphilis, arteriosclerosis, or history of trauma.
   B. Family history.
   C. Medical records showing evidence of preexisting diseases which result in aneurysms.
II. The physical assessment depends on the type and location of the aneurysm.
   A. Dissecting aneurysms. The most common site is in the thoracic aorta. The clinical picture is variable and includes:
      1. Excruciating pain in the back for aneurysms distal to the aortic arch; if proximal to the aortic arch, pain is in the anterior chest. Pain migrates as the dissecting aneurysm progresses along the aorta.

    2. Syncope.

    3. Neurologic symptoms.

    4. Hypertension with variation of blood pressure in both arms.

    5. Aortic diastolic murmur if the aneurysm is in the ascending aorta.

    6. Pallor and shock.

B. Fusiform and saccular aneurysms.

    1. These forms may give no symptoms and may be diagnosed by routine x-rays for other conditions.

    2. Expanding saccular aneurysms cause symptoms because of their compression and erosion into other tissues:

        a. Pain, dyspnea, cough, and atelectasis develop from compression on the left bronchus or lung when the aneurysm is in the thoracic aorta.

        b. Hemoptysis occurs if the aneurysm erodes into the bronchus.

        c. Hoarseness develops from compression on the left recurrent laryngeal nerve.

        d. Pulsation of mass occurs in abdominal aneurysms.

III. Diagnostic tests.

    A. A chest x-ray for thoracic aorta aneurysms may show notching of ribs.

    B. An aortogram will determine the extension and location of the aneurysm.

    C. An electrocardiogram is helpful in determining cardiac disease occurring concomitantly with the aneurysm.

    D. The blood urea nitrogen level (BUN) is helpful in determining renal function and renal disease.

    E. A pulsating abdominal mass helps to diagnose abdominal aneurysms.

    F. Comparison of blood pressures in the extremities helps to determine if an aneurysm is causing differences.

    G. Systolic bruit is heard over an aneurysm.

PROBLEMS

I. Excruciating pain with shocklike symptoms for dissecting aneurysms, requiring emergency surgery.

II. Anxiety of the patient who is facing a potential bleeding problem if the aneurysm ruptures.

III. Preparation of the patient for surgery.

GOALS OF CARE

I. Prevent rupture of the aneurysm.

II. Reestablish normal circulation of the aorta and its branches.

INTERVENTION

I. Resecting the aneurysm and replacing the segment with a graft. A Dacron graft or saphenous vein graft is used, doing end-to-end anastomoses. Surgery requires use of the heart-lung machine in order to maintain blood flow distal to the surgical site during the operative procedure.

II. Administer antihypertensive drugs for patients with dissecting aneurysms: chlorthiazide (Diuril), guanethedine (Ismelin) and methyldopa (Aldomet). This therapy not only decreases the blood pressure but also the force of ventricular contraction.

EVALUATION

I. Postoperatively, carefully evaluate vital signs and evidence of bleeding.

II. Evaluate whether symptoms related to aneurysms have been relieved.

REFERENCES

1. Earl Silber and Louis Katz, *Heart Disease,* The Macmillan Company, New York, 1975, p. 1079.

2. Ibid., p. 1080.

3. Albert Brest and John Moyer, *Cardiovascular Disorders,* F. A. Davis Company, Philadelphia, 1968, p. 894.
4. M. Falconer, M. Norman, H. R. Patterson, and E. Grestafson, *The Drug, The Nurse, The Patient,* W. B. Saunders Company, Philadelphia, 1970, p. 239.
5. L. Meltzer, R. Pinneo, and J. R. Kitchell, *Intensive Coronary Care: A Manual for Nurses,* 3d ed., Charles Press, Brady Company, Bowie, Md., 1977, p. 82.
6. Criteria Committee of the New York Heart Association, *Nomenclature and Criteria for Diagnosis of Diseases of the Heart and Great Vessels,* 7th ed., Little, Brown and Company, Boston, 1973, p. viii.
7. J. Willis Hurst and R. Bruce Logue, *The Heart: Arteries and Veins,* 2d ed., McGraw-Hill Book Company, New York, 1970, p. 1151.
8. Ibid., p. 1415.
9. Brest and Moyer, op. cit., p. 859.
10. Ibid., p. 860.
11. Joan Luckmann and Karen Sorenson, *Medical-Surgical Nursing: A Psychophysiologic Approach,* W. B. Saunders Company, Philadelphia, 1974.
12. Irene Beland and Joyce Passos, *Clinical Nursing: Pathophysiological and Psychosocial Approaches,* 3d ed., The Macmillan Company, New York, 1975, p. 542.
13. Luckmann and Sorenson, op. cit., p. 691.
14. Ibid., p. 824.
15. Ibid.
16. Brest and Moyer, op. cit.
17. Brest and Moyer, op. cit., p. 924.
18. Robert Rutherford (ed.), *Vascular Surgery,* W. B. Saunders Company, Philadelphia, 1977, p. 426.

BIBLIOGRAPHY

Beland, Irene, and Joyce Passos: *Clinical Nursing: Pathophysiological and Psychosocial Approaches,* 3d ed., The Macmillan Company, New York, 1975. A comprehensive text on clinical nursing with emphasis on the pathophysiologic and psychosocial aspects which relate to assessments and intervention.

Braunwald, Eugene (ed.): *The Myocardium: Failure and Infarction,* HP Publishing Co., Inc., New York, 1975. A thorough presentation of myocardial infarction and heart failure, including pathophysiology, assessment, and intervention.

Fowler, Noble (ed.): *Cardiac Arrhythmias: Diagnosis and Treatment,* 2d ed., Harper & Row, Publishers, Hagerstown, Md., 1977. A presentation of current diagnostic methods and current therapies applicable to cardiac arrhythmias commonly encountered in clinical practice.

Haimovici, Henry: *Vascular Surgery: Principles and Techniques,* Mc-Graw Hill Book Company, New York, 1976. A comprehensive presentation of all aspects related to vascular diseases and their surgical management.

Hurst, J. Willis, and R. Bruce Logue (eds.): *The Heart: Arteries and Veins,* 3d ed., McGraw-Hill Book Company, New York, 1974. A complete, thorough text on the medical aspects of the disorders of the heart, arteries and veins.

Juilian, Ormand, William Dye, Hushong Javid, James Hunter, and Hassan Najafi: *Cardiovascular Surgery,* 2d ed., Year Book Medical Publishers, Inc., Chicago, 1970. A handbook dealing with the technical aspects of operative procedures which are used to restore circulatory function in disease states and to correct congenital anomalies.

King, Ouida: *Care of the Cardiac Surgical Patient,* The C. V. Mosby Company, St. Louis, 1975. A concise presentation of the fundamentals of cardiac disease including embryology, physiology, pathology, and surgical techniques.

Luckmann, Joan, and Karen Sorensen: *Medical-Surgical Nursing: A Psychophysiologic Approach,* W. B. Saunders Company, Philadelphia, 1974. A text with a psychophysiologic approach to the broad scope of medical-surgical nursing. It is divided into three sections: general concepts basic to nursing practice, the psychophysiologic imbalances, and the clinical care of patients experiencing specific disorders of the various body systems.

Meltzer, Lawrence, Rose Pinneo, and J. Roderick Kitchell: *Intensive Coronary Care: A Manual for Nurses,* 3d ed., Charles Press, Brady Company, Bowie, Md., 1977. A basic textbook for nurses working in coronary care units or with coronary patients on general medical divisions. It includes nursing care related to acute myocardial infarction and its complications.

Rutherford, Robert (ed.): *Vascular Surgery,* W. B. Saunders Company, Philadelphia, 1977. A complete, well-written text on surgical management for vascular disorders.

Schwartz, Seymour (ed.): *Principles of Surgery,* vol. 1, McGraw-Hill Book Company, New York, 1969. A detailed text on general surgery with emphasis on techniques of the surgical procedures.

Silber, Earl, and Louis Katz: *Heart Disease,* The Macmillan Company, New York, 1975. This text is a thorough presentation of the physiology of circulation and pathophysiology of heart disease as it applies to the clinical care of the patient.

27

The Respiratory System

Dorothy L. Sexton and Mary E. Eddy

Adequate and effective oxygenation is contingent upon an intact respiratory system. When physiological changes occur, the actions of the respiratory structures are diminished. Such problems as obstruction, cellular proliferation, trauma, and infection can interfere with gas exchange and affect the body as a whole.

This chapter discusses common health problems that can affect respiration and oxygen–carbon dioxide exchange. Each problem is explored in terms of its overall impact on the individuals so afflicted. Patient care is discussed, using the vehicle of the standards of practice in order to develop a realistic plan of care for the client.

ABNORMAL CELLULAR GROWTH

Cancer of the Lung

Definition

A malignant neoplasm is an abnormal growth of new tissue that does not serve a useful purpose to the body and may metastasize to other tissues. Pulmonary neoplasms may be primary or secondary. The primary neoplasms include: (1) *squamous cell* carcinoma, which is more common in males and is almost always associated with cigarette smoking; (2) *undifferentiated* (anaplastic) carcinoma, which is more common in males and tends to metastasize early; (3) *adenocarcinoma,* which is usually peripheral and metastasizes particularly by the blood stream; (4) *bronchiolar* (alveolar cell) carcinoma, which is a rare tumor that involves the bronchiolar or alveolar lining.

While the cause of primary pulmonary neoplasms is unknown, the statistical relationship that exists between cigarette smoking and lung cancer indicates that bronchogenic carcinoma is 20 times more common in heavy cigarette smokers than in nonsmokers.

Secondary pulmonary neoplasms metastasize from other malignant tumors in body sites such as the breast, prostate, kidney, and bone.

Prevention

I. Medical evaluation of those with chronic cough and/or chronic respiratory infections.
II. Chest x-ray every 6 months for heavy smokers.
III. Abstinence from cigarette smoking.
IV. Decreasing exposure to pollution and irritants.

Assessment

I. Data sources.
   A. Patient.
   B. Family or significant other.
   C. Past medical records.
II. Health history.
   A. Age—varies, usually occurs during middle years or later.
   B. Sex—males seemed to be affected more than females. Recent research indicates an increase in females who smoke.
   C. Cultural background.
   D. Occupation (describe position)—investigate type of work and whether irritating pollutants are present, *e.g.,* asbestos.
   E. Socioeconomic status.
   F. Dietary (habits) history and assessment—if weight loss is reported, investigate food intake and appetite.
   G. Ingestion of alcohol should be investigated since a correlation between smoking and drinking may be present.

    H. Smoking habits—statistics seem to indicate a high correlation (80 to 90 percent) of lung cancer with smoking. Data should include:
1. Number of years individual has been smoking.
2. Number of cigarettes smoked per day.
3. Whether patient inhales smoke.

    I. History of cough—length of cough; time of cough (A.M. or P.M.); the amount and frequency of sputum production; and a description of sputum, e.g., blood-tinged.

    J. Blood type—identify.

    K. Sleep habits—amount of sleep as related to overall health habits.

    L. Life-style—identify potential stress; whether the individual lives alone; occupational investment; family construction and patient involvement in family; support system.

    M. Family history of cancer, especially lung cancer.

    N. Health perception—have the patient define health; identify factors that may influence health perception.

    O. Present condition of teeth—cancer may cause ulceration and bleeding of gums.

    P. The patient may complain of chest pain, which may be localized or affected by breathing. It can be mild to severe and referred to other body areas.

    Q. The patient may express fear of cancer or a general sense of anxiety, especially in the presence of such changes as hemoptysis or dyspnea.

III. Physical assessment.

    A. Examination of the chest may be normal or changes such as dullness on percussion (unilateral or bilateral); increased breath sounds; increased tactile fremitus and bronchial breath sounds may be heard. Use of a stethoscope is recommended for auscultation.

    B. If chest pain is severe, the patient may guard the affected side and decrease chest excursion (bilateral). Dyspnea may be present. It is aggravated by exertion.

    C. The patient may appear thin and apprehensive at the initial encounter. A complete physical examination will be required in order to assess the total effects of this problem.

    D. Careful palpation of lymph nodes together with other physiological changes may indicate metastatic spread of the disease.

IV. Diagnostic tests.

    A. Chest x-ray—will often indicate the presence of a lesion, a mass in the hilar region, pleural effusion, atelectasis, or erosion of the ribs or vertebrae.

    B. Sputum for cytology—done to examine abnormal cells contained in the sputum. The patient is asked to cough deeply in order to have a more accurate study. Malignant cells may be reported, depending on the stage of the lung cancer.

    C. Bronchoscopy—insertion of a fiberscope through the oral cavity into the bronchus in order to permit visualization of the area. In the lung cavity, direct visualization is not always possible. However, on occasion the tumor may be seen and a biopsy of this tissue can be done in order to confirm the diagnosis.

    D. Scalene fat pad biopsy—excision of tissue for examination.

    E. Mediastinoscopy—insertion of a mediastinoscope (through a skin incision) to examine the mediastinum for metastases.

    F. Pulmonary angiography—insertion of a dye, followed by x-ray, to assess the overall pulmonary status and to determine mediastinal involvement.

V. Other data sources.

    A. Referral note.

    B. Interview with family.

    C. Other records.

Problems[1]

I. Cough.

II. Blood in sputum.

III. Hemoptysis (does not always occur).

IV. Chest pain (severe, constant, unilateral).

V. Anxiety.

VI. Fatigue.

[1]Problems produced by pulmonary neoplasms vary. Symptoms depend upon the location and size of the tumor.

Diagnosis
    I. Respiratory dysfunction secondary to cellular proliferation and resulting lung obstruction.
   II. Alterations in comfort—pain, alteration in respiratory rate.
  III. Anxiety—mild.
  IV. Alteration in activity level, secondary to fatigue.

Goals of Care
    I. Immediate.
      A. Decrease anxiety.
      B. Provide reassurance and support during diagnostic workup.
      C. Prepare patient and family for treatment program, viz., radiation therapy, surgery, chemotherapy.
      D. Establish methods to help relieve pain.
   II. Long-range.
      A. Teach patient and family about medications, rest, and activity program.
      B. Promote adequate nutrition through diet counseling.
      C. Alert patient and family to additional symptoms that may develop and the need for medical evaluation.
      D. Counsel regarding abstinence from cigarettes.
      E. Provide spiritual counseling if desired by patient.

Intervention
    I. Counsel regarding smoking; develop a plan to limit smoking. This may include hypnosis or nonsmokers' group.
   II. Help patient and family deal with psychological trauma of cancer diagnosis. Provide support and counseling as needed. Answer questions honestly.
  III. Prepare the patient for diagnostic tests, e.g., bronchoscopy, sputum for cytology, or x-ray.
  IV. Administer tranquilizers as needed to help reduce anxiety.
   V. Oral hygiene should be performed frequently, especially if there is an increase in secretions. Potassium permanganate or half-strength hydrogen peroxide should be used.
  VI. Observe for signs of dehydration. Offer fluids as needed in order to maintain hydration.
 VII. Monitor vital signs; identify changes.
VIII. Prepare the patient for treatment program selected by the health team, e.g., surgery, radiation, medication (chemotherapy).
  IX. Reduce pain by administering analgesia, e.g., narcotic.
   X. Follow-up.

Evaluation
    I. Reassessment: complications.
      A. Pleural effusion (refer to Chap. 26).
      B. Metastasis—symptoms will depend upon site of metastasis.
   II. Intervention: surgery.
      A. Types of surgical intervention.
        1. Lobectomy—the surgical removal of one or more lobes of a lung.
        2. Pneumonectomy—the removal of an entire lung.
      B. Preoperative intervention.
        1. Decrease anxiety—provide an atmosphere to discuss surgery; offer support to family and patient.
        2. Spiritual counseling, if desired by patient.
        3. Digitalization (not always done)—this will depend upon cardiac status.
        4. Teach about postoperative expectations, e.g., chest tubes and drainage, turning, coughing, deep breathing.
      C. Postoperative intervention.
        1. Maintain adequate airway; position the patient to avoid the aspiration of fluids.
        2. Suction as needed.
        3. Provide humidified oxygen as needed. Mask or nasal oxygen may be used.
        4. Monitor vital signs—keep accurate records and note changes in blood pressure.
        5. Monitor chest drainage (amount, color, time); refer to "Trauma."

6. Position the patient to ensure optimum lung expansion.
7. Assist patient with the coughing, deep breathing, and mobilization routine. Splint chest as needed for maximum effect.
8. Decrease anxiety by discussing fears openly. If possible attempt to identify precipitating factors.
9. Oral hygiene to prevent halitosis; mouth care using glycerine swabs.
10. Hydration—maintain by IV fluids postoperatively. Maintain awareness of cardiac status and the threat of overhydration.
11. Accurate intake and output—chart frequently. Include chest drainage.
12. Assess pain; medicate as necessary. Care must be taken to avoid suppressing respirations.
13. Observe for:
    a. Bleeding along incision.
    b. Breathlessness, with or without exertion.
    c. Edema about head and neck.
    d. Amount of blood in chest drainage.
14. Gradual increase in food as tolerated to high-protein, high-carbohydrate diet.
15. Increase mobility; engage in range-of-motion (ROM) exercises as tolerated. Use elastic stockings while the patient is on bed rest.

D. Complications of surgery.
1. Respiratory failure—a condition in which the respiratory function is not adequate to maintain normal arterial blood gases, even during rest (refer to "Trauma").
2. Hemorrhage—the escape of excess blood via the great thoracic vessels or through the large incision.
3. Mediastinal shift—a condition in which the air enters the pleural space with each inspiration and becomes trapped; trapped air continues to build up pressure within the chest. As the tension increases it collapses the lung on the affected side and may shift the mediastinal contents (heart, trachea, esophagus, great vessels) to the unaffected side (refer to "Pneumothorax").
4. Interstitial emphysema—a condition in which air, which has escaped into the subpleural space, dissects along the pleura or vessels and may reach the mediastinum and spread to neck and chest.
5. Acute pulmonary edema—an accumulation of excess fluid in the extravascular spaces of the lungs (refer to Chap. 26).

III. Follow-up and reevaluation.

Laryngeal Cancer

Definition Laryngeal neoplasms may involve the true vocal cords or may extend to the supraglottic or subglottic areas. *Carcinoma in situ* is characteristically confined to the true vocal cord. *Verrucous cancer* (sessile appearance) is a laryngeal lesion that is histologically benign but is treated as malignant. Approximately 95 percent of laryngeal neoplasms are squamous cell, while the remainder are classified as sarcoma, adenocarcinoma, and metastatic. The incidence of laryngeal neoplasms is associated with smoking, excessive alcohol intake, and exposure to pollution and irritants.

Prevention I. Decrease exposure to irritants and noxious fumes.
II. Decrease alcohol intake and cigarette smoking.
III. Avoid voice abuse.
IV. Medical follow-up of patients with leukoplakia and laryngeal polyps.

Assessment I. Data sources (see "Cancer of the Lung").
II. Health history (see "Cancer of the Lung").
A. A prolonged period of hoarseness (chronic laryngitis) that does not improve over

time. (This is due to the presence of abnormal tissue around the vocal cords.) The patient should be asked to describe date of onset and accompanying factors, if any.

B. If metastases are present, complaints of weight loss, difficulty swallowing, dyspnea, and an odor to the breath may be described.

C. The patient may have problems maintaining adequate nutrition, and weight loss is not uncommon.

D. The presence of a cough (productive or nonproductive) should be investigated. Length of the cough as well as type and amount of sputum should be evaluated.

E. Age—cancer of the larynx tends to occur in individuals in late middle years or older and is associated with heavy smoking.

F. Patients may complain of the feeling of an obstruction (lump) in their throat.

G. Complaints of pain may vary, from a burning to pain upon swallowing.

III. Physical assessment.

A. Head and neck examination may reveal a painless lump.

B. Lymph nodes should be palpated. They may be enlarged, especially if met are present.

C. Examination of the larynx will usually reveal the initial lesion.

D. The patient is often apprehensive and may fear the diagnosis.

E. If the tumor has interfered with the patient's eating habits, weight loss may be apparent.

IV. Diagnostic tests.

A. Indirect laryngoscopy—use of a mirror to examine the larynx.

B. Direct laryngoscopy—visualization of the larynx through a laryngoscope.

C. Biopsy of lesion in order to analyze the tumor tissue.

D. Tomography to define the neoplasm's borders.

E. Barium esophagogram to define the neoplasm's borders. The patient is asked to swallow a barium substance and he or she is x-rayed.

V. Other data sources (see "Cancer of the Lung").

Problems

I. Hoarseness.

II. Pain and burning of the throat occurs in extrinsic cancer when drinking hot fluids or orange juice.

III. Lump in neck indicates metastasis.

IV. Cough.

V. Dysphagia.

VI. Late developing problems:

A. Dysphagia.   C. Weight loss.

B. Dyspnea.   D. Foul breath.

Diagnosis

I. Alterations in comfort—discomfort secondary to throat pain, cough, dysphagia.

II. Respiratory dysfunction.

III. Communication process impaired—secondary to the lesion at vocal cords.

IV. Potential nutritional alteration—secondary to decreased fluid intake.

V. Self-concept—alteration of body image secondary to physical changes of surgery.

Goals of Care

I. Immediate.

A. Promote physical and emotional rest.

B. Decrease discomfort localized at lesion.

C. Provide support during diagnostic tests.

D. Prepare for treatment plan—radiation, surgery, chemotherapy.

II. Long-range.

A. Help patient and family deal with the psychological impact of the diagnosis of cancer.

B. Help the patient deal with the altered mode of communication.

C. Teach about decreased exposure to pollution and irritants.

    D. Teach about food intake, management of laryngectomy tube or dressing (if needed).

    E. Counsel concerning abstinence from smoking.

    F. Refer to self-help groups such as New Voices (if needed).

    G. Counseling about being neck breather, need for altered communication, emergency intervention, crisis of surgery, and decreased alcohol intake.

Intervention

    I. Oral hygiene to relieve halitosis and prevent infection. Diluted hydrogen peroxide may used.

    II. Soothing steam inhalations to moisten mucosa and liquefy secretions.

    III. Provide fluids and food that are easy to swallow. Avoid acidic foods, e.g., orange juice.

    IV. Begin use of magic slate or notepaper for communication. Support the patient during this transition period.

    V. Provide support during diagnostic tests. Prepare the patient for each test to decrease fear.

    VI. Decrease anxiety. Promote an environment where the patient and family are free to discuss impending surgery.

    VII. Prepare for treatment plan—surgery, radiation, chemotherapy. Develop a teaching plan that includes all components of each therapy.

    VIII. Assess response to intervention.

    IX. Evaluate the patient's overall response to teaching; dietary changes; reduction in anxiety; and adaptation to changes in communication.

Evaluation

    I. Reassessment: complications. Poor response to other interventions or a decision following initial diagnostic work-up may result in surgery.

    II. Intervention: surgery (refer to Table 27-1).

        A. Preoperative intervention.

           1. Decrease anxiety by allowing the patient to verbalize fear of surgery.

           2. Provide reassurance and support during the period preceding surgery.

           3. Interpret surgeon's information (as needed) for patient and family in order to reduce misconceptions and clarify surgery.

           4. Provide spiritual counseling if desired.

           5. Prepare patient for breathing through tracheal opening. Tell patient what can be expected following the insertion of a tracheostomy tube.

           6. Plan means of communication for use after surgery.

           7. Discuss postoperative expectations—laryngectomy, tracheostomy tube, suctioning, Hemovac, tube feedings.

        B. Types of surgical intervention.

           1. Laryngofissure—an incision into the thyroid cartilage in order to excise the neoplasm. Usually only one true cord is excised (see Table 27-1). Postoperative intervention:

                a. Oral hygiene to reduce odor, prevent infection, and lubricate mucosa (see "Cancer of the Lung").

                b. Assess vital signs. Note changes and report as appropriate.

                c. Caution patient to restrict use of voice. Establish alternate means of communication.

                d. Teach patient to cover tracheostomy tube opening to speak.

                e. Use note pad, magic slate, or hand signals for communication.

                f. Monitor IV or gastric feeding.

                g. When tolerated, give sont foods (custard, gelatin) instead of liquids.

                h. Clean skin around tracheostomy tube (refer to Table 27-8).

                i. Clean tracheostomy tube as needed.

                j. Suction tracheostomy as needed.

                k. Observe operative site for:

                    (1) Bleeding.

                    (2) Subcutaneous emphysema.

l. Medicate with analgesic and/or narcotic for pain as needed. Monitor the patient's response to the drug.

2. Supraglottic laryngectomy—a horizontal incision above the true cords permits only the diseased tissue to be removed (see Table 27-1). Postoperative intervention:

    a. See postoperative intervention under point 1, above.

    b. Help patient to understand that cough will lessen when the ability to swallow improves.

    c. Observe operative site for:

    (1) Bleeding.

    (2) Subcutaneous emphysema.

    (3) Wound infection.

3. Total laryngectomy—removal of the thyroid cartilage, the hyoid bone, the cricoid cartilage, and two or three tracheal rings (see Table 27-1). Postoperative intervention:

    a. See postoperative intervention under point 1, above.

    b. Elevate head of bed to 30° to facilitate drainage and preserve the airway.

TABLE 27-1 / VARIATIONS OF SURGERY FOR LARYNGEAL TUMORS

Structures Removed	*Structures Left*	*Postoperative Condition*
Total Laryngectomy		
Hyoid bone	Tongue	Loses voice
Entire larynx (epiglottis, false cords, true cords)	Pharyngeal walls	Breathes through tracheostomy
Cricoid cartilage	Lower trachea	No problem swallowing
Two or three rings of trachea		
Supraglottic or Horizontal Laryngectomy		
Hyoid bone	True vocal cords	Normal voice
Epiglottis	Cricoid cartilage	May aspirate occasionally, especially liquids
False vocal cords	Trachea	Normal airway
Vertical (or Hemi-) Laryngectomy		
One true vocal cord	Epiglottis	Hoarse but serviceable voice
False cord	One false cord	Normal airway
Arytenoid	One true vocal cord	No problem swallowing
One-half thyroid cartilage	Cricoid	
Laryngofissure and Partial Laryngectomy		
One vocal cord	All other structures	Hoarse but serviceable voice; occasionally almost normal voice
		No airway problem
		No swallowing problem
Endoscopic Removal of Early Carcinoma		
Part of one vocal cord	All other structures	May have a normal voice
		No other problems

Source: William H. Havener, William H. Saunders, Carol Fair Keith, and Ardra W. Prescott, *Nursing Care in Ear, Eye, Nose and Throat Disorders,* 3d ed., The C. V. Mosby Company, St. Louis, 1974, p. 275.

     c. Maintain adequate airway. Be sure tracheostomy remains unobstructed.

     d. Provide moist air to tracheal opening; humidified oxygen can be administered as often as necessary.

     e. Clean skin around laryngectomy tube. Use ointment (Neosporin) to prevent crusting and skin breakdown.

     f. Suction as needed.

     g. Administer tube feedings. Teach patient how to handle abdominal distension if present. Provide additional amounts of water after tube feeding to prevent osmotic diuresis (refer to Chap. 29).

     h. Teach patient to place hand behind head to facilitate lifting it.

     i. Teach patient to modify oral hygiene (brush tongue, palate, inside of mouth).

     j. Provide psychological support and counseling.

4. Radical neck resection—removal of an extensive amount of facial tissue, nerves, bones, and lymph glands surrounding the lesion (refer to Table 27-2). Postoperative intervention:

     a. See postoperative intervention under point 3, above.

     b. Monitor Hemovac for the amount, color, and consistency of drainage.

     c. Observe operative site for:

          (1) Bleeding, hematoma.

          (2) Carotid rupture.

          (3) Wound infection.

C. Complications of surgery.

1. Hemorrhage—the escape of excess blood from the vessels of the neck or through the incision or stoma site.

TABLE 27-2 / STATEMENT OF OBJECTIVES AND STANDARDS FOR PATIENTS WITH RADICAL NECK RESECTIONS

The following objectives and standards cover the major areas of nursing care for patients undergoing radical neck resection.

Objective I: The patient is free of preventable complications.
    Standard A: The neck skin flaps are down and the wound is free of blood, fluid, and air.
    Standard B: The operative wound is free of infection.
    Standard C: Facial edema is minimal and circulation is maintained by positioning and activity.
Objective II: The patient's pain and discomfort are minimized.
    Standard A: The patient is positioned with the head of the bed elevated to promote comfort.
    Standard B: Pain and discomfort are reduced with the administration of medication.
Objective III: The patient's fear and anxiety related to illness and hospitalization are reduced.
    Standard A: The patient's level of anxiety is assessed continually and appropriate intervention is initiated.
    Standard B: The patient is provided with care that reduces the occurrence of physical symptoms unrelated to his pathophysiology.
Objective IV: The patient is prepared or arrangements are made for continuation of the necessary regimen of care after hospitalization.
    Standard A: The patient understands the physical limitations on him or her.
    Standard B: The patient knows that it is necessary to return for medical checkup at an appointed time.

Source: *Administrative Nursing Policy and Procedure Manual,* University of Iowa Hospitals and Clinics, Department of Nursing, Iowa City, 1971; Ardis J. O'Dell, "Objectives and Standards in the Care of the Patient with a Radical Neck Dissection," *Nursing Clinics of North America,* **8:**159–164, March 1973.

   2. Hematoma formation—a collection of blood beneath the suture lines.
   3. Rupture of the carotid artery—an interruption of the integrity of the carotid artery that is usually associated with radiation therapy.
   4. Wound infection—the response of the wound tissue to the presence of pathogens.
   5. Pharyngeal-cutaneous fistula—an opening that is caused by the leakage of secretions through breakdown in the pharyngeal suture line.
   6. Pneumonia—an acute infection of the alveolar spaces of the lung.
   7. Stenosis of stoma—a reduction in the size of the surgically created stoma due to fibrosis or infection.
   8. Slough of skin flap—a segment of necrotic tissue within the operative area.

III. Follow-up and reevaluation.

Sarcoidosis

Definition

Granulomas are tumors composed of granulated tissue. *Sarcoidosis,* a granulomatous reaction, has an undetermined etiology and pathogenesis. Its characteristic epithelioid cell tubercles involve multiple and varying organs or tissues. The most common sites include lymph nodes, lungs, liver, skin, eyes, spleen, and heart.

One suggested etiology involves a single agent (virus, fungus), while another suggested etiology includes a tissue response to a variety of agents (tuberculosis, other chronic infections). Sarcoidosis is universal in distribution, but has a particular predilection for blacks. The acute stage of sarcoidosis has a high incidence of complete and spontaneous remission in less than 2 years.

Assessment

I. Data sources (see "Cancer of the Lung").
II. Health history (see "Cancer of the Lung").
   A. Cultural background—seen more frequently in blacks.
   B. Family history—familial tendency observed.
   C. Increasing complaints of fatigue, dyspnea, and cough may be noted. (Description of cough, e.g., amount of sputum, frequency, etc., is essential).
   D. The patient may report a weight loss.
   E. Complaints of joint pain are not uncommon as the problem progresses.
III. Physical assessment.
   A. General appearance may indicate a significant loss of weight. The patient may appear tired and pale.
   B. Examination of the chest may indicate the auscultation of fine inspiratory rales. Shortness of breath (dyspnea) may be observed with varying degrees of activity.
   C. The skin may be warm to touch, especially if the patient has a fever. Erythema may be present along with plaques or papules. Subcutaneous nodules may be present, and edema is often palpated.
   D. Joint swelling and decreased movement may be observed.
   E. Palpation of the lymph glands will reveal a generalized lymphadenopathy.
   F. A complete physical examination will be needed in order to assess the complete impact of the problem (e.g., secondary cardiopulmonary changes, hepatic enlargement, visual changes, and enlargement of the spleen, etc.).
IV. Diagnostic tests.
   A. Chest x-ray will reveal:
      1. Mediastinal adenopathy.
      2. Bilateral hilar and right paratracheal adenopathy.
      3. Diffuse, symmetrical pulmonary infiltrates.
   B. Pulmonary function will demonstrate the following changes:
      1. Decreased compliance.
      2. Impaired diffusion of oxygen and carbon dioxide.
      3. Reduced vital capacity.

    C. Scalene fat pad biopsy will indicate positive nodes.
    D. Nickerson-Kveim test will yield local, papulonodular lesions in 4 to 6 weeks which should then be biopsied.
    E. Laboratory blood tests will demonstrate:
        1. Hyperglobulinemia.
        2. Elevated serum calcium.
        3. Elevated serum uric acid.
  V. Other data sources (see "Renal Tumors," Chap. 28).

Problems[2]

  I. Fever (may be low grade).   **IV.** Dyspnea.
  II. Weight loss.   **V.** Arthralgia.
  III. Cough.   **VI.** Fatigue.

Diagnosis

  I. Alterations in comfort—discomfort.
  II. Respiratory dysfunction—dyspnea, secondary to cell changes in lungs.
  III. Fatigue secondary to dyspnea and impaired cardiopulmonary status.
  IV. Depletion of body fluids; secondary to fever.

Goals of Care

  I. Immediate.
    A. Promote rest—decrease fatigue.
    B. Reduce fever.
    C. Maintain nutrition.
    D. Alleviate cough and dyspnea.
    E. Relieve arthralgias.
  II. Long-range.
    A. Teach patient about medication, activity levels, and avoiding pollution and irritants.
    B. Counsel about smoking.
    C. Prevent complications.

Intervention

  I. Lozenges and cough suppressants.
  II. Promote rest and relaxation—arrange planned rest periods to prevent overexertion.
  III. Provide high-protein, low-calcium diet. Plan menu with patient.
  IV. Administer analgesics to relieve pain. Use prednisone, antacids to help decrease the inflammation and joint involvement.
  V. Counsel about smoking (see "Cancer of the Lung").
  VI. Teach about medications dose, side effects and diet.
  VII. Follow-up.

Evaluation

  I. Reassessment: complications—cor pulmonale (refer to Chap. 26 for a complete discussion).
    A. Assessment:
        1. Dyspnea (increased).
        2. Wheezing—increased amount of rales noted on inspiration.
        3. Cough—more productive.
        4. Cyanosis—due to cardiovascular compromise.
        5. Loud pulmonic second sound.
    B. Intervention.
        1. Oxygen therapy—as needed.
        2. Rest—increase rest periods, control visitors, but be cautious about hazards of immobility.
        3. Sodium restriction.
        4. Diuretics (refer to Chap. 26 for a complete discussion).
        5. Digitalis (refer to Chap. 26 for a complete discussion).
  II. Follow-up and reevaluation.

[2] Problems may be minimal (or lacking), depending on organ localization.

Polyps

Definition

A *polyp* is a benign, epithelial tumor with a pedicle that attaches it to a mucous membrane. Polyps appear as a gray or pink grapelike lesion and are sometimes translucent. *Nasal polyps* (and sinus polyps) form, over time, from localized swellings of the nasal or sinus mucosa. Usually nasal polyps are multiple. Allergic rhinitis ("hay fever") is the most common predisposing factor. Polyps tend to recur when the underlying allergy is not well controlled. When polyps become large enough to occlude the airway, symptoms of nasal obstruction occur.

Assessment

I. Data sources (see "Cancer of the Lung").
II. Health history.
    A. Age—polyps can occur at any age.
    B. Occupation (describe position)—identify irritating pollutants.
    C. Habits—smoking (see "Cancer of the Lung").
    D. History of allergies, including chronic rhinitis; related problems, including drainage; and, on occasion, headache.
    E. Seasonal influence, e.g., hay fever.
    F. The patient complains of a problem with smelling.
III. Physical assessment—nasal exam with speculum or mirror will reveal:
    A. Thickened mucous membrane.
    B. Smooth, pink or gray, grapelike lesion in middle meatus.

Problems

I. Nasal obstruction.
II. Nasal discharge (usually clear mucus).
III. Headache.
IV. Anosmia.
V. Speech distortion—nasal hollow sound to the voice.

Diagnosis

I. Alterations in comfort—discomfort, secondary to headache; nasal discharge.
II. Respiratory dysfunction.
III. Sensory or perceptual alteration—smell.
IV. Alteration of sleep-rest pattern.

Goals of Care

I. Immediate.
    A. Alleviate headache.
    B. Reduce nasal obstruction and discharge.
    C. Provide foods with visual appeal.
II. Long-range.
    A. Teach about recurrent nature of problem.
    B. Counsel concerning identification of allergen and desensitization.

Intervention

I. Oral hygiene (see "Cancer of the Lung").
II. Moist inhalations to lubricate mucosa and prevent drying.
III. Antihistamines and decongestants to reduce secretions from the nasal passage.
IV. Analgesics (acetylsalicylic acid, ASA) to reduce inflammation of surrounding mucosa (ASA) and relieve headache.
V. Lubrication at nares entry to prevent skin breakdown.
VI. Foods that are colorful and appetizing to improve oral intake when patient is unable to smell.
VII. Teaching about:
    A. Medications—dose, side effects.
    B. Avoiding irritants.
VIII. Follow-up.

Evaluation I. Reassessment: complications.
    A. Nasal discomfort or fullness.
    B. Mouth breathing.
    C. Anxiety.
II. Intervention.
    A. Oral hygiene to reduce halitosis and prevent infection.
    B. Moist inhalations.
    C. Injection of steroid solution into polyp to help reduce inflammation.
    D. Surgery: polypectomy—surgical procedure to remove polyp obstructing the airway.
        1. Preoperative intervention.
            a. Decrease anxiety.
            b. Provide support and reassurance.
            c. Teach about postoperative expectations, e.g., mouth breathing, not to swallow secretions. Teach how to rid self of excess secretions following surgery.
        2. Postoperative intervention.
            a. Oral hygiene.
            b. Liquid diet (immediate)—as tolerated.
            c. Assess vital signs (rectal temperature).
            d. Observe for bleeding and disruptions in breathing. Check to see if nasal pack is in position.
        3. Complications of surgery.
            a. Hemorrhage.
            b. Infection.
III. Follow-up and reevaluation.

METABOLIC DISORDERS

Respiratory Failure

See "Obstructions."

Cystic Fibrosis

See Chap. 14.

INFLAMMATORY DISORDERS

Pneumonia

Definition *Pneumonia* is an inflammation of the air sacs in the lungs that causes consolidation of lung tissue as the alveoli fill with exudate. The four stages of the disease process, which may appear in a single lesion, include (1) edema, (2) red hepatization (arrival of erythrocytes and polymorphonuclear leukocytes), (3) gray hepatization (many leukocytes), and (4) resolution (Fig. 27-1).

The causative agent gains access to the respiratory tract by droplet infection or throurh contact with infected patients or carriers. Generally pneumonia begins in the right lower, right middle, or left lower lobes of the lungs, areas to which gravity is most likely to carry upper respiratory secretions aspirated during sleep.

Any pathology that represses the host's defense mechanisms could result in the development of pneumonia. Problems such as bronchial infections, depressed central nervous system (drugs, alcohol, head injury), immobility, superinfection, cancer, diabetes mellitus, cardiac failure, chronic obstructive lung disease (COLD), postsurgery, use of

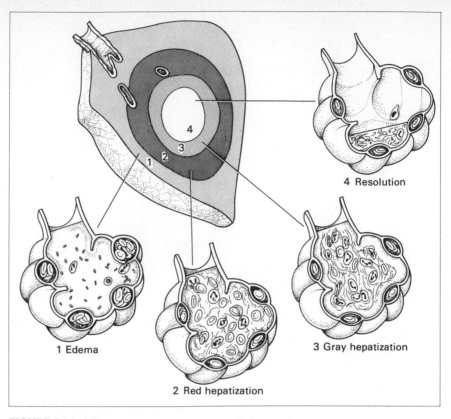

FIGURE 27-1 / Four stages apparent in a single lesion. Gross necropsy specimen clearly shows that all four stages of development, spreading in concentric rings, can be demonstrated in a single lesion. (*Adapted from Murray Wittner, Pneumoccal Pneumonia, Abbott Laboratories, Illinois, January 1974, p. 6.*)

steroids, or inhalation of a noxious gas may all contribute to the development of pneumonia. If a substantial portion of one or more of the lobes is involved, the disease is considered to be *lobar pneumonia. Bronchopneumonia* usually consists of diffuse patches of pneumonia scattered throughout the lungs. Pneumonia is generally classified according to causative agent: pneumococcal pneumonia, staphylococcal pneumonia, klebsiella pneumonia, and primary atypical pneumonia. Each is manifested by a variety of physical changes and is treated with a variety of antibiotics. Pneumococcal pneumonia, caused by gram-positive pneumococci, is outlined in detail below because it is the most common type of bacterial pneumonia and generally typifies pneumonia caused by an infectious agent.

Prevention

    I. Maintain natural resistance.
   II. Avoid upper respiratory infections (URI) and exposure to cold; treat colds and flu promptly.
 III. Vaccinate highly susceptible persons against influenza.
 IV. Maintain optimal respiratory function.
   V. Avoid obliteration of cough reflex and aspiration of secretions; check gag reflex (especially following surgery).
 VI. Ensure adequate bronchial hygiene by turning, coughing, and deep breathing frequently; suction when necessary, especially after surgery.
VII. Avoid medications that suppress bronchopulmonary defense mechanisms.
VIII. Place unconscious and semiconscious patients in an upright position.

IX. Provide frequent oral hygiene.

X. Prevent spread of infection by using appropriate medical asepsis.

XI. Assess each high-risk patient.

Assessment

I. Data sources.
   - **A.** Patient.
   - **B.** Family.
   - **C.** Significant others.
   - **D.** Medical records.

II. Health history.
   - **A.** Age—prognosis adversely affected in old age and infancy.
   - **B.** Sex—3 times more common in males than females.
   - **C.** Cultural background.
   - **D.** Occupation—type of job; pollutants.
   - **E.** Socioeconomic status.
   - **F.** Dietary habits—nutritional status.
   - **G.** Smoking, alcoholic intake, use of drugs.
   - **H.** Life-style—single, aged, health perception, health habits.
   - **I.** Incidence of colds in family—incidence of URI may predispose individual to pneumonia.
   - **J.** Season—increased susceptibility in winter.
   - **K.** Allergies—past history should be noted.
   - **L.** Patient will often complain of a cough and pleuritis; chest pain is not uncommon.
   - **M.** Muscle aches and pains along with headache are also reported.
   - **N.** History of recent surgery should be noted along with length of time under anesthesia.
   - **O.** Patient may complain of being short of breath, especially after coughing.

III. Physical assessment.
   - **A.** The patient will be warm to touch and usually have a fever (as high as 104 to 106°F).
   - **B.** The skin will appear pale, flushed, and dry. Skin turgor may be affected. The appearance of herpes simplex is not uncommon.
   - **C.** Nostril flaring may be seen and cyanosis of the nailbeds noted.
   - **D.** The patient will often be lying on the affected side and will guard the affected area when coughing (pleuritis pain).
   - **E.** The patient will have a productive cough. The sputum is often rust-colored and thick. Later, as the disease progresses, sputum will become yellow.
   - **F.** Severe chest pain is aggravated by chest excursion; therefore, chest movement may be limited.
   - **G.** Upon percussion the thoracic resonants will be diminished over the area(s) of infiltration.
   - **H.** Tactile fremitus is decreased initially and then will increase with consolidation.
   - **I.** Deviation of the trachea away from the affected lung may be noted.
   - **J.** Breath sounds will be diminished over the area of infiltration; pleuritic friction rub will become tubercular with fine crepitant rales present.
   - **K.** Nausea and vomiting along with jaundice may be noted in some cases. Abdominal distension may be observed.
   - **L.** Respirations are rapid and shallow and dypsneic; increase with consolidation is not uncommon. Tachycardia may be present.

IV. Diagnostic tests.
   - **A.** Sputum culture and sensitivity and selected blood tests are done to evaluate pathogen. Findings reveal:
     1. Leukocytosis (20,000 to 35,000 white blood cells per cubic milliliter).
     2. Decreased sodium, and increased bilirubin.
     3. Decreased chloride, and increased sedimentation rate.
     4. Thrombocytopenia.
     5. Leukopenia.
   - **B.** Blood gases may be altered depending upon the extent of the problem.

    C. Chest x-ray will demonstrate lung infiltration; areas of consolidation may be vague at first, but later become well defined.

    D. ECG—tachycardia may be present.

    E. Other data.
1. Referral.
2. Interview with family.
3. Medical records.

Problems[3]

I. Fever with chills and sweats.
II. Chest pain—sharp pleuritic; exacerbated by breathing or coughing.
III. Short dry hacking cough with rusty sputum.
IV. Increased pulse rate.
V. Shallow, rapid, labored respiration.
VI. Muscle aches and pains with headache.
VII. Nausea and vomiting with abdominal distension.
VIII. Skin breakdown (herpes simplex).
IX. Anxiety.

Diagnosis

I. Respiratory dysfunction (impairment of lung tissue).
II. Alteration in cardiac output.
III. Depletion of body fluid secondary to increased body temperature.
IV. Alterations in comfort—discomfort secondary to pleuritic pain, fever.
V. Disturbance in nutrition secondary to nausea and vomiting.
VI. Anxiety—mild to moderate, secondary to dyspnea and elevated body temperature.

Goals of Care

I. Immediate.
    A. Identify etiologic agent and treat with antimicrobial chemotherapy.
    B. Remove accumulated secretions from bronchi.
    C. Prevent spread of infection.
    D. Provide symptomatic and supportive care.
    E. Prevent complications and treat if present.
    F. Offer comfort.
II. Long-range.
    A. Teach patient and family about prevention, complications, and what actions are appropriate.
    B. Instruct patient and family about importance of follow-up and the purpose, dosage, frequency, and side effects of medications.
    C. Counsel regarding the use of cigarettes.

Intervention

I. Administer antibiotics—know purpose, dosage, frequency of administration, and side effects (penicillin is usually the drug of choice).
II. Administer cough suppressants, expectorants, analgesics, sedatives. Teach patient about importance of proper administration of cough medicines.
III. Collect and evaluate results of sputum and blood specimens.
IV. Assess vital signs and breath sounds frequently to evaluate patient progress.
V. Administration of oxygen may be necessary to assist respiration. (Should be humidified.) Mechanical ventilation may be needed if respiratory malfunction is severe.
VI. Assist with frequent coughing, deep breathing, teaching the patient how to cough. Chest splinting is important.
VII. Perform chest physiotherapy to assist with removal of secretions from lungs. Suctioning may be needed.
VIII. Promote rest; change position frequently. During the acute phase, patient may be given relaxant to promote sleep.

[3]Abrupt onset.

IX. Assist with normal activities of daily living (ADL).

X. Perform ROM exercises; help decrease side effects of immobility.

XI. Offer skin care; keep the patient warm and dry. Lubricate lips if dry and cracked.

XII. Provide oral hygiene—increase the amounts of fluids and use good mouth care to prevent infection.

XIII. Encourage well-balanced diet with good hydration; record intake and output of fluids.

XIV. Assist with intercostal block if necessary.

XV. Assess response to interventions; assess level of orientation.

XVI. Teach patient about:

    A. Methods to avoid spread of infection.

    B. Preventive measures for avoiding infection.

    C. Feeling weak and fatigued and being susceptible to colds for a while.

    D. Gradually increasing exercise.

    E. Continuing coughing and deep breathing exercises.

    F. Medications—purpose, dosage, frequency, and side effects.

    G. Importance of follow-up.

XVII. Follow-up.

Evaluation

I. Reassessment: complications.

    A. Atelectasis—area of lung that is collapsed, airless, and shrunken.

        1. Assessment.

            a. Pleuritic pain—increased over the affected area.

            b. Rapid respirations.

            c. Dyspnea—increase.

            d. Weakness—generalized malaise.

            e. Anxiety.

            f. Cyanosis.

            g. Increased temperature, pulse and blood pressure.

            h. Breath sounds absent over the affected area.

            i. Percussion—flat.

            j. Mediastinal shift toward affected side noted.

        2. Intervention.

            a. Assist with bronchoscopy.

            b. Assist with thoracentesis (the insertion of a tube into the chest cavity to remove fliid and to help reinflate the lung).

            c. Monitor condition after thoracentesis (see Fig. 27-5).

            d. Assess vital signs, breath sounds.

            e. Encourage coughing, deep breathing.

            f. Suction when necessary to help remove secretions.

            g. Position on unaffected side.

            h. Increase activity gradually.

            i. Perform chest physiotherapy.

            j. Administer antibiotics.

    B. Empyema—accumulation of purulent exudate in the pleural cavity.

        1. Assessment.

            a. Orthopnea.

            b. Localized chest pain; constant or on inspiration.

            c. Unequal chest expansion.

            d. Diminished or absent breath sounds over affected area.

            e. Percussion—dull over involved area.

            f. Productive cough.

         2. Intervention.

            a. Administer oxygen (humidify).

            b. Place in semi-Fowler's position.

            c. Assess vital signs, breath sounds, and chest expansion.

    d. Encourage coughing and deep breathing.
    e. Perform chest physiotherapy.
    f. Assist with thoracentesis.
    g. Monitor chest tubes (see "Trauma").
   C. Pleurisy (see "Pleurisy").
   D. Pleural effusion (see Chap. 26).
   E. Pulmonary edema (see Chap. 26).
   F. Lung abscess (see "Lung Abscess").
  II. Follow-up and reevaluation.

Chronic Bronchitis

Definition

Chronic bronchitis is a disorder chracterized by chronic cough and the production of sputum on most days for at least 3 months in the year for at least 2 years. It is an environmental disease that is associated with heavy smoking, cold, damp air, pollution, and industrial dusts. Long-term exposure to toxins hinders the function of cilia as well as causing excessive production of viscid mucus. Plugs of mucus obstruct the airways, creating an environment conducive to bronchopneumonia. During the healing process, fibrosis of tissues contributes to dilation or destruction of bronchioles. These changes contribute to the eventual development of chronic obstructive pulmonary disease.

Prevention

 I. Reduce exposure to persons with URI.
 II. Reduce exposure to pollution and occupational dusts.
 III. Abstain from smoking.

Assessment

 I. Data sources (see "Pneumonia").
 II. Health history (see "Pneumonia").
  A. Exposure to pollution and other irritants that may stimulate an inflammatory response.
  B. Sleep habits; number of pillows; amount of rest needed.
  C. Life-style—exposure to infection.
  D. Health perception—health maintenance patterns.
  E. Respiratory infections—identify chronic respiratory infections.
  F. History of recurrent cough that increases in persistence over many years.
  G. Increased production of sputum often reported upon rising, which may become tiring to the patient.
  H. Report of shortness of breath, especially upon exertion, and persistent weight loss.
 III. Physical assessment.
  A. Diminished chest excursion observed.
  B. Scattered moist rales noted upon auscultation over the affected areas.
  C. Wheezing may be auscultated. This problem intensified by inspiration of cold air. Musical rhonchi may also be heard especially if secondary to infection (URI).
  D. Dyspnea is present. Cough persistent. Sputum initially not present, but as the problem becomes more chronic, sputum becomes thicker and more productive.
  E. Clubbing of the fingers may be observed.
  F. The patient can be thin and pale. She or he may tire easily, and cyanosis around lips and nailbeds may be observed.
 IV. Diagnostic tests.
  A. Chest x-ray—allows visualization of the lungs and areas of infiltration.
  B. Bronchogram—allows for the viewing of the bronchial tree by way of the injection of a radiopaque dye. For chronic bronchitis, diverticula of the bronchioles with cylindrical dilatations may be noted. Small round terminal expansions of the bronchial tree may also be noted.
  C. Reid index[4]—indicates gradual enlargement of mucous glands.

[4]Reid index is a measure of mucous gland enlargement in relation to the thickness of the bronchial wall.

    D. Sputum culture—done to rule out superimposed infection and identify the pathogen.

    E. Sputum cytologic exam—the presence of eosinophils indicates underlying allergic disorder.

    F. Arterial blood gases—estimate progression of disorder. The more pulmonary obstruction, the more altered the blood gases.

    G. Lung function studies:

        1. Increased residual volume.

        2. Reduced vital capacity.

        3. Reduced maximum breathing capacity.

        4. Increased resistance to air flow.

  V. Other data sources (see "Pneumonia").

Problems

  I. Persistent cough (with spasms).

  II. Sputum production (mucoid or purulent).

  III. Sensation of heaviness in chest.

  IV. Fever (during episode).

  V. Dyspnea (does not always occur).

Diagnosis

  I. Respiratory dysfunction—mild to severe.

  II. Alteration in comfort—discomfort, secondary to respiratory changes.

Goals of Care

  I. Immediate.

    A. Promote movement of secretions by postural drainage, hydration, humidity, bronchodilators, and mucolytics.

    B. Improve ventilation.

    C. Promote comfort by oral hygiene, lozenges with topical anesthetic, and soothing inhalations.

  II. Long-range.

    A. Control progression of disease by preventing respiratory infections and complications.

    B. Teach about medications, diet, exposure to pollution and irritants.

    C. Counsel concerning smoking and being overweight.

Interventions

  I. Provide a quiet, nonstimulating environment.

  II. Promote a rest and activity program.

  III. Oxygen therapy (if needed).

  IV. Adminster bronchodilators, mucolytics, and prophylactic antibiotics to reduce inflammation, and promote liquefaction and removal of excess secretions.

  V. Give frequent oral hygiene to keep the patient hydrated and liquefy secretions.

  VII. Give soothing inhalations (humidify inspired air).

  VII. Provide lozenges with a topical anesthetic.

  VIII. Provide fluids and diet as tolerated.

  IX. Monitor vital signs (as needed).

  X. Teach about:

    A. Medications—dose, side effects.

    B. Diet—as needed to maintain health. Weight reduction as needed.

    C. Rest and activity to help maintain resistance to other infections.

    D. Preventing respiratory infections.

    E. Preventing exposure to pollution and irritants.

  XI. Counsel concerning nonsmoking and weight control.

  XII. Follow-up.

Evaluation

  I. Reassessment: complications.

    A. Bronchopneumonia (see "Pneumonia").

    B. Cor pulmonale (see Chap. 26).

    C. Chronic obstructive lung disease (see "Obstructions").

    D. Respiratory insufficiency.
      1. Assessment.
        a. Hypoxemia—decreased Pa_{O_2} (refer to Tables 27-10 and 27-11).
        b. Hypercapnia—increased Pa_{CO_2} (refer to Tables 27-10 and 27-11).
        c. pH—respiratory acidosis or normal.
        d. Restlessness.
        e. Headache.
        f. Shallow rapid respirations.
      2. Intervention.
        a. Suctioning as needed.
        b. Endotracheal intubation (if needed).
        c. Administer a nebulized bronchodilator, aminophylline, and mucolytics to reduce bronchospasm and increase bronchial dilatation.
        d. Administer humidified oxygen (as needed).
        e. Assist ventilation (as needed); teach intermittent positive pressure breathing (IPPB).
        f. ECG to to determine cardiac changes.
        g. Monitor arterial blood gases to evaluate effectiveness of treatment.
        h. Monitor electrolytes.
  II. Follow-up and reevaluation.

Pneumoconiosis

Definition   *Pneumoconiosis* implies a group of occupational lung diseases. The characteristic pulmonary abnormalities result from the inhalation and retention of dust particles. The inhaled particulate matter exerts harmful effects by various mechanisms. Organic materials (moldy hay) cause a hypersensitivity reaction and produce granulomas. Fiber dust (cotton) may produce allergic types of reactions. Particulate matter such as silica and asbestos may cause pulmonary fibrosis. A discrete, modular, less serious fibrosis results from 1- to 5-μm particles, while ultramicroscopic particles may cause a more diffuse fibrosis. As the fibrosis progresses, it will result in increased lung impairment and diminished pulmonary function.

Prevention
  I. Wear a mask when exposed to dusts and other particulate matter that could be inhaled.
  II. Implement standards to reduce hazardous dust levels.

Assessment
  I. Data sources (see "Pneumonia").
  II. Health history (see "Pneumonia").
    A. Continuous exposure to dusts and particulate matter.
    B. Occupation—e.g., stone cutter, miner.
    C. Patient will note increased shortness of breath over time, especially upon exertion.
    D. Persistent cough may be present.
    E. Chest pain may be present.
  III. Physical assessment.
    A. Examination of the chest will reveal areas of hypo- and hyperresonance, diminished intensity of breath sounds, and wheezing.
    B. Cough—expectoration of dark gray to black sputum observed.
    C. Breathlessness noted, especially upon exertion.
    D. Finger clubbing may be noted.
  IV. Diagnostic tests.
    A. Chest x-ray will show discrete nodular shadows distributed throughout lungs.
    B. Lung function tests reveal diminished vital capacity, diminished maximum breathing capacity, and decreased diffusion of oxygen–carbon dioxide.
  V. Other data sources (see "Pneumonia").

Problems I. Exertional dyspnea. IV. Prone to respiratory infections.
II. Cough. V. Sputum production.
III. Chest pain.

Diagnosis Respiratory dysfunction secondary to inhalation of free dust particles.

Goals of Care I. Immediate.
  A. Promote drainage of retained secretions.
  B. Improve ventilation.
  C. Reduce cough.
  D. Maintain general nutrition.
  E. Prevent respiratory infection.
  F. Determine if tuberculosis is present.
II. Long-range.
  A. Teach patient and family regarding smoking, prevention of infections, diet, activity level, and medications.
  B. Prevent complications.
  C. Counsel regarding safety standards and safety measures in occupational setting.
  D. Counsel regarding possible need to change occupations or retirement.

Intervention I. Administer purified protein derivative (PPD). (Pulmonary tuberculosis can be a complication of silicosis.)
II. Postural drainage with clapping or vibrating to help reduce congestion and consolidation of sputum (refer to Fig. 27-8).
III. Administer bronchodilators and mucolytic agents to allow for bronchodilatation and expulsion of secretion.
IV. Oral hygiene daily to prevent infection and increase comfort.
V. Hydration to liquefy secretions and hasten their removal.
VI. Teach regarding:
  A. Nutrition. C. Prevention of respiratory infections.
  B. Activity level. D. Medications—dose, side effects.
VII. Counsel regarding eliminating of smoking.
VIII. Counsel regarding methods of reducing occupational dust exposure to accepted safety limits.
IX. Counseling referral.
X. Assess response to interventions.
XI. Follow-up.

Evaluation I. Reassessment: complications—cor pulmonale (see Chap. 26).
II. Follow-up and reevaluation.

Tuberculosis

Definition *Tuberculosis* is a reportable, communicable, infectious, inflammatory, and chronic disease. The tubercle bacillus, *Mycobacterium tuberculosis,* is disseminated by droplets and enters the body by inhalation. The droplet nuclei become implanted on alveolar tissue, generally in the best ventilated portions of the lungs where the highest oxygen tension exists. After several weeks an allergy develops to the bacilli, which produces an inflammatory reaction. Soon leukocytes arrive, which are replaced by macrophages, that form a loose focus of infiltrated tissue (tubercle). Eventually the cells become compact, and necrosis of the control portion of the lesion occurs. If the necrotic tissue fails to liquefy, it persists as a yellowish cheesey mass called *caseous material.* The healing of tuberculosis lesions may involve resolution, fibrosis (scarring), or calcification.

A *primary infection* is usually well controlled by the body's defense systems so that generally no illness develops. When the primary lesion heals, spots of calcium are left that appear on x-rays. It is the hematogenous seeding of bacilli that accompanies the primary infection that sets the stage for chronic tuberculosis at a later date. *Chronic adult tuberculosis* is the result of the awakening of bacilli in dormant lesions when resistance is low. This stage of the disease is the most serious and contagious. Vigorous treatment is necessary to interfere with the multiplication of organisms. Persons with primary tuberculosis are rarely infectious because so few organisms are expelled.

The American Lung Association has developed a table of basic classification that assists in identifying the types of tuberculosis (see Table 27-3).

Tuberculosis occurs most often in the lungs, but lesions do develop in the kidneys, bones, lymph nodes, and meninges. Factors influencing the development of tuberculosis include (1) general physical debilitation, (2) constant exposure to acute tuberculosis, (3) malnutrition, and (4) lowered resistance. There is a higher incidence of tuberculosis in overcrowded, poorly sanitized, poorly ventilated institutions, in large general hospitals, and in slums, migrant work areas, and larger cities.

Prevention

I. Isoniazid (INH) is generally administered (dosage and frequency vary) to high-risk persons in order to prevent the development of active clinical disease. Such therapy is highly recommended for:
  A. Household contacts.
  B. Recent converters of any age (individuals whose skin tests for tuberculosis were originally negative but later became positive).
  C. Persons with inactive tuberculosis and positive reactions under 20 years of age.
  D. Individuals in special clinical situations who are highly susceptible.
II. Bacillus Calmette-Guérin (BCG) vaccine, which contains antigens, may be used to treat tuberculin-negative individuals. It is an attempt to produce increased resistance to clinical tuberculosis. Although it offers limited protection, it is not completely prophylactic. Because BCG changes tuberculin skin tests from a negative to a positive reaction, it interferes with case-finding programs.

Assessment

I. Data sources (see "Pneumonia").
II. Health history.
  A. Age—most susceptible are infants, adolescents, and those over 45.
  B. Sex—2 times more common in males than females.
  C. Race—4 times more common in nonwhites than whites.
  D. Occupation—crowded conditions; poor working situation, e.g., inadequate ventilation.
  E. Socioeconomic status—identify.
  F. Habits—dietary, alcoholic intake, recreation, smoking, life-style.
  G. Family history of tuberculosis.
  H. Health perception.
  I. Blood type—identify.
  J. Persistent cough may be present, but the amount of sputum produced is contingent upon the progression of the disease.
  K. Often the patient will complain of persistent weight loss, and fatigue; alterations in appetite will also be apparent.
  L. Initial contact with the patient may lead the examiner to believe the patient has the flu. However, after a careful health history and physical examination, other changes will be noted.
  M. Irregular menstrual periods may be reported.
III. Physical assessment.
  A. General appearance—patient may not appear ill but weight loss and pallor may be noted.
  B. Breath sounds—rales over affected lung after forced expiration can be auscultated. This is followed by a short cough and a quick deep inspiration.

TABLE 27-3 / BASIC CLASSIFICATION OF TUBERCULOSIS

0. *No tuberculosis exposure, not infected* (no history of exposure, negative tuberculin skin test).

I. *Tuberculosis exposure, no evidence of infection* (history of exposure, negative tuberculin skin test).

II. *Tuberculosis infection, without disease* [positive tuberculin skin test, negative bacteriological studies (if done), no roentgenographic findings compatible with tuberculosis, no symptoms due to tuberculosis]. *Chemotherapy status* (preventive therapy):
    A. None.
    B. On chemotherapy since (date).
    C. Chemotherapy terminated (date).
       1. Complete (prescribed course of therapy).
       2. Incomplete.

III. *Tuberculosis: infected, with disease.*
    A. *Location of disease* (predominant site; other sites if significant).
       1. Pulmonary.
       2. Pleural.
       3. Lymphatic.
       4. Bone or joint.
       5. Genitourinary.
       6. Miliary.
       7. Meningeal.
       8. Peritoneal.
       9. Other.
    B. *Bacteriological status.*
       1. Positive by:
          a. Microscopy only (date).
          b. Culture only (date).
          c. Microscopy and culture (date).
       2. Negative (date).
       3. Pending.
       4. Not done.
    C. *Chemotherapy status.*
       1. None.
       2. On chemotherapy since (date).
       3. Chemotherapy terminated (date).
          a. Complete (prescribed course of therapy).
          b. Incomplete.
    *D. *Roentgenogram findings.*
       1. Normal.
       2. Abnormal.
          a. Cavitary or noncavitary.
          b. Stable or worsening or improving.
    *E. *Tuberculin skin test.*
       1. Positive reaction.
       2. Doubtful reaction.
       3. Negative reaction.
       4. Not done.

Tuberculosis suspect (may be used until diagnostic procedures are complete but not for more than 3 months).

*These data are necessary in certain circumstances.
Source: *Diagnostic Standards and Classification of Tuberculosis and Other Mycobacterial Diseases,* American Lung Association, New York, 1974, pp. 34–36.

  C. Night sweating with a reportable temperature elevation may be noted (late afternoon).

  D. Indigestion, with accompanying nausea and vomiting, may be noted and may persist to the point of anorexia.

  E. Dyspnea on exertion may be noted.

  F. The patient may be irritable and aggravated by questioning.

IV. Diagnostic tests.

  A. Tuberculin tests (see Table 27-4 for interpretation of results).

    1. Mantoux (skin test), purified protein derivative (more specific product), or old tuberculin extract injected into forearm.

    2. Tine test, multiple puncture test (screening purposes).

    3. Jet injection used for screening purposes.

TABLE 27-4 / RECOMMENDED INTERPRETATION OF SKIN TEST REACTIONS

I. *Intracutaneous Mantoux and jet injection tests* (with standard test dose).

  A. *10 mm or more of induration = positive reaction.* This is interpreted as positive for past or present infection with *Mycobacterium tuberculosis* because reactions this large most likely represent specific sensitivity. The test does not need to be repeated for confirmation in ordinary circumstances, unless there is reason to question the validity of the test.

  B. *5 to 9 mm of induration = doubtful reaction.* Reactions in this size range reflect sensitivity that can result from infection with either atypical mycobacteria or *M. tuberculosis;* hence they are classed as doubtful. However, a person with a doubtful reaction who is known to have been in close contact with an infectious person, i.e., a subject with infectious sputum, or a person having radiographic or clinical evidence of disease compatible with tuberculosis, should be regarded as probably infected with *M. tuberculosis.* For all other persons, if an appropriate antigen for atypical mycobacteria is available, an intracutaneous test with such an antigen may be applied at the same time as a repeat tuberculin test.

  C. *0 to 4 mm of induration = negative reaction.* This reflects either a lack of tuberculin sensitivity, or a low-grade sensitivity that most likely is not caused by *M. tuberculosis* infection. No repeat test is necessary unless there is also suggestive clinical evidence of tuberculosis. If the person is the contact of a subject with tuberculosis, he should be followed up according to the established routine for contacts.

II. *Multiple-puncture tests.* In determining the size of induration, measure the diameter of the largest single reaction. If the reaction consists of discrete papules, the diameters of separate areas of induration should not be added. For screening tests, the following interpretation is suggested.

  A. *Vesiculation = positive reaction.* If vesiculation is present, the test may be interpreted as positive, in which case the management of the subject is the same as that for one classified as positive to the Mantoux test.

  B. *2 mm or more of induration = doubtful reaction.* Even though such reactions may be due to *M. tuberculosis,* a significant proportion of them may not be confirmed by a positive standard Mantoux test. This is particularly true of smaller reactions. Therefore, a standard Mantoux test should be done on all subjects in this group, and management should be based on the reaction to the Mantoux test or on the results of dual testing using PPD-tuberculin and PPD-B.

  C. *Less than 2 mm of induration = negative reaction.* There is no need for retesting unless the individual is a contact to a case of tuberculosis or there is clinical evidence suggestive of the disease.

Source: *Diagnostic Standards and Classification of Tuberculosis and Other Mycobacterial Diseases,* American Lung Association, New York, 1974, pp. 18–19.

    B. Chest x-ray.

    C. Sputum culture for acid-fast bacillus (AFB)—positive for tuberculosis. Often three or more specimens are examined to confirm diagnosis.

    D. Blood work (routine) will reveal:

        1. Increased sedimentation rate.

        2. WBC usually normal.

        3. Hemoglobin and hematocrit somewhat decreased.

Problems

    I. Fatigue.

    II. Weight loss.

    III. Anorexia, indigestion, vomiting.

    IV. Night sweating.

    V. Low-grade fever in early afternoon.

    VI. Productive cough.

    VII. Sputum—yellow, mucoid, blood-tinged; hemoptysis.

    VIII. Dyspnea.

Diagnosis

    I. Respiratory dysfunction—secondary to cough, dyspnea.

    II. Impairment of alveolar integrity—potential.

    III. Anxiety—mild to moderate.

    IV. Grief—secondary to diagnosis of long-term illness.

    V. Impairment of significant other's adjustment to illness.

    VI. Alteration in nutrition—secondary to indigestion, vomiting, cough.

    VII. Alteration in comfort—discomfort.

    VIII. Depletion of body fluids—potential, secondary to vomiting, diaphoresis, and fever.

    IX. Alteration in cardiac output—potential.

Goals of Care

    I. Immediate.

        A. Initiate chemotherapy and evaluate response.

        B. Control spread of infection.

        C. Offer support and assist with acceptance.

        D. Foster rehabilitation.

    II. Long-range.

        A. Educate patient and family about disease, treatment, medications, prevention, complications, and necessity of follow-up.

        B. Counsel regarding the use of cigarettes.

        C. Participate in case-finding programs.

Intervention

    I. Administer medications—know purpose, dosage, frequency, and side effects. Multiple drug therapy is usually used in treating active tuberculosis, with new medications introduced if the regime appears ineffective (see Table 27-5).

    II. Educate patient and family[5] about:

        A. Disease and necessity to continue treatment for a continuous period of time.

        B. Administration of medications, purpose, dosage, frequency, and side effects.

        C. Need for rest.

        D. Necessity of a good diet.

        E. Dangers of smoking and URI.

        F. Signs of complications.

        G. Actions to prevent spread of infection (see Table 27-6).

    III. Follow-up.

        A. Be aware of and participate in *tuberculosis control programs.*

        B. Referral of patients to agency for teaching; medical follow-up; case finding; referral to long-term care facilities, and prophylactic treatment for converters (family).

[5]A good source book is O. O. Stead, *Understanding Tuberculosis Today: A Handbook for Patients,* Milwaukee Press, Milwaukee, Wis., 1971.

TABLE 27-5 / ANTITUBERCULOUS DRUGS AND THEIR SIDE EFFECTS

Drug	Adult Daily Dosage	Side Effects	Monitoring*	Remarks
First-line Drugs				
Isonazid (INH)	5–10 mg/kg (300–600 mg)	Peripheral neuritis, hepatitis, hypersensitivity, convulsions	Symptoms, SGOT/SGPT (not routinely)	For neuritis, pyridoxine 25–50 mg prophylaxis; 50–100 mg as treatment
Ethambutol (EMB)	25 mg/kg for 60 days, then 15 mg/kg†	Optic neuritis (reversible with discontinuation of drug; very rare at 15 mg/kg), skin rash	Visual acuity, red-green color discrimination (Snellen chart)	Ocular history and funduscopic examination before use; contraindicated with optic neuritis; use with caution if serious ocular problem
Streptomycin (SM)	0.75–1.0 g daily (frequently given for initial 60 days with extensive disease)	Otic and vestibular toxicity, decreased hearing, vertigo, tinnitus (nephrotoxicity rare)	Gross hearing (ticking of watch), if abnormal, audiograms; if vertigo present, caloric testing; BUN, creatinine, SGOT/SGPT	More common in older patients; with renal insufficiency, decrease dose or avoid drug
Rifampin (RIF)	600 mg daily	Liver dysfunction rarely; hypersensitivity reactions	SGOT/SGPT	Extremely effective
p-Aminosalicylic acid (PAS)	12–15 g daily	Gastrointestinal, hypersensitivity (rash), hepatotoxicity, sodium load	SGOT/SGPT	For gastrointestinal irritation, temporarily reduce dose or use Ca, K, ascorbic acid, or resin combinations; avoid Na salt in elderly or patients with heart failure or renal disease

Second-line Drugs

Drug	Dose	Toxicity	SGOT/SGPT	Comments
Ethionamide	750–1000 mg	Gastrointestinal, hepatotoxicity, hypersensitivity (rash)	SGOT/SGPT	Temporarily stop or reduce dose with gastrointestinal irritation and hepatotoxicity
Pyrazinamide (PZA)	20–35 mg/kg (not over 3 g)	Hyperuricemia, hepatotoxicity, arthralgia	Uric acid, SGOT/SGPT	Benemid or allopurinol to reduce serum uric acid
Cyloserine	750 mg	Psychosis, personality changes, convulsions, rash	Drug blood levels if poor renal function	Pyridoxine, 50–300 mg/day, may help; mental problems more common with predisposition
Capreomycin	1 g daily for 60–120 days, then 1 g 2 to 3 times weekly	Nephrotoxicity, ototoxicity, hepatotoxicity hypersensitivity, hypokalemia	Same as streptomycin with SGOT/SGPT in addition	Effective newly released drug; frequent cross-resistance with viomycin, also kanamycin; not for pediatric use; also as for streptomycin
Viomycin	1 g every 12 h twice a week	Similar to streptomycin but nephrotoxicity more common, hypokalemia, hypocalcemia	As for streptomycin, plus urinalysis	As for streptomycin
Kanamycin	0.5–1 g daily, for streptomycin	As for streptomycin, greater nephrotoxicity	As for streptomycin	Rarely used; avoid concomitant ethacrynic acid, furosemide or mercurial diuretics and mannitol

*The most important monitoring device is an informed patient having ready access to medical care supplemented by a careful history and appropriate physical examination.
†FDA recommends 15 mg/kg for entire treatment period except for retreatment cases, when 25 mg/kg is recommended for the initial 60 days.
Source: Clarence Guenter, *Pulmonary Medicine*, J.B. Lippincott Company, Philadelphia, 1977, p. 341.

TABLE 27-6 / ADDITIONAL NURSING MEASURES FOR CARE OF THE PATIENT WITH TUBERCULOSIS

1. Instruct patient to cover nose and mouth with several layers of tissue when coughing, sneezing, or laughing; discard in appropriate place; wash hands and expectorate sputum in disposable sputum container; have patient wear mask if unwilling to cover nose and mouth while in the communicable phase of the disease.
2. Ensure adequate air ventilation; decontamination of air is achieved by noncirculating air conditioning or ultraviolet lighting.
3. Institute appropriate isolation techniques.
4. Collect and evaluate sputum specimens.
5. Offer oral hygiene.
6. Assess vital signs and breath sounds.
7. Provide restful environment; exercise as tolerated.
8. Encourage well-balanced diet with adequate hydration; measure fluid intake and output; check weight.
9. Manage cough and pain if present.
10. Encourage coughing, deep breathing.
11. Perform chest physiotherapy.
12. Assess emotional response of patient and family; provide support and encouragement.
13. Provide diversion—occupational therapy.
14. Assess response of interventions.
15. Inform patient of pre- and postoperative interventions, if necessary.

Evaluation

I. Reassessment: complications.
   A. Pleurisy (see "Pleurisy").
   B. Hemoptysis (see "Pneumonia" and "Trauma").
   C. Atelectasis (see "Pneumonia").
   D. Spontaneous pneumothorax (see "Trauma").
   E. Bronchopleural fistula—persistent communication between the pleural cavity and the bronchial tree. Intervention: surgery—performed if chemotherapy fails.
      1. Types of surgical intervention.
         a. Lung resection—removal of the diseased lobe(s) of the lung, or the lung itself in order to terminate the disease process and secondary effects.
         b. Decortication—removal of the lung covering (external).
      2. Preoperative intervention. (Refer to care of patients under "Trauma").
      3. Postoperative intervention. (Refer to care of patients under "Trauma").
II. Follow-up and reevaluation.

Lung Abscess

Definition

A *lung abscess* is a localized collection of pus within a cavity that has been formed by the necrosis of inflammatory tissue and lung tissue. Abscess formation is an attempt to wall off an infection. For a while the abscess remains somewhat isolated, but eventually it erodes and ruptures into a bronchus.

   The areas of the lung most often affected are the superior segment of the lower lobe or the lower part of the upper lobe. The right lung develops abscesses more often than the left lung. Occasionally, multiple abscesses occur. Events associated with aspiration, such as alcoholism and drug overdose, may lead to lung abscesses. Central nervous system disease and prolonged debility allow excess material from the mouth, nasopharynx, and stomach to reach the tracheobronchial system. Foreign bodies, infectious materials from the respiratory tract, and dental deposits are often aspirated. Classification of lung abscesses according to cause appears in Table 27-7.

TABLE 27-7 / CLASSIFICATION OF LUNG ABSCESSES ACCORDING TO CAUSE

I. Necrotizing infections.
    A. Pyogenic bacteria (*Staphylococcus aureus, Klebsiella,* group A streptococcus, *Bacteroides, Fusobacterium.* anaerobic and microaerophilic cocci and streptococci, other anaerobes. *Nocardia*).
    B. Mycobacteria (*Mycobacterium tuberculosis, M. Kansasii, M. intracellularis*).
    C. Fungi (*Histoplasma, Coccidioides*).
    D. Parasites (amebas, lung flukes).
II. Cavitary infarction.
    A. Bland embolism.
    B. Septic embolism (various anaerobes, *Staphylococcus, Candida*).
    C. Vasculitis (Wegener's granulomatosis, periarteritis).
III. Cavitary malignancy.
    A. Primary bronchogenic carcinoma.
    B. Metastatic malignancies (very uncommon).
IV. Other.
    A. Infected cysts.
    B. Necrotic conglomerate lesions (silicosis, coal miner's pneumoconiosis).

Source: John F. Murray, in George W. Thorne et al. (eds.), *Harrison's Principles of Internal Medicine,* 8th ed., McGraw-Hill Book Company, New York, 1976, p. 1365.

Prevention

I. Prevent aspiration.
II. Maintain oral hygiene; treat dental and periodontal disease.

Assessment

I. Data sources (see "Pneumonia").
II. Health history (refer to "Pneumonia").
    A. Sex—3 times more common in males than females.
    B. Season—secondary to URI, e.g., pneumonia.
    C. Can occur due to aspiration or swallowing of foreign object.
    D. History of pneumonia prior to onset of lung abscess not uncommon.
III. Physical examination (refer to "Pneumonia").
    A. Malodorous breath.
    B. Dental caries.
    C. Gingivitis.
    D. Periodontal infection.
    E. Chest percussion will reveal a dull area of consolidation and pleural thickening.
    F. Auscultation of breath sounds indicate cavernous sounds with rales heard over the involved area.
    G. Sputum will be prevalent and often dark brown in color. Hemoptysis may be present.
    H. If the lung abscess is chronic, anemia and weight loss may be observed.
    I. Clubbing of fingers and toes may be noted in chronic cases.
IV. Diagnostic tests.
    A. Chest x-ray—wall around lucent area must be present.
    B. Bronchogram and bronchoscopy will help isolate the abscess and surrounding cavity.
    C. Blood culture and related blood work may help to isolate the involved pathogen.
    D. Blood work will reveal:
        1. Leukocytosis.
        2. Anemia.
    E. Sputum, culture and sensitivity, helps to isolate pathogen.
    F. Needle aspiration is performed to remove liquid strainage and to culture its contents to isolate organism.
V. Other data sources (refer to "Pneumonia").

Problems
I. Chronic cough.
II. Purulent, bloody sputum.
III. Dyspnea.
IV. Fever, sweating, chills.
V. Malaise, anorexia, headache (flu symptoms).
VI. Pleuritic chest pain if pleura involved.
VII. Weight loss and anemia with chronic pulmonary abscess.
VIII. Anxiety.

Diagnosis
I. Respiratory dysfunction.
II. Impaired integrity of lung membrane.
III. Alteration in comfort—pain (pleuritic), cough, headache, fever.
IV. Depletion of body fluids secondary to inflammatory response.
V. Lack of understanding of preventive health measures.
VI. Anxiety—mild to moderate.
VII. Difficulty in coping, secondary to the diagnosis of a potentially chronic problem.
VIII. Alteration in nutrition (less than required), secondary to malaise, anorexia.

Goals of Care
I. Immediate.
   A. Establish adequate drainage.
   B. Eradicate infection.
   C. Utilize supportive measures during acute phase of illness.
   D. Prevent development of chronic condition.
   E. Offer emotional support.
II. Long-range.
   A. Stress importance of follow-up care.
   B. Make patient aware of steps of prevention, follow-up, signs of recurrence, and what actions are appropriate.
   C. Teach patient and family about medications.
   D. Counsel regarding use of cigarettes.

Intervention
I. Administer antibiotics; know purpose, dosage, frequency, and side effects (penicillin is usually the drug of choice).
II. Instruct patient how to cough effectively (refer to "Pneumonia").
III. Perform chest physiotherapy; suction if necessary (refer to "Pneumonia").
IV. Assist with bronchoscopy. Prepare the patient. Instruct the patient not to eat or drink after this test, because of the anesthetic effect.
V. Measure and record amount and color of sputum.
VI. Encourage well-balanced diet with adequate hydration to avoid reinfection.
VII. Provide rest.
VIII. Perform ROM exercises.
IX. Provide oral hygiene to help relieve malodorous breath. Use diluted hydrogen peroxide, lemon, glycerine, or other substances.
X. Assess response to interventions.
XI. Inform patient that it takes a long time for chest x-ray to clear and that good oral-dental hygiene is verh important.
XII. Follow-up.

Evaluation
I. Reassessment: complications.
   A. Chronic pulmonary abscess—development of abscess that is continuously present.
   B. Empyema.
   C. Shock (refer to Chap. 44).
   D. Bronchial-pleural fistula.
   E. Hemorrhage (refer to Chap. 44).
   F. Brain abscess (refer to Chap. 23).

II. Intervention: surgery. If the complications described above develop or no improvement is evident with medical treatment, surgery is performed.
  A. Types of surgical intervention.
    1. Thoracotomy (see "Trauma") is done to provide an exit for drainage and to promote healing of the cavity.
    2. Incision and drainage if patient is unable to tolerate thoracotomy.
  B. Preoperative intervention (see "Trauma").
  C. Postoperative intervention (see "Trauma").
III. Follow-up and reevaluation.

Pleurisy

Definition

Pleurisy is an acute or chronic inflammation of a small part or of the entire surface of the pleura. This condition may occur at the onset or during the course of many pulmonary diseases, such as pneumonia, tuberculosis, pulmonary embolus, lung abscess, pulmonary neoplasm, or following chest trauma or a thoracotomy. The inflammation usually resolves itself with subsidence of the primary disease. Pain develops when the two inflamed pleural walls rub together. *Fibrinous* (dry) pleurisy deposits a fibrinous exudate on the pleural surface. *Serofibrinous* (wet) pleurisy is due to an increase in nonpurulent pleural fluid and may result in pleural effusion.

Assessment

I. Data sources (refer to "Pneumonia").
II. Health history (refer to "Pneumonia").
  A. Pleurisy is often associated with a history of chest trauma, pulmonary infarction, or pericarditis.
  B. Pleurisy may develop suddenly and is characterized by pleuritic pain that must be differentiated from that due to pulmonary emboli.
III. Physical assessment
  A. General appearance—pallor, fever, malaise.
  B. Chest motion limited on affected side—decreased chest excursion.
  C. Lying on affected side—splinting; cough present.
  D. Pain—varies from intercostal tenderness to severe, sharp knifelike chest pain usually near the lower half of the thorax, especially on inspiration. The pain is augmented by coughing or sneezing and is minimal or absent when breath is held. It may be referred to upper abdomen and along costal margins. Neck and shoulder pain may be present with diaphragmatic pleurisy.
  E. Percussion—dullness due to the presence of increased fluid.
  F. Breath sounds—diminished; pleural friction rub heard 28 to 48 h after the onset of pleurisy. Auscultated on inspiration and expiration.
  G. Heart sounds—pleural-pericordial rub auscultated.
  H. Temperature—high fever is usually present.
IV. Diagnostic tests.
  A. Chest x-ray reveals areas of consolidation.
  B. Sputum examination—culture pathogen.
  C. Pleural biopsy—rule out metastases.
  D. Blood work—check increased WBC (leukocytosis); altered blood gases.
  E. Thoracentesis with removal of pleural fluid for examination.

Diagnosis

I. Alteration in comfort—pain secondary to pleurisy.
II. Respiratory dysfunction.
III. Anxiety—mild to moderate, intensified by pain and dyspnea.
IV. Impairment of pleural integrity.
V. Depletion of body fluids secondary to inflammatory response.

Goals of Care

I. Immediate.
  A. Discover and treat primary disease.
  B. Relieve pain.
  C. Offer emotional support.
II. Long-range.
  A. Teach patient and family about medication—know purpose, dose, frequency, and side effects.
  B. Prevent recurrences.
  C. Alert patient to signs of complication and what actions are appropriate.
  D. Counsel regarding use of cigarettes.

Intervention

I. Administer analgesics—know purpose, dosage, frequency, and side effects.
II. Assess vital signs.
III. Apply heat or cold over area of pain to reduce inflammation and to relieve discomfort.
IV. Encourage patient to cough and breathe deeply to rid the body of secretions.
V. Splint rib cage when patient coughs.
VI. Provide chest physiotherapy
VII. Provide restful environment—prevent stressful situations that may increase energy consumption.
VIII. Instruct patient to lie on affected side to prevent organisms from traveling to the unaffected side.
IX. Assist with procaine intercostal block—used to relieve pain.
X. Offer fluids for hydration and a well-balanced diet to maintain body weight and to help liquefy secretions.
XI. Provide reassurance—be supportive to relieve anxiety.
XII. Assess response to interventions.
XIII. Follow-up.

Evaluation

I. Reassessment: complications.
  A. Pleural effusion.
    1. Assessment.
      a. Shortness of breath.
      b. Localized chest pain.
      c. Decreased local expansion of chest wall.
      d. Increased pulse.
      e. Dull percussion; absence of breath sounds; pleural friction rub.
      f. Pallor.
      g. Prostration.
      h. High fever.
      i. Dry cough.
    2. Intervention.
      a. Assist with thoracentesis and insertion of intercostal drainage tube (Figs. 27-5 and 27-6).
      b. Monitor chest drainage.
      c. Check vital signs and breath sounds.
      d. Provide chest physiotherapy.
      e. Splint chest when coughing.
      f. Offer oral hygiene.
      g. Provide ROM exercises.
      h. Offer skin care.
      i. Encourage well-balanced diet with adequate hydration.
  B. Chronic adhesive pleuritis.
    1. Assessment: marked pleural thickening.
    2. Intervention: decortication—removal of thickened pleura.
II. Follow-up and reevaluation.

Rhinitis

Definition

Rhinitis is an acute or chronic inflammation of the mucous membrane of the nose. Common causes of rhinitis include infection, allergic reaction, or nonallergic reaction.

1. Infection—viral (common cold) or invasion of nasal mucosa in the course of a bacterial infection elsewhere in the body. Th engorgement of the blood spaces results in generalized hyperemia with enlargement of gland elements.
2. Allergic reaction.
3. Nonallergic reaction—chronic, intermittent nasal obstruction or nasal stuffiness resulting from nervous tension, repeated respiratory infections, exposure to noxious materials, deviated septum, or polyps.

Assessment

I. Data sources (see "Pneumonia").
II. Health history (see "Pneumonia" and "Polyps").
   A. Some burning and irritation with discharge and obstruction of nasal passage.
   B. General malaise, chills, slight fever, headache, sneezing, and watery eyes with cold.
   C. Catarrh, crusting of membrane with fetid odor (ozena), hoarseness, intermittent headache, and disturbed sense of smell.
III. Physical assessment.
   A. Inspection of nasal chamber reveals:
      1. Edematous mucous membranes—complaints of congestion.
      2. Nasopharynx smooth and glistening.
      3. Posterior turbinates enlarged and may be intruding into nasopharynx.
      4. Abnormal amount of connective tissue, hypertrophy of nasal septum, atrophy of membrane and cartilage (chronic rhinitis).
      5. Caseosa—accumulation of offensive cheeselike masses with serous purulent discharge.
   B. Headache, fever, and general malaise may be present.
   C. Tearing of the eyes may be present.
   D. The patient often is sneezing and drainage from the nose is usually clear.
   E. If fever is present, the patient may be warm to the touch.
   F. Disturbances of sense of smell may be reported.
IV. Diagnostic tests.
   A. Rhinoscopic exam—examination of the nasal chamber. This test will reveal reddened swollen membranes.
   B. Blood work when infection is present may indicate:
      1. Leukocytosis.
      2. A slight rise in sedimentation rate.
V. Other data sources (see "Pneumonia").

Diagnosis

I. Respiratory dysfunction.
II. Alteration in comfort—discomfort secondary to congestion.
III. Impairment of mucous membrane of nose.
IV. Alteration in sense of smell.
V. Depletion of body fluids: potential.

Goals of Care

I. Immediate.
   A. Relieve swelling and congestion of nasal passages.
   B. Provide hydration.
   C. Prevent herpes simplex of nares.
   D. Relieve discomfort.
II. Long-range.
   A. Teach patient about use of medications, prevention, and importance of follow-up care.
   B. Counsel regarding the use of cigarettes.

Intervention

I. Teach client to relieve nasal congestion by:
   A. Blowing the nose with mouth slightly open, through both nostrils at the same time, not too frequently or too hard.
   B. Using nose drops and knowing the purpose, dose, frequency, and side effects.
II. Provide rest, adequate fluids, well-balanced diet, medications—antipyretics, antihistamines, analgesics, and aspirin—for patient with a cold to help relieve inflammation and congestion.
III. See surgical interventions under "Polyps" and "Deviated Septum."
IV. Allergy interventions.

Evaluation

I. Reassessment: complications—pneumonia (see "Pneumonia").
II. Follow-up and reevaluation.

Sinusitis

Definition

Sinusitis is an inflammatory reaction of the sinus mucosa due to the retention of secretions or the presence of allergens or pathogens. The disorder is referred to as ethmoid, frontal, maxillary, or sphenoid sinusitis, or if all are involved—pansinusitis.

Inadequate drainage due to obstructions (polyps, deviated septum, enlarged turbinates), viral allergic rhinitis, dental infection, and changes in intranasal pressure are common causes of sinusitis. Because the nasal and sinus mucous membranes are continuous, infections spread rapidly from the nasal passages to the sinuses.

Prevention

I. Correction of deviated septum.
II. Removal of nasal polyps.
III. Allergen desensitization.
IV. Control of exposure to allergens.

Assessment

I. Data sources (see "Pneumonia").
II. Health history (see "Pneumonia").
   A. Dietary habits.
   B. Habits—smoking, snuff, drugs (cocaine).
   C. Recent dental work—injection of novacaine could stimulate an inflammatory response.
   D. Recent air travel.
   E. Seasonal nature (allergies).
   F. EENT disorders (nasal polyps, deviated septum).
III. Physical assessment.
   A. Nasal chamber examination may reveal:
      1. Inflamed mucosa.
      2. Deviated septum (not always present).
      3. Nasal polyps (not always present).
   B. Nasopharynx examination may reveal:
      1. Inflamed mucosa.
      2. Purulent secretions, often thick, green-yellow.
   C. Paranasal sinus examination may reveal:
      1. Tenderness over involved sinus.
      2. Swelling over involved sinus—right and/or left nasal cavity.
IV. Diagnostic tests.
   A. X-ray of sinuses reveals:
      1. Cloudy appearance.
      2. Air fluid level (not always seen).
   B. Transillumination of the sinuses—decreased light transmission may indicate mucosal thickening or the presence of fliid in the cavity.
   C. Culture and sensitivity of secretions to identify involved organisms.

Problems
    I. Pain (headache) over sinus involved.
    II. Purulent nasal discharge (if duct is patent).
    III. Anorexia, malaise.
    IV. Fever (low-grade).
    V. Mouth breathing.

Diagnosis
    I. Alterations in comfort—pain (headache severe at times).
    II. Respiratory dysfunction.
    III. Nutritional alteration—potential, secondary to anorexia, malaise, and purulent discharge.

Goals of Care
    I. Immediate.
        A. Relieve pain by administering analgesics.
        B. Promote sinus drainage.
        C. Reduce edema, congestion, and discomfort by steam inhalation, hydration, and medication (vasoconstrictor).
        D. Control infection by oral hygiene and administering antibiotics.
        E. Promote rest in a quiet, nonstimulating environment.
        F. Stimulate appetite by providing foods that are appealing and easy to eat.
    II. Long-range.
        A. Prevent recurrence by referral for surgery (nasal polyps, deviated septum) or desensitization.
        B. Teach proper method of blowing nose and caution regarding blowing nose too often or too vigorously.

Intervention
    I. Provide a quiet room for rest.
    II. Place in Fowler's position to promote drainage and relieve edema.
    III. Soothing steam inhalations.
    IV. Administration of medications (vasoconstrictors, analgesics, antibiotics).
    V. Oral hygiene and warm gargles.
    VI. Provide a diet that is easy to chew and swallow.
    VII. Teach proper way to blow nose.
    VIII. Assess response to interventions.
    IX. Follow-up.

Evaluation
    I. Reassessment: complications—chronic sinusitis.
        A. Assessment.
            1. Headaches.
            2. Purulent nasal discharge.
            3. Mouth breathing.
            4. Foul breath.
            5. Fever (low-grade).
            6. Malaise.
        B. Intervention.
            1. Analgesics.   3. Oral hygiene.
            2. Hydration.   4. Surgery.
                a. Types of surgical intervention.
                    (1) Antral irrigation—irrigation of the maxillary sinus.
                    (2) Incision and drainage of the sinus.
                    (3) Sinus resection.
                    (4) Ethmoidectomy—surgical removal of the ethnoid sinuses.
                    (5) Antrostomy—surgical opening into the antrum sinus to allow for drainage (radical or intranasal).
                b. Preoperative intervention.
                    (1) Decrease anxiety—offer a complete discussion of the surgery.
                    (2) Reassurance—support.

        (3) Spiritual counseling as needed.

        (4) Teach about postoperative expectations.

    c. Postoperative intervention.

        (1) Place in lateral position to promote drainage until consciousness returns.

        (2) Fowler's position to facilitate drainage and relieve dema.

        (3) Place ice bag on operative area to help reduce swelling.

        (4) Oral hygiene to promote comfort and prevent infection.

        (5) Assess vital signs and relieve pain by the use of analgesia.

        (6) Provide a liquid diet, progressing to soft, as tolerated by the patient.

        (7) Cool vapor inhalations to prevent drying of the nasal mucosa.

        (8) Teach patient to:

            (a) Breathe through the mouth.

            (b) Avoid blowing through the nose.

            (c) Expectorate secretions and avoid straining.

        (9) Observe patient for:

            (a) Hemorrhage at the operative site, often manifested by excessive swallowing.

            (b) Difficulty in breathing.

            (c) Excessive pain.

            (d) Dislodged packing.

    d. Complications of surgery.

        (1) Hemorrhage—the escape of excess blood from vessels in the nasal and sinus mucous membranes.

        (2) Wound infection—the response of the operative site to the presence of pathogens.

II. Follow-up and reevaluation.

Tonsillitis (Acute)

Definition

Tonsillitis is an inflammation of the tonsils or lymphatic tissue mass located on the lateral walls of the oropharynx and is usually caused by group A hemolytic streptococci. (Refer to Chap. 14 for additional information.)

Prevention

    I. Avoid contact with infected persons.

    II. Take prophylactic vitamin C.

Assessment

    I. Data sources (see "Pneumonia").

    II. Health history (see "Pneumonia").

        A. History of streptococcal infections—number per year and documentation via throat cultures.

        B. Family history of streptococcal infections.

        C. Complaint of sore throat, pain on swallowing, and viral symptoms, e.g., fever.

        D. Determine allergies, if any.

        E. Identify previous respiratory infections.

        F. Cardiac status—document with ECG and evaluation.

        G. Age—frequently occurs in children or adults who have not had tonsillectomies.

        H. Obtain previous history of throat surgery, e.g., tonsillectomy.

    III. Physical assessment.

        A. Pharynx and throat will reveal:

            1. Hyperemic and edematous tonsils.

            2. Presence of exudate on tonsils; yellow exudate sometimes drains from tonsil crypts.

            3. Hyperemia and edema of soft palate and posterior pharyngeal wall.

            4. White patching on the tonsil wall may be observed.

    B. Other changes may include:
        1. Anterior and posterior cervical lymphadenopathy.
        2. Fever (as high as 105 to 106°F).
        3. Pain referred to ear—aggravated by swallowing.
  IV. Diagnostic tests.
    A. Throat culture—done to identify causative organisms.
    B. WBC will usually show leukocytosis.
  V. Other data sources (see "Pneumonia").

Problems

  I. Sore throat.
  II. Fever, malaise.
  III. Pain radiating to ear.
  IV. Dysphagia.
  V. Anorexia.

Diagnosis

  I. Alteration in comfort—discomfort and throat pain.
  II. Nutritional alteration—potential secondary to dysphagia.
  III. Respiratory dysfunction.
  IV. Communication alteration—potential.
  V. Body fluid—depletion, secondary to fever and decreased appetite.

Goals of Care

  I. Immediate.
    A. Alleviate discomfort by gargles, lozenges, and analgesics.
    B. Reduce fever by medication (ASA).
    C. Reduce mucosal congestion by soothing inhalations and decongestants.
    D. Alleviate malaise with bed rest.
    E. Maintain hydration.
  II. Long-range.
    A. Teach about importance of throat cultures if there is a recurrence.
    B. Prevent recurrence.

Intervention

  I. Provide quiet, nonstimulating environment for rest.
  II. Oral hygiene (see "Pneumonia").
  III. Hot saline gargles to decrease inflammation and to provide temporary relief from discomfort.
  IV. Lozenges with topical anesthetic to decrease dysphagia.
  V. Ice collar to decrease inflammation.
  VI. Diet of fluids and soft foods as tolerated.
  VII. Administer analgesics, antipyretics, decongestants, and antibiotics, e.g., penicillin (Procaine). If an allergy to penicillin exists, another drug, e.g., ampicillin, may be selected.
  VIII. Teach regarding medications, dosage, side effects.
  IX. Assess response to interventions as demonstrated by relief of symptoms.
  X. Follow-up.

Evaluation

  I. Reassessment: complications.
    A. Peritonsillar abscess.
      1. Assessment.
        a. Severe throat pain and severe difficulty in opening mouth.
        b. Anterior or posterior cervical lymphadenopathy.
        c. Increased dysphagia.
        d. Increased temperature.
        e. Toxicity.
        f. Drooling.
        g. Visible closure of oropharynx.

    2. Intervention
      a. Administer narcotic.
      b. Throat irrigations (warm) to help relieve discomfort.
      c. Anesthetic sprays to decrease pain temporarily.
      d. Bed rest.
      e. Gargles.
      f. Systemic antibiotic.
      g. Antipyretic, e.g., aspirin, Tylenol.
      h. Oral hygiene must be stressed. Half-strength hydrogen peroxide can be used.
      j. Ice collar.
      k. Surgery may be needed to incise and drain the abscess.
  B. Acute otitis media (see Chap. 14 for a complete discussion).
  C. Pneumonia (see "Pneumonia").
  D. Acute rheumatic fever (see Chap. 26).
  E. Acute glomerulonephritis (see Chap. 28).
II. Intervention: surgery—tonsillectomy (see Chap. 14).
III. Follow-up care and reevaluation.

Acute Tracheobronchitis

Definition   *Acute tracheobronchitis* is an acute inflammation of the mucous membranes of the trachea and the bronchial tree. Usually the disorder is self-limiting with eventual complete healing and return of function. Tracheobronchitis may be caused by extension of an upper respiratory tract infection or exposure to pollution (dust, fumes, smoke). It occurs most often in the winter months and in persons who are cigarette smokers and/or who have chronic pulmonary disease. The precipitating factor causes temporary impairment of the cilia, permitting bacterial invasion and the subsequent accumulation of mucopurulent exudate and cellular debris. While tracheobronchitis may be a minor disorder for most persons, it can be life threatening to persons who have chronic pulmonary or cardiac disease.

Prevention   Avoid exposure to persons who have URI.

Assessment   **I.** Data sources (see "Pneumonia").
    II. Health history (see "Pneumonia").
      A. Occupation—exposure to dust, smoke or fumes may precipitate the problem.
      B. Recent history of an upper respiratory infection is not uncommon.
      C. Complaints associated with a viral infection may be present. (See "Tonsillitis.")
      D. Complaints of chest tightness are not uncommon.
    III. Physical assessment (see "Pneumonia").
      A. Erythema of pharynx—dryness and laryngitis may be present.
      B. Anterior cervical lymphadenopathy.
      C. Musical ronchi—cough may be productive, sputum may be thick.
      D. Wheezing with moist rales at the lung base.
      E. Fever and generalized malaise.
    IV. Diagnostic tests.
      A. A chest x-ray is done to rule out bronchopneumonia.
      B. Sputum cultures will identify pneumococci or beta-hemolytic streptococci and sensitivity to antibiotics.

Problems   **I.** Cough—repetitive, barking.
    II. Pleuritic pain.
    III. Sputum—mucopurulent.
    IV. Fever.

Diagnosis
    I. Respiratory dysfunction.
    II. Alterations in comfort—discomfort secondary to substernal tightness and pleuritic pain.
    III. Alteration in body fluids secondary to fever (101 to 102°F).

Goals of Care
    I. Immediate.
        A. Reduce discomfort by soothing steam inhalations.
        B. Alleviate cough by lozenges containing a topical anesthetic.
        C. Facilitate removal of secretions by hydration and postural drainage.
    II. Long-range.
        A. Prevent recurrence.
        B. Teach regarding medications.
        C. Alert patient to early symptoms and indicate appropriate actions to control the disorder.
        D. Counsel regarding smoking and exposure to pollution.

Intervention
    I. Promote bed rest. Keep patient free from pathogens in the environment.
    II. Provide for quiet, nonstimulating environment.
    III. Hydration (3000 to 4000 mL daily) to liquefy secretions and prevent dehydration. Offer the patient hot drinks and soft diet as tolerated.
    IV. Administer analgesics, antibiotics, bronchodilators (allergies to antibiotics should be identified).
    V. Prevent reinfection secondary to rapid rehabilitation.
    VI. Teach regarding:
        A. Medications—dose, untoward effects.
        B. Prevention of recurrence.
        C. Guidance of smoking.
        D. Decreasing exposure to pollutants in the environment.
    VII. Follow-up.

Evaluation
    I. Reassessment: complications—bronchopneumonia (see "Pneumonia").
        A. Assessment.
            1. Sharp pain in involved hemothorax.
            2. Paroxysms of coughing.
            3. Sputum, pink to rusty.
            4. Fever (101 to 105°F).
            5. Rapid respirations (25 to 45 per minute—dyspnea).
            6. Fine rales, suppressed breath sounds on auscultation.
            7. Pulmonary consolidation—lobar dullness heard over the affected area.
            8. Pleural friction rub (see Chap. 26).
            9. Nausea and vomiting.
            10. Leukocytosis.
        B. Intervention.
            1. Hydration—adequate fluid replacement (see "Acute Tracheobronchitis").
            2. Oxygen therapy as needed.
            3. Cultures—sputum and blood.
            4. Antibiotics, e.g., erythromycin.
            5. Steam inhalations to relieve congestion and liquefy secretions.
    II. Follow-up and reevaluation.

Herpes Simplex

Herpes simplex is a vesicular eruption, or "cold sore," on the lips and/or oral mucosa, that is associated with the herpes simplex virus type I. A small inflamed area develops which then evolves into a vesicle that ruptures. The lip lesion forms a crust, while the oral lesion presents as a shallow ulcer. Lesions generally last for 7 to 10 days. Secondary infection is a threat.

The primary infection usually occurs in childhood. After resolution the virus enters a latent stage. A high antibody titer remains, thereby limiting the degree of future responses to the virus. The herpes virus is apt to be activated when the person's resistance is lowered. Precipitants include dental trauma, abrasion of lips, sunburn, food allergies, fever, and the onset of menstruation.

Prevention

I. Use of sunscreens.
II. Lubrication of lips.
III. Filing down sharp areas on teeth.

Assessment

I. Data sources (see "Pneumonia").
II. Health history (see "Pneumonia").
   A. Allergies—history.
   B. Menstrual cycle.
   C. Stress response and history of coping patterns.
   D. History of previous herpes lesions.
III. Physical examination.
   A. Vesicle or crust formation on lip or shallow ulcer on oral mucosa.
   B. Erythema and local edema surrounding the lesion, pain and itching at site of lesion, or burning may be present.
   C. Cervical lymphadenopathy may appear 1 to 4 days after the onset (malaise and fever may be present).
IV. Diagnostic tests.
   A. Biopsy of the lesion.
   B. Culture of the lesion and exudate.
   C. Tzanck smear (multinucleate giant cells) to differentiate herpetic stomatitis from erythema multiforme, pemphigus, and drug eruptions.

Diagnosis

I. Alterations in comfort—pain.
II. Skin integrity, impairment of—actual.
III. Nutritional alteration—potential, secondary to difficulty in eating.

Goals of Care

I. Immediate.
   A. Reduce discomfort and pain.
   B. Prevent secondary infection.
   C. Promote healing.
   D. Provide suitable food and liquid.
II. Long-range.
   A. Dental care to decrease mechanical irritation.
   B. Teach regarding lubrication of lips and overexposure to sun.
   C. Alert persons to early signs and symptoms and explain the use of topical agents.

Intervention

I. Systemic antibiotics—not applicable to every situation.
II. Topical anesthetic (xylocaine gel) to provide local relief of pain.
III. Frequent oral hygiene—half-strength hydrogen peroxide.
IV. Analgesics to decrease pain and cool compresses to decrease discomfort.
V. Liquid or soft diet—avoid foods and liquids that are mechanically, thermally, or chemically irritating. Provide bland diet as tolerated.
VI. Antibiotic ointments to prevent secondary infection.
VII. Apply dyes (photoactive) that bind viral DNA.
VIII. Apply idoxuridine (Dendrid, Herplex, Stoxil) to inhibit DNA synthesis.

Evaluation

I. Reassessment: complications secondary to infection.
    A. Assessment.
        1. Increased cervical lymphadenopathy.
        2. Increased pain.
        3. Increased difficulty eating.
        4. Increased tissue erythema, edema, tenderness.
    B. Intervention.
        1. Identify cause and treat.
        2. Refer to "Intervention," above.
II. Follow-up and reevaluation.

Pharyngitis

Definition

Acute pharyngitis is a common throat inflammation that may be viral in origin or may be caused by streptococcal or staphylococcal infections. A sudden onset of symptoms with a white blood cell count over 12,000 per cubic millimeter is not unusual. It may arise by extension of infection from tonsils, nose, or sinuses or common cold, infected teeth, or other disorders involving the oral cavity.

Assessment

Refer to "Tonsillitis (Acute)."

Problems

I. Fever.	VII. Chills.
II. Severe sore throat.	VIII. Headache.
III. Hacking cough.	IX. Muscle-joint aches.
IV. Dysphagia.	X. General malaise.
V. Nasal congestion.	XI. Prostration.
VI. Hoarseness.	

Diagnosis

I. Alterations in comfort—pain.
II. Body fluid loss—potential.
III. Nutritional alteration—potential.
IV. Respiratory dysfunction.

Goals of Care

I. Immediate.
    A. Relieve pharyngeal mucosal congestion and discomfort.
    B. Reduce headache and muscle and joint pain.
    C. Promote rest in a warm, nonstimulating environment.
    D. Provide fluids and foods that are thermally, chemically, and mechanically nonirritating.
    E. Prevent potential sequelae—rheumatic fever, glomerulonephritis.
II. Long-range [refer to "Tonsillitis (Acute)"].
    A. Refer for counseling—become a nonsmoker.
    B. Counsel concerning possible need for tonsillectomy and/or adenoidectomy.

Intervention
[Refer to
"Tonsillitis
(Acute)"]

I. Nasal decongestants to relieve edema and congestion, e.g., Dimetapp, Chlor-Trimeton.
II. Cough syrup to help remove secretions.
III. Steam inhalation to moisten secretions and aid expectoration.
IV. Lubricant on lips to prevent cracking and skin breakdown.
V. Teach about:
    A. Medications—dose, side effects, method of administration, dietary constraints.
    B. Need for fluid intake—2500 mL daily (hourly intake of oral fluids to be stressed).
VI. Counsel regarding tonsillectomy and adenoidectomy, depending upon the number of streptococcal infections and whether the patient has his or her own tonsils.
VII. Follow-up.

Evaluation

I. Reassessment: complications.
    A. Otitis media [see discussion under "Tonsillitis (Acute)"].
    B. Sinusitis (see "Sinusitis").
    C. Rheumatic fever (see Chap. 26).
    D. Glomerulonephritis (see Chap. 28).
II. Follow-up care and reevaluation.

Laryngitis

Definition

Laryngitis is an inflammation of the larynx that may be associated with (1) an infection involving the vocal cords; (2) an upper respiratory infection; or (3) straining the voice.

Prevention

Avoid straining the voice.

Assessment

I. Data sources [refer to "Tonsillitis (Acute)"]. Information may be elicited by written communication if the patient cannot speak.
II. Health history [refer to "Tonsillitis (Acute)"].
III. Physical examination.
    A. An examination of the throat will reveal an engorged edematous mucosa.
    B. Exudate may be present.
    C. The patient's voice will be hoarse or aphonic due to impeded vocal cord movement.
    D. Anterior and posterior lymphadenopathy will be present.
IV. Diagnostic tests: indirect laryngoscopy (refer to "Laryngeal Cancer") will help confirm the diagnosis.

Diagnosis

I. Alterations in comfort—pain.
II. Nutritional alteration—potential.
III. Respiratory dysfunction—cough, secondary to increased secretions.
IV. Alteration in communication secondary to laryngeal edema.

Goals of Care

I. Immediate.
    A. Promote absolute voice rest.
    B. Reduce cough and discomfort in throat.
    C. Promote satisfactory mode of communication.
    D. Provide food and fluid that is not thermally, chemically, or mechanically irritating.
II. Long-range.
    A. Teach about influence of smoke and other irritants.
    B. Prevent recurrence.
    C. Counsel concerning becoming a nonsmoker.

Intervention

I. Counsel not to smoke to decrease irritation.
II. Counsel regarding voice rest in order to decrease strain on vocal cords.
III. Arrange for alternate mode of communication (use of pencil and pad, call bell).
IV. Steam inhalation—increased moisture will help loosen secretions and prevent dryness of the pharynx and pharyngeal area.
V. Lozenges with topical anesthetic.
VI. Oral hygiene—lubricate mucosa and prevent halitosis.
VII. Administration of antibiotics (if infection present)—check throat culture.
VIII. Administration of cough syrup.
IX. Bed rest in well-humidified room to lubricate mucosa and liquefy secretions.
X. Follow-up.

Evaluation

I. Reassessment: complications—chronic laryngitis.
    A. Assessment.
        1. Frequent cough.

        2. Voice fatigue.

        3. Ache in throat.

    B. Intervention.

        1. *Total* temporary voice rest.

        2. Nonmedicated steam inhalation.

        3. Abstinence from smoking.

  II. Follow-up and reevaluation.

TRAUMA

Chest trauma refers to those injuries sustained in major traffic or industrial accidents or in attempted suicide or homicide. Trauma may damage the chest walls, lungs, heart, great vessels, and other mediastinal structures and may be penetrating or nonpenetrating.

Trauma to the lung reduces oxygen and carbon dioxide exchange due to destruction of the parenchyma and respiratory units. This can lead to hypoxia and hypercapnia.

Pneumothorax

Definition

Pneumothorax refers to the collapse of a lung due to collection of air in the thorax. When air collects within the intrapleural space, it is called a *closed pneumothorax.* When air enters the intrapleural space through an opening in the chest wall, it is called an *open pneumothorax. Spontaneous pneumothorax* results when there is a rupture of an emphysematous bleb on the pleural surface. *Tension pneumothorax* occurs because of an open chest wound, with a flap that acts as a one-way valve; air entering on inspiration is unable to escape on expiration, and the lung collapses as intrathoracic tension increases. *Hemothorax* results from pulmonary laceration or torn intercostal blood vessels. This causes blood to accumulate in the chest cavity compressing the lung. A *flail chest* will result from multiple fractures of one or more ribs in different places (see Fig. 27-2).

Pneumothorax can result from penetrating chest wounds caused by stabbing, bullets, or any missile moving at a high speed. Nonpenetrating chest wall injuries include fractured ribs, electric shock, drowning, blast injuries, or alteration in barometric pressure. Unrelated health problems, e.g., head injury or metastatic tumors, can also contribute to pneumothorax (see Fig. 27-3).

Such injuries are potentially life threatening because multiple organs may be affected and the cardiopulmonary processes may be disturbed. Because the trauma results in pressure change, the expansion of the unaffected lung is affected and there may be shifting back and forth of the collapsed lung and mediastinum. This shifting interferes with the filling of the right side of the heart, which lessens cardiac output. Figure 27-4 illustrates the physiological events which may be caused by chest injuries.

Assessment

  I. Data sources (refer to "Pneumonia").

  II. Health history.

    A. Age—problem can occur at any age. Spontaneous pneumothorax often occurs in a young, healthy adult.

    B. Previous history of pneumothorax or other related health problems, e.g., malignancy, should be reported.

    C. Occupation—identify type of work setting and potential health hazards.

    D. Life-style—recreation, driving accidents. Accidental chest injury may be associated with youth. Traffic accidents and associated alcoholic ingestion should be noted.

    E. Habits—alcohol, drugs, smoking.

    F. Description of factors leading to incident should be obtained from the patient or another source.

    G. The patient may complain of chest pain and dyspnea, and a cough (with or without hemoptysis) may be present.

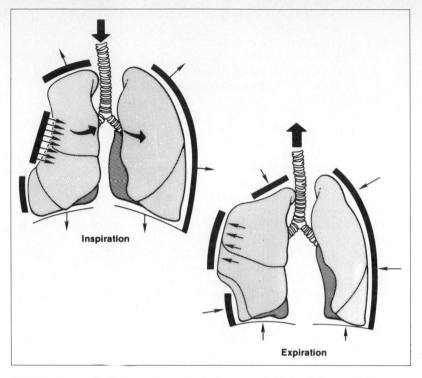

FIGURE 27-2 / Flail chest. (*From D. A. Jones et al., Medical-Surgical Nursing: A Conceptual Approach, McGraw-Hill Book Company, New York, 1978.*)

    H. Evaluation of level of consciousness and presence of shock should be assessed. (Refer to Chap. 44.)

    I. Anxiety may be apparent.

III. Physical assessment (for initial assessment and emergency care refer to Chap. 44).

    A. Inspection and observation.

        1. Determine the level of consciousness, emotional state, or degree of apprehension.

        2. Note the color of mucosa, nail beds, and the presence and degree of cyanosis or pallor.

        3. Evaluate the respiratory pattern and rate, and the use of accessory muscles of respiration.

        4. Note the status of cervical pulses and veins.

        5. Determine whether injury is closed or contused, and search for wounds of entrance and exit.

        6. Note character and amount of sputum or tracheal secretions.

        7. Observe chest for mediastinal shifting.

    B. Palpation and percussion.

        1. Determine equality and amplitude of all pulses.

        2. Determine cardiac size and point of maximal impulse (PMI).

        3. Evaluate chest expansion (excursion) and check for areas of hyperresonance or dullness.

        4. Determine areas of tenderness or pain, abnormal mobility of ribs or sternum, tracheal shift, or crepitation.

        5. Decreased chest movement should be noted along with the side affected.

    C. Auscultation.

        1. Evaluate breath sounds; sounds observed over collapsed lung.

2. Assess cardiac sounds; rales will be present on inspiration and do not clear with coughing.
3. Rhonchi heard on expiration but clear with coughing.
4. Determine blood pressure in arms and legs. Increased blood loss may be revealed by hypotension. However, in presence of anxiety or related health problems hypertension may be noted.

IV. Diagnostic tests.
  A. Chest x-ray will reveal collapsed lung.
  B. Blood gases indicate the adequacy of oxygen–carbon dioxide exchange.
  C. Blood work—electrolytes to assess fluid and electrolyte balance; hemoglobin and hematocrit to assess blood loss.
  D. ECG—identify cardiac changes.
  E. Lung biopsy—assess lung tissue.
  F. Mediastinoscopy—visualize the mediastinal pleural surfaces and the diaphragm.

Problems

I. Chest pain, especially upon movement.
II. Instability of ribs.
III. Crepitus (fluid and air in intrapleural cavity).
IV. Shallow or rapid respiration or dyspnea.
V. Anxiety—restlessness.
VI. Cough—varying degrees of productivity (hemoptysis).

FIGURE 27-3 / Pathogenesis of pneumothorax. (*From D. A. Jones et al., Medical-Surgical Nursing: A Conceptual Approach, McGraw-Hill Book Company, New York, 1978.*)

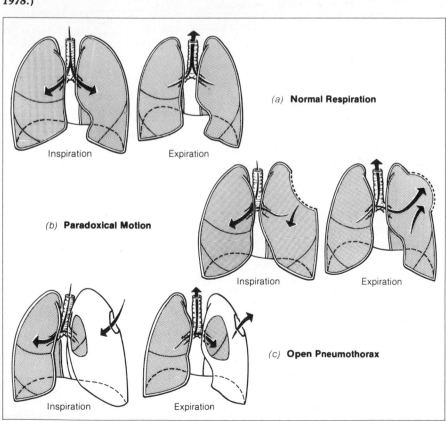

(a) **Normal Respiration**

Inspiration   Expiration

(b) **Paradoxical Motion**

Inspiration   Expiration

(c) **Open Pneumothorax**

Inspiration   Expiration

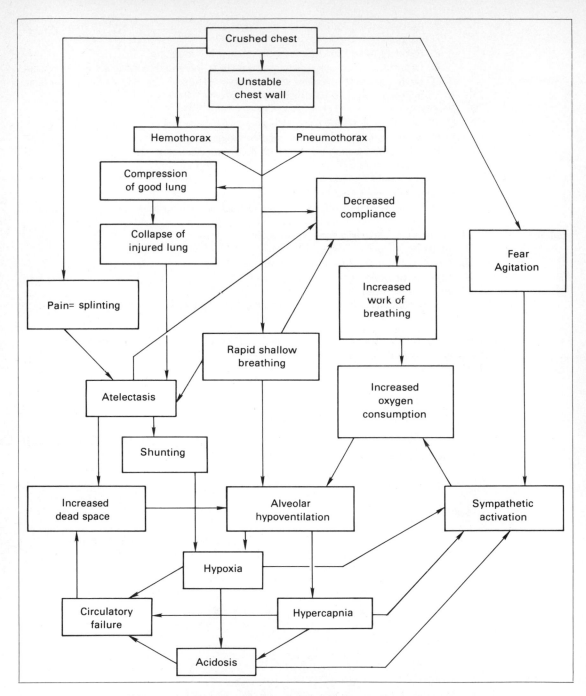

FIGURE 27-4 / Factors causing respiratory failure following crushed chest injuries. (*Adapted from H. H. Bendixin et al., Respiratory Care, The C. V. Mosby Company, St. Louis, 1965.*)

      VII. Diaphoresis (shock potential).

     VIII. Alteration in vital signs (elevated temperature).

      IX. Pallor or cyanosis.

Diagnosis
     I. Respiratory dysfunction secondary to thoracic trauma.

     II. Alterations of cardiac output secondary to thoracic trauma.

     III. Anxiety mild to severe, secondary to injury and blood loss.

     IV. Depletion of body fluids—dehydration, diaphoresis.

     V. Impaired lung tissue destruction of respiratory units.

     VI. Alteration in comfort—pain (thoracic).

Goals of Care
     I. Immediate.
- **A.** Maintain patent airway.
- **B.** Treat shock.
- **C.** Ensure adequate ventilation.
- **D.** Provide symptomatic care.
- **E.** Assist with diagnostic and therapeutic procedures.
- **F.** Offer emotional support.
- **G.** Prevent, observe, and treat complications.

     II. Long-range.
- **A.** Instruct patient about treatment, medications, signs of problems, and appropriate actions, prevention, and importance of follow-up.
- **B.** Counsel patient about use of cigarettes.

Intervention
     I. Continuous assessment of vital signs, breath sounds, chest expansion, and blood gases.

     II. Administer oxygen therapy. Humidified oxygen most effective.

     III. Place in semi-Fowler's position to facilitate drainage and ease the work of breathing.

     IV. Provide restful environment; keep dry and warm. Allow the patient to increase activity as tolerated.

     V. Perform ROM exercises and include chest physiotherapy to help decrease the hazards of immobility.

     VI. Administer analgesics and antibiotics. Know purpose, dosage, frequency, and side effects. Care should be taken to avoid suppressing the respiratory center with potent analgesia.

     VII. Avoid stretching or sudden movements as they could cause reoccurrence of the problems.

     VIII. Maintain diet and fluid intake as ordered or as tolerated; measure intake and output.

     IX. Assist with insertion of *closed chest drainage* in order to remove air and fluid from the thoracic cavity and facilitate lung reexpansion. Careful explanation to patient is critical to help reduce anxiety.
- **A.** A *thoracotomy* is done, and one or more chest tubes are inserted (see Fig. 27-5) above the area of the second or third rib.
- **B.** Each tube is connected to a closed drainage system; e.g., water seal drainage (see Fig. 27-6) or Pleur-evac.
- **C.** The nurse must carefully observe the drainage system to ensure its proper function. Care must be taken to avoid interruption in the airtight system via dislodgement of the tubing or bottle breakage.

     X. Tracheostomy care and suctioning should be provided as needed. (See Table 27-8 and Fig. 27-7.)

     XI. Intermittent positive pressure can be used to facilitate removal of secretions and aid in lung reexpansion.

     XII. Continued teaching about coughing and deep breathing important.

     XIII. Teach patient:
- **A.** Care of puncture area.
- **B.** Report signs of infections and URI.

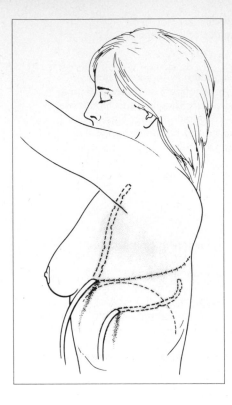

FIGURE 27-5 / Chest tube. (*From D. A. Jones et al., Medical-Surgical Nursing: A Conceptual Approach, McGraw-Hill Book Company, New York, 1978.*)

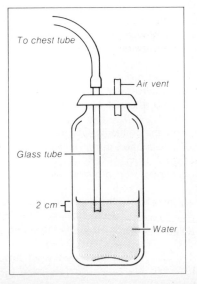

FIGURE 27-6 / Single-bottle, closed, water seal drainage system. (*From D. A. Jones et al., Medical-Surgical Nursing: A Conceptual Approach, McGraw-Hill Book Company, New York, 1978.*)

TABLE 27-8 / TRACHEOSTOMY CARE

1. Prior to care be sure the patient is well oxygenated.
2. Suction as needed to remove secretions (the use of humidified O_2 will help liquefy secretions).
3. Rest between suctionings.
4. Perform care at least every 6–8 h—more frequently, if needed.
5. Change dressing by sterile technique.
6. Utilize prepackaged tracheostomy kits, if available.
7. Be sure to secure new neck tapes before beginning the procedure.
8. Use a 3% hydrogen peroxide solution to clean the cannula.
9. Emergency tracheostomy set should be kept at the bedside in case the cannula slips out or is coughed out by the patient.
10. If emergency opening is necessary, a Kelly clamp, kept at the bedside at all times, may be used to keep the tracheostomy open until help arrives.
11. Cuffed tracheostomy tubes as well as endotracheal tubes need to be deflated frequently to prevent tissue necrosis at the tracheal site. Before deflating the cuff, the nurse should be certain that the patient has been adequately suctioned.

    C. Perform coughing and deep breathing exercises (see Table 27-9).
    D. Avoid persons with URI to prevent reinfection.
    E. Maintain well-balanced diet with adequate fluids to prevent reinfection.
    F. Balance activities and rest periods.
    G. Avoid strenuous exercise; especially contact sports.
    H. Avoid smoking.
    I. Stress importance of follow-up.

Evaluation
    I. Reassessment: complications.
      A. Wet lung syndrome—the presence of fluid in the lungs (mucus, blood, serum) as the result of severe chest injury and contusion of pulmonary tissue; causes an inability to cough, airway obstruction, and atelectasis.
      B. Respiratory distress syndrome (RDS, shock lung, postperfusion lung)—pathological changes that occur arise from either massive trauma elsewhere in the body (burns, crush injuries) or injuries from combat or changes arising from oxygen toxicity, fat embolism, rapid excessive transfusion, diffuse capillary leak syndrome, viral pneumonia, or any condition that results in severe shock. RDS is the result of changes that occur in the pulmonary vascular beds, plus an increased volume of interstitial fluid and an alteration in metabolic activity.
        1. Assessment.
          a. Dyspnea.
          b. Tachypnea.
          c. Diffuse bronchial breath sounds.
          d. Hypoxia.
          e. Altered cardiac output.
          f. X-ray—patchy infiltrates that progress to opacity.
        2. Intervention.
          a. Provide oxygen therapy.
          b. Assess and maintain mechanical support of respirations; utilize positive end expiratory pressure (PEEP) and intermittent positive pressure breathing (IPPB).
          c. Restrict fluids.
          d. Administer diuretics, steroids, and human serum albumin.
    II. Follow-up and reevaluation.

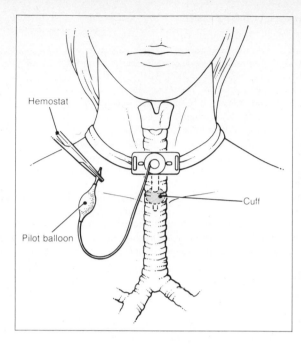

FIGURE 27-7 / Tracheostomy tube. (*From D. A. Jones et al., Medical-Surgical Nursing: A Conceptual Approach, McGraw-Hill Book Company, New York, 1978.*)

Fractured Nose

A *fractured* (broken) *nose,* with or without displacement, results from direct injury. Such trauma may cause bilateral nose bleeds. Generally, serious consequences do not arise but a deformity could lead to nasal obstruction, facial disfigurement, and chronic rhinitis.

Epistaxis

Ninety-five percent of *epistaxes*, or nosebleeds, arise from the anterior plexus of the blood vessels located in the mucosa of the nasal septum. Typically, bleeding is from only one naris and is only from one area. Bleeding from the posterior portion, involving the large vessels, is frequently profuse. Causes of epistaxis are numerous—trauma, the after effects of surgery, deviated septum, picking of nasal crusts, blowing the nose too hard, sclerotic blood vessels, hypertension, acute sinusitis, leukemia, high altitudes, and foreign bodies.

OBSTRUCTIONS

Pulmonary Embolus

Definition *Pulmonary emboli* are generally fragments of a thrombus that originated somewhere in the venous system, most often in the veins of the lower extremities, pelvic area, or in the right side of the heart. As the embolus travels, one or more of the pulmonary arteries may be obstructed. Other materials, such as tumors, amniotic fluid, air, bone marrow, fat, and a variety of foreign bodies, may also obstruct the arteries. The obstruction produces a zone of lung that is ventilated, not perfused. This increases pressure in the pulmonary artery, which in turn causes an increase in the volume and pressure in the great veins. The blood

TABLE 27-9 / EFFECTIVE COUGHING

Effective coughing requires a forward flexion motion and cannot be done while lying flat in bed.

The patient is first instructed to assume the "cough friendly" sitting position (head flexed, shoulders relaxed and slightly rolled forward, feet supported). A pillow may be placed on the patient's lap to assist in elevating the diaphragm.

Then the head drops, the chest sinks, and the patient slowly bends forward while blowing out through slightly parted or pursed lips with an expiratory airflow just below that which will cause collapse of the airways. Facial plethora or venous distension of the head or neck veins is an obvious sign of increased intrathoracic pressure and indicates the need to breathe out more slowly.

Sitting up, the patient is now told to sniff slowly, increasing aeration of the lung bases. Fast, gasping breaths do not aerate mucus-filled areas of the lung but are preferentially directed to the upper thorax and low-resistance areas of the lower thorax. A sufficient column of air behind the mucous plugs is necessary to propel them out of the airways.

After three or four repetitions (bending forward and sitting up), the patient may feel the mucus that has mobilized from the distal branches but is told to refrain from coughing until several additional repetitions have escalated even more secretions to the major bronchi. When the patient is ready to cough, she or he must first take a comfortably deep abdominal breath (feeling the abdomen push out against the pillow) and then bend forward to produce a soft, staged, staccato cough, generating an expiratory force sufficient to maintain maximum possible expiratory flow without airway collapse.

Source: Jeanne Lagerson, "Nursing Care of Patients with Chronic Pulmonary Insufficiency," *Nursing Clinics of North America,* **9:**165–179, March 1974.

volume in the left atrium is decreased, thus decreasing the stroke volume and leading to shock. Serotonin may be released from the platelets, causing pulmonary hypertension.

The mortality rate associated with this derangement is approximately 38 percent, half dying within $\frac{1}{2}$ h of onset, two-thirds within 1 h, and three-fourths within 2 h. The remaining patients with careful and continuous intervention recover from the problem. Situations associated with the occurrence of thromboembolism are trauma to the lower extremities, prolonged bed rest, the after effects of surgery, cold, obesity, varicose veins, congestive heart failure, myocardial infarction, pregnancy, polycythemia, high concentrations of estrogen, and prolonged sitting or standing.

Prevention
    I. Avoid immobilization and encourage early ambulation after surgery.
    II. Perform ROM and regular exercises for patients on complete bed rest.
    III. Do not let legs dangle without support, do not cross legs, and avoid prolonged sitting and standing.
    IV. Avoid wearing constricting clothing—garters, girdles.
    V. Avoid raising the bed below the knees; elevate legs 15 to 20°.
    VI. Inform females of the potential clotting effect of oral contraceptives.
    VII. Assess patients at risk of developing pulmonary emboli, e.g., postoperative patients; myocardial infarction.
    VIII. Administer anticoagulants prophylactically to susceptible patients.
    IX. Check length of time IV lines are in place—assess surrounding tissue.
    X. Identify consequences of smoking.

Assessment
    I. Data sources (refer to "Pneumonia").
    II. Health history (refer to "Pneumonia").
       A. Age—incidence of pulmonary emboli increases with age.

    B. Sex—occurs in both sexes.

    C. Occupation—e.g., does the job require continuous sitting with little position change.

    D. Habits—dietary, alcohol intake, smoking, drugs, caffeine.

    E. Life-style—sedentary, limited activity.

    F. Previous history of emboli; history of other health problems. Is the patient receiving anticoagulants or taking birth control pills?

    G. Complaints of shortness of breath and pleuritic pain which increases over time.

    H. Cough is present and the patient may have hemoptysis.

    I. The patient is often frightened by the pain and fears death.

    J. History of recent surgery.

III. Physical assessment.

    A. The patient's general appearance will be pale; cyanosis may be present.

    B. Appearance of neck veins, especially on inspiration, should be noted.

    C. Breath sounds—diminished; pleural friction rub may be heard along with rales, localized wheezing. Respirations rapid and gasping.

    D. The second heart sounds may be widely split; right ventricular gallop may be heard along with a grade II, III, or IV systolic ejection murmur.

    E. Cardiac changes—e.g., failure (see Chap. 26); tachycardia and arrhythmias may be present.

    F. Homan's sign—positive, but not a conclusive sign.

    G. Overt signs of peripheral phlebitis should be assessed—e.g., extremities.

    H. Skin may be wet (diaphoretic) and cold to touch, especially in the presence of shock.

    I. Assessment of vital signs may be altered by the presence of a fever and by difficulty in palpating peripheral pulses.

    J. The patient is usually anxious and frightened. This may be reflected by facial expression or changes in behavior.

    K. Chest expansion may be limited due to substernal chest pain.

    L. There may be alteration in level of consciousness and thought process due to cerebral anoxia.

IV. Diagnostic tests.

    A. Chest x-ray.

    B. Lung scan to localize area of obstruction.

    C. Angiography—definitive diagnosis.

    D. Ultrasound to help clarify diagnosis.

    E. Venography to help clarify diagnosis.

    F. ECG to assess cardiac changes secondary to pulmonary embolus. Changes noted often reveal:

        1. Right ventricular strain.

        2. Tachycardia.

        3. Premature ventricular contraction (PVC).

        4. Atrial fibrillation.

        5. Right bundle branch block.

    G. Blood gases (see Tables 27-10 and 27-11)—findings reveal:

        1. Hypoxia.

        2. Hypercapnia.

        3. Respiratory alkalosis.

    H. Blood work—findings reveal:

        1. Increased SGOT.

        2. Increased LDH.

        3. Increased serum bilirubin.

        4. Increased creatinine.

        5. Decreased phosphokinase.

TABLE 27-10 / OBSERVABLE SIGNS INDICATING CHANGE IN P_{O_2}* VALUE

Approximate P_{CO_2} Value, mmHg	Observable Signs
95–100	Normal.
80–95	Breathes with mouth open. Respiratory rate 25. (May be ambulatory but short of breath.)
75–80	Increased use of facial muscles (frontalis, nostrils). Creases in forehead with each breath. Telegraphic speech—short broken sentences, two to three words at a time. Tachycardia—pulse rate increased.
70	Mild duskiness. Respiratory rate 30–35.
60 and lower	Restless. Combative—may fight restraints, pull out tubes, etc. No response to morphine—patient cyanotic and more combative. Sweating, starting at forehead. Tugs on throat, trouble getting air in, coughs on respiration. Respirations more than 40. Gray cyanosis. Blood pressure decreases. Patient is within minutes of cardiac arrest.

*Partial pressure of oxygen in artery.
Source: Eleanor R. Murphy, "Intensive Nursing Care in a Respiratory Unit,"
Nursing Clinics of North America, **3**:423–436, September 1968.

Problems[6]

    I. Substernal or pleuritic pain.
   II. Shortness of breath.
  III. Tachycardia, palpitations.
   IV. Hypotension.
    V. Weakness, syncope.
   VI. Low fever.
  VII. Diaphoresis.
 VIII. Cough, hemoptysis.
   IX. Anxious, restless, and apprehensive.

Diagnosis

    I. Alteration in comfort—pain, cough.
   II. Interruption of circulation—potential.
  III. Alteration in cardiac output—decreased.
   IV. Anxiety—moderate to severe.
    V. Respiratory dysfunction secondary to obstruction of pulmonary vessels.
   VI. Depletion of body fluids secondary to diaphoresis, hemoptysis.
  VII. Confusion—potential, secondary to cerebral anoxia.

Goals of Care

I. Immediate.
   A. Treat shock and sustain life.
   B. Restore cardiopulmonary physiology.
   C. Assess response to interventions.
   D. Provide symptomatic and supportive care.
   E. Prevent recurrence and extension of thromboembolism.
   F. Offer support and encouragement.

[6] The effects of a pulmonary embolus are extremely variable and depend on the size and location of the embolus.

TABLE 27-11 / OBSERVABLE SIGNS INDICATING CHANGE IN P_{CO_2}* VALUE

Approximate P_{CO_2} Value, mmHg	Observable Signs
20	Tetany, cerebral deterioration.
35–45	Normal.
53	Headache, dizziness.
76	Dizziness, muscle twitching, unconsciousness.
110	Convulsions, coma.
200	Deep coma.

*Partial pressure of carbon dioxide in artery.
Source: William H. Havener, William H. Saunders, Carol Fair Keith, and Ardia W. Prescott, *Nursing Care in Ear, Eye, Nose and Throat Disorders,* 3d ed., The C. V. Mosby Company, St. Louis, 1974, p. 432.

II. Long-range.
    A. Instruct patient about treatment to be followed, signs of problems, what actions are appropriate, and *preventive* actions.
    B. Stress importance of follow-up.
    C. Counsel regarding use of cigarettes.

Intervention

I. Acute phase.
    A. Maintain IV line for administration of medications.
        1. Anticoagulants—heparin, coumadin.
        2. Analgesics, sedatives to decrease anxiety.
        3. Cardiotonics (see Chap. 26).
        4. Diuretics (see Chap. 26).
        5. Know purpose, dosage, frequency, and side effects.
    B. Place on bed rest in semi-Fowler's position to facilitate breathing.
    C. Administer oxygen therapy—assist with intubation and mechanical ventilation if necessary.
    D. Monitor vital signs, blood gases, ECG, and breath sounds.
    E. Provide emotional support to help relieve anxiety. Provide reassurance and clarification of situation.

II. Subacute phase.
    A. Provide elastic stockings.
    B. Encourage liberal intake of fluid; measure intake and output of fluids.
    C. Maintain rest, increasing activities gradually.
    D. Encourage ROM exercises.
    F. Administer skin care.
    G. Check the color, amount, and consistency of sputum.
    H. Provide oral hygiene.
    I. Avoid constipation.
    J. Adjust anticoagulation dosage to keep coagulation within therapeutic limits.
        1. Check coagulation, bleeding time, prothrombin time.
        2. Have appropriate antidote available (e.g., vitamin K or protamine sulfate).
        3. Assess for untoward bleeding following shaving, bleeding of gums, nosebleeds, bruises, and blood in stool or urine.
    K. Assess response to interventions.
    L. Teach patient about:
        1. Medication—purpose, dosage, frequency, and side effects.

        2. Preventive health measures.

        3. Reporting any faintness, dizziness, increased weakness, severe headaches, excessive menstrual flow.

        4. Informing dentist about medications currently being taken.

III. Follow-up.

Evaluation

I. Reassessment: complications—shock (refer to Chap. 44).

II. Intervention.

    A. Surgery—when anticoagulants cannot be used or when recurrent emboli of lower extremities occur despite anticoagulants.

        1. Embolectomy—removal of embolus.

        2. Ligation and plication to help trap emboli that may develop.

        3. Insertion of filter umbrella to filter blood and reduce clot formation.

    B. Medication.

        1. Urokinase to dissolve clot.

        2. Streptokinase to dissolve clot.

III. Follow-up and reevaluation.

Bronchiectasis

Definition

Bronchiectasis is a congenital or acquired disorder characterized by chronic dilatation of the medium-sized airways and destruction of bronchial elastic and muscular structures. Both obstruction and infection will, over time, cause the bronchi to dilate. The offending obstruction may be in the form of mucus, pus, or a foreign body, while the pulmonary infections are those that complicate influenza or measles.

Prevention

I. Evaluation of the cause of chronic coughs.

II. Prevention of severe respiratory infections.

III. Prompt and complete treatment of severe respiratory infections.

IV. Immunization against childhood diseases.

Assessment

I. Data sources (refer to "Pneumonia").

II. Health history (refer to "Pulmonary Embolus").

    A. History of childhood diseases (especially measles or pertussis complicated by respiratory infections).

    B. History of winter colds and URI.

    C. Occupation—describe; identify irritants and pollutants within the environment.

    D. Habits—smoking.

    E. Exposure to pollutants and irritants.

    F. History of chronic bronchitis and hemoptysis.

    G. Decreased appetite and weight loss.

III. Physical assessment.

    A. Chest examination will reveal:

        1. Limited chest expansion.

        2. Diminished breath sounds—absence over affected areas.

        3. Posttussive rales.

        4. Moist rales and rhonchi over lower lobes.

    B. Clubbing of fingers.

    C. General appearance—weak, pallor.

IV. Diagnostic tests.

    A. Bronchoscopy—findings reveal bronchial obstruction.

    B. Bronchogram—findings reveal:

        1. Expiratory bronchospasm.

        2. Distal saccular dilatation.

    C. Chest x-ray—may be normal.

Problems   I. Thick sputum containing pus (may be blood streaked).
II. Fetid breath.
III. Paroxysms of coughing.
IV. Exertional dyspnea.
V. Fatigue.
VI. Weight loss.
VII. Anorexia.

Diagnosis   I. Respiratory dysfunction.
II. Nutritional alteration—less than patient may require for normal maintenance.

Goals of Care   I. Immediate.
    A. Promote drainage of bronchial mucus.
    B. Promote liquefaction of bronchial secretions.
    C. Prevent superimposed infection.
    D. Reduce exposure to pollutants and irritants.
    E. Provide a restful environment.
    F. Maintain nutrition by providing foods that are appealing.
II. Long-range.
    A. Teach patient and family about prevention of respiratory infection and decreasing exposure to pollutants and irritants.
    B. Instruct patient in program of coughing and deep breathing.
    C. Counsel regarding becoming a nonsmoker.
    D. Plan a daily program of rest and exercise.

Intervention   I. Postural drainage to facilitate expectoration of secretion (see Fig. 27-8; a sitting position can also be used).
II. Hydration to liquefy secretions.
III. Oral hygiene—cleanse mouth; prevent infection.
IV. Administer bronchodilators, mucolytic agents and potassium iodide, antibiotics; facilitate drainage.
V. Daily rest and exercise periods to optimize health potential.
VI. Counsel regarding smoking (avoid).
VII. Teach regarding:
    A. Coughing and deep breathing.
    B. Medications—dose, side effects.
    C. Decreasing pollution exposure.
    D. Preventing respiratory infections.
VIII. Follow-up.

Evaluation   I. Reassessment: complications.
    A. Hemoptysis.
        1. Assessment.
            a. Expectoration—bright red, frothy blood.
            b. Apprehension.
            c. Discomfort in chest—burning or bubbling.
            d. Salty taste in mouth.
            e. Sensation in throat—tickling.
        2. Intervention.
            a. Reassurance.
            b. Bed rest.
            c. Monitor vital signs.
            d. Ice bag on chest.
            e. Advise patient not to talk and to breathe slowly.
            f. Suctioning as needed.
            g. Oral hygiene.

B. Cor pulmonale (see Chap. 26).

II. Intervention: surgery (if not controlled by medical intervention).

    A. Types of surgical intervention.

        1. Segmental resection—resection of one or more segments of a lung.

        2. Lobectomy—removal of entire lung.

    B. Preoperative intervention (refer to "Cancer of the Lung").

    C. Postoperative intervention (refer to "Cancer of the Lung").

    D. Complications of surgery.

        1. Hemorrhage—The escape of excess blood via the great thoracic vessels or through the large incision.

        2. Atelectasis (refer to "Pneumonia").

        3. Pneumothorax (refer to "Trauma").

        4. Respiratory insufficiency—condition in which respiratory function is not adequate to maintain normal arterial blood gases during minimal activity (refer to "Pulmonary Emphysema").

        5. Interstitial emphysema—A condition in which air, which has escaped into the subpleural space, dissects along the pleura or vessels and may reach the mediastinum and spread to neck and chest.

        6. Mediastinal shift—a condition in which the air enters the pleural space with each inspiration and becomes trapped, building up pressure within the chest. As the tension increases, it collapses the lung on the affected side and may shift the

FIGURE 27-8 / **Postural drainage. (a) Left lateral decubitus position. (b) Right lateral decubitus position. (From D. A. Jones et al., Medical-Surgical Nursing: A Conceptual Approach, McGraw-Hill Book Company, New York, 1978.)**

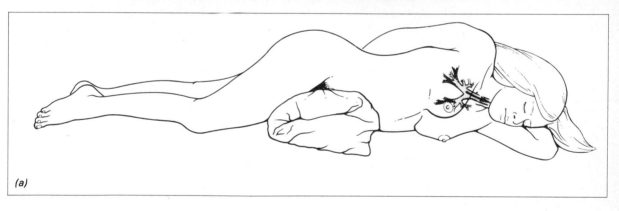

(a)

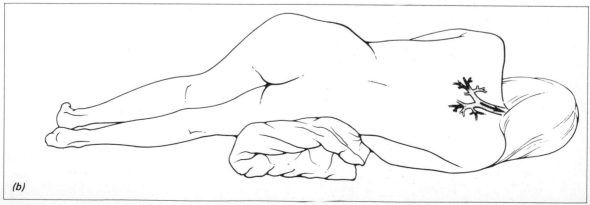

(b)

mediastinal contents (heart, trachea, esophagus, great vessels) to the unaffected side.
7. Wound infection.
III. Follow-up and reevaluation.

Deviated Septum

Definition

A *deviated septum* is a cartilaginous and bony septum containing rounded lumps or sharp projections that deflect from the midline of the nose. It may be bent or inclined to one side, or may encroach on the nasal chamber and sinus ostia. The deviation could cause nasal obstruction that increases with infections and allergic reactions. Great deviations might cause disturbances in breathing, interfere with paranasal sinus drainage, or produce irritation due to pressure on adjacent structures.

Assessment

I. Data source (refer to "Pneumonia").
II. Health history.
   A. Age—common in children and older adults.
   B. Family history—often congenital.
   C. Incident surrounding the problem—e.g., history of recent traumatic injury.
   D. Difficulty in breathing and complaints of postnasal drip.
   E. Headaches and occasional nasopharyngitis.
   F. Discomfort.
   G. Anxiety.
III. Physical examination.
   A. Visible alteration in the shape of the nasal chamber.
   B. Dry crusting mucosa.
   C. On occasion, evidence of bleeding.
IV. Diagnostic tests: routine preoperative tests are required.

Diagnosis

I. Respiratory dysfunction.
II. Alteration in gustatory and olfactory senses.
III. Impaired bone and cartilage structure of nose.
IV. Anxiety.

Goals of Care

I. Immediate.
   A. Maintain patent airway.
   B. Prepare for surgery to repair septum.
   C. Facilitate healing and anticipate complications.
   D. Decrease anxiety.
II. Long-range.
   A. Instruct client about home care of wound, medications, and importance of follow-up.
   B. Alert client to signs of problems and indicate what responses should be taken.
   C. Counsel regarding use of cigarettes.

Intervention

I. Surgery.
   A. Submucous resection.
   B. Nasal septum reconstruction.
II. Preoperative intervention.
   A. Explain recommended treatment.
   B. Teach postoperative expectations.
   C. Discuss anesthesia.
   D. Practice mouth breathing.
   E. Instruct not to cough vigorously or to swallow blood or to blow nose.

    F. Explain purpose of packing. Full feeling in nose is normal with packing. Packing will be checked periodically.

    G. Inform that discoloration and swelling around eyes may follow; final cosmetic result is not immediately evident.

III. Postoperative intervention.

    A. Assess vital signs (rectal temperature); slight temperature elevation is normal with packing.

    B. Check position of string attached to nasal packing; check mustache dressing.

    C. Check position of splint; observe underlying skin for evidence of pressure.

    D. Place in semi-Fowler's position.

    E. Provide oral hygiene.

    F. Foster appetite; provide liquids and food as tolerated. Explain why it is difficult to swallow.

    G. Assess discomfort. Offer sedative, analgesic—know purpose, dosage, frequency, and side effects.

    H. Apply ice compress over the nose.

    I. Assess response to interventions.

    J. Teach patient:

        1. Not to lift heavy weights for 2 weeks.

        2. Avoid pressure on nose from eyeglasses.

        3. Consult doctor about wearing contact lenses.

        4. Presence of tarry stools is normal.

        5. Utilize stool softener so as to avoid straining at stool.

IV. Follow-up.

Evaluation   Reassessment: complications. Hemorrhage—bleeding from nasal chamber (refer to "Epistaxis").

DEGENERATIVE DISORDERS

Pulmonary Emphysema

Definition   *Emphysema* is an irreversible condition characterized by destruction of lung tissue and structural changes within the lung, such as (1) overdistension of distant alveoli, (2) rupture of alveolar walls, and (3) destruction of the alveolar capillary bed. It may occur as the result of chronic bronchitis, asthma, or recurrent respiratory infections. *Pulmonary emphysema* is primarily a defect in the alveolar walls that may be caused by a variety of disorders. *Primary emphysema* is associated with years of chronic bronchitis and is described by two anatomic classifications: *centrilobular* involves destruction and dilatation of the respiratory bronchioles; *panlobular* is characterized by generalized destruction and dilatation of the terminal bronchioles throughout the lung. *Secondary emphysema* is caused by a condition that initiates scarring or fibrosis in the lung. These changes result in premature airway closure, loss of elastic recoil, and in trapping of air. This leads to hyperventilation and over time will result in increased lung volume, increased work of breathing, and decreased oxygen–carbon dioxide exchange.

Prevention   **I.** Early medical evaluation of respiratory disorders and avoiding persons with URI.

    II. Abstinence from cigarette smoking.

    III. Decrease exposure to air pollution.

    IV. Decrease occupational exposure to dusts, fibers, fumes, molds, and fungi.

    V. Early identification of population at risk.

Assessment   **I.** Data sources (refer to "Pneumonia").

    II. Health history (refer to "Pneumonia" and "Chronic Bronchitis").

A. Occupation—describe position, setting; identify protective measures used.
B. Dietary habits—history and assessment.
C. Habits:
   1. Alcohol.
   2. Smoking—number of years having smoked; number of cigarettes per day; inhalation of smoke; use of pipe, cigar; attempts to quit (evaluate success).
D. Exposure to pollution and irritants; response to allergens—dusts, mold.
E. Response to wet or dry climates.
F. History of respiratory infections—asthma, bronchitis, etc.
G. Family construction—history of COLD in family members.
H. Family history—e.g., α-antitrypsin deficiency.
I. History of chronic cough—productive, amount expectorated, frequency, color, etc.
J. Description of activity tolerance—fatigue, dyspnea on exertion, dyspnea without exertion.

III. Physical assessment.
A. Chest examination will indicate:
   1. Breath sounds are faint.
   2. Shallow, rapid respirations.
   3. Wheezing—sonorous rhonchi.
   4. Hyperinflation—hyperresonance.
   5. Prolonged expiration.
   6. Retraction of supraclavical fossae.
   7. Productive cough.
   8. Increased use of accessory muscles used in respiration.
   9. Barrel chest—increased anterior diameter of chest.
B. Additional changes include:
   1. Cyanosis of fingernail beds, lips, and ear lobes.
   2. Clubbing of fingertips and toes.
   3. Face ruddy to cyanotic (does not always occur).
C. General appearance.
   1. Fatigued.
   2. Air-hungry—patient found leaning forward.

IV. Diagnostic tests.
A. Chest x-ray—in relatively advanced state, results will show:
   1. Overaeration of lungs.
   2. Increased vascularity at lung peripheries.
   3. Abnormal heart size and position.
   4. Increased anteroposterior chest diameter.
   5. Low, flat diaphragm images.
   6. Widening of the intercostal spaces.
B. Fluoroscopy will show:
   1. Impaired expiration.
   2. Low, flat diaphragm.
C. Lung function tests (including vital capacity, forced vital capacity, forced expiration volume, and maximum volume) will show:
   1. Reduced maximum voluntary ventilation (MVV) capacity.
   2. Reduced forced expiratory volume (FEV).
   3. Slow maximal midexpiratory flow (MMF).
   4. Increased residual volume (RV).
   5. Reduced timed vital capacity (VC).
D. Arterial blood gases (refer to Tables 27-10 and 27-11) will show:
   1. Pa_{O_2} is reduced.
   2. Pa_{CO_2} is increased.
E. pH—normal or decreased.
F. α-Antitrypsin deficiency—change, flat alpha globulin curve with deficiency.

Problems	**I.** Shortness of breath—exertional and nonexertional.
	II. Expiration phase is prolonged and difficult.
	III. A sense of tightness in chest.
	IV. Chronic productive cough.
	V. Fatigue.
	VI. Apprehension.
	VII. Feeling of weakness.
	VIII. Lethargic.
	IX. Weight loss.
	X. Slowness in processing information.
	XI. Constipation.

Diagnosis

I. Respiratory dysfunction—moderate to severe.
II. Anxiety—mild to moderate, secondary to respiratory distress.
III. Bowel elimination, alteration in—constipation.
IV. Nutritional alteration—less intake than required.
V. Thought processes impaired secondary to decreased cerebral oxygenation.
VI. Fatigue secondary to cough; generalized weakness and loss of appetite.

Goals of Care

I. Immediate.
    A. Improve ventilation.
    B. Promote drainage of secretions from tracheobronchial tree.
    C. Reduce the work of breathing.
    D. Promote a program of activity and rest.
    E. Prevent complications.
    F. Provide an adequate diet that will not tire patient.
    G. Control cough.
II. Long-range.
    A. Arrange for desensitization of known allergens.
    B. Maintain existing lung function and prevent additional irreversible changes.
    C. Teach patient and family about medications, postural drainage, breathing exercises, effective coughing, activity level, diet, not smoking.
    D. Teach patient and family about exposure to pollution and irritants.
    E. Alert patient to be sensitive to factors that cause bronchospasm.
    F. Counsel about coping with a chronic illness.
    G. Alert patient to signs of respiratory infection or complications and indicate which responses are most appropriate.

Intervention

I. Provide humidified oxygen at 2 to 3 L if needed (use caution).
II. Provide bronchodilators by nebulizer or intermittent positive pressure breathing (IPPB) with Venturi mask.
III. Suction to help remove secretions if needed.
IV. Provide hydration to help liquify secretions and replace fluids.
V. Provide a diet of fluid and soft food in small amounts 4 to 5 times a day.
VI. Teach patient postural drainage with percussion and vibration (Fig. 27-8).
VII. Administer bronchodilators, mucolytics, and expectorants to dilate bronchioles and remove secretions.
VIII. Administer stool softeners and increase hydration to relieve constipation.
IX. Oral hygiene.
X. Provide program of activity and rest to assess tolerance levels (see Table 27-12).
XI. Monitor vital signs and arterial blood gases.
XII. Counsel: concerning limiting use of cigarettes.
XIII. Teach about:
    A. Medications—dose, side effects.   **C.** Limiting exposure to dusts and fumes.
    B. Modifying diet.   **D.** Effective coughing and deep breathing.

TABLE 27-12 / BASES FOR PREDICTING ACTIVITY TOLERANCE

Cardiovascular-respiratory status and stability and/or cardiac classification or medical prescription
Other diagnoses, physical impairments, time lapse since surgery
Sleeping or preexercise heart rate and rhythm, blood pressure
Body temperature
Hemoglobin and hematocrit level
Electrolyte and acid-base balance
Comfort level (pain)
Time lapse since last meal
Time since last use of tobacco, coffee, tranquilizers, sedatives, stimulants
Height-weight value (e.g., obesity)
Age, sex
Preillness activity level and current level tolerated
Emotional and motivational state

Source: Marjory Gordon, "Assessing Activity Tolerance," *American Journal of Nursing,* **76**:72–75, January 1976.

XIV. Assess response to interventions.
XV. Follow-up.

Evaluation

I. Reassessment: complications.
   A. Pneumothorax (refer to "Pneumothorax").
   B. Pneumonia (refer to "Pneumonia").
   C. Respiratory failure (refer to "Respiratory Failure").
   D. Cor pulmonale (refer to Chap. 26).
   E. Respiratory acidosis—an excessive retention of carbon dioxide. This is often due to chronic respiratory disease (refer to Tables 27-10 and 27-11).
      1. Assessment.
         a. Physical assesment.
            (1) Drowsiness, coma.   **(5)** Decreased, shallow respiration.
            (2) Irritability.   **(6)** Arrhythmias.
            (3) Depression.   **(7)** Muscular twitching—facial convulsions.
            (4) Hallucinations.
         b. Diagnostic test. Blood gasses will reveal:
            (1) Increased P_{CO_2}.
            (2) Decreased pH.
      2. Intervention.
         a. Control of respiratory problem—antibiotics, steroids, etc.
         b. Improve ventilation—intubation.
         c. Improve electrolytes—fluid replacement.
         d. Pulmonary physical therapy—respirators, postural drainage, bronchodilators.
         e. Administer O_2 with caution (CO_2 narcosis).
         f. Use of sodium bicarbonate and calcium gluconate.
   F. Respiratory alkalosis—the result of an excessive loss of hydrogen ions. The major factor is overstimulation of the respiratory center, e.g., from hyperventilation, anxiety, high altitudes, or aspirin poisoning.
      1. Assessment.
         a. Physical assessment.
             (1) Neuromuscular irritability.   **(3)** Increased respiration.
            (2) Hyperreflexes.   **(4)** Anxiety.
         b. Diagnostic tests. Blood gasses will reveal:
            (1) Decreased P_{CO_2}.
            (2) Increased pH.

    2. Intervention.
        a. Rebreathing carbon dioxide.
        b. Psychotherapy.
        c. Treat aspirin poisoning (gastric lavage).
II. Intervention: surgery—pulmonary resection (refer to "Tuberculosis" and "Cancer of the Lung").
III. Follow-up and reevaluation.

BIBLIOGRAPHY

American Hospital Association: "Guidelines on Tuberculosis Control Programs for Hospital Employees," *Journal of the American Hospital Association,* **49**:57–60, July 1, 1975. This article emphasizes the need for tuberculosis control programs to be a part of personnel health services in hospitals. Background information and guidelines for establishing such programs are provided.

Bushnell, Sharon Spaeth: *Respiratory Intensive Care Nursing,* Little, Brown and Company, Boston, 1973, Chap. 5, pp. 71–81. Contains discussion and pictures relevant to the techniques of chest physiotherapy and the appropriate postural drainage position.

Connor, George H., Dorothy Hughes, Martha J. Mills, Barbara Rittmanic, and Lisa V. Sigg: "Tracheostomy: When Is It Needed?" *American Journal of Nursing,* **72**:72–74, January, 1972. Includes information about the immediate and ongoing care, the complications and a guide to tube size.

Fitzgerald, Linda: "Mechanical Ventilation," *Heart and Lung,* **5**:939–949, November–December 1976. Classification of mechanical ventilation and the indications for principles and complications of mechanical ventilating a patient are presented, complete with figures and tables.

Fitzmaurice, Joan, and Arthur Sasahara: "Current Concepts of Pulmonary Embolism: Implications for Nursing Practice," *Heart and Lung,* **5**:209–218, March–April 1974. Sign and symptoms, diagnosis and treatment, and implications for nursing care for pulmonary embolism are outlined.

Kersten, Laurel: "Chest-Tube Drainage: Indications and Principles of Operation," *Heart and Lung,* **3**:97–101, January–February 1974. Discusses the indication for and principles of operation of chest tube drainage systems.

Keyes, Jack: "Blood-Gas Analysis and the Assessment of Acid-Base Status," *Heart and Lung,* **4**:239–255, March–April 1975. This article summarizes how the three variables of pH, P_{CO_2}, and HCO_3 concentration change in different kinds of acid-base disturbances. Rationale for the treatment of various disturbances is also outlined.

McCormick, Kathleen and Marion Bernbaum: "Acute Ventilatory Failure Following Thoracic Trauma," *Nursing Clinics of North America,* **9**:181–194, March 1974. Following a description of the pathophysiology involved with chest trauma, principles of nursing care of a patient with acute ventilatory failure are outlined.

Mechner, F.: "Patient Assessment: Examination of the Chest and Lungs, Part I," *American Journal of Nursing,* **76**:1–23, September 1976. This article is a programmed instruction of assessment techniques for examining the adult chest.

Owens, James: "Respiratory Failure After Injury: A Review and Plea for Accuracy," *Heart and Lung,* **6**:303–307, March–April 1977. Reviews clinical presentation, pathophysiology, and management of the adult respiratory syndrome.

Petty, Thomas L. (ed.): *Pulmonary Diagnostic Techniques,* Lea and Febiger, Philadelphia, 1975. A compilation of the practical approach to pulmonary diagnostic procedures such as lung function tests, fiber optic bronchoscopy, and mediastinoscopy.

Sedlock, Stephanie Ann: "Detection of Chronic Pulmonary Disease," *American Journal of Nursing,* **72**:1407–1411, August 1972. Elaborates on the specific observations relevant to the detection of chronic obstructive lung disease. A discussion of the complications of COPD is also included.

Traver, Gayle A. (ed.): "Symposium on Care in Respiratory Disease," *Nursing Clinics of North America,* **9**:97–207, March 1974. The articles in the symposium focus on clinical testing of lung function, the use of mechanical ventilators, and management of patients with chronic pulmonary insufficiency.

28

The Urinary System

Barbara A. Bihm

The optimal functioning of the genitourinary system is dependent upon the regulatory mechanisms and integrated functionings of the cardiovascular, nervous, and endocrine systems. A disturbance in excretory, regulatory, or secretory functionings of the kidney may result in a disturbance in other sections of the genitourinary system. Conversely, an obstruction of the free flow of urine or a disturbance in performance below the pelvis of the kidney may eventually result in destruction of nephrons. In addition, one must acknowledge that the genitourinary system may affect or be affected by alterations in the normal functionings of the above-mentioned systems.

In this chapter each phase of the nursing process is utilized in discussing various conditions. When applying this format to an actual patient situation, the reader must assess the patient's needs and delineate specific, appropriate, expected outcomes in terms of the individual patient. Though not in behavioral terms, the goals of care are ordered according to priority. The health history sections are by no means all inclusive. Here too, the reader must use sound professional judgment to delete or add to the items identified as essential areas of investigation.

ABNORMAL CELLULAR GROWTH

Renal Tumors

Definition

Masses in the kidney may be caused either by fluid-filled cavities, by *cysts,* or by solid tumors. Tumors of the kidney are rarely benign. Neoplasms of the kidney can be divided into three major categories: (1) tumors developing from embryonic tissues, (2) tumors originating in the renal parenchyma of the adult kidney, and (3) tumors developing in the renal pelvises or calycesof adults.

Nephroblastomas, or *Wilm's tumors,* the most common renal malignancies occurring in children, originate from embryonic tissues and contain epithelial and mesodermal elements. Rarely occurring bilaterally, this neoplasm appears in infancy or early childhood, usually before the age of 7.

Tumors of the renal parenchyma, often called *hypernephromas* or *adenocarcinomas,* are the most commonly seen neoplasms in the adult kidney and rarely occur before the age of 30. These tumors, usually unilateral, arise from epithelial tissue and are usually encapsulated. Men are more frequently affected than women. Some theories suggest a hormonal relationship. Growth of this renal neoplasm compresses surrounding renal tissue, and displaces and distorts the renal pelvis, calyces, and blood vessels (1). Invasion of the renal vein and metastasis to the liver, lungs, and long bones are characteristic of adenocarcinomas.

Tumors of the renal pelvis or calyces, *papillary carcinomas,* are far less common. Believed to be caused by carcinogens in the urine, these tumors arise from the epithelium of the renal pelvis. The neoplasms are often associated with bladder and ureteral tumors. Involvement of regional lymph nodes and the renal vein does occur; however, metastases to distant organs are uncommon.

Regardless of the origin of the renal neoplasm, obstruction of urinary drainage or destruction of renal tissue may eventually result. Most renal neoplasms grow insidiously and relatively fast. Many fail to produce distinctive symptoms early in the course of the disease.

Assessment

I. Data sources.
    A. Patient.   C. Significant others.
    B. Family.   D. Medical records, referral note.

II. Health history.
   A. Age.
   B. Sex.
   C. Marital status.
   D. Socioeconomic status.
   E. Occupation—possible exposure to carcinogens.
   F. Home environment.
   G. Height and weight (usual and present)—weight loss or gain; edema.
   H. Nutritional assessment—normal daily dietary pattern.
   I. Past health history—previous physical examinations, hospitalizations, and/or surgery.
   J. History of allergies (particularly to iodine) and blood type.
   K. History of drug use (particularly nephrotoxic agents and drugs, and anticoagulants). Include information about type of drug used, medically or self-prescribed, reason for taking the drug, length of time used, method and frequency of administration, and response to drug.
   L. Ascertain the perception of the patient and family regarding expectations of hospitalization and future, decision-making structure, and available support systems and resources.
   M. Describe motivation for self-care and adaptability to disruptions in health.
   N. Investigate nonurologic complaints that may be indicative of metastasis to surrounding or distant organs.
   O. Determine presence, location, intensity, quality, and precipitating or aggravating factors of pain (present in advanced cases).
   P. Determine agents or factors that aid in pain relief.
   Q. Determine voiding patterns and characteristics of urination, particularly intermittent or continuous painless hematuria, gross or microscopic.

III. Physical assessment.
   A. Palpable or visible mass in affected flank (not always present).
   B. Dull, aching, or dragging pain in affected costovertebral angle (not always present).
   C. Depending upon the extent of tumor invasion and/or metastasis the following may be present:
      1. Elevated temperature.
      2. If bleeding is present and anemia is noted, the patient will appear pale with poor capillary refill noted.
      3. Muscular weakness, malaise, lethargy.
      4. Painful or swollen femurs secondary to edema. Pathological fracture of long bones may occur if metastases are present.
      5. Dyspnea and/or cough.
      6. Edema in lower extremities.
      7. Distension of abdominal veins.
   D. Mild to moderate anxiety may be present, especially when a metastatic process is suspected.

IV. Diagnostic tests. There are a multiplicity of tests used to diagnose renal tumors. The following discussion focuses on some of the major ones. As with all diagnostic tests the patient will require a complete explanation of each procedure.
   A. Intravenous pyelogram (IVP)—a radiopaque substance is used to visualize the size and shape of the kidney and the urinary tract.
      1. The patient usually receives nothing by mouth from the midnight prior to the test.
      2. Usually the patient will receive a cathartic and/or enema prior to the x-ray in order to achieve a better view of the urinary structures.
      3. The patient should be observed for an allergic response to the dye; i.e., signs of redness, blotching, itching, and respiratory distress should be noted and treated immediately.
      4. At times a test dose is given to detect any serious side effect to the radiopaque substance.

     5. Following the test, the patient can be encouraged to force fluids to help flush out excess dye and prevent dehydration.

B. Retrograde pyelogram—back view of kidneys.

C. Renal angiogram—a radiopaque substance is introduced into a catheter, often placed in the femoral artery, so that the renal artery can be observed.

     1. The patient's preparation is similar to that done for an IVP.

     2. Following the procedure the patient should be observed for:

        a. Signs of bleeding from the catheter site.

        b. Reaction to the dye used.

        c. A decrease in pedal pulses.

D. Radiologic studies of the kidneys, ureters, and bladder (KUB)—an x-ray outlining the kidney and the urinary tract to observe changes in kidney structure, renal calculi, and other urinary tract components.

E. Nephrotomograms—tomographic x-ray of the kidney.

F. Renal scan—radiologic scanning of the kidneys and related structures.

G. Cystoscopy—inspection of the bladder through the use of a cystoscope, a metal instrument containing a tunnel opening for magnification and illumination of the bladder. It can be used to rule out the presence of satellite tumors in the bladder.

     1. The procedure is usually performed under general anesthesia, although a local anesthetic may be used.

     2. The patient receives nothing by mouth prior to the procedure, but fluids are given intravenously prior to the procedure so that specimens can be collected during the procedure.

H. Urinary cystologic examinations—the collection of urine specimens so that careful analysis of abnormal cells can be made.

I. Ultrasonography—x-ray scan of an area to isolate abnormalities, e.g., tumors.

J. Microscopic urinalysis to assess the presence of blood in the urine. Blood is seen in only a small percentage of patients with renal tumors.

K. Twenty-four hour urine specimens—bacteriologic study to determine presence of tuberculosis bacillus. (Tuberculosis tends to mimic cancer of the renal pelvis.)

     1. Procedures for collection of a 24-h urine should be completed according to a set procedure.

     2. Coagulation studies are also done.

L. Hematocrit and hemoglobin lowered the presence of bleeding.

M. Renal function studies to determine kidney function in unaffected kidney.

     1. Blood urea nitrogen (BUN).   **3.** Blood electrolytes.

     2. Creatinine.   **4.** Routine urinalysis.

N. Metastatic series (x-rays) to evaluate progression of the tumor and metastases to other areas.

Problems/
Diagnosis

I. Mild to moderate anxiety due to impending diagnostic studies and unconfirmed medical diagnosis.

II. Alteration in comfort due to dull dragging pain in affected costovertebral angle.

III. Muscular weakness, malaise, lethargy, and gradual unexplained weight loss due to neoplastic process.

IV. Generalized abdominal discomfort, anorexia, nausea, and vomiting due to invasion or displacement of organs in the adjacent gastrointestinal system.

V. Anemia due to intermittent or continuous, gross or microscopic, hematuria.

VI. Low-grade fever possibly due to metastatic brain lesion affecting the hypothalamus, renal infection, or the reabsorption of hematin or toxins from the tumor.

VII. Dyspnea or cough possibly due to metastasis to lungs.

VIII. Painful or swollen femurs and possible pathological fractures of long bones due to bony metastasis.

IX. Edema in lower extremities and distention of abdominal veins due to obstruction of the vena cava by expanding neoplasm.

Goals of Care

I. Immediate.
    A. Maintain fluid and electrolyte balance.
    B. Provide safe environment; prevent infection.
    C. Reduce effects of neoplasm on other systems.
    D. Minimize anxiety.
II. Long-range.
    A. Maintain maximal renal functioning.
    B. Develop with the patient appropriate rehabilitation goals.
    C. Limit the effects of increased cellular growth and proliferation.

Intervention

I. Develop therapeutic nurse-patient relationship. (Primary nurse seems to be ideal for the patient in an acute care setting or for those in a community setting.)
II. Provide avenue for patient and family or significant others to express concerns and anxieties regarding diagnostic studies and unconfirmed medical diagnosis.
III. Carry out teaching-learning transaction regarding rationale and physical and psychological preparation for diagnostic testing.
IV. Measure and correlate intake and output every 8 h. When possible teach the patient how to measure and record fluid intake and output.
V. Measure specific gravity and test urine for blood at every voiding; observe for presence of clots.
VI. Insert prescribed indwelling bladder catheter with continuous irrigation. Initiate measures to maintain a *sterile, closed system.* Care of the catheter should include:
    A. Insert catheter using strict aseptic technique.
    B. Anchor catheter securely to thigh, over the leg to drainage bag.
    C. Position the collecting bag below level of the bladder when patient is ambulating and lower than chair seat level when sitting (see Fig. 28-1).
    D. Position catheter and collection tubing to facilitate gravitational urinary drainage and prevent reflux of urine into the bladder (see Fig. 28-1).
    E. Avoid having tubing positioned below the point of entry into collection bag (see Fig. 28-1).
    F. Inspect skin carefully around the catheter and assess urinary drainage.
    G. Measure accurately and record intake and output of all fluids.
VII. Assess hematocrit and hemoglobin values every 24 h (more frequently if necessary) to evaluate degree of blood loss. Careful assessment of the patient for signs of anemia will be important.
VIII. Provide nutritional counseling to patient, spouse, and/or meal planner.
    A. Offer six small meals a day instead of three large ones to avoid fullness, improve digestion, and prevent vomiting.
    B. Provide requested snacks promptly. Keep preferred fruit juices readily available and at the proper temperature.
    C. Provide asthetic environment particularly at meal time to encourage and stimulate appetite.
IX. Weigh the patient daily—same scale, same time of day, same amount of clothing, preferably before breakfast—to assess fluid retention and weight gain.
X. Provide pain relief measures. Utilize information from assessment and reintervene if necessary.
    A. Administer prescribed analgesics.
    B. Provide back care.
    C. Provide distractors and selected activities if appropriate.
    D. Administer prescribed medications after meals or with milk if appropriate.
XI. Measure and assess vital signs every 4 h and more frequently if alterations are evident. Assess carefully for signs of systemic infection, especially if a Foley catheter is inserted.
XII. Provide atmosphere that fosters self-care and maximal independence.
    A. Encourage mild activity that is self-paced.
    B. Encourage frequent rest periods to avoid dyspnea.

XIII. If fluid retention is present, maintain bed in Fowler's or semi-Fowler's position.

XIV. Provide safe environment especially if the patient is elderly or heavily medicated.

    A. Orient the patient to his or her hospital environment.

    B. Initiate seizure precautions in the presence of elevated BUN levels.

    C. Provide physiologic body alignment with adequate pillow support to prevent pathological fractures.

    D. Turn the patient at least every 2 h.

XV. Unless contraindicated by dyspnea or other disease condition, elevate the foot of the bed on shock blocks to increase venous return from the lower extremities and to decrease abdominal vein distension.

Evaluation

REASSESSMENT: COMPLICATIONS

  I. Obstruction in lower urinary tract (bladder and/or urethra) due to blood clots or sloughed tumor tissue.

    A. Assessment.

      1. Blood clots or mucous threads or particles of tumor tissue in the urine.

      2. Oliguria with accompanying bladder distension.

      3. Increased pain.

      4. Altered vital signs especially increased blood pressure.

      5. Moderate to severe anxiety, restlessness, diaphoresis.

    B. Intervention.

      1. Insert prescribed indwelling bladder catheter with continuous irrigation (Refer to catheter care discissed in point VI under "Intervention," above. See Fig. 28-1.)

FIGURE 28-1 / Diagrams illustrating major points to consider when indwelling catheter is present.

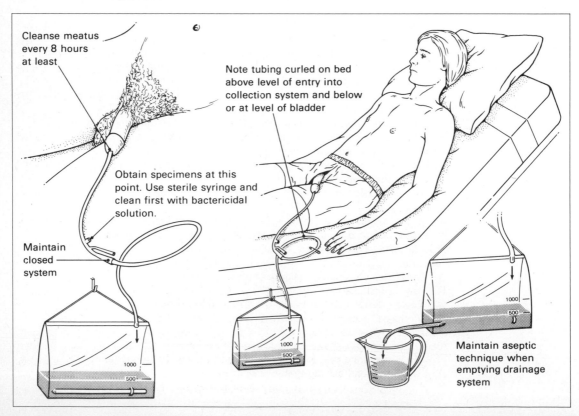

    2. Increase oral fluid intake for internal irrigation. Monitor and correlate intake and output.

    3. Administer prescribed antispasmodics and analgesics.

    4. Maintain blood volume; administer prescribed transfusions. Monitor and assess vital signs frequently.

    5. Offer reassurance and support.

    6. If unresolved, immediate surgery indicated. Begin preoperative preparation.

II. Obstruction in the upper urinary tract (ureter and/or kidney pelvis) due to abnormal cellular proliferation and/or blood clots (refer to "Obstructions").

III. Hemorrhage due to invasion of intravenal circulation.

  A. Assessment.

    1. Pallor, skin clamminess, diaphoresis.

    2. Hypotension, rapid thready pulse.

    3. Continuous gross frank hematuria.

    4. Increased pain in affected flank.

    5. Severe apprehension, restlessness.

  B. Intervention.

    1. Insert prescribed indwelling bladder catheter with continuous irrigation. Be sure to include irrigation fluids in the intake and output recordings.

    2. Monitor and assess vital signs every 15 min. Observe for signs of increasing hypovolemia.

    3. Maintain blood volume. Administer transfusions as prescribed.

    4. Maintain fluid and electrolyte balance; administer prescribed intravenous fluids.

    5. Institute measures to prevent hypovolemic shock (refer to Chap. 44).

    6. Monitor and assess hematocrit and hemoglobin.

    7. Monitor and correlate intake and output.

    8. If hemorrhage cannot be controlled, a nephrectomy may be performed regardless of the presence of metastasis. Begin preoperative preparation.

IV. Renal failure (refer to "Acute Renal Failure" and "Chronic Renal Failure").

INTERVENTION

I. Surgery.

  A. Types of surgical intervention.

    1. Lumbar nephrectomy—formation of a fistula within the pelvis of the kidney made through an incision in the loin.

    2. Transperitoneal nephrectomy—formation of a fistula within the pelvis of the kidney made through an incision made through the peritoneum.

    3. Transthoracic nephrectomy—formation of a fistula within the pelvis of the kidney made through the pleural cavity.

  B. Preoperative intervention.

    1. Decrease anxiety through reassurance and well-established nurse-patient relationship.

    2. Encourage support from family and significant others.

    3. Provide pastoral care and counseling, if appropriate.

    4. Teach regarding physical and psychological preparation for surgery.

    5. Teach regarding immediate and long-term postoperative expectations and activities including the intensive care unit, coughing and deep breathing exercises, intravenous fluids, and Foley catheter drainage.

    6. Reintroduce need to establish long-range rehabilitation goals.

  C. Postoperative intervention. In general the nursing care of a patient following a nephrectomy is similar to the care of a patient after major abdominal surgery.

    1. Assess for alterations in vital signs.

    2. Meticulous measurement and correlation of intake and output every hour.

    3. Assess dressings for serosanguineous drainage (measure the amount).

    4. Maintain fluid and electrolyte balance. Administer prescribed intravenous fluids.

    5. Assess for bladder distension.

    6. Provide meticulous indwelling bladder catheter care with prescribed continuous irrigation.

7. Assess urine for clots. Maintain adequate and safe outflow of urine through drainage system (see Fig. 28-1).

8. In the case of transthoracic nephrectomy, assess placement and drainage of catheter in pleural cavity.

9. Provide respiratory care, including deep breathing, coughing, and turning every hour. Splint operative area. Use caution if drains are present.

10. Administer pain relief measures: analgesics, massage, and/or moist heat.

11. Patient may have nothing by mouth (NPO) until peristaltic activity returns.
   a. Assess return of bowel sounds via abdominal auscultation.
   b. Gradually increase food according to tolerance.
   c. Provide oral hygiene when oral fluids are limited.

12. Encourage early mobility; ambulation within 24 h postoperatively. Utilize elastic knee-length stockings. Discourage sitting in a chair for long periods.

13. Provide reassurance and assistance in dealing with possible altered body image and loss of body part. If signs of grieving are apparent, the nurse should provide support (see Chap. 41).

14. Assess for signs and symptoms of infection. Examine the drainage and operative site for poor healing and signs of inflammation.

15. Administer prescribed antibiotics prophylactically. Change dressings according to orders.

16. Initiate teaching-learning transaction (include family and/or significant others) regarding:
   a. Medications, especially name, dosage, rationale, expected action, side effects, and signs of toxicity.
   b. Nutritional counseling.
   c. Signs and symptoms of urinary tract infections and appropriate responses.
   d. General health habits.
   e. Importance of health care follow-up. (Referrals for follow-up care should be initiated by the nurse and are essential to assessing metastasis.)

D. Complications of surgery. Reassessment of the patient following surgery should focus on reoccurrence of metastases.

1. Internal hemorrhage.
   a. Assessments.
      (1) Tachycardia, hypotension, shortness of breath.
      (2) Increased restlessness, changes in mental status.
      (3) Diaphoresis, cold clammy skin; changes in skin color (cyanosis).
      (4) Excessive drainage on dressing. Bleeding may be frank red or mixed in consistency.
      (5) Abdominal distension.
   b. Intervention.
      (1) Monitor and assess vital signs every 15 min. Administer oxygen as needed.
      (2) Administer blood replacements as prescribed; observe for volume overload.
      (3) Institute measures to prevent hypovolemic shock (refer to Chap. 44).
      (4) Assess hematocrit and hemoglobin; measure arterial blood gases.
      (5) Prepare for immediate surgical intervention. Terminate bleeding if possible.
      (6) Measure accurately fluid intake and output.

2. Reflex paralysis of intestinal peristalsis.
   a. Assessment.
      (1) Abdominal distension.
      (2) Nausea and vomiting.
      (3) Bowel sounds absent or hypoactive.
      (4) Increased difficulty in eating.
      (5) Complaining of feeling of fullness.

   b. Intervention.

   (1) Insert prescribed nasogastric tube with continuous aspiration of gastric contents (*e.g.*, Miller-Abbott tube).

   (2) Assess and replace electrolytes by administration of prescribed intravenous fluids and electrolytes.

   (3) Assess bowel sounds every 4 h. Observe for presence or absence of sounds and alteration in rate of activity.

   (4) Maintain on NPO status until peristaltic activity returns, then begin and gradually increase food according to tolerance.

3. Spontaneous pneumothorax (refer to Chap. 27).

   a. Assessment.

   (1) Sudden sharp chest pain.

   (2) Dyspnea; weak pulses (tachycardia may be present).

   (3) Acute anxiety and restlessness.

   (4) Increased diaphoresis.

   (5) Diminished chest movement; decreased or absent breath sounds on the affected side; presence of a mediastinal shift.

   b. Intervention.

   (1) Place patient in Fowler's position to improve respirations.

   (2) Encourage patient to remain quiet to avoid excess stress and decrease respiratory demand.

   (3) Administer oxygen as prescribed.

   (4) Prepare for chest x-ray.

   (5) Prepare for emergency thoracentesis. Chest tubes will be inserted to help regain normal pleural pressure. (Refer to Chap. 27 for a complete discussion.)

   (6) Encourage the patient to rest and discuss changes in order to reduce stress.

   (7) Evaluate pulse, blood pressure, and respiratory rate.

II. Medical management.

   A. Types of medical intervention.

   1. Radiation.

   2. Chemotherapy.

   B. Nursing intervention.

   1. Since irradiation and chemotherapy do not appear to be very effective, support patient, family, and/or significant others in dealing with the poor prognosis.

   2. Assist patient in developing realistic and attainable goals.

   3. Initiate teaching regarding untoward effects on treatment regimen. Assist patient and family in dealing with side effects of both radiation and chemotherapy.

   4. Initiate referral for follow-up home care.

Tumors of the Urinary Bladder

Definition   Tumors of the bladder occur more frequently in men than in women, and the incidence seems to increase with age. The etiology of the pathogenesis of tumors of the urinary bladder is obscure; however the ingestion, inhalation, or cutaneous application of certain chemical compounds is believed to cause bladder tumors. Chronic irritation and recurrent infections have also been suspected as causative factors.

Bladder tumors arising in the mucous membrane layer of the bladder wall constitute the majority of these genitourinary tumors. These tumors are papillary in nature.

Benign tumors protrude from the mucosal surface of the bladder wall as small outgrowths. They may undergo malignant degeneration with successive recurrences. *Nonepithelial infiltrating tumors* usually do not invade beyond the muscular layer of the bladder wall. They are malignant, but occur less frequently than papillary tumors. *Adenocarcinomas* and *sarcomas*, though rare, tend to penetrate deeply into the bladder wall and beyond.

Tumors of the urinary bladder generally originate near the bladder floor. Consequently, ureteral and urethral orifices are often obstructed by this abnormal cellular proliferation.

Assessment

I. Data sources (refer to "Renal Tumors").
II. Health history (refer to "Renal Tumors"). The health history, as well as the physical examination, should focus upon those changes that have occurred prior to and including hospitalization.
   A. History of recurrent urinary tract infections (particularly cystitis). Indicate the frequency with which they occur.
   B. Intermittent or continuous gross *painless hematuria* (present in 60 to 80 percent of patients) should be identified.
   C. Voiding patterns and characteristics of urine, particularly frequency, urgency, nocturia, and dysuria, must be identified.
   D. Presence, location, intensity, quality, and precipitating or aggravating factors of pain. Investigate factors that aid in analgesia. Pain is not always present. Pain in bladder, rectum, pelvis, flank, back, or legs is usually present in advanced disease process.
III. Physical assessment.
   A. Palpable suprapubic mass (rare).
   B. Edema in lower extremities may be noted. This often indicates venous obstruction caused by invasive tumor.
   C. Fever and severe flank pain may be observed. This may indicate renal infection. Elevation in serum white blood counts and urinalysis may be present.
   D. Uremic symptoms may be present secondary to impaired renal function (refer to "Acute Renal Failure" and "Chronic Renal Failure").
   E. Hematuria is noted; anemia may be present.
IV. Diagnostic tests.
   A. Cystoscopy (refer to "Renal Tumors"). Ultraviolet cystoscopy may be used to outline the bladder lesion.
   B. Biopsy of bladder wall.
   C. IVP—filling defect may indicate presence of bladder tumor. (For a complete discussion refer to "Renal Tumors.")
   D. Excretory urogram—radiological viewing of the urinary tract showing excretion of intravenous fluids or opaque dye.
   E. Bimanual pelvic examination to estimate degree of tumor invasion.
   F. Urinary cytologic examination to study cell composition of the urine.
   G. Microscopic urinalysis, specifically for hematuria. A "clean catch" urinalysis or sterile urine collection is often used.
   H. Renal function studies—usually normal unless obstruction has resulted in damage to renal parenchyma (refer to "Renal Tumors").
   I. Hematocrit and hemoglobin to evaluate blood loss.
   J. Coagulation studies to rule out predisposition to bleeding.
   K. Blood typing and cross-matching.
   L. Metastatic series, including bone scan to assess metastases.

Problems/ Diagnosis

I. Anemia due to gross painless hematuria resulting from the presence of the bladder tumor acting as a foreign body.
II. Alteration in comfort (pain) due to abnormal cellular proliferation and/or invasion of surrounding tissue.
III. Frequency, urgency, and dysuria due to development of an infectious process secondary to development of tumor of the bladder.
IV. Mild to moderate anxiety due to impending diagnostic studies, unconfirmed medical diagnosis, and alteration in voiding patterns.
V. Possible obstruction of the vesical outlet due to abnormal cellular proliferation and or blood clots.
VI. Muscular weakness, malaise, lethargy, gradual unexplained weight loss, and elevated temperature due to neoplastic process and/or severe infection.
VII. Edema in lower extremities due to venous obstruction by the expanding malignancy.

Goals of Care	Refer to "Renal Tumors."
Intervention	Refer to "Renal Tumors."
Evaluation	**REASSESSMENT: COMPLICATIONS**

      I. Obstruction of lower urinary tract outlet due to abnormal cellular proliferation and/or blood clots. (See "Obstructions" for complete discussion.)

    II. Hydronephrosis (see "Hydronephrosis" for discussion).

   III. Renal failure (see "Hyperactivity and Hypoactivity").

INTERVENTION

  I. Surgery.

    A. Transurethral resection and fulguration—*transurethral resection* involves the resection of the prostate by using an instrument called a resectoscope which enters the area via the urethra; *fulguration* is the process of destroying tissue that is thought to be malignant by the use of electric current.

      1. Preoperative intervention (refer to "Renal Tumors").

      2. Postoperative intervention.

        a. Measure and correlate intake and output every 4 h for first 24 h, progressing to every 8 h when appropriate.

        b. Test urine for blood at each voiding if no indwelling catheter present; if catheter present, test urine at least every 2 h. (Urine may be pink-tinged, and gross bleeding may be intermittent.) Hemoglobin and hematocrit levels should be checked to assess suspected blood loss.

        c. Observe urine for clots. *Maintain free unobstructed flow of urine.* Irrigate as needed according to doctor's orders.

        d. Provide meticulous and safe indwelling bladder catheter care. (Refer to discussion under "Renal Tumors.")

        e. Maintain oral fluid intake between 2500 and 3000 mL per 24 h.

        f. Administer prescribed blood replacements, i.e., transfusions, intravenous fluids, and electrolytes.

        g. Administer prescribed analgesics and antispasmodics for pain and complaints of spasm. A sitz bath or moist heat may provide relief from bladder spasms.

        h. Observe for signs of infection. Administer prescribed prophylactic antibiotics, and assess temperature frequently.

        i. Initiate teaching-learning transaction (include family and/or significant others) regarding:

          (1) Medications, especially name, dosage, rationale, expected action, side effects, and signs of toxicity.

          (2) Nutritional counseling: e.g., counseling is needed concerning decreased bladder capacity following the removal of the urethral catheter.

          (3) Continued intake of approximately 3000 mL per 24-h period. (The patient should be told to space oral intake.)

          (4) Need for follow-up and cystoscopic examination every 3 months for 1 year, then every 6 months thereafter.

        j. Initiate referral for follow-up care. Include a planned appointment for discharge evaluation.

      3. Complications of transurethral resection and fulguration.

        a. Hemorrhage. If hemorrhage cannot be controlled, surgical reintervention may be necessary.

        b. Obstruction in lower urinary tract (refer to "Obstructions"). Radical cystectomy with pelvic lymph node dissection and urinary diversion. For the male patient this involves radical prostatoseminal vesiculectomy.

    B. Segmental resection of the bladder.

      1. Preoperative intervention (refer to "Renal Tumors").

      2. Postoperative intervention (see point I A 2, above).

    a. Monitor and assess drainage from cystostomy tube and indwelling bladder catheter. Include cystostomy drainage in total urinary output.

    b. Offer reassurance that bladder capacity will gradually increase. Immediate postoperative bladder capacity may not be more than 60 mL. This may increase from 200 to 400 mL over time.

    c. Instruct patient on how to time ingestion of fluids to prevent frequent urination due to decreased bladder capacity.

        (1) Consume large amounts of fluids at one time.

        (2) Limit fluids at least 2 h before going out.

        (3) Consume no fluids after 6 P.M.

        (4) Assist patient in dealing with possible altered body image and self-esteem. Offer the patient an opportunity to discuss issues that may be of concern regarding the surgery. The nurse can be supportive to the patient by being reassuring whenever possible.

        (5) Follow up and evaluate the effectiveness of each intervention in light of the patient's overall progress. Include patient teaching whenever possible.

  3. Complications of segmental resection (see point I A 3, above).

C. Cystectomy—the complete removal of the bladder. This type of surgical procedure is usually performed after assessing the size of the lesion, the depth of tissue involvement, the patient's general health status, and whether the cellular growth is curable. This type of surgery will result in permanent *urinary diversion*. There are several procedures that can be performed and each will require special management following surgery.

  1. Types of urinary diversion.

    a. Rectal bladder—formation of a sigmoid colostomy with implantation of the ureters into the rectum (Fig. 28-2*a*).

    b. Ureterosigmoidostomy—transplantation of the ureters into the intact colon (Fig. 28-2*b*).

    c. Ureterileostomy (ileal conduit, Bricker procedure)—transplantation of ureters into an isolated section of ileum which is sutured closed at one end; the open end is brought to the skin (Fig. 28-2*c*).

    d. Cutaneous ureterostomy—implantation of the ureters directly into abdominal skin (Fig. 28-2*d*).

  2. Preoperative intervention (see the discussions under points I A and I B, above).

    a. Psychological preparation for urinary diversion is vital. Changes in body image may be of much concern to the patient. Offer reassurance, encouragement, and support.

    b. Anxiety can be relieved by creation of an atmosphere that fosters open discussion.

    c. A bowel preparation is usually given to the patient several days prior to surgery and includes a cathartic, an enema, and a sulfonamide such as neomycin.

    d. The patient is given a clear liquid diet (for 3 days) and vitamins B and K may be given if a deficiency is suspected. Fluid supplements via intravenous therapy may be suggested.

  3. Postoperative intervention.

    a. Label catheters. Maintain their patency. Irrigations may be prescribed as frequently as every 2 h. Measure, assess, and correlate fluid intake and output hourly.

    b. Maintain unobstructed flow of urine. Observe for edema around stoma. If a collection bag is attached, it should be emptied frequently to prevent backflow.

    c. Observe for signs of infection. Measure temperature at least every 2 h. Peritonitis can occur through escape of feces into peritoneal cavity.

    d. Administer pain relief measures. Initiate measures to prevent postoperative complications.

    e. Observe for distension of lower abdomen, particularly with ileal conduit since distension can cause tension on the suture line and can result in rupture. Frequently a nasogastric tube is used after surgery to reduce bowel distension.

f. Observe for electrolyte disturbances, especially following ureterosigmoidoscopy because of reabsorptive powers of the sigmoid.

g. Provide meticulous skin care around stoma. Consult enterostomal clinical nurse specialist. Utilize protective devices and preparations. Assess response to interventions. The stoma should be measured carefully and the size of the opening accurately determined. The bag used should fit firmly and not exert pressure on the stoma.

h. Depending on the type of urinary diversion performed, initiate early teaching regarding use of ostomy equipment, *only if appropriate.* This intervention may be inappropriate depending on the patient. Assess anxiety level and readiness to learn.

FIGURE 28-2 / Urinary diversion. (*From D. A. Jones et al., Medical-Surgical Nursing: A Conceptual Approach, McGraw-Hill Book Company, New York, 1978.*)

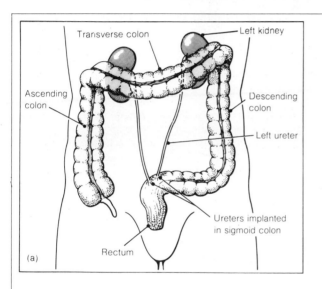

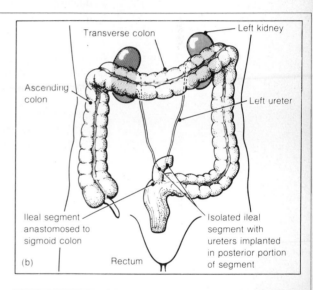

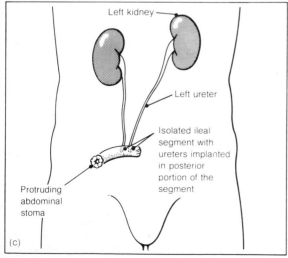

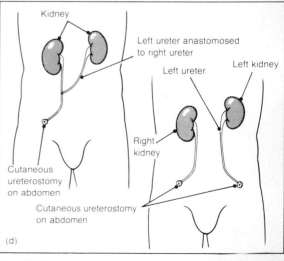

   i. Begin discharge teaching and planning early. Instruct patient, family member, or significant other if appropriate, regarding care of the stoma, activity, diet, etc. Be specific.

   j. Assist patient in accepting altered body image. Communicate concern and interest. Offer reassurance, support, and encouragement. Be patient but firm. Maintain aesthetic environment. Encourage interaction with others.

   k. Refer to American Cancer Society or Ostomy Association for group support and guided demonstrations.

   l. Maintain environment that fosters maximal self-care.

    (1) Allow patient time to adjust to urinary diversion progressing to total independence.

    (2) Assist patient in developing realistic rehabilitation goals.

    (3) Refer for vocational and sexual counseling.

    (4) Initiate referral for follow-up home care.

   m. Follow-up and reevaluate.

  4. Complications of urinary diversion.

   a. Peritonitis (see Chap. 29).

   b. Urethritis, pyelonephritis (see "Urethritis" and "Pyelonephritis").

   c. Obstruction of urinary outlet (see "Obstructions").

   d. Renal failure (see "Acute Renal Failure" and "Chronic Renal Failure").

II. Medical management.

 A. Intracavity irradiation—introduction of radioactive isotopes contained in the balloon of a Foley catheter. Nursing interventions include:

  1. Increase oral fluid intake.

  2. Administer prescribed urinary antiseptics and antispasmodics.

  3. Observe for signs of cystitis (the most frequent complication).

  4. Avoid excessive exposure to patient. Initiate radiation precautions.

 B. External irradiation.

 C. Combination therapy (external irradiation and surgery).

Carcinoma of the Prostate

Definition   *Carcinoma of the prostate* is the most common type of the malignant tumor of the genitourinary tract. Men over 55 years of age appear to be more frequently affected; however, this condition is not limited to that age group. Blacks are more frequently affected than any other ethnic group. Prostatic carcinoma arises in the periurethral and posterior portions of the prostate, which is adjacent to the rectum. Most prostatic carcinomas are classified as adenocarcinomas. Benign prostatic hypertrophy, though unrelated, frequently occurs simultaneously with prostatic carcinoma. Both of these conditions eventually result in obstruction of the bladder outlet. Patients with prostatic cancer usually remain asymptomatic until late in the course of the disease.

Assessment   **I.** Data sources (refer to "Renal Tumors").

 II. Health history (refer to "Renal Tumors").

  A. Race.

  B. Family history of cancer. History of venereal disease.

  C. Sexual history and contraceptive devices.

  D. Time of last voiding.

  E. Difficulty in starting and maintaining urinary stream.

  F. Diminished caliber and force of stream and "dribbling" or urine after micturition completed.

  G. Frequency, urgency, nocturia, and burning on urination.

  H. Hematuria (late manifestation).

  I. Presence, location, intensity, quality, and precipitating or aggravating factors of pain. Investigate factors that aid in analgesia. (Pain in bony structures may indicate metastasis.)

III. Physical assessment.
    A. Palpation of small firm fixed nodule in the posterior or lateral portions of the gland on rectal examination if the lesion is advanced. Nodule is not fixed if detected early.
    B. Bladder distension (present in acute/or chronic urinary retention).
    C. Dyspnea and cough (not always present; may indicate lung metastasis).
IV. Diagnostic tests.
    A. Prostatic biopsy (necessary to confirm diagnosis).
    B. Cystoscopy and IVP to rule out associated renal pathology (refer to discussion under "Renal Tumors").
    C. Excretory urogram.
    D. Metastatic series—x-ray examination of skeletal structures, especially pelvis, spine, ribs, and skull.
    E. Electrocardiogram.
    F. Renal function studies.
    G. Serum acid phosphatase—elevated when prostatic carcinoma has penetrated its capsule.
    H. Serum alkaline phosphatase—elevated when bony metastasis present.
    I. CBC and electrolyte determinations.
    J. Microscopic urinalysis, urine cultures, and antibiotic sensitivities.
    K. Coagulation studies to rule out potential bleeding tendency.
    L. Blood typing and cross-matching.

Problems/Diagnosis   See "Benign Prostatic Hypertrophy."

Goals of Care   See "Benign Prostatic Hypertrophy."

Intervention
    I. Refer to "Renal Tumors" and "Tumors of the Urinary Bladder".
    II. Support and reassure the patient and his family.
    III. This patient could benefit from a primary care nurse.
    IV. If metastasis has occurred, intervention should center around symptomatic management of the involved systems.

Evaluation

REASSESSMENT: COMPLICATIONS
    I. Insertion of urethral catheter may be impossible due to complete urethral obstruction. Suprapubic cystostomy necessary.
    II. Metastasis (refer to appropriate sections of this text to manage problems involving other systems).
    III. See "Benign Prostatic Hypertrophy" for complications resulting from obstruction of the bladder outlet.

INTERVENTION
    I. Surgery.
        A. Types of surgical intervention. Radical resection of the prostate gland—removal of the entire prostate gland, prostatic capsule, seminal vesicles, and adjacent tissue. Perineal and retropubic approaches are utilized most frequently. If the retropubic approach is utilized, a lymphadenectomy may be done. Orchidectomy and/or estrogen therapy may be used in conjunction with surgery.
        B. Preoperative intervention (refer to "Renal Tumors").
        C. Postoperative intervention.
            1. Observe dressing for drainage (usually less drainage than following prostatectomy for benign prostatic hypertrophy).
            2. Avoid dislodging urethral catheter since it serves as a splint for urethral anastomosis.
            3. Encourage use of perineal exercises (incontinence is common).

    4. Assist patient in rebuilding self-esteem and positive body image.

    5. Initiate sexual counseling since impotence follows this radical procedure.

II. Management of inoperable neoplasms.

  A. Types of medical intervention.

    1. Huggins treatment—the elimination of androgens by orchidectomy and/or administration of estrogenic hormones, usually diethylstilbesterol (2).

    2. Bilateral adrenalectomy.

    3. Hypophysectomy—experimental at this point in time.

    4. Cryosurgery—reduces the size of the obstructive lesion by freezing of the prostatic tissue.

    5. Transurethral resection may be performed to relieve immediate obstruction.

    6. Suprapubic cystostomy drainage if transurethral resection cannot be done.

    7. Radiation therapy—utilized to decrease tumor size. Frequently relieves pain of bony metastasis.

  B. Nursing intervention.

    1. Administer prescribed estrogenic hormones (usually diethylstilbesterol). Corticosteroids may be utilized to alleviate recurring symptoms. These give symptomatic relief but do not affect tumor growth.

    2. Observe for signs of hormonal imbalances.

    3. Observe for signs of side effects of medications. (Gynecomastia is a common side effect of estrogen therapy.)

    4. Support, reassurance, and encouragement needed. Realistic approach useful. Show genuine concern.

    5. Assist patient in capitalizing on the positive aspects of his life.

    6. Initiate referral for vocational and/or sexual counseling.

    7. Following orchidectomy, assist in redefining role and rebuilding self-esteem and positive body image.

    8. Assist patient and family in dealing with diagnosis and prognosis.

HYPERACTIVITY AND HYPOACTIVITY

Acute Renal Failure

Definition

Renal failure may be classified as either "acute or chronic according to the length of time required for the development of the condition and whether it is short-lived or prolonged" (3). *Acute renal failure* is a sudden severe reduction of renal function resulting in the accumulation of metabolic waste products in the blood and a disturbance in fluid and electrolyte concentrations. Acute renal failure, acute tubular necrosis, and acute tubular insufficiency are synonymous terms. When the kidneys are unable to eliminate body wastes and maintain fluid and electrolyte balance, the patient develops *azotemia*.

The many causes of acute renal failure have been classified as *prerenal causes,* conditions which decrease renal blood flow; *renal causes,* conditions resulting from primary damage to the kidney; and *postrenal causes,* conditions involving the distal portion of the urinary tract (4). Many other classification systems have been devised; however, prerenal, renal, and postrenal appear to be the most popular.

Acute renal failure typically has three clinical phases.

1. The first is the *oliguric phase* when urinary output is less than 400 to 600 mL per 24-h period. The oliguric phase may persist from 10 days to 3 weeks, in which time clinical features of uremia develop.

2. In the *diuretic phase,* the second clinical phase, urinary output gradually increases to 2 to 6 L per day, and BUN levels gradually fall and stabilize to within normal range.

3. The third phase is the *period of convalescence,* which may last from 6 to 12 months. During this time renal functioning is restored (5).

Regardless of the specific cause of acute renal failure, tubular epithelium is damaged. Renal ischemia leads to a decreased glomerular filtration and tubular necrosis, resulting in oliguria.

The prognosis of acute renal failure is variable depending on the length of the oliguric phase, the severity of the underlying causative disease process, and the rate of urea production. If acute renal failure continues unabated, *chronic uremia*, a clinical syndrome, develops.

Assessment

I. Data sources (refer to "Renal Tumors").
II. Health history. Since renal failure, both acute and chronic, is an extremely complex condition all body systems must be assessed. The following areas should be investigated in detail with each patient. This is not intended to be an exhaustive list of items to include in a nursing health history. Each patient is an individual; therefore, the nurse must individualize the health history by expanding or deleting certain areas.
   A. Age.
   B. Sex.
   C. Marital status.
   D. Occupation.
   E. Socioeconomic status, educational background, intelligence level.
   F. Family structure and significant others, life-style, religion, ethnic background, description of home environment (explore family resources).
   G. Level of consciousness—mental and emotional status.
   H. Height and usual weight, present weight.
   I. Family history of renal disease.
   J. Previous medical history.
      1. Discuss previous health problems that may be of significance, e.g., diabetes mellitus, systemic lupus erythematosus, streptococcal pharyngitis, gout, etc.
      2. Investigate previous hospitalizations, surgery, radiation, and medical/nursing care.
      3. Investigate for congenital malformation of the ear, spinal cord anomalies, imperforate anus, or genital anomalies. (Congenital renal anomalies and these defects frequently occur in the same patient.)
   K. Complete and detailed nutritional assessment (include history of anorexia, diarrhea, nausea and vomiting; food preferences and dislikes; dietary restrictions, self- or medically imposed).
   L. History of allergies; drug use (e.g., nephrotoxic drugs).
   M. Activity, rest, and sleep patterns. Activities of daily living.
   N. Voiding patterns and characteristics of urine including decreased volume.
      1. *Oliguria* is defined as 24-h total of approximately 500 mL.
      2. *Anuria* is defined as 24-h total of approximately 250 mL.
   O. Sexual history and contraceptive practices.
      1. Development of secondary sexual characteristics.
      2. A discussion of actual or perceived alterations in sexual drive and/or functioning should be included.
      3. With female clients investigate history of menstrual cycle.
   P. Alteration in body image and/or self-esteem. Assess response to illness, motivation for self-care, body image disturbances, role disturbances, and coping mechanisms.
III. Physical assessment.
   A. Enlarged kidney(s) palpable.
   B. Elevated blood pressure—renin-angiotensin system may be involved.
   C. Weight gain due to edema and decreased removal of body fluids.
   D. Skin—pallor due to anemia, urate crystals, pruritis, dry and cracked mucous membranes. Assess skin turgor.
   E. Eye changes—retinal hemorrhages, papilledema (not always present; usually associated with markedly elevated blood pressure).

F. Mouth—halitosis (due to acidosis), urinous breath, odor resulting from urea that is secreted into saliva breaking down to ammonia.

G. Edema in face, abdomen, and extremities. Pitting edema may be palpated in presence of decreased urinary output.

H. Muscular twitching may be present.

I. Elevated body temperature (not always present).

J. *Assess all body systems for deviations from the norm.*

IV. Diagnostic tests.

A. IVP (refer to "Renal Tumors").

B. Chest x-ray.

C. Electrocardiogram (refer to Chap. 26).

D. Renal arteriography.

E. Renal biopsy, renal scan, radioactive renogram.

F. Blood studies.

1. Nonprotein nitrogen.
2. Plasma alkaline phosphatase.
3. BUN (usually elevated).
4. Serum creatinine (usually elevated).
5. Serum magnesium.
6. Serum uric acid.
7. Serum chloride.
8. Serum potassium.
9. Serum calcium (usually decreased).
10. Serum sodium.
11. CO_2 content (usually low).
12. Inorganic serum sulfates.
13. Arterial blood gases (refer to Chap. 27).

G. Blood coagulation studies to rule out predisposition to bleeding.

H. Hematocrit and hemoglobin—anemia almost always present.

I. White blood cell differential count—leukocytosis usually present.

J. Blood typing and cross-matching.

K. Urine culture and antibiotic sensitivities.

L. Microscopic urinalysis—usually with low fixed specific gravity, some proteinuria, casts, hematuria, and cellular debris. Urine osmolarity has a tendency to be maintained at the same osmolarity as plasma (1.010). This is called *isosthenuria*.

V. Other data sources.

A. Referral note.

B. Previous available medical records.

Problems/ Diagnosis

I. Urinary elimination—impairment in excretion of end products of protein metabolism due to damaged renal tissue.

II. Body fluids—disruption in electrolyte (sodium, potassium, calcium, magnesium) and fluid balance due to damaged renal tissue.

III. Susceptibility to infections due to azotemic state.

IV. Alterations in cardiovascular status—hypertension, systemic edema, congestive heart failure, pericarditis, and pulmonary edema due to retention of sodium and consequent retention of fluid.

V. Circulation—anemia due to failure of kidneys to secrete erythropoietin, and to decreased life span of red blood cells in uremic environment.

VI. Urinary elimination—metabolic acidosis due to inability of the kidneys to excrete acid and reabsorb bicarbonate.

VII. Discomfort—parotitis or stomatitis due to decreased salivary flow, dehydration, and mouth breathing, which occurs in acidosis.

VIII. Possible renal osteodystrophy due to *osteomalacia* ["softening of the bones due to failure of calcium salts to be deposited in newly formed osteoid tissue" (6)], *osteitis fibrosa* ["reabsorption of calcium salts from the bone and replacement of these salts by fibrous tissue" (7)], and *osteosclerosis* ["abnormal hardening of bone characterized by areas of increased bony density" (8)].

IX. Self-concept—male libido and potency depressed; female libido, ovulation, and menstruation suppressed due to disturbance of endocrine system. (Onset of puberty may be delayed for several years.)

X. Confusion—psychological disturbances and central nervous system dysfunction due to azotemic state. "Degree of severity of psychological disturbances is usually proportional to severity of azotemia" (9).

Goals of Care

I. Immediate.
  A. Identify and remove initial cause of renal failure, if possible.
  B. Maintain as normal a fluid and electrolyte balance as possible.
  C. Prevent infection.
  D. Prevent overhydration.
  E. Decrease workload of the kidneys; reduce level of serum toxic materials.
  F. Prevent acidosis and minimize protein catabolism.
  G. Prevent further renal damage and decrease in function.
  H. Maintain adequate nutritional status but decrease metabolic demands.
  I. Control hypertension.

II. Long-range.
  A. Restore renal function.
  B. Patient compliance with treatment regimen.

Intervention

I. Assist in determining and eliminating the cause of acute tubular necrosis.

II. Dietary restrictions:
  A. Administer prescribed diet, which is usually nonprotein and low in potassium and sodium. Diet usually high in carbohydrates (at least 100 g) and fat. This diet reduces endogenous protein catabolism and helps to prevent ketosis.
  B. Enforce fluid restrictions. (Rule of thumb: fluid intake of 400 mL plus amount of total output on the previous day.)
  C. Serve food at the proper temperature.
  D. Allow patient choice in food whenever possible. Allow her or him to choose from exchange list.
  E. Allow patient to choose distribution of fluid restriction.
  F. Help allay thirst with wet cloth to suck to keep mouth moist; ice chips. (Include in total oral intake.)
  G. Meticulous and accurate measurement of fluid intake and output every hour.
  H. Daily weight on same scale (preferably a bed scale), same amount of clothing, same time of day, preferably before breakfast. [Weight should not increase or decrease over 0.45 kg per day (10).]
  I. Referral to nutritionist.
  J. Teaching (include family, food preparer) regarding the reading of labels on processed foods and avoiding the use of salt substitutes (most are low in sodium but high in potassium).
  K. Maintain reassuring supportive attitude. Allow the patient an opportunity to discuss feelings related to surgery and perceived changes in body image.
  L. Intravenous hypertonic carbohydrate solution may be administered if oral intake impossible.

III. Prevention of infection.
  A. Meticulous attention to all sterile procedures.
  B. Environmental asepsis is vital. Patient should be in private room.
  C. Avoid exposing patient to any kind of infection.
  D. Recognize and report signs of infection. (Patient may have hypothermia even in presence of infection; may also have leukocytosis without infection.)
  E. Administer prescribed antibiotics if infection does occur. Continue to protect from infection. Avoid use of *potassium penicillin*.

     F. Avoid chilling, but maintain carefully ventilated room.

     G. Avoid unnecessary instrumentation of any kind. If indwelling bladder catheter used, seek order for continuous irrigation with antibiotic solution.

     H. Turn frequently. Administer pulmonary care to prevent pneumonia.

     I. Reverse precautions sometimes necessary.

     J. Instruct patient about good personal hygiene and avoiding contact with individuals who have an upper respiratory infection.

IV. Activity restrictions to decrease metabolic rate.

     A. Encourage strict bed rest in acute phase.

     B. Provide diversional activity if appropriate. Consult the patient. Enlist aid of family and/or significant others.

     C. Passive and active exercises to prevent muscle atrophy.

     D. During diuretic phase assist and encourage progressive ambulation.

V. Electrolyte imbalance and fluid disturbance.

     A. Monitor ECGs for arrhythmias and/or heart block. Patient should be on cardiac monitor.

     B. Monitor and assess central venous pressure hourly until condition stabilizes.

     C. Monitor and assess vital signs every hour. Assess radial and apical pulses.

     D. Observe for signs of sudden or severe hypotension. Measure postural signs.

     E. Assess heart sounds. Listen for friction rub and tachycardia. Watch for signs of developing effusion and cardiac tamponade. Be prepared for emergency pericardiocentesis.

     F. Assess pulmonary status (lung sounds). Assess for Kussmaul's respirations, which are present in acidotic state.

     G. Observe for congestive heart failure, chest pains, pericarditis, and pulmonary edema (see Chap. 26).

     H. Observe for signs of *hyperkalemia* (flaccid paralysis, slow respirations, anxiety, convulsions, and cardiac arrest).

     I. Initiate measures to reduce hyperkalemia. Administer prescribed medications:

        1. Cation exchange resins—this increases potassium excretion from the bowel. Acidosis may result as a side effect.

        2. Insulin and glucose intravenously—insulin promotes removal of potassium from extracellular fluid.

        3. Intravenous calcium gluconate or calcium chloride—this protects the heart from the effects of hyperkalemia but does not reduce serum potassium.

        4. Intravenous sodium bicarbonate—this assists in combating acidosis.

        5. Observe for signs for hypokalemia.

     J. Administer prescribed aluminum hydroxide gel with meals to reduce absorption of phosphorus thus causing an increase in serum calcium. (Gels with magnesium are avoided because of danger of magnesium toxicity.)

     K. Observe for signs of hypernatremia during oliguric phase and hyponatremia during diuretic phase.

        1. *Hypernatremia*—characterized by fluid retention, weight gain, and systemic edema. Restrict sodium intake.

        2. *Hyponatremia*—characterized by dry mouth, loss of skin turgor, and hypotension. Administer prescribed sodium supplements.

     L. Administer prescribed diuretics during early acute renal failure. (Mannitol is frequently used.)

     M. Observe for signs of developing or increasing acidosis. Administer prescribed medications. Watch for development of side effects.

     N. Observe for signs of hypocalemic tetany and convulsions if acidosis is corrected. Administer prescribed medications.

VI. Skin care and oral hygiene.

     A. Oral hygiene before each meal. Sour balls help to alleviate metallic ammonium halitosis. Vinegar (0.25% acetic acid) neutralizes ammonium.

B. Keep nasogastric tube free of encrustations.

C. Special skin care required. Use bland soaps that do not contain perfume.

D. If uremic frost present, bathe patient frequently to remove crystals. It is not necessary to use soap because the skin is dry enough.

E. Systematically examine bony prominences every 4 h.

F. Turn the patient every 2 h. Utilize nondrying agents to massage bony prominences. Prevent decubitus ulcers.

VII. Environmental conditions

A. Keep noise to a minimum. Maintain calm, quiet atmosphere. Plan rest periods.

B. Allow for self-care and maintain independence as much as possible. Assist with hygiene as needed.

C. Institute seizure precautions. Utilize padded tongue blade, airway, suction, oxygen, and padded side rails.

D. Environmental safety necessary.

VIII. Combat anemia and bleeding tendency.

A. Avoid unnecessary trauma. Keep patient's fingernails trimmed.

B. Instruct patient on safety. Use soft toothbrush, avoid constipation, avoid vigorous nose blowing, rough contact sports, etc.

C. Observe for evidences of bleeding.

D. If blood administered, observe for signs of reaction. (Washed packed red cells frequently used because transfusions may add to potassium level.)

IX. Psychological status.

A. Explain to the patient and family that periods of confusion are expected outcomes of the disease process. Reorient the confused patient. Responses may be slowed. Allow time for patient response; avoid requiring complex choices to be made.

B. Offer reassurance, support, and encouragement.

C. Reassess level of consciousness and mental status every 4 h.

D. Keep bed in low position and side rails elevated.

X. General nursing considerations.

A. Observe for drug toxicity.

B. Monitor and assess all blood values.

C. Initiate referral for sexual and vocational counseling.

D. Keep avenues open to allow patient to discuss anxieties, fears, concerns, and apprehensions regarding alteration in sexual patterns. Include spouse in conferences.

E. Initiate social service and nutritional consultation.

F. Initiate teaching-learning transaction (include family and/or significant others) regarding:

  1. Nature of the disease process.

  2. Dietary allowances and restrictions.

  3. Medications especially name, dosage, rationale, expected action, side effects, and signs of toxicity.

  4. Symptoms that require medical attention.

  5. Symptoms of infection, fluid retention, and hypertension.

  6. General health care practices.

  7. Importance of health care follow-up.

G. Initiate referral for follow-up care.

H. Follow-up and evaluation.

Evaluations

REASSESSMENT: COMPLICATIONS

Reassess need for either peritoneal dialysis or hemodialysis (see "Peritoneal Dialysis" and "Hemodialysis").

INTERVENTION

See "Chronic Renal Failure."

Chronic Renal Failure

Definition

Chronic renal failure is the progressive irreversible deterioration of renal functioning that may develop insidiously over a period of years or following an unresolved bout of acute renal failure. The nephrons are gradually destroyed until uremia develops, resulting in death if dialysis and/or kidney transplantation is not part of the treatment plan.

Uremia is a complex clinical syndrome associated with the end stages of renal disease. Uremia results from acute or chronic renal failure. The uremic syndrome is characterized by markedly elevated blood urea nitrogen, elevated serum creatinine (which is less affected by external variables than the BUN), increased serum sodium, serum potassium, serum magnesium, serum phosphate, and serum sulfate. Serum calcium and serum chloride levels will be decreased.

Assessment

I. Data sources (refer to "Renal Tumors").
II. Health history (refer to "Acute Renal Failure").
III. Physical assessment.
    A. Uremic frost; skin discoloration due to retained urinary chromogen.
    B. Periorbital edema; edematous extremities.
    C. Arterial hypertension.
    D. Halitosis (ammonia odor).
    E. Frothy urine.
IV. Diagnostic tests (refer to "Acute Renal Failure").

Problems/ Diagnosis

I. Decreased urinary elimination—retention of toxic materials, and the disturbance of fluid, electrolyte, and acid-base balances (uremia).
II. Sensory perceptual alteration—impaired functioning of central nervous system due to accumulation of toxic materials (peripheral neuropathy).
III. Hypertension due to excessive secretion of renin, causing increased aldosterone levels, resulting in retention of fluids and electrolytes.
IV. Cardiac output—bilateral accumulation of fluid in the lungs due to possible coexisting heart failure and/or the direct result of toxic materials on lung tissue.
V. Nutritional alteration—secondary to a disturbance in the normal functioning of the gastrointestinal system (stomatitis, esophagitis, gastritis, peptic ulcers, colitis, pancreatitis, parotitis) due to uremic state.
VI. Cardiac output—blood volume alteration due to reduction in secretion of erythropoietin, malfunction of platelet factor 3, and loss of blood caused by intestinal bleeding.
VII. Potential disruption of skin integrity (pruritis, defective nails) due to disposition of toxic materials on the skin.
VIII. Thought process—impaired due to retention of toxins.
IX. Anxiety—mild to severe because of emotional impact of chronic illness.

Goals of Care

I. Immediate (see "Acute Renal Failure").
    A. Preserve renal function.
    B. Improve fluid and body chemistry balance.
    C. Reverse alterations in other body organs.
    D. Postpone or eliminate the need for dialysis and transplantation.
    E. Improve the quality of life and provide comfort.
II. Long-range.
    A. Restore renal functioning to as normal a level as possible.
    B. Evaluate patient compliance with treatment regimen.
    C. Evaluation of patient for dialysis.

Intervention
(see "Acute Renal Failure")

I. Administer diet according to blood electrolyte and chemistry levels and the clinical status of the patient.
    A. Provide appropriate motivation for staying on prescribed diet. Offer praise for a

job well done. Refer patient and family to organized groups with similar dietary restrictions.

   B. Rigid salt restrictions vital (400 to 2000 mg per day) in the oliguric or anuric patient.
   C. Strict restriction in dietary potassium (usually restricted to 1000 to 2000 mg daily).
   D. Assess need for vitamin supplements.
   E. Keep caloric intake at 2000 to 2500 cal per day. The ratio of nonprotein to protein kilocalories should be 5:1.
   F. Enforce fluid restriction during advanced stages to avoid overhydration, but avoid dehydration.
   G. Administer prescribed alkaline salts to combat acidosis. (Caution: Patients with far advanced renal disease cannot tolerate sodium bicarbonate because of possibility of hypernatremia.)
   H. Administer prescribed diuretics to decrease circulating fluid volume and decrease hypertension. Initiate measures to control hypertension to prevent further renal damage.

II. Psychological considerations.
   A. Allow patient time to mourn loss of an important bodily function.
   B. Assist patient, family, and significant others in accepting and dealing with this chronic illness.
   C. Assist in planning future and in realizing potential decisions to be made.
   D. Early discussion of use of dialysis and/or transplantation is vital.
   E. Allow patient and family to consider changes in occupation, residence, and finances.
   F. Provide an atmosphere for open discussion of problems with family and patient.

III. Initiate teaching-learning transaction (include patient, family, and/or significant others) regarding:
   A. Positive aspects of patient's condition. Encourage family to avoid overprotectiveness.
   B. Medication and dietary information should be given in written form as well as orally.
   C. Avoidance of any medication without the consent of a physician.
   D. Self-care practices.
   E. Development of self-observational skills: e.g., patient should note daily weight, note development of edema, and measure fluid intake and output.
   F. Nursing consideration: Emotional response to illness will require multiple repetitions and repeated reinforcements of material taught.

IV. During period of conservative management, assess patient's ability and willingness to cooperate in chronic hemodialysis and/or transplantation.

V. Initiate referral for vocational and exual counseling.

VI. Seek dietary and social service consultations if necessary.

VII. Follow-up and evaluation—vital aspect of patient compliance with treatment regimen.

Evaluation

REASSESSMENT: COMPLICATIONS
If patient is not a candidate for dialysis or transplantation, nursing interventions are related to terminal care.

INTERVENTION
Dialysis   Dialysis is the physical movement of solutes from an area of greater concentration through a semipermeable membrane into an area of lesser concentration of the same solutes until the concentration of both areas is equal. This differential diffusion for the removal of endogenous or exogenous toxins and other substances can be achieved either by extracorporeal means (hemodialysis) or by intracorporeal means (peritoneal dialysis). Either of these types of treatment may be used in acute renal failure to sustain life until the damaged kidney can repair itself and regain function. Additionally, either form of dialysis

may be employed to overcome uremia and/or physically prepare a patient for transplantation (11). The goals of dialysis therapy include:

1. Removal of toxic substances and metabolic wastes (end products of protein metabolism).
2. Regulation of fluid balance; removal of excessive body fluid.
3. Maintenance of serum electrolyte balances.
4. Correction of acid-base imbalances.

Peritoneal dialysis In peritoneal dialysis the principles of osmosis, diffusion, and filtration are utilized to move low-molecular-weight substances such as urea, glucose, and electrolytes through the peritoneum, which acts as an inert semipermeable membrane. These substances move between the dialyzing solution, which is introduced into the peritoneal cavity, and the blood vessels of the abdominal cavity. When the concentrations of solutes in the dialyzing solution and the blood are equal, the dialyzing solution (dialysate) is drained from the peritoneal cavity by the use of gravity. Additional dialysate may be utilized to remove excess nitrogenous products and to restore normal fluid and electrolyte balance.

Peritoneal dialysis may be utilized in both acute and chronic renal failure. Frequently, chronic renal failure patients are maintained on peritoneal dialysis while being evaluated for chronic hemodialysis or transplantation (12). The value and feasibility of long-term peritoneal dialysis is not clearly established.

I. Intervention before dialysis.
  A. The nurse should explain:
    1. The purpose of the procedure.
    2. Insertion of the catheter.
    3. Cycling of fluid.
    4. Allowed activity during dialysis.
    5. Expected length of procedure (usually 36 to 72 h, but if BUN levels are high, longer periods will be required).
  B. Provide a reassuring, supportive attitude. Assess patient's anxiety level and intervene appropriately. (Some patients desire and need only minimal information, while other patients desire and benefit from exact and detailed information.)
  C. Allow patient avenue for expressing fears and anxities. Offer reassurance. Allow time for questions.
  D. Informed written consent is necessary.
  E. Ask patient to void. If he or she cannot, a urethral catheter may be inserted to ensure the bladder is empty. This decreases the likelihood that it will be perforated during insertion of the trocar into the peritoneum.
  F. Measure weight for baseline information. Bed scale should be used.
  G. Measure vital signs for baseline information.
  H. Assist in physically preparing the trocar insertion site and the actual insertion of the catheter.
II. Intervention during dialysis (see Fig. 28-3).
  A. Adhere to time schedule for cycling as prescribed by physician. Optimum dialyzing rate is approximately 2.5 L/h.
    1. Connect two bottles of dialysate to Y-administration tubing. (This reduces chance of contamination by half by reducing the number of required bottle changes.)
    2. Dialysate should be warmed to 37°C before infusion. (This helps increase peritoneal clearance, helps the patient maintain a constant body temperature, and appears to be more comfortable for the patient.) Overheating of the dialysate can cause damage to abdominal organs.
    3. Heparin may be added to dialysate to prevent formation of fibrin plugs.
    4. Infuse dialysate according to time specifications of physician (usually 10 to 20 min). Do not allow air to enter tubing as this can result in abdominal discomfort and drainage difficulties. Clamp administration tubing.
    5. Wait for equilibration to occur per physician's orders (usually 30 to 45 min).

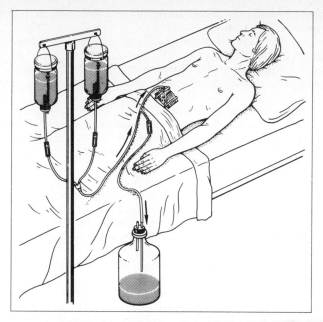

FIGURE 28-3 / Diagram illustrating peritoneal dialysis. Note that 2 L of dialysate are connected at one time to reduce risk of infection. Direction of arrows indicates direction of the flow of dialysate. Inflow clamps open during instillation while outflow clamps are closed. The reverse is true during outflow. Note presence of sterile dressing over entry site of catheter.

6. Allow fluid to drain from peritoneal cavity and close outflow valve. Time is specified by physician (usually 20 min).
7. Observe color of outflow fluid. Normally it is clear, pale yellow, and may be blood tinged during first few cycles because of traumatic insertion of catheter. If it is blood-tinged after first few cycles, suspect abdominal bleeding.
8. If drainage of dialysate is difficult, check for kinks in tubing, "milk" the tubing, have the patient change positions, apply firm pressure using both hands, and/or irrigate the peritoneal cavity with heparinized saline. If these measures do not increase drainage, notify the physician. A new catheter may need to be inserted.

B. Maintain dialysis flow sheet.
1. Record type of dialysate, medications added, amount of dialysate infused and drained, precise timing of inflow and outflow, observations regarding outflow dialysate, net fluid balance of each cycle, and cumulative net fluid balance.
2. Notify physician of fluid balance at least every 8 h. Significant changes in fluid balance must be reported immediatelh.
3. Monitor and assess all other forms and amounts of intake and output. Diet may be higher in protein than diet before dialysis since protein is lost in the dialysate.

C. Monitor and compare vital signs with baseline readings.
1. Vital signs should be measured every 15 min during the first exchange and every 1 to 4 h thereafter.
2. Patient should be on a cardiac monitor. Evaluate apical pulse and observe for arrhythmias.

D. Measure weight every 24 h after beginning dialysis. Patient should be weighed at the same point in the dialysis cycle each time. (One liter of dialysate weighs approximately 2.2 lb.)

E. Monitor and assess blood electrolyte determinations every 12 h or more frequently, if necessary.

F. Test urine for glucose, ketones, specific gravity, protein, blood, pH, etc., at each voiding.

G. Observe for hyperglycemia, hypotension, hypovolemia, infection, overhydration, hyponatremia, and hypoproteinemia. (Protein lost is approximated at 0.2 to 0.8 g/L.)

H. Provide necessary comfort measures.

    1. Equilibration and outflow periods are best for baths, backrubs, and other hygienic measures. If movement interferes with drainage, activity should cease. Movement is most uncomfortable during the inflow phase.

        a. Diversional activity is needed since the procedure is very time-consuming.

        b. Encourage self-care as much as possible.

        c. Physician's order is required for the patient to be allowed out of bed for short periods of time.

    2. If pain occurs during inflow phase, infuse dialysate at a slightly slower rate. Analgesics and local anesthetics can be used.

I. Maintain environmental asepsis.

    1. Change dressing at catheter site every 8 h. Use strict aseptic technique. (Reverse isolation precautions may be used.)

J. Observe for signs of peritonitis. If suspected, send dialysate outflow for culture and sensitivity. Signs of peritonitis include abdominal pain, tenderness, abdominal rigidity, fever, leukocytosis, and cloudy drained dialysate.

K. Observe for signs of perforated bowel (pain and fecal material in outflow dialysate). Stop dialysate and notify physician.

L. Observe for signs of pulmonary edema (rapid respiratory rate; rales; tachycardia; markedly reduced respiration depth due to fluid in the peritoneal cavity pushing the diaphragm upward). Stop inflow phase. Elevate the head of the bed. Notify the physician.

M. Observe for signs of leakage of dialysate into abdominal tissues, chest cavity, and scrotum. If this occurs, change the dressing around the catheter site and notify the physician.

N. Provide constant reassurance and support. Maintain therapeutic nurse-patient relationship. Provide avenue for expression of frustrations and anxieties. Assist patient in maintaining self-esteem and body image.

O. Observe for behavioral changes that may accompany dialysis disequilibrium.

P. Provide for safety needs.

III. Intervention after dialysis.

A. After removal, send catheter tip for culture.

B. Continue to monitor vital signs every 2 to 4 h, especially temperature.

C. Maintain aseptic technique when changing sterile dressing at catheter site.

D. Continue to measure and correlate all intake and output. Daily weights vital.

E. Monitor and assess renal function studies and electrolyte determinations.

F. Carry out frequent periodic total physical assessments.

G. Psychological aspects of peritoneal dialysis are discussed under "Hemodialysis."

IV. Complications of peritoneal dialysis.

A. Loss of the catheter into the abdomen. Removed by laporoscopy.

B. Perforation of the bowel (refer to Chap. 29).

C. Perforation of the bladder (refer to "Trauma to the Bladder").

D. Peritonitis.

E. Wound infection.

F. Arrhythmia due to removal of potassium (refer to Chap. 26).

G. Hyperglycemia (refer to Chap. 24).

H. Hypernatremia.

I. Hyperosmolarity.

J. Reactive hypoglycemia—sometimes occurs 24 to 48 h after dialysis, most often in diabetics.

Hemodialysis   Hemodialysis is a complex mode of therapy that is extremely expensive and psychologically and physically demanding. Extracorporeal dialysis (hemodialysis) utilizes the same physical principles described in peritoneal dialysis. In hemodialysis blood is removed from the patient's radial or brachial artery and pumped through a semipermeable cellophane membrane while the dialysate flows on the outside of the membrane. The waste products of metabolism, water, and electrolytes flow freely across the semipermeable membrane from the blood into the dialysate. Since end-stage renal disease has both reversible and irreversible oiochemical components, long-term dialysis can only partially serve as a substitute for normal renal function (13).

Hemodialysis is indicated for use in patients with acute renal failure when very rapid or frequent dialysis is necessary or when peritoneal dialysis is contraindicated, e.g., in cases of poisoning or severe uremia. Since the facilities for hemodialysis are limited and the cost is prohibitive, the selection of candidates for hemodialysis is often a complex process. The nurse frequently brings valuable information to a multidisciplinary conference for evaluating the feasibility and value of long-term hemodialysis.

I. Assessment (refer to "Acute Renal Failure").
  A. Before dialysis.
    1. General condition. Observe gait, facial expressions, tone of voice, dress, posture, nonverbal communications, etc.
    2. Accurate weight vital.
    3. Baseline vital signs. Take blood pressure standing and lying. These parameters are used to evaluate the patient during and following dialysis.
    4. Condition of the shunt site.
      a. Cannula (arteriovenous shunt).
        (1) Inspect and evaluate the condition of the dressing.
        (2) Remove the dressing and inspect for signs of clotting. Note color of blood and pulsation. Maintain aseptic technique. (Note: Follow the policies and procedures of your institution. Many agencies allow only the "dialysis nurse" to carry out cannula care.)
        (3) Observe for signs of infection. Note areas of redness, edema, and/or drainage.
        (4) Evaluate need for further instruction regarding care of the cannula.
      b. Subcutaneous arteriovenous shunt (arteriovenous fistula) (see Fig. 28-4).
        (1) Inspect area for signs of thrombophlebitis.
        (2) Note any edema or discoloration.
    5. Date of previous dialysis.
    6. History of bleeding.
    7. General psychosocial condition. Patients' families are valuable in providing this information, particularly if the patient is uremic.
    8. Information regarding compliance with dietary regimen.
  B. During dialysis. It is not within the scope of this book to explain in detail the nursing management of a patient during hemodialysis. Special instruction is needed before a nurse should assume this responsibility. The reader is referred to the bibliography if additional information is desired.
  C. After dialysis.
    1. Vital signs—expect a decline from blood pressure before dialysis; temperature may be elevated.
    2. Accurate weight.
    3. Fluid intake and output. If patient had some urine output prior to dialysis, expect oliguria since water and waste products have been eliminated from the blood.
    4. Observe for signs of cerebral edema (dialysis disequilibrium).
    5. Observe for bleeding tendency. Heparinization is necessary for dialysis.

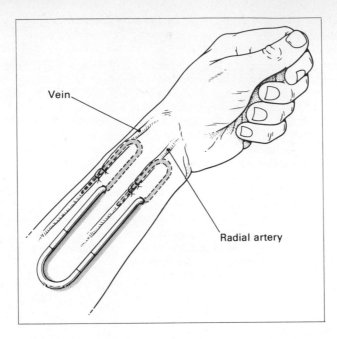

FIGURE 28-4 / Schematic representation of a silastic shunt. This cannula allows easy access to both the artery and vein without repeated venipuncture. [*Adapted from B. J. Fellows, "The Role of the Nurse in a Chronic Dialysis Unit," Nursing Clinics of North America, 1(4):259, 1966.*]

II. Problems. Obviously the nursing problems identified in acute and chronic renal failure apply to the patient prior to initiating dialysis. Additional problems may include:
  A. Noncompliance with dialysis regimen due to denial of the gravity of the medical diagnosis and prognosis.
  B. Marital discord due to serious sexual impairment.
  C. Failure to resume active life due to lack of motivation and/or extreme dependency.
  D. Suicidal behavior due to impact of stresses associated with long-term dialysis.
  E. Severe economic difficulties due to high cost of long-term dialysis and possible decreased family income.
  F. Marked alteration in psychological status (fear of death, projection, displacement, suppression, distortion, rage, denial, guilt, hostility, anxiety, and dependency) due to permanency of treatment regimen.
III. Goals of care. The goals identified and discussed under "Acute Renal Failure" are applicable here. In addition, the patient's psychosocial and sociocultural needs will be addressed in more detail here.
  A. Immediate.
    1. Compliance with dialysis regimen.
    2. Acceptance of medical diagnosis and the realization of the full impact of the prognosis.
    3. Appropriate use of body defense mechanisms.
  B. Long-range.
    1. Realistic adaptation to dialysis regimen.
    2. Total independence by utilization of home dialysis.
IV. Intervention.
  A. Unless the patient's defense mechanisms are clearly destructive or maladaptive, the nurse should support the patient. Acceptance of the patient's attitudes is essential.

Assist the patient to mourn the loss of health, independence, financial stability, and possibly employment. Assist in developing and exploring interests and hobbies.

B. Observe for signs of severe depression. Noncompliance such as improper cannula care, ingesting foods high in potassium, etc., may be a manifestation of depression. Insomnia (physical response to dialysis) can also contribute to depression.

C. Assist the patient and her or his family to develop realistic expectations and to avoid overprotectiveness. Maintain and encourage independence. Encourage responsibility for maintenance of therapy regimen within the realistic limitations of his or her condition.

D. Counsel both the patient and the spouse regarding decreased libido and impotence. Marital stability before dialysis carries through the stresses of dialysis. Role reversal is common.

E. Assist the family in supporting the patient. Use of denial by the family may be destructive. The family should be allowed avenues for expressing anxiety, hostility, and guilt. The nurse must be supportive, nonjudgmental, and objective in achieving this goal.

F. Support development of and participation in family-patient dialysis groups. This helps combat social isolation and provides avenue for teaching and sharing common experiences.

G. Staff must recognize and deal with their own reactions. Health team attitudes are communicated to patients. Consistency of a multidisciplinary team is vital. Staff conferences with a psychologist or psychiatrist will aid staff in dealing with their personal reactions to dialysis.

H. Assist patient in dealing with financial difficulties. Refer to appropriate agencies.

I. Initiate appropriate referrals for vocational rehabilitation, social services, and follow-up home care.

J. Evaluate feasibility of home dialysis.

K. Follow-up and evaluation.

V. Evaluation: complications of hemodialysis.
  A. Hyper- or hypovolemia.
  B. Hemolysis.
  C. Dialysis disequilibrium syndrome.
  D. Transfusion hazards.
  E. Psychological dysfunction.
  F. Continuation of uremic problems despite dialysis.
    1. Anemia.
    2. Hypertension.
    3. Peripheral neuropathy.
    4. Renal osteodystrophy.
    5. Reproductive system abnormalities such as gynecomastia and menorrhagia.

Renal transplantation Renal transplantation involves the surgical transfer of a human kidney from one individual to another. Organs may be obtained from two sources: (1) a living donor or (2) a cadaver. Regardless of the source of the organ, the donor kidney is placed in the iliac fossa and the donor renal artery is anastomosed end to end to the recipient's hypogastric artery while the donor renal vein is anastomosed to the recipient's internal iliac vein. The donor ureter is implanted into the bladder wall in such a way as to prevent reflux (14). Prior to transplantation a nephrectomy (bilateral) may be performed.

I. Goals of care. With regard to preoperative preparation, these are similar to those for patients undergoing renal surgery. Heavy emphasis should be placed on the psychological as well as the physical preparation for both the donor and the recipient.

II. Intervention.
  A. Preoperative intervention: recipient.
    1. Answer questions honestly regarding the actual surgery, immediate postoperative period, and discharge plans.

    2. Encourage maintenance of self-car and maximal independence. Allow patient to express fears.

    3. Psychotherapy may be necessary to prevent development of severe emotional disturbances.

    4. Intervention includes management of chronic renal failure (refer to "Intervention" under "Chronic Renal Failure").

    5. Identify and support medical treatment of any and all infectious processes. Prepare the patient for reverse isolation postoperatively.

    6. Assist in the collection of specimens to ascertain tissue compatibility.

B. Preoperative intervention: donor.

    1. Physical preparation similar to the patient undergoing abdominal surgery. Assist in the collection of specimens to ascertain tissue compatibility.

    2. Psychological preparation.

        a. Identify motivation for donating kidney.

        b. Assist with psychiatric and physical evaluations of the donor.

        c. Donor should be well informed of risks involved. Answer questions openly and honestly. Clarify misconceptions.

        d. Allow patient avenue for refusing to be a donor. Let him or her know that it is all right to say no.

C. Postoperative intervention: recipient.

    1. Immediate reverse isolation is necessary for recipient only. Usually recipient does not go to the recovery room, because few recovery rooms are equipped to manage reverse precautions. Care is similar to any patient recovering from general anesthesia.

    2. Maintain flui balance and renal functioning.

        a. Hourly urine outputs. Inspect and monitor composition of urine.

        b. Monitor and assess serum electrolyte and renal function values every 24 h, progressing to 3 times a week as condition stabilizes.

        c. Monitor vital signs hourly, including central venous pressure (CVP).

        d. With a return to normal function in 48 to 72 h, urine output may exceed 2000 mL/h. Observe for bladder spasms resulting from use of previously underused urinary tract.

        e. Collect 24-h urine specimen for creatinine clearance and sodium, potassium, and protein excretion.

        f. After 24 h, monitor vital signs evry 4 h and fluid intake and output every 8 h.

        g. Daily weights essential.

    3. Early mobility to maintain optimal pulmonary functioning.

        a. Begin ambulation 24 h after surgery. When in bed, patient may lie on operative side. Elevate head of the bed 30 to 45°.

        b. Instruct patient to avoid sitting for extended periods (may cause kinking of ureter, tension on anastomosis, or rotation of the graft.)

    4. Prevent infection.

        a. Administer prescribed immunosuppressive drugs (usually azathioprine) and corticosteroids. Administer prescribed antacids with corticosteroids.

        b. Monitor daily white blood counts.

        c. Strict aseptic precautions must be maintained. Careful handwashing vital. Avoid exposure to anyone with infections.

        d. Meticulous catheter care.

        e. Obtain routine cultures of likely signs of infection.

    5. Initiate teaching-learning transaction (include family and/or significant others) regarding:

        a. Self-assessment and self-care—measuring fluid (intake and output, recording weight, taking blood pressure, collecting urine specimens, etc.)

        b. General health habits and activity levels. Oral and personal hygiene essential.

        c. Dietary counseling.

        d. Signs and symptoms of infection and/or rejection.

        e. Importance of follow-up care.

    6. Assist patient in dealing with "new" body image and emotional feelings of obligation to the donor. Allow patient avenues to express fears of rejection, etc. Emphasize positive aspects of her or his life.

  D. Postoperative intervention: donor.

    1. Physical care is similar to that for a patient following major abdominal surgery.

    2. Assist the donor in working through depression and feelings of not being adequately regarded for personal sacrifice.

    3. In cases of rejection reactions, assist the patient in working through feeling of guilt.

  E. Initiate referral for follow-up and reevaluation.

  F. Staff must deal with their own reactions as well as the family's pre- and posttransplantation reactions.

III. Evaluation—complications of transplantation.

  A. Rejection—depending on the severity of the reaction, interventions are supportive and similar to those employed in acute renal failure with the use of corticosteroids. Hemodialysis may be necessary.

    1. Assessment.

        a. Anorexia, malaise.

        b. Fever, edema, and tenderness at the site of the transplant.

        c. Decreased urinary volume.

        d. Elevated BUN levels and creatinine values.

        e. Hypertension.

        f. Weight gain.

    2. Intervention.

        a. Record and report suspect signs immediately.

        b. Assist patient with depression following rejection reaction.

  B. Spontaneous rupture of the graft.

  C. Primary renal disease such as glomerulonephritis.

INFLAMMATORY DISORDERS

Urethritis

Definition

Urethritis, inflammation of the urethra, may be of an acute nature or it may be a long-standing chronic condition. In either case the inflammation is generally limited to the epithelial and subepithelial layers of the urethra. Urethritis may be *nonspecific* in that no organism can be identified as the causative agent. Exposure to chemicals such as bubble baths and some spermicidal jellies have been identified as etiological factors. However, in the majority of instances urethritis is due to bacteria, especially *Neisseria gonorrhoeae,* which is transmitted by direct sexual contact. In addition, exposure to other organisms (such as viruses, fungi, and protozoa) from the vagina and/or rectum may be the cause.

Assessment

  I. Data sources (refer to "Renal Tumors").

  II. Health history (refer to "Renal Tumor," points II A to II M).

    A. Past history of urinary tract infections, location, frequency of recurrence, severity, duration, and mode of treatment.

    B. Question hygienic self-care practices (particularly use of bubble baths, perfumed soaps and/or feminine hygiene deodorant sprays).

    C. Identification of possible causative factor(s).

    D. Sexual history and contraceptive practices (particularly use of spermicidal jellies).

    E. Actual and/or perceived alteration in sexual drive and/or function.

    F. Alteration in body image and/or self-esteem.

    G. Voiding patterns and characteristics of urination (particularly frequency, nocturia, urgency, burning upon *initiating* micturition).

III. Physical assessment.
   A. Elevated body temperature.
   B. Edema and erythema around urinary meatus.
   C. Creamy white discharge from urethra (usually present in males, but not always in females).
   D. Pain in urethra upon movement.
IV. Diagnostic tests.
   A. Culture and antibiotic sensitivities of urethral discharge.
   B. Urine culture and antibiotic sensitivities.
   C. Microscopic urinalysis.
   D. Visual inspection of several urine specimens in glass receptacles. (Only the first voided specimen will contain purulent material and/or mucous shreds.)
   E. White blood cell differential count.
   F. Serological test for syphilis.

Problems/ Diagnosis

I. Urinary impairment—alteration in voiding patterns (frequency, nocturia, urgency, burning on initiating micturition) due to presence of inflammatory process in the urethra.
II. Alteration in comfort (pain) due to inflammatory process in the urethra.
III. Increased body temperature due to inflammatory process.
IV. Mild to moderate anxiety due to alteration in voiding patterns, body image, and/or sexual functioning.
V. Possible extension of inflammatory process due to urinary stasis.
VI. Potential transmission of causative organism (if of infectious origin) due to urethral discharge.
VII. Possible recurrence of urethritis due to unidentified causative factor(s).

Goals of Care

I. Immediate.
   A. Prevent transmission of causative organism (if of infectious origin).
   B. Eradicate the existing inflammatory/infectious process.
   C. Prevent urinary stasis.
   D. Reduce pain and discomfort.
   E. Reduce elevated temperature.
   F. Reduce anxiety.
   G. Identify and remove causative factor(s).
II. Long-range.
   A. Prevent extension of inflammatory/infectious process.
   B. Prevent recurrence through patient education.

Intervention

I. Initiate precautionary isolation measures. (Linen, towels, clothing, etc. should be treated as contaminated items. Particular caution is necessary in discarding contaminated urine.)
II. Administer prescribed antibiotics (usually broad-spectrum). Penicillin used if urethritis if from gonorrhea. Tetracycline antibiotic used if patient allergic to penicillin.
   A. Assess urethral discharge for response to antibiotics.
   B. Continue and monitor periodic culture and antibiotic sensitivities of urethral discharge.
III. Increase fluid intake to 3000 mL per 24-h period (unless contraindicated by other coexisting physical condition).
IV. Insert prescribed urethral catheter. Administer prescribed antibiotic solution (not always done). Maintain adequate and safe outflow of urine through urinary irrigation drainage system (see Fig. 28-5). Provide meticulous indwelling catheter care.
V. Monitor and assess correlation between intake and output.
VI. Encourage sitz baths or warm tub baths 3 or 4 times daily.
VII. Administer prescribed analgesics and other appropriate pain relief measures.

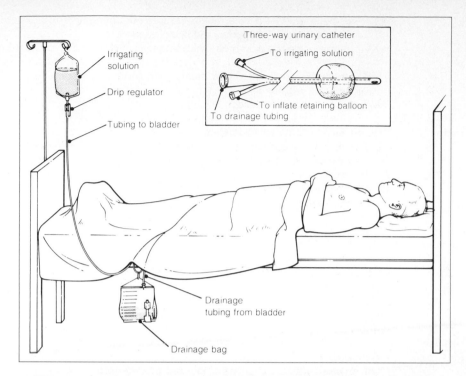

FIGURE 28-5 / Urinary irrigation drainage system. (*From D. A. Jones et al., Medical-Surgical Nursing: A Conceptual Approach, McGraw-Hill Book Company, New York, 1978.*)

VIII. Monitor and assess temperature every 4 h (more frequently if indicated by marked deviation from the norm).

IX. Cleanse urinary meatus and surrounding area with prescribed solution at least every 4 h.

X. Provide environment that promotes improvement of general physical and psychological health.

XI. Prevent *unnecessary* urinary tract instrumentation.

XII. Offer reassurance that voiding patterns will return to state before urethritis (barring any complications).

XIII. Decrease anxiety regarding sexual concerns by presenting a supportive atmosphere.

XIV. Initiate teaching-learning transaction (include family and/or significant others) regarding:

  A. Home care of linen, towels, clothing, etc., until infectious process has been successfully treated.

  B. Avoidance of sexual intercourse to prevent transmission of the infection. Alcohol should be temporarily discontinued since it may prolong the acute phase (15).

  C. Hygienic practices, particularly in reference to proper cleansing after urination and defecation and avoidance of bubble baths. (See "Cystitis" for more information.)

  D. Continued utilization of warm tub baths for relief of discomfort.

  E. Medications, desired effects, and side effects.

   1. Alert the patient that some medications cause discoloration of urine.

   2. Advise continuation of full course of medications despite cessation of symptoms.

F. Note signs of a recurrence and indicate appropriate responses to these signs.

G. Avoidance of any other identified cause.

XV. Referral for evaluation of alternative means of contraception if spermicidal jellies are utilized.

XVI. Counseling and referral of sexual partner(s) for investigation and treatment of causative organism.

XVII. Follow-up and evaluation.

Evaluation

REASSESSMENT: COMPLICATIONS

I. If urethritis is of gonorrheal origin, sequelae of gonorrhea may develop (see Chap. 30).

II. Cystitis (see "Cystitis").

III. Prostatitis (see "Prostatitis").

IV. Seminal vesiculitis.

V. Urethral stricture (see "Urethral Stricture").

Cystitis

Definition

Cystitis, inflammation of the wall of the urinary bladder, may occur as a primary condition; however, it is more frequently associated with an infectious process elsewhere in the urinary tract. Cystitis may also be related to the obstruction of the free flow of urine (urethral obstruction). Females are more frequently affected than males. In females with cystitis, nonspecific urethritis may also be present. Cystitis may result from vaginal trauma and often occurs 36 to 72 h following sexual intercourse. Contamination of the urethra from the rectum and vagina may also be the cause. Cystitis in males is usually associated with urinary retention caused by an enlarged or infected prostate gland.

Chronic cystitis may develop when the underlying cause or predisposing factors are not eliminated. Urine cultures may reveal no growth of organisms in the chronic state. Chronic cystitis may be asymptomatic.

Interstitial cystitis, also known as *Hunner's ulcer,* most frequently affects middle-aged women. In this condition there is decreased bladder capacity and actual splitting of the epithelium in the presence of bladder distension. The etiology remains obscure. The treatment of interstitial cystitis is extremely difficult; however, fulguration of the bleeding ulcer (under general anesthesia) has been successful in the past.

Assessment

I. Data sources (refer to "Renal Tumors").

II. Health history (refer to "Renal Tumors," points II A to II M). Data collected in the health history are of critical importance since recurring bladder infections should be carefully documented for further follow-up.

A. Voiding patterns and characteristics of micturition (particularly frequency, nocturia, urgency, tenesmus, and burning throughout voiding or at the end of micturition).

B. Description and characteristics of urine (particularly purulence, hematuria, and/or malodor).

III. Physical assessment.

A. Elevated body temperature.

B. Suprapubic pain.

C. Cloudy, malodorous urine.

D. Abdominal discomfort upon palpation and fullness in abdominal cavity.

IV. Diagnostic tests.

A. Microscopic urinalysis—specimens will show alkaline pH, albuminuria (common in chronic cases), and hematuria.

B. Urine culture and antibiotic sensitivities.

C. Visual inspection of several urine specimens in glass receptacles (random specimens will contain sediment).

D. White blood cell differential count.

Problems/
Diagnosis

I. Urinary elimination—alteration in voiding patterns (frequency, nocturia, urgency, tenesmus, and burning throughout voiding or at the end of micturition) due to presence of inflammation of the bladder wall.

II. Alteration in comfort (suprapubic pain) due to inflammation of the bladder wall.

III. Increased body temperature due to inflammatory process in the urinary bladder.

IV. Mild to moderate anxiety due to alteration in voiding patterns, body image, and/or sexual functioning.

V. Possible extension of infectious process to upper urinary tract due to stasis of urine.

VI. Potential transmission of causative organism due to improper handling of urine.

VII. Possible recurrence of cystitis due to patient's lack of information regarding causative and preventive factor(s).

Goal of Care

I. Immediate.
   A. Prevent transmission of causative organism.
   B. Eradicate the existing infection.
   C. Prevent urinary stasis.
   D. Reduce pain and discomfort.
   E. Reduce body temperature to normal limits.
   F. Prevent fecal contamination of the urinary meatus.
   G. Reduce anxiety.
   H. Identify and remove underlying cause.
II. Long-range.
   A. Prevent extension of inflammatory/infectious process.
   B. Prevent recurrence through patient education.

Intervention

I. Initiate urine isolation precautions to prevent transmission of infecting organism (not appropriate in all cases).

II. Administer prescribed broad-spectrum antibiotics, urinary antiseptics, and/or urinary analgesics.
   A. If methanamine mandelate (Mandelamine) is used, increase the acidity of the urine, but increased fluid intake is not indicated.
   B. In some cases, an alkaline urine relieves symptoms.
   C. Invading organisms are not visible in acidic urine (pH of 5.5 or less).
   D. Assess urine cultures and antibiotic sensitivities to determine response to chemotherapy.
   E. Encourage fluid intake (oral and parenteral) of at least 3000 mL per 24-h period to reduce residual urine (unless contraindicated by medications, coexisting disease conditions, and/or complete obstruction of the flow of urine).
   F. Insert indwelling bladder catheter and instillation of prescribed antibiotic solution. Assess for residual urine (refer to Fig. 28-5). Provide perineal care as needed.
   G. Encourage mild to moderate activity to prevent urinary stasis. (Some restrictions are imposed during the acute phase.)
   H. Assist in dilatation of urethra to drain urethral abscesses (not always done).
   I. Administer prescribed antispasmodics to reduce tenesmus.
   J. Encourage warm sitz baths or tub baths at least 3 or 4 times daily. Hot water bottle to perineum and/or cotton ball with witch hazel to the urethral orifice.
   K. Administer prescribed analgesics and/or other measures to relieve pain.
   L. Monitor and assess temperature every 4 h and more frequently as indicated by marked deviation from the norm. Provide comfort measures.
   M. Offer support and reassurance that voiding patterns will return to precystitis state (barring complications).
   N. Provide environment that fosters maintenance of self-esteem and positive body image.
   O. Establish nurse-patient relationship that encourages discussion of anxieties regarding sexual activity.

P. Initiate referral for marriage and/or sexual counseling.

Q. Initiate teaching-learning transaction (include appropriate family members and/or significant others) regarding:

    1. Hygienic self-care practices (16).

        a. Voiding after sexual intercourse.

        b. Cleansing anus after bowel movement. (Women should clean from front to back.)

        c. Suggest that women switch from nylon to cotton underwear.

        d. Women should avoid panty hose, tight slacks, and/or damp swim suits.

        e. Avoid strong powders and bleaches when washing clothes. Rinse thoroughly.

        f. Avoid use of bubble baths, perfumed soaps, and/or feminine hygiene sprays.

        g. Chlorinated drinking water may irritate urinary tract. Use of large quantities of spring water may be helpful.

    2. Continued utilization of warm tub baths for relief of mild discomfort.

    3. Know signs of a recurrence. Indicate appropriate responses to these signs.

    4. Medications, desired effects, and side effects, etc.

        a. Alert patient that some medications used cause discoloration of urine.

        b. Advise patient to continue full course of medication despite cessation of symptoms.

    5. Emphasize need for follow-up care including examination of urine specimens. (Asymptomatic infections may develop and eventually result in irreversible kidney damage.)

III. Follow-up and evaluation.

Evaluation

REASSESSMENT: COMPLICATIONS

I. Chronic cystitis.

  A. Assessment (refer to "Assessment," above).

    1. Tendency toward depression.

    2. Method of coping.

    3. Marital difficulties associated with this illness.

    4. Financial or occupational difficulties associated with this illness.

    5. Limited social activities because of persistent distressing symptoms.

  B. Intervention.

    1. Observe for signs of superimposed infection if antibiotics used for prolonged periods (particularly *Monilia* vaginitis).

    2. Provide patient with avenue for venting fears and fristrations.

    3. Establish caring empathetic relationship.

    4. Discuss sexual concerns in competent professional manner.

    5. Referral for counseling.

    6. Follow-up and reevaluation.

II. Bladder calculi (refer to "Obstructions").

III. Contracture of the neck of the bladder (refer to "Obstructions").

IV. *Ureteritis,* acute or chronic inflammation of the ureter, which usually coexists with pyelonephritis. The medical and nursing interventions implemented to alleviate the pyelonephritis also apply to ureteritis. In chronic ureteritis, fibrosis and strictures of the ureter may develop.

V. Pyelonephritis (refer to "Pyelonephritis").

VI. Septicemia—usually gram-negative septic shock (refer to Chap. 44).

Pyelonephritis

Definition

Acute pyelonephritis is an inflammation of one or both kidney pelvices caused by a bacterial infection. This inflammation "involves the pelvocalycal system as well as the renal interstitlum" (17), particularly the medulla. Gram-negative enteric bacilli are the most commonly encountered organisms that enter the urinary system. *Escherichia coli* is frequently the causative organism. In addition to developing from an ascending infection in the lower urinary tract, acute pyelonephritis may be caused by a blood-borne infection such as streptococcus.

Females, particularly girls under the age of 10 and women in their early childbearing years, are more frequently affected than males. Individuals with diabetes mellitus and females in the first trimester of pregnancy appear to have a particular predisposition to pyelonephritis.

Of prime concern in dealing with acute pyelonephritis is the possible cessation of symptoms with the persistence of an asymptomatic infection that eventually develops into destruction of the kidneys.

Assessment

I. Data sources (refer to "Renal Tumors").
II. Health history. Because of the nature of the predisposing factors associated with acute pyelonephritis, the reader should review the nursing health history outlines related to the obstruction of the free flow of urine due to any cause and/or infection in any part of the urinary tract. In addition the nurse should investigate:
   A. Onset of symptoms and treatment to date. (Onset is usually manifested by violent chills.)
   B. Presence, location, intensity, quality, and precipitating or aggravating factors of pain. Determine agents and/or factors that aid in analgesia.
   C. Voiding patterns and characteristics of urination—particularly frequency, urgency, nocturia, and burning on urination.
   D. Description and characteristics of urine—particularly malodorous, cloudy, or bloody urine.
III. Physical assessment.
   A. Elevated body temperature.
   B. Tenderness in affected costovertebral angle (may be bilateral).
   C. Enlarged kidney may be palpable (possibly bilaterally).
   D. Slightly rigid abdomen.
   E. Lethargy and malaise.
IV. Diagnostic tests.
   A. Review of diagnostic studies is utilized to rule out obstruction of urine due to any cause and infections of the urinary tract distal to the kidney pelvis.
   B. An IVP will detect dilatations of urinary pelvis.
   C. Cystoscopy is used to view the bladder and related structures.
   D. Renal biopsy.
   E. Microscopic urinalysis is done to isolate organisms involved.

Problems/ Diagnosis

I. Alteration in comfort (flank pain) due to infection of the kiny pelvis.
II. Elevation in body temperature due to infectious process in the kidney pelvis.
III. Alteration in voiding patterns (frequency, nocturia, urgency, and burning on urination) due to infection of the kidney pelvis and/or along the urinary tract.
IV. Mild to moderate anxiety due to alteration in voiding patterns.
V. Possible stasis of urine due to obstruction of the free flow of urine.
VI. Potential damage to renal tissue due to extension of infectious process.
VII. Possible transmission of causative organism due to improper handling of urine.
VIII. Possible recurrence of pyelonephritis due to unidentified causative factors and/or patient's lack of education regarding preventative factors.

Goals of Care

I. Immediate.
   A. Reduce pain and discomfort.
   B. Permanently eradicate existing infection.
   C. Prevent transmission of causative organism.
   D. Relieve obstruction of flow of urine (if present).
   E. Prevent urinary stasis.
   F. Maintain urinary output of at least 1500 mL per 24-h period.

G. Reduce body temperature.

H. Prevent fecal contamination of urinary meatus.

I. Reduce anxiety.

II. Long-range.

A. Prevent permanent renal damage.

B. Prevent recurrence through patient education.

Intervention

I. Institute urine isolation precautions to prevent transmission of infecting organism (not appropriate in all cases). Consult nurse epidemiologist.

II. Administer prescribed analgesics and/or other measures to relieve pain. Back massages helpful.

A. Assess response to pain relief measures.

B. More vigorous nursing/medical measures may be needed.

III. Administer prescribed broad-spectrum antibiotics (determined by urine cultures and antibiotic sensitivities).

IV. Assess urine cultures and antibiotic sensitivities to determine response to chemotherapy. Reculture urine after antibiotics are discontinued and periodically for 1 year after infection.

V. Encourage fluid intake (oral and parenteral) to at least 3000 mL per 24-h period to reduce residual urine and prevent stasis (unless contraindicated).

VI. Monitor and assess correlation of intake and output every 4 h (more frequently if indicated). Urinary output should be maintained at *no less* than 30 to 40 mL/h.

VII. Test urine for specific gravity, protein, pH, and hematuria every 2 h.

VIII. Prevent unnecessary instrumentation of urinary tract.

IX. Observe for signs of obstruction—drainage of urine proximal to obstruction may be necessary. Nephrostomy, ureterostomy, cystostomy, urethral catheterization, or surgery to repair congenital anomalies and defects may be necessary.

A. Ensure unobstructed urine flow through urinary drainage system to prevent reflux and/or stasis.

B. Provide meticulous catheter care. (Refer to "Renal Tumors.")

X. Monitor and assess vital signs especially temperature every 4 h or more frequently as indicated by marked deviation from the norm.

A. Carry out comfort measures during periods of hyperpyrexia (tepid sponge baths, fresh dry linen, and bed clothes, etc.).

B. Administer prescribed medications to reduce temperature.

C. Assess response to interventions.

XI. Encourage strict bed rest during acute phase; however, avoid total immobility to prevent stasis of urine.

XII. Weigh patient daily. (Same scale, same amount of clothes, same time of day, preferably before breakfast and after voiding.)

XIII. Monitor and assess renal function studies and electrolyte determinations especially blood urea nitrogen, sodium, chloride, and serum creatinine.

XIV. Assist patient in determining possible causative factors.

XV. Establish therapeutic nurse-patient relationship that encourages discussion of anxieties and concerns regarding diagnostic testing and treatment regimen.

XVI. Provide environment that fosters maximal self-esteem and self-care activities despite initial restrictions.

XVII. Initiate teaching-learning transaction (include family and/or significant other). (Refer to "Renal Tumors.")

Evaluation

REASSESSMENT: COMPLICATIONS

I. Chronic pyelonephritis—believed to be related to multiple episodes of acute pyelonephritis which cause healing with the formation of large scars, fibrosis, and tubular dilatation characteristic of chronic disease. Generally, the glomeruli are spared injury except in advanced cases.

    A. Assessment.

      1. Most patients have a history of repeated attacks of acute pyelonephritis or chronic bacteriuria.

      2. The patient may complain of dull flank pain (unilateral or bilateral), low-grade fever, fatigue, headache, and anorexia often accompanied by weight loss and lethargy.

      3. Decreased specific gravity of urine (indicative of kidney failure to adequately concentrate urine), polyuria, and excessive thirst may also be noted.

      4. If the problem remains untreated, hyperchloremic acidosis, hyponatremia, and symptoms of uremia may result.

    B. Intervention. Refer to discussion under "Chronic Renal Failure" for nursing interventions that promote psychological adjustment to chronic condition.

II. Bacteremic shock (refer to Chap. 44).

III. Renal failure (refer to "Acute Renal Failure" and "Chronic Renal Failure").

Acute Glomerulonephritis

Definition   *Acute glomerulonephritis* is a disease in which the glomeruli of both kidneys are seriously damaged and partially destroyed by an inflammatory process that originates as an allergic or autoimmune response. This allergic or autoimmune response is stimulated by a beta-hemolytic streptococcus infection which precedes the glomerulonephritis by 2 or 3 weeks. The exact mechanism of this response is not known. The pathology is characterized by diffuse inflammatory changes in glomeruli and an increase in permeability of the systemic capillary bed. All renal tissues are affected to varying degrees, and nephrotic changes result in the formation of increasing amounts of scar tissue, resulting in atrophy and complete destruction of the nephrons.

    Males are more frequently affected than females. This disease most often affects children and young adults.

Assessment   **I.** Data sources (refer to "Renal Tumors").

    II. Health history (refer to "Acute Renal Failure").

      A. History of beta-hemolytic streptococcal infections (particularly of the throat).

      B. Visual disturbances (due to retinal edema), weakness, nausea, anorexia, headaches, and dizziness.

    III. Physical assessment.

      A. Enlarged kidneys palpable.

      B. Periorbital edema and dependent edema.

      C. Papilledema and/or retinal hemorrhage (not always present).

      D. Elevated temperature; elevated arterial blood pressure (renin-angiotensin system may be involved).

      E. Tenderness in costovertebral angles.

    IV. Diagnostic tests.

      A. IVP or retrograde pyelograms.

      B. Appropriate cardiovascular and pulmonary function tests.

      C. Antistreptolysin (ASO) titer and C-reactive protein (CRP)—both elevated during the course of glomerulonephritis.

      D. Blood chemistry determinations, e.g., serum electrolytes.

      E. Renal function studies—elevated blood urea nitrogen and serum creatinine; decreased plasma protein; phenolsulfonphthalein and creatinine clearance test may show decreased excretion in urine specimens.

      F. Hematocrit and hemoglobin—anemia may be present because of hematuria and disturbance of the hemopoietic mechanism.

      G. Microscopic urinalysis—oliguria or anuria; hematuria almost always present; color is smoky brown or mahogany; low specific gravity (1.020 to 1.025); leukocytosis; many casts; large amounts of albumin; pH usually acid).

Problems/
Diagnosis

   I. Disturbance of fluid and electrolyte balance due to damaged renal tissue.
  II. Hypertension due to presence of renal disease.
 III. Fluid and electrolyte alterations (edema, proteinuria, and oliguria) due to malfunctioning glomeruli.
  IV. Moderate to severe anxiety due to extensive treatment plan and medical diagnosis.
   V. See "Renal Failure" for additional nursing diagnoses applicable to the patient with glomerulonephritis.

Goals of Care (See "Acute Renal Failure" and "Chronic Renal Failure")

   I. Immediate.
     A. Diminish rate of nephron destruction.
     B. Preserve renal functioning.
     C. Decrease metabolic demands.
     D. Control hypertension and infection.
     E. Early recognition and treatment of complications.
  II. Long-range.
     A. Restore renal functioning.
     B. Reduce anxiety and apprehension.

Intervention (See "Acute Renal Failure")

     I. Administer prescribed antibiotics.
    II. Provide safe environment. Initiate seizure precautions. (Uremic seizures may develop.)
   III. Provide and encourage total physical and psychological rest. Bed rest essential during acute phase. Activity may increase as renal function improves. Provide reassurance, encouragement, and support. Provide avenue for expression of anxieties.
   IV. Measure and assess vital signs every 4 h.
    V. Measure daily weight and assess water retention.
   VI. Massage skin and change position every hour. Encourage and carry out passive and active range of motion exercises. Assess condition of skin and surface membranes. Oral hygiene essential.
 VII. Administer prescribed diet. Foods high in carbohydrates and fats allowed. Carbohydrates provide energy and reduce catabolism of protein. Diet is usually low in protein (depending on BUN levels) and limited in sodium and potassium. Fluid restriction usually 1200 mL per 24-h period. Initiate teaching.
VIII. Meticulous measurement and assessment of intake and output.
     A. Measure total amount and frequency of voided urine.
     B. Test specific gravity, hematuria, and albumin at each voiding or every 2 h if catheter present.
   IX. Maintain strict aseptic technique.
    X. Initiate teaching-learning transaction (include family and/or significant others) regarding:
     A. Avoiding overexertion and exposure to drafty environment.
     B. Avoiding exposure to any and all acute and chronic infections. If infectious process does develop, prompt attention and treatment necessary.
     C. Prophylactic immunizations to prevent secondary infections.
     D. Early prenatal care (if appropriate).
     E. General health care practices.
   XI. Initiate social service consultation (necessary because of prolonged convalescence). Economic problems frequently develop.
 XII. Initiate referral for follow-up home care.
XIII. Follow-up and evaluation.

Evaluation

REASSESSMENT: COMPLICATIONS
  I. Cerebral edema due to excessive fluid retention (see Chap. 23).
 II. Pulmonary edema due to excessive fluid retention (see Chap. 26).

III. Cardiac failure due to rapid development of arterial hypertension (see Chap. 26). Mercurial diuretics are contraindicated in acute glomerulonephritis.

IV. Nephrotic syndrome (see "Nephrotic Syndrome").

V. Subacute glomerulonephritis. This condition may develop insidiously without dramatic features.

VI. Chronic glomerulonephritis.

INTERVENTION

I. See "Acute Renal Failure."

II. Peritoneal dialysis and hemodialysis may be used (see "Dialysis" under "Chronic Renal Failure").

Tuberculosis of the Urinary Tract

Definition   *Mycobacterium tuberculosis* is the causative organism of tuberculosis of the urinary tract. This disease process (unilateral or bilateral) originates from a pulmonary or gastrointestinal lesion and reaches the kidney via the bloodstream.

Lesions in the renal parenchyma gradually erode into the renal pelvis, and eventually large cavities develop with complete destruction of the kidney. The infection usually descends via the ureters into the bladder, causing symptoms similar to cystitis and urethritis. Development of fibrous tissue and urethral strictures is not uncommon.

Complaints of gross hematuria, frequency, burning on urination, and dull flank pain accompanied by fatigue and gradual weight loss should alert the nurse to suspect tuberculosis. In addition to urine cultures and skin testing to confirm the diagnosis, identification of the primary sources of the disease is vital.

Assessment   Refer to "Cystitis" and to the discussion of tuberculosis in Chap. 27.

Problems/   Refer to "Cystitis" and to the discussion of tuberculosis in Chap. 27.
Diagnosis

Goals of Care   Refer to "Cystitis" and to the discussion of tuberculosis in Chap. 27.

Intervention   I. Administer anti-tuberculosis medications—specifically isoniazid, sodium PAS, and cycloserine. Streptomycin, kanamycin, ethionamide, rifampin, and viomycin may be used if drug resistance or intolerance to previously mentioned medications develops.

II. Initiate precautions to prevent transmission of the organism. Urine precautions. Initiate teaching regarding use of protective devices (condom) during sexual intercourse to prevent transfer of organism. Continue until urine cultures negative.

III. Assist patient in dealing with actual, perceived, or self-imposed social isolation.

IV. Initiate teaching-learning transaction (include family and/or significant others) regarding:

A. Disease process and treatment regimen.

B. General health care measures (adequate rest and avoidance of overexertion).

C. Medications.

D. Importance of routine health care follow-up.

V. Support medical management of primary lesion. Preoperative teaching should be planned as needed.

VI. Initiate referral for occupational therapy, social service, and follow-up home care.

VII. Initiate referral for screening of family members, contacts, etc.

VIII. Follow-up and evaluation.

Evaluation   Continuous reassessment is essential in order to evaluate the patient's long-term compliance with therapy.

Nephrotic Syndrome (Nephrosis)

Definition

Nephrotic syndrome is not an actual disease entity, but rather a group of symptoms that develop along with an increased permeability of the glomerulus to plasma protein. The nephrotic syndrome is frequently found in association with glomerulonephritis, systemic lupus erythematosus, nephrotoxic reactions, pregnancy, and diabetic glomerulosclerosis. The etiology remains obscure in 80 percent of the cases that develop in children. Although the younger age group is more frequently affected, any age group may develop this condition. (Refer to Chap. 18.)

Assessment

I. Data sources (refer to "Renal Tumors").
II. Health history (refer to "Acute Renal Failure" and "Acute Glomerulonephritis").
III. Physical assessment.
   A. Generalized edema—particularly around the eyes, neck, genitalia, and lower extremities. Ascites frequently develops.
   B. Foamy urine; color deeper than usual; oval fat bodies present.
   C. Skin—waxy pallor due to edema.
IV. Diagnostic tests.
   A. Plasma albumin levels [concentration less than 1 g per 100 mL and reversed albumin/globulin (A/G) ratio].
   B. Serum cholesterol—hyperlipidemia.
   C. Electrolyte determinations—particularly hypernatremia.
   D. Renal function studies—elevated BUN, creatinine, etc., reflecting underlying renal pathology).
   E. Renal biopsy to determine potential response to corticosteroids.

Problems/

See "Acute Glomerulonephritis."

Goals of Care

See "Acute Glomerulonephritis."

Intervention

The nursing interventions for a patient with nephrosis are the same as those identified in "Acute Glomerulonephritis" with *one exception,* dietary management. A diet high in protein is indicated because of excessive losses in the urine. In addition, sodium may be only moderately restricted.

Evaluation

See "Acute Glomerulonephritis."

TRAUMA

Trauma to the Kidneys

Definition

The kidneys are afforded a great deal of protection by the rib cage and the heavy muscles that line the back. Trauma to the kidneys may be due to penetrating wounds, crushing injuries, or blunt blows directly to the flank or abdomen. In addition to causing renal damage, these types of trauma usually involve other viscera as well.

Kidney trauma "may be classified as *contusions* (minor bruising of parenchyma and capsule or major bruising with rupture of parenchyma and perirenal hematoma formation), *laceration* (a tear in the renal parenchyma with or without rupture of the drainage system), and *rupture* of vascular pedicle, which is the most serious" (18). Following injury, the presence of a local mass may be due to extravasation of blood and/or urine. There may be leakage of urine from an open wound.

Assessment

    I. Data sources (refer to "Renal Tumors").

    II. Health history (refer to "Renal Tumors").

       A. Identification of circumstances surrounding the injury, what and how it happened, and the anatomical location of the traumatic blow.

       B. Past history of conditions that affected urinary tract.

       C. Voiding patterns and characteristics of urination prior to injury.

       D. Health perception and identification of response patterns to crisis situations.

    III. Physical assessment.

       A. Tenderness and/or pain in affected costovertebral angle and/or abdominal quadrant.

       B. Expanding mass in affected costovertebral angle due to extravasation of blood and/or urine.

    IV. Diagnostic tests (refer to "Renal Tumors").

       A. Radiologic tests of the kidneys, ureter, and bladder.

       B. IVP (absolutely essential).

       C. Renal arteriogram.

       D. Microscopic urinalysis (specifically for hematuria).

       E. Urine culture and antibiotic sensitivities.

       F. Hematocrit and hemoglobin.

       G. Renal function studies.

       H. Blood typing and cross-matching.

    V. Other data sources.

       A. Emergency room records.

       B. Previous available medical records.

Problems/ Diagnosis

    I. Possible undetected extensive renal damage due to traumatic injury.

    II. Possible rupture of liver and/or spleen due to traumatic injury.

    III. Alteration in comfort (flank pain) due to traumatic injury.

    IV. Moderate to severe anxiety of patient, family, and/or significant other due to traumatic injury.

Goals of Care

    I. Immediate.

       A. Early recognition of extension of damage at the site of injury.

       B. Maintain unobstructed flow of urine.

       C. Prevent introduction of organisms into already traumatized urinary tract.

       D. Reduce pain and anxiety.

       E. Prevent hemorrhagic shock.

    II. Long-range.

       A. Return renal function to previous state.

       B. Educate the patient, family, and/or significant others regarding signs that require medical attention.

Intervention

    I. Insertion of indwelling bladder catheter. Prevent unnecessary instrumentation.

       A. Meticulous catheter care (refer to "Renal Tumors").

       B. Provide safe and unobstructed flow of urine.

    II. Test specific gravity of urine at least every 2 h.

    III. Test urine for blood at least every 2 h.

       A. Inspect for presence of clots.

       B. Prevent obstruction of urinary drainage by clots.

    IV. Administer prescribed intravenous fluids and/or blood transfusions.

    V. Administer prescribed diet. (Patient is usually on NPO status until condition stabilizes; then feeding gradually increases according to tolerance.)

    VI. Measure and correlate fluid intake and output every 2 h.

       A. More frequently oliguria and/or gross hematuria develops.

       B. Oral and parenteral intake of fluids should be sufficient to provide internal irrigation but not beyond functional renal capacity.

    VII. Enforce strict bed rest. Take measures to prevent complications of bed rest. Activity increases as condition stabilizes.

  VIII. Administer prescribed prophylactic antibiotics and analgesics. (Narcotics and analgesics may mask abdominal symptoms.)

    IX. Monitor and assess vital signs every hour unless otherwise indicated.

    X. Monitor hematocrit, hemoglobin, and renal function studies every 24 h (more frequently if indicated).

    XI. Assess hematoma and/or mass for any increase in size. Abdominal girths should be checked every 4 h.

   XII. Provide support and reassurance to patient, family, and/or significant others during time of crisis. Assist patient in dealing with possible alteration in body image.

  XIII. Initiate teaching-learning transaction (include family and/or significant others) regarding:
    A. Need for follow-up care.
    B. Signs that require attention of the health care team.
    C. Home care activities, medications, diet, etc.

  XIV. Follow-up and evaluation.

Evaluation **REASSESSMENT: COMPLICATIONS**

    I. Shock due to torn pedicle, extensive intraperitoneal hemorrhage and/or retroperitoneal hemorrhage (see Chap. 44). If hemorrhage cannot be controlled, emergency surgery is indicated. Frequently the kidney can be repaired; however, if the laceration is extensive, a nephrectomy may be necessary.

   II. Perirenal abscess.
    A. Assessment.
      1. A sudden onset of fever, chills, and pain in affected flank.
      2. Palpable tenderness and gradual onset of low-grade fever.
      3. Malaise, anorexia, and gradual weight loss.
      4. Leukocytosis may be present.
    B. Intervention.
      1. Surgical intervention.
        a. Drainage of the abscess.
        b. Removal of the kidney (nephrectomy) if it is not functioning.
      2. Preoperative intervention.
        a. Monitor and assess vital signs everh 2 h (especially temperature).
        b. Administer prescribed analgesics, antibiotics, and antipyretics.
        c. Maintain fluid and electrolyte balance.
        d. Administer prescribed intravenous fluids.
      3. Postoperative intervention—similar to that employed following a lumbar nephrectomy (see "Renal Tumors").
      4. Complications of surgery.
        a. Reflex paralytic ileus due to retroperitoneal hemorrhage.
        b. Traumatic renal failure (see "Acute Renal Failure" and "Chronic Renal Failure").

Trauma to the Urinary Bladder

Definition   *Trauma to the urinary bladder* is most frequently caused by a fracture of the symphysis pubis. A distended bladder may be easily ruptured by blunt trauma, such as a light kick or blow to the lower abdomen. In addition, accidental injuries during surgery and from penetrating missiles may result in a ruptured bladder.

Assessment   **I.** Data sources (refer to "Renal Tumors").

   II. Health history. The health history required of clients with suspected trauma to the bladder is basically the same as in kidney trauma (refer to "Trauma to the Kidneys"). In addition, the time of the last voiding prior to the injury should be ascertained.

III. Physical assessment.
    A. Diffuse abdominal pain on palpation.
    B. Urine draining from an open wound.
    C. Free fluid in peritoneal cavity on palpation.
    D. Abdominal distension; abdominal rigidity may indicate intraperitoneal rupture.
IV. Diagnostic tests.
    A. Cystogram; excretory urogram.
    B. Radiologic tests of the kidneys, ureter, and bladder.
    C. IVP (not the definitive diagnostic study).
    D. Microscopic urinalysis (particularly for hematuria).
    E. Urine culture and antibiotic sensitivities.
    F. Hematocrit and hemoglobin.
    G. Blood typing and cross-matching.

Problems/Diagnosis   See Chap. 44.

Goals of Care   See Chap. 44.

Intervention   See Chap. 44 for nursing care during the acute emergency phase. Surgical intervention is usually immediate.

Evaluation   REASSESSMENT: COMPLICATIONS
    I. Peritonitis (refer to Chap. 29).
    II. Hemorrhage and shock (refer to Chap. 44).

INTERVENTION
Repair of lacerated bladder with or without insertion of suprapubic cystostomy tube (refer to "Benign Prostatic Hypertrophy").

Obstructions

Urethral Stricture

Definition   *Urethral strictures* may be either congenital or acquired. The urethral canal may be obstructed by a flap of mucosal tissue that acts as a valvelike obstruction. The lumen of the urethra may be narrowed by scar tissue formation, which eventually results in contracture.

Urethral strictures frequently develop following the healing of an infectious process or following traumatic instrumentation. Fibrous tissue fills the site of injury or infection, causing gradual reduction in the lumen of the urethra. Males are particularly susceptible following repeated episodes of venereal disease, especially gonorrhea.

Assessment   I. Data sources (refer to "Renal Tumors").
    II. Health history.
        A. Age.
        B. Sex.
        C. Occupation.
        D. Marital status.
        E. Recent history of injury to the urethra, urethral catheterizations, and/or history of urinary tract infections (particularly gonorrhea).
        F. Investigate possible cause of stricture and evaluate severity of obstruction.
        G. Voiding patterns and characteristics of urination (particularly difficulty in starting urinary stream, decreased caliber and force of urinary stream, frequency, and "dribbling" at the end of micturition).
        H. Alterations in body image and/or self-esteem.

      I. Motivation for self-care and adaptability to extended treatment plan.

      J. Perceptions of the patient and family regarding expected outcomes, future decisions, and available support systems and resources.

III. Physical assessment—palpation above the symphysis pubis may reveal distended bladder.

IV. Diagnostic tests.

    A. Urethrogram.

    B. Voiding cystourethrogram.

    C. Cystoscopy (may not be done).

    D. IVP (not always done).

V. Other data sources.

    A. Referral note.

    B. Previous available medical records (past history of urinary tract infections, urethral catheterizations, or trauma to the urethra).

Problems/ Diagnosis

I. Urinary elimination—obstruction of free flow of urine resulting in retention and stasis of urine due to urethral stricture.

II. Mild depression and discouragement due to extensive plan of treatment.

III. Self-concept—altered body image and/or self-esteem due to alteration of voiding patterns and characteristics.

Goals of Care

I. Immediate.

    A. Restore free flow pattern of urine.

    B. Prevent urinary retention and consequently urinary stasis which may result in calculi and infection.

II. Long range.

    A. Restore body image and self-esteem.

    B. Reduce anxiety associated with long-term treatment.

    C. Retain adequate renal functioning.

Interventions

I. Develop therapeutic nurse-patient relationship.

II. Assist in insertion of indwelling urethral catheter or urethral sound.

    A. Maintain adequate and safe outflow of urine through drainage system.

    B. Provide meticulous indwelling catheter care (refer to "Tumors of the Urinary Bladder").

III. Maintain adequate oral fluid intake according to patient tolerance for internal irrigation.

IV. Measure and correlate intake and output of urine every 8 h.

V. Encourage mild to moderate activity to prevent urinary stasis.

VI. Assess for signs and symptoms of complications of urinary retention and/or stasis.

VII. Assess for bladder distension.

VIII. Provide avenue for patient to express concerns and anxieties regarding extensive treatment plan.

IX. Carry out teaching-learning transaction regarding physical and psychological preparation and expectations of treatment plan.

X. Assist patient in dealing with altered body image.

XI. Provide atmosphere that fosters self-care and maximal independence.

XII. Offer support, reassurance, and encouragement. Include family and/or significant others.

XIII. Alert patient that any difficulty in voiding should be reported immediately.

XIV. Follow-up and evaluation.

Evaluation

REASSESSMENT: COMPLICATIONS

I. Acute urinary retention due to obstruction of the urethra by stricture.

    A. Assessment.

        1. Oliguria with accompanying marked bladder distention.

        2. Bladder spasms.

        3. Altered vital signs (especially hypertension).

        4. Diaphoresis.

        5. Moderate to severe anxiety; restlessness.

    B. Intervention.

        1. Medical management.

            a. Types of medical management.

                (1) Dilatation of the urethra with metal instruments (sounds) of increasing size for an indefinite period of time.

                (2) Dilatation of the urethra by insertion of a series of indwelling bladder catheters of increasing size over a period of time.

            b. Nursing intervention.

                (1) Assist with insertion of prescribed indwelling transurethral catheter, sound, or bougie.

                (2) Increase oral intake for internal irrigation.

                (3) Administer prescribed antispasmodics and analgesics.

                (4) Monitor and assess vital signs, especially blood pressure.

                (5) Monitor, assess, and correlate fliid intake and output.

                (6) Offer reassurance and support. Include family and/or significant others if appropriate.

        2. Surgery.

            a. Types of surgical intervention.

                (1) Cystostomy may be done prior to reconstruction to ensure adequate urinary drainage.

                (2) Urethrotomy—incision of the urethral stricture.

                (3) Urethroplasty—reconstructive surgery of the urethra.

            b. Preoperative intervention (refer to "Benign Prostatic Hypertrophy").

            c. Postoperative intervention (refer to "Benign Prostatic Hypertrophy").

II. Urinary tract infection (see "Cystitis").

III. Urinary calculi (see "Nephrolithiasis").

IV. Hydronephrosis and/or hydroureter (see "Hydronephrosis").

V. Renal failure (see "Acute Renal Failure" and "Chronic Renal Failure").

Benign Prostatic Hypertrophy

Definition   *Benign prostatic hypertrophy* is a term utilized to describe the most commonly occurring tumor of the prostate. The incidence of this condition increases with age, and approximately one out of every ten 40-year-old males is affected (19). The etiology remains unknown; however, an endocrine imbalance has been suspected. Since the prostate encircles the urethra directly below the bladder, as the periurethral tissue of the gland hypertrophies, it extends upward into the bladder, forming a reservoir that results in incomplete emptying of the bladder and stasis of urine.

    In addition to tte hyperplastic tissue moving upward, there is an inward compression of the walls of the prostatic urethra that may partially or completely obstruct the flow of urine. Nodules appear under the epithelium of the posterior urethra. The nodules enlarge concentrically, thus compressing the normal prostatic tissue against the prostatic capsule. Since this condition develops slowly, many men attribute the alteration in voiding patterns to advancing age, thus delaying active seeking out of medical attention.

Assessment   **I.** Data sources (refer to "Renal Tumors").

    II. Health history (refer to "Renal Tumors").

        A. Seasonal conditions—acute urinary retention occurs more frequently after exposure to cold.

        B. Nutritional assessment—spicy foods and alcohol may precipitate acute congestion of enlarged lobes.

        C. Time of last voiding.

        D. Voiding patterns and characteristics of urination—difficulty in starting and maintaining urinary stream, diminished caliber and force of stream and "dribbling" of urine after urination, frequency, urgency, nocturia, hematuria, and burning on urination.

    III. Physical assessment.

        A. Enlarged prostate on rectal examination.

        B. Bladder distension due to acute/chronic urinary retention.

    IV. Diagnostic tests.

        A. Cystoscopy and panendoscopy.

        B. IVP (necessary to evaluate structural changes due to enlarged prostate).

        C. Urethrograms (not always done).

        D. Excretory urogram.

        E. Renal function studies.

        F. CBC and electrolyte determinations.

        G. Coagulation studies to rule out potential bleeding tendency.

        H. Microscopic urinalysis (particularly for hematuria).

        I. Urine culture and antibiotic sensitivities.

        J. Blood typing and cross-matching.

        K. Catheterization following voiding to evaluate residual urine.

Problems/Diagnosis

    I. Urinary elimination—acute urinary retention due to obstruction of bladder outlet by enlarged prostate.

    II. Urinary elimination—alteration in voiding patterns (hesitancy, diminished caliber and force of stream, "dribbling" at the end of micturition, frequency, urgency, nocturia, hematuria, and burning on urination) due to obstruction of bladder outlet by enlarged prostate.

    III. Mild to moderate anxiety due to alteration in voiding patterns and diagnostic and/or treatment procedures.

    IV. Alteration in self-esteem (and possibly in body image) due to alteration in voiding patterns and diagnostic and/or treatment procedures.

Goals of Care

    I. Immediate.

        A. Relieve acute irinary retention.

        B. Prevent urinary complications secondary to prolonged obstruction of the free flow of urine.

    II. Long-range.

        A. Reduce anxiety associated with altered voiding patterns and diagnostic and/or treatment procedures.

        B. Restore positive body image and self-esteem.

        C. Maintain optimal renal functioning.

Intervention

    I. Offer reassurance and maintain unhurried atmosphere (patients often are elderly). Assist older patient to adjust to hospital environment.

    II. Maintain matter-of-fact approach.

    III. Assist with insertion of urethral catheter (considered a medical intervention if a catheter with a stylet, a coudé woven catheter, or metal catheter with prostatic curve is utilized). Interval irrigation may be prescribed.

    IV. Assess and maintain patency of catheter and drainage system.

    V. Maintain adequate and safe outflow of urine through drainage system. "Milk" tubing if flow is obstructed. Provide meticulous catheter care.

    VI. Reassess bladder distension.

    VII. Maintain fluid intake between 2500 to 3000 mL per 24-h period (unless contraindicated by coexisting medical diagnosis).

    VIII. Measure and assess fluid intake and output.

    IX. Observe urine for hematuria and blood clots (possibly due to traumatic insertion of urethral catheter).

X. Prevent too rapid emptying of bladder. If residual urine is over 100 mL, it should be removed at a slow rate to prevent shock (approximately 100 mL/h).

XI. Assess renal functioning. Monitor renal function studies.

Evaluation

REASSESSMENT: COMPLICATIONS

I. Bladder diverticula—irregular outpouchings of the bladder wall.

II. Renal and bladder calculi (see "Nephrolithiasis").

III. Cystitis (see "Cystitis").

IV. Hydronephrosis (see "Hydronephrosis").

V. Renal failure (see "Acute Renal Failure" and "Chronic Renal Failure").

VI. Complete urethral obstruction—insertion of urethral catheter may be impossible due to complete obstruction of the urethra. Suprapubic cystostomy necessary.

   A. Assessment.

      1. Marked bladder distension.

      2. Increased suprapubic pain.

      3. Increased blood pressure, pulse, and respirations.

      4. Diaphoresis.

      5. Moderate to severe apprehension.

   B. Intervention.

      1. Medical management.

         a. Urinary antiseptics used concurrently with prostatic massage to relieve congestion of enlarged lobes.

         b. Nursing intervention.

            (1) Offer reassurance and support to patient, family, and/or significant others.

            (2) Monitor and assess vital signs frequently.

            (3) Initiate preoperative preparation and teaching regarding postoperative expectations and activities (include family and significant others).

            (4) Suprapubic cystostomy—surgical incision through the abdominal wall into the bladder is done to drain urine. A suprapubic catheter will probably be left in place to prevent another episode of acute retention.

               (a) When prescribed, clamp catheter for 4 h and unclamp for 15 to 30 min.

               (b) Assess patient's ability to void while catheter is clamped.

               (c) Catheter is removed per physician's orders afterpatient is able to void while suprapubic catheter clamped.

               (d) Once removed, place sterile dressing over suprapubic catheter site.

            (5) Follow-up and reevaluation every 6 months.

      2. Surgery.

         a. Types of surgical intervention.

            (1) Transurethral resection—removal of the prostate with instruments introduced transurethrally. No incision is needed.

            (2) Suprapubic prostatectomy—removal of the hypertrophied prostate gland through an abdominal incision that extends into the bladder.

            (3) Perineal prostatectomy—removal of the prostate through a perineal resection. Postoperative wound contamination, incontinence, and impotence are likely sequelae.

            (4) Retropubic prostatectomy—removal of the prostate gland through an incision between the pubic arch and the bladder. No incision is made into the bladder.

         b. Preoperative intervention.

            (1) Initiate teaching-learning interaction regarding postoperative activities and expectations.

               (a) Avoid attempting to void around catheter.

               (b) Avoid straining when having a bowel movement (may cause prostatic hemorrhage).

(*c*) Perineal exercises to decrease incontinence.

(2) Encourage patient to discuss possibility of impotence with wife and physician. Be supportive during this conference.

(3) Carry out prescribed bowel preparations.

c. Postoperative intervention.

(1) Administer prescribed analgesics and antispasmodics. Wean patient off antispasmodics 24 h before removal of urethral catheter.

(2) Maintain free unobstructed flow of urine. Inspect catheter(s) for signs of obstruction from blood clots and occasionally a piece of tissue. Continuous irrigation frequently ordered. Monitor and assess drainage from wounds and catheter sites.

(3) Observe closely for signs of hemorrhage. Some hematuria expected. Test urine for blood. Measure specific gravity. Monitor and assess vital signs, particularly blood pressure and *oral* temperature.

(4) Maintain strict aseptic technique at all times.

(5) Maintain fluid intake (oral and parenteral) between 2500 and 3500 mL per 24-h period (unless contraindicated by coexisting condition).

(6) Monitor and correlate intake and output every 2 h immediately postoperatively, progressing to every 8 h as condition stabilizes.

(7) Avoid taking rectal temperatures, using rectal tubes, or administering enemas (particularly following perineal resection).

(8) Initiate preventative measures to prevent postoperative complications, i.e., turning every 2 h, passive and active range of motion exercises, early ambulation, and antiembolism stockings. Although coughing is encouraged, *vigorous* coughing should be avoided.

(9) Review preoperative teaching plan, particularly review of perineal exercises and instructions not to attempt to void around catheter. Perineal exercises should be started two to three days postoperatively.

(10) Seek order for laxative or stool softener 3 to 4 days postoperatively.

(11) Provide nutritional information to avoid constipation postdischarge.

(12) Instruct patient to avoid vigorous exercises and heavy lifting for at least 3 weeks postoperatively. Instruct patient:

(*a*) That any sign of bleeding should be reported to member of the health care team immediately (physician or nurse).

(*b*) About signs of developing urethral strictures and infection.

(*c*) That abstinence from sexual activity for at least 4 weeks is essential.

(*d*) That high oral fluid intake is to be continued following discharge.

(13) Initiate referral for vocational and sexual counseling. (Postoperative incontinence may be a problem; impotence may create marital discord.)

(14) Reassure, encourage, support patient, family, and/or significant others. Depression common because of inability to regain bladder control immediately. Encourage diversional activity. Elicit assistance from the family.

(15) Follow-up and reevaluation.

d. Complications of surgery.

(1) Hemorrhage.

(*a*) In addition to interventions listed (refer to "Renal Tumors"), the *physician* may apply gentle traction on the urethral catheter to provide pressure on the prostatic arteries.

(*b*) Nursing responsibilities are to maintain the amount of traction, continue to assess for signs of hemorrhage, and assess response to interventions.

(2) Water intoxication. Because of the large amounts of irrigating fluid utilized during a transurethral resection, the patient may develop water intoxication, which is manifested by hyponatremia and/or circulatory overload.

          (*a*) Assessment.
              (i) Extreme irritability progressing to coma if undetected.
              (ii) Hypertension followed by hypotension.
              (iii) Decreased sodium.
              (iv) Polyuria.
          (*b*) Intervention.
              (i) Administer prescribed sodium replacements.
              (ii) Assess vital signs.
              (iii) Observe for pulmonary edema and cardiac failure.
              (iv) Monitor and assess fluid intake and output.
      (3) Obstruction in lower urinary tract (see "Urethral Stricture").
      (4) Cystitis (see "Cystitis").
      (5) Pyelonephritis (see "Pyelonephritis").
      (6) Renal failure (see "Acute Renal Failure" and "Chronic Renal Failure").

Nephrolithiasis

Definition

Urinary calculi may develop in the kidney, ureter, bladder, or urethra and may be multiple and bilateral. Ninety percent of urinary calculi are composed of calcium salts, while nearly all the rest are urate stones. *Cystine stones* develop in patients with a rare hereditary metabolic disorder. Like uric acid stones, they develop in an acidic environment. Infection, urinary stasis, and high urinary concentration predisposes to precipitation of the urinary salts. Middle-aged individuals and males have a higher incidence.

    Calcium stone formation can be caused by hyperparathyroidism (this causes excretion of calcium), excessive ingestion of vitamin D, Cushing's syndrome, acute osteoporosis due to immobilization, or acute renal tubular acidosis. Alkaline urine causes calcium to come out of solution and crystallize.

    Uric acid stones are formed only in an acidic urine (pH of less than 5.5). Increased excretion of uric acid due to gout or a persistently acidic urine result in the formation of uric acid stones.

    The size of calculi varies from small sandy particles (gravel) to large staghorn stones that may occupy the entire renal pelvis. *Silent calculi* are large stones that remain in the renal pelvis and produce no symptoms (see Fig. 28-6). These stones may remain in the kidney pelvis (usually the large ones) or they pass down through the ureters into the bladder and eventually are excreted through the urethra. *Renal colic* may develop if urinary calculi are unable to pass through the narrow lumen of the ureters.

Assessment

  I. Data sources (refer to "Renal Tumors").
 II. Health history (refer to "Renal Tumors").
    A. Race—blacks are affected less frequently than other races.
    B. Geographical residential area—southeastern, southwestern, and the Great Lakes region of the United States are considered the "stone belt."
    C. Family history—cystine stones are of genetic etiology.
    D. Past history of any condition predisposing to stasis of urine (extended periods of immobilization, infections, etc.).
    E. Comprehensive nutritional assessment.
    F. Past history of urinary calculi, method of treatment, etc.
    G. Voiding patterns and characteristics of urination (particularly frequency, urgency, hematuria, and intermittent stream).
    H. Presence, location, frequency, intensity, quality, and precipitating or aggravating factors that aid in relief of pain.
    I. Health perception and identification of response patterns to crisis situation.

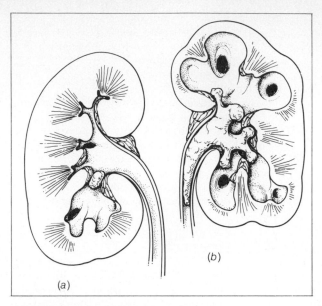

FIGURE 28-6 / (a) Single calculus obstructing and dilating the lower renal calyx. (b) "Staghorn" calculus obstructing and dilating all the renal calyces. [Adapted from R. H. Flocks, "Urology," in R. D. Liechty and R. T. Soper (eds.), Synopsis of Surgery, 2d ed., The C.V. Mosby Company, St. Louis, 1972.]

III. Physical assessment.
  A. Sharp excruciating pain radiating from affected flank toward groin and testes or labia.
  B. Tenderness over involved kidney and ureter on palpation.
IV. Diagnostic tests.
  A. Microscopic urinalysis—particularly interested in albuminuria, pH, and hematuria.
    1. Alkaline urine associated with stones of calcium slats.
    2. Acidic urine associated with uric acid and cystine stones.
  B. Urine culture and antibiotic sensitivity.
  C. Sulkowitch test for calcium (positive).
  D. Twenty-four hour urine specimen for calcium and uric acid.
  E. Blood studies—serum calcium, serum phosphorus, and serum uric acid.
  F. Renal function tests—blood urea nitrogen, creatinine, and creatinine clearance.
  G. Radiologic studies—IVP, cystogram, KUB, cystoscopy with retrograde pyelography (uric acid stones not radiopaque).
V. Other data sources.
  A. Referral note.
  B. Previous available medical records—past history of urinary calculi, method of treatment, and chemical analysis of stone.

Problems/
Diagnosis

I. Obstruction of the free flow of urine due to presence of urinary calculi.
II. Alteration in comfort (severe pain) due to urinary calculi causing obstruction of free flow of urine.
III. Moderate to severe anxiety associated with severe pain and alteration in voiding patterns.
IV. Potential urinary tract infection due to stasis of urine.
V. Potential destruction of renal tissue due to obstruction of free flow of urine.
VI. Altered body image and/or self-esteem due to response to acute severe pain and alterations in voiding patterns.

Goals of Care

I. Immediate.
   A. Relief of obstruction of urinary flow.
   B. Relief of pain and reduce anxiety.
   C. Symptomatic relief of urinary colic.
   D. Control of urinary tract infection (prevent if possible).
   E. Preserve renal function.
   F. Restore positive body image and self-esteem.
II. Long-range.
   A. Identify cause of stone formation.
   B. Prevent further stone formation.

Intervention

I. Develop therapeutic nurse-patient relationship.
II. Reassure and support patient, family, and/or significant others.
III. Provide avenue for patient to verbalize concerns and anxieties regarding his or her reaction to severe pain.
IV. Assist patient in dealing with altered body image and self-esteem.
V. Observe for spontaneous passage of stone. Strain all urine at each voiding. Remain with the patient as long as needed.
VI. Observe urine for hematuria. Measure specific gravity at each voiding to assess renal function.
VII. Monitor and assess vital signs (particularly temperature) every 4 h.
VIII. Observe for signs and symptoms of urinary complications resulting from retention and/or stasis.
IX. Initiate pain relief measures, e.g., analgesics, antispasmodics, moist heat, and sitz bath.
X. Insert prescribed indwelling bladder catheter.
XI. Increase fluid intake to 3000 mL per 24-h period (unless contraindicated by coexisting condition). Calculi re-formers should have fluid intake around the clock.
XII. Monitor and assess intake and output every 8 h (more frequently if necessary).
XIII. Encourage moderate activity to prevent stasis of urine.
XIV. Monitor and assess renal function studies.
XV. Nutritional counseling. See Table 28-1 for specific information.

TABLE 28-1 / DIETARY MANAGEMENT FOR NEPHROLITHIASIS

Type of Stone	Dietary Management	pH Maintenance
Calcium oxalate stones	Avoid excessive consumption of dairy products, green leafy vegetables, Vitamin D. Increase water intake.	Form in any urine pH.
Calcium phosphate stones	Same as above. Also avoid poultry, fish, nuts, whole grain cereals.	Form in any urine pH.
Uric acid stones	Avoid milk; fruits except cranberries, plums and prunes; vegetables, especially legumes and green vegetables. Increase fluid intake.	Maintain alkaline urine. pH = 7.0–7.5.
Cystine stones	Increase water intake. Restrict intake of methionine, an essential amino acid. Limit amount of dairy products, eggs, poultry, fish, and nuts.	Maintain alkaline urine. pH = 7.0–7.5.

Evaluation

REASSESSMENT: COMPLICATIONS
    I. Infection in any structure proximal to the calculi (see "Inflammatory Disorders").
    II. Hydronephrosis (see "Hydronephrosis").
    III. Renal failure (see "Acute Renal Failure" and "Chronic Renal Failure").
    IV. Acute ureteral colic.

INTERVENTION
If the patient is unable to spontaneously pass the stone the following medical interventions may be employed. Medical treatment is dependent upon the position, location, and size of the stone. Of course, the patient's general condition and coexisting conditions must also be considered.
    I. Types of surgical intervention.
        A. Ureteral catheter into renal pelvis by cystoscopy.
        B. Cystolithectomy—removal of stone from the bladder.
        C. Ureterolithotomy—removal of a stone that is lodged in the ureter.
        D. Pyelolithotomy—removal of a stone lodged in the kidney pelvis.
        E. Nephrolithotomy—removal of a stone from the kidney through an incision into the kidney.
        F. Litholapaxy—crushing of a stone in the bladder followed by immediate washing out of the crushed fragments through a catheter (see Fig. 28-7).
        G. Nephrectomy may be necessary if kidney is functionless. (See "Renal Tumors" for preoperative and postoperative intervention.)

FIGURE 28-7 / **Litholapaxy: removal of stone by crushing forceps. [*Adapted from R. D. Liechty and R. T. Soper (eds.), Synopsis of Surgery, 2d ed., The C.V. Mosby Company, St. Louis, 1972.*]**

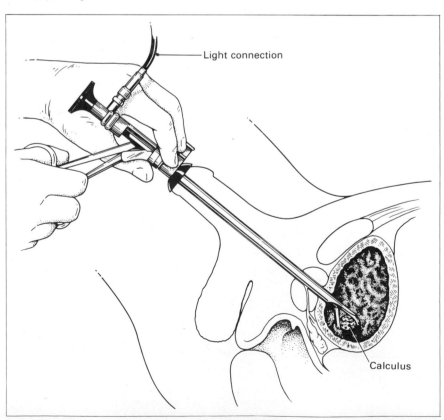

Light connection

Calculus

II. Preoperative intervention (see "Renal Tumors").
III. Postoperative intervention.
    A. Following ureteral surgery. The nursing care of a patient following ureteral surgery is similar to that of any patient who has undergone abdominal surgery under general anesthesia. (Review medical-surgical nursing text.) In addition, the following nursing measures should be considered.
        1. Offer reassurance, support, and understanding. The abdominal incision will drain urine for approximately 3 weeks.
        2. Prevent dressing from being constantly wet with urinary drainage. Initiate appropriate measures.
        3. Initiate meticulous care of the skin utilizing protective powders, ointments, etc. (See discussion on urinary diversion under "Tumors of the Urinary Bladder.")
        4. Encourage free fluid intake to decrease urine concentration.
        5. Maintain odorless environment.
        6. Observe incision for signs of infection.
        7. Maintain patency of ureteral catheter for adequate drainage. Intermittent irrigation may be necessary. Check physician's orders. (Note: The kidney pelvis normally holds between 3 and 5 mL of fluid; therefore, extreme care should be utilized in irrigating ureteral catheters.)
    B. Following flank (kidney) incision.
        1. Assess for alterations in vital signs.
        2. Meticulous measurement and correlation of fluid intake and output every 2 h. Assess color of urine. Observe for clots. Meticulous catheter care. Intake 3000 mL per 24 h.
        3. Assess dressing for serosanguineous drainage.
        4. Maintain fluid and electrolyte balance.
            a. Administer prescribed intravenous fluids.
            b. Monitor and assess blood electrolytes.
        5. Provide vigorous respiratory care, including deep breathing, coughing, and turning every 2 h. Splint the operative area. (Incision is directly below the diaphragm.) Oral hygiene as needed.
        6. Assess response to interventions. Respiratory therapy consultation may be necessary.
        7. Administer prescribed narcotic analgesics; utilize back massage as pain relief measure. Assess response to interventions.
        8. Encourage early mobility; perform passive and active range of motion exercises. Ambulation started 24 h postoperatively. Utilize elastic knee-length stockings.
        9. Discourage sitting in chair for long periods.
      10. Assess for signs of infection and administer prescribed antibiotics to prevent infection.
      11. Provide nephrostomy tube care (see Fig. 28-8).
            a. Maintain adequate drainage of urine.
            b. Ensure patency of nephrostomy tube.
            c. When positioning patient, support nephrostomy tube with pillows, etc., to prevent kinking of tubing.
      12. Initiate teaching-learning transaction (include patient, family, and/or significant others) regarding:
            a. Medications, especially name, dosage, rationale, desired effects, side effects, and signs of toxicity.
            b. Nutritional counseling (adjust to culture and food preferences). Also depends on chemical analysis of stone.
            c. Continued intake of large amounts of fluids (2500 to 3000 mL per 24 h) unless contraindicated by coexisting condition.
            d. Prevention of urinary tract infection. Detection of signs of urinary tract infections and appropriate responses.
            e. Avoidance of long periods of immobilization.

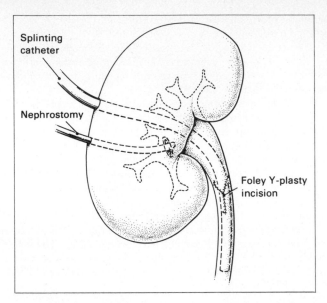

FIGURE 28-8 / Schematic representation showing the placement of a nephrostomy tube. The nephrostomy tube is used to drain urine while the splinting catheter is used to support the Y incision. (*Adapted from K. N. Shafer, J. B. Sawyer, A. M. McCluskey, E. L. Beck, and W. J. Phipps, Medical-Surgical Nursing, 6th ed., The C.V. Mosby Company, St. Louis, 1975.*)

        f. Possible vocational counseling if present occupation predisposes patient to dehydration through excessive perspiration.
    13. Initiate referral for follow-up care.
    14. Follow-up and reevaluation.
IV. Complications of surgery.
    A. Reflex paralytic ileus.
    B. Hemorrhage.
    C. Pyelonephritis (see "Pyelonephritis").
    D. Septic shock (see Chap. 44).

Hydronephrosis

Definition

Hydronephrosis is the distension of the pelvis of the kidney (may be bilateral) and its calyces beyond their normal capacity of 3 to 10 mL. Hydronephrosis is caused by a gradual, partial, or intermittent obstruction of the free flow of urine. As discussed earlier, any interference with the flow of urine (stasis) can result in infection that may produce narrowing and further obstruction. If obstruction is intermittent but frequent, there may be an increase in pressure and the renal parenchyma begin to atrophy in a retrograde manner. The collecting tubules dilate and atrophy. Fibrous tissue replaces the dilated, muscular wall of the kidney pelvis. If the obstruction is located in the bladder or urethra, hydronephrosis may develop bilaterally; however, if the obstruction is in the ureter, hydronephrosis may develop in the related kidney.

Problems/
Diagnosis

I. Urinary stasis due to obstruction of the free flow of urine.
II. Potential development of infection due to stasis of urine.
III. Decreased renal function due to obstruction of the free flow of urine.

Intervention

I. Support medical interventions to identify and relieve underlying cause of urinary stasis.
   A. Initiate care of nephrostomy tube—may be inserted to drain the kidney pelvis when high ureteral obstruction present (only a temporary measure). (See Fig. 28-8.)
      1. Assess for bleeding or drainage from cutaneous nephrostomy site.
      2. Because of the limited fluid capacity of the kidney pelvis, *never* clamp the nephrostomy tube.
      3. Exercise extreme caution when performing *prescribed* irrigations. (Must be done gently. Follow policies of individual institution. May be considered a medical intervention.)
   B. Initiate care for ureteral catheter—inserted if nephrostomy tube insertion contraindicated. Exercise extreme caution to prevent dislodging. Label the catheter as *ureteral*. (Catheter will exit the body through the urinary meatus.) Tape catheter to the shaved thigh. (Note: Irrigation of ureteral catheter is not considered a nursing function.)
II. Refer to appropriate sections in this chapter for nursing interventions regarding specific causes of obstruction.
III. See "Pyelonephritis," which may develop as a result of obstruction and the subsequent stasis of urine.
IV. Initiate preoperative interventions. (Surgery may be indicated if conservative management cannot relieve the underlying cause of obstruction.)
V. See "Acute Renal Failure," which may develop if obstruction is of acute onset with sudden cessation of renal function.

REFERENCES

1. Sylvia Whitehead, *Nursing Care of the Adult Urology Patient,* Appleton-Century-Crofts, New York, 1970, p. 223.
2. Chester C. Winter and Alice Morel, *Nursing Care of Patients with Urologic Diseases,* 4th ed., The C.V. Mosby Company, St. Louis, 1977, p. 310.
3. Dorothy J. Brundage, *Nursing Management of Renal Problems,* The C.V. Mosby Company, St. Louis, 1976, p. 15.
4. Ibid.
5. Lillian Sholtis Brunner and Doris Smith Suddarth: *The Lippincott Manual of Nursing Practice,* J.B. Lippincott Company, Philadelphia, 1974, p. 473.
6. Joan DeLong Harrington and Etta Rae Brener, *Patient Care in Renal Failure,* W.B. Saunders Company, Philadelphia, 1973, pp. 53–54.
7. Ibid.
8. Ibid.
9. Ibid., p. 54.
10. Brunner et al., op cit., p. 476.
11. Brundage, op cit., pp. 77–78.
12. Ibid., p. 111.
13. Ibid., p. 83.
14. Winter and Morel, op. cit., p. 245.
15. Brunner et al. op cit., p. 507.
16. Evelyn R. Anderson, "Women and Cystitis," *Nursing '77,* **7:**50–53, April 1977.
17. Chester S. Keefer, and Robert W. Wilkins (eds.), *Medicine: Essentials of Clinical Practice,* Little, Brown and Company, Boston, 1970, p. 810.
18. George L. Nardi and George D. Zuidema (eds.), *Surgery: A Concise Guide to Clinical Practice,* Little, Brown and Company, Boston, 1972, p. 881.
19. Joan Luckmann and Karen Sorensen, *Medical-Surgical Nursing: A Psychophysiologic Approach,* W.B. Saunders Company, Philadelphia, 1974, p. 1394.

BIBLIOGRAPHY

Brundage, Dorothy J.: *Nursing Management of Renal Problems,* The C.V. Mosby Company, St. Louis, 1976. Renal failure is the major problem that this book addresses. Entire sections are devoted to exploring the numerous causes of renal failure, acute and chronic. Dialysis and transplantation are discussed in some detail with an equal distribution of emphasis on physical and psychological needs. Concrete and practical suggestions are given for comprehensive nursing management of a patient with renal failure. Excellent reference for comprehensive understanding of renal failure.

Cameron, Stewart, Alison Russell, and Diana Sale: *Nephrology for Nurses,* Medical Examination Publishing Co., Inc., Flushing, N.Y., 1976. This book can serve as a good reference for the basic pathophysiology of renal diseases. Dialysis, transplantation, and dietary management of renal disease are covered extensively. Pharmacological agents are discussed only briefly. Social and ethical problems are discussed in relation to dialysis and transplantation.

Hansen, Ginny L. (ed.): *Caring for Patients with Chronic Renal Disease: A Reference Guide for Nurses,* Rochester Regional Medical Program and University of Rochester Medical Center, Rochester, N.Y., 1972. Detailed and comprehensive coverage of the management of the patient with chronic renal failure is the emphasis of the publication. Dietary management, dialysis, and related nursing care, including a teaching plan for home dialysis are included. Tables provide the reader with patient assessment tools that can be used at various stages in the treatment program. Information about renal transplantation is not included in this book.

Harrington, Joan DeLong, and Etta Brener: *Patient Care in Renal Failure,* W.B. Saunders Company, Philadelphia, 1973. This publication can provide any level reader with clear, comprehensive and practical information related to the clinical care of patients with renal failure. Basic anatomy, physiology, and pathophysiology are included in the introductory chapters. The conservative treatment of renal disease, peritoneal dialysis, hemodialysis, and renal transplantation are the major sections of the book. Practical and concrete suggestions for nursing care are provided for "routine" and complex patient situations with emphasis on the application of physiological principles.

Metheny, Norma, and W.D. Sively, Jr.: *Nurses' Handbook of Fluid Balance,* 2d ed., J.B. Lippincott Company, Philadelphia, 1974. This book is included in the bibliography because it provides information about fluid and electrolyte balances and imbalances in numerous patient conditions. In addition to being helpful to the beginner, this book can provide the experienced nurse practitioner with information that can be applied to complex patient situations.

Sachs, Bonnie: *Renal Transplantation: A Nursing Perspctive,* Medical Examination Publishing Company, Inc., Flushing, New York, 1977. This publication provides comprehensive yet basic information regarding all aspects of nursing care through each phase of transplantation. One of the most positive aspects of this book is the chapter on the multidisciplinary approach to patient care, complete with case studies. The appendix provides the reader with a teaching guide that can be adapted to various situations.

Whitehead, Sylvia: *Nursing Care of the Adult Urology Patient,* Appleton-Century-Crofts, New York, 1970. Nursing care of the patient with various dysfunctions of the genitourinary system is addressed. Particular emphasis is paid to infectious processes, calculi, benign prostatic hypertrophy, and neoplastic processes in the prostate, testicles, kidneys, and bladder. This book also includes a section on tuberculosis of the kidney, urologic equipment, and basic anatomy and physiology.

Winter, Chester C., and Alice Morel: *Nursing Care of Patients with Urologic Diseases* 4th ed., The C.V. Mosby Company, St. Louis, 1977. This book concerns itself more with genitourinary problems than with renal problems. Although major renal dysfunctions are briefly addressed, the strength of the book lies in the presentation of basic nursing considerations of genitourinary problems. A review of urinary and renal diagnostic studies, urologic equipment, and its care, and a consideration of basic anatomy and physiology is included.

29

The Gastrointestinal System

Mary Marmoll Jirovec

Effective functioning of the body's gastrointestinal components is essential for adequate body metabolism. Disruptions in such components as ingestion, digestion, absorption, and elimination can alter gastrointestinal function and contribute to a variety of health problems. The following chapter will focus upon concept areas as outlined in the introduction to Part 4 and will discuss major and minor health problems related to each area in terms of nursing assessment, diagnosis, intervention, and evaliation and revision of care.

ABNORMAL CELLULAR GROWTH

Oral Cancer

Definition
Of all human cancer, 5 percent occurs in the oral cavity, and 90 to 95 percent of this is squamous cell (epidermoid) carcinoma (1). Extraoral cancer usually occurs on the lower lip and is thought to be related to exposure to intense sunlight. The tongue is the most common site for intraoral cancer, followed by the gingiva, floor of the mouth, buccal mucosa, and soft and hard palates. Intraoral cancer is often associated with the use of tobacco or snuff, poor oral hygiene with bacterial irritation, syphilitic glossitis, excessive alcohol ingestion, and leukoplakia. The prognosis for oral cancer is generally good if detected early. The speed of metastasis varies with the type and location of the lesion. Oral cancers usually spread by direct invasion, with the submaxillary and cervical lymph nodes the first to become involved.

Assessment
The nursing assessment findings will vary according to the location of the oral cancer.
  I. Data sources.
   A. Patient.   **C.** Previous medical records.
   B. Family.   **D.** Significant others.
  II. Health history. During the health history the patient may complain of a roughened area or area of overgrowth or ulceration. The lesions are often painless although local tenderness may be present. The patient may have also noted swelling, numbness, or a loss of feeling in part of the mouth.
   A. Cancer of the *tongue* usually begins with an area of hyperkeratosis which progresses to an ulcerated lesion. When the posterior half of the tongue is involved, the patient may experience dysphagia and pain on swallowing, halitosis, and weight loss. As the cancer invades muscle, the pain increases; there are soreness, when hot or seasoned foods are eaten, and limited tongue motion. If untreated, neighboring structures become invaded and the patient will salivate more, speech will become slurred, and the sputum may be blood-tinged. Extensive invasion can result in trismus (tonic contraction of the muscles used for mastication), the inability to swallow, and constant pain in the ears, face, and teeth.
   B. Patients with *gingival* cancer often describe a mass or slight tenderness with loose teeth. With more extensive involvement, the lesion may ulcerate and bleed, mastication may be affected, and the mandibular nerve may become involved.
   C. The initial complaints of a patient with cancer in the *floor of the mouth* are minimal. As the lesion spreads, however, the patient experiences pain, difficulty eating and speaking, and a swollen tongue.
   D. Cancer of the *buccal mucosa* usually begins with an ulcer and spreads locally.
   E. When the lesion is in the *hard palate,* the patient often notes a painless mass which becomes tender with time.
   F. *Soft palate* lesions most frequently result in pain and dysphagia.

III. Physical assessment. In the case of the patient with oral cancer, the physical assessment must focus on the entire patient as well as the oral cavity itself. There are several major physical changes that can be noted. These include assessment of the following.

A. The patient's overall appearance, body build, and weight should be determined. A patient with long-standing cancer often appears wasted with a significant weight loss noted when compared to a previous weight record.

B. All structures in the oral cavity should be examined. A tongue blade and flashlight should be used to adequately visualize the structures.

1. All surfaces should be examined for any roughness, white, patchy areas, abnormally pigmented areas, redness, or ulcerations. Any lesion that has not healed in 3 weeks should be suspect. Lesions may appear as small swellings, ulcerated areas (Fig. 29-1), or overgrowths (Fig. 29-2).

2. Oral structures should be examined for symmetry. Any swelling should be palpated and tenderness noted.

3. The teeth should be palpated to detect any looseness.

4. The patient's ability to speak and swallow should also be noted.

5. Surfaces in the oral cavity should be evaluated for loss of sensation by lightly touching areas bilaterally with the tongue blade.

C. The lymph nodes in the head and neck should be carefully palpated to determine the extent of any metastatic spread.

IV. Diagnostic tests. To confirm a diagnosis of oral cancer, all diagnostic tests involved include examination of the oral tissues. These tests involve the use of dyes, biopsy, and scrapings of tissue.

A. If a lesion is suspected but only a reddened area is noted, a *dye* such as toluidine blue can be applied to the area to enhance visualization of the lesion.

B. The cells of a lesion can be examined through *exfoliative cytology* by scraping cells from the lesion with a spatula and spreading them on a slide.

FIGURE 29-1 / Squamous carcinoma of the lateral border of the middle third of the tongue. The lesion is deeply invasive and much larger than the area of ulceration would indicate. The curled, raised border is characteristic. (*From S. I. Schwartz et al., Principles of Surgery, McGraw-Hill Book Company, New York, 1974.*)

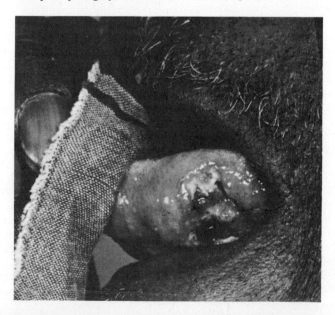

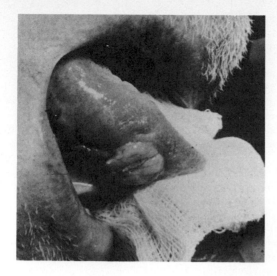

FIGURE 29-2 / Squamous carcinoma of the tip of the tongue. An exophytic, fairly superficial lesion which histologically shows a well-differentiated structure. The prognosis for such a lesion is excellent. (*From S. I. Schwartz et al., Principles of Surgery, McGraw-Hill Book Company, New York, 1974.*)

C. A definitive diagnosis is made by *biopsy*. This can usually be easily accomplished on an outpatient basis. The area is cleansed with an antiseptic that contains a small amount of local anesthesia. A small piece of tissue is then removed using a skin punch. Bleeding can be controlled with local pressure for a short period following the biopsy. Any ulcer, sore area, or white patchy spot in the mouth that has not healed in 2 to 3 weeks should be biopsied.

Problems   Nursing problems may vary depending on the extent and location of the lesion. Frequently, patients with oral lesions may experience one or more of the following problems.

   I. Pain.
  II. Halitosis.
 III. Dysphagia.
 IV. Excess salivation and drooling.
  V. Difficulty chewing.
 VI. Difficulty speaking.
VII. Anxiety.

Diagnosis   Nursing diagnosis is made on the basis of individual problems. Thy can include the following.

   I. Pain may be experienced in the area of the lesion or surrounding tissue. The pain will worsen secondarily to extended involvement of the ears, face, or teeth.
  II. Complaints of mouth odors noticed by self and others as a result of tissue degeneration.
 III. Increased salivation, and drooling secondary to difficulty in swallowing and possible increase in saliva or exudate.
 IV. Difficulty chewing foods due to lesion or pain.
  V. Difficulty speaking due to slurring of speech caused by abnormal growth.
 VI. Patient is anxious and concerned with fears of cancer and death, changes in body image due to surgery, and prolonged illness interfering with family and work responsibilities.
VII. Patient is embarrassed due to continuous breath odor, drooling, or speech changes.

Goals of Care   I. Immediate.
    A. Maintain patent airways (immediate priority).
    B. Control the pain.

    C. Eliminate mouth odors.
    D. Promote adequate nutrition.
    E. Prevent aspiration.
    F. Foster communication with family and others.
    G. Arrest the abnormal cellular growth.
II. Long-range.
    A. Promote adequate nutrition and maintenance of normal body weight.
    B. Prevent reoccurrence of abnormal growth.
    C. Foster a positive self-image, and encourage patient to function up to optimal level.
    D. Promote family involvement in the patient's adjustment.

Intervention

I. Surgical intervention. The most common treatment for oral cancer is surgery, involving excision of the cancerous area and radical neck dissection, if necessary. The excision will often include wide resection. Radiation may also be used with some types of cancer, either alone or in combination with surgery.
    A. *Glossectomy* (*hemiglossectomy*)—removal of all (part) of the tongue.
    B. *Mandibulectomy*—removal of part of the mandible.

II. Preoperative intervention. Before surgery, nursing procedures are planned to alleviate problems most disturbing to the individual.
    A. Pain can generally be controlled with medication.
    B. To control halitosis, frequent mouthwashes with oxidizing agents such as potassium permanganate (1:10,000) or half-strength hydrogen peroxide should be used. Oral lavages and power sprays aid in cleaning lesions and removing necrotic tissue. If the patient is a mouth breather, glycerine, mineral oil with lemon juice, or milk of magnesia swabs are helpful. The room should be well ventilated.
    C. Patients with dysphagia should be watched closely when eating and drinking to prevent aspiration. The diet should be bland and in soft or liquid form. A teaspoon or straw may be helpful in taking only small amounts. Suction equipment should be kept at the bedside. Use of local anesthetics should be used with caution to avoid disrupting the function of the gag reflex.
    D. Patients who salivate excessively may need frequent suctioning. The patient should be positioned to prevent aspiration. A wick with one end placed in the mouth and the other in a basin is often helpful (refer to Chap. 27 for discussion of suctioning).
    E. Patients should be given an opportunity to ventilate fears, ask questions, and interact with others. Questions should be answered honestly without destroying all hope. Referrals for counseling should be made as appropriate. The family should be supported in interacting with the patient. Social services should be contacted to assist with economic difficulties.

III. Postoperative intervention.
    A. The patient should be positioned to *prevent aspiration* and maintain a *patent airway.*
        1. The patient should be kept prone, lateral, or supine with the head turned.
        2. Often a tracheostomy will be performed because postoperative edema can interfere with respirations (refer to Chap. 27).
        3. Oral suctioning should be done gently to prevent trauma to the suture line.
    B. *Pain* is usually controlled with analgesics. Mild sedation may be used to reduce anxiety.
    C. Initially, the patient will be unable to take anything orally, and *nutritional needs* will be met through intravenous and nasogastric fluids. Depending on the extent of the surgery, a gastrostomy tube may be used. As healing occurs, oral fluids will be reinstituted.
    D. *Oral hygiene* must be performed meticulously and frequently to prevent infection and promote comfort. Gentle lavage with a power spray or mouth irrigations using normal saline, diluted hydrogen peroxide, a weak sodium bicarbonate solution, or an alkaline mouthwash is helpful. Occasionally, an antibiotic solution may be used.
    E. *Speech* will often be temporarily or permanently affected. A means of communicating

with the patient after surgery should be planned preoperatively. Long-term speech rehabilitation may necessitate speech therapy and/or a prosthesis.

F. Patients must deal with an *altered body image.* The patient may be disfigured or have difficulty communicating. Social interaction should be encouraged and the family helped to adjust to the change. Fear, anger, and grief are normal reactions the patient should be helped to deal with.

G. A teaching plan should be instituted to ensure the patient's knowledge and understanding of any special mouth care, nutritional needs, and the avoidance of infection. Special equipment may be needed for home suctioning. The patient or a family member should be taught the proper use and technique. The importance of avoiding the use of tobacco, snuff, or alcohol should be impressed upon the patient.

Evaluation

I. Reassessment.

   A. Reassessment of the patient following oral surgery should focus on any reoccurrence or metastases as well as the patient's adjustment to the physical changes.

   B. The patient's self-care ability and level of nutrition should be determined. If problems are identified, a new teaching plan should be instituted.

   C. The patient's and family's psychological adjustment should also be assessed, and individual, family, or group counseling instituted, if necessary.

   D. Any speech problems not being dealt with should be referred to the proper resource person, such as a speech therapist or a dentist.

II. Complications. Hemorrhage may occur during the postoperative period (up to several days). Observations of frank bleeding as well as continuous swallowing may suggest active bleeding. Local pressure should be applied, blood loss assessed, and the patient returned to surgery.

III. Regular follow-up care is essential to detecting reoccurrence or metastases. The importance of frequent visits, especially in the first 2 years, should be emphasized.

Leukoplakia

Definition

Leukoplakia is the most common precancerous lesion. It can occur anywhere in the mouth or on the lips and is found most frequently in men over 40 years of age. In fair-skinned individuals, it often occurs on the lip. It appears to be a reaction to long-term chemical, thermal, or physical irritation and has been associated with heavy smoking, tobacco chewing, and ill-fitting dentures. It consists of a painless, dry, inflamed area that is usually white or blue. The plaque is slightly raised and irregular, with sharp borders. After many years leukoplakia can hypertrophy or degenerate into fissures or ulcers.

Problems

The lesion itself can potentially become malignant, and any irritations should be removed.

Intervention

I. Because the lesion is premalignant, it should be watched closely and a biopsy taken if any changes are noted.

II. Any initiating factors such as tobacco use should be minimized and dentures evaluated for proper fit.

III. Good oral hygiene should be maintained.

IV. Vitamin A may also be given.

V. Follow-up care is essential.

Salivary Tumors

Tumors of the salivary glands are most frequently benign. Adenocarcinoma is the most common malignant growth and usually occurs in the sixth decade. It is a slow-growing tumor that spreads widely through both lymph and blood vessels. Mucoepidermoid carcinoma is seen most frequently in the parotid gland. Its degree of malignancy and rate of growth varies. Squamous cell carcinomas are rapidly growing, highly invasive tumors. Malignant tumors initially cause enlargement of the gland involved. As the growth spreads, pressure on sensory and motor nerves results in varying degrees of pain and paralysis.

Problems

I. Patients with salivary tumors are usually in pain and may have to cope with some oral motor impairment that makes chewing, swallowing, or talking difficult.
II. Changes in body image due to surgery are often a major concern to the patient.

Intervention

I. Treatment involves surgical excision of the malignancy. Because of the proximity of the facial nerve during surgery, damage to it can easily result. If possible, the nerve is preserved. During a *parotidectomy,* the mandibular branch of the facial nerve is most often damaged, causing paralysis. This is, however, often temporary, and the nerve regenerates with a return of function in 18 to 24 months.
II. Some salivary malignancies are radiosensitive, and irradiation will be coupled with surgical intervention.

Esophageal Tumors

Definition

Benign tumors of the esophagus are rare. Malignant neoplasms are more common and are responsible for 2 percent of all cancer deaths. Squamous cell carcinomas are most common. Cancer of the esophagus is seen in men more often than women. Its peak incidence is in the sixth and seventh decades. Its cause is unknown, but it has been associated with esophageal damage from lye, achalasia, and the use of alcohol and tobacco. It is thought that genetic differences and chemicals in the diet may also play a role.

The cancer spreads by lymph channels via regional lymph nodes, by blood to the liver and lungs, and through direct invasion, although seldom entering the stomach. Signs and symptoms appear late, and spread so quickly that early detection is difficult. Initially, the patient experiences only slight dysphagia and transient difficulty passing food through the esophagus. As the dysphagia progresses, the patient has trouble swallowing solids. then semisolid food, and finally liquids. As the tumor spreads, there is pain on swallowing and vague, burning, retrosternal pain. As food intake diminishes, weight loss occurs. Halitosis develops, the patient has a bad taste in the mouth, and regurgitation occurs. With obstruction of the esophagus, the patient may aspirate, and severe coughing episodes often develop.

Problems

I. Dysphagia.
II. Pain.
III. Weight loss.
IV. Oral hygiene.
V. Potential aspiration.

Intervention

All interventions should focus on relieving the problems and arresting the malignant growth. Whatever the specific treatment selected, the cure rate is low.
I. *Surgical excision* and *irradiation* may be used alone or in combination. Some physicians use preoperative irradiation. The type of surgical procedure will depend on the cancer and the patient's condition. It is often difficult to resect all the cancer. Therefore, the goal of any intervention is to prolong the patient's ability to eat normally. This may be accomplished with an esophagectomy and/or implanting an artificial esophagus, using a segment of colon as the esophagus, creating a channel through the tumor, or bringing the stomach into the mediastinum to anastomose the ends of the esophagus. Radiation therapy may also be used as a palliative procedure to reduce the size and slow the growth of the tumor.
II. *Pain* following surgery may be controlled with medication (analgesia).
III. Within the limits of the individual situation, the *diet* should be made as nutritional as possible. When oral intake is delayed, hyperalimentation may be used. Frequent *mouth care* will improve the patient's appetite and foster nutrition.

IV. Because aspiration is a danger, the patient should be cautioned to take small bites and chew food thoroughly. Eating alone should be avoided, and a suction machine should be kept at the bedside.

V. *Tracheoesophogeal fistulas* may develop postoperatively and prolong the patient's hospitalization period.

Gastric Tumors

Definition Of all gastric tumors, 95 percent are malignant. The most common types are adenocarcinoma, lymphoma, and leiomyosarcoma. While the incidence of gastric cancer is decreasing in the United States, it is the fourth leading cause of cancer deaths in men. It is seen in men twice as frequently as women, has its peak incidence between 50 and 69 years of age, and occurs in blacks and orientals twice as often as in whites. Its cause is unknown, but it has been associated with genetic factors, polyps, changes in the gastric mucosa (i.e., chronic gastritis), and peptic ulcer disease.

Gastric cancer spreads by direct invasion (usually into the pancreas), through lymphatic channels (which occurs early), via the bloodstream to the liver, lungs, and bones, and by growing across the peritoneum. While spread occurs early, symptoms appear late and are often vague. Anorexia often develops, and weight loss is common. The pain can vary in intensity. The patient often describes a feeling of rapid filling after eating. Vomiting occurs in about half the patients, and if the cancer is high in the stomach, dysphagia may develop. The patient often fatigues easily. Occult bleeding is common, and anemia can develop.

Problems
I. Anorexia.
II. Vomiting.
III. Dysphagia.
IV. Weight loss.
V. Pain.
VI. Fatigue.
VII. Blood loss.

Intervention Nursing care should focus on arresting the malignant growth, improving nutrition, relieving pain, and correcting the anemia.
I. The most effective treatment is surgery with complete excision. This usually involves some type of *subtotal gastrectomy*. Total gastrectomy is seldom indicated. (See "Peptic Ulcer" for a complete discussion of gastric surgery.)
II. Irradiation for gastric cancer has not been tried much. Chemotherapy using 5-fluorouracil
III. Follow-up care is essential.

Small Bowel Tumors

Definition Both benign and malignant tumors are infrequent in the small bowel. Malignant neoplasms account for less than 1 percent of gastrointestinal cancers in the United States. The most common types are adenocarcinomas, lymphomas, and leiomyosarcomas. Small bowel cancer spreads to the liver and local lymph nodes. While its cause is not known, it is associated with chronic small bowel disease (i.e., regional enteritis). Genetic factors have also been implicated.

Patients usually experience malaise, anorexia, weight loss, and abdominal pain. Bleeding is frequent as the lesion ulcerates. Depending on its location in the small intestine, malabsorption, biliary obstruction, or intestinal obstruction can occur.

I. Anorexia.
II. Malnutrition.
III. Weight loss.
IV. Pain.
V. Fatigue.
VI. Hemorrhage.
VII. Biliary obstruction and its problems.
VIII. Intestinal obstruction.

Intervention   Nursing care should focus on arresting the abnormal growth, promoting adequate nutrition, relieving pain, preventing anemia, and relieving any obstructions.

    I. *Surgical excision* is the most effective treatment, although the survival rate still remains low.

    II. *Irradiation, alkalating agents, nitrogen mustard,* and *corticosteroids* may be helpful in treating lymphomas.

    III. Follow-up care and continuous evaluation are important.

Rectocolonic Tumors

Definition   Rectocolonic cancer comprises 15 percent of all cancers and accounts for 20 percent of cancer deaths. Carcinoma is the most frequently occurring tumor of the colon or rectum. It usually occurs after the age of 55 and is seen in both men and women. Rectal cancer is more common in men, while cancer of the colon is found in women more frequently. Its incidence has been associated with environmental factors, such as a diet low in fiber and high in refined carbohydrates, diets high in animal meats and fats, genetic factors, and ulcerative colitis.

    Rectocolonic cancer can spread by direct invasion, often into the bladder or vagina, via the regional lymphatics, through the blood to the liver, lungs, kidneys, or bone, and by multiple peritoneal implants. Signs and symptoms usually vary with the location. The usual presenting symptom is a significant change in bowel habits. The patient often experiences increasing constipation or constipation alternating with diarrhea and colicky lower abdominal pain. The pain often increases when climbing stairs or bending over. Blood is often present in the stool and may be visible if the tumor is on the left side. Anorexia, nausea, and/or vomiting may be present, and weight loss is common. The patient often describes a feeling of fullness in the bowel after defecation.

Problems   I. Varying degrees of bowel obstruction.
    II. Weight loss.
    III. Pain.
    IV. Rectal bleeding.

Intervention   Nursing care should focus on arresting the tumor growth, relieving obstruction, promoting adequate nutrition, alleviating pain, and preventing anemia.

    I. *Surgical resection* is the most effective treatment and may be curative or palliative. It involves large bowel resection with anastomosis of healthy ends or resection and the formation of a colostomy. (See "Intestinal Obstruction" for a more complete discussion.)

    II. *Radiotherapy* and *chemotherapy* (5-fluorouracil used most frequently) have not been used extensively but may prove beneficial when used in conjunction with surgery.

Tumors of the Liver

Definition   Both malignant and benign tumors of the liver are rare. Malignant tumors account for only 1 to 2 percent of all cancers in North and South America and Europe. In Africa and Asia, however, where hepatic carcinogens are found in the food, hepatic carcinoma accounts for 20 to 30 percent of all malignancies. In the United States, tumors of the liver are most frequently associated with hepatic cirrhosis. Metastatic tumors of the liver are usually from lung, gastrointestinal, or breast carcinomas.

    Many of the effects of hepatic carcinoma are similar to those of cirrhosis. For this reason its development may be overlooked in the severely ill patient with cirrhosis. It may be distinguished by the fact that it is painful (usually moderate upper abdominal pain), causes bloody ascitic fluid, and results in a friction rub or bruit over the liver. Palpation usually reveals massive hepatomegaly, tenderness, and multiple nodes. Jaundice may occur, depending on the type of cancer. When cancer metastasizes to the liver, in the absence of previous liver pathology, the liver will become enlarged, the abdomen will swell, and pain and jaundice will develop.

Problems   Patients with tumors of the liver may present nursing problems associated with hepatic cirrhosis. These often include:

I. Pain.   IV. Jaundice.
II. Blood loss.   V. Malnutrition.
III. Ascites.

Intervention   Nursing care should focus on relieving the many problems associated with hepatic failure (see "Hepatic Cirrhosis") and arresting the abnormal growth.

I. Surgery may be tried if the patient is young, a good surgical risk, and spread of the cancer is not extensive. The procedure used usually involves a *partial hepatectomy*. Liver transplantation has been of limited value.
II. Chemotherapy may be used as a palliative measure to relieve pain.

Pancreatic Tumors

Definition   Pancreatic masses most frequently result from cysts or carcinoma. *Pancreatic cysts* consist of a collection of fluid that is encapsulated. Retention cysts arise from dilatation of pancreatic ducts within the gland. Pseudocysts are collections of pancreatic juice and cellular debris that can develop 3 to 4 weeks after an attack of acute pancreatitis. They usually cause aching pain and form a tender, palpable mass. Because of the danger of rupture, surgical drainage will usually be employed.

Pancreatic cancer is the fourth leading cause of cancer death in the United States. It affects men twice as frequently as women and is usually seen after 50 years of age. It can affect the head or the body and tail of the pancreas and rapidly spreads by direct invasion into the rest of the pancreas, liver, biliary tract, and duodenum. Quickly adhering to adjacent structures, metastases are carried by lymphatic and blood vessels. Its incidence has been associated with chronic pancreatitis, heavy alcohol use, and diabetes mellitus.

Physical and behavioral symptoms will vary with the location of the tumor. Usually pain is present and may be severe, radiating into the mid back if the body or tail are involved. With biliary tract involvement, jaundice develops. Weight loss is common, and digestive disturbances may include anorexia, an aversion to food, nausea, vomiting, gastric fullness, flatulence, constipation, or diarrhea in some. When the body or tail are involved, the patient often experiences emotional disturbances with depression and a feeling of doom.

Problems   I. Pain.   V. Gastrointestinal disturbances.
II. Jaundice.   VI. Disturbances in glucose metabolism.
III. Itching.   VII. Emotional difficulties.
IV. Weight loss.

Intervention   Nursing care should focus on relieving pain, minimizing pruritus, preventing skin breakdown, promoting adequate nutrition, and relieving anxiety.

I. Prognosis for pancreatic carcinoma is usually poor, and death is often swift. Because fewer than a quarter of cases can be surgically resected (carcinoma of the body or tail almost never), palliative surgery to relieve obstruction may be the only feasible alternative.
II. Irradiation and chemotherapy has not proven effective but may also be employed for palliation. Testolactose and 5-fluorouracil have been most useful.
III. A sound, nutritionally balanced diet may be coupled with insulin therapy and pancreatic enzyme replacement.
IV. Narcotics will be needed to relieve pain.
V. Long-term care will be required.

HYPERACTIVITY AND HYPOACTIVITY

Peptic Ulcer

Definition

A *peptic ulcer* is a clearly defined break in tissue involving the mucosa, submucosa, or musculature of the gastrointestinal track. Of all North Americans, 10 percent have a chronic peptic ulcer at some time (2). The problem occurs most frequently in the stomach or duodenum but can occur in any area exposed to gastric acid, such as the esophagus or the jejunum, after gastric surgery. A peptic ulcer develops when the digestive ability of the gastric secretions exceeds the mucosal defenses. This occurs when hydrochloric acid secretion is excessive or when mucosal resistance is decreased by poor circulation, inadequate tissue regeneration, or inadequate mucous production.

Gastric ulcers are associated with normal or low levels of acid production. The mechanism involved may be related to acid diffusing back into the gastric mucosa, causing damage. While they can occur at any age, gastric ulcers are generally found in older persons, with men affected twice as frequently as women (3).

Duodenal ulcers are associated with excess acid production and tend to be found more frequently in young and middle-aged males. *Stress* may be a factor in their development. Emotional, psychologic, or physical stress stimulates the vagus nerve which increases acid production. The physical stress of a severe burn can result in *Curling's ulcer,* while a central nervous system lesion can lead to *Cushing's ulcer.* Acute stress ulcers have also been associated with surgery, trauma, sepsis, anoxia, and radiation therapy.

Assessment

I. Data sources (refer to "Oral Cancer").
II. Health history. The patient's medical records should also be examined for any previous history of peptic ulcer or chronic indigestion, and blood type should be determined. Peptic ulcer occurs more frquently in persons with type O blood.
   A. The patient should be questioned about the use of drugs known to predispose to ulceration by increasing acid secretion or decreasing mucosal resistance. These include salicylates, corticosteroids, reserpine, histamine, indomethacin, cinchophen, and phenylbutazone. The use of alcohol, caffeine, or cigarettes is also associated with peptic disease.
   B. Genetic factors have been implicated in the development of peptic ulcers, and a family history should be sought.
   C. The patient's occupation and work routine should be discussed. Persons with duodenal ulcers are often nervous, competitive, compulsive workers in demanding positions.
   D. *Pain* is a frequent complaint of a person with peptic ulceration. It may be described as burning, gnawing, aching, sharp, stabbing, cramplike, a fullness, a "sinking" feling, or "gas" pain. It is usually felt in the area of the epigastrium and behind the xiphoid cartilage. With duodenal ulcers the pain may be felt over much of the abdomen with increased intensity in the upper right quadrant. Abdominal pain associated with gastric ulcers is usually left of the midline and localized. Peptic ulcer pain often radiates behind the lower sternum.

   The patient should be questioned about the rhythmicity of the pain and its relation to meals. Usually, pain occurs when the stomach is empty and may often wake the patient at night. The pain of duodenal ulcers is usually decreased for 1 to 4 h after eating, while gastric ulcer pain is relieved for $\frac{1}{2}$ to $1\frac{1}{2}$ h.
   E. The patient may also complain of *nausea, vomiting,* or *pyrosis* (a burning sensation coupled with the regurgitation of acid fluid into the throat)
   F. The patient's life-style and coping mechanisms should be explored. Stresses should be identified and their relation to pain determined.
III. Physical assessment. For the patient with peptic ulcer, the physical assessment will not reveal significant findings unless complications have developed.
   A. The patient often appears nervous and anxious.

   B. The abdominal examination should be given special attention. There is often a superficial tenderness in the epigastrium. Occasionally, this is associated with cutaneous hyperesthesia.

   C. Weight loss may be significant, depending upon the duration of the symptoms.

IV. Diagnostic tests. There are a variety of diagnostic tests used to establish the diagnosis of peptic ulcer. Thse may include some of the following.

   A. A *barium swallow* is often utilized to visualize the ulcer. The patient is given barium, a radiopaque substance, orally or through a nasogastric tube, and x-rays are taken which visualize the ulcer. A laxative or enema may be given subsequently to prevent fecal impaction by the barium.

   B. To directly visualize the ulcer, *gastrointestinal endoscopy* may be done. The patient should take nothing orally for several hours preceding the test. After applying a local anesthetic to the pharynx, a long, flexible, lighted fiberscope is passed through the mouth into the stomach. The ulcer can be visualized and specimens for cytology can be taken.

   C. The gastric secretions may be analyzed during a *gastric analysis.* After an 8-h fast the gastric secretions are withdrawn via a nasogastric tube and examined for acidity. Subsequently, another analysis may be done, stimulating gastric secretion with histamine. In both analyses, acid secretion is higher than normal with duodenal ulcers.

   D. Stools and gastric secretions are also examined for *occult blood* which may be indicative of blood loss from the ulcer.

Problems

I. Pain, often present prior to ingestion of food.
II. Nausea and vomiting.
III. Weight loss.
IV. Anxiety.
V. Stress.

Diagnosis

I. Complains of pain in the epigastric regions which may radiate to the back. May be secondary to increased production of hydrochloric acid, decreased mucosal resistance, etc.
II. Is frequently nauseous, and may vomit several hours after eating.
III. Has experienced weight loss over past few weeks.
IV. Anxiety associated with concern about family and work responsibilities, and worries about own health.
V. Inability to cope satisfactorily with daily stress.

Goals of Care

I. Immediate.
   A. Promote complete physical, emotional, and psychologic rest.
   B. Reduce stress in the internal and external environment.
   C. Neutralize acidity to alleviate nausea, vomiting, and pain and to prevent their reoccurrence.
II. Long-range.
   A. Heal the ulceration and prevent its reoccurrence or the development of complications.
   B. Reduce stress at home and work.
   C. Develop healthy coping strategies to handle stress.
III. *Priorities of care* should initially focus on neutralizing the acidity, which will relieve the pain, nausea, and vomiting.

Intervention

I. *Diet therapy* may vary according to individual preferences. Traditionally, frequent feedings of bland foods were used, but more liberal diets have evolved which allow the patient to eat a fairly normal diet while eliminating from the diet those foods that are not well tolerated. This often includes foods that may be *chemically irritating,* such as spicy foods, foods that may be *thermally irritating,* such as very hot foods; or foods that may be *mechanically irritating,* such as popcorn. With severe pain, the patient may be given milk and an antacid on an alternating schedule every $\frac{1}{2}$ h before being progressed to three meals a day with between-meal and bedtime snacks. If the patient is experiencing night pain, he or she should be awakened once or twice during the night and given milk or an antacid (see below).

II. *Medications* are used which neutralize acid, decrease gastric secretion and mobility, and reduce anxiety.

  A. Nonsystemic *antacids,* which are not absorbed, are used to buffer gastric acid. Some tend to be constipating, such as calcium carbonate and aluminum hydroxide (Amphogel), while those that include magnesium salts (Maalox) may cause diarrhea. Antacids that combine these groups afford fewer complications. These include Gelusil and Delcid. An alternating schedule of the two types will also decrease ill effects. The nurse should observe the contents of antacids, as some are high in sodium (Mylanta) and may affect patients on low sodium diets.

  B. *Anticholinergic drugs* are used to decrease gastric motility and secretion but are associated with toxic side effects. These include mouth dryness, nausea and vomiting, decreased visual acuity, and urinary retention.

  C. *Sedatives* may be used to decrease anxiety and restlessness, allowing physical and psychologic relaxation.

  D. Recently, the use of synthetic histamine H_2-receptor antagonists, prostaglandins, and gastrointestinal hormones and related peptides which decrease hydrochloride secretion has been investigated. Carbenoxolone, which is a licorice extract, and bismuth, both increase peptic ulcer healing, but their mechanism of action is not known (4).

III. Once diet and medication therapy is begun, patients often become symptom-free within a week. Therapy must be continued for 4 to 6 weeks until the ulcer is healed. A comprehensive *teaching plan* should be instituted to ensure the patient's understanding and cooperation.

  A. Patients should be taught the rationale for medications, their schedule of adminis-tration, likely side effects, and adverse effects that should be reported. Patients should be cautioned against the abuse and overuse of antacids as they can predispose an individual to acid-base imbalances.

  B. Dietary teaching should include the frequency and timing of meals and foods to be avoided. The primary food preparer should be included in the teaching and the emphasis should be placed on what can rather than what cannot be eaten. Coffee, tea, and cola drinks should be avoided because of their stimulatory effects. Alcohol intake should also be minimized, although a relaxing drink taken with milk or an antacid is not contraindicated.

  C. Patients should be encouraged and supported to decrease or stop smoking. The nervous tension that will be associated with this must be weighed against the effect smoking has in enhancing gastric secretion and the patient should be advised accordingly.

IV. Everyday *stressful situations* should be explored with the patient and family. Ways to decrease stress should be sought, and the patient should be helped to develop alternate coping mechanisms. The patient should be given a list of drugs known to predispose to ulceration and cautioned against taking any drug without prior approval.

V. If the ulcer pain is intractable and recurrent, and the patient is severely ill with associated disease that makes surgery too great a risk, *irradiation* may be used. The radiation to the stomach serves to destroy parietal and chief cells, thus decreasing the secretion of pepsin and hydrochloric acid.

VI. Frequent *follow-up care* is mandatory for 4 to 6 weeks to ensure ulcer healing and detect any complications (see below). After the ulcer has healed, the patient should receive regular checkups to assess coping strategies and detect reoccurrence.

Evaluation   At any time during the course of peptic ulcer disease, if the therapeutic regimen fails, dietary indiscretions become excessive, or stress and emotional tension mount, complications can occur. The patient should be periodically reassessed to detect their development.

  I. If the ulceration penetrates an artery, vein, or capillary bed, hemorrhage can develop.

A. Nursing assessment to detect hemorrhage may include the appearance of hematemesis or melena; nausea; a decrease in pain, as the blood lost buffers acid; and indications of developing shock. The latter may include restlessness, tachycardia, weakness, hypotension, and diaphoresis.

B. Interventions focus on stopping the bleeding and replacing lost blood volume.

   1. Blood volume is expanded with intravenous solutions that often include whole blood and plasma. The hematocrit and hemoglobin levels will be utilized to assess the patient's blood loss.

   2. The patient may be sedated to decrease apprehension and anxiety.

   3. A nasogastric tube (see Fig. 29-3) will be inserted, and *gastric lavage* with iced saline will be begun to stop the bleeding. Often, milk and antacids will be administered through the nasogastric tube after the bleeding has subsided. A large-bore *Ewald tube* may be used to facilitate clot removal.

   4. Once the stomach is emptied of blood and clots, a gastric balloon may be inserted and *gastric cooling* can begin. A cooling solution is circulated through the balloon to promote vasoconstriction and temporarily depress secretions. This is often used as an interim measure until surgery can be considered. A *Levin tube* is used to aspirate stomach contents while the balloon is in place.

   5. The patient's vital signs and urinary output should be closely monitored, and appropriate measures should be instituted to combat shock.

   6. *Gastric surgery* is indicated when the bleeding is not countered by blood transfusions after 12 h, bleeding persists after 24 h, or the bleeding reoccurs while the patient is in the hospital. Common surgical procedures include a *gastric resection* (a portion of the stomach removed), a *subtotal gastrectomy* (70 to 80 percent of the stomach removed; see Fig. 29-4a) and *vagatomy* (dividing

FIGURE 29-3 / Nasogastric tube to suction. (*From D. A. Jones et al., Medical-Surgical Nursing: A Conceptual Approach, McGraw-Hill Book Company, New York, 1978.*)

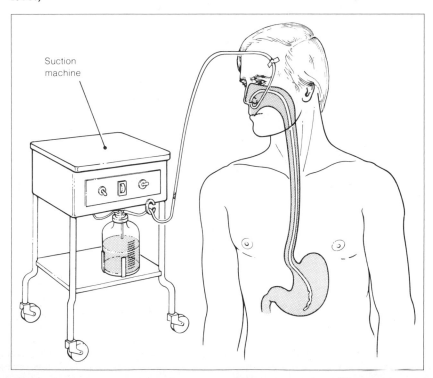

Suction machine

branches of the vagus nerve), *suturing of the ulcer, pyloroplasty* (repair of the pylorus), and *antrectomy* (excision of walls of the antrum; see Fig. 29-4*b*).

7. Postoperative care.
   a. Following gastric surgery the patient should be watched in the *immediate postoperative period* for bleeding. The initial drainage from the nasogastric tube will be bright red but should turn dark red after 12 h and greenish yellow in 36 h. After several days the patient will be given clear liquids, and as tolerated, the nasogastric tube will be removed and the diet progressed.
   b. Following gastric surgery, about 50 percent of patients develop a *dumping syndrome* which usually subsides in 6 to 12 months. This involves the rapid emptying of the gastric contents into the intestines, which draws fluid into the intestinal lumen and causes a decrease in the circulating blood volume. The patient experiences a feeling of fullness and nausea with diaphoresis, pallor, dizziness, a feeling of warmth, headache, and palpitations. Because of excess insulin secretion at this time, patients experience weakness, tremors, diaphoresis, and an anxious feeling 2 to 3 h after eating. A high-protein, high-fat, low-carbohydrate diet consisting of small, frequent meals is helpful. Fluids should be avoided around mealtimes. Lying down after eating and eating while semirecumbent are also helpful.

II. The most serious complication of peptic ulcer is *perforation*. It is frequently associated with emotional stress or fatigue. It generally results in *peritonitis,* an inflammation of the peritoneum that results from the chemical irritation of the gastric and duodenal contents.
   A. *Nursing assessment* will reveal an acutely ill patient complaining of sudden severe epigastric pain that spreads through the abdomen and is worse in the right lower quadrant. The patient is often prostrate with the knees drawn up. The abdominal examination will find an extremely tender, rigid, boardlike abdomen with rebound tenderness evident. The patient may be nauseous and vomit, and as fluid is lost to the peritoneal cavity, hypovolemia and shock may develop. Paralytic ileus often occurs and will be evidenced by an absence of bowel sounds. The patient will be extremely apprehensive, and respirations may be rapid and shallow.
   B. Treatment for perforation always involves *surgical repair.* Usually, a patch of omentum is used to close the perforation. Depending on the patient's condition, more definitive procedures, discussed under hemorrhage, may also be performed.
   C. Prior to surgery a nasogastric tube with suctioning will be used to empty the stomach, pain medication will be given, and symptoms of hypovolemia will be combatted.

III. Inflammation and edema around the pylorus can result in *pyloric obstruction*. Gastric emptying decreases, resulting in gastric dilatation.
   A. During nursing assessment the patient will complain of classic ulcer pain, distension after eating, anorexia, weight loss, and vomiting of undigested food. The abdominal examination will reveal a distended abdomen with visible peristalsis. A succussion splash, evidencing fluid and air in the stomach, will be noted.
   B. To relieve gastric distension, a nasogastric tube will be inserted through the nares, pharynx, and esophagus into the stomach. Intermittent suction will be applied to empty the stomach. The obstruction often subsides in 48 h. Until liquids can be taken orally, fluid and nutritional needs will be met with administration of intravenous fluids (refer to Fig. 29-3).
   C. If the obstruction does not subside or if the pyloric opening is significantly narrowed, surgery will be considered and pyloroplasty performed.

Achalasia

Definition   *Achalasia* (cardiospasm) is a condition characterized by the failure of swallowed food to pass from the esophagus into the stomach. It is thought to result when esophageal peristalsis is feeble or absent and the cardiac sphincter fails to relax after swallowing. As food accumulates in the esophagus, its terminal end dilates (*megaesophagus*). It is thought to be related to impairment of cholinergic innervation, but the cause is not known. Occasionally, it is precipitated by emotional stress such as a death of someone close or feelings of guilt after sex. It occurs most frequently in women between the ages of 20 and 40.

The course of achalasia is usually chronic and progressive with remissions and exacerbations. The patient experiences mild dysphagia which increases with excitement or tension. There is a feeling of fullness that is relieved after a while as the food passes into the stomach. A dull ache or pain radiating to the base of the neck, left shoulder, or scapular area may be experienced. The patient is unable to belch, loses weight, and often has a mild esophagitis. Halitosis is usually a problem. With megaesophagus, pressure on the trachea and/or blood vessels can cause difficulty.

Problems
    I. Difficulty swallowing.
    II. Weight loss.
    III. Pain or discomfort.
    IV. Halitosis.
    V. Possible aspiration.
    VI. Tracheal obstruction.
    VII. Circulatory impairment.

Intervention
Nursing care should focus on promoting esophageal emptying, minimizing stress, and preventing respiratory difficulties.
    I. Treatment usually focuses initially on dilating the cardiac sphincter (see Fig. 29-5) and, if unsuccessful, surgically cutting it (*esophagocardiomyotomy*) to promote passage of food into the stomach. The patient will often be taught self-dilatation (*bougienage*) and instructed to do it every 3 to 7 days.

FIGURE 29-4 / (*a*) Billroth I. (*b*) Billroth II.

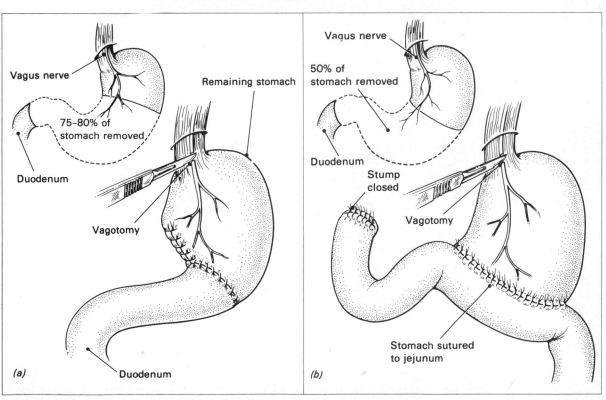

(a) Vagus nerve — 75–80% of stomach removed — Remaining stomach — Duodenum — Vagotomy — Duodenum

(b) Vagus nerve — 50% of stomach removed — Duodenum — Stump closed — Vagotomy — Stomach sutured to jejunum

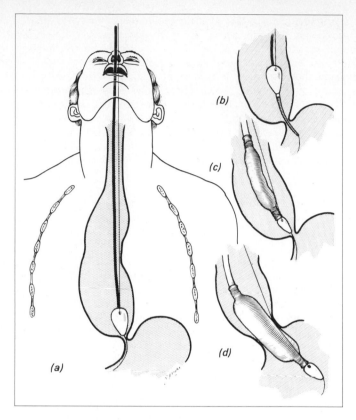

FIGURE 29-5 / Hydrostatic dilatation of the lower esophagus to relieve achalasia. An olive-tipped bougie is passed to the stomach (*a*). A sound is passed through the sphincter guided by a previously swallowed flexible wire (*b*). The hydrostatic dilator is then passed through the sphincter (*c*) and distended (*d*) to dilate the sphincter. (*From S. I. Schwartz et al., Principles of Surgery, McGraw-Hill Book Company, New York, 1974.*)

II. Food passage can be further facilitated by encouraging a soft diet and teaching the patient to eat slowly, chew all food well, take fluids while eating, and arch the back, strain, and flex the chin to the sternum after swallowing. Patients should avoid eating at night or when emotionally stressed, and the patient should remain upright after meals.

III. Small doses of sedatives may be given to relieve emotional stress, and smooth muscle relaxants may be tried. The latter are associated with adverse side effects.

Constipation

Definition   *Constipation* may be defined as a failure of the rectum to evacuate its contents normally. As this occurs, stool accumulates in the rectum, which becomes chronically distended. As water is absorbed from the stool, making it dehydrated, *fecal impaction* of hard, puttylike stools results. Constipation can result from mechanical obstruction, decreased colonic contractility (i.e., paralytic ileus and megacolon), or most frequently, when the defecation reflex fails. Dietary changes, inactivity, muscle weakness, overuse of laxatives, chronic suppression of the urge to defecate, and motional stress can all contribute to its development.

Constipation often results in anorexia, a bloated feeling, belching, flatus, malaise, weakness, headache, dizziness, and mild abdominal distension. If fecal impaction develops, watery diarrhea occurs as stool passes around the impaction, and crampy lower abdominal pain ensues.

Problems	**I.** Inadequate nutrition. **IV.** Fatigability.
	II. Discomfort. **V.** Diarrhea.
	III. Headache.

Intervention Nursing care should focus on relieving the constipation and preventing its reoccurrence.

    I. To empty the rectum, the following may be used in combination or individually: tap water enema, soapsuds enema, Fleet enema, stool softeners, and mild laxatives.

    II. Fecal impactions may be softened with an oil retention enema and then removed with a tap water enema or digitally broken and removed by the nurse.

    III. Diet therapy is the most effective way to prevent reoccurrence. High-fiber foods should be encouraged. Prune juice with breakfast is often helpful, and fresh fruits and vegetables should be eaten liberally. Ingestion of fluids, including water, should be encouraged. The use of laxatives should be discouraged.

METABOLIC DISORDERS

Obesity

Definition In areas of the world where the food supply is good, obesity is the most common type of metabolic disorder. It is estimated that about 20 percent of the United States population over 30 is overweight, with women affected more frequently than men. Approximately 15 to 30 percent of school-age children are thought to be obese (5). Simply defined, obesity involves an excess accumulation of fat that occurs when the caloric intake exceeds the energy requirements (6).

Obesity can be caused by either endogenous or exogenous factors. *Endogenous obesity* results when there is a disturbance within the individual, such as a hypothalamic lesion in the ventromedial nucleus or a hormonal imbalance. *Exogenous obesity* occurs when external factors lead to overeating. These include psychologic, sociocultural, economic, and physical influences. People are often psychologically conditioned to think that eating relieves stress. Cultural practices often include eating as a means of celebration. Certain social groups have a higher incidence of obesity than others. In a mechanized society, physical inactivity can also contribute to weight gain. Weight gain often increases with age because the basal metabolic rate and physical activity decrease while the usual caloric intake is continued.

Assessment **I.** Data sources (refer to "Oral Cancer").

    II. Health history.

        A. Have the patient recall what was eaten in the last 24 h, few days, or week. Special attention should be given to the type and amount of food eaten, when and where it was eaten, activity just before and during eating, and feelings before, during, and after eating.

        B. The patient should be questioned about the onset of obesity and other obese family members. There is an increased chance of being obese if one or both parents are overweight.

        C. The patient's health record should be examined for any history of diabetes mellitus, gout, gallbladder disease, atherosclerosis, or coronary artery disease, all of which have been associated with obesity.

    III. Physical assessment. Examination of the person who is obese usually reveals visible evidence of fat accumulation. People accumulate body fat differently. Women tend to develop adiposity below the waist, while men will often carry excess fat on their trunks. Some fat is evenly distributed throughout the body, while other adipose tissue may be localized. Depending on body build, occasionally a person will be obese without obvious visible evidence.

A. The patient should be weighed and the result compared to standard height and weight tables (see Table 29-1). A person who is 10 percent over her or his desired weight is considered overweight, while one who is 20 percent or more over is obese.

B. A complete physical examination should be given to detect a concomitant disease associated with obesity. Auscultation through adipose tissue diminishes the sounds, making breath, heart, and bowel sounds difficult to hear. Palpating through fat is also more difficult. Pulses may be difficult to find, and the abdominal examination may be uninformative. Percussion sounds will be duller.

C. Vital signs of the severely obese patient often evidence tachycardia, hypoventilation, and/or mild hypertension.

D. Because obesity often results in pendulous fatty skin aprons, skin folds should be examined for evidence of excoriation, breakdown, and/or infection.

IV. Diagnostic tests. There are a few significant tests which may help elicit data relative to obesity.

A. The use of *calipers* is an effective way to estimate obesity. This involves the measurement of the thickness of skin folds in different parts of the boy. Comparing the results with normal values presents a fairly accurate estimate of obesity.

B. Several laboratory tests may be used to detect the development of any of the medical problems commonly associated with obesity. These may include fasting blood sugar, glucose tolerance test, and tests of glycosuria and ketonuria to detect diabetes, serum cholesterol for atherosclerosis, an electrocardiogram to evaluate cardiac functioning, and tests of gallbladder function, among others.

Problems

I. Overeating.
II. Inactivity.
III. Dyspnea on exertion.
IV. Skin breakdown.
V. Hygiene problems.
VI. Poor psychologic adjustment.

TABLE 29-1 / DESIRABLE WEIGHT, IN POUNDS, FOR ADULTS 25 AND OVER (INDOOR CLOTHING)

Height (in Shoes)		Small Frame	Medium Frame	Large Frame	Height (in Shoes)		Small Frame	Medium Frame	Large Frame
ft	in				ft	in			
Men					*Women*				
5	2	112–120	118–129	126–141	4	10	92–98	96–107	104–119
5	3	115–123	121–133	129–144	4	11	94–101	98–110	106–122
5	4	118–126	124–136	132–148	5		96–104	101–113	109–125
5	5	121–129	127–139	135–152	5	1	99–107	104–116	112–128
5	6	124–133	130–143	138–156	5	2	102–110	107–119	115–131
5	7	128–137	134–147	142–161	5	3	105–113	110–122	118–134
5	8	132–141	138–152	147–166	5	4	108–116	113–126	121–138
5	9	136–145	142–156	151–170	5	5	111–119	116–130	125–142
5	10	140–150	146–160	155–174	5	6	114–123	120–135	129–146
5	11	144–154	150–165	159–179	5	7	118–127	124–139	133–150
6		148–158	154–170	164–184	5	8	122–131	128–143	147–154
6	1	152–162	158–175	168–189	5	9	126–135	132–147	141–158
6	2	156–167	162–180	173–194	5	10	130–140	136–151	145–163
6	3	160–171	167–185	178–199	5	11	134–144	140–155	149–168
6	4	164–175	172–190	182–204	6		138–148	144–159	153–173

Source: G. W. Thorn and G. F. Cahill, Jr., "Gain in Weight. Obesity," in G. W. Thorn et al. (eds.), *Harrison's Principles of Internal Medicine,* 8th ed., McGraw-Hill Book Company, New York, 1977.

Diagnosis

I. Eats in excess, often consuming high-calorie low-protein foods (this may be secondary to anxiety, stress, or depression).
II. Is sedentary and tires quickly with minimal exertion (this may be secondary to increased weight).
III. Unable to tolerate even moderate activity without becoming short of breath.
IV. Has reddened and raw areas in skin folds.
V. May have difficulties with body odor.
VI. Eats to satisfy psychologic needs and tends to isolate self.

Goals of Care

I. Immediate.
   A. Decrease caloric intake.
   B. Increase activity without shortness of breath.
   C. Heal skin breakdown.
   D. Promote good hygiene.
II. Long-range.
   A. Attain and maintain ideal body weight by permanently modifying eating habits.
   B. Exercise moderately and daily.
   C. Promote psychologic well-being by meeting needs in ways other than eating.
III. *Priorities of care* should focus on initial weight reduction, healing areas of broken skin, and promoting hygiene.

Intervention

I. Nursing care.
   A. *Diet therapy* is the cornerstone of therapy for obese patients. The diet should include modest caloric reduction with a low-fat, high-protein content. Protein tends to increase satiety and decrease the blood glucose level. The low fat content may constipate the patient, and fresh fruit and bulk foods should be encouraged. A stool softener may be needed. At the onset the patient should understand that some diet restriction will be necessary as a lifelong activity. Interventions should focus on identifying behaviors that lead to overeating and modifying them.
   B. *Group therapy* with long-term reinforcement is helpful. Programs that focus on behavior modification rather than supportive care have been especially therapeutic. Lay groups such as TOPS (Take Off Pounds Sensibly), Fattys Anonymous, and Weight Watchers have also been of value.
   C. *Starvation diets* are not recommended for long-term care because they are associated with loss of protein tissue. In severely obese patients fasts may be used initially because the weight loss associated with such an approach gives encouragement to the patient. A fast 1 day a week may also be used.
   D. While a feasible *exercise* regimen suitable for an overweight patient has little caloric effect, it is excellent for promoting circulation and should be encouraged.
   E. *Drugs* that depress the appetite may be used but are generally discouraged. The weight loss associated with them is usually temporary. The most common are the amphetamines which produce a feeling of euphoria but also cause nervousness and sleeplessness and are habit forming.
   F. *Skin care* should focus on cleaning and drying skin folds. Cotton inserted into the fold to absorb moisture and taping the fold of tissue up to expose the area to the air are both helpful.
   G. Sound *hygiene* practices should be encouraged. Because of the physical difficulty in moving when severely obese and the trapping of body secretions in folds, odor is often a problem. Daily baths or showers and more frequent cleansing of the armpits and perineum should be suggested.
II. *Surgical bypass* of the intestine is an extreme procedure that may be considered if the patient's life is threatened from respiratory or cardiac failure, in cases of severe hypertension, or in cases of severe peripheral edema with ulceration. The most common procedure is the *jejunoileal shunt* in which about 6 m of the ileum and jejunum are resected, and the remaining jejunum and ileum are anastamosed end to end. In effect, a malabsorption syndrome is created, and diarrhea which may last into the second

postoperative year is a result. Complications following intestinal bypass can include fatty infiltration of the liver, vitamin deficiencies, hypomagnesemia, and iron deficiency. Patients should understand that due to surgery oral medications are not likely to be absorbed (including birth control pills). Because of liver complications, alcohol should be avoided.

III. *Follow-up care* for the overweight person is especially important because relapses are the rule rather than the exception. Weight gains should be handled with a forthright, nonpunitive approach, and weight losses should be praised. Behavior that minimizes overeating should be reinforced, and reasons for "eating binges" and "indiscretion" should be sought out and discussed.

Evaluation
I. Severely obese patients must be continually reassessed for the onset of medical problems commonly associated with obesity. These include diabetes mellitus, respiratory and cardiac difficulties, and osteoarthritis.

II. Occasionally, extreme obesity will result in the development of *pickwickian syndrome*. This is a hypoventilation syndrome that results from the weight of the chest wall decreasing chest expansion. It is characterized by hypoventilation, somnolence, polycythemia, and cyanosis.

Anorexia Nervosa

Definition
Anorexia nervosa is a chronic, psychoneurotic disorder characterized by self-induced weight loss, amenorrhea, and psychopathology. It occurs most frequently in young girls around the time of puberty, and is rare in boys. Its cause is not known. It is associated with a hypothalamic disorder that causes the menstrual changes. Psychologic conflicts regarding puberty and adolescence are common, and a relation between self-image and culturally determined attitudes about body size have been implicated in its genesis.

The patient with anorexia nervosa fears becoming fat and avoids food, especially carbohydrate foods. Self-induced vomiting and the abuse of purgatives are not uncommon. Weight loss occurs, and if it is severe, emaciation with apathy, weakness, and marked depression develop. The patient is often impatient and irritable.

Problems
I. Weight loss and malnutrition.
II. Psychologic problems.
III. Susceptibility to infection.
IV. Hypokalemia from vomiting.
V. Susceptibility to cold.

Intervention
Nursing care must focus on improving the nutritional intake and providing psychologic support.

I. Adequate dietary intake must be fostered. Initially, a 1500-cal diet will be given, which after a week will progress to a 3000- to 5000-cal diet. A sound, trusting nurse-patient relationship should be established, and the patient should be gently supervised at each meal. The use of purgatives should be terminated, and vomiting should be made difficult by supervision and support. As weight is gained, the patient should be complimented.

II. Long-term psychiatric therapy is indicated as relapses are common.

Malabsorption Syndromes

Definition
Malabsorption syndromes are a complex of conditions characterized by inadequate absorption of one or more substances by the small intestine. There are a wide variety of conditions that result in a malabsorption syndrome. Their classification usually includes inadequate digestion (e.g., pancreatic insufficiency), inadequate bile salts (e.g., cholestasis), inadequate absorptive surface (e.g., intestinal bypass), lymphatic obstruction (e.g., Whipple's disease),

cardiovascular disorders (e.g., congestive heart failure), absorptive defects of the mucosa of inflammatory origin (e.g., tropical sprue), mucosal absorptive defects of biochemical origin (e.g., nontropical sprue), and endocrine or metabolic disorders.

Physical symptoms usually consist of severe weight loss, malnutrition, anorexia, abdominal distension, borborygmi, muscle wasting, and diarrhea. Stools are often light yellow to gray and are greasy and soft. As malnutrition becomes severe, various protein, vitamin, and electrolyte disturbances occur. Table 29-2 summarizes the signs and symptoms observed and their pathophysiologic bases.

Problems   Nursing problems are widespread and will depend on the degree of malnutrition.
    I. Weight loss.
    II. Diarrhea.
    III. Weakness.
    IV. Fluid and electrolyte imbalance.
    V. Bone pain.
    VI. Anemia.
    VII. Hemorrhage.
    VIII. Vitamin-associated inflammations.

Intervention   Nursing care should focus on improving nutrition and preventing fluid ad electrolyte imbalances.

TABLE 29-2 / PATHOPHYSIOLOGIC BASIS FOR SYMPTOMS AND SIGNS IN MALABSORPTIVE DISORDERS

Symptom or Sign	Pathophysiology
Generalized malnutrition and weight loss	Malabsorption of fat, carbohydrate, and protein → loss of calories
Diarrhea	Impaired absorption or increased intestinal secretion of water and electrolytes; unabsorbed dihydroxy bile acids and fatty acids → lowered absorption of water and electrolytes; excess load of fluid and electrolytes presented to the colon may exceed its absorptive capacity
Nocturia	Delayed absorption of water; hypokalemia
Anemia	Impaired absorption of iron, vitamin B_{12}, and folic acid
Glossitis, cheilosis	Deficiency of iron, vitamin B_{12}, folate, and other vitamins
Peripheral neuritis	Deficiency of vitamin B_{12}
Edema	Impaired absorption of amino acids → protein depletion → hypoproteinemia
Amenorrhea	Protein depletion and "caloric starvation" → secondary hypopituitarism
Bone pain	Protein depletion → impaired bone formation → osteoporosis
	Calcium malabsorption → demineralization of bone → osteomalacia
Tetany, paresthesias	Calcium malabsorption → hypocalcemia; magnesium malabsorption → hypomagnesemia
Hemorrhagic phenomena	Vitamin K malabsorption → hypoprothrombinemia
Weakness	Anemia; electrolyte depletion (hypokalemia)
Eczema	Cause uncertain

Source: N. J. Greenberger and K. J. Isselbacher, "Disorders of Absorption," in G. W. Thorn et al. (eds.), *Harrison's Principles of Internal Medicine,* 8th ed., McGraw-Hill Book Company, New York, 1977, p. 229.

I. Specific treatment varies with the type of malabsorption syndrome. For instance, one of infectious origin, such as tropical sprue, is treated with a broad-spectrum antibiotic, while adult celiac disease (nontropical sprue) responds to a gluten-free diet.

II. Depending on the particular syndrome, patients are often managed with one or more of the following: calcium, magnesium, iron, fat-soluble vitamins, folic acid, vitamin B_{12}, vitamin B complex, pancreatic supplements, broad-spectrum antimicrobials, salt-poor human albumin, immune serum globulin, corticosteroids, antidiarrheal agents, cholestryamine, caloric supplements, and/or antiparasitic agents.

III. Reassessment and long-term care are essential.

INFLAMMATORY DISORDERS

Ulcerative Colitis

Definition

Ulcerative colitis is a diffuse inflammation involving the mucosa and submucosa of the rectum and colon. It begins in the rectum, spreading proximally into adjacent bowel and may involve all or part of the colon. Multiple ulcerations and crypt abscesses develop and are often replaced by scar tissue. When only the rectum is involved, it is called *proctitis*. If all of the colon is involved, the term used is *pancolitis*. The course of the disease can be intermittent or continuous, although most frequently it is characterized by remissions and exacerbations.

The peak incidence for ulcerative colitis is between 20 and 25 years and 50 and 60 years of age. It occurs more frequently among women, and Jews and blacks are only one-third as susceptible as whites to its development (7). About 10 to 20 percent of families with ulcerative colitis have multiple cases within the family (8).

The cause of ulcerative colitis is not known, although several factors have been implicated. These include infection, autonomic stimulation, genetic predisposition, immunologic and autoimmune mechanisms, excessive enzymes, basement membrane changes, hypersensitivity reactions, and psychogenic factors. An intolerance to cow's milk is frequently found in these patients. The onset of the disease or an exacerbation is frequently precipitated by a traumatic emotional experience. The etiologic mechanism involved may prove to be a combination of factors.

Assessment

I. Data sources (refer to "Oral Cancer").

II. Health history. The patient will usually relate a health history whose primary feature is diarrhea. The patient's health record should be examined for any past difficulty with elimination and any occurrence of colitis within the patient's family should be elicited.

   A. There is wide variation in patient's descriptions of diarrhea. Some describe a sudden onset, while its development is gradual in others. The difficulty can range from a few semisoft stools a day to several liquid stools often coming every 30 min to 1 h. The feces often contains blood, mucus, and pus. An occasional patient will be incontinent. In more severe cases, patients experience *tenesmus* (spasmatic contraction of the anal sphincter that is accompanied by pain and urgency).

   B. Most patients describe a mild, cramping, lower abdominal pain that is worse before defecation and may be referred to the back.

   C. Patients should be asked about their energy level; malaise and fatigue are common complaints.

   D. The patient's personality structure and coping strategies should be explored. About half the patients with ulcerative colitis exhibit characteristic feelings of helplessness and hopelessness in coping with stress. They often have difficulty with interpersonal relationships and have an underlying hostility. The patient and family should be questioned about any emotional stresses that may have occurred in the past months, as they often are associated with onset of the disease.

   E. Any changes in appetite should be explored. Anorexia is a frequent complaint.

III. Physical examination frequently reveals a patient who appears thin and weak. In severe cases the patient will have a wasted, emaciated appearance.

A. The weight should be taken and compared with a previous recording in the past history to detect weight loss, which is common.

B. Findings on the abdominal examination vary according to the severity of the inflammation. The abdomen may appear flat with visible peristalsis. Bowel sounds are often increased. As the inflammation worsens, the abdomen can become distended. There may be guarding and tenderness on palpation, especially along the descending colon and in the left lower quadrant.

C. During the rectal examination, redness and excoriation around the anus may be noted. During digital exploration, the rectum is usually found to be empty, anospasm may be felt, and the presence of fissures or abscesses may be noted.

D. The temperature should be taken, as fever is a common finding.

E. With severe diarrhea, dehydration can develop. Vital signs should be checked frequently and evaluated for indications of hypovolemia. Tissue turgor should be tested, the mucous membranes examined, and the eyeballs palpated for softness.

F. Infrequently, patients will evidence inflammatory processes in various parts of the body which parallel the activity in the bowel. Skin lesions such as *erythema nodosum,* which are common in women, and *pyoderma gangrenosum* which occur on the legs and ankles, may be noted (refer to Chap. 33). The eyes may appear reddened, pupil reactions may be sluggish, and pupil size small. The patient often complains of blurred vision. These changes may be due to a variety of ocular inflammations such as episcleritis, iritis, uveitis, or keratitis (refer to Chap. 23). The liver can become infiltrated with fat, which is evidenced by jaundice. Joint manifestations are the most common of theseinflammations, occurring in 10 to 20 percent of ulcerative colitis patients (9). It usually involves an acute arthritis of the knees, hips, and/or ankles that is of short duration, recurrent, and not deforming.

IV. Diagnostic tests.

A. There are a variety of *laboratory examinations* which will aid in evaluating the patient with ulcerative colitis. The red blood cells are usually decreased, depending on the blood loss. White blood cells may be slightly increased. The erythrocyte sedimentation rate is usually elevated, and the serum albumin may be depressed. Serum chemistries may show electrolyte disturbances from the fluid loss. Stools should be cultured and examined for blood, pus, or mucus.

B. *Barium enema* is frequently used with ulcerative colitis patients. The usual bowel preparations, however, are often too rigorous, and the colon is usually sufficiently cleansed with a high fluid intake (240 mL/h for 8 to 10 h) and a mild cathartic (10). Barium, a radiopaque substance, is instilled into the rectum and visualized with a fluoroscope.

C. To directly visualize the rectum and sigmoid colon, *sigmoidoscopy* may be done. The colon is cleansed prior to the examination, but, again, something less than strong cathartics and enemas may be indicated. An inflexible, straight instrument is then inserted. The patient will experience some cramping and discomfort during the procedure.

D. A *colonoscopy* involves direct visualization of the entire colon through the use of a flexible fiberscope. The procedure and preparation is similar to sigmoidoscopy. The patient is often given clear liquids for a few days prior to the procedure. Biopsies are often taken at the same time. Because these patients are often tense, the nurse must be most supportive when preparing the patient for each test. Careful, clear explanations may be helpful.

Problems

I. Diarrhea.
II. Pain.
III. Fever.
IV. Fatigue.
V. Anorexia.

VI. Malnutrition.
VII. Dehydration.
VIII. Extracolonic manifestations.
IX. Inability to cope with stress.

Diagnosis
I. Complains of cramping pain in lower abdomen that worsens before bowel movements.
II. Experiences frequent loose stools, often containing blood, mucus, and pus. (This can occur secondary to stress, ingestion of food, etc.)
III. Has a moderately elevated temperature (secondary to inflammation and/or dehydration).
IV. Feels tired and is unable to maintain normal activity level (secondary to poor appetite and anemia).
V. Has no appetite and tends to avoid eating because of subsequent diarrhea.
VI. Alteration in nutrition: loses significant weight and is malnourished.
VII. Alteration in fluid balance: with severe diarrhea may cause dehydration.
VIII. May evidence inflammation in the eyes, joints, or skin, and/or may have liver involvement.
IX. Feels helpless in stressful situations and does not have strong, supporting, interpersonal relationships.

Goals of Care
I. Immediate.
A. Relieve the diarrhea.
B. Alleviate the pain.
C. Decrease the body temperature.
D. Increase energy level.
E. Prevent dehydration.
F. Relieve extracolonic inflammation.
II. Long-range.
A. Promote adequate nutrition with weight gain.
B. Prevent exacerbations of diarrhea attack.
C. Promote healthful coping strategies.
III. *Priorities of care* should focus on relieving the diarrhea to minimize fluid losses and prevent dehydration.

Intervention
I. Nursing care.
A. *Antiinflammatory drugs* are used to control the inflammation. Salicylazosulfapyridine (Azulfidine) is used most frequently although its mode of action is not known. When use of this fails or if diarrhea is severe, corticosteroids may be used. They have the added effect of relieving the noncolonic inflammations.
B. Initially, the patient will be given nothing by mouth. Calories, electrolytes, and vitamins will be supplemented intravenously. As the patient improves, fluids and then food will be given orally. Serum electrolytes should be monitored, and the patient should be watched for signs of dehydration.
C. *Anticholinergics* may be given to decrease spasm and pain. *Antidiarrhetics* to increase the stool consistency may be utilized. The use of immunosuppressants is being investigated, but results have been variable (11).
D. Adequate *rest* is important for the patient, as physical activity increases intestinal motility. The amount varies with the severity. A tranquilizer may promote general body relaxation.
E. Analgesics may be necessary to help reduce pain, but opiates should be avoided because of their addicting effect. A hot water bottle to the abdomen may promote comfort. If the anus is sore and excoriated, a cortisone-containing ointment may be used. The patient should be kept clean, and sitz baths may be soothing.
F. When blood loss is significant, blood transfusions may be needed. The nurse must assess the patient while he or she is receiving a blood transfusion and be alert to signs of a transfusion reaction (e.g., rash, urticaria).
G. Because of the protein losses from the bowel, adequate nutrition is imperative. In severely ill patients, *hyperalimentation* may be used.
1. Hyperalimentation is a procedure whereby additional nutrients are administered to the patient through an indwelling catheter placed into the superior vena cava. This procedure is frequently used when the patient has a problem (e.g., esophogeal stricture or fissure) that prevents oral ingestion of nutrients for a prolonged period of time. Special solutions are prepared throughout the 24 h.

Each institution varies in the actual technique of administration, but all procedures should include:

  a. Absolute sterile technique (including the use of gowns, masks, and gloves).
  b. Changing of all external tubing at least every other day.
  c. Careful observation of the patient for signs of inflammation, including redness, pain, and swelling at the catheter site and body temperature elevation. If drainage is present, culture the infection site.
  d. Changing dressing daily or as the institution prescribes.
  e. Cleaning skin around catheter site and using an antibiotic ointment (Betadine) as prescribed.
  f. Covering the catheter with a sterile dressing and securing carefully.
  g. Weighing the patient daily.

  2. After the acute stage, the diet can be progressed, and diet teaching should be instituted. A high-calorie, high-protein, low-residue diet should be explained. Roughage is avoided to minimize mechanical irritation. Chemically irritating foods should be avoided. Patients with a history of milk intolerance should restrict their milk intake. Iron may also be supplemented orally.

H. Psychologic aspects of care can be complex. During the acute phase, explanation and reassurance should be offered. Emotional stress should be minimized. Psychiatric consultation may be indicated, and individual, group, or family therapy may be beneficial. Occasionally, antidepressant drugs may be given.

II. Surgical intervention.

A. About 15 to 40 percent of patients hospitalized for ulcerative colitis require surgery. Surgical intervention will often be considered in the event of hemorrhage, obstruction, perforation, toxic megacolon, or failure of the patient to respond to treatment.

B. The procedure is usually permanent and involves total *proctocolectomy* and ileostomy. The colon and rectum are removed with the end of the ileum to create an opening to the abdomen (Fig. 29-6). More recently, an ileostomy with an intraabdominal pouch and an artificial sphincter has been developed (see Fig. 29-6e).

C. *Preoperative care* involves building up the patient's resistance with blood, albumin, electrolytes, vitamins, diet, and/or hyperalimentation as needed, and cleansing the bowel. Some physicians use oral antibiotics in an effort to "sterilize" the bowel. Patients should be prepared for the drastic change in elimination. Often a visit from a patient with an ileostomy is helpful.

FIGURE 29-6 / **Various procedures for fecal diversion. (*From D. A. Jones et al., Medical-Surgical Nursing: A Conceptual Approach, McGraw-Hill Book Company, New York, 1978.*)**

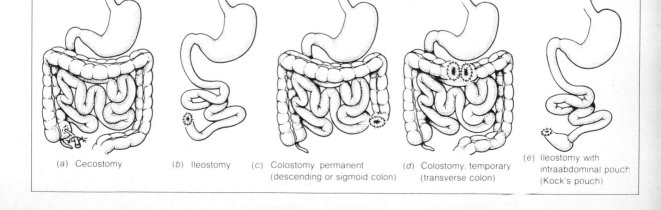

(a) Cecostomy   (b) Ileostomy   (c) Colostomy permanent (descending or sigmoid colon)   (d) Colostomy, temporary (transverse colon)   (e) Ileostomy with intraabdominal pouch (Kock's pouch)

D. *Postoperative care* should focus on the usual threats following surgery, namely, infection, fluid losses and/or hemorrhage, and respiratory difficulties. The patient will have an abdominal wound, the stoma, and a perineal wound. Nothing will be given orally, and a nasogastric tube will be in place until bowel sounds return. Measures to relieve pain should also be implemented.

1. When ready to learn, the patient should be taught to care for the ileostomy. Because of the digestive action of the ileal secretions, the skin around the stoma will be susceptible to breakdown. It should be cleaned, rinsed, and dried well and a protective covering such as sterculia powder or rings applied.

2. The patient should be fitted with a close-fitting appliance after the stomal edema has subsided. Drainage from an ileostomy is generally semiliquid to soft and continuous, making a permanent appliance necessary.

3. No specific dietary restrictions are necessary. However, patients should avoid foods that had a laxative effect prior to surgery. It is often best to add foods to the diet one at a time so that intolerance can be pinpointed and the offending food eliminated.

4. After the convalescent period, the patient with an ileostomy can resume normal activities of work and socialization.

E. *Follow-up care* for the patient with an ileostomy should focus on the patient's ability to manage the ostomy. The physical management and psychologic and family adjustment should be evaluated. The patient's financial ability to obtain equipment should also be assessed.

Evaluation

I. Patients with ulcerative colitis should be reassessed at intervals for the development of exacerbations or any complications.

A. Patients with the disease for 10 years or longer are more susceptible to the development of cancer of the colon. Regular sigmoidoscopy will aid in detecting malignant change.

B. A small percentage of patients develop toxic megacolon, an extreme dilatation usually involving the transverse colon.

C. Because the colitis thins the bowel, perforation and peritoitis can occur.

D. Anorectal complications are common. *Rectal fissures* (a cracklike, ulcerous sore), *rectal fistulas* (a tubelike passage from the rectum into surrounding tissue), *rectal abscesses* (collection of pus), and/or hemorrhoids occur and will be found on rectal examinations.

E. Other complications include strictures and pseudopolyps.

II. Severe complications such as cancer, megacolon, and perforation will require surgical intervention (refer to discussion of colostomy under "Intestinal Obstruction").

Cholecystitis

Definition

Cholecystitis is an inflammation of the gallbladder that usually results from the presence of gallstones (*cholelithiasis*). Most commonly a stone becomes impacted in the neck of the gallbladder or cystic duct, interfering with gallbladder emptying and resulting in inflammation. Initially, the inflammation is chemical, resulting from the action of bile. The normal bacterial flora soon proliferate, and infection ensues. The associated edema causes vascular congestion with the development of thromboses and eventual infarction. The pressure of the gallstone itself results in ischemia, necrosis, and ulceration.

Cholecystitis can occur at any age, but is most frequent during middle age (12). Obese persons develop cholecystitis significantly more frquently than those of average weight. Diet may be a significant factor, with diets high in fat implicated in the genesis of gallbladder disease.

Assessment

During nursing assessment, the patient may be found to be having mild attacks of cholecystitis during which the calculi are dislogd and the discomfort relieved, or the patient may experience an acute attack during which the symptoms do not remit.

I. Data sources (refer to "Oral Cancer")

II. Health history. This will vary according to the severity of the attack. The patient and/or health record should be consulted for any history of cholelithiasis or cholecystitis. A dietary history should be taken and the fat content in the diet estimated. Patients should be questioned about the onset of discomfort. It is often related to ingestion of a heavy, fatty meal.

    A. The pain associated with cholecystitis is termed *biliary colic.* Initial episodes are often mild, characterized by a constant epigastric ache or mild indigestion. As the inflammation becomes acute, the pain steadily increases in severity. The patient often complains of extreme pain that is worse in the right upper quadrant and may radiate to the shoulder or subscapular area.

    B. Patients are frequently anorexic and may complain of nausea and/or vomiting.

    C. Patients should be questioned about any changes in the color of their urine or stools. With common bile duct obstruction, the urine will darken and stools will become clay colored.

III. Physical assessment. Examination of the patient with acute cholecystitis will reveal a patient in extreme distress.

    A. The severity of the abdominal pain may cause the patient to be guarded, making the abdominal examination difficult. The patient will experience discomfort with fist percussion over the liver. The gallbladder may be palpable as a tender mass. When the inflammatory process is extensive, paralytic ileus can develop and is evidenced by abdominal distention and an absence of bowel sounds.

    B. The skin and sclera of the eye should be examined for evidence of jaundice. A slight icterus is common, but more severe jaundice usually indicates obstruction of the common bile duct by calculi or edema.

    C. The patient's temperature should be taken, as it usually becomes elevated with infection. Vital signs will show a mild degree of tachycardia and hypotension if complications have not developed.

    D. The severe pain often causes the patient to splint during respirations, and rales may be heard at the bases of the lungs.

    E. The patient should be weighed and the result compared with weight norms, as cholecystitis has been associated with obesity.

IV. Diagnostic tests.

    A. *Oral cholecystography* is often used to visualize the gallbladder. The patient is given an oral radiopaque substance, such as isopanoic acid (Telepaque), sodium ipodate (Oragrafin), or sodium tyropanoate (Bilopaque), which concentrates in the gallbladder making it visible on x-ray. Usually, six tablets are given the evening before, although the test must often be repeated for adequate visualization. Some authorities recommend giving six tablets 2 days before and again the day before testing, for a total of 12 tablets (13). Others prefer a procedure modification that involves giving the six tablets the day before over a 6-h period and preceding their administration with a meal containing fat to maximize absorption (14). Nonvisualization after the second test is indicative of impairment in bile excretion.

    B. In the interest of time, acutely ill patients will often be tested using *intravenous cholangiography.* A dye containing iodine is injected intravenously and the gallbladder visualized.

    C. With *percutaneous cholangiography,* the dye is injected directly into a bile duct using a long, spinal-type needle. Fluoroscopy shows ductal filling and localizes any obstructions.

    D. During *endoscopic retrograde cholangiopancreatography* (ERCP), a flexible fiberscope is inserted into the small intestine and a cannula passed through the scope to the ampulla of Vater and into the bile duct. Obstructions can be directly visualized.

    E. *Ultrasonic scanning* may be used to detect calculi.

    F. Several *laboratory tests* contribute to the assessment data base. The leukocyte count is usually elevated reflecting the inflammation. There also may be a slight hyperbilirubinemia. The serum alkaline phosphatase is elevated, as are the serum glutamic-oxaloacetic transaminase (SGOT) and lactate dehydrogenase (LDH) levels. Urine bilirubin levels may be elevated and the urobilinogen in the feces decreased.

Problems

I. Abdominal pain.
II. Anorexia, nausea, and vomiting.
III. Fever.
IV. Shallow respirations.
V. Jaundice.
VI. Apprehension.

Diagnosis

I. Complains of pain, often severe, especially in the right upper quadrant and radiating to the shoulder.
II. Alteration in nutrition: loses appetite, tolerates fatty foods poorly, and often feels nauseous with occasional vomiting.
III. Temperature is elevated with occasional chills (secondary to an inflammatory response).
IV. Breathing is shallow causing chest congestion (secondary to abdominal pain).
V. Slight jaundice making the skin susceptible to breakdown. With more pronounced jaundice, experiences itching.
VI. Apprehension about worsening pain, and fear of possible surgery.

Goals of Care

I. Immediate.
  A. Alleviate the pain.
  B. Prevent nausea and vomiting.
  C. Arrest the infection.
  D. Promote removal of respiratory secretions and prevent respiratory infection.
  E. Prevent skin breakdown.
  F. Relieve itching.
  G. Alleviate fears and promote psychologic comfort.
II. Long-range.
  A. Promote adequate nutrition.
  B. Attain normal weight.
III. *Priorities of care* should focus on relieving the pain, nausea, and vomiting, with interventions then instituted to prevent respiratory infection and skin breakdown and decrease the inflammation.

Intervention

I. Nursing care.
  A. To minimize gallbladder stimulation, the patient will usually be given nothing by mouth. A nasogastric tube (see Fig. 29-3) may be inserted to relieve nausea and vomiting and keep the stomach empty. Antiemetics may also be given for nausea and vomiting. With bed rest, 75 percent of cases will remit in 1 to 4 days, and intake can be gradually advanced to a high-carbohydrate, high-protein, low-fat diet. Patients experiencing intolerance to fatty food, while encouraged to avoid them, may be given replacement therapy with oral bile salts. The fat-soluble vitamins are also frequently supplemented.
  B. Parenteral fluids will be given to meet nutritional needs and replace fluid losses from the edema, nasogastric tube, diaphoresis, and kidney.
  C. Pain is controlled with parenteral meperidine rather than morphine, as the latter has a stronger spasmogenic effect on the bile duct.
  D. Anticholinergic drugs may be given to decrease secretion and muscle spasm.
  E. Antibiotics that concentrate well in the biliary tract, such as ampicillin, tetracycline, or a cephalosporin, are usually given to decrease infection.
  F. The patient should be encouraged to take deep breaths and cough. Splinting the abdomen may help reduce added pain. Position should be changed frequently to prevent respiratory congestion and skin breakdown.
  G. Patients should be discouraged from itching. Cholestyramine resin may be helpful in lessening the pruritus. Frequent skin care will also be helpful.
  H. An experimental form of treating cholelithiasis involves the administration of

chenodeoxycholic acid to dissolve cholesterol stones (15). More recent investigations have combined chenodeoxycholic acid an β-sitosterol (16) and cholic acid and lecithin (17).

II. Teaching should focus on a decrease in fat intake, avoidance of fatty foods, and weight reduction as needed.

III. Authorities disagree as to the indications for *surgery*. Some prefer the more conservative approach outlined previously, while others advocate immediate surgical intervention.

A. The most common procedure involves removal of the gallbladder (*cholecystectomy*). This is often accompanied by exploration and drainage of the common bile duct (*choledochotomy*). *Cholecystotomy* (removal of stones from the gallbladder) is performed if the patient is unable to tolerate a more extensive procedure.

B. Postoperatively the patient often has drains to determine if any bile is leaking. These are removed after 4 or 5 days. A T tube (Fig. 29-7) is often placed in the common bile duct and left in place for 7 to 10 days to insure patency of the duct. The skin around the T tube should be protected from breakdown.

C. Following cholecystectomy patients continue to produce bile, but it is discharged into the intestine at a somewhat constant rate. For this reason, patients should be taught to avoid fatty meals. Th fat-soluble vitamins may also have to be supplemented because of the decrease in fat absorption. If the patient is overweight, weight reduction should be encouraged.

IV. Complications after gallbladder surgery are not common. Follow-up care should ensure adequate wound healing, an understanding of dietary restrictions, and adherence to a weight reduction program.

Evaluation If patients have not been treated surgically, reoccurrence of an acute attack is a possibility.

I. Patients should be evaluated regularly to assess any episodes of pain, indigestion, etc. A patient's adherence to a low-fat diet should be determined. Any indications of reoccurrence should be referred for treatment.

II. Patients with cholecystitis need to be watched regularly for ensuing complications. These can include acute perforation with peritonitis, subacute perforation with abscess formation, biliary fistula formation, or pancreatitis.

III. On occasion, small stones may be left in the common bile duct, and several weeks after

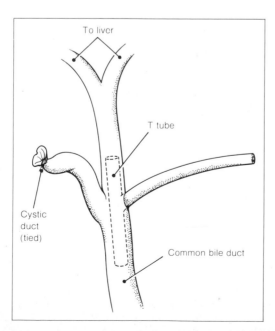

FIGURE 29-7 / The T tube. (*From D. A. Jones et al., Medical-Surgical Nursing: A Conceptual Approach, McGraw-Hill Book Company, New York, 1978.*)

surgery the patient may begin to manifest symptoms similar to those presented prior to surgery. When possible, the stones are identified through x-ray, and attempts are made to dissolve the stones. However, if this fails, surgery may be necessary.

Acute Pancreatitis

Definition

Acute pancreatitis is a sever, incapacitating illness characterized by inflammation of the pancreas. Its genesis involves the activation of pancreatic proteolytic and lipolytic enzymes within the pancreas resulting in autodigestion of pancreatic tissue. Initially, the inflammation results in edema, but as venous congestion develops, pancreatic necrosis results. As enzymatic action destroys tissue, vessels can become involved and hemorrhage can occur. Lipases are liberated from the pancreas and fat necrosis often develops (Fig. 29-8). It usually involves the pancreas and surrounding fatty tissue, but can become widespread. As necrotic tissue builds up, infection becomes an increasing danger.

The exact mechanism involved in the development of acute pancreatitis is not known, although several etiologic factors have been implicated. These include pancreatic duct obstruction, biliary tract disease, infection, ischemia, drugs, hypersensitivity reactions, autoimmune phenomena, alcoholism, mumps, and trauma. In 10 to 15 percent of cases no apparent cause is evident (18). It can occur in adults of any age but is seen more frequently after 40 years of age and affects both sexes equally.

Assessment

I. Data sources (refer to "Oral Cancer").
II. Health history. The primary feature of the health history will be pain.
   A. The patient usually describes an intense, upper abdominal pain in the area of the epigastrium or in the left or right upper quadrant. The pain is usually steady and may be referred to the area of the twelfth thoracic vertebra. Initially, the pain is localized but after a time may diffuse to the back, chest, or lower abdomen. The patient may be too distressed to respond to questions, and the family may have to be questioned regarding onset. The pain often develops after a large meal or significant alcohol intake.
   B. Vomiting is a second common feature. The patient often relates episodes of forceful vomiting which continue even after the stomach is empty and increase the pain.
   C. The patient, family, and/or health record should be consulted for any history of gallbladder disease, alcoholism, mumps, or trauma. Any drugs the patient has taken in the recent past should be identified.
III. Physical assessment. Examination will reveal a restless, distressed, and apprehensive patient.
   A. The patient may obtain pain relief by curling up with both arms over the abdomen, making the abdominal examination difficult. At best there will be guarding in the epigastrium. The abdomen will appear distended and will be tender to deep palpation. Rebound tenderness will also be present. As the inflammation becomes more widespread, boardlike rigidity of the abdominal wall develops. Bowel sounds will be diminished or, if paralytic ileus has developed, absent.
   B. Signs of hypovolemia and shock will become evident as fluid losses to the edema are marked. The skin often appears mottled and feels cold and moist. Tachycardia is present, and the blood pressure falls.
   C. Hemorrhage can develop 3 to 6 days after onset and may be evidenced by Turner's sign, a blue-green-brown discoloration in the flanks from blood accumulation, or Cullen's sign, a similar discoloration around the umbilicus.
   D. Respirations are often shallow and rapid. Rales may be heard in the lower lobes, and pleural effusion, especially on the left side, may develop.
   E. The temperature should be taken, as fever is usually present after a few days.
   F. If edema compresses the common bile duct, jaundice will become evident and the urine will darken. Stool specimens ar often difficult to examine because constipation is present.

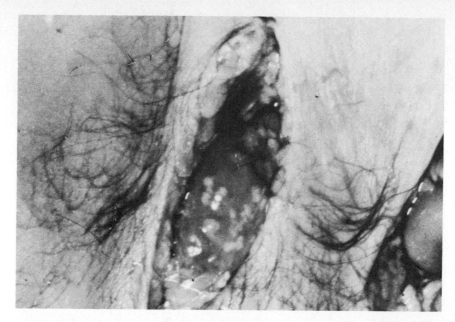

FIGURE 29-8 / Fat necrosis on the external surface of a femoral hernia sac in a patient who died of acute pancreatitis. (*From A. Bogoch, Gastroenterology, McGraw-Hill Book Company, New York, 1973.*)

IV. Diagnostic tests. None are specific for pancreatitis.
  A. A common finding, however, is an increase in the serum amylase, above 250 Somogyi units, which begins to return to normal after 48 h. The serum lipase will also be elevated.
  B. With widespread fat necrosis, hypocalcemia and signs of tetany can develop. The liberated lipases break fat into glycerol and fatty acids. Some of these fatty acids unite with calcium to form soap, thus depleting the serum calcium.
  C. With islet cell damage, the blood glucose becomes elevated.
  D. Fluid losses to the edema lead to hemoconcentration and an increase in the hematocrit.
  E. Other laboratory tests include an increase in white blood cells.
  F. X-ray of the abdomen will reveal gaseous distension, and calcification of the pancreas from previous inflammations may be seen.
  G. Chest x-ray will show an elevation on the left side of the diaphragm, and left pleural effusion may be seen.

Problems

  I. Abdominal pain.
  II. Vomiting.
  III. Hypovolemia.
  IV. Respiratory congestion.
  V. Inflammation.
  VI. Infection.
  VII. Altered nutritional status.
  VIII. Hypocalcemia.
  IX. Hyperglycemia.

Diagnosis

  I. Complains of constant, severe, upper abdominal pain, due to pancreatic inflammation, that radiates to the back.
  II. Has experienced forceful vomiting with retching that increases the pain.
  III. Fluid loss to the edema causes restlessness, dizziness, tachycardia, and hypotension. Hemorrhage may contribute to hypovolemia.
  IV. Chest expansion is restricted, secondary to pain, resulting in shallow respirations.
  V. Has massive inflammation with abdominal distension (secondary to pancreatic inflammation).

     VI. Has developed infection with fever.

    VII. Nutrition is altered because of a decrease in pancreatic enzymes secreted into the intestine.

   VIII. May become hypocalcemic with tetany developing.

    IX. Has an elevated blood glucose level secondary to metabolic changes in glucose.

     X. Feels general apprehension (mild to severe) and anxiety due to pain.

Goals of Care

     I. Immediate.
      A. Relieve the pain.
      B. Control the vomiting.
      C. Prevent shock.
      D. Prevent pulmonary infection.
      E. Decrease the inflammation by decreasing the action of the pancreatic enzymes.
      F. Control the infection.
      G. Prevent tetany.
      H. Prevent ketoacidosis.

    II. Long-range.
      A. Maintain adequate nutritional status.
      B. Prevent reoccurrence.

   III. *Priorities of care* should focus on preventing shock and respiratory embarrassment and controlling the pain and vomiting.

Intervention

     I. Nursing care.

      A. Blood volume will be maintained with plasma, human serum albumin, and electrolyte solutions. The amounts will be titrated to the hematocrit, central venous pressure, and urine output results, which will be monitored frequently. The blood pressure and pulse will also be followed carefully to evaluate the extent of hypovolemia. If hemorrhage has occurred, whole blood may be given. The patient is often placed on a cardiac monitor to observe for changes in cardiac rhythms (see Chap. 26).

      B. Pain is usually controlled with meperidine because it causes less spasm of the sphincter of Oddi than the opiates. Pentazocine may also be used. If maximum doses of meperidine are not effective, morphine must be considered. Positioning the patient on one side with the knees and back flexed is often helpful. A sedative, given in conjunction with the analgesic, is often helpful. On rare occasions, a nerve block is used to relieve the pain.

      C. Pulmonary congestion should be avoided by having the patient take deep breaths, cough, and change position frequently. Intermittent, positive-pressure breathing may be helpful.

      D. To relieve distension and decrease gastric acid stimulation of pancreatic secretions, a nasogastric tube with intermittent suction will be used to keep the stomach empty. The patient will receive nothing by mouth. Antacids may be administered through the tube to further decrease gastric acidity.

      E. Various drugs may be used to affect the pancreatic secretions. Acetazolamide (Diamox), a carbonic anhydrase inhibitor, decreases the volume and bicarbonate concentration of pancreatic secretions. Anticholinergics may also be used to decrease pancreatic secretion. Aprotinin (Trasylol), an antiproteolytic substance which inhibits kallikrein, chymotrypsin, and trypsin, is currently being investigated (19).

      F. Antibiotics will be given to treat infection.

      G. The serum calcium level should be monitored. Calcium gluconate will be given intravenously for hypocalcemia.

      H. Intravenous corticosteroids may be given if the shock does not respond to intravascular volume replacement.

      I. The urine and serum glucose levels should be monitored. Insulin will be given to control hyperglycemia.

      J. Glucagon may be given because it tends to suppress pancreatic secretion and increase blood flow to the intestines. The use of insulin-glucose infusions is also being investigated (20).

K. After the initial fasting period, as the patient improves, sips of water will be allowed. If tolerated, the diet will be advanced to carbohydrate drinks. After the pain has subsided for at least a week, the diet will be progressed to a low-fat intake of small, frequent meals. The avoidance of alcohol and caffeine should be stressed. If pancreatic destruction has been extensive, supplementation with enteric-coated pancreatic digestive enzymes may be indicated.

L. Patients should be cautioned of the danger of diabetes mellitus. Signs and symptoms to watch for should be taught and the importance of avoiding a high-carbohydrate diet with concentrated sweets and refined sugar stressed.

II. *Surgery* is avoided unless the patient fails to improve or complications develop. Procedures may involve cleaning the peritoneal cavity, draining the area of the pancreas, or relieving compression in the biliary tract. More extensive procedures include opening the pancreatic duct and anastomosing it to the jejunum or removing part or almost all of the pancreas (*pancreatectomy*).

III. *Follow-up care* should focus on preventing reoccurrence by ensuring adherence to diet restrictions and promoting adequate nutrition. If the patient has lost a significant amount of pancreatic tissue, diabetes mellitus will be a threat and should be watched for.

Evaluation

I. Complications must be watched for so that appropriate interventions can be instituted.
A. About 3 to 4 weeks after onset, abscesses from infection or pseudocysts can form.
B. Frank diabetes mellitus can develop at any time and may be temporary or permanent.

II. Small pseudocysts may resolve spontaneously. Surgery may be needed to drain an abscess or large pseudocyst.

Chronic Pancreatitis

Definition

Chronic pancreatitis is a long-term inflammation of the pancreas. It usually begins after 30 to 40 years of age and is found in men more often than women. Many factors have been implicated as causative agents. The most common of these is chronic alcohol ingestion; other causes include biliary tract disease and trauma.

Symptoms usually develop in two stages. Initially, the inflammation causes an acute episode with attacks of abdominal pain. As chronicity develops, the pain becomes constant. Significant portions of the pancreas are destroyed, and its production of endocrine (insulin and glucagon) and exocrine hormones (pancreatic enzymes) becomes impaired. Digestion is incomplete, with azotorrhea and steatorrhea characterized by bulky, frothy, glistening, foul-smelling stools. Weight loss occurs, and complaints of nausea, vomiting, a feeling of fullness, and abdominal distension are common. Diabetes mellitus results from the endocrine disorder.

Problems

I. Weight loss with vitamin deficiencies.
II. Foul, loose stools.
III. Pain.
IV. Impaired glucose metabolism.

Intervention

Nursing care and treatment during an acute attack is similar to that during acute pancreatitis.
I. Care during chronic disease must focus on avoidance of alcohol.
II. A bland, low-fat diet will be given, and pancreatic extracts will be used to improve digestion.
III. Overating should be avoided, and anticholinergics may relieve pain.
IV. Because of the chronic nature of the disease, narcotics should be avoided.
V. Vitamin and electrolyte supplements will be given as needed.
VI. Diabetes mellitus will be treated, if present (refer to Chap. 24).
VII. Follow-up care is essential.

Hepatitis

Definition

Hepatitis may be defined as an inflammation of the liver. When caused by a substance that is toxic to the liver, it is called *toxic* or *drug-induced hepatitis*. Some of the offending agents include industrial toxins such as carbon tetrachloride and yellow phosphorus, the toxin associated with mushroom poisoning, halothane, diphenylhydantoin, α-methyldopa, chlorthiazide, and oxyphenisatin.

The more common type of hepatitis involves *viral infection*. The most common types ar hepatitis A and hepatitis B. A third viral type, sometimes referred to as type C or non-A, non-B hepatitis, has recently been discovered (21). It appears to be associated with blood transfusions, has a variable incubation period (usually 6 to 7 weeks), and is less severe than type B hepatitis (22). The pathologic changes observed in all hepatitis involve inflammation of the liver with hepatic cell necrosis, regenerative activity, Kupffer cell hyperplasia, and varying degrees of bile stasis.

Type A viral hepatitis may be called infectious hepatitis, short-incubation hepatitis, MS-1 hepatitis, or epidemic hepatitis. The type A virus is usually transmitted through the fecal-oral route, although parenteral transmission can occur. After entry into the body, its incubation period is 15 to 50 days before symptoms begin. Type A occurs throughout the world, but is most commonly found in areas with poor sanitation facilities. It occurs more often in the fall and early winter and is more frequent in children and young adults.

Type B viral hepatitis has been called serum hepatitis, long-incubation hepatitis, MS-2 hepatitis, and Australia antigen-positive hepatitis. The incubation period for type B is 50 to 180 days. It is most frequently transmitted when the blood of an infected person comes in contact with the blood or mucous membrane of another person. This can occur with transfusions, needle puncture, skin cut, sexual intercourse, hemodialysis, kissing, etc. Type B hepatitis can also be transmitted through the fecal-oral route.

Types A and B hepatitis differ in onset. With type A it is often sudden and febrile, while the prodromal phase in type B is usually insidious and fever is seldom evident. The morbidity and mortality is greater with Type B.

Assessment

The accuracy of a good health history and physical examination cannot be stressed enough in the patient with hepatitis, as the information presented will give the health team much data critical to good health care.

I. Data sources (refer to "Oral Cancer").
II. Health history. During the health history it should be remembered that symptoms of hepatitis usually progress through three phases: prodromal phase, icteric stage, and recovery period.
   A. The *prodromal phase,* sometimes referred to as the preicteric phase, usually lasts 3 to 4 days but may extend to 2 weeks or more. Initially, the patient often complains of anorexia, fatigue, malaise, and lassitude. As the inflammation spreads, nausea, vomiting, and diarrhea often develop, and the patient may have an aversion to food and distaste of cigarettes. Arthralgia, myalgia, and headache may occur. The patient often describes a fullness or discomfort in the epigastrium or right upper quadrant late in this phase. Fever and flulike symptoms may be evident, especially with type A. Occasionally, the patient experiences skin rash, urticaria, angioneurotic edema, or polyarthritis. During the last few days of this stage the patient may note the urine darken, a lighter stool color, and some itching.
   B. The *icteric phase* is characterized by jaundice, which becomes maximum in 1 to 2 weeks and lasts 6 to 8 weeks. During this phase the patient will feel better, with the gastrointestinal symptoms and fever decreasing. Infrequently, a patient with hepatitis will never become jaundiced (anicteric hepatitis).
   C. The *recovery period* lasts 3 to 4 months, during which the patient will find that he or she fatigues easily.
   D. The patient and family should be questioned about any contact with jaundiced persons, camping trips, shellfish ingestion, traveling outside of the country where

sanitation is poor, blood transfusions in the last 6 months, ear piercing, tattooing, and the like, which may be indicative of possible hepatitis. The patient's health record should be consulted for past parenteral therapy and any history of hepatitis. The type of work the patient does, living quarters, and drugs taken should all be elicited.

III. Physical assessment. Findings are usually not remarkable.

    A. The patient's temperature may be mildly elevated during the prodromal phase.

    B. The patient should be weighed and the results compared with a previous weight record. Weight loss commonly occurs.

    C. During the abdominal examination, the liver is usually tender and palpable 2 to 3 cm below the costal margin. The liver size begins to decrease 1 to 2 weeks after the onset of jaundice.

    D. Jaundice is a prominent feature of the physical examination and is best observed in the sclera of the eyes.

IV. Diagnostic tests. Several laboratory tests are used to evaluate the patient with hepatitis. The significance of liver function tests may be found in Table 29-3.

    A. The most definitive test distinguishes type A from type B hepatitis. During the incubation and early acute phase, 80 percent of patients with type B hepatitis have hepatitis B antigen (HBsAg, Australia antigen) circulating in their serum.

    B. Other laboratory test results include elevations in the SGOT and SGPT 7 to 14 days prior to jaundice, an increase in the direct and indirect bilirubin, Bromsulphalein retention, a mild increase in serum alkaline phosphatase, mild hypoalbuminemia, slight increases in globulin, and leukopenia if fever develops.

    C. Examinations of the urine and stool show the urine urobilinogen usually normal initially and later increased, the urine bilirubinincreased, and the stool bilirubin and urobilinogen both decreased.

    D. The serum of patients who have had hepatitis A will contain antibody to the hepatitis A antigen (anti-HA). The anti-HA titer increases late in the course of hepatitis A but is not a definitive diagnostic tool.

Problems

I. Anorexia, nausea, and vomiting.
II. Fatigue.
III. Pain.
IV. Fever.
V. Jaundice.

VI. Itching.
VII. Weight loss.
VIII. Possible spread of infection.
IX. Irritability.
X. Boredom.

Diagnosis

I. Alteration in nutrition: has a poor appetite, dislikes food, and may occasionally feel nauseous and vomit.
II. Tires easily and is unable to meet work requirements.
III. Complains of epigastric discomfort and may ache in muscles or joints.
IV. Has a mild fever, secondary to infection.
V. Is jaundiced, making skin susceptible to breakdown.
VI. Widespread itching that is difficult to relieve (secondary to jaundice).
VII. Has lost weight over the last few weeks due to decreased appetite.
VIII. Is infectious and can potentially infect others.
IX. Is angry with restrictions and feels irritable.
X. Is unable to fill the time during the day without becoming bored.

Goals of Care

I. Immediate.

    A. Prevent spread of the infection to others.

    B. Promote adequate nutrition.

    C. Promote rest and prevent fatigue.

    D. Relieve any pain and discomfort.

    E. Prevent skin breakdown.

    F. Foster interactions, and relieve boredom.

TABLE 29-3 / TESTS OF LIVER FUNCTION

Test	Normal	Comment
Blood Clotting and Blood Cell Count		
Prothrombin time	12–15 s	Prothrombin time most important test in assessing liver pathology. In liver disease, blood takes longer to clot owing to decreased ability of the liver to synthesize the protein prothrombin. Also, there is decreased absorption of vitamin K which is essential for prothrombin synthesis. Failure of the liver to return the prothrombin time to normal in presence of vitamin K indicates clinically significant liver cell damage. The degree of liver impairment can fairly accurately be estimated by the degree of prothrombin abnormality.
Hematocrit	35–45%	
WBC	5000–10,000 cells/mm^3	Normal early in cirrhosis and hepatitis. Leukopenia with enlarged, overactive spleen. Leukopenia accompanies fever in hepatitis.
Clearance Studies		
Indocyanine green (ICG) Bromsulphalein (BSP)	Less than 5% remaining in serum 45 min after injection of 5 mg/kg body weight	Procedure: Patient fasts for 12 h before test. Dose is reduced if clinical symptoms already present. Dye retained in liver cell damage.
Serum Enzyme Studies		
SGPT SGOT LDH	5–35 U/mL 5–40 U/mL 400 U/mL (varies with method used)	Damage to liver cells causes release of these enzymes into blood, but the increased levels in the serum do not directly correlate with the amount of liver impairment. Elevations occur in other diseases. Blood withdrawn from vein.
Alkaline phosphatase	2–5 Bodansky units (varies with method)	Synthesized in liver, bone, and kidney and excreted in the biliary tract. A measure of biliary obstruction.
γ-Glutamyl transpeptidase		Enzyme found in biliary tract and not in cardiac or skeletal muscle. Elevated in hepatitis. More sensitive in detecting hepatic disease than alkaline phosphatase.
Special Tests		
Hepatitis B surface antigen (HBsAg)		HBsAg is normally absent from the serum and, if present, is diagnostic for vital hepatitis, type B. Tests for HBsAg include counterelectrophoresis and radioimmunoassay. Not found in serum of patients with type A viral hepatitis.
Liver scan		Through the injection of a radioactive substance, the therapist can visualize the size and shape of the liver. Serves as a guide for liver biopsy.
Liver biopsy		Used to determine microscopic, cellular pathology of liver cells.
Hepatic hemodynamic studies (in patients with suspected cirrhosis)		Splenoportogram is used to determine the adequacy of portal blood flow. Diminished in cirrhosis. Endoscopy to view esophageal varices. Measurement of portal vein pressure.

TABLE 29-3 / TESTS OF LIVER FUNCTION (Continued)

Test	Normal	Comment
Metabolic Studies		
Protein metabolism:		Serum proteins are synthesized by the liver. Serum albumin is markedly decreased in liver cellular damage. Gamma globulin is usually elevated in liver disease and markedly elevated in chronic active liver disease.
Serum albumin	3.5–5.5 g/100 mL	
Plasma fibrinogen	10.2–0.4 g/100 mL	
Serum globulin	2.5–3.5 g/100 mL	
Total protein	6–8 g/100 mL	
Serum protein electrophoresis	50–65% of total	
Albumin	4–7.5%	
α_1 globulin	4–7.5%	
α_2 globulin	7–12%	
α_2 globulin	7–12%	
β globulin	10–20%	
γ globulin		
Ammonia	30–70 μg/100 mL	In liver disease, less ammonia is converted to urea, and thus the serum ammonia concentration increases.
Carbohydrate metabolism:		
Galactose or glucose tolerance tests	Removed from blood in 1–2 h	Injected intravenously, and serial samples are drawn from the vein. If serum galactose remains elev after 75 min, liver function is impaired. If serum glucose remains elevated after 1–2 h, the liver cells are damaged or utilization of glucose by body tissues is impaired.
Fat metabolism:		Blood drawn after low-cholesterol diet. Cholesterol esters 70% of total cholesterol. Lipids decreased in liver parenchymal cell damage, elevated in biliary duct obstruction.
Serum cholesterol	150–250 mg/100 mL	
Serum phospholipids	125–300 mg/100 mL	
Triglycerides	30–135 mg/100 mL	
Bilirubin metabolism:		Venous blood drawn. Bilirubin is a product of RBC hemoglobin breakdown, and elevation may cause jaundice. Total bilirubin measures both direct and indirect bilirubin. Direct bilirubin elevated with obstructed biliary ducts or impaired excretion of conjugated bilirubin. Indirect bilirubin elevated with accelerated erythrocyte hemolysis, absence of glucuronyl transferase, and/or damaged liver cells.
Serum bilirubin	0.2 mg/100 mL	
Direct (conjugated, soluble)	0.8 mg/100 mL	
Indirect (not conjugated, not water soluble)	1.0 mg/100 mL	
Total bilirubin		
Urine bilirubin	None	A measure of conjugated bilirubin. If bilirubin present in urine, shaking the specimen results in a yellow tint in the foam. Urinary and fecal urobilinogen decrease with bile duct obstruction. Antibiotics reduce the urobilinogen levels. Fecal urobilinogen seldom measured.
Urobilinogen		
Urine	0–4 mg/24 h	
Feces	40–280 mg/24 h	

Source: I. B. Alyn, "Disturbances in Hepatic Function," in D. A. Jones et al. (eds.), *Medical-Surgical Nursing: A Conceptual Approach,* McGraw-Hill Book Company, New York, 1978.

II. Long-range.
A. Complete recovery from hepatitis.
B. Prevent relapse.
C. Promote weight gain.
III. *Priorities of care* must initially focus on preventing spread of the infection.

Intervention

I. *Nursing care* should be established to prevent spread of the infection.
A. Any avenue of entrance from the gastrointestinal or parenteral route must be considered.
B. Procedures should include hand washing, isolation of linen, separate toilet facilities, separate or disposable dishes, no communal items such as washcloths or toothbrushes, no sexual contact, and the use of disposable needles.
C. The family should be included in all discussions whenever possible.
D. Human immune serum globulin (ISG), if given to persons exposed to type A hepatitis during the incubation period, will stimulate antibody production and provide immunity for 6 to 8 weeks. Usually, 0.02 to 0.05 mL per kilogram of body weight is given.
II. *Treatment* for hepatitis is supportive and symptomatic in nature.
A. Adequate rest is important, and bed rest with bathroom privileges is usually recommended. Stress should be minimized.
B. Adequate nutrition is essential for the liver to heal and regenerate. Usually, a high-calorie (3000-cal), high-carbohydrate, high-protein diet, in small, frequent feedings, is recommended. Fat is usually restricted because of intolerance. Alcohol should be avoided for at least 6 months following the onset of hepatitis.
C. Drug therapy may include the use of corticosteroids to decrease the inflammation in severe cases. Sedatives and analgesics should be used cautiously; those eliminated through the kidney are preferable. If the prothrombin time is prolonged, vitamin K may be given parenterally.
III. Most patients recover in 4 to 12 weeks. Relapses, however, occur in 5 to 25 percent of adult patients during the first 4 months.
A. *Follow-up care* should focus on the patient's steady recovery. If any indications of relapse become evident, laboratory values should be checked promptly and supportive measures instituted.
B. Patients with Type A and B hepatitis generally have a lasting immunity to the specific type. Patients, however, have been known to develop a second case, and it is thought that there may be more than one type A virus.

Evaluation

During the recovery period patients should be evaluated for the development of posthepatitis syndrome.
I. *Posthepatitis syndrome* is characterized by a complex of vague symptoms that may include fatigue, weakness, malaise, anorexia, vague upper abdominal discomfort, and poorly defined gastrointestinal symptoms and often lasts 6 to 12 months. Continued rest and good nutrition are critical in the prevention of secondary infection.
II. Infrequently, hepatitis can result in postnecrotic cirrhosis. After recovery, patients should be watched for its development.

Oral and Perioral Inflammations

Definition

There are a variety of inflammations that occur in or around the oral cavity. These include gingivitis, Vincent's angina, periodontitis, stomatitis, aphthous stomatitis, and herpes simplex.
I. *Gingivitis* is an inflammation of the gums. It can result from infectious origin because of poor dental hygiene, such as food debris in the mouth, or excessive dryness of the mouth, or as a manifestation of systemic disease. There is also a chronic, desquamative gingivitis that occurs in postmenopausal women.

II. *Vincent's angina* (trench mouth) is an infectious gingivitis thought to be caused by bacteria that are normally found in the mouth. Local trauma, poor oral hygiene, nutritional deficiencies, and debilitation have been implicated as precipitating factors. It is a malodorous infection with painful ulcers found along the margins of the gums. The ulcers have a punched-out appearance. Regional lymph nodes are often enlarged, salivation is increased, and fever is present. Occasionally, the infection will spread to the cheeks, lips, tongue, palate, and/or pharynx.

III. *Periodontitis* involves inflammation of the gums as well as structures in the periodontal pockets that support the teeth. As the inflammation destroys tissue, the teeth loosen.

IV. *Stomatitis* is an inflammation of the mouth. Its most common causes are mechanical (e.g., jagged teeth), chemical, or infectious (e.g., virus, bacteria, yeast, mold). It is usually associated with a loss of appetite, halitosis, and increased salivation. *Stomatitis medicamentosa* can develop as a reaction to drugs, such as iodides, barbiturates, antibiotics, sulfonamides, salicylates, and cytotoxic drugs. *Stomatitis venenata* is a contact stomatitis that can be caused by cosmetics, mouthwashes, toothpaste, drugs, or snuff.

V. *Aphthous stomatitis* (canker sores) is the most common mouth inflammation and can occur on the lips, gums, inner surface of the cheeks, palate, tongue, or labia. It is associated with small, reddened macules that form vesicles, necrose, and ulcerate, leaving a lesion with a gray, white base and reddened halo. The lesions are usually painful and heal spontaneously in 1 to 2 weeks. The cause is not known, but it is most common in young women, often recurs rhythmically, and may be preceded by emotional or physical stress.

VI. *Herpes simplex* is an inflammation of the mouth caused by the herpes simplex virus, usually consisting of cold sore(s) and fever blister(s). It is often preceded by fever, headache, and malaise. Vesicular lesions develop and progress to multiple, small ulcers with red bases. The lesions are painful and may form on the lips, gums, inner cheeks, tongue, and/or oropharynx. The fever and pain last for about 1 week, and the regional lymph nodes are often tender and enlarged. The ulcers usually crust over and heal without scarring in about 2 weeks. Herpes simplex will often recur in the same spot and may be precipitated by fatigue, fever, emotional stress, or an irritant (e.g., sunlight).

Problems

I. Pain.
II. Disinterest in eating.
III. Halitosis.
IV. Fever.
V. Excess salivation.
VI. Malaise.

Intervention

Nursing care should focus on symptomatic care until definitive treatment, if any, relieves the inflammation.

I. Frequent oral hygiene with the use of mouthwashes should be instituted and the patient taught the importance of this.

II. All local and systemic factors that predispose to the inflammation should be removed. This includes local physical irritants. Penicillin and/or antispirochetal agents may be used for infections.

III. Nutrition should be encouraged with a soft, bland diet, and supplemental multivitamins may be given.

IV. Topical medications may include steroids, silver nitrate, or local anesthetics.

V. Estrogen supplements may be given in cases where menopausal changes may have contributed to the inflammation.

VI. Referral for dental care is critical in cases where tooth structures are involved.

Inflammation of the Salivary Glands

Definition

While any of the salivary glands can become inflamed, *parotitis* (inflammation of the parotid glands) is the most common. The best known of these is *epidemic parotitis* (mumps), an acute and highly contagious infection, usually seen in children, which can affect the salivary glands (especially the parotid), testes, pancreas, meninges, and/or central nervous system. It is caused by a virus whose incubation period is 8 to 28 (18) days. The person is contagious from several days before to 10 days after the onset of symptoms. It is characterized by anorexia, malaise, fever, a sore throat, and parotid tenderness. Treatment is symptomatic. With the development of a mumps vaccine, its incidence has decreased.

More frquently seen in adults is an *acute suppurative parotitis* that is usually caused by *Staphylococcus aureus* and may develop as a complication of severe illness. Debilitation and dehydration are thought to contribute to its development. The parotids become swollen and tender with local pain, fever, and chills. If the swelling is severe, facial paralysis can develop.

Problems

I. Pain.
II. Fever.
III. Dehydration.

IV. Contagion.
V. Facial paralysis.

Intervention

Nursing care should focus on preventing dissemination of the bacteria and healing the infection.
I. Antibiotics will be given to fight the infection.
II. The patient's fluid status must be carefully monitored and dehydration prevented to ensure adequate secretion by the salivary glands.
III. Heat may be applied locally to foster vasodilatation and hasten healing.
IV. If the swelling is severe and unrelieved, the gland may be incised and drained.

Esophagitis

Definition

Esophagitis is an inflammation of the esophagus that can result from esophageal trauma (discussed below), gastric reflux, or systemic conditions, such as scleroderma or tuberculosis. *Peptic* (reflux) *esophagitis* is the most common and results from the backflow of gastric secretions into the lower esophagus. While it can occur at any age, its incidence increases from 40 to 60 years of age. Reflux esophagitis has been associated with hiatus hernia, pregnancy, obesity, straining, peptic ulcer disease, gastroesophageal surgery, persistent vomiting, intubation, and severe systemic infection. It causes a generalized inflammation that can erode and ulcerate, eventually healing with fibrosis and scar tissue formation.

Esophagitis causes retrosternal, epigastric pain that may radiate to the throat, jaws, arms, or back. It generally begins a few minutes after eating and persists for a couple of hours. Belching may offer some relief. The patient often has difficulty swallowing and complains that food "sticks" in the lower esophagus. The dysphagia is worse when eating solids and at the beginning of a meal. Coughing and choking may be evident, especially at night or in the recumbent position. If bleeding occurs, it is usually mild and chronic.

Problems

I. Pain.
II. Dysphagia.
III. Aspiration.

IV. Weight loss.
V. Anemia.

Intervention

Nursing care should focus on minimizing the inflammation, alleviating pain, preventing aspiration, and promoting good nutrition.
I. A bland diet, with four or five small feedings, eaten slowly and well chewed, is recommended. Because dietary indiscretions (e.g., spicy foods) and alcohol are associated with exacerbations, they should be avoided. Keeping the head elevated after eating is also helpful. Obese patients should be encouraged to lose weight.
II. Milk and antacids are often given every 1 to 2 h. For severe pain an anesthetic/antacid preparation may be given. A constant intraesophageal drip of antacid may also be used.

III. Barbiturates are sometimes given to decrease spasm. Anticholinergics should be avoided because they tend to increase reflux.

IV. Emotional stress should be minimized as it can cause painful esophagospasm.

Acute Gastritis

Definition   *Acute gastritis,* inflammation of the stomach, can result from a variety of causes that include acute alcoholism, thermal, chemical, or bacterial irritants, infiltrative diseases, food poisoning, various drugs, acute illness, heavy metal poisoning, uremia, and shock. It usually results in anorexia, nausea, and vomiting with epigastric pain and fever. If severe, hemorrhage can develop. The inflammation can last several hours to days and usually heals spontaneously.

Problems

I. Nausea and vomiting.   IV. Pain.
II. Fluid and electrolyte imbalance.   V. Possible shock (refer to Chap. 44).
III. Fever.

Intervention

I. Nursing care is usually supportive and often includes antacids to neutralize stomach acid, antispasmodics, and a bland diet.
II. Any offending agent (e.g., alcohol) should be eliminated.
III. If the inflammation causes erosion with hemorrhage, iced saline lavage, gastric cooling, and/or gastric resection may be necessary.
IV. Prevention of dehydration is important. Monitor urinary output and fluid intake. Intravenous therapy may be required in severe cases of fluid imbalance.
V. Check vital signs frequently.

Chronic Gastritis

Definition   *Chronic gastritis* is found more frquently in older people and may involve inflammatory or atrophic changes. Its cause is unknown, but its occurrence is associated with chronic alcoholism, aspirin use, endocrine disorders, pernicious anemia, carcinoma, polyps, gastric ulcer, and chronic debilitating disease. Often it is asymptomatic but may cause occasional nausea and anorexia. Vomiting occurs after eating, and the patient often awakes with a bad taste in her or his mouth. Dull epigastric discomfort may be felt.

Problems

I. Lack of appetite.   III. Discomfort.
II. Weight loss.   IV. Possibility of gastric carcinoma.

Intervention

I. Nursing care should focus on promoting nutrition with frequent small feedings of a bland diet.
II. Antacids may offer some relief.
III. Any possible precipitating factors should be eliminated or treated.
IV. Avoid stress.

Regional Enteritis

Definition   *Regional enteritis* (Crohn's disease) is a chronic inflammatory disease of the small bowel. The terminal ileum is involved in 40 percent of cases, although occasionally the colon, rectum, and (rarely) the stomach are involved. It is a problem seen more frequently in young people, although any age group can be affected. While many factors have been implicated, the cause is not known.

Its onset is insidious, with malaise, loss of appetite, mild episodes of diarrhea, intermittent pain, weight loss, and fever developing slowly. The stool usually contains occult blood, and anemia is common. The pain is felt most frequently around the umbilicus and in the right lower quadrant. Cramping is often increased after eating and lessened with defecation. The formation of rectal fissures, fistulas, and abscesses may occur.

Problems	I. Severe weight loss. V. Anemia.

Problems

I. Severe weight loss.
II. Diarrhea.
III. Fluid and electrolyte imbalances.
IV. Pain and cramping.

V. Anemia.
VI. Fever.
VII. Debilitation.

Intervention

Nursing care for the patient with regional enteritis is similar to that discussed under "Ulcerative Colitis."

I. A well-balanced, high-calorie, high-protein diet is encouraged.
II. The pain, cramps, and diarrhea are treated symptomatically.
III. Surgical intervention is not popular because recurrence of the enteritis after surgery occurs in 50 percent of patients.

Dysentery

Definition

Dysentery refers to a variety of intestinal disorders that are characterized by inflammation of the gastrointestinal tract. They can be of bacterial, viral, protozoal, parasitic, or chemical origin. Salmonella infections are the most common bacterial cause. Viral infections are often referred to as "intestinal flu."

Dysentery is associated with some degree of diarrhea. This can range from moderately loose stools to frequent, watery stools that contain blood and pus. Flatulence is often present and colicky, abdominal pain experienced. Fever is usually evident. Bacterial and viral infections are usually associated with *gastroenteritis* (inflammation of the stomach and intestine) and often result in nausea, vomiting, and malaise as well as diarrhea.

Problems

I. Nausea and vomiting.
II. Diarrhea.
III. Pain.
IV. Lethargy.

V. Fever.
VI. Fluid and electrolyte losses.
VII. Contagion (often).

Intervention

Nursing care should focus on symptomatic relief, eradicating the offending agent, and preventing fluid and electrolyte imbalances.

I. Diarrhea is often controlled with antidiarrheal agents, anticholinergic drugs, and/or narcotics.
II. Appropriate antimicrobial agents will be employed to eliminate the offending organism.
III. Fluid and electrolyte status should be monitored and losses replaced orally or parenterally.

Diverticulitis

Definition

Diverticula are small outpouchings that can occur anywhere in the gastrointestinal tract. They are not common in the esophagus and occur rarely in the stomach. The most common type found in the small intestine is *Meckel's diverticulum,* which is a developmental anomaly that usually does not cause difficulties. Diverticula are found most often in the colon. The occurrence of multiple diverticula is called *diverticulosis.* Of all persons over 50 years of age in the United States, 20 percent are thought to have diverticulosis. The cause is not known, but it may be associated with colonic hypermotility. Diets high in fiber tend to decrease its occurrence.

Diverticulosis is most often a silent condition that does not cause difficulty. About one-fifth of cases, however, become inflamed (*diverticulitis*). This is thought to develop as the pouches do not empty completely and food and bacteria collect. Lower abdominal pain that often lasts 1 to 10 days results. The pain is worse after eating, and guarding may be evident. Some degree of constipation and abdominal fullness develops, and fever is usually present. Chronic blood loss may also occur. If the diverticulum ruptures, peritonitis, ileus, and shock will quickly develop.

Problems

I. Pain.
II. Constipation.
III. Weight loss.
IV. Fever.
V. Anemia.

Intervention

Nursing care should focus on decreasing the infection, promoting adequate hydration, and fostering normal elimination.

I. Bed rest is indicated until the infection is controlled.
II. A broad-spectrum antibiotic will be given and liquids encouraged.
III. Anticholinergic drugs are often used to decrease pain.
IV. Initially, a liquid diet and tool and softener will be given to minimize mechanical stimulation. As the inflammation subsides, diet teaching should focus on a diet high in vegetable and fruit fiber. Supplemental unprocessed bran and/or bulk laxatives may also be indicated.
V. In severe cases, where medical management fails or attacks occur repeatedly in the same area, surgical intervention may be considered (refer to "Intestinal Obstructions").

TRAUMA

Esophageal Trauma

Definition

The esophagus can be injured in several ways. The most common of these is a burn from the ingestion of corrosive or hot liquids. Foreign bodies can also lodge in the esophagus, traumatizing tissue. Last, the esophagus can be injured from external trauma such as during an esophagoscopy. This discussion will be limited to chemical burns of the esophagus (*acute corrosive esophagitis*).

The agents involved in chemical burns are usually alkalis (e.g., ammonia, washing soda, bleach, lye, drain cleaners, and dishwashing detergents) or acids (e.g., toilet bowl cleaners, rust removers, iodine, silver nitrate, and sulfuric, nitric, hydrochloric, acetic, or oxalic acid). Both types of agent result in intense inflammation with mucosal edema and esophagospasm. Areas of necrosis develop and are surrounded by intensely inflamed areas. With sloughing of necrotic tissue, ulcers form. Fibrous healing then occurs, and strictures often develop. Because of the esophagospasm, entrance of the agent into the stomach is limited, decreasing injury to the gastric mucosa. Burns caused by alkalis are usually deeper than acid burns.

Assessment

I. Data sources (refer to "Oral Cancer").
II. Health history. Following ingestion of corrosive materials the patient will be in severe distress and may be unable to give an accurate health history.
  A. A description of the type and amount of substance ingested should be sought from the patient or family. Ideally, a sample of the substance should be obtained for analysis, especially if the nature of the substance is in question.
  B. The family should be questioned about any attempts at first aid and whether any vomiting occurred.
  C. Any past history of psychiatric difficulties may be illuminating if the ingestion was intentional.
  D. Pain will be the patient's primary complaint. It is usually an intense, violent pain, behind the sternum and often referred to the back and neck. It may be accompanied by vomiting which will increase injury to the pharynx, mouth, and lips.
III. Physical assessment. Examination will reveal an acutely ill, severely distressed patient.
  A. Respiratory status should be carefully assessed. Edema in the throat often decreases patency of the airway. As it becomes occluded, stridor will become evident.

      B. Vital signs should be evaluated, as the fluid losses associated with edema often result in hypovolemia and shock (refer to Chap. 44).

      C. The oral cavity should be carefully examined. Burns of the lips and mouth are often noted. Salivation is increased, and the patient may experience pain and/or difficulty with swallowing.

      D. Vomiting may lead to retching, and the vomitus usually contains blood and mucus.

      E. The temperature should be taken, as fever is often present.

   IV. Diagnostic tests. After the acute inflammation has subsided, *esophagoscopy* may be performed to determine the extent of injury.

Problems

   I. Pain.
   II. Dysphagia, with decreased nutrition.
   III. Airway obstruction.
   IV. Hypovolemia.
   V. Possible infection.
   VI. Psychiatric problems.

Diagnosis

   I. Complains of severe retrosternal pain that radiates to the neck and back.
   II. Has difficulty swallowing which is painful, limiting nutritional intake.
   III. Can potentially develop respiratory difficulties if laryngeal edema causes airway obstruction.
   IV. May become dehydrated with hypovolemia developing secondary to decreased ingestion of food.
   V. Has large aras of open lesions which can become infected.
   VI. May be emotionally ill, if ingestion was intentional.

Goals of Care

   I. Immediate.
      A. Maintain patent airway.
      B. Prevent shock.
      C. Alleviate pain.
      D. Prevent infection.
   II. Long-range.
      A. Promote adequate nutrition.
      B. Foster mental health.
   III. *Priorities of care* should focus on maintaining a patent airway, preventing shock, and alleviating the pain.

Intervention

   I. Nursing care *during the acute phase* should be aimed toward neutralizing the chemical and preventing complications.

      A. The corrosive chemical should be neutralized within a few minutes with alkaline agents. The patient should be given milk, water, fruit juice, dilute vinegar, 2% acetic acid, or lemon juice. Acidic chemicals can be diluted with milk, water, sodium bicarbonate, or 1 tbsp of milk of magnesia in 1 cup of water. Areas that are accessible should be washed with copious amounts of water.

      B. Vitals signs and urine output should be monitored frequently to detect the development of hypovolemia. Parenteral fluids are usually given to replace fluid losses.

      C. During the acute phase, laryngeal edema can develop. The patient should be watched closely, and a tracheostomy set should be kept at the bedside (refer to Chap. 27).

      D. The patient's pain is often severe, and analgesic medication will be necessary.

      E. Corticosteroids are usually given for 4 to 6 weeks. They act to decrease the inflammation and, therefore, subsequent scar tissue formation.

      F. Prophylactic antibiotics are given to prevent secondary infection.

      G. Fluid and nutritional requirements are often met intravenously during the acute phase. After a few days, if the patient can swallow, does not have a fever, and there is no danger of perforation, clear liquids and milk will be given orally.

   II. *After the acute phase,* the development of strictures with esophageal obstruction becomes a danger.

      A. A nasogastric tube (refer to Fig. 29-3) will be initially inserted to maintain patency of the esophagus during the acute inflammation.

B. About a week after ingestion of the chemical, esophageal dilatation will be started in an attempt to decrease stricture formation. The procedure involves passing a well-lubricated, small-caliber bougie daily and gradually increasing its size until the lumen of the esophagus is stable. Some physicians use an olive-shaped metal dilator for the same purpose (refer to Fig. 29-5).

C. After the burns have healed, if stricture formation prevents dilating the esophagus through the above method, retrograde passage may be employed. A string is passed through the nose and esophagus into the stomach and brought out through a gastrostomy tube. The two ends are joined making a continuous loop. Dilators can then be attached and pulled through from the stomach.

III. *Follow-up care* should focus on the patient's nutritional status and mental health.

A. The patient's diet may be restrictive, especially if strictures have formed. The weight should be monitored. The diet should be reviewed with the patient. Depending on the esophageal lumen, the diet may range from a normal consistency to liquids only.

B. The patient who intentionally ingested the corrosive agent should be referred for long-term psychiatric help.

Evaluation

I. About two-thirds of patients who survive esophageal burns develop esophageal stenosis, and increased dysphagia should be watched for. This often occurs 3 to 6 weeks after the ingestion. Severe cases of stricture formation that do not respond to bougienage may require surgery. The procedure usually involves resection of the esophagus or replacement of it with a piece of colon or jejunum.

II. Occasionally, if gastric injury has occurred, pyloric stenosis can develop and should be watched for. (Refer to Chap. 16 for a complete discussion.)

OBSTRUCTIONS

Intestinal Obstruction

Definition

Intestinal obstruction occurs when the intestinal contents fail to progress through the small and/or large intestine. It can be caused by mechanical or nonmechanical factors. Some of the mechanical factors include gallstones, worms, adhesions, hernias, volvulus (a twisting of the bowel upon itself), intussusception (slipping of part of the intestine into the part below it), and tumors. Nonmechanical factors can result in an adynamic (paralytic) ileus or a dynamic (spastic) ileus. A dynamic ileus occurs most frequently in response to trauma (i.e., surgery), peritoneal irritation, hypoxia, or metabolic changes (i.e., hypokalemia), while dynamic ileus is uncommon and is often associated with toxic conditions. Table 29-4 summarizes some of the causes of intestinal obstruction.

Uncomplicated intestinal obstruction has a 15 percent mortality rate; 9000 deaths per year in the United States can be attributed to it (23). It causes widespread pathophysiologic changes that make the patient severely ill. As obstruction occurs, air and fluid accumulate in the proximal intestine, and distension develops. About 70 to 80 percent of the gaseous distension is attributed to swallowed air. Fluid accumulates primarily from that produced by the intestines. Normally about 8 L of fluid is produced and reabsorbed. As obstruction occurs, not only is this production increased, but reabsorption is decreased, increasing further the fluid losses to the intestinal lumen. In the first few hours after obstruction, the intestine attempts to "push past" the obstruction by increasing peristalsis. As the bowel dilates, however, motility decreases, and eventually atony develops.

As distension increases, pressure decreases the venous return to the intestinal wall. Fluid from the intestinal capillaries is lost to the lumen, bowel wall, and peritoneal cavity. As the splanchnic circulation becomes inadequate, intramural hemorrhage and necrosis occur. The bowel wall becomes permeable, and fluid as well as bacteria is lost to the peritoneal cavity. The fluid losses into the intestinal lumen and peritoneal cavity eventually cause dehydration. If the intraluminal pressure is unrelieved, the bowel will eventually burst. These changes are usually gradual, but can develop rapidly if an obstruction strangulates part of the intestine.

TABLE 29-4 / CAUSES OF SMALL BOWEL OBSTRUCTION

I. Mechanical occlusion of lumen.
  A. Intrinsic defects of intestine.
    1. Congenital defects.
      a. Errors in rotation of intestine.
      b. Duplications and cysts.
      c. Meckel's diverticulum.
    2. Inflammatory lesions.
      a. Regional enteritis.
      b. Tuberculosis.
      c. Diverticulitis.
      d. Eosinophilic granuloma.
    3. Tumors.
      a. Benign.
      b. Malignant.
    4. Traumatic lesions.
      a. Strictures.
      b. Hematomas.
    5. Intussusception.
    6. Radiation strictures.
    7. Endometriosis.
    8. Pneumatosis intestinalis.
  B. Obturation obstruction.
    1. Gallstones.
    2. Bezoars.
    3. Foreign bodies.
    4. Enteroliths.
    5. Worms.
    6. Balloons of intestinal tubes.
  C. Volvulus.
    1. Primary.
    2. Secondary.
      a. Associated congenital abnormality.
      b. Secondary surgical artifact.
      c. Secondary bands, adhesions, stenosis, or obturation.

  D. Extraintestinal lesions.
    1. Adhesions and bands.
    2. Hernia.
      a. Extraabdominal: inguinal, femoral, umbilical, ventral, diaphragmatic, lumbar, epigastric, interstitial, prevesical, obturator, sciatic, perineal, Richter's or Littre's.
      b. Intraabdominal: paraduodenal, foramen of Winslow, paracecal, intersigmoid, through omental or mesenteric defect, or through broad ligament.
    3. Compression by extraintestinal mass.
      a. Carcinomatosis.
      b. Intraperitoneal abscess.
      c. Adjacent tumor.
      d. Pregnancy.
      e. Foreign body.
      f. Superior mesenteric artery duodenal obstruction.
      g. Annular pancreas.
      h. Wandering spleen.
  E. Obstruction secondary to surgical operation (other than adhesions).
    1. Intraperitoneal abscess.
    2. Wound dehiscence.
    3. Anastomotic obstruction (stricture or edema).
    4. Anastomotic leak.
    5. Obstruction at external stoma.
    6. Hernia through peritoneal defect.
    7. Volvulus about fixed point.
II. Obstruction with open lumen.
  A. Paralytic ileus.
  B. Spastic ileus.
  C. Mesenteric vascular occlusion.

Source: A. Bogoch, *Gastroenterology,* McGraw-Hill Book Company, New York, 1973.

Assessment

I. Data sources (refer to "Oral Cancer").
II. Health history. During the health history the patient, family, and/or health record should be consulted for any history of cancer, polyps, chronic inflammatory conditions such as diverticulitis or ulcerative colitis, and abdominal operations.
  A. Indications of chronic obstruction should be elicited. Complaints may include increasing constipation, vague, diffuse pain, lower abdominal cramps, and/or occasional abdominal distension.
  B. Patients with mechanical obstruction usually describe a rhythmical, colicky pain that reaches a peak and then subsides. In small bowel obstruction the pain is usually in the mid abdomen, while the pain associated with large bowel obstruction is frequently located in the lower abdomen and is less severe.
  C. Patients with adynamic ileus usually do not experience pain until the distension becomes severe and the abdomen tight.
  D. Nausea and vomiting commonly occur with obstruction. Th higher the obstruction is located, the earlier they occur and with increasing severity. The patient initially will vomit the stomach contents, then the intestinal contents, so that the vomitus eventually becomes fecal in character.

E. Once the intestine distal to the obstruction is empty, absolute constipation (obstipation) will occur.

III. Physical assessment. This should focus on the abdominal and rectal examinations.

    A. The patient's abdomen will appear distended. The lower the obstruction, the worse the distension. Early in the obstruction, peristalsis may be visible, and as the proximal intestine contracts, high-pitched gurgling and eventually tinkling sounds will be heard on auscultation. As motility decreases and eventually ceases, so do bowel sounds. With adynamic ileus, bowel sounds are diminished or absent from the onset. Percussion of the abdomen will reveal tympany, and with mechanical obstruction guarding and abdominal tenderness are present during palpation.

    B. A careful rectal examination should be performed, as obstructions in the rectum can often be felt.

    C. The vital signs and fluid status should be carefully watched for indications of dehydration, shock, or sepsis. If the obstruction is strangulated and becomes gangrenous, the pain will worsen, tachycardia will develop, the temperature will rise, and the blood pressure will fall. If a strangulated obstruction becomes perforated, sepsis will ensue, manifested by pallor, sweating, cold, clammy extremities, tachycardia, hypotension, and disorientation.

IV. Diagnostic tests.

    A. The most useful diagnostic test is a flat, film x-ray of the abdomen. It usually will show the gas-filled intestines.

    B. A *sigmoidoscopy* or *proctoscopy* may be attempted to visualize a low obstruction. The procedure is very painful and uncomfortable for patients with obstruction since it involves the insertion through the rectum of an inflexible tube. Through this tube the bowel can be visualized and biopsies taken (see "Ulcerative Colitis"). The patient is forced to assume a jackknife type of position for the duration of the test in order to make the visualization of the bowel more accessible.

    C. A *barium enema,* carefully done, may be attempted if colonic obstruction is suspected. This will occasionally correct obstructions caused by volvulus or intussuception. (See "Ulcerative Colitis" for discussion of procedure.)

Problems

I. Pain.
II. Abdominal distension.
III. Nausea and vomiting.
IV. Fluid and electrolyte imbalances.
V. Anxiety.

Diagnosis

I. Complains of colicky pain that may be centered in the mid or lower abdomen (secondary to distension and obstruction).
II. Abdomen is distended, increasing pain and limiting respiratory expansion.
III. Occasionally vomits fecal material secondary to obstruction.
IV. Has lost large amounts of fluid to the abdomen and from vomiting, and can potentially develop hypovolemia.
V. Is extremely apprehensive, and is having difficulty comprehending what is happening.
VI. Fears disruption in body image secondary to radical surgery.

Goals of Care

I. Immediate.
    A. Relieve pain.
    B. Prevent fluid and electrolyte imbalances.
    C. Alleviate vomiting.
    D. Decrease distension.
    E. Remove obstruction, and restore gastrointestinal integrity.
    F. Promote adequate nutrition.
    G. Relieve anxiety.
II. Long-range.
    A. Promote regular bowel habits.
    B. Prevent recurrence.
III. *Priorities of care* should focus on relieving the distension and alleviating the pain.

Intervention

I. *Nursing intervention* should initially be aimed toward decompression of the distended bowel, relief of pain, and replacement of fluid losses.

    A. A *nasogastric tube* (see Fig. 29-3) attached to intermittent suction is the simplest method for decompression if the obstruction is high in the intestine. Some physicians prefer inserting a tube to the point of obstruction. This is accomplished by inserting a long *intestinal tube* with a weighted tip through the nose and into the stomach. The weighted tip, then, allows it to be advanced by peristalsis. Once in the intestine, the tube will be advanced by the nurse at regular intervals, until it reaches the point of obstruction. The location of the tube should be frequently checked during insertion by x-ray or fluoroscopy. It will usually be attached to gravity or low, continuous suction. When intestinal tubes are used, a nasogastric tube will also be necessary to keep the stomach empty.

    B. Patients with mechanical obstruction will require *medication for pain*. As the intestinal distension is relieved, the pain will lessen.

    C. If the obstruction is strangulated, sepsis becomes a threat, and broad-spectrum *antibiotics* may be given.

    D. Fluid losses should be replaced with *intravenous fluids*. The amount is usually determined by the urine output, central venous pressure, and hematocrit. Unless the obstruction is very high, acidic fluids from the stomach and alkaline fluids from the intestines are both lost, and acid-base imbalances do not develop. Saline intravenous fluids with added potassium chloride will usually meet the patient's needs.

    E. Until the obstruction is relieved, the patient will be given *nothing by mouth*. Nutritional needs will be met by intravenous glucose solutions with supplemental vitamins.

    F. For patients with *paralytic ileus*, symptomatic care and/or removing the causative factor often will effect a return of peristalsis. For example, hypoxia should be reversed or hypokalemia corrected. Occasionally, a medication regimen will be tried where the patient is first given a sympathetic blocking agent to decrease the antiperistaltic effect and then given a cholinergic drug to promote the parasympathetic effect of increasing motility.

    G. During the acute phase, patients will be apprehensive and should be reassured. Explanations should be offered frequently and the patient allowed to ventilate fears.

II. *Surgery* is needed to relieve most mechanical obstructions. Several procedures may be employed.

    A. *Surgical decompression* is a palliative measure that may be employed if the patient is too ill to undergo more extensive surgery. It involves the insertion of a *cecostomy* tube in an opening in the bowel. The tube is then brought out through the abdominal wall (see Fig. 29-6a).

    B. A *bowel resection* will be done if the diseased portion of the bowel can be removed and the ends anastomosed.

    C. A *colostomy* involves creating an avenue for bowel excretion by opening the colon and bringing it to the abdominal wall (see Fig. 29-9).

        1. A *temporary colostomy* is done when there is hope that the lower (distal) portion of the colon will heal and normal elimination can be restored (e.g., trauma, diverticulitis). It is usually kept 3 to 6 months and involves bringing a loop of bowel to the abdominal surface and creating two holes. One will allow the proximal intestine to empty and the second will communicate with the distal portion of the colon (Fig. 29-6d).

        2. A *permanent colostomy* is most frequently done when there is cancer close to the anal sphincter. The colon is opened and brought to the surface, while the rectum and distal section are removed (Fig. 29-6c).

            a. *Preoperative care* should focus on cleaning the intestine and preparing the patient psychologically. Continuous support is critical. For all surgeries that involve opening the bowel, special attention will be given to cleaning the intestines. Cleansing enemas will be given, and often poorly absorbed

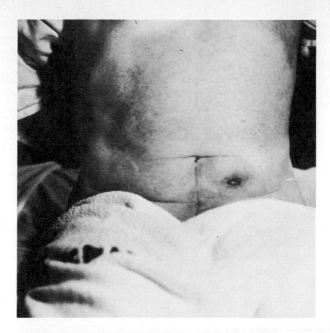

FIGURE 29-9 / Colostomy stoma. (*From D. A. Jones et al., Medical-Surgical Nursing: A Conceptual Approach, McGraw-Hill Book Company, New York, 1978.*)

antibiotics are used in an attempt to sterilize the bowel. The nature of the surgery should be fully discussed with the patient, and time should be provided for questions and concerns. Where possible, the family should be included in the discussions. Often a visit preoperatively from a patient with a colostomy helps to alleviate some anxiety and provides the patient with an additional opportunity to discuss pertinent issues.

  b. *Postoperative care* will initially focus on the usual concerns following surgery: hemorrhage, atelectasis, thrombophlebitis, and infection. When the patient is ready, physically and psychologically, he or she should be taught to care for the colostomy. Patients with colostomies often can be trained to perform regular evacuation of soft to formed stool with suppositories, irrigations, or finger dilation. Appliances should be properly fitted and community resources made available. Dietary restrictions will be minimal and are usually dictated by the patient's needs. If diarrhea is a problem, residue should be decreased. For constipation, patients should be taught to increase residue. In general, flatus can be partly controlled by avoiding gas-forming foods. Patients must adjust to a significant change in body image and should be given support in this process.

III. *Follow-up care* after intestinal obstruction will depend on the cause and treatment. Adynamic ileus is not likely to recur unless the cause recurs. Because most mechanical obstructions are treated surgically, patients should be watched for adequate healing and any recurrence of obstruction. Patients with a colostomy should be evaluated in terms of their ability to cope both physically and mentally with the change.

Evaluation

The mortality rate for intestinal obstruction increases to 35 to 40 percent if complications develop (24). The patient's general condition, vital signs, and response to treatment should be continually reassessed to detect any of the following complications. Immediate interventions should be instituted to reverse the problem.

  I. *Strangulation* occurs when the blood supply to a segment of bowel is cut off. Gangrene can develop.

II. With strangulation or severe distension, *perforation* can occur, spilling intestinal contents into the peritoneal cavity, which may lead to peritonitis and possible sepsis.

III. If fluid losses are severe and not corrected, *hypovolemia* and *shock* can develop (refer to Chap. 44).

IV. As the bowel becomes increasingly inflamed and necrotic areas appear, *infection* can occur (refer to "Inflammatory Disorders").

V. As the abdominal distension presses on the diaphragm, lung expansion decreases and *pneumonia* can develop (refer to Chap. 27).

VI. Vomiting can result in *aspiration pneumonitis*.

VII. Follow-up care is essential.

Hernias

Definition A *hernia* is a projection (rupture) of the abdominal contents through a weakness in the muscular wall that encloses the peritoneal cavity. Penetration of the intestines through the opening can be constant or intermittent. If the intestines can be returned into the peritoneal cavity, the hernia is *reducible*. If this is not possible, it is considered *irreducible* or *incarcerated*. When the size of the abdominal opening compromises the blood supply to the protruding intestine, the hernia is *strangulated*. Hernias result from a defect in the abdominal wall that can be caused by a congenital weakness, trauma, aging, or increased intraabdominal pressure. The latter can be caused by obesity, pregnancy, heavy lifting, coughing, or trauma.

Hernias occur in a variety of sites. Among the more common are *indirect inguinal hernias,* that pass through the inguinal ring into the canal and can descend into the scrotum; *direct inguinal hernias,* that pass through a weakness in the abdominal wall; *femoral hernias,* that pass through the femoral ring; *hiatus hernias,* that result in the stomach partially entering the thorax through a weakness in the diaphragm; *umbilical hernias,* seen more frequently in children; and *incisional hernias.*

Problems Nursing problems are usually minimal.

I. Often the patient experiences only a lump that disappears when lying down.

II. Vague discomfort and epigastric pain may be felt.

III. If the hernia becomes strangulated, however, the pain will increase and the patient will become acutely ill (refer to "Intestinal Obstruction").

Intervention I. Nursing care should focus on preoperative and postoperative care, as surgical repair is recommended because of the danger of strangulation and intestinal obstruction.

II. If surgery is not a viable alternative, the patient should be taught to keep the hernia reduced with a belt, truss, or well-fitting corset. A pad or sponge may be placed over the hernia.

III. The patient should be instructed to avoid heavy lifting both before and after surgery.

Hemorrhoids

Definition *Hemorrhoids* are varicosities of the hemorrhoidal venous plexus that occur in the anorectal area. They are considered external if covered by skin and internal if covered by mucous membrane. They have been associated with standing erect for long periods, anorectal sepsis, straining, rectal cancer, pregnancy, portal hypertension, and diarrhea. If uncomplicated, hemorrhoids are usually asymptomatic. Acute episodes can develop, however, if they become thrombosed, causing severe pain. Internal hemorrhoids may bleed and can prolapse through the anus, predisposing to thrombosis.

Problems I. Pain, especially on defecation.

II. Bleeding.

III. Anemia (occasionally).

Intervention
    I. Nursing care should focus on symptomatic relief until the thrombosis resolves. This may include bed rest with the foot elevated to increase venous return, analgesics, suppositories (Anusol), sedation, good anal hygiene, witch hazel compresses, and a laxative such as milk of magnesia.

   II. After the acute attack, sitz baths and a low-residue diet may be considered, with evacuation of the clot in external hemorrhoids or hemorrhoidectomy for internal hemorrhoids.

DEGENERATIVE DISORDERS

Hepatic Cirrhosis

Definition
    Hepatic cirrhosis is a chronic, diffuse liver disease that involves hepatic cell loss and necrosis with fibrosis, scar tissue formation, and regeneration. The most common type of cirrhosis is that caused by chronic alcoholism (*Laennec's cirrhosis, alcoholic cirrhosis, fatty cirrhosis*). Laennec's cirrhosis is often preceded by an alcoholic hepatitis and is associated with fatty infiltration of the liver. Malnutrition is a contributing factor and may, in combination with alcohol, cause the hepatic changes. Laennec's cirrhosis occurs in both sexes and all ages but is found more frequently in men about 50 years of age after 5 to 15 years of alcoholic abuse (25).

    While alcoholic abuse is the most frequent cause of cirrhosis, it can also result from other factors. *Postnecrotic cirrhosis* can follow the liver damage caused by viral infections of the liver, chemical intoxications, or hepatic infections. *Biliary cirrhosis* results from bile duct obstruction or intrahepatic cholestasis of unknown etiology. *Hemachromatosis* leads to liver damage and cirrhosis as hemosiderin is deposited in hepatic tissue. *Congestive heart failure* can lead to vena caval hypertension, increasing pressure in hepatic circulation and causing cirrhosis. Hepatic cirrhosis has also been associated with metabolic disorders, infectious diseases, infiltrative diseases, and gastrointestinal disorders.

    All types of hepatic cirrhosis result in widespread disruption of liver function. Metabolic functions, such as the conversion of carbohydrates, fats, and proteins into various nutrients and substances, the storage of vitamins A, D, and E, as well as carotene, and the synthesis of albumin, are diminished. The liver's ability to detoxify ammonia, estrogen, the antidiuretic hormone aldosterone, adrenocorticosteroids, and various drugs, poisons, and heavy metals is decreased. Storage of vitamin B_{12} and iron is impaired, as is vitamin K storage and the synthesis of fibrinogen, prothrombin, and factors V, VII, and X. The ability of the liver to remove bilirubin from the circulation is also diminished.

    As cirrhosis in the liver becomes widespread, the hepatic microcirculation becomes disrupted, and pressure increases in the portal vein. With increasing pressure, collateral circulation develops primarily around the anus (causing hemorrhoids), the esophageal gastric junction (causing esophageal varices), and the abdominal wall and periumbilical area. The pressure from portal hypertension is also communicated to the spleen, causing splenomegaly.

Assessment
    I. Data sources (refer to "Oral Cancer").

   II. Health history. The health history may be obtained from the patient if she or he is coherent and not intoxicated. Often a relative or friend and the previous medical record must be consulted.

       A. Generalized weakness, lassitude, and easy fatigability are common complaints. The patient may also complain of vague upper abdominal discomfort or a dull ache in the upper right quadrant. Anorexia and nausea are common, and the patient may complain of gagging and retching in the morning.

       B. The patient should be questioned about any episodes of slight jaundice, ankle edema, changes in the color of urine or stool, and itching (seldom occurs).

       C. The female patient's menstrual history should be taken, and any changes in sexual function in the male determined. A decreased libido and impotence are common, and women often develop amenorrhea or irregularity.

      D. The patient's use of alcohol should be explored with both the patient and family members. Any history of hepatic infections, biliary disease, cardiac disease, metabolic disorders, or gastrointestinal problems should be elicited. Any drugs the patient takes or chemicals he or she was exposed to should be determined.

  III. Physical assessment. The onset of hepatic cirrhosis is insidious, and changes on physical assessment usually appear late because of the liver's ability to maintain function with loss of up to 75 percent of its mass. After 4 or 5 years, however, the changes are usually obvious on examination.

      A. Weight loss may be visible. Some patients appear emaciated. The weight should be taken and compared with a previous record to document the weight loss.

      B. The skin surfaces of the entire body should be examined.

         1. The characteristic yellow color of jaundice is usually noted and is best observed in the sclera of the eyes.

         2. Because of the decreased synthesis of clotting factors, purpura and bruises are occasionally present.

         3. As estrogen detoxification is decreased, males often lose body hair (alopecia), pubic hair and auxiliary hair are decreased, enlarged breasts (gynecomastia) may be noted, and spider angiomas (spider nevi) are often seen.

         4. The hands should be examined for a mottled redness of the palms (palmar erythema), clubbing of the finger, and Dupuytren's contracture (flexion of the ring and little fingers into the palm).

         5. The skin is dry and there is musculoskeletal wasting.

         6. The tongue may be swollen and red.

      C. The patient's temperature should be taken. An intermittent, low-grade fever without chills is seen in 25 to 50 percent of patients.

      D. Any abnormal collections of fluid should be noted. Initially, ascites occur, but it is soon followed by peripheral edema. The abdominal girth should be measured. Serial measurements usually reveal a gradual increase in size.

      E. Special attention should be given the abdominal examination.

         1. Observation usually reveals spider nevi, distension, and dilated periumbilical veins (caput medusae).

         2. The extent of fluid in the peritoneum can be estimated by testing for shifting dullness and by performing the puddle examination.

         3. Vascular bruits may be heard over the upper abdomen.

         4. The liver will be enlarged, and the edge will feel round and firm.

         5. The spleen may be palpable because of the splenomegaly.

      F. During the rectal examination, hemorrhoids are usually noted and palpation often reveals prostatic atrophy from the estrogenic effect. Testicular atrophy may also be noted.

  IV. Diagnostic tests.

      A. Liver function can be evaluated using *dye clearance studies*. After a 12-h fast, a dye such as Bromsulphalein (BSP) or indocyanine green (ICG), which is removed from the serum by the liver, is injected intravenously. Any retention of the dye in the blood indicates hepatic dysfunction.

      B. Because the liver stores vitamin K and synthesizes various clotting factors, the *prothrombin time* is often prolonged.

      C. Anemia often results from blood loss from esophageal varices, folic acid deficiency, hypersplenism (overactivity of the spleen), and the toxic effect of alcohol on the blood. It is reflected in the hemoglobin, hematocrit, and red blood cell count.

      D. Folic acid deficiency, hyperinsulinism, and the toxic effect of alcohol also result in leukopenia and thrombocytopenia.

      E. Because ammonia is converted to urea by the liver for elimination by the kidney, the *serum ammonia* level is increased.

      F. *Serum alkaline phosphatase,* some of which is synthesized by the liver, is excreted in the biliary tract and will be elevated.

      G. Bilirubin is conjugated by the liver and eliminated in the bile. With hepatic dysfunction *indirect bilirubin* (unconjugated) and *total bilirubin* will be increased. If biliary excretion is impaired, direct bilirubin (conjugated) will also be elevated.

H. *Urine bilirubin* and *urobilinogen* will be increased.

I. *Serum enzymes* such as serum glutamic-oxaloacetic transaminase (SGOT) and serum glutamic-pyruvic transaminase (SGPT), which are liberated during hepatic damage, will be elevated but are not specific indicators of hepatic damage.

J. Because the liver synthesizes many fats, *serum cholesterol, serum phospholipids,* and *triglycerides* will be decreased.

K. The *serum albumin* which is synthesized by the liver will be decreased, and the serum globulins, especially IgG, will be elevated.

L. A *liver scan* is infrequently done to visualize the size of the liver and is used as a guide to liver biopsy. It involves the injection of a radioactive substance. More often a *photoscan* (Scintiscan) will be utilized to outline the liver.

M. A *liver biopsy* may be done to evaluate the microscopic cellular hepatic changes. The procedure involves the insertion of a needle intercostally into the liver and the aspiration of hepatic cells through it. Because of the liver's vascularity, bleeding is a problem. The prothrombin time should be checked prior to the test and vitamin K should be given as needed. Following the biopsy, the patient's vital signs should be closely monitored until all chance of bleeding has passed. The patient should be kept supine or lying on the right side. This latter position causes the abdominal contents to fall against the liver, applying a slight pressure.

N. *Radiography* may be used to evaluate the circulatory changes associated with portal hypertension. The procedures involve the injection of a radiopaque dye into a vessel and subsequent x-ray or fluoroscopy to examine the flow of blood. Studies may include splenoportography, hepatoportography, or celiac arteriography.

O. To directly visualize esophageal varices and/or the gastric mucosa, *esophagoscopy* or *esophagogastroscopy* may be used. The procedure involves the insertion of a flexible tube with a lighted tip and lens into the esophagus and, at times, through to the stomach.

Problems

I. Anorexia, nausea, and vomiting.
II. Weight loss.
III. Fatigue.
IV. Anemia.
V. Malnutrition and vitamin deficiencies.
VI. Fluid retention and ascites.
VII. Electrolyte imbalances.
VIII. Dyspnea.
IX. Jaundice.
X. Pruritus.
XI. Abdominal pain.
XII. Infection.
XIII. Neurologic changes.
XIV. Altered body image.

Diagnosis

I. Alteration in nutrition: loses appetite, occasionally is nauseous, and may vomit in the morning.
II. Has lost weight, which is especially noticeable in a decreased muscle mass, secondary to malnutrition.
III. Fatigues easily and is unable to maintain normal activity level (secondary to anemia).
IV. Is severely malnourished, and is beginning to show signs of vitamin deficiency.
V. Alteration in fluid balance: retains fluid, noticeable in pitting pedal edema and ascites.
VI. Is prone to hyponatremia and hypokalemia due to electrolyte imbalance.
VII. Because of the abdominal distension, is unable to fully expand chest and easily becomes short of breath.
VIII. Is jaundiced, making skin susceptible to breakdown.
IX. Experiences itching over entire body, secondary to jaundice.
X. Complains of mild upper abdominal pain.
XI. Alteration in level of consciousness: is occasionally disoriented and has a heightened response to sedatives, hypnotics, barbiturates, and narcotics, secondary to decreased liver detoxification capability.
XII. Is concerned and embarrassed about abdominal distension, enlarged breasts, hair loss, and sexual difficulties.

Goals of Care   **I.** Immediate.

    A. Correct nausea and vomiting.

    B. Promote adequate nutrition and prevent vitamin deficiency.

    C. Prevent fatigue.

    D. Reverse anemia.

    E. Decrease fluid retention.

    F. Prevent electrolyte imbalance.

    G. Promote adequate ventilation.

    H. Prevent skin breakdown.

    I. Relieve pruritus.

    J. Alleviate abdominal pain.

    K. Prevent disorientation and oversedation.

    L. Foster positive body image.

II. Long-range.

    A. Attain and maintain ideal body weight with healthy muscle mass.

    B. Prevent complications.

    C. Eliminate alcohol abuse.

III. *Priorities of care* should focus on fluid and electrolyte imbalances, neurological and nutritional problems, and changes in oxygenation.

Intervention   **I.** If hepatic cirrhosis is not associated with neurologic or hemorrhagic complications (discussed below), *nursing care* can often be instituted to reverse the problems.

    A. If there is no indication of neurologic involvement, a high-protein (1 g per kilogram of body weight), high-calorie (2000 to 3000 cal) diet will be given in three to four small feedings with nutritional supplements between meals such as eggnog or ice cream. Liquid protein supplements may be used initially. Supplemental multivitamins will be given, and all alcohol will be restricted.

        1. The patient should be encouraged to eat and the environment made conducive to an appetite.

        2. Frequent oral hygiene and minimal movement may help decrease nausea and vomiting. If necessary, antiemetics may be given.

        3. Diet teaching should be done to ensure adequate nutrition after hospitalization.

    B. The fluid retention that results from the portal hypertension (increasing portal hydrostatic pressure), the hypoalbuminemia (decreasing the vascular colloid osmotic pressure), and the sodium and water retention are usually treated with a combination of sodium and water restriction, diuretic therapy, and the intravenous administration of salt-poor albumin. The patient's intake and output should be monitored, and the patient should be weighed daily to assess fluid changes. A daily measurement of the abdominal girth will monitor changes in ascitic fluid retention. Elevating edematous extremities will promote fluid return and decrease retention.

    C. Bed rest will decrease fatigue and improve the patient's overall condition, although the exact reason for this is not clear.

    D. Anemia is usually treated with adequate nutrition, iron supplements, and vitamin B_{12} therapy. Patient teaching should include these medications.

    E. Because the patient is prone to infection, possible sites should be watched closely. Cutdown sites and skin breaks should be cleansed regularly. Personal hygiene should be encouraged. The temperature should be monitored, and exposure to infections should be minimized.

    F. Because of jaundice and pruritus, skin breakdown is a potential problem. To control itching, cholestyramine (Cuemid) may be given. Other nursing procedures should include decreasing anoxia which increases itching (i.e., correcting anemia), minimizing perspiration, decreasing anxiety and emotional stress, avoiding overexertion, minimizing scratching, and avoiding dry skin. The patient's skin should be assessed regularly and the patient turned frequently to avoid skin breakdown.

    G. The route of elimination of all medications given to the patient should be noted;

those eliminated through the liver should be used judiciously. Narcotics, sedatives, hypnotics, and barbiturates should be avoided, if possible.

    H. The body image changes faced by the patient should be discussed, and the likelihood of their resolution should be explained. The patient should be given an opportunity to ventilate concerns.

II. If the ascites is severe enough to cause respiratory embarrassment, hernia, or severe distension, *paracentesis* may be performed.

    A. The procedure involves the insertion of a trocar with an obturator and the removal of fluid from the peritoneal cavity.

    B. Because the ascitic fluid is rich in albumin, it has a depleting effect on the patient. For this reason it is done only when absolutely necessary, and rarely is more than 100 mL removed.

    C. Following the procedure, the patient should be monitored until vital signs are stable and a sample of the fluid sent to the laboratory.

III. *Follow-up care* for the patient with cirrhosis should focus on abstinence from alcohol. This is an extremely difficult goal to attain, and all resources should be considered. This may include individual, family, and/or group therapy. Lay groups such as Alcoholics Anonymous and Al-Anon should especially be considered.

Evaluation

Complications are common in severe cirrhosis, and throughout the treatment period patients should be regularly reassessed to detect their development.

I. As hepatic function fails, ammonia builds up in the blood and interferes with normal brain metabolism. The result is *hepatic coma* (hepatocerebral intoxication, ammonia intoxication, portal-systemic encephalopathy).

    A. Initially, the patient experiences slight apathy and/or euphoria with incoordination which progresses to forgetfulness, confusion, and an inversion of the normal sleep rhythm. The patient becomes restless, untidy, and behaves inappropriately, with picking at the bedclothes. Lethargy and stupor ensue, and finally coma develops. Rarely, the patient develops seizures, but rigidity, hyperreflexia, and a characteristic flapping tremor (*asterixis*) of the hands are usually present. The patient will also have a musty breath odor (*fetor hepaticus*), and changes will be seen on the electroencephalogram.

    B. In an attempt to decrease ammonia absorption from the gastrointestinal tract, a low-protein diet, high in calories to minimize endogenous protein breakdown, will be given.

    C. Because blood is a source of protein, gastrointestinal bleeding should be controlled, and any blood in the stomach should be aspirated. A large-bore Ewall tube is often utilized so large clots can be removed. Laxatives and/or an enema is used to empty the colon of nitrogenous products.

    D. Neomycin is a poorly absorbed antibiotic used to decrease intestinal bacteria. It is their action on protein that produces ammonia.

    E. Lactulose is often given because it acidifies the colon and decreases ammonia absorption.

    F. Because hypokalemia increases ammonia reabsorption by the kidneys, the potassium level is monitored and supplements are given.

    G. For severe cases, heroic measures such as exchange blood transfusions, hemodialysis, plasmapheresis, cross-circulation with humans or animals, extracorporeal pig liver perfusion, charcoal hemoperfusion, and liver homotransplant are being investigated (26).

    H. L-Dopa therapy may be useful in controlling symptoms until the ammonia level is decreased.

II. Patients should also be watched for the development of hemorrhage. As *esophageal varices* become overextended, they often bleed. Control of this bleeding can be complicated if the liver pathology has resulted in clotting defects.

    A. The patient's vital signs and skin temperature should be carefully *monitored for indications of hypovolemia and shock.* If the blood loss is slow, the first indication may be black, tarry stools. All stools should be tested for the presence of blood (guaiac). With rapid blood loss the patient usually vomits bright red or coffee ground emesis (hematemesis).

B. Initial treatment should focus on controlling the bleeding and preventing shock. Blood loss will be replaced intravenously. *Intravenous vasopressin* may also be used to control hypotension and decrease bleeding. The latter occurs because of its vasoconstricting effect on the splanchnic blood flow. Vitamin K will be given if the prothrombin time is prolonged (refer to Chap. 44).

C. *Gastric lavage* with iced saline is often used to control the bleeding initially and remove blood from the stomach. It will be done continuously until the fluid begins to clear.

D. A *Sengstaken-Blakemore tube* is usually inserted to compress bleeding varices. It consists of a three-lumen tube, one going to the stomach for suctioning, one ending in a gastric balloon, and one in an esophageal balloon. After insertion the correct positioning is determined by x-ray, and the two balloons are inflated (see Fig. 29-10). Continuous pressure is then applied to keep the gastric balloon against the cardioesophageal junction. To prevent necrosis the balloons are deflated (esophageal balloon first) in 24 h. After 48 h, if no further bleeding occurs, they are removed. Dislodgment and airway obstruction are constant dangers while using this tube, and scissors should be kept at the bedside.

E. If medical management does not control the hemorrhage, surgery utilizing a *portosystemic shunt* may be considered. The procedure involves diverting blood from the portal vein so that pressure is relieved and esophageal varices are thus

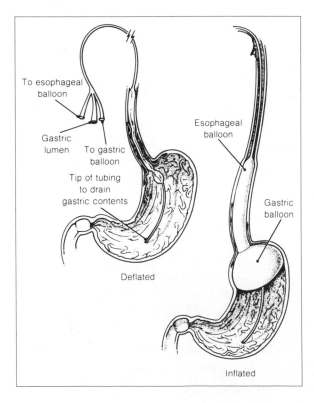

FIGURE 29-10 / Sengstaken-Blakemore tube for bleeding esophageal varices. (From D. A. Jones et al., Medical-Surgical Nursing: A Conceptual Approach, McGraw-Hill Book Company, New York, 1978.)

drained (Fig. 29-11). Because the procedure diverts splanchnic blood from the liver, the ammonia absorbed from the intestine is not detoxified as readily by the liver and hepatic encephalopathy can develop.

    F. Cover the catheter with a sterile dressing and secure carefully.

    G. Weigh the patient daily.

III. Follow-up after complications are treated is essential in order to evaluate long-term response to and compliance with therapy.

FIGURE 29-11 / **Diagrammatic representation of major portal-systemic shunts.** (*From S. I. Schwartz, Surgical Diseases of the Liver, McGraw-Hill Book Company, New York, 1964.*)

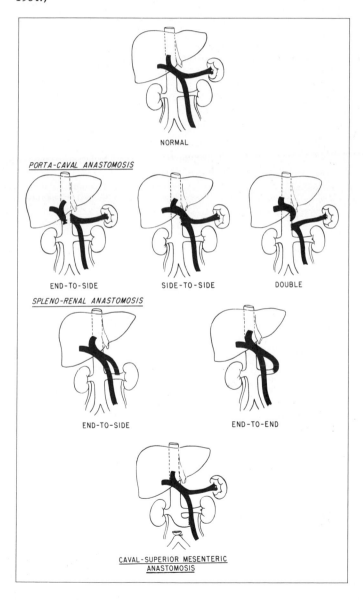

REFERENCES

1. Paul Goldhaber, "Oral Manifestations of Disease," in G. W. Thorn et al. (eds.), *Harrison's Principles of Internal Medicine,* 8th ed., McGraw-Hill Book Company, New York, 1977, p. 204.
2. A. Bogoch, R. Wilson, S. Fishman, M. Kliman, G. Trueman, and G. Norton, "The Stomach and Duodenum," in A. Bogoch (ed.), *Gastroenterology,* McGraw-Hill Book Company, New York, 1973, p. 367.
3. Ibid., p. 368.
4. M. I. Grossman, P. H. Guth, J. I. Isenberg, E. P. Passaro, B. E. Roth, R. Sturdevant, and J. H. Walsh, "A New Look at Peptic Ulcer," *Annals of Internal Medicine,* **84:**57—67, January 1976.
5. C. H. Robinson, *Normal and Therapeutic Nutrition,* The Macmillan Company, New York, 1972, p. 418.
6. Ibid., p. 10.
7. J. Lemanske, "Helping the Ileostomy Patient to Help Himself," *Nursing 77,* **7:**34–39, January 1977.
8. J. T. LaMont and K. J. Isselbacher, "Diseases of the Colon and Rectum," in G. W. Thorn et al. (eds.), *Harrison's Principles of Internal Medicine,* 8th ed., McGraw-Hill Book Company, New York, 1977, p. 1553.
9. Ibid., p. 1558.
10. R. Miller, "The Clean Colon," *Gastroenterology,* **70:**289, February 1976.
11. A. D. McKenzie and R. A. Palmer, "Diseases of the Colon, Rectum, and Anus," in A. Bogoch (ed.), *Gastroenterology,* McGraw-Hill Book Company, New York, 1973, p. 653.
12. R. E. Robins, G. E. Trueman, and A. Bogoch, "The Gallbladder and Extrahepatic Bile Ducts," in A. Bogoch (ed.), *Gastroenterology,* McGraw-Hill Book Company, New York, 1973, p. 880.
13. H. J. Burhenne and W. G. Obata, "Single-Visit Oral Cholecystography," *New England Journal of Medicine,* **292**(12):627–628, March 20, 1975.
14. C. E. Shopfner, "Letter: Cholecystographic Modifications to Improve Initial Study Opacification," *Journal of the American Medical Association,* **234**(5):479–480, November 3, 1975.
15. R. G. Danzinger, A. F. Hofmann, L. J. Schoenfield, and J. L. Thistle, "Dissolution of Cholesterol Gallstones by Chenodeoxycholic Acid," *New England Journal of Medicine,* **286**(1):1–8, January 6, 1972.
16. A. Gerolami and H. Sarles, "Letter: β-Sitosterol and Chenodeoxycholic Acid in the Treatment of Cholesterol Gallstones," *The Lancet,* **2**(7937):721, October 11, 1975.
17. J. Toouli, P. Jablonski, and J. Watts, "Gallstone Dissolution in Man Using Cholic Acid and Lecithin," *The Lancet,* **2**(7945):1124–1125, December 6, 1975.
18. H. R. Robertson and A. Bogoch, "Diseases of the Pancreas," in A. Bogoch (ed.), *Gastroenterology,* McGraw-Hill Book Company, New York, 1973, p. 948.
19. K. J. Worthington and A. Cuschieri, "Estimation of Plasma Esterolytic Activity and Its in Vitro Inhibition by Proteinase Inhibitors during Acute Pancreatitis in the Human," *British Journal of Experimental Pathology,* **57**(2):165–169, April 1976.
20. "Management of Acute Pancreatitis," *British Medical Journal,* **4**(5995):488, November 29, 1975.
21. J. H. Hoofnagle, R. J. Gerety, E. Tabor, S. Feinstone, L. Barker, and R. Purcell, "Transmission of Non-A, Non-B Hepatitis," *Annals of Internal Medicine,* **87:**14–20, July 1977.
22. R. H. Purcell, H. J. Alter, and J. L. Dienstag, "Non-A, Non-B Hepatitis," *Yale Journal of Biology and Medicine,* **49**(3):243–250, July 1976.
23. D. B. Allardyce and F. Johnstone, "Bowel Obstruction," in A. Bogoch (ed.), *Gastroenterology,* McGraw-Hill Book Company, New York, 1973, p. 1152.
24. Ibid., p. 1153.
25. J. T. LaMont and K. J. Isselbacher, "Cirrhosis," in G. W. Thorn et al. (eds.), *Harrison's Principles of Internal Medicine,* 8th ed., McGraw-Hill Book Company, New York, 1977, p. 1605.
26. J. Eschar, "The Case for Intensive Care in Hepatic Coma," *Heart and Lung,* **4**(5):781, September–October 1975.

BIBLIOGRAPHY

Alexander, M. and M. S. Brown: "Physical Examination," *Nursing 76,* **6:**65–70, January 1976. Very good discussion that focuses on the abdominal examination.
Altshuler, A. and D. Hilden: "The Patient with Portal Hypertension," *Nursing Clinics of North America,* **12**(2):317–329, June 1977. Discusses esophageal bleeding with good overview of surgical management.

Baranowski, K., H. Greene, and J. Lamont: "Viral Hepatitis," *Nursing 76*, **6**(5):31–38, May 1976. Excellent discussion of type A and B hepatitis and related nursing care.

Bogoch, A.: *Gastroenterology,* McGraw-Hill Book Company, New York, 1973. Excellent discussions on all aspects of gastrointestinal disease with most current research incorporated throughout.

Brunner, L.: "What to Do (and What to Teach Your Patient) about Peptic Ulcer," *Nursing 76*, **6**(11):27–34, November 1976. Excellent comprehensive discission of peptic ulcer.

Connors, M.: "Ostomy Care: A Personal Approach," *American Journal of Nursing*, **74**(8):1422–1425, August 1974. Includes author's experiences and suggestions regarding appliances, care, and irrigations.

Cullen, P. P.: "Patients with Colorectal Cancer: How to Assess and Meet Their Needs," *Nursing 76*, **6**(9):42–47, September 1976. Good discussion of caring for patients with colorectal cancer during various phases of the disease.

Daniel, E.: "Chronic Problems in Rehabilitation of Patients with Laennec's Cirrhosis," *Nursing Clinics of North America*, **12**(2):345–356, June 1977. Good discussion of long-term management of encephalopathy and ascites.

Dolan, P. O., and H. Greene: "Conquering Cirrhosis of the Liver and a Dangerous Complication," *Nursing 76*, **6**(11):44–53, November 1976. Excellent discussion of esophageal hemorrhage with pathophysiology and treatment.

Gillies, D., and I. Alyn: "How Well Do You Understand Cirrhosis?" *Nursing 75*, **5**(1):38–43, January 1975. Contains excellent multiple choice questions for self-evaluation.

Given, B. A., and S. J. Simmons: *Gastroenterology in Clinical Nursing,* The C.V. Mosby Company, St. Louis, 1975. Good discussions focusing on pre- and postoperative care and specific disorders of the gastrointestinal tract.

Jackson, B.: "Ulcerative Colitis from an Etiological Perspective," *American Journal of Nursing*, **73**(2):258–261, February 1973. Overviews theories of causation for ulcerative colitis.

Jirovec, M. M.: *Metabolism,* Boston University Press, Boston, 1974. A learning package covering peptic ulcer, ulcerative colitis, hypothyroidism, hyperthyroidism, diabetes mellitus, and hepatic cirrhosis. An excellent tool for individualized instruction.

Jones, D., C. F. Dunbar, and M. M. Jirovec: *Medical-Surgical Nursing: A Conceptual Approach,* McGraw-Hill Book Company, New York, 1978. Excellent general medical-surgical text with pathophysiology, physical assessment, and preventative, ambulatory, and acute care incorporated throughout. Metabolic disorders are covered in depth.

Keough, G., and H. Niebel: "Oral Cancer Detection—A Nursing Responsibility," *American Journal of Nursing*, **73**(4):684–686, April 1973. Excellent focus on assessment for early detection.

Literte, J.: "Nursing Care of Patients with Intestinal Obstruction," *American Journal of Nursing*, **77**(6):1003–1006, June 1977. Good discussion focusing on nurse's role.

Mansell, E., S. Stokes, J. Adler, and N. Rosensweig: "Patient Assessment: Examination of the Abdomen," *American Journal of Nursing*, **74**(9):1679–1702, September 1974. Excellent programmed instruction.

McConnell, E.: "All about Gastrointestinal Intubation," *Nursing 75*, **5**(9):30–37, September 1975. Excellent review of nasogastric tubes, their uses, and care.

Shahinpour, N.: "The Adult Patient with Bleeding Esophageal Varices," *Nursing Clinics of North America*, **12**(2):331–343, June 1977. Discusses patient management during active bleeding and complications associated with esophageal varices.

Sweet, K.: "Hiatal Hernia," *Nursing 77*, **7**(8):36–43, August 1977. Excellent discussion of etiology, effects, diagnosis, treatment, and care of hiatal hernia.

Watt, R.: "Colostomy Irrigation: Yes or No?" *American Journal of Nursing*, **77**(3):442–444, March 1977. Good discussion of available ways to manage colostomy with special section on controlling odor.

Wentworth, A., and B. Cox: "Nursing the Patient with a Continent Ileostomy," *American Journal of Nursing*, **76**(9):1424–1428, September 1976. Very good discussion of postoperative care and management of internal ileostomy pouch.

30

Gynecology and Andrology

Nancy E. Reame

ABNORMAL CELLULAR GROWTH

Cervical Carcinoma

Definition   Cancer of the cervix is one of the most common tumors in women, being second only to breast cancer in frequency (1). The area where the cervix meets the portio vaginalis is known as the *squamocolumnar junction* and is usually located just inside the external opening of the cervix. Here there is a change from a single layer of tall, columnar epithelium, which covers the cervix, to several layers of stratified squamous epithelium, which covers the vaginal mucosa. The most common site of origin of cervical cancer is in this transitional zone (Fig. 30-1). The largest numbers of malignancies in the uterine cervix are squamous cell carcinomas, meaning that abnormal cell maturation, organization, and growth has occurred in the squamous epithelium.

It is generally believed that squamous cell cancer of the cervix passes through precursor stages, characterized by progressive disturbances of maturation of the squamous epithelium (dysplasia). These premalignant changes progress to carcinoma in situ, a preinvasive cancer that does not extend beyond the basement membrane of the surface epithelium, is asymptomatic, and has a 100 percent 5-year survival rate (2).

As the disease advances, it spreads to the vaginal wall, to the uterine body, and in its late stages to the bladder. Through the lymphatic vessels, cervical carcinoma may metastasize to the external iliac and hypogastric nodes. In most cases, cervical cancer is confined to the pelvic region. The disease is staged according to internationally established conventions, from stage 0 (carcinoma in situ) progressively through stage IV (invasion of the bladder or rectum) (3).

Symptoms do not generally appear until the later stages, at which time abnormal discharge, bleeding, pelvic pain, or difficulty with urination may be noticed. In the final stages, renal failure and uremia occur, which are the most common causes of death.

Depending on stage of disease, treatment of cervical cancer generally involves surgery and/or radiation initially, followed by more radical surgical technique and/or chemotherapy for treatment of recurrent, persistent cancer.

Cervical cancer appears to be more common in women who become sexually active at an early age and who have children. Herpesvirus type 2 infection has been implicated as an etiological factor (4).

Assessment   I. Health History.
        A. Age.
        B. Marital status.
        C. Menstrual, obstetrical, and sexual history.
        D. Personal hygiene habits.
        E. Previous cervical problems, symptoms, herpes.
        F. Use of vaginal antibiotics.
        G. Date of last Papanicolaou (Pap) smear.
        H. Family history of cancer.
    II. Physical assessment. Pelvic examination will reveal:
        A. Normal external genitalia.
        B. No remarkable change in vaginal mucosa or cervix.

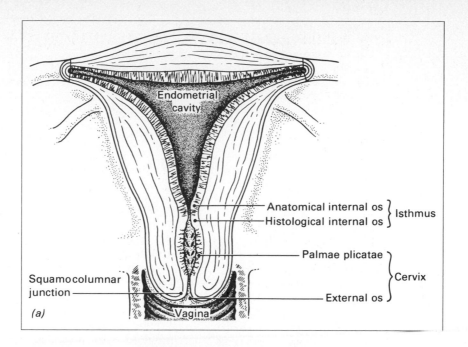

(a)

Endometrial cavity

Anatomical internal os
Histological internal os
} Isthmus

Palmae plicatae
} Cervix

Squamocolumnar junction

External os

Vagina

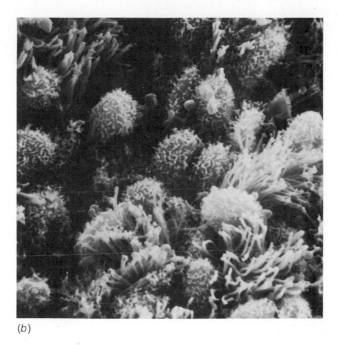

(b)

FIGURE 30-1 / The transition zone (squamocolumnar junction) is a common site for cervical cancer. (*a*) Anatomy of the cervix. (*b*) Area above the squamocolumnar junction (endocervix) composed of a single layer of ciliated and secretory cells. (*Adapted from S. L. Romney et al., Gynecology and Obstetrics: The Health Care of Women, McGraw-Hill Book Company, New York, 1975.*)

    III. Diagnostic tests.
        A. Pap smear—positive class IV, probably malignant.
        B. Colposcopy—no suspicious or atypical lesions.
        C. Punch biopsy—histology reveals less than invasive cancer.
        D. Cone biopsy—stage Ia, carcinoma strictly confined to cervix; preclinical squamous cell cancer.
    IV. Other data sources—previous lab findings.

Problems

    I. Physiological—patient is asymptomatic.
    II. Psychosocial—patient lacks knowledge, understanding of cancer disease process, measures for treatment, and absolute need for vigilant follow-up.

Diagnosis

    I. Altered self-concept, i.e., implications of surgery on body image, sexuality, fertility.
    II. Anxiety, fear of cancer, dying.

Goals of Care

    I. Immediate—reduce anxiety, fear of surgery.
    II. Long-range.
        A. Assist patient to live with cancer diagnosis.
        B. Reduce risk of recurrence.

Interventions

    I. Types of surgical intervention.
        A. Simple total hysterectomy.
        B. Radical hysterectomy.
    II. Preoperative intervention.
        A. Teach (patient, family, patient groups) concerning:
            1. Definition of hysterectomy.
            2. Anesthesia.
            3. Preoperative procedures, hospital routines.
            4. Postoperative procedures, treatments, pain, activity, diet.
            5. Intercourse, menstruation, old wives' tales.
        B. Counseling concerning:
            1. Sexuality, femininity, frigidity, infertility.
            2. Cancer, dying.
        C. Provide preoperative hysterectomy care.
        D. Arrange for spiritual counseling if desired.
    III. Postoperative intervention.
        A. Assess: vital signs, pain, intake, and output, vaginal drainage, incision drainage.
        B. Promote rest, relaxation, relief of pain.
        C. Promote healing, return to homeostasis.
        D. Assess for complications of abdominal surgery, i.e., postoperative infection, hemorrhage.
        E. Evaluate preoperative teaching and counseling.
        F. Promote understanding of need for regular follow-up screening and evaluation.
        G. Refer for counseling about problems of depression, sexuality, self-image.
        H. Provide information on self-help groups for cancer patients, posthysterectomy patients.

Evaluation

    I. Complications.
        A. Recurrence, vaginal vault.
            1. Assessment.
                a. Suspicious Pap smear (class III).
                b. Rectal and vaginal palpation reveals parametrial lump.
                c. Punch biopsy of vaginal vault reveals invasive carcinoma.
                d. Anxious, fearful.

2. Intervention.
   a. Prepare for pelvic radiation therapy by teaching about purpose, side effects, and treatment of side effects.
   b. Provide emotional support during radiation therapy sessions to reduce anxiety.
   c. Assess malaise, nausea, skin irritation.
   d. Promote rest and healing.
   e. Referral to visiting nurse, American Cancer Society patient groups.
   f. Promote frequent return visits.
B. Recurrence, bladder.
   1. Assessment.
      a. Backache, urinary discomfort.
      b. Blood in urine.
   2. Intervention.
      a. Prepare patient for further diagnostic tests, i.e., intravenous pyelogram, bone scan, liver enzymes, barium enema.
      b. Prepare patient for pelvic exenteration (total, anterior, posterior) by:
         (1) Teaching patient, family about:
             (a) Purpose, alternatives of surgery.
             (b) Preoperative procedures, routines.
             (c) Changes in body image and in excretory and sexual function.
             (d) Changes in daily routines.
         (2) Evaluate emotional stability, family support systems, financial situation, facilities for home care, need for nursing care in home.
         (3) Preparation of bowels for surgery: antibiotics, laxative, enemas, intestinal tube, abdominal preparation.
         (4) Assist in intravenous placement of central venous pressure line.
      c. Evaluate immediate postoperative condition by assessing cardiac changes, signs of shock, kidney function.
      d. Promote return of physiological homeostasis and healing.
      e. Reduce anxiety, discomfort.
      f. Postoperative teaching of patient and family concerning dressing changes, stoma care.
      g. Postoperative counseling and support concerning grief over bodily mutilation, extent of surgery, change in body functions and life-style, fear of sudden death, relapse.
      h. Promote continuity of care and support during convalescence by visiting nurse referral and visit in hospital, periodic calls to patient at home, continued teaching, counseling at physician's visits concerning sexual function and new problems, referral for sexual counseling for couple if desired.
C. Metastasis to spine.
   1. Assessment.
      a. Backache.
      b. Weight loss, fatigue.
      c. Depression, despair.
   2. Intervention.
      a. Prepare patient for chemotherapy.
         (1) Maintain nutritional and health status.
         (2) Teach about purpose, procedure, side effects, and treatment of side effects.
         (3) Counsel and provide emotional support.
      b. Reduce discomfort of side effects, i.e., pain, nausea, vomiting, mouth bleeding, skin irritation, diarrhea.
      c. Reduce risk of infection.
      d. Promote family support and environment for expression of feelings.
      e. Observe for signs of drug tolerance.

Breast Carcinoma

Definition

Breast carcinoma is now the most common malignancy and a leading cause of death in women (5). Although not considered a gynecological disorder in the true sense, the woman with breast cancer usually presents herself to her gynecologist with a lump in the breast. The most common type of invasive breast carcinomas arises from the epithelium of the mammary ducts. Tumor cells spread via the lymphatics and bloodstream. Common sites of metastasis are the skeletal system, lungs, and the liver.

The etiology of breast cancer is unknown, but an increased risk of disease exists for women who have never been pregnant, whose mother or sister had breast cancer, who have had a history of benign breast disease, and who have had menstrual cycles for 30 years or more (6). Breast feeding does not appear to influence the incidence.

In spite of newer surgical techniques and diagnostic methods, the cure rate for breast cancer has not improved dramatically since the 1920s. If the primary tumor is small (less than 2 cm in diameter), and if there is no lymph node involvement, then the patient has an 80 percent chance of living 5 years (7).

Surgery, whether simple or radical mastectomy, represents the principal therapy for initial treatment. Radiation and chemotherapy are commonly used for treatment of advanced disease.

Assessment

I. Health history.
    A. Age.
    B. Occupation.
    C. Marital status.
    D. Menstrual, obstetrical, and sexual history.
    E. Family health history.
    F. Previous breast disease.
    G. Hormonal therapy.
    H. Breast-feeding currently.

II. Physical and behavioral assessment.
    A. Breast examination may reveal:
        1. Serous or bloody discharge.
        2. Hard, ill-defined lump that is not movable.
        3. Eczematoid patch around nipple.
        4. Redness, hyperthermia, patchy edema.
        5. Asymmetrical breast contour (Fig. 30-2).
    B. Behavior—anxious.

III. Diagnostic tests.
    A. Mammography.
    B. Thermography.
    C. Biopsy.

IV. Other data sources—previous mammographic, thermographic reports.

Problems

I. Physiological—patient is asymptomatic.
II. Psychosocial.
    A. Disbelief, unable to accept diagnosis of cancer.
    B. Angry, confused, depressed.

Diagnosis

I. Lacks appropriate knowledge about mastectomy procedures, effects on body image, sexual function, daily living activities.
II. Altered self-concept, i.e., fear of death, loss of femininity, body disfigurement.
III. Impairment of relationships with family, husband.

Goals of Care

I. Immediate—assist patient to accept cancer diagnosis and loss of breast.
II. Intermediate—promote postoperative healing.
III. Long-range.
    A. Assist patient and family to adapt to altered self-concept and impact of cancer on wife-husband, mother-children roles.
    B. Reduce risk of recurrence of disease.

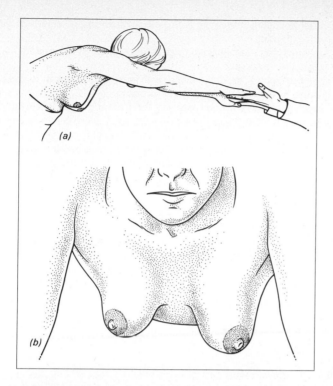

FIGURE 30-2 / (a) Position for detecting asymmetry in breast contour. **(b)** Right breast is fixed with lateral deviation of nipple, indicative of tumor in upper quadrant. [*Adapted from L. Parsons and S. Sommers (eds.), Gynecology, W. B. Saunders Company, Philadelphia, 1962.*]

Intervention

I. Types of surgical intervention.
   A. "Lumpectomy"—local excision only.
   B. Subcutaneous mastectomy—nipple and skin are left intact.
   C. Simple or total mastectomy—all mammary tissue removed; muscles and axilla preserved.
   D. Radical mastectomy—breast, skin, deep fascia, muscles, and axillary lymph nodes are removed.
II. Preoperative intervention.
   A. Teach patient and family about surgical procedures, routines, postoperative appearance of chest, common feelings after mastectomy, pain, activity, reconstructive mammoplasty.
   B. Routine preoperative care for mastectomy patient.
   C. Assist patient and family to express feelings, fears, concerns.
III. Postoperative intervention.
   A. Immediate.
      1. Reduce pain, discomfort.
      2. Promote healing.
      3. Prevent lymphadema.
   B. Intermediate.
      1. Prevent injury to desensitized area.
      2. Assist patient to accept body image, responsibility for care.
      3. Reinforce preoperative teaching and counseling.

4. Support patient in dealing with pathological report, extent of disease, need for further therapy.

5. Assess coping mechanisms, grieving processes, and emotional support systems.

C. Long-range.

1. Promote return to daily living activities, i.e., referral to Reach-to-Recovery groups, sexual counseling, breast prosthesis.

2. Maintain effective communication for fostering rigid follow-up screening, e.g., return visit every 3 months for 3 years, then every 6 months up to 5 years, and then annually.

3. Teach self-examination of remaining breast and incision area.

Evaluation

I. Complications.

A. Local recurrence.

1. Assessment.

a. Lump in chest wall at site of incision.

2. Intervention.

a. Prepare patient for further diagnostic tests, e.g., metastatic series, estrogen receptor assay, mammogram of remaining breast.

b. Assist in preparation for radiation therapy (Fig. 30-3) (see "Evaluation" under "Cervical Carcinoma").

B. Metastasis to other organs.

1. Assessment.

a. Backache, fatigue.   c. Urinary discomfort, bowel problems.

b. Weight loss.   d. Depression, despair.

FIGURE 30-3 / **Postmastectomy patient being prepared for radiation therapy.** (*Adapted from N. Tapley and E. Montague, "Elective Irradiation with the Electron Beam after Mastectomy for Breast Cancer," American Journal of Roentgenology, 126:127–134, 1976.*)

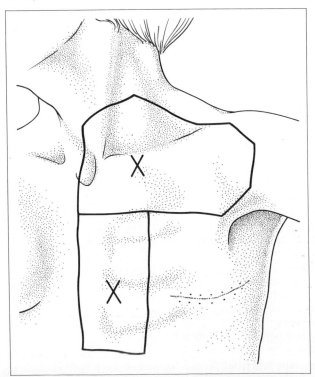

2. Intervention.
   a. Reduce pain, discomfort.
   b. Prevent fractures of spine.
   c. Assist in preparation for chemotherapy (see "Evaluation" under "Cervical Carcinoma").

Other Malignant Tumors of the Reproductive Tract

Most malignant tumors of the reproductive tract require hysterectomy, generally in association with bilateral *salpingo-oopherectomy* (removal of oviducts and ovaries). Radiation therapy and chemotherapy may be alternative or additional choices of treatment. To the patient undergoing such procedures, the gynecological nurse provides invaluable physical and emotional support as educator, counselor, and mediator. Because of the nature of the disease and its highly specialized treatment regimens, the gynecological nurse may represent an important link in the chain of gynecologist, surgeon, radiologist, medical social worker, and family.

Vulvar Carcinoma

Vulvar carcinoma is a rare malignancy most commonly seen in women over 60 years of age. Leukoplakia vulvitis and prolonged vulvar itching are symptoms that may be attributed to other minor disorders, uncleanliness, or aging. Delay in obtaining medical attention may be due to embarrassment and reluctance to submit to a pelvic examination.

Vulvar cancer may initially appear as small nodules with eroded surfaces localized on the labia majora. This type of cancer grows slowly, with a 5-year survival rate of 70 percent if it is diagnosed before spread to the inguinal lymph nodes has occurred (8).

Removal of the external genitalia (*vulvectomy*) is the treatment of choice. Postoperative nursing procedures generally include dressing changes, sitz baths, catheter irrigations, and preventive care against leg edema. Vulvectomy patients may require special counseling in dealing with body disfigurement and the effects on sexuality.

Carcinoma of the Vagina

Vaginal cancers account for only a small percentage of genital malignancies, being more common after menopause. Recently, a rare form of malignant tumor of the vagina has been reported in young women whose mothers had been treated with diethylstilbestrol (DES), a synthetic estrogen, in early pregnancy (9). It is believed that these women, who were exposed in utero to this drug, are at risk to develop the benign condition known as *vaginal adenosis,* the abnormal appearance of glandular epithelium, which may then give rise to clear cell adenocarcinoma. Normally, in young women squamous epithelium is found in the vagina, and gland cells are confined to the cervix.

Early lesions do not generally cause symptoms. Later manifestations include painless bleeding, leukorrhea, itching, and constipation. Biopsy is required to confirm diagnosis and rule out secondary spread of other genital tumors. Radical hysterectomy and/or radiation therapy is associated with a 5-year survival rate of 38 percent (10).

For the young girl admitted to a DES screening program, the nurse must be aware of the emotional and physical factors at work in both patient and mother. Fear of the pelvic exam, maternal guilt, and threat of cancer may all be important issues which the nurse can address with appropriate explanation, counseling, and education.

Cancer of the Uterus (Corpus Carcinoma)

Endometrial carcinoma or cancer of the uterine lining follows mammary and cervical cancer as the third most frequent malignancy of the reproductive organs in women (11). It is most prevalent in postmenopausal women, especially in association with obesity, hypertension, diabetes, and abnormal estrogen production. There is current controversy regarding an increased risk of uterine cancer in premenopausal women who have taken the sequential type of oral contraceptive (12).

The most common site of the primary lesion is the uterine fundus and the area of insertion of the oviducts. The malignant tissue later fills the uterine cavity and eventually involves the myometrium, serosa, and adjacent pelvic organs. In the advanced stage, the pattern of lymphatic infiltration is the same as for cervical cancer with distant metastasis to the lungs, liver, skeleton, and brain.

Endometrial cancer appears to be the result of progressively abnormal changes in both uterine glands and stroma. Depending on the degree of atypia, lesions are considered either reversiole (cystic glandular hyperplasia) or irreversible and premalignant (dysplasia, adenomatous hyperplasia).

The history of a patient with endometrial cancer often includes dysfunctional bleeding: generally, a serosanguinous *metrorrhagia* (bleeding unrelated to the menstrual cycle) in younger women or postmenopausal bleeding after normal menses has ceased. Pain, contractions, and increased pressure may also be present. A Pap smear is usually not as reliable a method for diagnosis of endometrial cancer as it is for cervical cancer, because exfoliated malignant cells are liable to degenerate inside the uterine cavity. Curettage is a more accurate method of diagnosis.

For cancerous lesions, three types of treatment are available: (1) surgery, (2) radiation, or (3) a combination of surgery and radiation. Surgery usually involves total abdominal hysterectomy with bilateral salpingo-oophorectomy, since spread frequently occurs along the lymphatics of the ovarian vessels into the vagina, parametria, uterus, and ovaries, Hormone therapy, specifically progestogens in massive doses, may be used for suppression of advanced disease.

Choriocarcinoma of the Uterus   This reproductive disease is a malignant neoplasm arising from the trophoblastic epithelium of the embryo. Pregnancies in rapid succession and protein deficiency are believed to be predisposing factors (13). Clinical symptoms may mimic signs of abortion or dysfunctional bleeding.

Although the disease is rare, choriocarcinoma is the outstanding example of a malignancy that can be successfully treated with chemotherapy. Methotrexate is used in conjunction with total hysterectomy or alone in low-risk patients. It blocks the conversion of folic acid to tetrahydrofolic acid, thus interrupting the life cycle of the malignant cell by inhibiting DNA synthesis (14). The drug's side effects include gastric bleeding, ulcers, and bone marrow depression.

Carcinoma of the Fallopian Tubes   Cancer of the oviduct is a rare malignancy. Most cancers occur in nulliparous, postmenopausal women (15). Pain or bleeding does not usually occur until the lesion is well established, so that early diagnosis is difficult. Metastatic tumors of the oviduct are more common than primary cancers, often occurring secondarily to ovarian, endometrial, or mammary carcinoma.

Ovarian Cancers   Because the ovary is composed of several histological structures, a variety of malignant and premalignant tumors can arise. The incidence of ovarian cancer appears to be rising, possibly due to an increased life expectancy since the peak incidence occurs after age 60 (16). The signs and symptoms of early ovarian carcinoma are nonspecific but will include postmenopausal vaginal bleeding in about one-third of the cases. Because growth and spread to other organs is rapid, symptoms may also include abdominal pressure, ascites, and gastrointestinal distress. If the tumor is derived from hormone-producing tissue, symptoms of masculinization or hyperestrogenism may occur. Exploratory laparoscopy with tissue biopsy is the most accurate diagnostic method. If diagnosed early, the 5-year survival rate may reach 60 percent (17).

Benign Lesions of the Reproductive Tract

With the exception of the oviducts, reproductive organs including the breast are especially susceptible to the proliferation of normal cells of muscle, glands, and connective tissue. Unlike malignancies, benign lesions have a limited growth potential, remain localized, and are usually not life-threatening. Genital lesions have been classified according to tissue of origin, gross features, cell type, and degree of proliferation. Several types appear to be dependent and responsive to the reproductive hormones that have been used in suppressive therapy.

The signs and symptoms of abnormal growth depend on the size and location of the lesion. Many are found incidentally on gynecological examination or in hysterectomy specimens. Inappropriate uterine bleeding is the most common manifestation of benign and malignant tumors. In women of childbearing age, symptoms of benign growth may sometimes be mistaken for pregnancy. Pain does not generally occur unless the growth is large enough to produce tension on surrounding structures. Treatment usually involves surgical removal, ranging from curettage to hysterectomy.

Some of the more common sites of benign lesions are shown in Fig. 30-4.

Cervical Polyps
Cervical polyps, an excessive growth of the endocervical epithelium, may appear as reddish blue, soft lesions that may have an ulcerated surface. Oral contraceptives may be a predisposing factor.

Endometriosis
Endometriosis, the occurrence of localized areas of functional endometrium outside the uterus, is believed to be primarily caused by a regurgitation of menstrual blood through the oviducts into the peritoneal cavity. The ovaries are the most common site of implantation. Progressive dysmenorrhea occurs, but the degree and frequency of symptoms are extremely variable.

Fibroids
Uterine fibroids (myoma, fibromyoma) are slow-growing tumors of smooth muscle and fibrous connective tissue which usually occur in multiple sites. Although benign, their association with pain, pressure, irregular uterine bleeding, and abdominal enlargement makes this disorder the most common indication for hysterectomy (18); however, controversy regarding the necessity for hysterectomy has encouraged a more conservative approach to treatment. A myomectomy may be the choice of treatment for women who desire future pregnancies, although cesarean section delivery and the risk of uterine rupture are possible consequences.

Ovarian Cysts
Because the ovary undergoes a monthly cycle of follicular growth, ovulation, and corpus luteum formation, it is especially susceptible to the development of abnormal structures due to defects in any of these ovulatory processes. The resulting lesions, known as *functional*

FIGURE 30-4 / **Common sites of benign lesions of the female reproductive tract.**

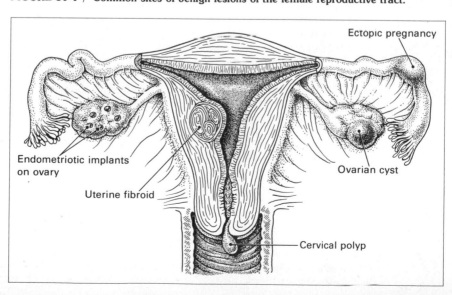

or *retention cysts,* may occur without symptoms and undergo spontaneous resorption. If rupture occurs, the associated symptomatology of pelvic pain and tenderness, nausea, or vomiting, may mimic that of ectopic pregnancy and/or appendicitis.

Ectopic Pregnancy

An *ectopic pregnancy* is one which occurs as a result of implantation of a fertilized ovum at a site other than the uterine cavity. The majority occur in the fallopian tube but may also arise at abdominal, ovarian, and cervical sites. It is believed that a delay in transport of the ova through the oviduct may predispose to tubal implantation.

INFLAMMATORY DISORDERS

Vaginitis

Definition

Vaginitis is an inflammation of the vagina generally caused by an irritation or infection that disturbs the normal physiology and homeostasis of the vaginal environment. A change or increase in the vaginal discharge is usually the most common symptom. The normal pH of the vagina is approximately 4.0, and it is maintained primarily by lactic acid produced by Doederlein bacillus (*Lactobacillus*), a gram-positive nonmotile rod. The moist, acidic milieu of the vagina is essential to the growth of beneficial vaginal bacteria. It also provides protection against invasion by other microorganisms and their upward progression through the reproductive tract. Vaginitis may be a consequence of any of the following etiological factors:

1. Suppression of the cyclic estrogenic stimulation of the vaginal epithelium as in menopause, during oral contraceptive therapy, or in children prior to puberty.
2. Change in acidity. Acidity may be destroyed by the excessive use of deodorants and vaginal douches.
3. Inhibition of growth of Doederlein bacilli. A side effect of antibiotics is the destruction of the normal vaginal flora.

The most common organisms causing symptomatic vaginitis are *Trichomonas vaginalis* and *Candida albicans,* which produce characteristic vaginal discharges and require specific antibacterial therapy. Infection may be transmitted to sexual partners.

Assessment

I. Data sources (refer to "Oral Cancer").
II. Health history.
    A. Age.
    B. Menstrual history.
    C. Sexual history.
    D. History of diabetes, birth of a large baby, debilitating disease.
    E. Medication history—type and route.
    F. Personal hygiene habits—vaginal deodorants, douche, bubble bath, type of undergarment worn.
    G. Type of vaginal discharge—amount and odor.
    H. Recent emotional stress.
III. Physical assessment.
    A. Pelvic examination will reveal:
        1. Abnormal vaginal discharge (color, amount, odor, consistency).
        2. Vaginal and/or vulvar reddening, swelling, tenderness.
        3. Foreign body.
    B. Specific findings for *Trichomonas* vaginitis (Fig. 30-5):

FIGURE 30-5 / Specific findings in diagnosing the causative agent for vaginitis. (*a*) *Trichomonas* as viewed by the light microscope. (*b*) The spores and hyphae of *Candida albicans* as seen microscopically with potassium hydroxide suspension. (*From S. L. Romney et al., Gynecology and Obstetrics: The Health Care of Women, McGraw-Hill Book Company, New York, 1975.*)

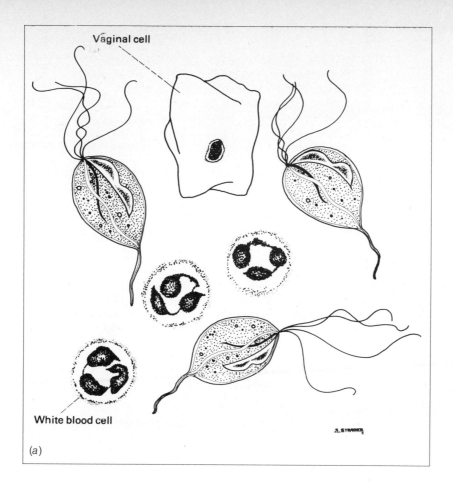

Vaginal cell

White blood cell

(a)

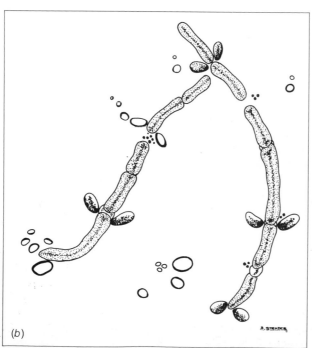

(b)

        1. Frothy, greenish yellow, foul-smelling discharge.
        2. Reddened vaginal mucosa, multiple red papules.
     C. Specific findings for moniliasis (*C. albicans*):
        1. White, cheesy vaginal discharge.
        2. White patches on vaginal mucosa.
  IV. Diagnostic tests.
     A. Microscopic examination of wet smear[1] (urine or vaginal secretion) mounted on a glass slide.
        1. Presence of moving trichomonads confirms diagnosis of *Trichomonas* vaginitis.
        2. Presence of branching hyphae and buds confirms diagnosis of moniliasis.
     B. Pap smear.
     C. Organism culture.
  V. Other data sources.
     A. Family, especially if young child.
     B. Old record.

Problems

  I. Physiological.
     A. Complains of profuse, foul-smelling vaginal discharge.
     B. Complains of vulvar and vaginal itching, burning and tenderness.
  II. Psychosocial—Complains of painful intercourse and is anxious about feelings of sexual partner.

Diagnosis

  I. Impairment of skin and mucous membrane integrity.
  II. Impairment of relationships with others.

Goals of Care

  I. Immediate.
     A. Reduce itching, swelling, tenderness of vaginal mucosa.
     B. Promote return of vaginal milieu to normal pH and floral environment.
  II. Long-range.
     A. Prevent reinfection or recurrence of inflammation.
     B. Promote sexually satisfying relationship.

Intervention

  I. Provide explanation of mechanism of action, use, and insertion of medication specific for vaginitis.
  II. Promote rest of vaginal mucosa.
  III. Provide teaching, counseling as to personal hygiene habits, predisposing factors to vaginitis, alternate forms of contraception.
  IV. Encourage health examination and treatment of sexual partner and use of condom to prevent cross-infection.
  V. Encourage follow-up visit to assess success of treatment.

Evaluation

  I. Complications.
     A. Multiple causes of reproductive tract infection (*see* "Gonorrhea," "Vulvitis," "Cervicitis," and "Syphilis").
     B. Secondary spread of vaginal infection to upper reproductive tract.

Gonorrhea

Definition

Gonorrhea is the most common infectious disease in the United States (19). The apparent lack of immunity to this disease is a major reason why it remains endemic. This venereal disease is caused by a gram-negative diplococcus, *Neisseria gonorrhoeae* (Fig. 30-6*a*). Gonococci invade columnar secretory epithelium, but the squamous epithelium of the

[1]Normal saline for *Trichomonas* vaginitis; potassium hydroxide for candidiasis (moniliasis).

vagina is relatively resistant. The infantile vagina, however, is susceptible to gonococcal inflammation. Virulent gonococci have hairlike appendages (pili) on their surfaces that are believed to enable gonococci to stick to host cells and to avoid being washed away. These pili may also protect the gonococci from ingestion by white blood cells. In addition, gonococci have been shown to secrete an enzyme that cleaves IgA, the antibody secreted by mucosal surfaces, and thus interfere with possible defense mechanisms against reinfection. The increased use of the condom in Sweden, England, and Norway has been associated with a significant decline in gonorrhea incidence (20).

Infection occurs almost exclusively during intercourse. With acute infection, 60 percent of women are asymptomatic (21). The initial sites of infection are the urethra, the Bartholin gland ducts, and the cervical mucosa. Infection of the cervix may result in acute cervicitis with infectious, purulent discharge. Bartholin gland abscesses are typical manifestations (Fig. 30-6b). Gonorrhea may spread to the endometrium during or after menstruation, abortion, or delivery. The organism spreads easily from the endometrium to the oviducts, causing acute salpingitis. A chronic pelvic inflammatory reaction may then result due to secondary infection by other organisms, commonly *Escherichia coli.*

Assessment

I. Health history.
   A. Age.
   B. Occupation.
   C. Marital status.
   D. Menstrual history.
   E. Sexual history.
   F. Previous history of reproductive tract infection.
   G. Incidence of venereal disease in sexual partner.
   H. Drug allergies.
II. Physical assessment.
   A. Purulent, greenish yellow discharge from external os of cervix.
   B. Milking of Skene's glands induces discharge from urethra.
   C. Unilateral, edematous reddening at opening of Bartholin duct.
   D. Rectal discharge.
III. Diagnostic tests.
   A. Microscopic examination of gram-stained cervical and urethral secretions will show gram-negative intracellular diplococci.
   B. Organism culture from cervical, urethral secretions, rectum, and throat.
   C. Measurement of antibody titer to gonococcal pili.
   D. Serological studies to rule out syphilis, other venereal diseases.

Problems

I. Physiological.
   A. Complains of change in length of menstrual periods, occasional abnormal spotting, increased vaginal discharge.
   B. Complains of dysuria, frequency, urgency to void.
   C. Complains of perineal tenderness especially with intercourse.
   D. May be asymptomatic in early acute stage.
II. Psychosocial—Is very anxious and concerned about social stigma attached to diagnosis of venereal disease, effect on relationship with sexual partner, future fertility, and sexuality.

Diagnosis

I. Impairment of skin and mucous membrane integrity.
II. Impairment of urinary elimination.
III. Impairment of reproductive function.
IV. Impairment of relationships with others.
V. Altered self-concept.
VI. Lack of knowledge concerning disease process, treatment and long-term effects.

Goals of Care

I. Immediate—reduce urinary discomfort, local tenderness, and cervical discharge.
II. Long-range.
   A. Prevent recurrence and spread of disease.
   B. Prevent development of problems with sexuality, self-esteem.

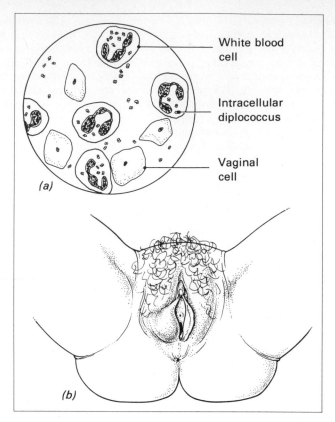

White blood cell

Intracellular diplococcus

Vaginal cell

(a)

(b)

FIGURE 30-6 / Possible diagnostic findings for gonorrhea. (a) Microscopic evidence of gonococci. Gram-negative diplococci may be taken up by white blood cells. (b) Bartholin abscess. The opening of the Bartholin gland may become inflamed and occluded, resulting in swelling of the labia due to collection of purulent exudate. (*Adapted from F. K. Beller et al., Gynecology: A Textbook for Students, Springer-Verlag, New York, 1974.*)

Intervention

  I. Explain rationale for type, dosage, and length of treatment regimen.
  II. Promote rest and healing of vaginal and cervical mucosa.
  III. Provide teaching regarding disease process, spread, preventive measures, personal hygiene.
  IV. Assess need for counseling referral regarding sexuality.
  V. Explain importance of follow-up visits to assess disease recurrence, especially if pregnant.

Evaluation

  I. Complications.
    A. Acute salpingitis—pelvic inflammatory disease.
      1. Assessment.
        a. Malaise, chills, fever (temperature greater than 101°F), rapid pulse.
        b. Intense, lower abdominal pain.
        c. Local heat, swelling, rebound tenderness.
        d. Loss of appetite, nausea.
        e. Cervix tender on palpation.
        f. Spotting, leukorrhea, dyspareunia.
        g. High sedimentation rate (50 to 60 mm/h) and WBC (20,000 to 30,000 per cubic millimeter).

2. Intervention.
   a. Reduce pain, nausea, fever.
   b. Promote rest and healing.
   c. Reduce risk of peritonitis.
   d. Prepare patient for diagnostic procedures to assess tubal damage, patency, and future fertility.
      (1) Rubin test.
      (2) Hysterosalpingogram.
      (3) Laparoscopy, culdoscopy.

B. Infertility due to tubal occlusion.
   1. Assessment.
      a. Unable to become pregnant in association with ovulatory menstrual cycle characteristics and normal male fertility work-up.
      b. Rubin test reveals inadequate CO_2 insufflation of oviducts, i.e., no referred shoulder pain, pressure above 150 to 200 mmHg.
      c. Laparoscopic examination reveals periadnexal adhesions and/or entrapment of contrast media in tubes.
   2. Intervention.
      a. Assist in explanation of surgical procedures to improve patency of oviducts. Types of tuboplasty:
         (1) Salpingolysis—the separation of peritubal adhesions.
         (2) Salpingoplasty—opening of the occluded distal end of the tube.
         (3) Midsegment reconstruction.
         (4) Resection and reimplantation into the uterus.
      b. Reduce preoperative anxiety.
      c. Assist in routine preparation for surgery.
      d. Promote postoperative healing.
      e. Reduce risk of adhesion formation.
      f. Reduce risk of postoperative infection.
      g. Counsel, teach concerning methods for pregnancy enhancement (see Chap. 5).

C. Chronic salpingitis.
   1. Assessment.
      a. Low-grade fever; malaise.
      b. Persistent abdominal aching, low backache.
      c. Weight loss.
      d. Enlarged, immobile adnexal mass (usually bilateral).
      e. Rebound tenderness absent.
      f. Bulging cul de sac due to abscess.
      g. Retroverted uterus.
   2. Intervention.
      a. Prepare patient for diagnostic procedures:
         (1) Cul de sac aspiration.
         (2) Blood and culture studies to determine invading secondary organism.
      b. Promote healing.
      c. Reduce risk of rupture of hydrosalpinx.
      d. Counsel, teach about prevention of reinfection.
      e. If indicated, prepare patient for bilateral salpingoopherectomy or total hysterectomy (see "Cervical Carcinoma").

Vulvitis

Inflammation of the vulva may be caused by a local manifestation of a dermatological or systemic infectious disease or by a secondary infection of the genital tract. Common symptoms include itching or pruritus, followed by prolonged scratching and trauma to the skin. The inguinal lymph nodes may be enlarged and tender. Soap, detergent, and antiseptic solutions either applied directly or used in laundering underwear may cause a local allergic reaction. Excretion through the urine of drugs such as antibiotics and sulfonamides may also be responsible. Herpes genitalis (herpes simplex type 2) and condyloma acuminatus (venereal warts) are viral diseases that cause vulvar lesions and are transmitted via sexual contact (Fig. 30-7). Herpes genitalis is considered carcinogenic in the cervix, so Pap smears should be performed every 6 months following a primary infection.

The nurse should attempt to identify the causative agent or etiologic factor for the vulvitis by obtaining a comprehensive health history in conjunction with diagnostic evaluation of the lesions or discharge. Specific nursing interventions would include the relief of local pain and itching, and teaching appropriate personal hygiene measures to prevent the spread of infection and cross-infection.

Cervicitis

The main symptom of inflammation of the cervix is increased cervical discharge, although cervical mucorrhea may be seen under physiological as well as pathological conditions. Secretions of the cervical gland are increased under the influence of estrogen, as at the time of ovulation or in pregnancy. Excess mucous production also occurs normally in the newborn and in adults, as a result of sexual or other emotional stimulation. Oral contraceptives produce cervical mucous properties similar to those seen during the luteal (progestogenic) phase of the menstrual cycle.

Cervicitis is common after vaginal delivery due to subsequent infection of cervical lacerations. Gonorrhea produces an acute cervicitis which may become chronic due to secondary infection by streptococci. Other factors in the pathogenesis of cervicitis are poor hygiene, decreased resistance to infection, irritation by foreign bodies, and neoplastic disease of the upper genital tract.

The acute inflammatory reaction of the cervix is characterized by a thick, purulent, whitish discharge with an acrid odor. Dysuria may also be present. The general well-being of the patient is unaffected. Chronic infection of the cervix results in hyperactivity of the cervical gland cells, resulting in excess secretions, hypertropy and hyperplasia. There is a forward

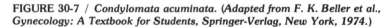

FIGURE 30-7 / *Condylomata acuminata. (Adapted from F. K. Beller et al., Gynecology: A Textbook for Students, Springer-Verlag, New York, 1974.)*

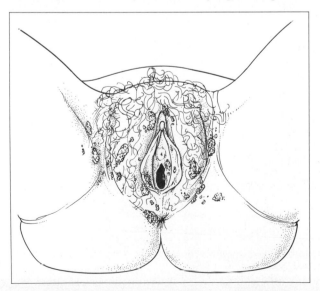

growth or displacement of the squamocolumnar junction, producing an eversion and redness about the external os with new cervical glands developing where they do not normally exist. Chronic cervicitis is a major etiologic factor in infertility, dyspareunia, and abortion (22).

As with other inflammatory disorders of the reproductive tract, a complete health history should be obtained to aid in the identification of the source(s) of infection. Specific medical treatment will depend on the infectious agent, age of the patient, her desire for pregnancy, and the severity of cervical involvement. Cervical cauterization or electrocoagulation (to destroy diseased gland tissue) is indicated when erosion and infection are extensive.

Syphilis

Although the occurrence of syphilis has been increasing in recent years, it is still less common than gonorrhea (23). It is transmitted by sexual contact with a person who has an open lesion containing *Treponema pallidum*. The spirochetes can be transmitted transplacentally to the fetus. Syphilis is usually described in terms of primary, secondary, and latent stages (24). The primary and secondary stages are considered the transmissive or infectious periods, lasting up to 2 years. The latent stage begins after 2 years of infection and is considered noninfectious.

The primary syphilitic lesion is called a *chancre* or ulcer and usually involves the vulva, posterior vaginal wall, cervix, or mouth. The average incubation period prior to chancre formation is 3 weeks. The inguinal lymph nodes may become enlarged and tender, indicating the entry of spirochetes into the circulation.

Manifestations of secondary syphilis generally do not appear for 6 to 9 weeks, during which time the primary chancre heals spontaneously. In the secondary stage, a generalized skin rash occurs that does not itch and extends over the palms of the hands and soles of the feet. Loss of scalp and eyebrow hair may occur. Moist, grayish lesions known as *condylomata lata* may appear on the vulva, anus, or corners of the mouth and are highly infectious. Serological tests for syphilis are positive for the first time at this stage. Symptoms will disappear within 2 to 6 weeks of onset but may reoccur as primary or secondary lesions during the next 2 years. After this period, untreated disease causes no further symptoms in a majority of the cases. In the remainder, the tertiary stage involves noninfectious granulomatous lesions (gummas) in skin, bone, and liver; degenerative changes in the central nervous system; and cardiovascular lesions, all caused by immunological reactions with the organisms.

Because of the insidious nature of the disease and its resemblance to other dermatological conditions in the initial stages, syphilis may go undiagnosed. All obstetrical and gynecological patients should therefore be screened for syphilis at the initial visit, if gonorrhea is diagnosed or if a venereal disease contact has been made, and especially during the last 6 weeks prior to delivery to prevent infant morbidity or congenital syphilis. Even in the latent stages of the disease, a pregnant woman may infect her unborn child.

Once syphilis has been diagnosed, treatment generally involves intramuscular penicillin therapy, abstinence from intercourse, and repeated serological tests 1, 3, and 12 months after diagnosis, until the disease is cured.

The nurse may prove most valuable as a counselor or teacher to promote knowledge of the disease process and of transmission and prevention and to encourage treatment of all sexual contacts for infectious syphilis.

REPRODUCTIVE DISORDERS IN WOMEN

Amenorrhea after Discontinuation of Oral Contraceptives

Definition It is estimated that over 20 million women in the world are using some form of birth control pill, making oral contraceptive therapy a major reason for a gynecological visit (25). Currently, in the United States, oral contraceptives contain either a combination of synthetic estrogens and progestogens varying in type and dosage, or a lower dose of a progestogen-only compound. The "combination" pill prevents pregnancy mainly by suppressing the midcycle release of pituitary gonadotropins, an essential trigger for ovulation (26). This suppressive effect of oral contraceptives on gonadotropin secretion may result in amenorrhea and anovulation when the pill is discontinued, especially in women with a prior history of menstrual irregularities (27). Spontaneous resolution of the problem tends to occur within 6 to 12 months after stopping the pill, but it can pose an emotional stress to the patient who is attempting to conceive during this time. There appears to be no relationship between the dosage or duration of pill usage and the duration of amenorrhea after discontinuation of usage (28).

Assessment
I. Health history.
    A. Age.
    B. Menstrual and obstetrical history.
    C. Sexual history.
    D. Medical history—headache, dizziness, liver disease, diabetes, renal disease, breast disease, phlebitis, thromboembolism, sickle cell disease, heart disease, hypertension.
    E. Family history—genital or breast cancer, stroke, heart disease.
    F. Medication history.
    G. Smoking.
II. Physical and behavioral assessment.
    A. Pelvic examination will reveal normal external, internal genitalia and organs.
    B. Breast examination will reveal:
        1. No palpable masses.
        2. No complaints of tenderness.
    C. Behavioral—intelligent, alert.
III. Diagnostic tests.
    A. Pap smear.
    B. Venereal disease reaction level (VDRL).
    C. Urinalysis, complete blood count (CBC), chest x-ray.
    D. Blood pressure.

Problems
I. Physiological—complains of menstrual cramps relieved by aspirin.
II. Psychosocial.
    A. Dissatisfied with condom method of contraception.
    B. Wishes to avoid pregnancy but continue sexual activity.

Diagnosis
I. Impairment of menstrual function which interferes with normal activity.
II. Impairment of relationships with others.
III. Lack of knowledge concerning methods of contraception.

Goals of Care
I. Reduce risk of pregnancy.
II. Reduce anxiety regarding sexual activity.
III. Reduce menstrual discomfort.

Intervention
I. Teach about methods of contraception, advantages, risks, side effects, route of administration, reproductive physiology.
II. Encourage regular follow-up visits to evaluate satisfaction with therapy and side effects.

Evaluation
I. Complications.
    A. Amenorrhea and infertility and discontinuation of oral contraceptives.
        1. Assessment.
            a. Desires pregnancy.
            b. Has not had a period for 4 months after discontinuing oral contraceptives.
            c. Is using no other form of contraception but is sexually active.
            d. No cyclic changes in breast.
            e. No complaints of cramps, premenstrual edema.
            f. Pelvic examination normal.

g. Husband's fertility work-up is normal (see Chap. 5).

2. Intervention.

a. Provide explanation of amenorrhea occurring after discontinuance of oral contraceptives.

b. Provide explanation of hormone treatment regimen to stimulate ovulation:
   (1) Climiphene citrate.
   (2) Human menopausal gonadotropin (HMG), gonadotropin-releasing hormone (GRH).

c. Demonstrate use of basal body temperature (BBT) record sheet and thermometer.

d. Explain other diagnostic tests used to determine ovulatory cycles, e.g., cervical mucous fern test, Simms-Huhner test, endometrial biopsy, serum luteinizing hormone (LH) and estrogen measurement, vaginal smear.

Menopausal Syndrome

Menopause, or the cessation of menstruation, is the period of a woman's life that marks the end of reproductive function and may be associated with a variety of physiological and psychological disorders known as the *menopausal syndrome.* The most common symptoms associated with the menopausal syndrome include fatigue, hot flashes, dizziness, headache, depression, and irritability. Although all women experience the cessation of menses, the incidence and severity of menopausal disturbances are extremely variable (29). Married women with only primary education, of low income, who had completed their childbearing at an early age, and who experience premenstrual depression are more likely to develop menopausal disorders (30). Although many theories have been proposed to explain the menopausal syndrome, it is unclear how much of the symptomatology is attributable to biological, psychological, or cultural factors (31).

The gradual disappearance of growing follicles in the ovary is associated with ovulation failure, decline in estrogen secretion, and irregular uterine bleeding. Menopause is considered complete after one full year of amenorrhea, which generally occurs between the ages of 45 and 50. Atrophy of the vaginal mucosa may occur with estrogen deficiency and interfere with sexual pleasure at a time when the fear of pregnancy has been alleviated. Surgical removal of the ovaries can produce a sudden drop in estrogen levels and without replacement therapy produces a premature menopause. In addition to somatic complaints, menopause may be diagnosed by measuring the levels of luteinizing hormone (LH) in either the blood or urine. In menopausal women, LH secretion is elevated as a result of a decreased negative feedback effect of estrogen from the ovary on the hypothalamus and pituitary.

Much controversy exists regarding the benefits of estrogen replacement therapy in the treatment of menopausal syndrome. Although symptoms generally improve, there are possible, long-term, carcinogenic side effects of estrogen treatment that remain to be explored (32). Estradiol valerate, which is administered after hysterectomy, and conjugated equine estrogens (Premarin, which is given orally in doses of 0.3, 0.6, or 1.25 mg per day) are the main drugs used for treatment of symptoms. Nausea, abdominal bloating, and breast tenderness may be signs of overdosage. Uterine bleeding is rare. Tranquilizers have also been used in conjunction with estrogen therapy.

Nurses need to be aware of the possible psychological implications associated with the loss of reproductive capacity for a patient with menopausal symptoms. If the patient's purpose in life has centered around her childbearing functions, she may need support in developing a new role and life-style.

Although pregnancy is unlikely, contraceptive measures should be continued until 4 years after the last menstrual period. However, oral contraceptives are not advised for women over 40 because of their suspected association with heart disease (33). In addition, women taking birth control pills may not recognize the onset of menopause, since regular bleedings usually continue while estrogen and progesterone are taken cyclically.

When pregnancy does occur in premenopausal women, both maternal and fetal complication rates increase (34). Antepartum care for women in their late reproductive years should include amniocentesis for the detection of chromosomal mutations in the fetus, since certain birth defects appear to be related to aging effects in the oocyte (35).

REPRODUCTIVE DISORDERS IN MEN

Andrology, the counterpart to gynecology, is the study of disorders of the male reproductive system. Clinical andrology has been neglected primarily because of the lack of relevant, accurate laboratory methods for functional analysis, as well as the erroneous belief that the male factor was relatively unimportant in the etiology of reproductive failure. Little is known about the effects of diet, diseases, environmental factors, and drugs in male reproduction.

Although andrological nursing is not as yet considered an area of specialty, the nurse who practices in an infertility clinic or family planning center should be knowledgeable about male-related reproductive disorders, their effects on infertile couples, diagnostic procedures, and treatments. As the concept of male contraception becomes a reality, nurses may one day be faced with a whole new population of family planning clientele. The most common disorders that have been shown to affect male reproductive function are described below.

Genital Infections

Microbial infections of the male genitourinary tract are associated with decreased fertility (36). The presence of pus cells and bacteria in semen interfere with sperm production, motility, and viability. Urethral stricture is a frequent complication of gonococcal infection in the male which predisposes to recurrent urinary tract infections especially due to *Escherichia coli,* a potent spermicidal pathogen. *Mycoplasma,* organisms that have been associated with infection in the reproductive tracts of both men and women, are believed to be a causative agent in habitual abortion (37). Infection of the epididymus may cause ductal obstruction and the inhibition of sperm transport, resulting in *oligospermia,* a condition in which sperm numbers are insufficient to produce a successful fertilization. The fertility of a couple may also be impaired when the male has a chronic, silent infection that triggers an immune response to sperm in the female. The marked depression in sperm production associated with acute viral illnesses (e.g., mononucleosis, hepatitis) may be due to the accompanying high fever rather than the disease itself.

Clinical evaluation of patients with urogenital tract infections must include diagnostic laboratory procedures, since the history and physical examination may be unremarkable or reveal only complaints of low backache. Urethritis and prostatitis can be diagnosed indirectly by debris and a white blood cell count greater than 20 per high-power microscopic field in fresh semen (38).

Abnormal Cellular Growth

Defects in testicular development may result in abnormalities of sperm at various stages of maturation (*spermatogenesis*) or in the malfunction of the Leydig cells, which produce testosterone. The descent of the testes from the abdominal cavity into the scrotum may also be impaired (*cryptorchidism*) and cause spermatogenic arrest. The defect in cell development and growth may be at the level of the hypothalamic pituitary axis, resulting in hypogonadotropic hypogonadism, a condition in which spermatogenesis is suppressed due to inadequate stimulation of the testes by the gonadotropin hormones, LH and FSH (follicle-stimulating hormone).

Obstructions of the male reproductive tract may be of congenital origin and suppress fertility by inhibiting sperm transport and altering the physical and biochemical characteristics of seminal fluid. Thus an obstruction of the ejaculatory ducts may be characterized by an ejaculate with reduced volume, low sperm count and fructose levels, and an acidic pH. Obstructions may occur anywhere along the course of the reproductive tract and account for almost one-half of all conditions associated with the absence of sperm in the seminal fluid (azoospermia) (39). Although rare until the late reproductive years, obstructions may also be due to benign or malignant tumors in any of the reproductive organs, with the prostate gland being a common site of abnormal growth (40).

Any of these types of abnormal cell growth can result in infertility. Chromosomal abnormalities appear to be one etiologic factor in genital tract anomalies affecting fertility (41). The majority of chromosomal aberrations involve the sex chromosomes (e.g., Klinefelter's syndrome), but the incidence of defects involving autosomes has been shown to be 3 times greater in subfertile men than in the normal population (42).

Depending on the cause of the defect in development or growth, management of the infertile male may include hormone therapy to stimulate spermatogenesis and secondary sex characteristics or surgical intervention to remove, repair, or bypass a specific anomaly (Figure 30-8).

Vascular Changes

Varicocele (dilated scrotal veins) is a common cause of male infertility and appears to be due to increased pressure on the valves of the internal spermatic venous system, resulting in retrograde flow from the renal vein into the scrotal circulation. Although varicocele usually occurs on the left side because of differences in venous anatomy, both gonads can be affected because of the presence of cross-venous circulation in the testes. It is postulated that blood carrying a high concentration of toxic metabolic substances can reach both testicles and affect sperm production (43). Varicocelectomy is one of the most successful surgical procedures in the treatment of male infertility, if all varicosities are removed so that retrograde flow is completely arrested.

Male Contraception

For purposes of fertility inhibition, the vulnerable sites in the male reproductive system include:

1. The hypothalamic-pituitary-gonadal axis to affect hormone production.
2. The testes to affect spermatogenesis.
3. The epididymis to affect sperm maturation.
4. The ejaculatory ducts to affect sperm transport.
5. The seminal fluid to affect sperm viability (Fig. 30-9).

To date, the most successful methods of male contraception act by inhibiting sperm transport either temporarily (condom) or permanently (vasectomy).

Interruption of the hypothalamic-pituitary-gonadal axis via steroid therapy has achieved only limited success. Different classes of steroid compounds produce sperm suppression, but almost all of them also have an effect on Leydig cell function and cause alterations in libido and potency. Therefore, any male contraceptive method based on hormonal suppression of spermatogenesis must also be combined with testosterone replacement therapy. In addition, optimal dosage, type, and effect of long-term treatment with steroids remain to be clearly defined.

The *condom* is a safe, nonsystemic, coitally related method of birth control. Because of improvements in durability, viscosity, and shelf life, recent failure rates range from 1.6 to 4.8 per 100 woman-years when used properly, but can be as high as 28 failures per 100 woman-years with poor motivation (44). A recent upsurge in its popularity with younger contraceptive users may reflect its use as a barrier against gonorrhea and other venereal diseases.

Vasectomy, or removal of a portion of the vas deferens, which connects the epididymis to the urethra, is considered a relatively permanent method of contraception since its surgical reversal (*vasovasostomy*) results in only a low postoperative conception rate (45). Although sperm numbers in the ejaculate are essentially reduced to zero (*aspermia*) approximately 8 weeks after surgery, hormone production, spermatogenesis, and the ejaculate volume ar not affected, so that normal androgen balance, sexual desire, and the capacity for erection

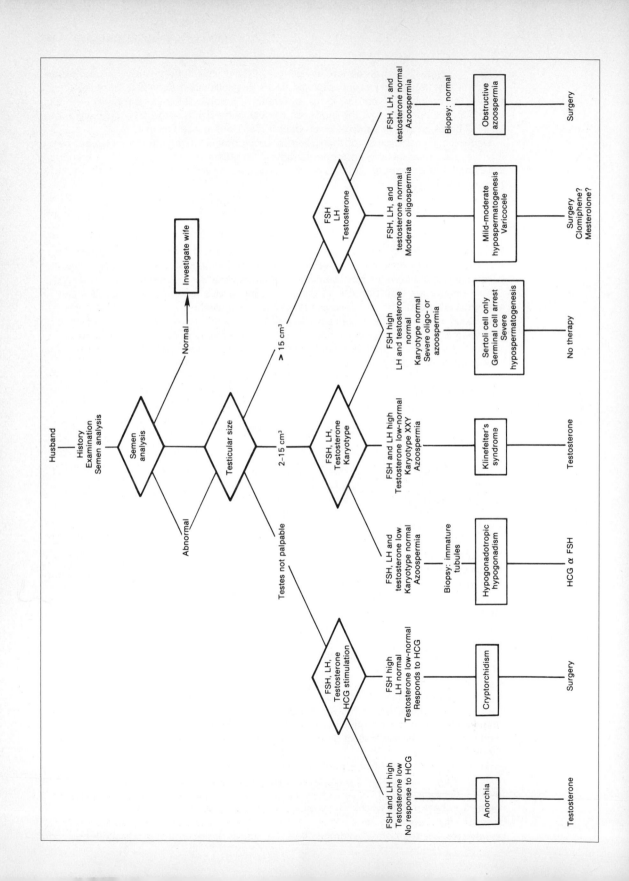

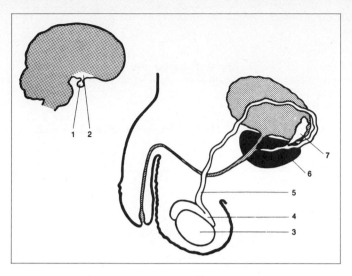

FIGURE 30-9 / Possible sites of fertility regulation within the male reproductive system: *1,* pituitary control and steroid negative feedback; *2,* steroid negative feedback; *3,* sperm formation in testis; *4,* sperm maturation in epididymis; *5,* sperm transport in vas; *6* and *7,* seminal fluid biochemistry. (*After S. L. Romney et al., Gynecology and Obstetrics: The Health Care of Women, McGraw-Hill Book Company, New York, 1975.*)

and ejaculation are maintained (46). An autoimmune response may develop after vasectomy since sperm agglutinating antibodies have been found in the blood of a large number of men up to 10 years after sterilization (47, 48). What long-term effects these immunological changes may have remain to be defined. To date, no systemic dysfunctions attributable to vasectomy have been reported (49). Emotional trauma and sexual dysfunction are not common postoperative complications in most men without a previous history of psychiatric disorder (50).

Assessing the couple's eligibility for vasectomy in terms of reason for sterilization and psychological stability may be an important function of the family planning nurse. Prevasectomy counseling should include a discussion of possible emotional reactions such as regret, anxiety, and guilt in both the husband and wife that may occur during the immediate postoperative period. The couple also needs to plan for the use of other birth control methods until aspermia in the ejaculate has been attained.

REFERENCES

1. UICC Committee on Professional Education, *Clinical Oncology,* Springer-Verlag, New York, 1973, p. 212.
2. F. K. Beller, K. Knorr, C. Lauritzen, and R. Wynn, *Gynecology: A Textbook for Students,* Springer-Verlag, New York, 1974, p. 315.
3. Cancer Committee (FIGO), "Classification and Staging of Malignant Tumors in the Female Pelvis," *International Journal of Gynecology and Obstetrics,* **9:**172–179, 1971.
4. W. E. Rawls et al., "Herpes Virus Type 2: Association with Carcinoma of the Cervix," *Science,* **161:**1255–1256, 1968.

FIGURE 30-8 / Course of management of reproductive disorders in the male. FSH = follicle-stimulating hormone; LH = luteinizing hormone; HCG = human chorionic gonadotropin. [*Adapted from E. J. Keogh, H. B. Burger, D. M. de Kretser, and B. Hudson, "Surgical Management of Male Infertility," in E. S. E. Hafez (ed.), Human Semen and Fertility Regulation in Men, The C. V. Mosby Company, St. Louis, 1976.*]

5. UICC Committee on Professional Education, op. cit., p. 203.
6. Ibid.
7. Ibid., p. 211.
8. Ibid., p. 232.
9. A. I. Herbst, H. Ulfelder, and D. Poskanzer, "Adenocarcinoma of the Vagina: Association of Maternal Stilbestrol Theraph with Tumor Appearance in Young Women," *New England Journal of Medicine,* **284:**878–881, 1971.
10. Beller et al., op. cit., p. 289.
11. Ibid., p. 322.
12. J. L. Marx, "Estrogen Drugs: Do They Increase the Risk of Cancer?" *Science,* **191:**838–840, 1976.
13. UICC Committee on Professional Education, op. cit., p. 222.
14. R. D. Bloomfield, "Current Cancer Chemotherapy in Obstetrics and Gynecology," *American Journal of Obstetrics and Gynecology,* **109:**487–528, 1976.
15. Beller et al., op. cit. p. 327.
16. Ibid., p. 339.
17. UICC Committee on Professional Education, op. cit., p. 227.
18. A. Altchek, "Guidelines for Hysterectomies, Non-cancerous Conditions Requiring Surgery," *The Female Patient,* March 1976, pp. 68–73.
19. L. K. Huxall, "VD: The Equal Opportunity Disease" *Journal of Obstetrical, Gynecological and Neonatal Nursing,* **4:**16–22, 1975.
20. G. B. Kolata, "Gonorrhea: More of a Problem but Less of a Mystery," *Science,* **192:**244–247, 1976.
21. J. F. Porter and P. Kane, "Sexually Transmitted Diseases," *Research in Reproduction,* **7:**1, 1975.
22. R. C. Benson, *Handbook of Obstetrics and Gynecology,* Lange Medical Publications, Los Altos, Calif.; 1971, p. 500.
23. Huxall, op. cit., p. 16.
24. Ibid.
25. C. I. Meeker and M. J. Gray, "Birth Control, Abortion and Sterilization," in S. L. Romney et al. (eds.), *Obstetrics and Gynecology: The Health Care of Women,* McGraw-Hill Book Company, New York, 1975, p. 552.
26. E. Diczfalusy, "Mode of Action of Contraceptive Drugs," *American Journal of Obstetrics and Gynecology,* **100:**136–163, 1968.
27. R. P. Shearman, "Prolonged Secondary Amenorrhea after Oral Contraceptive Therapy," *Lancet,* **2:**64–66, 1971.
28. F. W. Hanson, "Safety of Contraceptive Methods: Amenorrhea," *Journal of Reproductive Medicine,* **15:**153–157, 1975.
29. S. J. Tucker, "The Menopause: How Much Soma and How Much Psyche?" *Journal of Obstetrical, Gynecological and Neonatal Nursing,* **6:**40–48, 1977.
30. L. Jaszmann, N. D. van Lith, and J. C. A. Zaat, "The Perimenopausal Symptoms: The Statistical Analysis of a Survey," *Medical Gynecological Society,* **4:**268–275, 1969.
31. Tucker, op. cit., p. 46.
32. Marx, op. cit., p. 838.
33. J. I. Mann, W. H. W. Inman, and M. I. Thorogood, "Oral Contraceptive Use in Older Women and Fatal Myocardial Infarction," *British Medical Journal,* **2:**445–447, 1976.
34. E. S. E. Hafez and T. N. Evans, *Human Reproduction, Conception and Contraception,* Harper & Row Publishers, Incorporated, New York, 1973, p. 193.
35. G. B. Talbert, "Effect of Maternal Age on Reproductive Capacity," *American Journal of Obstetrics and Gynecology,* **10:**451–455, 1968.
36. D. Dahlberg, "The Lethal Factor in Infertility: An Immunological Reaction in the Vaginal Environment," in A. Centaro and H. Carretti (eds.), *Proceedings of the First International Congress of Infertility,* Excerpta Medica, Amsterdam, 1973.
37. H. W. Horn, R. B. Kundsin, and T. S. Kosasa, "The Role of Mycoplasma Infection in Human Reproductive Failure," *Fertility and Sterility,* **25:**380–389, 1974.
38. F. C. Derrick and B. Dahlberg, "Male Genital Tract Infections and Sperm Viability," in E. S. E. Hafez (ed.), *Human Semen and Fertility Regulation,* The C. V. Mosby Company, St. Louis, 1976, p. 389.
39. J. M. Pomerol and S. Marina, "Congenital and Postinflammatory Obstructions of the Male Reproductive Tract," in E. S. E. Hafez (ed.), *Human Semen and Fertility Regulation,* The C. V. Mosby Company, St. Louis, 1976, p. 398.
40. UICC Committee on Professional Education, op. cit., p. 248.

41. N. E. Reame and E. S. E. Hafez, "Hereditary Defects Affecting Fertility," *New England Journal of Medicine,* **292:**675–681, 1975.

42. A. C. Chandley, "Cytogenetics of Infertile Men," in E. S. E. Hafez (ed.), *Human Semen and Fertility Regulation,* The C. V. Mosby Company, St. Louis, 1976, p. 419.

43. S. S. Schmidt, R. Schoysman, and B. H. Stewart, "Surgical Approaches to Male Infertility," in E. S. E. Hafez (ed.), *Human Semen and Fertility Regulation,* The C. V. Mosby Company, St. Louis, 1976, p. 476.

44. M. J. Free and N. J. Alexander, "Male Contraception without Prescription," in E. S. E. Hafez (ed.), *Human Semen and Fertility Regulation,* The C. V. Mosby Company, St. Louis, 1976, p. 556.

45. F. C. Derrick, W. Yarbrough, and J. D'Agostino, "Vasovasostomy Results of Questionnaire of Members of the American Urological Association," *Journal of Urology,* **110:**556–557, 1973.

46. N. J. Alexander, "Vasectomy: Morphological and Immunological Effects," in E. S. E. Hafez (ed.), *Human Semen and Fertility Regulation,* The C. V. Mosby Company, St. Louis, 1976, p. 308.

47. N. J. Alexander, B. J. Wilson, and G. D. Patterson, "Vasectomy: Immunological Effects in Rhesus Monkeys and Men," *Fertility and Sterility,* **25:**149–156, 1974.

48. R. Ansbacher, "Bilateral Vas Ligation: Sperm Antibodies," *Contraception,* **9:**227–237, 1974.

49. Alexander et al., op. cit., p. 308.

50. J. E. Davis, "Vasectomy," *American Journal of Nursing,* **72:**509–513, 1972.

BIBLIOGRAPHY

Amelar, R. D., and L. Dubin: "Stimulation of Fertility in Men," in E. S. E. Hafez (ed.), *Human Reproduction, Conception and Contraception,* Harper & Row, Publishers, Incorporated, New York, 1973, pp. 645–668. This chapter provides the pathophysiological basis and specifics of clinical manifestations, diagnosis, and treatment of male infertility.

Avery, W., C. Gardner, and C. Palmer: "Vulvectomy," *American Journal of Nursing,* **74:**453–455, 1974. This article focuses on nursing management of the postvulvectomy patient.

Beller, F. K., L. Knorr, C. Lauritzen, and R. M. Wynn: *Gynecology: A Textbook for Students,* Springer-Verlag, New York, 1974, pp. 279–357. A student-oriented presentation of gynecological disorders. The chapters on gynecological infections and neoplasms of the genitalia are most relevant to this discussion.

Benton, B. D. A.: "Stilbestrol and Vaginal Cancer," *American Journal of Nursing,* **74:**900–901, 1974. This article presents a concise review of the etiology of this disorder and focuses on nursing management of the adolescent patient with vaginal cancer.

Britt, S. S.: "Fertility Awareness: Four Methods of Natural Family Planning," *Journal of Obstetrical, Gynecological and Neonatal Nursing,* **6:**9–18, 1977. This article provides the physiological rationale and a clear description of each method of natural family planning.

Dyche, M. E.: "Pelvic Exenteration: A Nursing Challenge," *Journal of Obstetrical, Gynecological and Neonatal Nursing,* **4:**11–19, 1975. This article focuses on the problems and nursing management of the cancer patient undergoing pelvic exenteration.

Foreman, J. R.: "Vasectomy Clinic," *American Journal of Nursing,* **73:**819–821, 1973. This article explains the procedure and describes nursing management of the postvasectomy couple.

Gribbons, C. A. and M. A. Aliapoulios: "Treatment for Advanced Breast Carcinoma," *American Journal of Nursing,* **72:**678–682, 1972. This article presents medical and nursing problems related to the patient with recurrent breast cancer.

Hafez, E. S. E.: *Human Semen and Fertility Regulation,* The C. V. Mosby Company, St. Louis, 1976. This book has been written by the leading experts in the new field of *andrology* and provides an in-depth understanding of fertility regulation in the male.

Hebert, P., I. Welch, and B. Jackson: "Colposcopy—What Is It?" *Journal of Obstetrical, Gynecological and Neonatal Nursing,* **5:**29–32, 1976. This article presents a review of the procedure, its indications, and role of the nurse in preparing the patient for colposcopy.

Huxall, L. K.: "VD: The Equal Opportunity Disease. Part II. The 'Social Diseases'—Gonorrhea and Syphilis," *Journal of Obstetrical, Gynecological and Neonatal Nursing,* **4:**16–22, 1975. This article provides a good review of the etiology, symptomatology, diagnosis, and treatment of the two most common types of venereal disease.

Katzman, E. M.: "Common Disorders of Female Genitalia from Birth to Older Years: Implications for Nursing Interventions," *Journal of Obstetrical, Gynecological and Neonatal Nursing,* **6:**19–21, 1977. The author discusses common disorders in children, adult women, and older women. Principles for prevention and nursing intervention are offered.

Quirk, B.: "VD: The Equal Opportunity Disease. Part I. This is VD Too?—Moniliases, Trichomoniases

Vaginalis, Herpes Simplex, Condylomata Accuminata," *Journal of Obstetrical, Gynecological and Neonatal Nursing,* **4:**13–15, 1975. This article reviews the less commonly considered types of venereal disease and discusses the nursing role in their management.

Romney, S. L., M. J. Gray, A. B. Little, J. A. Merrill, E. J. Quilligan, and R. Stander: *Gynecology and Obstetrics: The Health Care of Women,* McGraw-Hill Book Company, New York, 1975. The authors present not only an in-depth description of obstetrical and gynecological medicine but also deal with contemporary problems of health care delivery and extramedical issues concerned with population growth, contraception, abortion, and sexual mores.

Tucker, S. J.: "The Menopause: How Much Soma and How Much Psyche?" *Journal of Obstetrical, Gynecological and Neonatal Nursing,* **6:**40–48, 1977. The author reviews the clinical and experimental literature on the menopause, describes menopausal syndrome, and presents the diverse biological, psychological, and cultural views on its etiology.

UICC Committee on Professional Education: *Clinical Oncology,* Springer-Verlag, New York, 1973. This manual for clinicians presents a concise description of neoplasia, organized by organ systems and classified according to stage, survival rate, and treatment.

Wahl, T. P. and J. G. Blythe: "Chemotherapy in Gynecological Malignancies—and Its Nursing Aspects," *Journal of Obstetrical, Gynecological and Neonatal Nursing,* **5:**9–14, 1976. This article describes the indications, applications, and complications of cancer chemotherapy, and the role of the gynecological nurse as an educator, listener, and friend.

Woods, N. F.: "Influences on Sexual Adaptation to Mastectomy," *Journal of Obstetrical, Gynecological and Neonatal Nursing,* **4:**33–37, 1975. This nursing article focuses on the problems in sexuality faced by the postmastectomy patient.

Zeitz, A. N.: "Oral Contraceptives: Women's Rights, Nurses' Responsibilities," *Journal of Obstetrical, Gynecological and Neonatal Nursing,* **5:**54–55, 1976. This author discusses concerns about preparing nurses for the role of counselor on birth control—specifically, what the clients should know in order to make informed choices.

31

The Musculoskeletal System

Phyllis J. Gale

The effective functioning of an intact musculoskeletal system provides support and structure to the body and allows for individual mobility and independence. When disruptions occur within skeletal structures due to problems associated with trauma, degeneration, inflammation, or abnormal cellular growth, a multiplicity of problems develops. These include pain, immobility, loss of independence, and changes in one's ability to perform activities of daily living at optimal levels.

The following pages will discuss disruptions in musculoskeletal functioning and related changes. Using the standards of nursing practice, nursing care plans will be developed for each problem discussed.

ABNORMAL CELLULAR GROWTH

Bone Tumors

Definition

Abnormal cellular growth in bone may be primary or secondary in nature and benign or malignant. When bone injury or fracture occurs, there may be a local overgrowth of bone, which may be present for a long period of time, producing a benign, tumorlike lesion. *Osteogenic sarcoma,* a primary malignant tumor arising from bone cells, is predominantly a lesion found in children and adolescents. It may also occur in later life as a complication of a preexisting health problem such as Paget's disease or after deep radiotherapy. The distal portion of the femur and the proximal portions of the tibia and fibula are the most common sites. Metastases usually involve the lungs.

Osteoclastoma or *giant cell tumor* occurs in adults between 20 and 50 years of age. The tumor arises in the end of the long bone, later infiltrating into the shaft of the bone. Common tumor sites are the distal portions of the femur and radius and the proximal portion of the tibia.

Metastatic bone tumors are the most common bone tumors. They arise from tissues other than bone, metastasize, and produce localized bone destruction. The tumors which most frequently metastasize are carcinomas of the breast, prostate gland, lungs, kidneys, thyroid, and ovary. Pathologic bone fractures can result from bone cancer.

Most bone tumors that are primary or secondary malignant lesions often spread to other body parts and can result in death. Newer therapy used to treat cancer today may help arrest or alleviate the problems.

Assessment

I. Data sources
   A. Patient.
   B. Family.
   C. Previous medical records.
   D. Significant others.
II. Health history of an individual with a bone malignancy may suggest:
   A. Age: specific bone tumors affect different age groups.
   B. Past history: may suggest a primary lesion from which a secondary site has developed.
   C. Complaints of limb pain and reduction of use of the affected part.
   D. Decreased nutritional intake.
   E. Generalized weakness.

  III. Physical examination may reveal:
   A. Increased body temperature.
   B. Measurable increase in limb size when compared bilaterally.
   C. Decreased range-of-motion activity.
   D. Pain, which varies. Some early pain may be localized. Later it will be more diffuse.
   E. Anxiety will be manifested in a variety of ways, and the nurse should be aware of behavioral changes.
  IV. Diagnostic tests (refer to Table 31-1) usually include:
   A. A complete x-ray of the involved area.
   B. Biopsy of the lesion.
   C. Frozen sections.
   D. Bone marrow aspiration.
   E. Bone scan.
   F. Bence-Jones protein, 24-h (refer to Chap. 28).

Diagnosis

  I. Alteration in comfort: pain and local swelling moderate to severe.
  II. Nutritional alteration: less than required.
  III. Impairment of mobility: potential, secondary to decreased limb movement.

TABLE 31-1 / COMMON DIAGNOSTIC TESTS AND PROCEDURES PERFORMED FOR PATIENTS WITH ORTHOPEDIC PROBLEMS

 I. Blood.
  A. Complete blood count.
  B. Latex fixation.
  C. Lupus erythematosus (LE) preparation.
  D. Sedimentation rate.
  E. Serum salicylate level.
  F. Electrocardiogram.
  G. Blood coagulation studies.
  H. Uric acid.
  I. Alkaline phosphatase.
 II. Radiography.
  A. Tomography, body section radiography which focuses on certain tissues, eliminating or blurring surrounding tissue.
  B. Arteriography, an injection of a radiopaque substance into the arterial system of a given region and the subsequent taking of radiographs to study bone, joints, or bone lesions.
  C. Arthrography, introduction of air or a radiopaque material into a joint space, outlining joint structures and detailing views of the joint surface on a radiograph.
  D. Discography, the injection of a radiopaque solution into the nucleus pulposus of an intervertebral disk to view the internal disk structures.
  E. Myelography, injection of air or an opaque material into the subarachnoid space to view filling defects associated with herniated disks and tumors in the spinal column.
 III. Cinefluoroscopy, film recording of skeletal motion.
 IV. Arthroscopy, insertion of a lighted instrument, via a small incision, to view the internal structure of a joint.
 V. Arthrostomy, a temporary opening into a joint for drainage purposes.
 VI. Bone scanning, intravenous injection of a radioisotope material having a special affinity to bone and emitting penetrating gamma rays to detect, locate, and outline bone lesions.

    IV. Disruptions in fluid balance, secondary to fever.

    V. Alteration in body image: potential amputation.

    VI. Anxiety: mild to moderate, secondary to fear of surgery.

    VII. Fear of death: potential.

Intervention

    I. Administer medications for pain relief (analgesics and narcotics) and chemotherapy [methotrexate (MTX) and citrovorum]. Observe the drug effects, and report them accordingly.

    II. Reduce fever.

      A. Antipyretic drugs and force fluids.

      B. Minimal covering; provide a cool external environment.

      C. Tepid water sponge baths or hyperthermia, as needed.

    III. High-caloric diet (high carbohydrate, high protein) to maintain the healthy state.

    IV. Engage in frank discussion about disease, treatment, and prognosis, and listen for and explore cues (verbal or behavioral) indicating anxiety from underlying stressors.

    V. Assist patient in working through loss and grief, especially if loss of a limb is anticipated.

    VI. Make referrals for appropriate counseling.

    VII. Explain all procedures, including biopsy and nature of surgery (refer to "Osteoarthritis" for a complete discussion).

    VIII. Teach patient and family about radiation and chemotherapy and common, expected outcomes from these, including:

      A. General malaise.

      B. Weakness.

      C. Alopecia.

      D. Skin integrity disruptions.

      E. Susceptibility to infection.

      F. Stomatitis.

      G. Alterations in blood.

      H. Gastrointestinal disturbances, including anorexia.

      I. Adjustments in work load.

    IX. Provide supplemental health care, including nutritional counseling, mouth care, planned rest periods, and prevention of upper respiratory and other related infections.

Evaluation

    I. Reassessment.

    II. Complications: may include a secondary infection, hemorrhage, and metastatic progression of the primary lesion.

Multiple Myeloma

Definition

Multiple myeloma is an osteocytic malignant disease of the plasma cells that can proliferate throughout the entire skeleton and infiltrate soft tissue. Common bone sites are the spine, skull, ribs, sternum, and pelvis; the lymph nodes, kidneys, liver, and spleen may also become involved. Although the disease is fatal, symptoms can be relieved and the disease may be held in abeyance for several years. Characteristically, multiple myeloma affects men over 40 years of age.

Problems

    I. Constant, severe bone pain (especially back pain).

    II. Hemorrhagic tendency.

    III. Dehydration.

    IV. Further tumor invasion (metastasis).

Intervention (Refer to "Bone Tumors")

    I. Anticipate movement and activity: give pain medication $\frac{1}{2}$ h prior to planned activity.

    II. Careful handwashing and other medical aseptic techniques.

    III. Encourage to decrease secondary infection. Assist with mobility and ambulation: permit patient to move at own speed with planned, smooth, supported movements. This should be done to help decrease pain upon movement and stimulate movement.

    A. Support extremities at joints.

    B. Use turning sheets.

    C. Jacknife position provides comfort.

    D. Back brace may be used.

IV. Assess patient for dehydration (monitor urine pH) and blood electrolytes.

V. Administer medication for chemotherapy: phenylalanine (Melphalan) or cyclophosphamide (Cytoxan), with prednisone as needed.

VI. Assess for bleeding (hematomas, ecchymoses, hemorrhagic areas in buccal membrane, and blanching of finger nail beds), especially if patient is receiving prednisone. Monitor hemoglobin and hematocrit.

Evaluation

I. Reassessment.

II. Complications.

    A. Infection (developed as a result of decreased resistance to infection).

        1. Leukopenia.

        2. Reddened areas.

        3. Fever.

        4. Pain.

    B. Renal failure (see Chap. 28).

        1. Decreased urinary output.

        2. Increased blood serum calcium.

    C. Severe anmia: decreased platelets, hemoglobin, and hematocrit (refer to Chap. 25).

    D. Fractures (see "Fractures").

        1. Cracking sound.

        2. Abnormal positioning of extremity.

        3. Pain.

METABOLIC DISORDERS

Gout

Definition

Gout is a metabolic disorder caused by the overproduction and accumulation of uric acid (increased purine metabolism) in the blood (*hyperuricemia*) and by the deposition of sodium urate crystals in and around joints, cartilage, epiphyseal bone, and periarticular structures. Physiologically, there is abnormal metabolic degradation of purine (a product of protein metabolism) resulting in reduced urinary secretion of urates and increased accumulation of uric acid in the blood. Because of the low solubility a precipitate forms, depositing masses of crystals or *tophi* at sites where the blood flow is least active, particularly in the large toe, the knuckles, and the ears. *Synovitis* (inflammation of a joint) results, and the cyclic process continues, causing an acute inflammatory process in which there are red, warm, swollen, and painful joints.

Primary gout (gouty arthritis) appears to be a genetic defect in purine metabolism, affecting men over 30 years of age and postmenopausal women.

Secondary gout may be associated with multiple myeloma, polycythemia vera, and granulocytic leukemia, and with patients who have had prolonged usage of certain thiazide diuretics. Onset of the disease can occur after recent surgery, recent ingestion of purine-rich foods, excess alcohol intake, and with acute infection and emotional trauma.

Pseudogout may present similar symptoms, affecting the larger joints in which calcium pyrophosphate crystals are present in the synovial fluid. Pseudogout does not respond to colchicine.

Gout often begins in one joint and heals within several weeks. However, the problem can return at any time and may affect more than one joint.

Assessment	**I.** Data sources (refer to "Bone Tumors").

I. Data sources (refer to "Bone Tumors").
II. Health history.
  A. Age: males above 30, females after menopause.
  B. Sex: males affected more; females are affected after menopause.
  C. Occupation: should be identified, often not significant.
  D. Dietary habits.
    1. Assess recent intake: alcohol may influence the problem.
    2. Assess diet for caloric and protein composition.
  E. Recent life experience:
    1. Infection.
    2. Emotional trauma: stress may precipitate problem.
    3. Other illness (e.g., leukemia, polycythemia) or pregnancy.
  F. Family history.
  G. Health perception.
  H. Previous history of gout: note familial tendency.
  I. Time of onset of symptoms (usually early a.m.).
  J. Describe pain: usually increased with weight bearing.
  K. Anorexia and malaise often common complaints.
III. Physical and behavioral assessment.
  A. General physical examination, including weight distribution.
  B. Agonizing pain appearing in the first joint of large toe (later appears in other joints of foot).
  C. Pain may subside or disappear later in day and evening, but returns at night.
  D. Joints are swollen, red, warm, tender (appearance remains, although pain may have subsided); decreased range of motion; increased pain with weight bearing.
  E. Increased pain when weight, e.g., linen, is applied.
  F. Fever and general malaise may be present.
  G. Trophi nodules (deposits of sodium acid urate crystals) may be palpated over bones, joints, and cartilage. Kidneys may also be affected.
  H. Tachycardia may be auscultated, palpated.
  I. Gastrointestinal disturbances: vomiting, diarrhea, constipating.
  J. General appearance; restlessness, anxiety, and stress assessment should be noted.
IV. Diagnostic tests (refer to Table 31-1).
  A. Elevated serum uric acid above 5 mg per 100 mL of serum.
  B. Elevated sedimentation rate.
  C. Synovial fluid from affected joints: presence of sodium urate crystals.
  D. Radiograph findings suggest gout.
  E. Complete blood count: leukocytosis present.
  F. Rheumatoid factor test and lupus erythematosus (LE) preparation both negative.

Problems

I. Painful joints.
II. Fever may be present.
III. Gastrointestinal disturbances.
IV. Diet modifications.
V. Repeated, acute gout attacks.
VI. Side effects of medication.

Diagnosis

I. Alteration in comfort: joint pain.
II. Changes in body temperature: fever.
III. Alteration in nutrition: potential.
IV. Impairment of mobility: increased in early morning.
V. Anxiety: mild to moderate.

Goals of Care

I. Immediate.
  A. Reduce acute discomfort.
  B. Reduce hyperuricemia and uric acid crystal deposits.
  C. Evaluate effectiveness of treatment.
  D. Identify precipitating causes, e.g., stress; secondary causes.

II. Long-range.
  A. Prevent recurring gout episodes.
  B. Prevent development of chronic gouty arthritis, renal calculi, and renal damage.
  C. Weight reduction, if indicated.

Intervention

I. Bed rest during acute phase to relax joints and reduce stress on affected body part.
II. Provide quiet environment to help relieve precipitating factor.
III. Foot boards or cradle to prevent weight of sheets and blankets on the affected joint.
IV. Position involved joints in semiflexion to prevent contractures.
V. Heat or cold applications to involved joints to facilitate movement and reduce inflammation.
VI. Administer medication for pain: analgesics and narcotics, as well as antiinflammatory agents, e.g., indomethacin and phenylbutazone. ACTH may be given.
VII. Administer medication to reduce hyperuricemia, e.g.:
  A. Colchicine orally every hour until pain subsides or until onset of gastrointestinal disturbances, and then daily (Colchicine can be administered intravenously.)
  B. Probencid (Benemid) or allopurinol (Zyloprim).
VIII. Low-fat, low-purine diet to help reduce precipitating cause.
IX. High fluid intake to increase urinary output and prevent the position of urate crystals in the kidney.
X. Observe for gastrointestinal disturbances secondary to medication.
XI. Observe for urolithiasis and renal colic. Assess the patient for flank pain. Teach patient to sift urine for crystals. (Refer to Chap. 27.)
XII. Discharge planning.
  A. Follow-up care and referrals.
  B. Teaching especially related to:
    1. Establishing regular habits of eating, exercise, and rest periods.
    2. Modified dietary regimen, i.e.:
      a. *Encourage* eggs, fat-free milk, cottage cheese, cereals, fruits, and vegetables.
      b. *Limit* kidney, liver, sweetbreads, squab, meats, fowl, beans, mushrooms, peas, and spinach.
      c. *Discourage* meat extracts, glandular meats, roe, shellfish, sardines, and brain.
XIII. Teach about medications: Colchicine and other uricosuric agents.
  A. Aspirin in large doses counteracts uricosuric agents.
  B. Gastrointestinal disturbances and bleeding may indicate drug intolerance.
  C. Discourage fasting and ingestion of alcohol, as these changes may stimulate attacks of gout and/or enhance drug reactions.

Evaluation

I. Reassessment.
  A. Evaluate response to medications as manifested by a decrease in joint swelling, decreased joint pain, and increased mobility.
  B. Revise plan with onset of gastrointestinal symptoms or pain relief.
  C. Compliance concerning medications, activity, diet.
II. Complications.
  A. Deformities secondary to joint destruction.
  B. Cartilage damage, e.g., bony ankylosis.
  C. Development of trophi bodies in cartilage.
  D. Increased frequency of attacks.
  E. Progressive renal dysfunction (see Chap. 28).
III. Intervention: Surgery may be needed to correct bone deformities that may develop as a result of joint damage (refer to "Osteoarthritis").
IV. Follow-up and reevaluation.

Osteoporosis

Definition

Osteoporosis is a metabolic bone dysfunction in which bone resorption supersedes bone formation, resulting in bone demineralization. The disease is characterized by a reduction in bone density and tensile strength. Defects in osteoplasts result from (1) reduced stress and strain normally caused by physical activity, (2) prolonged immobility, and (3) a decrease in estrogen and androgen levels. Although osteoporosis is most common in postmenopausal women, it can occur in older men (approximately 50 to 70 years). Other causes of osteoporosis are liver disease, deficiencies of calcium, phosphorus, and protein, hyperthyroidism, hyperparathyroidism, Cushing's disease, and bone marrow disorders. Prevention of physical trauma may help prevent further damage.

Assessment

I. Data sources (refer to "Bone Tumors").
II. Health history often reveals changes presented by older individuals, most frequently fair-skinned, light-weight females.
    A. Complaints include difficulty in walking and pain (usually low back pain).
    B. There is a susceptibility to fractures, especially of the proximal femur, ribs, vertebrae, and distal radius (see "Fractures").
III. Physical and behavioral assessment.
    A. Joint pain elicited by palpation over an affected area.
    B. Loss of body stature.
    C. Instability and unsteady gait.
    D. Pain elicited by activities (e.g., bending).
    E. Changes in an individual's self-concept related to musculoskeletal changes may also be apparent.
IV. Diagnostic tests.
    A. Radiography.
    B. Blood serum calcium, phosphorous, and alkaline phosphatase levels are normal.

Intervention

I. Encourage physical activity, increasing over a planned period of time.
II. Continue exercise regimen established in physical therapy, or consult with physical therapist about appropriate exercises.
III. Provide ambulatory assistance: crutches, canes, walker, or corset, as needed.
IV. Teach techniques to avoid possible falling and trauma. Avoid heavy lifting. Teach patients effective body mechanics.
V. Explore verbal and nonverbal cues of self-image, dependence, other stresses.
VI. Adequate diet with increased calcium, phosphorus, proteins, vitamins, and minerals.
VII. Administer hormone therapy. This may be done only after careful assessment of each individual's health status.
VIII. Observe for and teach possible occurrence of vaginal bleeding with estrogen therapy and report to physician.
IX. Discharge planning includes information about all of the above.
X. Follow-up health care referral.

Paget's Disease

Definition

Osteitis deformans or *Paget's disease* is a metabolic health problem associated with aging. The disease develops insidiously, usually affecting men. Physiologically there is hypertrophy and bowing of the long bones and marked thickening and irregular deformities of the flat bones. The process usually begins in the skull, tibia, or vertebral column and may eventually involve the entire skeleton. Pain is usually experienced first in the shins and is often attributed to the aging process. The problem may be associated with cardiovascular and pulmonary disorders. Progressive bone dysfunction accompanied by fractures is not uncommon.

Assessment

I. Data sources (refer to "Bone Tumors").
II. Health history (refer to "Bone Tumors").
    A. Pain, usually in the shins.
    B. Cardiovascular and pulmonary problems should be identified.
    C. History of fractures should be elicited.
    D. Age (common in aged).
III. Physical examination.
    A. Reduction in stature and an increase in head size; one usually becomes aware that a hat no longer fits. There is marked enlargement of the cranium; the face appears small and triangular in shape, although it retains its normal configuration.
    B. Involvement of the spine, thorax, trunk, and legs may be manifested by a noticeable change in posture and stature (up to 30 cm), giving the person an "ape-like" appearance; the gait becomes labored and waddling.
    C. Complaints of weakness are not uncommon.
    D. Although the involved bones become massive, they are extremely brittle, and fractures occur frequently.
IV. Diagnostic tests.
    A. Radiography.
    B. Serum alkaline phosphatase: elevated.

Intervention

I. Modified exercise regimen to prevent additional bone trauma.
II. Promote self-care in activities of daily living.
III. Assistive devices for ambulation (e.g., cane, etc.)
IV. Provide continuity of therapy established by physical and occupational therapists.
V. Administer pain medications such as analgesics and salicylates.
VI. Teach:
    A. Planned, careful movements (body mechanics).
    B. Recognition of increased possibility of fractures (see "Fractures").
VII. Provide nursing care consistent with other existing health problems.
VIII. Listen to verbal and nonverbal cues about self, health problem, family, finances, and independence, and explore these with the patient.
IX. Counsel about body image alterations and other stresses.
X. Make referrals if additional counseling is needed.
XI. Follow-up referrals.

Osteomalacia

Definition

Adult rickets or *osteomalacia* is a disorder of calcium and phosphorus metabolism caused by a deficiency in vitamin D. The disease process is usually manifested throughout the skeleton and results from the failure of calcium salt deposition in the bone matrix. Bones become soft, flattened, and deformed.

This health problem occurs in women between 20 and 30 years of age, many of whom have had frequent, repeated pregnancies and lactation, and in patients with gastrointestinal disorders in which calcium and phosphorus are inadequately absorbed. These disorders include sprue, celiac disease, chronic biliary tract obstruction, and pancreatitis, as well as small bowel resections or shunts. Renal disorders and hyperparathyroidism may also cause osteomalacia.

Prevention of pathologic fractures, dietary replacement of vitamin D, and increased ingestion of calcium and phosphate may help relieve the problem and its related problems.

Assessment

I. Data sources (refer to "Bone Tumors").
II. Health history (refer to "Bone Tumors").
III. Physical and behavioral assessment.
    A. Pain in affected bones.

  B. Deformed postures associated with softening of bone structures; these changes may contribute to fractures.

  C. Body image alterations may be present.

IV. Diagnostic tests.

  A. Radiography.

  B. Laboratory findings.

   1. Serum phosphorus: reduced.

   2. Serum calcium: reduced.

   3. Serum alkaline phosphatase: increased.

Intervention

I. Careful, active exercise to counteract atrophy and disease.

II. Adequate diet, including protein, calcium, phosphorus, and dietary supplements of calcium salts, phosphates, and vitamin D.

III. Cesarean section at term, if pregnant.

IV. Discourage lactation in the postpartum period.

V. Teaching plan to include:

  A. Diet (high calcium, protein, phosphorus).

  B. Planned, less frequent pregnancies.

  C. Protection from trauma, with body exercise and planned activity periods.

INFLAMMATORY DISORDERS

Osteomyelitis

Definition

Osteomyelitis is an acute or chronic infection in or around bone usually caused by *Staphylococcus aureus*. The infection is often blood-borne from another infection point or can develop directly as a result of a compound fracture. The infection tends to remain medullary, progressing to cancellous and cortical bone. When the suppurative process reaches the periosteum, erosion occurs and a soft-tissue abscess forms. If the infection invades the bone itself, the bone undergoes necrosis and has a tendency to retain the infection, resulting in retardation of the healing process. The necrotic area can become a potential focal point for reinfection. The *sequestrum* or necrotic bone can be surgically separated from normal bone and, following this procedure, new bone begins to form as the body attempts to repair itself. However, some remaining sequestrum may be covered by new bone, and although healing seems to occur, the remaining sequestrum becomes chronically infected and is prone to repeated abscess formation. Prevention of this problem is the most critical factor in eliminating osteomyelitis.

Assessment

I. Data sources (refer to "Bone Tumors").

II. Health history.

  A. Age: problem can occur in any age group.

  B. History of recent health problems, e.g., fracture.

  C. Complaints of fever and malaise not uncommon.

III. Physical assessment.

  A. Local pain and tenderness upon palpation.

  B. Swelling of affected area; if the extremities are involved, bilateral measurements are unequal.

  C. Area involved is red and warm to the touch.

  D. Patient will have an elevated temperature with chills.

  E. Tachycardia may be present.

  F. Signs of dehydration may be apparent.

  G. Immobility of the affected limb.

  H. Wound odor may be present if the lesion is open.

IV. Diagnostic tests (refer to Table 31-1).

  A. Leukocytosis.

         B. Elevated sedimentation rate.
         C. Blood cultures may grow out of the affecting pathogen.
         D. X-ray of the affected limb.

Problems
   I. Fever.
  II. Pain.
 III. Immobilization of affected body part.
 IV. Compound fracture may or may not be present.
  V. Acute, chronic infectious process.
 VI. Behavioral manifestations: boredom, apathy, low morale.

Diagnosis
   I. Alteration in comfort: pain.
  II. Impairment of mobility, secondary to bone pain and infection.
 III. Impairment of skin integrity: potential.
 IV. Disruption in bone integrity: potential.
  V. Elevation in body temperature, secondary to infection.
 VI. Behavioral changes, e.g., anxiety, boredom, secondary to long-term immobility.

Goals of Care
   I. Immediate.
     A. Identify cause of infection.
     B. Reduce body temperature.
     C. Relieve anxiety.
     D. Relieve pain discomfort.
     E. Treat and improve infection site.
  II. Long-range.
     A. Regain complete skin integrity.
     B. Complete healing of fracture and inflammatory site.
     C. Prevent recurrence of the problems.
     D. Regain complete mobility.

Intervention
     I. Bed rest to reduce stress on extremity.
    II. Administer antipyretics to reduce inflammation.
   III. Cool environment to help relieve body temperature.
   IV. Cast or splint on affected body part to control fracture site and to provide rest for the bone.
    V. Support extremity, especially at joints, to reduce stress on the affected part.
   VI. Maintain proper body alignment to reduce deformity.
  VII. Apply heat to affected areas to increase circulation to the affected area and to hasten removal of pathogen.
 VIII. Administer antibiotics. Be sure that a culture is made and that sensitivity is tested so that the correct drug will be used. Observe for side effects and allergic reactions to drugs used.
   IX. Apply nonstick dressings (Telfa or Vaseline) using aseptic technique.
    X. Wound precautions may or may not be necessary depending upon the presence of wound drainage; drain culture if necessary.
   XI. Use room deodorant, if necessary.
  XII. Skin care as necessary and continuously. Observe for other infected sites, e.g., abscess and necrosis.
 XIII. Provide sensory stimulation during prolonged mobility, and create diversional activities for the patient.
 XIV. Evaluate care on daily basis, and revise nursing care plan, if indicated.
  XV. Allow for expression of fear and anxiety.
 XVI. Be supportive, and explain things to the patient.
 XVII. Follow-up health care referrals.

Evaluation
   I. Reassessment.
  II. Complications.
     A. *Bone necrosis:* massive antibiotic therapy.
        1. Surgery may be necessary (e.g., amputation) if blood vessels are involved.
        2. Skin grafts may also be necessary.
     B. Septicemia may also be present (refer to Chap. 44).

Ankylosing Spondylitis

Definition
    Ankylosing spondylitis is a systemic disease resulting from inflammatory involvement, causing pain and stiffness of the intervertebral, sacroiliac, and costovertebral joints (1). As the disease progresses, there is ossification and fixation (*ankylosis*) of the joints, thorax, and the entire spine. This health problem, predominant in men, may develop either *without* pain or *with* severe nerve root pain.

Assessment
    I. Pain may or may not be present.
   II. Deformity of spine and thorax.
  III. Limitation of functional movement.
  IV. Body image alterations.
   V. Continuation of disease process.

Intervention
     I. Administer medications: indomethacin, phenylbutazone.
    II. Teach patient to maintain erect posture.
   III. Continue prescribed exercises established by physical therapist.
   IV. Use a firm mattress and bed board to maintain posture.
    V. Establish specific rest periods to be spent on flat, firm surface.
   VI. Teach and provide adaptations for activities of daily living.
  VII. Explore cues about body image changes and changes in life-style.
 VIII. Make appropriate referrals, e.g., counseling, vocational rehabilitation,
   IX. Follow-up health care referral.

Bursitis

Definition
    Bursitis, an acute or chronic inflammation of a bursa, results from trauma, infection, irritation, or calcareous deposits which form within the bursal walls. The bursae, saclike spaces found between bones, muscles, or tendons, are lined with synovium and contain a small amount of synovial fluid. Usually this fluid cushions joints and permits muscular movements with the least amount of friction. With inflammation, the bursa fills with fluid, causing a joint to become swollen and resulting in restricted joint movement. The most commonly involved joint is the shoulder, although the elbows, knees, and ankles can also be involved. Pain, causing marked disability, is provoked by specific abduction movements and causes a problem commonly referred to as "frozen shoulder."

Assessment (Refer to "Osteomylitis")
     I. Joint pain; swelling; hot, tender area.
    II. Restricted joint mobility, especially in abduction.
   III. Dependence in activities of daily living.
   IV. Occupational causation, e.g., jobs involving excessive stress on joints.
    V. May be precipitated by other problems, e.g., connective tissue disorders (refer to Chap. 32).
   VI. May be associated with such physical activities as tennis.

Intervention

I. Immobilize affected joint by using pillows, splints, and/or sling.
II. Administer pain medication: analgesics or narcotics (e.g., codeine with or without aspirin).
III. Provide the patient with muscle relaxants, e.g., Valium, to prevent muscle spasms.
IV. Patients may be given steroids to help reduce inflammation and secondary swelling.
V. Assist with procaine block if indicated, preparing patient for procedure. Novacaine injected into joint for temporary relief of pain.
VI. Apply moist heat or cold packs to decrease inflammation and swelling.
VII. Continue active exercises prescribed by physical therapist, as tolerated (range-of-motion exercises).
VIII. Teach energy conservation through modifications in activities of daily living.
IX. Refer for vocational counseling if bursitis is job-related.
X. Follow-up health care referral.

Rheumatoid Arthritis

Rheumatoid arthritis is a major health problem associated with inflammation and has been discussed in Chap. 21. Surgical intervention has assisted patients toward well-being and functional independence. Refer to "Osteoarthritis" for nursing care associated with disabling arthritis and surgical intervention.

Tuberculosis of the Bones and Joints

Definition

Characteristically monarticular in nature, *tuberculous arthritis* can involve a vertebra, an elbow, a hip, or a knee. During the acute phase of this disease, *cold abscesses* are produced. Destruction of the joint may occur, resulting in hip deformity or "hunchback." Sinus pathways from a tuberculous joint are known to extend for long distances. In more than half of the affected patients, there is evidence of pulmonary tuberculosis. The symptoms of pain, wasting of adjacent muscle, weight loss, fever in conjunction with a positive history of tuberculosis, and the monarticular involvement, usually suggest the diagnosis. Tuberculous arthritis, as well as *tenosynovitis* (inflammation of the tendon and tendon sheath) and *bursitis,* can be caused by *Mycobacterium tuberculosis.* (Refer to Chap. 27 for a complete discussion of tuberculosis.)

Assessment

I. Joint and bone pain.
II. Fever; elevation seen later in the day.
III. Progressive infectious process.
IV. Pulmonary tuberculosis may or may not be present.
V. Weight loss.
VI. Dependency, secondary to chronic illness.

Intervention

I. Bed rest for several weeks.
II. Administer pain medication: analgesics.
III. Administer antibiotics and specific chemotherapy for tuberculosis. Usually two of the following are selected (refer to Chap. 27):
   A. Isoniazid (INH).
   B. Rifampin (RM).
   C. Ethambutol (EMB).
   D. Streptomycin or another antibiotic.
IV. Observe for toxic effects of medications, e.g., hepatitis.
V. Specific isolation for pulmonary tuberculosis, if present.
VI. Implement progressive muscle exercises planned in collaboration with physical therapist.

VII. Provide assistive devices for mobility and ambulation, e.g., trapeze, cane, walker.
VIII. Accept patient and his or her behavior and listen for cues of stress.
IX. Assist patient in working through dependency, and encourage self-care.
X. Teach patient:
    A. Need for initial bed rest.
    B. Progressive exercises.
    C. About medications and toxic effects.
XI. Follow-up referral.

TRAUMA

Fractures

Definition

A *fracture* can be described as a break in the continuity of a bone. There are several types of fractures; these are discussed in Chap. 44. As the bone begins to heal, it progresses through a stage of hematoma formation, beginning regrowth of new tissue, bone and callus formation, and ossification and bone remolding. (2). This section deals with the care of the patient after emergency treatment has been given. Refer to Chap. 44 for discussion of emergency care.

Assessment

Refer to Chap. 44.

Problems

I. Pain: usually subsides after bone is set and swelling is decreased.
II. Immobility.
III. Anxiety about cast, bed rest.
IV. Adequate nutrition and fluid intake.
V. Bowel and bladder elimination.
VI. Skin breakdown: decubiti.
VII. Edema.
VIII. Dependence.

Diagnosis

I. Alteration in comfort: pain.
II. Anxiety: mild, moderate, severe; secondary to pain; dependence.
III. Alteration in bowel elimination: constipation.
IV. Impairment of mobility: bed rest, cast, etc.
V. Alteration in ability to perform self-care activities.
VI. Complications (e.g., infections): potential.
VII. Alteration in nutrition: potential.
VIII. Respiratory an circulatory dysfunction: potential.

Goals of Care

I. Immediate.
    A. Stabilize respiratory and circulatory functioning.
    B. Immobilize bone to facilitate healing and proper alignment.
    C. Prevent circulatory and/or nerve impairment.
    D. Relieve pain.
    E. Provide cast care to prevent complications.
    F. Prevent constipation: improve fluid intake.
II. Long-range.
    A. Maintain cast integrity.
    B. Promote self-care.
    C. Maintain adequate nutrition and fluid intake.
    D. Prevent complications of immobility.
    E. Prepare patient for ambulation.
    F. Prevent recurrence of fracture.

Intervention

I. Medical intervention.

   A. Emergency care of a fracture may include *reduction* of the fracture by closed (manipulative) or open method, and casting.

      1. In a *closed reduction,* bone fragments are brought into apposition by manipulation and manual traction. A cast is usually applied to immobilize the fracture fragments and to support the injured parts.

      2. *Open reduction* involves surgery on the injured area in order to remove debris, remove bone fragments, or place bones in proper alignment (see "Hip Fractures" for a complete discussion).

      3. *Casts* can be applied to the extremities, the complete torso, and the upper torso to include the head and neck. *Spica casts* are applied to immobilize extremities and are used with shoulder and hip fractures; spica casts can be bilateral, depending on the areas involved. Casting usually includes the joints above and below the fracture. Currently there are two types of cast material:

         a. Plaster of Paris.

         b. Rigid plastic material such as Lightcase cast.

   B. *Traction* is the maintenance of a steady pull on a body part by means of a force to keep two bone fragments in alignment, just touching each other. With traction, there is a forward force produced by weights; *counterbalance* or *countertraction* is produced by the backward force of the muscles and the frictional force between the patient's body and the bed. Counterbalance is also achieved by elevating the body part placed in traction and by raising the bed on wooden blocks or by traction pull against a fixed body part [i.e., with the use of a *Thomas splint* (see Fig. 31-3), the proximal ring presses against the ischial tuberosity]. The most effective traction will have an equal amount of traction and counterbalance. When this occurs, the traction is considered *balanced.*

      1. The purposes of traction are:

         a. To immobilize a reduced fracture.

         b. To alleviate or eliminate muscle spasm and pain.

         c. To prevent or correct deformities.

         d. To permit and/or promote healing to an inflamed joint or extremity by means of immobilization.

      2. Types of traction.

         a. *Skin traction:* the pulling force is exerted directly on the skin and indirectly on the bone (see Figs. 31-1 and 31-2).

            (1) Buck's extension.

            (2) Russell's traction.

            (3) Pelvic or cervical traction.

         b. *Skeletal traction:* the force is applied directly to the bone by means of a metal pin or wire which is inserted directly into or through the bone.

            (1) Kirschner wire.

            (2) Steinmann pin.

            (3) Crutchfield tongs.

            (4) Thomas splint and Pearson attachment are usually used in conjunction with skeletal traction for fractures of the femur (see Fig. 31-3).

      3. Specific nursing intervention for patients in traction.

         a. Monitor attachment of traction frame with the bed in low position, then raise bed (prior to transfer to unit).

         b. Use firm mattress with bed board and trapeze prior to transfer to unit to facilitate movement.

         c. Position in recumbent supine position throughout traction duration, unless specified otherwise.

         d. Assess respiratory functioning to prevent pneumonia secondary to immobility.

         e. Assist with insertion of Kirschner wire (see Chap. 23) and care for wires using sterile technique.

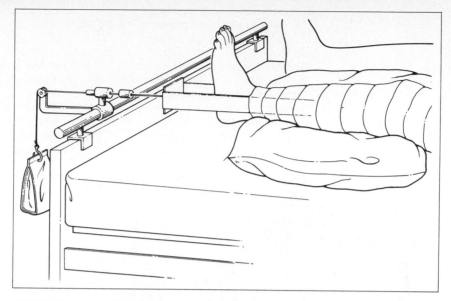

FIGURE 31-1 / Buck's extension. (*Adapted from D. Jones et al., Medical-Surgical Nursing: A Conceptual Approach, McGraw-Hill Book Company, New York, 1978.*)

FIGURE 31-2 / Russell's traction. (*Adapted from D. Jones et al., Medical-Surgical Nursing: A Conceptual Approach, McGraw-Hill Book Company, New York, 1978.*)

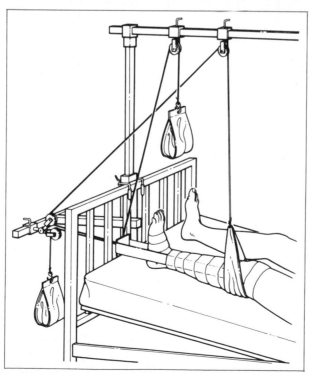

f. Examine traction apparatus daily.
   (1) Maintain ropes and pulleys in straight alignment.
   (2) Keep weights hanging free.
   (3) Ropes should be unobstructed and not touching patient.
   (4) Keep the heel of affected limb off bed and hip flexion at 20°.
   (5) Use adhesive materials that will not slip out of place.
g. Administer medication to relieve pain.
h. Maintain the patient on a well-balanced diet and provide adequate fluid intake to aid in tissue healing and to prevent problems of elimination.
i. Assess for pressure at popliteal space of the affected limb.
j. Assess for positive Homan's sign on both legs to evaluate potential of phlebitis (see Chap. 26).
k. Assess for foot drop in affected limb: use foot board to prevent changes.
l. Assess for circulatory and nerve impairment.
m. Maintain active exercises to unaffected body parts and muscle strengthening exercises for ambulation. Use isometric exercises for affected limb.
n. Inspect skin integrity.
   (1) Give skin care to back, coccyx, scapulae.
   (2) Massage bony prominences every 2 to 3 h.
   (3) Examine skin adjacent to traction apparatus.
o. Rewrap elastic bandages daily to prevent potential embolus formation, and reapply elastic stocking twice each day.
p. Encourage visitors to distract patient, provide social interest, and decrease boredom and social isolation.

FIGURE 31-3 / Balanced, suspended traction with a Thomas splint and Pearson attachment. (*Adapted from D. Jones et al., Medical-Surgical Nursing: A Conceptual Approach, McGraw-Hill Book Company, New York, 1978.*)

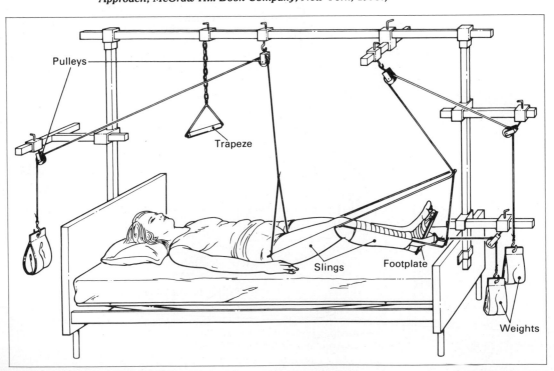

q. Explore verbal and nonverbal cues of anxiety. Have the patient freely discuss the impact of immobility, and explore diversions.

r. Implement teaching plan. Include:

(1) Use of trapeze.

(2) Limitation of movement to that tolerated.

(3) Exercise program.

s. Allocate time for diversional activities and therapeutic communication.

t. Discharge planning and referral for follow-up.

II. General nursing intervention for patients with fractures.

A. Monitor vital signs frequently to assess early signs of infection.

B. Deep breathing and coughing every 2 h to prevent respiratory problems.

C. Support wet cast with pillows, and expose cast to air for at least 24 to 48 h to facilitate drying.

D. Manipulate cast with palms of hands, rather than fingers, to prevent cracking of cast.

E. Use fan to increase circulation of air to cast. If the weather is damp, drying may take a longer period of time.

F. Elevate injured part with pillows to level of heart or above.

G. Medication for pain should be given as needed: e.g., analgesia, narcotics.

H. Apply ice bags to injured region to help reduce swelling for the first 24 h after injury.

I. Remove plaster crumbs with moist cloth, and petal cast with adhesive tape if edges are rough or unfinished to prevent skin breakdown.

J. Use plastic wrap to line edge near genital portion of cast to prevent the cast from becoming damp following excretion and/or urination.

K. Massage red areas around bony prominences to prevent tissue breakdown.

L. Inspect cast for drainage and inspect under cast edges for lesions.

M. Assess odors emitted from cast and observe for "hot spots" (hot areas over a particular point of the cast that may indicate infection).

N. Assess toes for pallor, blanching, tingling, numbness, temperature differences, cyanosis, edema, and pain.

O. Palpate peripheral pulses that are accessible, and evaluate frequently.

P. Provide well-balanced diet—high in protein, caloric content, and vitamins D and C—to aid in wound healing.

Q. Adequate fluid intake to prevent dehydration and maintain urinary output.

R. Use fracture bedpan for elimination, and schedule elimination similar to patterns prior to hospitalization.

S. Have patient participate in isometric exercises to affected limb.

T. Active exercises for unaffected extremities for ambulation conditioning.

U. For ambulation, transfer patient to side of bed opposite affected side.

V. Skin care:

1. Inspect and massage bony prominences.

2. Apply cream to skin directly under cast, using fingers or swabs, to stimulate circulation to the area.

3. Turn the patient every 2 h to prevent skin breakdown.

W. Encourage self-care to help decrease dependence. Provide support and encouragement to patient and family.

X. Teaching plan:

1. Explain need for elevation of extremity in cast.

2. Stress that nothing should be placed inside cast.

3. Teach isometric exercises.

4. Prepare for ambulation through muscle strengthening program.

5. Encourage use of trapeze to facilitate movement (refer to Fig. 31-3).

6. Instruct in use of crutches or other assistive devices. Provide instruction on gaits to be used when walking with the assistance of crutches.

7. Inform of cast removal procedures, need for support to unstable limb after cast removal, and skin care of affected limb.

Y. Discharge planning and evaluation of teaching should include:
1. Written directions for patients, e.g., exercises, diet, cast care, and medication.
2. Return demonstration of teaching: reactivity, exercise, crutch walking.

Z. Follow-up referral.

Evaluation

I. Reassessment: evaluate compliance.

II. Complications.

A. Hypovolemic shock secondary to fluid or blood loss, may develop.
1. Assessment (see Chap. 44).
   a. Decreased blood pressure and pulse.
   b. Increased respirations; may be shallow.
   c. Restlessness can be associated with blood loss.
   d. Acute anxiety, fear of injury.
   e. Complaints of severe pain.
   f. Alteration in level of consciousness.
2. Intervention.
   a. Keep patient warm, conserve heat.
   b. Monitor vital signs.
   c. Provide oxygen, if necessary.
   d. Check hemoglobin and hematocrit to evaluate blood loss. Evaluate serum sodium, chloride, and potassium levels.
   e. Replace or maintain blood volume by transfusion or intravenous fluids. Assess blood reactions.
   f. Relieve pain, since it may contribute to hypovolemia.
   g. Splint injury to avoid fluid loss and shock.

B. Thromboembolism (refer to Chap. 26).

C. Fat embolism: usually occurs in first few days after injury; often follows fractures of long bones due to release of fatty substances into bone matrix.
1. Assessment.
   a. Presence of petechiae in buccal membrane, conjunctival sacs, neck, shoulder, and chest.
   b. Tachycardia and chest pain (e.g., precordial) may be assessed.
   c. Fever.
   d. Increased respiratory rate, especially if embolus lodges in the lung; cyanosis and dyspnea may accompany the problem. A productive, blood-tinged cough may be experienced, and the presence of basal rales or rhonchi may suggest the beginning of pulmonary edema.
   e. Altered state of consciousness.
2. Intervention.
   a. Reduce shock.
   b. Position for maximum respiration; provide oxygen therapy.
   c. Use heparin to prevent additional clot formation.
   d. Measure arterial blood gases to assess oxygen and carbon dioxide exchange and perfusion.
   e. Give intravenous fluids and glucose to prevent hypovolemia; Dextran may be given as a volume expander.
   f. Antibiotics, as needed.
   g. Monitor urinary output: assess venal perfusion and evaluate cardiovascular status.
   h. Assess neurological signs, especially level of consciousness.
   i. Provide a quiet environment to promote rest.
   j. *Do not turn* patient: keep patient stable to prevent dislodgment of emboli.
   k. Intravenous corticosteroids to decrease vascular inflammation.
   l. Allay apprehension: provide information to the patient about tests, answer patient's questions, and create an atmosphere for open discussion. Support is essential.

D. Circulatory impairment: arterial and venous impairment.
  1. Assessment.
      a. Pallor or blanching of toes.
      b. Numbness and tingling.
      c. Coldness to touch.
      d. Pain not relieved by narcotics; the pain intensifies with motion of toes.
      e. Peripheral pulses unequal.
      f. Venous impairment may be manifested by cyanosis and edema.
  2. Intervention.
      a. Assess for tightness of cast.
      b. Monitor vital signs.
      c. Assess peripheral pulses.
      d. Report to physician.
      e. Open bivalve cast and reapply.
      f. Elevate limb (venous impairment).

E. Nerve impairment.
  1. Assessment.
      a. Tingling or numbness in the affected limb, e.g., the elbow.
      b. Decreased ability or inability to move previously functioning toes.
      c. Decreased feeling or lack of feeling in toes (*paresthesia*).
      d. When the *perineal* nerve is involved, the foot and lateral aspect of the ankle are affected.
  2. Intervention.
      a. Assess for edema; monitor peripheral pulses.
      b. Assess for cast tightness, and release cast (bivalve).
      c. Monitor vital signs.
      d. Change traction, if necessary.

F. Infection.
  1. Assessment.
      a. The presence of an open, contaminated wound (usually a compound fracture).
      b. If infection is deep, gas gangrene or tetanus may develop.
      c. Drainage from cast: note color, odor, and amount.
      d. Pain may be localized or diffuse.
      e. So-called hot spots may be palpated over an affected area of the cast.
      f. If gas gangrene is present, cellulitis, fever, tachycardia, discoloration of tissue, and alteration in hemoglobin will be noted.
  2. Intervention.
      a. Culture drainage from wound; note the amount.
      b. Inspect skin under cast, and remove cast if necessary.
      c. Note drainage, encircle drainage area on the cast, and monitor frequently.
      d. If gangrene is present, open wound to air, facilitate drainage, irrigate, and apply dressing changes using sterile technique.
      e. Give oral antibiotics, e.g., penicillin or tetracycline; check drug allergies.
      f. Monitor vital signs.
      g. Cast reapplication may be necessary.
      h. Administer analgesics and/or narcotics to reduce pain.
      i. Window cut in cast to assess site of infection.

G. Delayed union or nonunion.
  1. Assessment.
      a. Radiography: nonunion, lack of callus formation.
      b. False motion (pseudoarthrosis).
      c. Refer to assessment of fractures.
  2. Intervention.
      a. Surgery (open reduction).
      b. Postoperative cast care.
      c. Braces.

H. Orthostatic hypotension (refer to Chap. 26).
  1. Assessment.

      a. Weakness, diaphoresis, and dizziness upon elevation.

      b. Syncope upon elevation.

      c. Hypotension.

  2. Intervention.

      a. Place in dorsal recumbent position.

      b. Gradually increase elevation over a period of days.

      c. Elastic compression bandages and abdominal binder, prior to elevation and ambulation.

      d. Active exercises.

      e. Monitor vital signs in supine and Fowler's positions and while affected extremity is dangling.

Hip Fractures

Definition

The highest incidence of *hip fracture* is with elderly women and occurs as a result of falling accidents. While carrying out activities of daily living, the person turns or twists, breaking a bone, and then falls. Hip fractures are caused primarily by (1) degenerative and osteoporotic changes and (2) a decreased resistance to normal stresses. Concomitantly there may be normal physiologic changes in balance and perception that may occur with senescence. Hip fractures may be *intracapsular,* involving the head and neck of the femur, or *extracapsular,* in which the trochanteric portion of the femur is involved. The characteristic position of a suspected hip fracture is hip abduction and external rotation accompanied by shortening of the affected leg. Also present are muscle spasm and pain. Intracapsular fracture of the femur can easily disrupt the blood supply to the area, and nonunion of the fracture fragments may occur, despite the fact that perfect reduction may have been achieved. Management of the patient with a hip fracture is further complicated if there is a history of chronic disease.

Assessment

    I. Data sources (refer to "Bone Tumors").

   II. Health history (refer to "Fractures").

     A. Age: tendency for this problem to occur in the elderly. Common in women.

     B. Occupation may predispose the individual to injuries.

     C. Dietary habits: depressed calcium, especially in early development.

     D. History of falling, previous fractures, "accident-prone".

     E. Presence of associated diseases (e.g., malignancy, pathological fracture).

  III. Physical assessment (refer to Chap. 44 and "Fractures").

     A. Changes in vital signs may indicate presence of or impending shock.

     B. Specific findings upon examination of injured site:

       1. Affected hip in abduction and external rotation.

       2. Affected leg is shorter than unaffected leg.

       3. Pain aggravated by movement.

       4. Muscle spasm intensified by movement.

       5. Localized or peripheral edema.

       6. Limitation of movement.

       7. Temperature inference: affected extremity and toes may be cold.

  IV. Diagnostic tests (refer to Table 31-1).

     A. Radiograph of affected hip.

     B. Chest plate.

     C. ECG to assess cardiac changes.

     D. CBC: decreased hemoglobin and sedimentation rate.

     E. Others, specifically related to any accompanying illness.

   V. Other data sources.

     A. Emergency care report.

     B. Referral from local physician.

     C. Old records.

Problems   Refer to "Fractures."

Diagnosis   Refer to "Fractures."

Goals of Care (Refer to "Fractures")
  I. Immediate.
   A. Stabilize and maintain adequate health status prior to and after surgery.
   B. Maintain extension of affected hip.
   C. Prepare patient from surgery.
   D. Prevent complications.
   E. Meet psychosocial needs.
  II. Long-range.
   A. Restoration of health.
   B. Independence in activities of daily living.
   C. Prepare patient for mobilization.
   D. Teach patient how to achieve maximum functional stability of affected hip.
   E. Assist patient in transition to home care.

Intervention (Refer to "Fractures")
  I. Use a flotation mattress and trapeze on bed prior to transfer from emergency room.
  II. Transfer to bed with one person assigned to support affected leg. Apply manual traction, if indicated.
  III. Monitor vital signs, e.g., pulse; temperature; evaluate changes.
  IV. Initiate coughing, deep breathing exercises.
  V. Assess need for pain medication and muscle relaxants; administer as necessary.
  VI. Assist with application of Buck's extension (Fig. 31-1) and explain its purpose.
  VII. Elevate affected leg on pillow; elevate bed 25°.
  VIII. Check alignment of traction every 2 h; use trochanter rolls or sandbags if needed to maintain internal rotation.
  IX. Range-of-motion exercises to unaffected limbs.
  X. Inspect toes for circulatory and nerve impairment.
  XI. Muscle strengthening exercises to upper extremities, abdomen, and unaffected leg.
  XII. If patient is not placed in traction prior to surgery, the following turning and positioning techniques can be utilized. Turn every 2 h, using turning sheets.
   A. Supine position.
    1. Pillow under affected limb from knee to heel.
    2. Trochanter roll or sandbag to maintain internal rotation and extension.
    3. Head of bed elevated only if necessary.
   B. Side lying.
    1. Position pillow between legs from groin to ankle.
    2. Bring patient close to side of bed.
    3. Turn to side with one person always assigned to support affected leg.
    4. Partial turn to 45° may or may not be tolerated on affected hip.
    5. Pillows:
     a. To back.
     b. Additional pillow may be necessary to keep hip joint in alignment.

Evaluation   **I.** Reassessment.
  II. Surgery.
   A. Preoperative nursing intervention: routine.
   B. *Open reduction* or *internal fixation* may be performed to expose, realign, and immobilize the hip and related structures in place by means of a metallic device. A metal device, usually vitallium or stainless steel, is nontoxic, inert, nonporous, nonpyrogenic, and nondegradable in the body (refer to Fig. 31-4). Surgical intervention with hip fractures permits early weight bearing and mobility. Bone union usually occurs 4 to 6 months postoperatively.

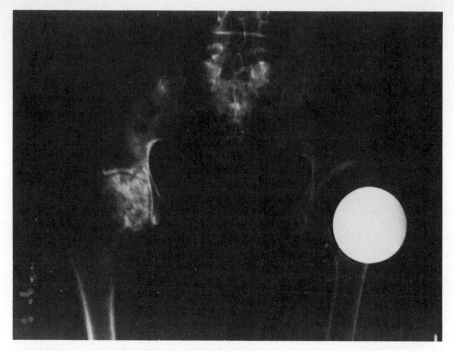

FIGURE 31-4 / X-ray showing vitallium cup prosthesis for intracapsular fracture.
(*Courtesy of Radiation Sciences Department, Bunker Hill Community College, Charlesburg, Mass.*)

    C. Postoperative nursing intervention.
        1. Prevention of complications (refer to "Osteoarthritis" and see the discussion of complications under "Fractures").
        2. Support involved limb; handle gently and carefully.
        3. Maintain body alignment while in bed; maintain hip extension.
        4. Encourage self-care in activities of daily living; encourage patient to move on own.
        5. Continue range-of-motion and active exercises, and begin active assistive exercise in collaboration with physical therapist.
        6. Ambulate as soon as possible. When ambulating:
            a. Apply elastic bandages to both lower extremities.
            b. Get out of bed on unaffected side.
            c. Assist patient in moving slowly, to attain sitting position, and to maintain dangling position until balance is attained (monitor vital signs).
            d. Weight bearing on affected leg may be limited.
            e. Use of crutches or walker is important to provide assisted ambulation.
        7. Discharge planning.
            a. Prepare for home care or for transfer to rehabilitation center.
            b. Teaching plan to include:
                (1) Adaptation to activities of daily living.
                (2) Removal of potential hazards at home.
                (3) Adequate lighting in darkened areas and at night.
                (4) Slow, purposeful movements, and achievement of balance prior to getting out of bed or chair.
                (5) Need for continuity of care.
        8. Referral for follow-up care (e.g., visiting nurse). Extended care facility should be considered.

    D. Assess response to outcomes of therapeutic regimen, and revise nursing care plan as recovery progresses.

    E. Complications of surgery (see complications discussed under "Fractures" for appropriate intervention).

       1. Delayed union or nonunion.
       2. Disuse phenomena from immobility.
       3. Nerve and circulatory impairment.
       4. Respiratory complications.
       5. Cardiovascular complications.
       6. Wound infection.
       7. Alterations in mental acuity.

Lower Back Pain

Definition

Lower back pain is one of the most common health problems in our society today. It results in great discomfort, disability, and loss of time from work. Among the causes are muscle strains, tension, lack of physical exercise, poor posture, and certain systemic diseases. As people grow older, lower back pain becomes more chronic in nature and results from the degenerative processes occurring in the disks and vertebral joints. The therapeutic course is treatment of symptoms.

Assessment

  I. Pain, severe at times.
 II. Muscle spasm which may intensify pain.
III. Immobility due to pain.
 IV. Muscle weakness, unsteady gait.
  V. Associated health problem .

Intervention

   I. Use of firm mattress and bed board; the floor may be used.
  II. Applications of warm heat (heating pad).
 III. Rest in Fowler's position.
  IV. Administer medication for pain (e.g., Darvon, Tylenol, codeine) and for muscle relaxation (e.g., Valium).
   V. Continue exercises initiated in physical therapy.
    A. Maybe abdominal muscle-strengthening exercises.
    B. Maybe exercises to attain mobility of spine.
  VI. Teaching plan:
    A. Daily physical exercise (avoid strenuous exercises).
    B. Correct posture; good use of effective body mechanics.
    C. Firm mattress and hard plywood board under mattress at home.
    D. Avoid straining or lifting heavy objects.
    E. Avoidance of sleeping in prone position.
    F. Avoidance of prolonged sitting, standing, walking, and driving.
    G. Referral for follow-up care.
 VII. Traction may be necessary (refer to "Fractures").

Evaluation

 I. Reassessment.
II. Complications.
   A. Chronic lower back pain syndrome.
   B. Nerve blocks and other surgical intervention (refer to Chap. 23).
   C. Fracture of spine (refer to Chap. 23).
   D. Sprains, strains, discolorations (refer to Chap. 44).

OBSTRUCTIONS

Peripheral Vascular Disease (Refer to Chap. 26)

Definition

Peripheral vascular disease occurs when local cells cannot receive their nutritional requirements because blood supply to the leg is greatly diminished. This may result from peripheral vascular insufficiency caused by athrogenesis and arteriosclerotic changes. A reduction in blood supply to a lower extremity can result in infection, ischemia, and gangrene. All measures to restore circulation are usually attempted before *amputation* is decided upon (refer to Chap. 26).

Assessment (Refer to Chap. 26)

I. Include oscillometric readings.
II. Skin, temperature changes.

Problems

I. Pain caused by deficiency of blood supply in area (ischemia).
II. Infection may be present.
III. Fear of surgery (preoperative).
IV. Anxiety.

Diagnosis

I. Alteration in comfort: pain.
II. Anxiety: mild to severe.
III. Grieving: anticipatory, secondary to a lost limb.
IV. Alteration in ability to move effectively: state of dependence.
V. Self-concept: alteration in body image, secondary to amputation.
VI. Impairment of skin integrity, secondary to immobility.
VII. Alteration in elimination: potential.
VIII. Alteration in sensory perception: motor loss.
IX. Impairment of significant others' adjustment to loss of limb.

Goals of Care

I. Immediate.
 A. Alleviate pain.
 B. Prevent infection.
 C. Allay fears.
II. Long-range.
 A. Full ambulation to optimal level of function with prosthesis.
 B. Eliminate pain and discomfort.
 C. Help patient retain independence.

Intervention (Refer to Chap. 26)

I. Surgery: *Amputation,* the surgical removal of a diseased limb, body part, or organ.
 A. Major reasons for amputation:
  1. Trauma or complication resulting from trauma.
  2. Acute disease processes such as cancer of the bone, infections, and peripheral vascular disease and its complications (e.g., arteriosclerosis, diabetes mellitus, and Buerger's disease).
  3. Congenital anomaly.
 B. Types of amputation (see Fig. 31-5):
  1. *Disarticulation*—removal by resection of an extremity through a joint, hip, or ankle.
  2. Amputation above the knee.
  3. Amputation below the knee.
  4. *Guillotine* or *open*—amputation in which the surface of the wound is not covered by skin.
  5. *Metatarsal*—amputation occurring in the foot.
II. Preoperative intervention.
 A. Place foot board or cradle on bed; elevate head of bed with wooden blocks.
 B. Relieve pain with specified narcotics and/or analgesics.
 C. Prepare the patient for surgery; discuss feelings of loss openly.
 D. Maintain upper extremity strength through exercises, especially to muscles of the affected limb.
III. Postoperative intervention.
 A. Either a soft dressing is applied to the stump, or a rigid dressing, which is a cast to

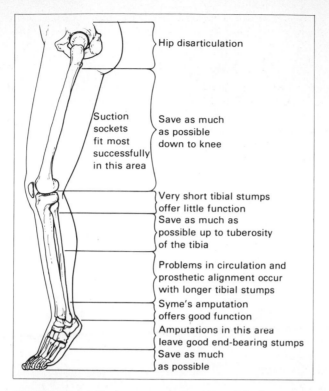

Hip disarticulation

Suction sockets fit most successfully in this area

Save as much as possible down to knee

Very short tibial stumps offer little function
Save as much as possible up to tuberosity of the tibia

Problems in circulation and prosthetic alignment occur with longer tibial stumps

Syme's amputation offers good function

Amputations in this area leave good end-bearing stumps

Save as much as possible

FIGURE 31-5 / **Common amputation sites of the lower extremities. (***Adapted from Richard Warren and Eugene Record, Lower Extremity Amputation, Little, Brown and Company, Boston, 1967.***)**

which a pylon and foot piece are attached, is applied. This immediate postoperative "prosthesis" reduces edema, shapes the stump, and permits early weight-bearing ambulation.

B. Prevent stump edema, elevate tump (e.g., pillows), and prevent contractures.

C. Stump bandaging (see Fig. 31-6).

1. Use two or three elastic bandages sewn together (4-in total length for amputation below the knee; 6-in length for amputation above the knee).
2. Hip should be flexed about 24°.
3. Clean bandage every day.
4. Rewrap 4 times a day.
5. Apply before patient gets out of bed.

D. Stump conditioning after healing.

1. Wash stump and dry carefully each day.
2. Inspect for irritation, pressure.
3. Massage stump.
4. Push stump into soft pillow, progressing to firm pillow, and finally to hard surface.
5. Small amount of powder over stump (not incisional site).
6. Apply stump sock.
7. Apply heat, and change position for muscle spasm.

E. Facilitate movement as tolerated; use trapeze over bed and foot cradle (for unaffected leg).

F. Monitor vital signs: prevent shock (hypovolemia); assess and measure drainage from dressings; use Hemovac.

G. Help the patient and family members deal with loss of the limb. Accept behavior demonstrated, be supportive, and offer the individual and family an opportunity to

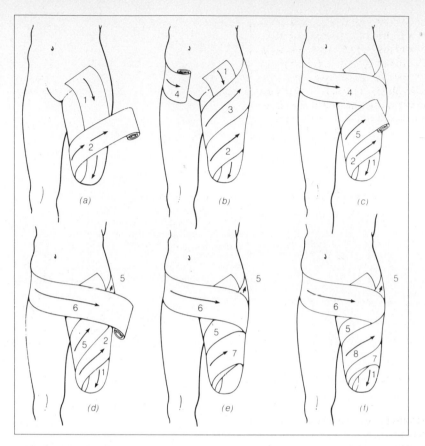

FIGURE 31-6 / Applying a stump bandage. (*From D. Jones et al., Medical-Surgical Nursing: A Conceptual Approach, McGraw-Hill Book Company, New York, 1978.*)

share feelings. Explore feelings of grief and dependence, and perception of body image.

H. Teaching plan for patients and families.
1. Procedure for alleviating muscle spasm (e.g., warmth, applications).
2. Diet to avoid obesity.
3. Physical care of remaining extremity includes inspection, hygiene, nail care, etc.
4. Stump care, conditioning, and bandaging (refer to Fig. 31-6).
5. Modifications of self-care activities if confined to wheelchair.
6. Crutch walking or other ambulatory adaptations.
7. Phantom pain sensations, an annoying phenomenon, decrease with activity. Provide analgesia and/or distraction.
8. Associated health problems to prevent complications.
9. Exercise.
    a. Range of motion.
    b. Tricep sitting and strengthening.
    c. Push-up exercises (wheelchair).
    d. Hip extension and adduction exercises.
    e. Teach balancing exercises. With the nurse or a family member standing close to prevent falling, have the patient:
        (1) Arise from chair to standing position.
        (2) Stand on toes while holding onto chair.

(3) Bend knees while holding onto chair.

(4) Balance on one leg without support.

(5) Hop on one leg while holding onto chair (3).

Evaluation

I. Reassessment. Nursing care plan should be revised as patient progresses toward discharge. Constant evaluation of the patient's health status will alert the nurse to complications.

II. Complications.
   A. Hemorrhage from surgical site (refer to Chap. 44).
   B. Infection of wound.
   C. Wound separation.
   D. Contracture formation.
   E. Stump lesions.
   F. Phantom pain.
   G. Delayed grieving.

III. The nurse should refer to the literature for the care of patients with *upper extremity* amputations and for information about prostheses, if appropriate.

DEGENERATIVE DISORDERS

Osteoarthritis

Definition

Osteoarthritis is a noninflammatory disease affecting the joints. Deterioration and abrasion occur in the articulating cartilage, as well as in the new bone at the articular surface. Osteoarthritis may be idiopathic, occurring with normal use and aging. Structural damage to the joints in an earlier, developmental stage of life can provoke osteoarthritis as one approaches middle age or early senescence.

Osteoarthritis is a localized process found most commonly in the weight-bearing joints of the lower extremities, in the lumbar vertebrae, and in the hands. With aging, the cartilage loses water content and elastic abilities, resulting in softening, separation, and fraying of cartilage. As the cartilage thins and erodes, new bone is stimulated to grow on the articular surface, producing *bony spurs* that interfere with the mechanical function of the joint. As osteoarthritis progresses, bones, with their eroded cartilage surfaces, come in direct contact with each other, producing pain and restricted motion. As a result, muscle spasms and contractures are common outcomes. *Heberden's nodes,* bony nodules occurring on the dorsolateral aspects of the distal finger joints, are chronic manifestations of osteoarthritis in the fingers.

Assessment

I. Data sources (refer to "Bone Tumors").

II. Health history.
   A. Age: usually over 50 years.
   B. Sex: more women than men affected.
   C. Cultural background.
   D. Environmental, occupational, financial, educative, recreational, and spiritual information relating to *habits* and *social and work roles.*
   E. Description of pain.
      1. Date of onset.
      2. Causative factors.
      3. Methods of relief.
   F. Associated health problems, current and past.
   G. Pharmacological history.
      1. Current medication.
      2. Use of steroids and salicylates.
      3. Allergies.
   H. Nutritional history and dietary habits.

       I. Relevant family history, e.g., arthritis associated with aging.

       J. History of trauma (fall on affected joint).

III. Physical assessment.

  A. Assess range-of-motion limitations.

  B. Position and appearance of extremities: note deformities in affected joints.

  C. Joints: tenderness on palpation and pain on motion; some edema may be present.

  D. Sensory perception and circulation may not be affected. May be secondary to this problem.

  E. Muscle strength: palpation grip test limited.

  F. Appearance of affected joints should be normal except for bony enlargement, pain, stiffness, restricted motion, Heberden's nodes.

  G. Presence of crepitus on motion: note in affected joints.

  H. Vertebral column involvement: motor weakness and paresthesia may be present.

  I. Gait unsteady and guarded.

  J. Fatigue may be noted, and tolerance (muscle, etc.) may be diminished.

  K. Assess general physical health status, including cardiopulmonary status, weight, mental activity.

IV. Diagnostic tests (see Table 31-1).

  A. Arthroscopy.

  B. Synovial fluid analysis: normal.

  C. Serology: negative.

  D. Arthrography and radiographs of affected joints.

    1. Narrowing of joint space.

    2. Bony sclerosis.

    3. Bony spur formation.

  E. Radiographs of vertebral column reveal spaces between vertebrae are narrowed.

V. Other data sources.

  A. Previous health records.

  B. Consultation, referral notes.

Problems

I. Pain.

II. Decreased joint mobility: potential contracture formation.

III. Altered nutritional state: obesity or cachexia.

IV. Altered gait patterns.

V. Difficulty in carrying out activities of daily living.

VI. Anxiety.

Diagnosis

I. Alteration in comfort: discomfort, pain.

II. Immobility, secondary to restricted joint mobility.

III. Alteration in nutrition: more or less than required.

IV. Alteration in ability to move effectively; dependence.

V. Alteration in ability to perform self-care activities.

VI. Alteration in sensory and motor perception.

VII. Associated health problems: potential.

VIII. Anxiety: mild to severe.

Goals of Care

I. Immediate.

  A. Reduce or alleviate pain.

  B. Maintain or improve joint mobility.

  C. Reduce stresses on affected joints.

  D. Identify cause of joint pain and eliminate.

II. Long-range.

  A. Remove source of stress on joint, e.g., weight reduction.

  B. Maintain or improve mobility, and return patient to optimal level of functioning.

  C. Prevent or control pain.

  D. Prevent trauma to weight-bearing joints.

    E. Restore maximum joint functioning.

    F. Prepare for surgery, if needed.

Intervention

    I. Heat applications to affected joint for edema.

    II. Administer medications to reduce pain:

      A. Corticosteroids to reduce joint inflammation.

      B. Analgesics and/or salicylates to reduce pain and joint inflammation.

      C. Muscle relaxants to reduce muscle spasm.

    III. Explain local intraarticular injections, e.g., cortisone, to patient and support during injection.

    IV. Assist in diet selection, considering likes and dislikes; control weight, and plan diet accordingly.

    V. Encourage self-care and other physical activities.

    VI. Continue exercise regimen and use of assistive devices, initiated in physical and occupational therapy.

    VII. Refer to counseling for vocational rehabilitation, if applicable.

    VIII. Teaching plan:

      A. Understanding and cooperation in weight reduction.

      B. Reduction of joint strain.

      C. Rationale and side effects of medication, e.g., steroids, salicylates.

      D. Modification of activities to perform within physical limits and stress on joints; plan physical activity as tolerated.

      E. Rest periods twice per day in recumbent position; encourage periods of sitting.

      F. Proper body mechanics; plan exercise program for continuation at home.

    IX. Continuity of health care and follow-up referral.

Evaluation

    I. Reassessment.

      A. Pain not reduced.

      B. Progression of joint stiffness with increase in muscle spasm and contracture formation.

      C. Complications from side effects of medications:

        1. Hemorrhagic tendency from salicylates.

        2. Stress ulcer from corticosteroids.

        3. Allergies.

    II. Intervention.

      A. Trial of other medications and evaluate response.

      B. Alterations in exercise program.

      C. Surgery.

        1. Synovectomy—removal of the synovial membrane.

        2. Total knee replacement.

        3. Osteotomy—surgical section of a bone, e.g., subtrocanteric.

        4. Reconstructive finger and elbow surgery.

        5. *Total hip arthroplasty* (total hip replacement): a surgical procedure in which the acetabular cartilage and head of the femur are replaced with a prosthesis (see Fig. 31-7).

          a. The goals of surgery, in conjunction with the health team treatment regimen, are:

            (1) To restore, improve, or maintain joint function.

            (2) To provide greater stability of the hip joint.

          b. Preoperative intervention.

            (1) Teaching plan.

              (a) Patient and family participation in mobility regimen.

              (b) Postoperative exercise program.

              (c) Techniques in hip abduction.

              (d) Use of urinal and bedpan in recumbent position.

              (e) Postoperative respiratory exercises.

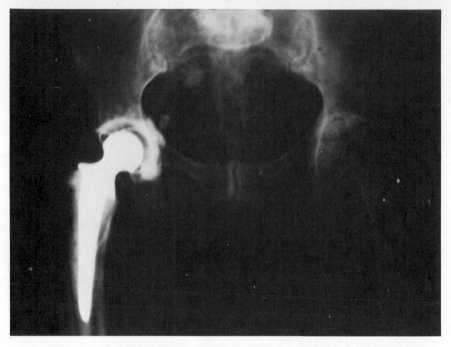

FIGURE 31-7 / Total hip arthroplasty with Charney-type prosthesis. (*Courtesy of Radiation Sciences Department, Bunker Hill Community College, Charlestown, Mass.*)

      (2) Demonstrate balanced suspension traction apparatus and use of trapeze (*see* Fig. 31-3).
      (3) Administer systemic antibiotic and anticoagulant therapy.
      (4) Perform bacteriostatic skin scrub preparation: usually pHisoHex and/or Bedadine is used.
      (5) Explore verbal and nonverbal cues of emotional stress.
      (6) Explain and perform routine preoperative procedures.
   c. Postoperative intervention.
      (1) Use flotation mattress, traction apparatus, and trapeze on bed.
      (2) Monitor vital signs.
      (3) Provide for adequate respiratory functioning.
      (4) Maintain integrity of hip prosthesis:
         (*a*) Maintain hip in abduction *at all times;* use wedge-shaped abduction pillow between legs.
         (*b*) Turn every 2 h: supine, to unaffected side, keeping hip in abduction.
         (*c*) Elevate affected extremity on pillows.
         (*d*) Limit head of bed elevation to 45°.
      (5) Assess circulatory and nerve functioning of affected leg every hour.
      (6) Initiate exercise program early, in collaboration with physical therapist.
         (*a*) Affected leg: isometric exercises.
         (*b*) Active exercises to unaffected extremities, using foot board.
         (*c*) Discourage sitting for prolonged periods.
      (7) Monitor alignment of traction 3 to 4 times per day.
      (8) Observe incisional dressing for drainage, bleeding; Hemovac may be present.
      (9) Assess patient for signs of infection in operative site.
   (10) Assess patient for thrombophlebitis and possible emboli.
         (*a*) Use antiemboli stockings, Ace bandages.

(b) Leg exercises.

(c) Frequent turning.

(11) Assess for dislocation (subluxation) of hip prosthesis.

    (a) Severe pain.

    (b) External rotation of hip with noticeable shortening of leg.

    (c) Bulge can be palpated over head of femur.

(12) Assess bony prominences for skin breakdown.

    (a) Use of air mattress.

    (b) Artificial sheepskin.

    (c) Skin care every 2 h.

(13) Discharge planning.

    (a) Progressive exercise program.

    (b) Follow-up in ambulatory health care setting.

REFERENCES

1. Lillian S. Brunner and Doris S. Suddarth, *Textbook of Medical-Surgical Nursing,* 3d ed., J. B. Lippincott Company, Philadelphia, 1975, p. 1010.
2. Ibid., p. 968.
3. Ibid., p. 993.

BIBLIOGRAPHY

Beyers, Marjorie, and Susan Dudas: *The Clinical Practice of Medical-Surgical Nursing,* Little, Brown and Company, Boston, 1977. A new comprehensive book detailing pathophysiology, patient needs, and nursing care of patients who have common health problems; applicable to the clinical setting.

Buck, Barbara and Allen D. Lee: "Amputation: Two Views," *Nursing Clinics of North America,* **11:** 641–657, December, 1976. A patient's personal account of amputation and a nurse's discussion of the nursing care involved with this patient.

"How to Negotiate the Ups and Downs, Ins and Outs of Body Alignment," *Nursing '74,* **4:**46–51, October 1974. A photographed account of how to prevent some of the effects of prolonged bed rest.

Jennings, Kate R.: "The Cheerful Operation: Total Hip Replacement," *Nursing '76,* **6:**32–37, July 1976. An informative discussion about pre- and postoperative care of the person undergoing total hip replacement.

Jungreis, Sidney W.: "Exercises for Expediting Mobility in Bedridden Patients," *Nursing '77,* **7:**47–51, August 1977. Planning and implementing a program to promote mobility.

Long, Barbara C., and Patricia S. Buergin: "The Pivot Transfer," *American Journal of Nursing,* **77:** 980–982, June 1977. Illustrated information about moving patient with one non-weight-bearing leg safely from bed to chair.

McClinton, Virginia S.: "Nursing of the Upper Extremity Amputee and Preparation for Prosthetic Training," *Nursing Clinics of North America,* **11:**671–677, December 1976. A discussion of the nursing care after surgery and during prosthetic fitting and initial training.

O'Dell, Ardis, J.: "Hot Packs for Morning Joint Stiffness," *American Journal of Nursing,* **75:**986–987, June 1975. A nursing research study that presents information about nursing management of patients with arthritis.

Orthopedic Nurses' Association and American Nurses' Association Division on Medical-Surgical Nursing: *Standards of Orthopedic Nursing Practice,* American Nurses Association, Kansas City, 1975.

Pasnau, Robert O. and Betty Pfefferbaum: "Psychological Aspects of Post-Amputation Pain," *Nursing Clinics of North America,* **11:**679–685, December 1976. A discussion of the nursing management of patients who are affected by phantom limb pain.

Pfefferbaum, Betty, and Robert O. Pasnau: "Post-Amputation Grief," *Nursing Clinics of North America,* **11:**687–690, December 1976. A discussion of the acute grieving process accompanying the loss of a limb and the role of the professional staff in assisting a patient during the grief process.

Pitorak, Elizabeth F.: "Rheumatoid Arthritis: Living with It More Comfortably," *Nursing '75,* **5:**33–35, December 1975. A personal account of a nurse coping with an alteration in body image.

Staudt, Annamay R.: "Femur Replacement," *American Journal of Nursing,* **8:**1347–1348, August 1975. Adolescents with osteogenic sarcoma are given a new perspective for life with femur replacement.

Stein, Alice M., Delaine Mandell, and Jacqueline Ferguson: "Multiple Fractures: How to Prevent the Pulmonary Complications," *Nursing '74,* **4:**26–32, November 1974. Deals with the complications of immobility, especially emboli.

32

The Immunologic System

Mackey P. Torbett

DEFENSE SYSTEM

The first section of this chapter deals with the defense system of the body and how it resists disease. The major function of the defense system is to identify substances which are not "self" (foreign substances) and enact mechanisms to render them harmless to the body.

I. The noxious substances that incite a defense reaction originate either externally or internally.
   A. External substances.
      1. Bacteria and their products.
      2. Viruses may not directly cause a reaction, but indirectly, via necrosis of tissue, they may.
      3. Protein, e.g.:
         a. Egg white.
         b. Milk.
      4. Allografts.
         a. Kidney.   d. Liver.
         b. Skin.   e. Lung.
         c. Heart.
      5. Insect venom.
         a. Bee sting.
         b. Spider bite.
      6. Drugs, e.g.:
         a. Penicillin.   c. Codeine.
         b. Horse serum.   d. Aspirin.
      7. Thermal injuries.
   B. Internal substances.
      1. The exact causal agent in these reactions in most cases has not yet been determined.
      2. Some theoretical substances are:
         a. Collagen.
         b. Native DNA (N-DNA).
         c. Basement membranes.
II. Resistance mechanisms.
   A. Nonspecific mechanisms.
      1. Skin acts as a mechanical barrier.
      2. Mucous membranes.
         a. Mucus traps bacteria.
         b. In the respiratory tract, specialized cilia sweep bacteria toward exterior.
      3. Inflammatory response (see Fig. 32-1). The components of inflammatory response due to vascular changes include:
         a. Blood vessels dilate, increasing blood supply to the area and causing *redness*.
         b. The enlarged vessels become more permeable, allowing fluid to flow into tissues, and resulting in localized *swelling*.
         c. Increased blood flow to the area causes increased *heat* in involved tissues.
         d. If nerves are stretched by swelling, *pain* occurs.
      4. Other mechanisms.
         a. Difference between pH favorable for invading organism and that of organs under attack (e.g., vagina, bladder).
         b. Natural bacteria flora (e.g., in intestine).

B. Specific mechanisms of immune system. There are four components that make up this system.

    1. Phagocytosis ("cell eating"): engulfing and destruction or inactivation of foreign substances by body cells.

        a. Cellular involvement (see Table 32-1 for complete classification of leukocytes).

            (1) Neutrophils [polymorphonuclear (PMN) and granular cells].

                (a) Origin in white blood cells derived from bone marrow.

                (b) Exerts automicrobial effect in conjunction with other components such as antibody and complement system.

                (c) Abnormal defects are of two types: decrease in number and defect in the cell structure and/or function.

                (d) Active in acute infections.

            (2) Monocytes.

                (a) Origin in white blood cells derived from bone marrow.

                (b) Mononuclear agranulocyte cells.

                (c) Found in circulation, bone marrow, and tissues. They mature to

FIGURE 32-1 / Summary of the nonspecific local inflammatory response to infection.
(From Arthur J. Vander, James H. Sherman, and Dorothy S. Luciano, Human Physiology, 2d ed., McGraw-Hill Book Company, New York, 1975, p. 487.)

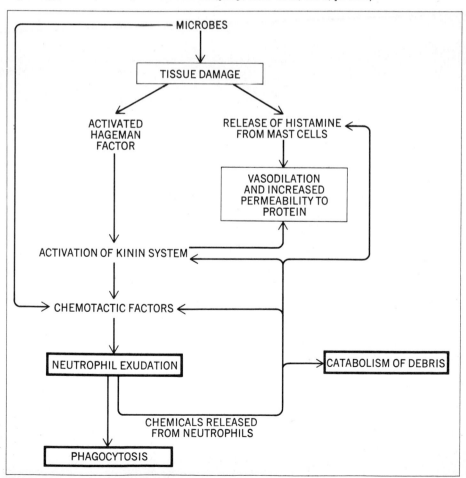

macrophages in lung, Kupffer cells in liver, and macrophages in spleen, lymph nodes, and other organs.

(d) May act as back-up system for neutrophils in acute infections. They play a larger role in chronic infections.

  b. Modes of action.
    (1) Chemotaxis:
      (a) Phagocytic cells are attracted to the area of the invading pathogen.
      (b) Complement chemotactic factors are C3a and C5a.
      (c) Thymus-dependent lymphocytes (T cells) secrete lymphokines such as migration inhibitory factor (MIF) that attract macrophages to area of inflammation.
    (2) Opsonization. Bacteria are made more susceptible to action of macrophages by antibody response and/or combination of antibody and complement mechanisms.
    (3) Ingestion (see Fig. 32-2). The neutrophil or macrophage cell extends its cell membrane, which surrounds the foreign or invading matter and pulls it into the interior of the cell.

TABLE 32-1 / CLASSIFICATION OF LEUKOCYTES

Cell	Normal Blood Concentration	Description	Formation Site	Function
Total leukocytes	5000–9000/mL			
Granular leukocytes:				
Polymorphonuclear neutrophils (PMN)	62–65% of total leukocytes	Fine granules in cytoplasm; two- to three-lobed nucleus	Bone marrow (myeloblast)	Phagocytosis
Polymorphonuclear eosinophils	2–4% of total	Large granules in cytoplasm; bilobed nucleus	Bone marrow (myeloblast)	Weak role in phagocytosis; increased concentration in the presence of foreign protein, perhaps a detoxifying function; increased in parasitic infection
Polymorphonuclear basophils	0.2–0.5% of total	Large granules in cytoplasm; bilobed nucleus	Bone marrow (myeloblast)	Complete function unknown; resemble mast cells in the release of histamine and heparin; increased during inflammation
Nongranular leukocytes:				
Lymphocytes	25% of total	Nongranular cytoplasm; large globular nucleus	Bone marrow (lymphoblasts) go to thymus and bursal-equivalent lymphoid tissue to differentiate into thymic (T) and bursal (B) lymphocytes	T cells responsible for cellular immunity; B cells produce large lymphocytes and plasma cells which form the antibodies of humoral immunity
Monocytes	5–7% of total	Nongranular cytoplasm; large, deeply indented nucleus	Bone marrow (monoblasts)	Phagocytosis; form tissue macrophages (histiocytes) that also participate in phagocytosis

Source: Adapted from Russell M. DeCoursey, *The Human Organism*, 4th ed., McGraw-Hill Book Company, New York, 1974, p. 329; and Maxwell Wintrobe, *Clinical Hematology*, Lea & Febiger, Philadelphia, 1974, pp. 228–229.

(4) Killing.

    (a) Certain bacteria are acted on by neutrophils.

    (b) Those that survive the attack by PMN cells are acted on by the macrophages.

    (c) The exact mechanism for destruction is not well understood.

2. Antibody-mediated immunity (humoral).

    a. Development (see Fig. 32-2).

      (1) Bone marrow- or bursa- (B cell–) derived lymphocytes develop from common stem cells.

      (2) B cells, when stimulated by an antigen, proliferate into plasma cells.

      (3) Plasma cells secrete antibodies specific to antigen. Antibody or immunoglobulin (Ig) types are described in Table 32-2.

        (a) IgG. The major immunoglobulin class in quantity. Crosses placenta to provide protection for the infant for 6 months after birth. Protects against infections such as pneumonia, sinusitis, and bronchitis.

        (b) IgM. Seems to be active in chronic diseases and autoimmune reactions such as systemic lupus erythematosus.

        (c) IgA. Found in secretions such as those from nasopharynx, gastrointestinal tract, and urinary tract. It is thought that this immunoglobulin protects against pathogens that invade through the mucous membrane (1).

        (d) IgE. Active in type I allergic reactions. Has an affinity for mast cells and basophils which release such mediators as histamine. Slow-reacting substance of anaphylaxis (SRSA) eosinophilic chemotactic factor.

        (e) IgD. Has been isolated but function has not been determined.

    b. Modes of action:

      (1) Antibody itself is not destructive.

      (2) Factors that cooperate to cause destruction are:

        (a) Classic complement pathway.   **(c)** T-cell lymphocytes.

        (b) Alternate complement pathway.   **(d)** Phagocytosis.

3. Cell-mediated immunity (direct attack by mediators which stimulate activity of lymphocytes to destroy or inactivate foreign substances).

    a. Development.

      (1) Stem cells originate in bone marrow.

      (2) Lymphocytes designated to be T cells (thymus-dependent) are acted upon by thymus.

      (3) Released into circulation and peripheral lymph tissue.

    b. Modes of action (see Fig. 32-2).

      (1) When T cells are stimulated by foreign antigen, they are destructive to the antigen via direct contact and by production and release of lymphokines.

      (2) A number of lymphokines have been identified. Some are inhibitory and others are augmenters. Of the better described lymphokines, four are:

        (a) Lymphotoxin lysis, the target cell.

        (b) MIF, which inhibits migration of macrophages.

        (c) Transfer factor, which is capable of transferring delayed hypersensitivity.

        (d) Interferon, which defends against viral infections.

4. Complement. This is a series of proteins which stimulate cellular activities (via reactions with antibody-antigen complexes) essential to immune responses.

    a. Classic pathway involves 11 serum proteins initiated by IVGG or IgM (see Table 32-3 for description of complement activities).

      (1) Recognition unit: C1, having three components (C1q, C1r, and C1s); C2, and C3.

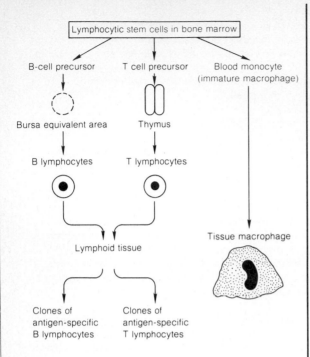

I. **Maturation pathways for antibodies, sensitized lymphocytes and macrophages**

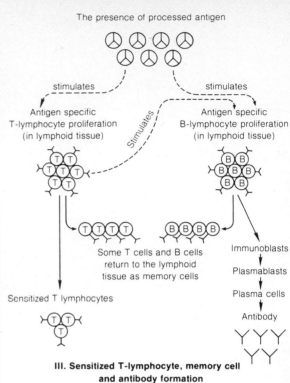

III. **Sensitized T-lymphocyte, memory cell and antibody formation**

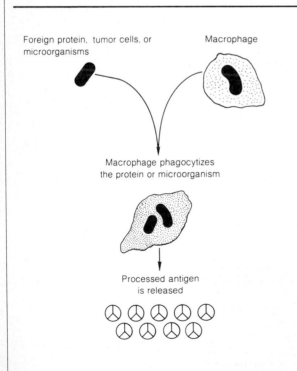

II. **Role of the macrophage in stimulating the immune response**

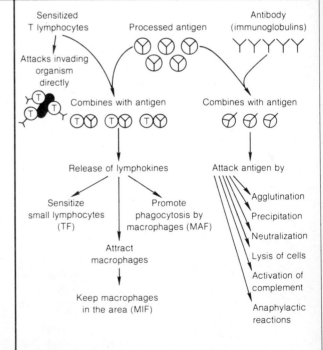

IV. **Cellular (cell-mediated) and humoral (antibody) immunity**

TABLE 32-2 / CLASSIFICATION OF IMMUNOGLOBULINS

Class	Quantity	Location	Function
IgG	About 75% of total immunoglobulins	Plasma and interstitial fluid	Produces antibodies against bacteria, viruses, and toxins; largely responsible for secondary immune response reactions; activates the complement system
IgA	About 15% of total	Large quantities in tears, saliva, milk, and other exocrine secretions; small quantities in serum	Functions in mucous membrane protection and defense of exposed body surfaces, particularly from infectious agents
IgM	About 10% of total	Serum	In combination with IgG, has specific antitoxin action; provides the "natural" antibodies that include the rheumatoid factor and the ABO isoantibodies; largely responsible for the primary immune response reaction; activates the complement system
IgD	Less than 1% of total	Serum	Unknown
IgE	Less than 1% of total	Serum and interstitial fluid; present also in exocrine secretions	Allergic reactions: atopy and anaphylaxis

Source: Dorothy A. Jones, Claire F. Dunbar, and Mary M. Jirovec, Medical-Surgical Nursing: A Conceptual Approach, McGraw-Hill Book Company, New York, 1978.

     (2) Activation unit: C4, C2, and C3, which has two fragments (C3a and C3b).

     (3) Membrane attack unit, which causes lysis of the cell, includes C5, C6, C7, C8, and C9. C5 has two fragments (C5a and C5b).

   b. Alternate or properdin pathway.

     (1) This is initiated by contact of cell and factor I.

     (2) Then there is cooperation with :

        (a) C3b.

        (b) Serum factor B.

        (c) Serum factor D.

     (3) Properdin stabilizes this complex.

     (4) After properdin, the pathway is the same as the classic pathway.

III. Hypersensitivity reactions (allergic states).

   A. Type I reaction: anaphylactic. Components of immune systems involved:

     1. Antibody IgE.

     2. No complement involvement.

     3. Reaction mediators are basophils and mast cells which release histamine and SRSA.

   B. Type II reaction: Cytotoxic. Components of immune systems involved:

     1. Antibody IgG or IgM.

     2. Complements C1 through C9.

     3. Reaction mediators are complement lysis and mononuclear phagocytosis.

FIGURE 32-2 / Immune response sequence. [*Adapted from Herman Eisen, Immunology, Harper and Row, Hagerstown, Md., 1974, p. 461; and John O. Nysather et al., "The Immune System: Its Development and Function," American Journal of Nursing, 76(10):1617–1618, October 1976.*]

TABLE 32-3 / BIOLOGICAL EFFECTS OF ACTIVATION PRODUCTS OF COMPLE-MENT SYSTEM

Complexes and Components Involved	Activities
C1, 4	Neutralization of herpes simplex virus together with IgM
C1, 4, 2	Possible generation of kinins, increase in vascular permeability
C3b	Leukocyte phagocytosis; immune adherence, C3b on the RBC, WBC, or platelet adheres to normal RBC—agglutination (in vitro); viruses coated with Ig and complement adhere to platelets or RBC, resulting in removal by phagocytes
C3a	Leukocyte chemotaxis; anaphylotoxin (contraction of smooth muscle, increased vascular permeability, and histamine release)
C5a	Leukocyte chemotaxis; anaphylatoxin
C5, 6, 7	Leukocyte chemotaxis
C8, 9	Cytotoxic effect

Source: D.M. Weir, *Immunology for Undergraduates*, 3d ed., Churchill Living-stone, Edinburgh, 1973.

    C. Type III reaction: immune complex–mediated. Components of immune systems involved:
        1. Antibody IVGG or IgM.
        2. Complement C3a and C5a chemotactic factors and anaphylatoxins.
        3. Reaction mediated by neutrophil (lysosome) enzymes.
    D. Type IV reaction: delayed (cell-mediated).
        1. No antibody involvement.
        2. No complement involvement.
        3. Mediated by lymphocytes (lymphokines) and macrophages.

ANAPHYLAXIS

DEFINITION

An *anaphylactic reaction* is a type I immediate hypersensitivity response to a foreign antigen. This is a systemic response that can result in death due to respiratory obstruction or vascular collapse. The reaction involves the combining of the antigen with IgE antibody on mast cells. This releases histamine and SRSA. (Also refer to the discussion of shock in Chap. 44.)

ASSESSMENT

  I. Physical assessment. In this situation, a *quick* assessment of the patient's condition may be vital to save the patient's life, and therefore should be completed before time is taken to acquire the health history.
    A. Respiratory system.
        1. Dyspnea.   **3.** Rhinorrhea.
        2. Wheezing.   **4.** Itching of nose.
    B. Cardiovascular system.
        1. Hypotension and shock due to vasodilatation and increased permeability.
        2. Arrhythmias.
        3. Palpitations.
    C. Gastrointestinal system.
        1. Nausea.   **3.** Abdominal pain.
        2. Vomiting.   **4.** Diarrhea.
    D. Neurologic system.
        1. Convulsions.
        2. Loss of consciousness.

    E. Skin.
        1. Urticaria.
        2. Erythema.
        3. Angioedema.
II. Health history.
    A. Data sources.
        1. Patient.   **3.** Witnesses to patient's collapse.
        2. Family.   **4.** Significant others.
    B. Sensitivity to:
        1. Foods.
           a. Nuts.   *c.* Seafood.
           b. Berries.   *d.* Egg albumin.
        2. Insect venom.
           a. Honeybees.
           b. Hornets.
           c. Wasps.
        3. Drugs.
           a. Penicillin and some other antibiotics.   *e.* Vaccines.
           b. Salicylates.   *f.* Horse serum.
           c. Sulfonamides.   *g.* Enzymes.
           d. Local anesthetics.
    C. Occupation (may help to identify causative agent).
    D. Location of home (identify proximity to possible causative agents).
    E. Smoking (affects respiratory component of response).
    F. Drinking (possible component in hypersensitivity).
    G. Response pattern to stress (identify precipitating factors of anaphylaxis).
    H. Family allergies (possible contributing factors).
III. Diagnostic tests.
    A. Radiographic.
    B. Contrast media.

PROBLEMS

  I. Hypoxia due to: **III.** Cardiac arrhythmias.
    A. Laryngeal edema.   **IV.** Skin eruptions.
    B. Bronchospasm.   **V.** Anxiety due to fear of death.
    C. Obstruction.   **VI.** Unconsciousness.
  II. Hypovolemia.

GOALS OF CARE

  I. Immediate (save the patient's life).
    A. Maintain open airway.   *C.* Prevent hypovolemia.
    B. Prevent hypoxia.   *D.* Prevent cardiac arrest.
  II. Long-range.
    A. All efforts should be made to determine the allergen that caused the reaction.
    B. Prevent recurrence.
    C. Hyposensitization.

INTERVENTION

  I. Immediate.
    A. Give oxygen. Cardiopulmonary resuscitation (CPR) may be necessary if cardiac arrest occurs.
    B. Give 1000 to 2000 mL physiologic saline or 5% glucose in saline rapidly and intravenously (2). Plasma expanders or whole blood may be necessary.
    C. Epinephrine, 1:1000, 0.2 to 0.5 mL IM (3).
    D. Monitor blood pressure, pulse, and respiration.

II. Long-range.
   A. Teach patient and family how to avoid allergen.
   B. Teach patient and family about allergic reaction.
   C. Alert family and significant others to possible recurrence and actions to take.
   D. Counsel for hyposensitization.

EVALUATION
I. Death usually occurs within minutes after onset of reaction unless condition is reversed.
II. In some cases, shock may persist.
   A. Respiratory and cardiac failure must be prevented (refer to Chaps. 26 and 27).
   B. Irreversible brain damage may result.
III. Repeat assessment to ascertain probability of preventing recurrence.

IMMUNODEFICIENCY DISEASES

DEFINITION
I. T-cell deficiencies (cell-mediated).
   A. DiGeorge's syndrome (thymic hypoplasia).
      1. Symptoms appear immediately following birth.
      2. Associated with hypoparathyroidism.
      3. If there is survival beyond the neonatal period, frequent and chronic infections ensue.
   B. Chronic mucocutaneous candidiasis.
      1. Associated with a selective deficit of T-cell immunity resulting in increased susceptibility to candidal infections.
      2. Infections may involve:
         a. Skin.   c. Mucous membranes.
         b. Nails.   d. Vagina.
      3. May or may not be associated with endocrine pathologies, such as:
         a. Hypoparathyroidism.
         b. Addison's disease.
         c. Diabetes.
II. B-cell deficiency disorders (antibody).
   A. X-linked agammaglobulinemia.
   B. Acquired.
      1. Associated with repeated infections in the adult.
      2. May develop many disorders, such as:
         a. Hemolytic anemia.
         b. Eczema.
         c. Rheumatoid arthritis.
   C. Increased IgM with deficient IgG and IgA.
   D. IgM deficiency.
   E. IgA deficiency.
III. Phagocytic dysfunctions. These disorders account for 1 percent of immunodeficiency disorders (4).
   A. Chronic granulomatous disease.
   B. Chédiak-Higashi syndrome.
   C. Job's syndrome.
   D. Lazy leukocyte syndrome.
   E. Glucose 6-phosphate dehydrogenase (G6PD) deficiency.
   F. Splenic deficiency.
   G. Defective leukocyte chemotaxis.
IV. Complement system disorders. There can be a deficiency in:
   A. C1q, C1s, C1r.   D. C4.
   B. C2.   E. C5.
   C. C3.

V. Combined T- and B-cell disorders.
   A. Ataxia-telangiectasia.
   B. Eczema and thrombocytopenia (Wiskott-Aldrich syndrome).
   C. Thymoma.
   D. Short-limbed dwarfism.
   E. Graft-versus-host (GVH) disease.

ASSESSMENT
   I. Data sources.
      A. Family.
      B. Patient.
      C. Old records.
  II. Health history.
      A. Age (young and older individuals are more apt to develop disorders).
      B. Sex.
      C. Dietary habits (malnourishment is a possible predisposing factor).
      D. Frequency of infection.
      E. Duration of infection.
      F. Unexpected complications of infection.
      G. Frequent diarrhea or vomiting.
      H. History of surgery, radiation therapy, chemotherapy, and alcohol or drug abuse (possible iatrogenic and autogenic causes).
 III. Physical assessment.
      A. General appearance.   E. Ears.
      B. Joints.   F. Nose.
      C. Skin.   G. Throat.
      D. Eyes.
  IV. Diagnostic tests.
      A. CBC and differential (leukopenia).   D. Chest x-ray.
      B. Bone marrow (pancytopenia).   E. Skin tests (allergic response).
      C. Lateral x-ray of pharynx.

PROBLEMS
   I. Fever.   III. Nausea and vomiting.
  II. Joint pain.   IV. Diarrhea.

GOALS OF CARE
    I. Relieve discomfort from generalized symptoms.
   II. Education.
       A. Disease process.
       B. Good health habits.
       C. Prevention of infection.
  III. Decrease fever.
   IV. Relieve pain.
    V. Regulate iet.
   VI. Psychologic support.
  VII. Provide clean environment.
 VIII. Encourage good hygiene.
   IX. Prevent recurrence of infection.
    X. Prepare for diagnostic procedures.

INTERVENTION
    I. Damp dust equipment and furniture in patient's room with disinfectant solution: dry dusting scatters pathogens.
   II. Dehumidify air: reduce number of moisture-laden microorganisms.
  III. Use disposable equipment whenever possible.

IV. Arrange nursing assignments so that immunologically depressed patients receive care first: reduce transmission of pathogens from other patients.

V. Do not assign personnel with infections to these patients.

VI. Careful hand-washing technique should be followed by nursing and other medical personnel and visitors.

VII. Provide meticulous skin care to prevent entry of pathogens.

VIII. Aseptic technique should be used with all procedures and equipment.

IX. Turn frequently to prevent decubitus ulcers.

X. Encourage passive and/or active joint exercise to prevent friction injuries.

XI. Change linens immediately when soiled.

XII. Avoid sunburn and any other possible sources of direct trauma to the skin.

XIII. Encourage frequent deep breathing and coughing to prevent respiratory infections.

XIV. Provide protective isolation to prevent transmission of pathogens to patient.

XV. Provide balanced nutrition and encourage adequate rest to enhance resistance to infection.

XVI. Teach patient and family safety, self-protection procedures, signs of infection, skin care, etc.

EVALUATION

I. Chronicity may result: will necessitate preparing patient and family to cope with long-term involvement.

II. Death may be imminent: support for patient, family, and others.

AUTOIMMUNITY

Autoimmunity is a pathologic immune response to one's own tissue, thus causing irreversible damage in many cases.

Organ-specific Disease

Thyroiditis
Arthritis

I. Self-antigen is thyroglobulin.

II. Diffuse enlargement of thyroid may be present.

III. May be associated with symptoms of systemic inflammatory response.

IV. Thyroid function may be normal or diminished.

V. Thought to be a T-cell response.

Generalized Systemic Diseases

Rheumatoid (Hashimoto's Disease)

DEFINITION

Rheumatoid arthritis is a chronic systemic disease that is more prevalent in females and affects 5 million Americans (5). With the discovery of the rheumatoid factor (RF), it is now thought to be a type III immune complex reaction. Refer to Chap. 31 for a complete discussion; juvenile rheumatoid arthritis is discussed in Chap. 21.

ASSESSMENT

I. General health history.

A. Age.
B. Sex.
C. Occupation.
D. Dietary habits.
E. Bowel habits.
F. Reaction to stress.
G. Recent stressful events.

H. Infections.
  1. Frequency.
  2. Type.
  3. Time of most recent infection.
I. Recreation.
J. Illnesses of family (often occurs within same family).
K. Allergies.

II. Specific health history.
  A. Joints.
    1. Stiffness.
    2. Redness.
    3. Aching.
    4. Swelling.
    5. Warmth.
    6. Involved joints:
      a. Asymmetry.
      b. Stiffness on awakening in the morning.
      c. Migration.
  B. Constitutional symptoms.
    1. Easily fatigued.
    2. Loss of appetite.
    3. Weight loss.
    4. Unexplained fever.
III. Physical assessment (see Fig. 32-3 for summary of clinical features).
  A. General appearance. Patient may be pale due to anemia; also may have drawn features due to chronic discomfort.
  B. Skin: subcutaneous nodules, especially around the olecranon process.
  C. Joints (see Fig. 32-4 for joint changes).
    1. Inflammation.
    2. Deformity.
    3. Asymmetry.
    4. Pain on movement.
  D. Musculature. Test range of motion to identify tendon and muscle involvement.
  E. Renal system. Urinalysis to test for presence of blood cells or protein.
  F. Gastrointestinal system.
    1. Epigastric pain.
    2. Nausea.

FIGURE 32-3 / Common clinical features of rheumatoid arthritis. (*From Dorothy A. Jones, Claire F. Dunbar, and Mary M. Jirovec, Medical-Surgical Nursing: A Conceptual Approach, McGraw-Hill Book Company, New York, 1978, p. 381.*)

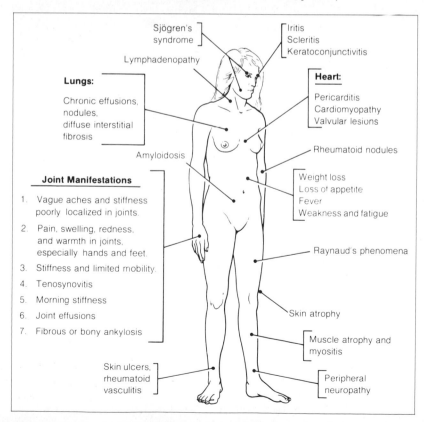

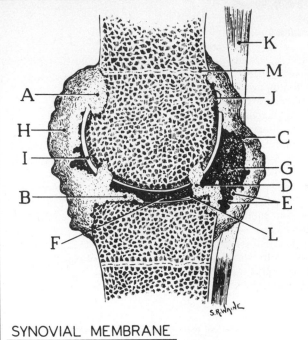

SYNOVIAL MEMBRANE

 A - Invasion of Subchondral Bone
 B - Erosion of Articular Cartilage (Pannus)
 C - Fibrotic Area
 D - Fibrous Adhesions
 E - Multiple Villi

JOINT SPACE

 F - Narrowed
 G - Loculated Effusion

 H - Laxity of Thickened Capsule and Ligaments
 I - Articular Cartilage
 J - Subchondral Bone
 K - Muscle
 L - Fibrocartilage
 M - Old Epiphyseal Plate

FIGURE 32-4 / Some changes in a synovial joint in rheumatoid arthritis. (*From D. Hamerman, J. Sandson, and M. Schubert, "Biochemical Events in Joint Disease," Journal of Chronic Disease, 16:837, 1963.*)

  3. Vomiting.
  4. Tarry stools. This is particularly important after treatment has been started.
 G. Lungs.
  1. Congestion.
  2. Pain.

IV. Diagnostic tests.
   A. X-rays.
   B. Red blood cells (RBC).
   C. Hemoglobin: decreased.
   D. Sedimentation rate: elevated.
   E. Latex agglutination to determine presence of rheumatoid factor (RF).

PROBLEMS
I. Pain.
II. Mobility.
III. Adjustment to chronic disease.

GOALS OF CARE
I. Control pain.
II. Proper regimen for rest and exercise.
III. Maintain present life-style as nearly as possible.
IV. Support from family and/or significant others.

INTERVENTION
I. Teach patient and family concerning:
   A. Drugs, especially side effects, e.g., with:
      1. Salicylates.
      2. Steroids.
      3. Gold salts.
   B. Quackery.
   C. Pathology of disease.
II. Plan with patient and family a routine that includes proper exercise and rest periods, support for inflamed joints.
III. Provide emotional support.
IV. Diet instruction: avoid obesity to reduce weight supported by involved joints.
V. Instruct patient to avoid extreme cold and stressful events when possible, to reduce precipitating factors to exacerbations.
VI. Consistency in follow-up. Should see same health team members to establish rapport and trust.

EVALUATION
I. Reassessment.
   A. Follows drug regimen without side effects.
   B. Minimal joint deformities.
   C. Relief of pain.
   D. Activities tolerated without increase in pain.
   E. Continues to maintain life-style similar to that prior to illness or has adjusted to change.
II. Follow-up.
   A. Clinic visits.
   B. Home visits: very important for supportive and informative follow-up.
   C. Telephone calls.

Systemic Lupus Erythematosus

DEFINITION
Systemic lupus erythematosus (SLE) is a chronic inflammatory disease (with occasional exacerbations) of connective tissues associated with lesions in vascular system, dermis, and serous and synovial membranes.

ASSESSMENT
I. Data sources.
   A. Patient.
   B. Family.
   C. Significant others.

II. Health history (include family history: tends to occur in certain ethnic groups and among immediate relatives, especially an identical twin).

III. Physical assessment.
   A. May complain first of constitutional symptoms:
      1. Generalized aching.
      2. Weakness.
      3. Malaise.
      4. Low-grade fever.
      5. Chills.
      6. Weight loss.
      7. Present medications: SLE can be drug-induced.
   B. Skin.
      1. Butterfly rash.
      2. Discoid lesion.
      3. Any skin reaction to sun.
   C. Musculoskeletal system.
      1. Nonerosive arthritis.
      2. Arthralgias.
   D. Central nervous system.
      1. Seizures.
      2. Psychosis.
      3. Cranial nerve involvement.
   E. Cardiopulmonary system.
      1. Chest pain on breathing: pleurisy.
      2. Substernal or precordial pain aggravated by movement may indicate pericardial involvement.
   F. Renal system.
      1. Blood cells and protein in urine.
      2. Elevated blood pressure on several different readings.

IV. Diagnostic tests.
   A. Lupus erythematosus cell preparation.
   B. Antinuclear antibody.
   C. Complement testing.
   D. False-positive serology for syphilis.

PROBLEM
   I. Pain.
   II. Immobility.
   III. Fatigue.
   IV. Decreased appetite.
   V. Constipation.
   VI. Anxiety and/or depression.
   VII. Low-grade fever.
   VIII. Dermal lesions.
   IX. Cardiopulmonary dysfunction.
   X. Renal dysfunction.
   XI. Bruising and/or bleeding.
   XII. Central nervous system involvement.

GOALS OF CARE
   I. Prevent exacerbations.
   II. Maintain life-style and activity.
   III. Promote adequate nutrition.
   IV. Relieve pain.
   V. Promote adequate rest.
   VI. Reduce depression.

INTERVENTION
   I. Teach patient, family, and significant others about:
      A. Pathology of disease.
      B. Possible course of disease.
      C. Medications and side effects.
      D. Warning signs which indicate flare-up, i.e., constitutional symptoms.
   II. Explain emotional involvement to patient and family, mood swings.
   III. Plan activity and rest schedule.
   IV. Discuss possible effects of stress and different ways to cope.
   V. Explain to employer the disease process and patient's need to continue to be productive.
   VI. Antiinflammatory medications: aspirin, nonsteroids (Indocin).
   VII. Skin lesions: antiinflammatory creams; skin care; avoid trauma, sunburn, antimalarial medications.

  VIII. Joint inflammation: salicylates, exercise regularly.

  IX. Gastrointestinal upset: aspirin, prednisone, antiemetics, laxatives, bland diet.

  X. Cardiopulmonary dysfunction: regulate exercise, monitor vital signs, observe for signs of pneumonia and other secondary lung infections.

  XI. Vascular involvement: observe for tarry stools, abdominal pain and distension, abnormal bowel sounds.

  XII. Renal problems: monitor blood pressure and temperature, observe for edema in lower extremities, weigh daily (indications of fluid retention).

  XIII. Central nervous system involvement: observe for ptosis, diplopia, seizures, alterations in consciousness.

  XIV. Vascular spasms: signs of Raynaud's syndrome (sensitive, ulcerative, or gangrenous digits).

  XV. Hematologic problems: observe for malaise, chills, and fever; check urine for hematuria; check for back and abdomen pain.

  XVI. Bruising and petechiae: observe for blood in stools and gastric secretions, nosebleeds, or any other bleeding.

  XVII. Corticosteroid therapy.
- **A.** Observe for toxic effects: diabetes, peptic ulcers, secondary infections, necrosis.
- **B.** Provide for adequate rest and nutrition: control inflammation.

  XVIII. Provide support in handling stress: reduce susceptibility to secondary infections.

  XVIX. Immunosuppressant therapy: uncertain action; observe for possible toxic effects.

EVALUATION

  I. Reassessment.
- **A.** Remission of symptoms.
- **B.** Follows drug regimen.
- **C.** Follows routine for rest and activity.
- **D.** Continues life-style prior to illness as nearly as possible.
- **E.** Return to normal laboratory values.
- **F.** No indication of further systemic involvement.

  II. Follow-up.
- **A.** Acute phase.
  1. Clinic visits should be determined on individual basis.
  2. Depends on severity of symptoms.
  3. Support of family.
  4. Adjustment of patient.
- **B.** Chronic phase.
  1. The patient must be followed by health team for remainder of life.
  2. Consistency of health team members of utmost importance.
  3. Group therapy with other patients or involvement in Lupus Club may be beneficial.

GRAFT REJECTION

DEFINITION

Unless an organ for transplantation is secured from an identical twin, the immune system must be suppressed to prevent rejection. There have been many different organs transplanted in humans, including the lung, liver, heart, and kidney. Of these, the most common and perhaps the most successful to transplant has been the kidney. Regardless of the organ transplanted, the immune response is the same. This section describes that response. When a specific example is needed, the patient receiving a kidney transplant is considered.

1. Types of rejection.
   a. Type II: cytotoxic.
   b. Type IV: delayed hypersensitivity.

2. Immunosuppressants.
   a. Cytotoxic drugs.
   b. Corticosteroids.

ASSESSMENT (AFTER TRANSPLANTATION)

I. Wound inspection.
  A. Pain.
  B. Infection.
II. Signs that organ is not functioning properly, e.g., kidney:
  A. Decreased urinary output.
  B. Elevated serum creatinine.
  C. Elevated blood urea nitrogen (BUN).
III. Side effects of immunosuppression: bone marrow suppression.
  A. Infection.
  B. Anemia.
  C. Bleeding.

PROBLEMS

I. Infection.   V. Restricted intake.
II. Bleeding.   VI. Special diet.
III. Anxiety.   VII. Decreased output.
IV. Isolation.

GOALS OF CARE

I. Prevent infections.   III. Rehabilitation.
II. Prevent emotional isolation.   IV. Psychologic support.

INTERVENTION

I. Before transplant. Teach patient and family:
  A. Side effects of drugs.   C. Limitation of visitors.
  B. Reverse isolation procedure.   D. Rejection signs.
II. After transplant.
  A. Enforce reverse isolation.
  B. Monitor signs of infection.
  C. Monitor vital signs.
  D. Monitor fluid intake and output.
  E. Monitor signs of severe bone marrow depression.

EVALUATION

Transplant patients take the chance of losing their lives to complications of immunosuppression.
I. Follow-up on any indication of complications.
II. The patient must be very aware of rejection and complications.
III. Readjustment of life-style if transplant is a success.
IV. Acceptance of rejection.

TUMOR IMMUNOLOGY[1]

DEFINITION

Treatment of cancer by immunotherapy is still experimental. The basic premise is that the immune system (both T and B cells) is responsible for keeping cancer cells from overwhelming the body. However, in many cases, for some unknown reason this system fails or is overcome. Thus, a neoplastic growth progresses uncontrolled. The therapy is aimed at stimulating the immune system to resist growth of the neoplastic lesion. Types of therapy include:

1. Active immunotherapy.
  a. Specific: involves injection of tumor-specific antigen and is still in experimental stages.

[1] Elaboration on specific cancer nursing can be found in appropriate chapters.

   b. Nonspecific: an antigen other than cancer is injected to stimulate a generalized immune response. Bacillus Calmette-Guérin (BCG) is an example of this type of therapy and has been used with some success in the treatment of melanoma.
2. Passive immunotherapy. This involves transferring the antitumor antibody from a person who has been cured of the cancer to one with active growth. This is still experimental and carries with it some hazardous side effects at this time.

ASSESSMENT
I. Pathology.
II. Anatomical involvement.
III. Patient's knowledge and understanding of disease.
IV. Family's knowledge and understanding of disease.

GOALS OF CARE
I. Decrease anxiety.
II. Minimize side reactions.

INTERVENTION
I. Teach objective of therapy.
II. Teach possible side effects.
III. Teach advances in research to provide hope.

EVALUATION
I. Reaction of patient to therapy.
   A. Physical.
   B. Mental.
II. Reaction of family to patient. Rejection or support.

REFERENCES

1. Morton L. Hammond, "Clinical Evaluation of the Immunologically Involved Patient," *The Journal of the Florida Medical Association,* **64:**633–643, September 1977.
2. H. H. Fudenberg et al. (eds.), *Basic and Clinical Immunology,* Lange Medical Publications, Los Altos, Calif. 1976, p. 440.
3. Ibid., p. 440.
4. Walter L. Henley, "Immunodeficiency Disorders," *Pediatric Annals,* **5:**418–429, July 1976.
5. 1976 Annual Report, The Arthritis Foundation, Atlanta, Ga., 1976.

BIBLIOGRAPHY

Bochow, Alyson: "Cancer Immunotherapy: What Promise Does It Hold?" *Nursing 76,* **6:**50–56, October 1976. Discusses types of immunity and the treatment of cancer.
Bonforte, Richard: "Evaluation of the Child with Repeated Infections," *Pediatric Annals,* **5:**431–438, July 1976. Physical and laboratory assessment in immune diseases.
Boyse, Edward A., and Harvey Cantor: "Surface Characteristics of T-Lymphocyte Subpopulations," *Hospital Practice,* **12:**81–88, April 1977. Different surface characteristics of helper, suppressor, and killer T cells.
Cathcart, Edgar. S.: "Current Concepts in Management of Lupus Nephritis," *Hospital Practice,* **12:** 59–67, May 1977. Options of steroid, cytotoxic, and thymic hormones are discussed as therapy.
Dharan, Murali: "The Immune System: Immunoglobulin Abnormalities," *The American Journal of Nursing,* **76:**1626–1628, October 1976. Discusses all globulins and hyper- and hypogammaglobulinemias.
Donadio, James V.: "Systemic Lupus Erythematosus and Lupus Renal Disease: Diagnosis and Management," *Geriatrics,* **29:**39–44, December 1974. Early diagnosis necessity and results with steroid therapy.

Donley, Diana L.: "The Immune System: Nursing the Patient Who Is Immunosuppressed," *The American Journal of Nursing,* **76:**1619–1625, October 1976. Agents that suppress the system, laboratory findings, and specific nursing care.

Fudenberg, H. Hugh, et al. (eds.): *Basic and Clinical Immunology,* Lange Medical Publications, Los Altos, Calif. 1976. Contains 40 chapters on all aspects of immunology.

Hammond, Morton L.: "Clinical Evaluation of the Immunologically Involved Patient," *Journal of the Florida Medical Association,* **64:**633–643, September 1977. The immune system and reaction types.

Henley, Walter L.: "Immunodeficiency Disorders," *Pediatrics Annals,* **5:**418–429, July 1976. Discusses symptoms, prognosis, and treatment.

Johnson, P. M., and W. Page Faulk: "Rheumatoid Factor: Its Nature, Specificity, and Production in Rheumatoid Arthritis," *Clinical Immunology and Immunopathology,* **6:**414–430, November 1976. A review of rheumatoid factor in rheumatoid arthritis.

Katz, David H.: "Genetic Controls and Cellular Interactions in Antibody Formation," *Hospital Practice,* **12:**85–99, February 1977. Discussion of genes that code for immune response, suppression, and cell interaction.

Kimishige, Ishizaka: "Structure and Biologic Activity of Immunoglobulin E," *Hospital Practice,* **12:** 57–67, January 1977. The structure an activities of all identified immunoglobulins, with emphasis on IgE.

McKhann, Charles F, and Melvin A. Yarlott, Jr.: *Tumor Immunology,* Professional Education Publication Pamphlet, American Cancer Society, Chicago, 1975. Cancer and immunity: interaction of components in the system.

Muller-Eberhard, Hans J.: "Chemistry and Function of the Complement System," *Hospital Practice,* **12:**33–43, August 1977. Describes the action of complement components in both classic and alternate pathways.

Nysather, John O., et al.: "The Immune System: Its Development and Function," *The American Journal of Nursing,* **76:**1614–1618, October 1976. Humoral and cellular immunity and the steps in their response.

Old, Lloyd J.: "Cancer Immunology," *Scientific American,* May 1977, pp. 62–79. Discusses how cancer cells escape destruction by the immune system.

Rodman, Gerald P. (ed.): *Primer on the Rheumatic Diseases,* 7th ed., The Arthritis Foundation, New York, 1973. In some sections discusses immunology of autoimmune diseases.

Seidenfeld, John J., and Hal B. Richerson: "Basics of Pulmonary Immunology and Hypersensitivity Pneumonitis (Extrinsic Allergic Alveolitis)," *Heart and Lung,* **6:**439–443, May–June 1977. Basics of pulmonary immunology, hypersensitivity reactions, and pneumonitis.

Torbett, Mackey P., and Judy C. Ervin: "The Patient with Systemic Lupus Erythematosus," *American Journal of Nursing,* **77:**1299–1302, August 1977. Clinical article on nursing care of systemic manifestations of systemic lupus erythematosus.

Warren, Stanley: "A New Look at Type I Immediate Hypersensitivity Immune Reactions," *Annals of Allergy,* **36:**337–341, May 1976. Detailed discussion of the process in type I reactions.

Weigle, William L.: "Immunologic Tolerance and Immunopathology," *Hospital Practice,* **12:**71–80, June 1977. Discusses different tolerance requirements of T and B cells.

33

The Integumentary System

Meredith Censullo

An intact integumentary system is vital in maintaining body temperature, protecting the body against infectious pathogens, preserving body fluids, and contributing to an individual's personal appearance. Disruptions of the integument can be precipitated by such things as trauma, abnormal cellular growth, and inflammation. When these disturbances occur, they result in a variety of behavioral and pathophysiologic changes within the body. This chapter discusses common health problems which alter an individual's integumentary system, identifies related psychosocial and physiological effects, and discusses the nursing care that can be applied to each health problem.

ABNORMAL CELLULAR GROWTH

Skin Tumors

Definition Skin tumors include all benign, precancerous, and cancerous lesions of the skin. The depth of cutaneous layers involved and pattern of growth can be indicative of potential malignancy. Prompt reporting and treatment of any suspicious lesions are strongly encouraged.

  I. *Basal cell epithelioma* affects the epidermis, grows laterally, and rarely metastasizes.
  II. *Squamous cell epithelioma* arises in the epidermis, grows peripherally and inwardly, and spreads rapidly if the tumor is located at the mucocutaneous junction (refer to point V, below).
  III. *Basal cell epithelioma* is found in the epithelial layer of the skin in locations of greatest sebaceous gland concentration. It is the most common skin cancer, but rarely metastasizes. It can slowly invade underlying tissues, specifically if found around the nose, eyes, mouth, or ears. The initial lesion is a papule, which enlarges laterally. Over a period of several months it will progress to an ulcer, with a shiny, translucent border and *telangiectasis*. The lesion bleeds easily. The majority are found on the face between the hairline and upper lip. After excision, other lesions may occur.
  IV. *Squamous cell cancer* or *epidermoid carcinoma* develops from the prickle cells of the epidermis. It begins as a yellowish pink papule or plaque. It grows peripherally and inwardly. The tumor spreads rapidly if located at the mucocutaneous junction. The original lesion may ulcerate, leaving a crusted ulcer with a hard, firm base. Frequently the lesions are found on the mucous membranes as well as the skin of sites exposed to *chronic irritation,* e.g., the mouth of a pipe smoker and the glans penis in an uncircumsized male.
  V. *Nevi* or *moles* are circumscribed, pigmented papules or macules, composed of nevus cells, specialized epithelial cells containing melanin. *Intradermal* or *common moles* are benign lesions. The melanocyte is located in the corium rather than the epidermal layer of the skin. Hairy moles are usually intradermal. *Functional nevi* can be benign or precancerous. The melanocyte is contained at the junction of the dermal and epidermal layers of the skin. The lesion is flat or slightly elevated, dark brown or black.
  VI. *Melanoma* is the most malignant skin tumor, but it accounts for a small percentage of all skin cancers. *Malignant melanomas* are rare before puberty and occur most frequently in patients 40 to 70 years of age. Melanoma usually arises from suspicious, precancerous, pigmented nevi, which occur in clusters at the junction of the dermis and epidermis. They are characteristically flat, soft, brown, and hairless. Nevi located on feet, genitals, palms of the hands or at sites of chronic irritation, are susceptible to malignant changes. Sudden increase in size, alteration in color by darkening, speckling, or forming a halo

of pigment around their base, indicate serious change. The tumor can invade surrounding tissue and become painful. Metastasis then occurs rapidly through the lymph and blood systems so early detection is essential.

Assessment

I. Data sources.
 A. Patient.
 B. Family member.
 C. Previous medical record.
II. Health history.
 A. Age at time of onset (varies).
 B. Occupation pertinent if establishes history of chronic irritant.
 C. Environment. Establish history of irritant, i.e., sun, specialized clothing, boots, pipe, helicopter pilots in World War II exposed to constant wind on side of face.
 D. Coping pattern, patient's perception of disease, available human and medical resources. Data important in planning care for the chronically or terminally ill patients.
 E. Patients will often complain of a suspicious lesion which does not heal over time. Instead it changes its characteristics, begins to grow rapidly, gets darker, becomes painful, ulcerates or bleeds.
III. Physical assessment: Refer to "Definition," above. Additional information should include the following:
 A. Evaluation of the direction and rate of cellular growth.
 B. Observation and description of the lesion, including details, onset, location, size, shape, margins, growth rate, color and changes in color, and presence or absence of pain.
 C. Palpation of the lesion for hardness, softness, flatness, or elevation.
 D. Identification of telangiectasis, crusting, ulceration, bleeding, or irritation.
IV. Diagnostic tests: Biopsy of tissue (lesion) to evaluate tissue composition.

Problems

I. Fear of cancer.
II. Presence of a potentially cancerous growth.
III. Pain.
IV. Cosmetic concerns, especially related to facial lesions.

Diagnosis

I. Impaired skin integrity, secondary to lesion.
II. Anxiety: mild to moderate; fear of death.
III. Alteration in comfort: pain.
IV. Self-concept: alteration in body images, secondary to diagnosis.

Goals of Care

I. Immediate.
 A. Identify cause of cellular growth.
 B. Offer support and provide teaching.
 C. Reduce symptoms of pain, pruritus.
 D. Reduce anxiety.

II. Long-range.
 A. Restore skin integrity.
 B. Prevent metastasis.
 C. Prevent infection.

Intervention

I. Supportive counseling throughout diagnostic period and long-term follow-up. Reassurance and careful explanation of each problem essential.
II. Basal cell epithelioma.
 A. Preparation of patient and supportive counseling throughout treatment and biopsy.
 B. Tumor excised by electrodesiccation, curettage, x-ray therapy, surgery, or cryosurgery.
III. Squamous cell epithelioma.
 A. Preparation of patient and support throughout treatment and biopsy.
 B. Irradiation by superficial or deep x-ray; surgical excision.
 C. Identify external irritant and remove when possible.

IV. Suspicious nevi.
   A. Preparation and support throughout procedure.
   B. Lesion excised with wide margins and biopsied.
V. Malignant melanoma.
   A. Preoperative and postoperative care throughout procedure of surgical excision of lesion and regional lymph nodes (routine).
   B. Care of cancer patient receiving cytotoxic drugs and radiation. (Various cytotoxic drugs under investigation and use at this time regimented under close scrutiny and reevaluation.)
   C. Long-term counseling for the patient coping with a chronic terminal illness.
   D. Provide support in helping the patient through the loss and grieving process.
VI. Prevent future lesions, plan with patient to remove chronic irritants.
VII. Emphasis on prevention.

Evaluation

I. Reassessment.
   A. Encourage routine yearly skin checkups along with a complete physical.
   B. Assess effectiveness of intervention.
   C. Reevaluate for noncompliance, i.e., biopsy.
II. Complications.
   A. Secondary infection.
   B. Metastasis.

Warts (Verruca)

Definition

A *wart* is a benign contagious epithelial tumor caused by the papilloma virus. It is spread by autoinoculation. The course of infection is erratic and over half the infections spontaneously clear. Warts are classified as common, plantar, flat, and venereal.

I. *Common warts* (Fig. 33-1) appear as yellowish pink papules that grow over several weeks, increasing in discoloration.
II. *Plantar warts* (Fig. 33-2) are firm, elevated or flat lesions that interrupt natural skin folds. Red or black capillary dots are seen. They can form a mosaic, a group of multiple warts in one large, flat lesion.
III. *Flat warts* are yellowish pink or tan, soft papules found on the face, neck, extensor surfaces of forearms and hands.
IV. *Venereal warts* (condylomata acuminata) occur in clusters in warm, moist, intertriginous areas, usually in the anogenital region. They are sexually transmitted and may appear up to 6 months following exposure. Therefore, the patient under treatment should be followed for 6 months to be checked for previously undetected lesions.

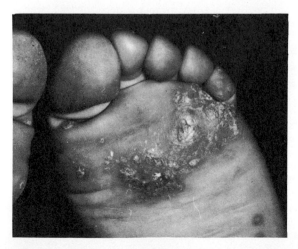

FIGURE 33-1 / Common warts. [*From T. B. Fitzpatrick et al. (eds.), Dermatology in General Medicine, McGraw-Hill Book Company, New York, 1971.*]

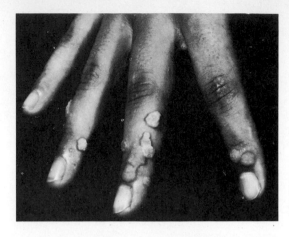

FIGURE 33-2 / Plantar warts.
[*From T. B. Fitzpatrick et al. (eds.),
Dermatology in General Medicine,
McGraw-Hill Book Company, New
York, 1971.*]

Assessment

I. Data sources (see "Skin Tumors").
II. Health history.
   A. Identify occupation: significant if it requires standing in the patient complaining of severe plantar warts.
   B. Stress responses should be evaluated in relation to the appearance of the lesion.
   C. Sexual history should be taken.
   D. Complaints of pain may be noted as the problem intensifies and the wart enlarges.
   E. Previous history of warts important, along with treatment implemented to remove wart.
III. Physical examination.
   A. Common and plantar warts are elevated or flat lesions; may be painful.
   B. Capillaries may be seen over the surface of the warts.
   C. Flat warts may be seen over face or arms.
   D. Venereal warts are seen in the genital regions. They are yellowish pink, "cauliflower" papules which may be singular or in groups.
   E. Warts in general have clearly defined borders.
   F. Tenderness may appear upon palpation of wart.
   G. Continued observation and description of the location, distribution, color, site, and number of lesions.
IV. Diagnostic tests: not specific; rule out venereal disease.

Problems

I. Pain if lesion is in pressure site, i.e., palmer surfaces of feet, genitalia.
II. Anxiety related to alteration of physical appearance.

Diagnosis

I. Impairment of skin integrity; potential infection.
II. Alteration of comfort: pain.
III. Alteration in self-concept: potential.

Goals of Care

I. Immediate.
   A. Reduce pain.
   B. Identify precipitating cause of warts (where possible).
II. Long-range.
   A. Restore skin integrity.
   B. Prevent recurrence.

Intervention

I. Prepare and support patient through electrodesiccation (dithermal destruction of small skin lesions), curettage.
II. Freezing with liquid nitrogen then painting with 0.25% podophyllin. Instruct patient to

wash medication off 6 h after application. Since the medication is very irritating, it should not be allowed to drip on surrounding tissue.

III. Prepare patient for a long course of treatment, as removal of warts may require several follow-up visits.

IV. Caution patient against overzealous self-treatment, as it may be harmful to surrounding tissue and could affect healing.

V. Emphasize follow-up. Compliance is necessary for successful treatment. However, since warts may return even with compliance, the patient may become frustrated easily. Reassurance and encouragement will be needed.

Evaluation

I. Reassessment.

II. Complications.
- **A.** Excoriation of healthy skin, pain from overtreatment. Discontinue plasters.
- **B.** Secondary infection.

HYPERACTIVITY AND HYPOACTIVITY

Psoriasis[1]

Definition

Psoriasis is a classic example of hyperactivity. It is a chronic, recurrent epidermal disease which begins usually in early adult life. It is an inherited polygenic trait thought to be caused by an overproduction of keratin. Hormonal influence has also been associated with psoriasis. The problem is characterized by rapid cell proliferation of the epidermis (which is replaced in 4 days, compared to 28 days in normal skin). The epidermal cells of psoriatic lesions synthesize DNA and divide more rapidly, producing a thick, dry, silvery, scaly epidermis. The course is prolonged and unpredictable. For most patients the disease is localized. In severe cases it can cover the whole body. Spontaneous clearing is rare, although it has been reported temporarily to clear with pregnancy. Unexplained exacerbations are common. Topical treatment temporarily clears up most lesions. Since psoriasis is not life-threatening, systemic treatment with the related risk of side effects is reserved for severe cases that are resistant to topical therapy. A small percentage of psoriatic patients develop arthritis of the distal, interphalangeal joints. Cosmetic and psychological effects for some patients can be socially disabling. Unaesthetic lesions can be associated with disfigurement, contagion, or uncleanliness, leading to social isolation. This disease dictates the occupational, social, and sexual life of the patient. This stress, combined with additional stress and anxiety, frequently precedes exacerbations.

Assessment

I. Data sources (refer to "Skin Tumors").

II. Health history: onset slow but continuous.
- **A.** Scaling lesions, pruritus; in severe cases the patient may shiver while warm.
- **B.** Psoriatic arthritis presents with tenderness, morning stiffness, pain in small joints of hands and feet in early stages.
- **C.** Later, intense pain in large joints, cervical and lumbar spine.
- **D.** Anxiety associated with physical appearance.
- **E.** History of psoriasis in family members (inherited autosomal traits).
- **F.** Age: psoriasis usually appears late in childhood, in adolescence, and in middle-aged adults.
- **G.** Occupation. Assess presence of mechanical injury. Identify environmental problems.
- **H.** Identify stress factors within the individual's environment, as this may aggravate the condition.

III. Physical examination.
- **A.** Lesion is erythematous, consisting of sharply circumscribed plaques and papules,

[1]The author acknowledges the assistance of Carol Buttercase, R.N., M.S., and Joan Clark, R.N., in reviewing the manuscript of this section.

covered by silvery white scals. Localized to elbows, scalp, knees, sacrum, and behind the ears (see Fig. 33-3).
   B. Lesions are dry, and pruritus may be present.
   C. Pitting, plating, ridging, or total destruction of fingernails and toenails.
   D. Bilateral symmetry of the lesion observed.
   E. Lesions can appear at sites of injury, scratches, surgical scars, sunburn.
   F. Acute psoriatic arthritis, distal phalanges have sausagelike appearance, with swollen, erythematous, painful distal joints.
   G. Depending upon the extent of the lesion or the multiplicity of lesions, the patient's general appearance may be changed. The patient may appear withdrawn.
IV. Diagnostic tests.
   A. Sedimentation rate: elevated.
   B. Rheumatoid factor: negative.

Problems
   I. Flaking scales.
   II. Pruritus.
   III. Aesthetically unappealing lesions.
   IV. Joint pain in severe cases.
   V. Anxiety stress reaction.

Diagnosis
   I. Impaired skin integrity; potential infection.
   II. Self-concept, altered body image, secondary to psoriatic lesions.
   III. Social isolation, secondary to skin lesion.
   IV. Alterations in comfort: pain and pruritus.
   V. Anxiety: mild to moderate, secondary to physical appearance.

Goals of Care
   I. Immediate.
      A. Restore skin integrity.
      B. Restore self-esteem.
      C. Remove aggravating factors.
   II. Long-range.
      A. Relieve pruritus pain.
      B. Decrease social isolation.
      C. Control the itching and scaling.

Intervention
   I. The choice of outpatient or inpatient treatments depends on the extent, location, and degree of discomfort. Patients are hospitalized until condition is under control.
   II. Administer and teach patient use of medications.
   III. The choice of medication depends on the patient's response to previous therapy, location of lesions, and the extent of the body surface involved.
      A. Coal tar ointment (Psori-Gel, Estar). Used at night and rubbed into lesions. Apply

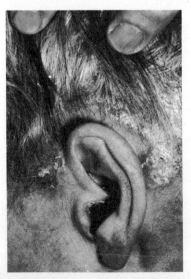

FIGURE 33-3 / Psoriasis (hairline). [*From T. B. Fitzpatrick et al. (eds.), Dermatology in General Medicine, McGraw-Hill Book Company, New York, 1971.*]

thin film in intertriginous areas to avoid irritation. Enhances effectiveness of ultraviolet light (B wavelength) therapy.

B. Fluorinated corticosteroids (Valisone, Synalar, Halog, Lidex, Hydrocortisone). These medications are used in varying strengths and preparations, and the method of application depends on the stage of treatment. *Creams,* in a water base, usually are used first because they alleviate dryness, remove scales, and allow the medication to penetrate the skin. *Ointments* have a petrolatum base, are greasy, and also remove scales, enhancing absorption.

Long-term use of topical steroids can lead to irreversible skin changes and systemic absorption. Topically, skin thins, atrophies, forms striae, and becomes hypopigmented. Systemically, steroids can cause atrophy of the adrenal cortex, resulting in a decreased response to stress. Preoperatively, patients may be given supplemental medications. The nurse should be alert to side effects of topical steroids used to treat chronic dermatologic problems and should document their use.

IV. Application.

A. The medications are applied 3 times a day to local lesions, with occlusive dressings at night.

1. Teach patient application of airtight dressings at home.
2. Wash area well while skin is *moist;* rub medication thoroughly into the lesion.
3. Cover area with plastic wrap (e.g., Saran Wrap).
4. Seal edges with airtight paper tape..
5. Corticosteroids are used in combination with coal tar. Because of the required nightly use, treatment is very costly. The dressings are awkward, and patients need encouragement for continued use. Occlusive dressings with ointment can cause folliculitis.
6. Psoralen and ultraviolet light (A wavelength), PUVA. Drug taken in pill form with excellent results, still being tested.

B. Administration of ultraviolet light (B wavelength). This intervention is used alone and in conjunction with topical medications. It should be used for restricted time periods, with a timer and eye protection. Usually exposure is desired until minimal erythema is attained. The dose is gradually increased.

C. The patient should be taught good scalp care. The scalp can be washed with a mild shampoo, with vigorous scrubbing to remove scales. The hair is parted and a kerolytic agent (phenol and sodium chloride solution, or Kerolytic Gel) can be applied. The patient should be instructed to remove all medication before reapplication. Sometimes the medication may remain on overnight. Thoroughly wash hands after application of medication (very irritating to healthy skin).

D. The patient will require constant encouragement. Th nightly somewhat messy dressing and expensive medication are a constant source of discouragement. In addition, the physical changes in personal appearance can be frustrating. The nurse should emphasize that the disease can be controlled with consistent care. Support and encouragement will be needed throughout the course of treatment.

E. Teach, evaluate, and reteach home care as needed. The importance of appropriate use of medications and application of dressings cannot be overemphasized.

F. Family members hould be included in all stages of treatment. Encourage the patient and family to touch the skin without fear.

G. Provide an opportunity for patients to express their feelings regarding self-image, verbalize discouragements, and ask questions regarding tte treatment and expectations of improvement.

H. Explore stress factors within the patient's environment, and select possible solutions to decrease them.

I. Refer to counseling if patient is socially disabled by illness and the alterations of physical appearance.

J. Support patient during quiescent periods to continue skin care nightly and apply emollients faithfully (Eucerin, Alpha-Keri, bath oil without perfumes).

K. Patients require strong support due to chronic course of illness and the continual demand for constant care and attention. Psoriasis patients have formed mutual support groups in various parts of the country. Write the National Psoriasis Foundation for further information.

Evaluation

I. Reassessment.
  A. Evaluate for signs of decreased lesions.
  B. Monitor for signs of exacerbations.
  C. Observe for complications; lack of improvement due to noncompliance. Reevaluate nursing process.
II. Complications.
  A. Continued skin breakdown.
  B. Secondary infection (refer to Chap. 32).
III. Follow-up and reevaluation.

INFLAMMATORY DISORDERS

Acne Vulgaris

Definition

Acne vulgaris is a chronic inflammatory condition of the pilosebaceous structures (sebaceous follicles), usually involving the face, shoulders, back, chest, and upper arms. The problem results when excessive sebum is secreted into the follicle. Bacteria (e.g., *Corynebacterium acnes*) then break up the fatty acid of the sebum and keratin increases. This substance is irritating to the skin and its presence results in the formation of *comedones* (blackheads), formed by increased compaction of keratin, or *milia* (whiteheads), which result from closure of the follicular opening and trapping of oil in the skin.

These lesions may be cystic, papular, or pustular. They usually affect people from the age of puberty to middle years (age 40). There may be periods of remission, or the problem can be aggravated by a particular season of the year, menstrual problems, gastrointestinal disturbances, hormonal changes (e.g., ACTH), or stress.

There are a variety of lesions that characterize acne. These can be noninflammatory and/or chronic (see Fig. 33-4), or an acute inflammatory response which results in pitting and facial scarring (see Fig. 33-5). These physical changes in appearance may lead to social withdrawal and isolation.

Assessment

I. Data sources (refer to "Skin Tumors").
II. Health history.
  A. Complaints of chronic eruptions on face, back, shoulders, arms, chest.
  B. Assess previous history in relation to skin lesion.
  C. Age: onset of problem common around puberty to middle years.
  D. History of menstrual, gastrointestinal, or hormonal health problems.
  E. History of increased hormonal intake, e.g., estrogen, ACTH.
  F. Stress response: identify issues within the environment that may be stress-producing; identify coping patterns.
  G. Elicit socialization pattern and interactions with age group.
  H. Evaluate occupation in terms of continued exposure to dirt, and review hygiene habits.
III. Physical examination.
  A. Examine scalp, skin, hair for oily appearance.
  B. Examine lesions for drainage, and note color and odor of discharge.
  C. Examine face, back, arms, chest, and shoulders for the presence of comedones.
  D. Closed follicles (comedones) will appear white or pale, slightly elevated; upon stretching the skin they are more easily observed.
  E. Open comedone will be slightly raised with a central black or brown appearance due to the collection of keratin.

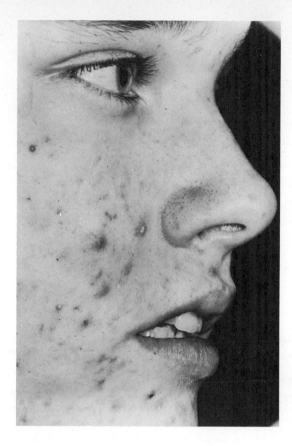

FIGURE 33-4 / Milk acne. [*From T. B. Fitzpatrick et al. (eds.), Dermatology in General Medicine, McGraw-Hill Book Company, New York, 1971.*]

    F. Pruritus and complaints of pruritus may be present.
    G. Upon palpation the lesion may feel cystic, papular, or pustular (see Fig. 33-5).
IV. Diagnostic tests.
    A. Occasionally there will be a positive culture for *Staphylococcus*.
    B. X-ray on occasion may demonstrate local calcium deposits.

Problems

I. Pruritus and/or pain.
II. Self-consciousness, developmentally difficult in adolescence when self-image is in transition.
III. Long, discouraging course of illness.
IV. Increased skin oil, aggravated by stress, hormonal changes, etc.
V. Scar formation feared, especially on the face.

Diagnosis

I. Impaired skin integrity.
II. Self-concept: altered self-image, secondary to lesions.
III. Alteration in comfort: pruritus and/or pain.
IV. Alterations in socialization: withdrawal, secondary to physical appearance.

Goals of Care

I. Immediate.
    A. Relieve pruritis, pain.
    B. Restore self-esteem, positive self-image.
    C. Reduce factors that precipitate the problem.
II. Long-range.
    A. Restore skin integrity.
    B. Increase social interaction.

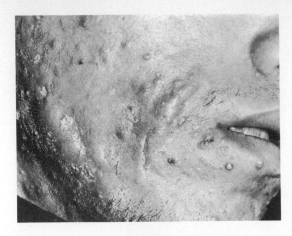

FIGURE 33-5 / Cystic acne. [*From T. B. Fitzpatrick et al. (eds.), Dermatology in General Medicine, McGraw-Hill Book Company, New York, 1971.*]

Intervention

I. Encourage patient conscientiously to follow instructions for treatment throughout exacerbations and remissions.

II. Teach self-care; purpose is to decrease oil accumulation on the skin.
   A. Cleanse face with abrasive soaps (Pernox, Fostex, Neutragina soap or cream). Caution against overtreatment to avoid further irritation.
   B. Apply drying preparations both day and night (e.g., Benoxyl and Microsyn). The purpose of these medications is to achieve mild drying and erythema without discomfort.
   C. Systemic antibiotics. Tetracycline, 250 mg, is the drug most commonly used. Tetracycline prevents new lesions from forming but does not affect those already present. It is the least expensive antibiotic. Patients should be told not to expect results until 4 to 6 weeks after treatment begins. When the patient is receiving tetracycline, he or she should be taught to take the drug 1 h before or after meals, without milk or milk products. Monilia vaginitis can occur as a side effect of tetracycline therapy.

III. Ultraviolet light may be used to dry lesions. Midday sun is also good. When a sun lamp is used at home, the patient should be encouraged to protect eyes always, never use when sleepy, and use a timer to prevent facial burns.

IV. The use of estrogen has been associated with production of sebum. Encourage good hygiene, keep face and hair clean and free of oil, shampoo as often as necessary.

V. Encourage patients to verbalize feelings toward acne, self-image, and treatment. The nurse should be supportive and create an atmosphere in which this problem can be discussed.

VI. Encourage consistent follow-up; counseling may be needed with severe acne as the patient may be withdrawn and depressed.

Evaluation

I. Reassessment.
   A. Assess effectiveness of intervention (look for signs of improvement).
   B. Observe for signs of complications; inflammatory lesions cause scarring in severe cases.

II. Surgery.
   A. Acne surgery relieves pressure and prevents the progression of the lesion. The procedure involves incision and drainage of cysts, intralesional injection of steroids, cryosurgery, and dermabrasions (removal of epidermis and upper dermis) for scarring.
   B. Plastic surgery.

III. Follow-up and reevaluation are continuous.

Dermatophytosis

Definition

Dermatophytosis infections are contagious, superficial, fungal infections, classified as *tinea corporis* (ringworm of body), *tinea capitis* (ringworm of the scalp; see Fig. 33-6), *tinea cruris* (ringworm of the inguinal area, or jock itch), and *tinea pedis* (ringworm of the feet or athlete's foot). Tineas gradually expand areas of scaling and mild erythema without treatment. With specific antifungal treatment along with prevention the problem can be totally eliminated.

Assessment

I. Data sources (refer to "Skin Tumors").
II. Health history.
   A. Assess recent exposure to pools, woods, pets, or locker rooms.
   B. Determine recent exposure to fungus (e.g., tinea capitis), in a school population; in a day-care center, from other family members, etc.
   C. Patient complains of pruritic, spreading lesions.
   D. Loss of hair may be a response to fungus (tinea capitis).
   E. Poor hygiene and lack of foot care often noted in history.
   F. Age: this problem can occur in any age group (tinea capitis is more often observed in children).
   G. Heredity may be involved in the development of this problem (particularly, tinea pedis), e.g., sweating and immunological reactions.
   H. Men may be more affected than women (tinea pedis).
III. Physical examination.
   A. Tinea pedis.
     1. Acute inflammatory response involving one or both feet. A red rash is often observed in the interdigital spaces and on soles of feet.
     2. Lesions are vesicular in nature with scaling.
     3. Toenails may be involved in the inflammatory reaction. When this occurs, the nails become brittle and break easily, and brownish discoloration may be observed.
     4. Itching is not uncommon, and this can contribute to generalized swelling. If there are breaks in the skin, cellulitis may occur.

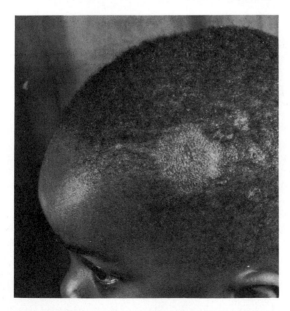

FIGURE 33-6 / Tinea capitis.
[*From T. B. Fitzpatrick et al. (eds.), Dermatology in General Medicine, McGraw-Hill Book Company, New York, 1971.*]

          5. Another form of tinea pedis may lead to fissures developing between the toes. Laceration of the skin may be observed.

    B. Tinea corporis.
          1. Skin lesions are usually vesicular, with redness and scaling.
          2. Lesion can begin as a red papule and spread peripherally with central healing.
          3. The outer borders of the lesion are sharply defined and may appear in clusters.
          4. Lesions are often observed on the scalp, hair, nails.

    C. Tinea capitis.
          1. Most commonly found in the scalp, hair.
          2. Granulomatous lesions on scalp, red macules (raised lesions, crusting may be noted) (see Fig. 33-6).
          3. Hair loss may be observed. Hair becomes brittle (temporarily).
          4. Seen in children most often.

    D. Tinea cruris.
          1. Aggravated by obesity, increased sweating, friction; seen more frequently in men.
          2. Sharp, symmetric eruptions observed in groin and thigh, and may spread to buttocks.
          3. Pustules are present at margin of lesions. Scaling and brownish discoloration observed.

IV. Diagnostic tests.
    A. Microscopic examination of scraping of lesion reveals hyphae of fungi.
    B. Culture for fungi (scraping on a slide for direct visualization).
    C. Wood's lamp in tinea capitis: affected hairs fluoresce.

Problems

I. Experiencing pruritis (especially in area directly affected).
II. Extending lesions: redness, inflammation.
III. Transmissible disease (physical contact).
IV. Reinfection unless prevented or treated thoroughly.

Diagnosis

I. Impaired skin integrity, secondary to obesity.
II. Alteration in comfort: pruritus.
III. Potential risk of spreading infection.

Goals of Care

I. Immediate.
    A. Prevent transmission.
    B. Relieve pruritus.

II. Long-range.
    A. Restore skin integrity.
    B. Prevent reinfection or secondary infection.

Intervention

I. Instruct patient on self-care, proper use of medication, course of illness, cause.
II. Administration of antifungal medications used *topically,* such as Lotrimin, Mycatin, and Halotex. In severe cases *systemic* treatment: griseofulvin should be taken orally with meals (the presence of fat enhances absorption). Side effects include epigastric pain, nausea, and leukopenia.
III. Teach patient to decrease moisture in affected areas, as this will facilitate treatment and reduce chance of reinfection. Encourage the patient to wear cotton next to skin and to change clothing and socks whenver wet to avoid accumulation of moisture. Rubber-soled shoes and tight clothing should also be avoided.
IV. Shave head in affected area for tinea capitis. Remaining scales can be removed with mild shampoo before medication applied (e.g., Whitfield's ointment).
V. The nurse should teach the patient and family members to protect themselves and others by wearing shoes in public showers, not sharing personal articles, i.e., towels, combs, in order to reduce transmission of these problems. Pets should be checked and treated if fur has moth-eaten appearance, as they may be the source of the problem.
VI. All contacts should be screened and referred for treatment if symptomatic.

VII. Follow the patient and family members until infection has cleared.

VIII. Use drying powder (Lotrimin) after infection has cleared to prevent reinfection.

Evaluation

I. Reassessment: Observe and describe changes in lesions, distribution, erythema, and edema. Assessment of external borders and patterns of spreading is important.

II. Complications: Secondary infection, e.g., cellulitis and lymphadermatitis; administer appropriate antibiotic after cultures.

III. Follow-up and reevaluation should continue until the problem is eliminated.

Dermatosis: Atopic Dermatitis

Definition

Atopic dermatitis, or *eczema,* is a superficial inflammation of the skin. Although the etiology is unknown, it is thought to be due to sensitization to particular substances. Usually there is a familial history of some type of allergy. The lesion often results in itching and scratching, and leads to secondary infection and lichenification, triggering the "scratch-itch cycle." Typical lesions are found in local areas of the body, usually flexor surfaces, around the eyes, and the hands, but there may be total body involvement. The course of the disease is periodic, unpredictable, and discouraging, with exacerbations and partial remissions. Exacerbations occur often during periods of psychological or physical stress. Certain factors trigger the itch. This condition is often worse in the winter, intensified by extremes in temperature, and irritated by substances such as wool or silk clothing, oil, soaps, and detergents.

Assessment

I. Data sources (refer to "Skin Tumors").

II. Health history.
  A. Intense pruritic, scaling, erythematous patches described.
  B. Obtain a personal or family history of past allergies. Determine if home treatment has been initiated.
  C. May occur at any age.
  D. Factors which precipitate the problem should be determined (e.g., season, stress).

III. Physical examination.
  A. Erythema and scaling progressing to excoriations secondary to itching.
  B. Lesions may appear anywhere on the body. Often noted (in adults) on face, neck, upper chest, and flexures of the arms and legs.
  C. Scratching leads to dry, lichenified, hyperpigmented, or hypopigmented plaques.

Problems

I. Severe pruritus.
II. Scratch-itch cycle.
III. Stress, anxiety.
IV. Chronic course.
V. Danger of secondary infection.

Diagnosis

I. Impaired skin integrity, potential infection.
II. Alteration in comfort: discomfort secondary to pruritus.
III. Disturbed sleep-rest pattern.
IV. Condition aggravated by stress.
V. Anxiety: mild to moderate.

Goals of Care

I. Immediate.
  A. Reduce pruritus, stop scratch-itch cycle.
  B. Decrease stress.
  C. Promote rest.

II. Long-range.
  A. Restore skin integrity.
  B. Prevent secondary infection.

Intervention

I. Support patient through long, discouraging course of treatment by consistent, positive approach throughout the interaction.

II. Prepare patient for treatment by explaining rationale for interventions, expectations, application of medications. Consistently reevaluate patient compliance, which can be measured by the condition of the skin.

III. Identify stresses causing exacerbations (job, family, or situational crisis), and help patient eliminate the problem or improve ability to cope with specific problems.

IV. Suppress scratch-itch cycle by:
   A. Keeping skin moist and supple by using compresses with emollients or tub baths with antipruritic additives (e.g., Aveena).
   B. Administering topical corticosteroids (e.g., Valisone, Synalar, Lidex, Aristocort). (See "Psoriasis" for caution with topical steroid use.) Teach patient to apply small amounts on damp skin. Medication is expensive. May use occlusive dressings at night.

V. Caution patient against excessive bathing and high humidity; these may aggravate the symptoms. Prevent contact with wool, silk, and other trigger factors.

VI. Identify real or potential causes of anxiety, and promote rest by decreasing pruritus and creating a quiet environment. Antihistamines sometimes used (Atarax, 10 to 25 mg; caution patient that it causes sleepiness: avoid driving).

VII. Explain to the patient that initially useful medications may become ineffective for periods of time and the patient may need to change medications.

VIII. Alert patient not to receive or be exposed to recent smallpox vaccinations, active herpes simplex infections, or chickenpox, as these may exacerbate symptoms.

IX. Encase hands in mittens at night if necessary to prevent scratching and skin abrasion.

X. Follow-up: urge consistency, observe effectiveness of treatment, and note any change in the skin condition.

Evaluation

I. Reassessment: Assess effectiveness of treatment and status of skin integrity.
II. Complications: secondary infection. Administer antibiotics after culture.

Dermatosis: Contact Dermatitis

Definition

Contact dermatitis is a superficial inflammation which results from a sensitization of the skin due to skin contact with natural or synthetic substances (nonallergic). Reactions may be immediate or delayed, with symptoms occurring within hours or weeks. *Allergic contact dermatitis* is delayed hypersensitivity to exposure to contact allergens by sensitized people, e.g., poison ivy, poison oak. Primary irritants in contact dermatitis are plants, trees, chemicals, therapeutic agents, cosmetics, fabrics, and metals (nickel). Successful intervention and removal of the precipitating irritant should relieve the symptoms.

Assessment

I. Data sources (see "Skin Tumors").
II. Health history (see "Dermatosis: Atopic Dermatitis").
   A. Screen for irritant.
   B. Identify home remedies that relieve symptoms.
   C. Description of the onset of the symptoms.
III. Physical examination.
   A. Erythema, vesicles, ulcers, edema, and oozing observed.
   B. Chronic exposure may lead to fissuring of the skin with dryness and thickness. Burning may be noted.
   C. Distribution of contact dermatitis is significant. Usually has sharp, straight borders, due to direct contact with primary irritant. Skin thickness is noted in prolonged cases.
   D. Hemorrhagic bullae may develop in more severe cases.

Problems

I. Severe pruritus, edema.
II. Oozing lesions, pain.
III. Inflammation continues until irritant is removed.
IV. Risk of secondary infection.

Diagnosis See "Dermatosis: Atopic Dermatitis."

Goals of Care
I. Immediate (see "Dermatosis: Atopic Dermatitis").
II. Long-range.
   A. Prevent recurrence through teaching.
   B. Identify precipitating cause.

Intervention
I. Treatment of contact dermatitis depends on stage of the problem and related symptoms.
   A. Acute (mild to moderate) contact dermatitis: apply compresses of Burow's solution directly to vesicles. These can be followed by applying a soothing, drying solution (e.g., calamine). Oral steroids may be used. After vesiculation decreases, topical corticosteroids may be applied.
   B. During the *chronic stage* use tar compounds in combination with steroids and occlusive dressings.
II. Decrease pruritus.
   A. Teach the patient or family member the application of compresses.
   B. Administer antihistamines if indicated (e.g., Chlor-trimeton or Benadryl).
   C. Poison ivy may continue to present symptoms up to 10 days following exposure.
   D. Continued use of topical solutions as well as medication to decrease itching will help support the patient during this difficult period.
III. Prevention of recurrence is important. The patient should be taught to limit exposure to abrasives and detergents and to wear rubber gloves to protect the skin.
IV. Follow-up is important until the problem has cleared.
V. After a case of poison ivy, the patient or family member should be told to wash clothing or sneakers, as resin remains on inanimate objects (and also on pets).
VI. If an allergen is a suspected cause of the problem, skin testing may be suggested to isolate the cause.

Evaluation
I. Reevaluation.
II. Complications: secondary infection. Administer appropriate antibiotic after cultures.

Seborrheic Dermatitis

Definition An acute, inflammatory dermatosis of oily skin, *seborrheic dermatitis* is usually found in those parts of the body containing large sebaceous glands. The lesions are pruritic and characterized by dry, moist, or greasy scales and crusted yellowish plaques; when located in the scalp, it is known as dandruff. Clinical course of exacerbations and remissions.

Assessment
I. Data sources (see "Dermatosis: Contact Dermatitis").
II. Health history (see "Dermatosis: Atopic Dermatitis").
   A. History of present illness.
   B. Pruritus, scaling, oily scalp.
III. Physical examination.
   A. Lesions located at hairline with mild erythema.
   B. Fine, dry scaling on scalp, eyebrows, postauricular folds, and beard is noted.
   C. In distinct borders, can form greasy yellow scales.
   D. Irritation may occur in men in hairy areas of the chest.

Problems
I. Scaling, pruritic lesions.
II. Oily skin and scalp.

Diagnosis See "Dermatosis: Atopic Dermatitis."

Goals of Care
I. Decrease oil.
II. Relieve pruritus.

Intervention I. Teach patient the administration of topical medications to control skin inflammation. Use of a steroid, e.g., hydrocortisone creme or lotion, on the scalp may help relieve the problem.

II. Instruct patient to scrub scalp with mild shampoo; remove crusts and previous medications before reapplication of a shampoo. Sebulex, Nu-flow, Zincon, available in drugstores, may be used for this purpose.

III. Follow-up until the condition improves, as this problem may become chronic.

Evaluation I. Reassessment.

    A. Observe for signs of improvement, e.g., decreased scaling and itching.

    B. Observe for recurrence at a future time.

II. Complications: secondary infection.

Scabies

Definition *Scabies* is a parasitic skin infection, characterized by fine, superficial burrows and intense pruritus. The disease is caused by the burrowing itch mite, *Sarcoptes scabiei*. Scabies is readily transmissible by intimate contact. The burrows are a result of female mites entering the supernicial layers of skin and depositing eggs. Symptoms appear when larvae hatch, up to 3 weeks after exposure. Lesions are generally found on the interdigital webs of the hands, wrists, intertriginous spaces, lower abdomen, around nipples, genitalia, and ankles, and usually not on the scalp or back (see Fig. 33-7).

Assessment I. Data sources (refer to "Skin Tumors").

II. Health history.

    A. Environmental exposure: increased incidence in areas with substandard hygienic conditions.

    B. Contacts, e.g., dogs, cats, small animals, sexual contacts.

    C. Intense itching, worse at night. Obtain history of the medication or treatment already started at home.

III. Physical examination.

    A. Upper skin layer involved, e.g., fingers (digital folds), wrists, elbows, axilla, penis.

    B. Erythema and papules at the end of fine, wavy grey lines. (See better by holding flashlight to taut skin.)

    C. Develop pustules, and excoriations from scratching observed.

IV. Diagnostic tests: Scraping of lesions and microscopic confirmation.

Problems I. Pruritus. III. Potential risk for secondary infection.

II. Transmissible disease. IV. Anxiety.

Diagnosis I. Impaired skin integrity; potential infection.

II. Alteration in comfort: discomfort, secondary to pruritus.

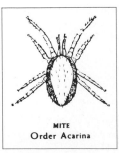

MITE
Order Acarina

FIGURE 33-7 / Mite (scabies). [*From T. B. Fitzpatrick et al. (eds.), Dermatology in General Medicine, McGraw-Hill Book Company, New York, 1971.*]

    III. Altered sleep patterns.
    IV. Transmissible via contact: potential.

Goals of Care
    I. Immediate.
        A. Reduce pruritus.
        B. Promote rest.
        C. Refer contacts for treatment.
    II. Long-range.
        A. Restore skin integrity.
        B. Prevent recurrence: remove original source.

Intervention
    I. Explain course of disease, cause, treatment to the patient and family members.
    II. Teach patient application of 1% Kwell (lotion or creme, and shampoo). Instruct the patient to apply in areas from neck down and to leave for 24 h. Reapply in areas where lotion may be removed, i.e., hands, genitalia. While medication is in use, launder clothing, bed linen. Dry cleaning may be helpful, as well as detergents (e.g., Lysol).
    III. Caution patient to follow all instructions so that the scabies may be totally eliminated. If the medication is irritating, instruct the patient to wait 7 to 10 days before reapplication. If pruritus continues after treatment is completed, use an emollient (e.g., Aveeno) for relief.
    IV. Promote rest by proper use of medication. Pruritus may not be relieved immediately. Explain scratch-itch cycle. Encourage patient to utilize distractions, physical activity to break cycle. Antihistamines may be orally administered.
    V. Contacts should be treated prophylactically and simultaneously, as scabies is contagious.
    VI. Reassure the patient that the use of medication will relieve the problem. Be supportive during this time, and reassure the patient to help reduce anxiety.

Evaluation
    I. Reassessment. Follow up if treatment is not successful; check compliance carefully. Due to 3-week incubation period, it is wise to recheck patient 3 to 4 weeks following treatment
    II. Complications: secondary infection.
        A. Administer appropriate antibiotics after skin culture is taken.
        B. Stop scabicide.
        C. Utilize starch baths to decrease pruritus, apply soothing lotion or emollient (e.g., calamine).
        D. Be careful to avoid overtreating the patient initially, as this can lead to skin breakdown and infection.

Erythema Multiforme

Definition
    Erythema multiforme is an inflammatory as well as hypersensitivity reaction. The problem may begin similarly to a viral illness. Symptoms usually begin a few days after a febrile onset. The course of the problem generally lasts 2 to 3 weeks in mild cases and 6 to 8 weeks in a more severe form. (The severe form is sometimes called Stevens-Johnson syndrome.) Many factors, e.g., drugs, barbiturates, penicillin, malignancy, endocrine changes, viral illness, and most often herpes simplex, can precipitate the occurrence of this illness. The problem can be terminated with treatment but may reoccur. In severe forms the problem may be life-threatening due to infection. Secondary blindness may develop if eyelids are involved. Leakage of fluid into the dermis (caused by blistering) can lead to tissue necrosis.

Assessment
    I. Data sources (see "Skin Tumors").
    II. Health history.
        A. Complaints associated with an upper respiratory infection. Fever is not uncommon.
        B. Initial eruption may be symptomless. Some patients complain of stinging and burning.
        C. Dietary changes may be noted if oral mucosa is involved.
        D. History of herpes simplex is not uncommon.
        E. Identification of the precipitating cause is critical.

      F. The problem is rarely observed before the age of 2 or after age 50.

      G. It is often precipitated by the cold weather, increasing in incidence in December, January, and February.

  III. Physical examination.

      A. Lesions are red blotches which erupt suddenly (see Fig. 33-8). They are symmetrically distributed.

      B. The face, neck, legs, dorsal surface of the hands, forearms, feet, and oral mucosa may be affected.

      C. The iris may also be a target for lesions.

      D. The lesion often appears as a white central vesicle, surrounded by alternating concentric rings.

      E. In severe forms the patient will have generalized lesions that blister, with bullae and hemorrhage.

      F. The skin becomes dusky as the lesions progress (age). As fluids leak into the dermis (e.g., from blisters), they can cause tissue necrosis.

      G. Oral mucous membranes may be involved, with drainage.

      H. Body temperature may be increased.

  IV. Diagnostic tests.

      A. CBC: anemia may be present.

      B. Leukocytosis may be observed.

      C. Serology tests.

      D. Chest x-rays to rule out pneumonia and malignancy.

      E. Liver function tests to rule out hepatitis, mononucleosis.

      F. Skin tests (Mantoux).

      G. Rule out mycoplasmic infections and histoplasmosis.

      H. Culture wounds to rule out *Staphylococcus.*

Problems

   I. Painful, draining lesions.
   II. Impaired oral intake.
  III. Fever.

  IV. Precipitating cause, e.g., viral infection.
   V. Anxiety.

Diagnosis

   I. Impairment of skin integrity; potential necrosis and infection.
   II. Alteration in nutrition, secondary to oral mucosa involvement.
  III. Potentially life-threatening problem.
  IV. Alteration in comfort: pain.
   V. Anxiety: mild to moderate.
  VI. Self-concept: alteration in body image, secondary to lesions.

Goals of Care

   I. Immediate.
     A. Maintain intake (oral).
     B. Identify precipitating cause.
     C. Reduce pain.
     D. Reduce anxiety.

  II. Long-range.
     A. Restore skin integrity.
     B. Prevent serious complications.
     C. Prevent recurrence.

Intervention

   I. Reassure patient, explain treatment, provide physical and emotional comfort, and offer support to patient and family.

   II. Administer steroids orally to reduce inflammation; antibiotics are used when infection is present or suspected.

  III. Apply open wet compresses to bullae and erosive lesions to help reduce inflammation and promote comfort.

  IV. Oral hygiene: mouthwash for cleanliness (3% hydrogen peroxide), Dyclone solution, viscous Xylocaine for pain (used topically) in order to reduce halitosis and to limit infection.

   V. Provide bland diet to make oral intake possible and to promote comfort while eating.

  VI. Administer analgesics: aminosalicylic acid (ASA), 600 mg as circumstances require.

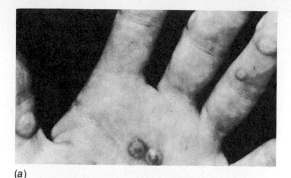

(a)

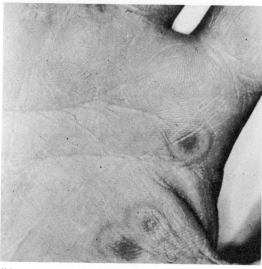

(b)

FIGURE 33-8 / Erythema multiforme: (a) target lesions; (b) major lesions. [*From T. B. Fitzpatrick et al. (eds.), Dermatology in General Medicine, McGraw-Hill Book Company, New York, 1971.*]

VII. With severe cases, monitor IV fluids, oral hygiene, and eye care. Administer prednisone to help reduce inflammation.
VIII. Create an environment in which patients can discuss fears and apprehension, especially if the cause of the problem is unknown.
IX. Observe closely, record changes.
X. Encourage follow-up of diagnostic tests.

Evaluation
    I. Reassessment: check for observable results for improvement of lesions.
   II. Complications.
      A. Secondary infection.
      B. Blindness (refer to Chap. 23).
      C. Toxic reaction to tissue necrosis.
      D. Kidney damage. (refer to Chap. 28).
      E. Malignancy: suspected when lesions appear after the age of 50.

TRAUMA

The most common wounds or injuries to the skin are burns. Therefore, most of the following section will focus on nursing care of the burn patient. The reader is referred to Chap. 44 for a complete discussion of the immediate care of a burn patient.

Burns

Definition   *Burns* are a profound trauma to the skin that interrupt the normal skin function. As a result there is an ineffective barrier against infection, loss of body fluids, disruption in temperatire control, destruction of sweat and sebaceous glands, and an alteration in sensory receptors. The causes of burns include prolonged exposure to flames, hot liquids, chemicals, electricity, and radiation. Burns are classified as first, second, and third degree, depending on depth of skin traumatized. *First-degree burns* are superficial injuries of the epidermis resulting in localized erythema and edema. *Second-degree burns* are partial thickness injuries involving the epidermis and part of the dermis. Erythema, edema, and bullae appear. Sebaceous glands, sweat glands, and hair follicles remain intact. Pain is often severe. *Third-degree burns* are full thickness injuries that destroy all layers, leaving necrotic tissue. No regeneration can occur. These burns destroy the skin appendages, nerve endings, fascia, and blood supply. Skin grafting is required for healing since no new epithelialization can occur. The area is painless because of nerve destruction.

I. When an individual sustains a burn there is initial fear, pain, and anxiety (neurogenic shock). (See Chap. 44.)

II. Physiologically, vasodilatation and increased capillary permeability occur.

III. Extracellular fluid shifts to the site of injury accompanied by sodium and protein. The escape of these substances into the wound causes edema and blister formation, or loss through the open wound.

IV. Fluid is also depleted from the circulating blood as fluid extravasates into deeper tissues. Half of the extracellular fluid can shift from the interstitial spaces and the bloodstream to the site of a severe burn.

V. Plasma also seeps into the tissue.

VI. Hypovolemic shock (refer to Chap. 44) results, accompanied by a fall in blood pressure and inadequate kidney perfusion (leading to anuria). Pump failure, hormonal disturbances, and cerebral anorexia result.

VII. The shock stage is accompanied by dehydration, hyperproteinemia, electrolyte imbalance, and increased stress on the kidney due to decreased blood volume and increased by-products of hemolyzed cells being excreted.

VIII. Blood potassium elevates due to decreased urinary output, and cardiac arrhythmias may be seen.

IX. Anemia develops because red blood cells are trapped in the burn site and destroyed.

X. Heat is lost through open wounds by evaporation, increasing the metabolic rate and leading to weight loss.

XI. Adrenocortical activity increases in response to the generalized stress.

XII. Respiratory distress is a problem for head and neck injuries or when a substance (e.g., smoke) is inhaled.

XIII. After the first 24 to 36 h, fluid shifts from the extravascular space and returns to the vascular system. Caution at this stage to avoid fluid overload by carefully monitoring cardiac output, renal output, and intravenous intake cannot be overemphasized.

XIV. The next stage of physiologic change is the period of burn slough and infection. The burned necrotic tissue or eschar separated from underlying viable tissues leaves an open wound with a high risk for infection. Before repair can begin, the eschar must be removed. If some of the original layer of skin remains, the skin will regenerate. If all the layers are destroyed, only granulation tissue remains to form unsightly scars. Therefore, skin grafting is utilized to prevent scarring and promote early healing.

The homeostatic mechanisms of the severely burned patient are disturbed. Most victims of second-degree burns and all victims of third-degree burns, inhalation burns, and burns of the face and neck require hospitalization. The psychological toll on the patient is devastating. Physiologically, death may occur during any period of treatment; therefore, care becomes most demanding. Depending upon the severity of the injury, rehabilitation may require many months or even years of nursing and medical care. Long-term nursing interventions are needed for patients with chronic health problems, and referral to a variety of health resources will be required, again depending upon the depth of the burn and the extent of tissue involvement. Permanent alteration in body image may necessitate counseling.

Assessment

I. Data sources.
   A. Patient.   *C.* Previous records.
   B. Family.   *D.* Witnesses at the site of injury.
II. Health history (may be obtained from family or friend if patient is unable to talk).
   A. Age: Developmentally significant, especially if disfigurement is anticipated. Age is also significant in determining treatment (e.g., fluid replacement).
   B. Occupation: Was the injury job-related? If so, was there an explosion? Identify the materials that were burning and the source of the fire.
   C. Complete medical history: Screen the patient for cardiac or renal diseases, diabetes, ulcers, allergies, and factors that may complicate treating the burn, e.g., emotional illness, alcoholism, or epilepsy.
   D. History of the injury.
      1. Identify the material that directly burned the patient, materials that were inhaled, and length of time patient was exposed to burning substance.
      2. Identify when and where first aid was given, the treatment given, and whether or not tetanus toxoid was given prophylactically.
      3. Identify the amount and type of fluid replacement instituted, if any.
      4. Question if other losses were involved in the fire, e.g., home or family members.
   E. Personal history: Identify the patient's relationships, previous coping patterns, personal needs, needs of family and significant others, life-style, sleep patterns, nutritional habits, and educational background.
   F. Socioeconomic factors: Assess financial status and insurance benefits, as long-term care may be costly.
   G. Assess current health status (prior to injury). Evaluate past health perceptions.
III. Physical assessment (for initial assessment, refer to Chap. 44).
   A. A complete physical examination is necessary in order to assess whether there are other injuries (e.g., fractures and internal trauma).
   B. General appearance: Observe for alertness, anxiety, vital signs, blood pressure, signs of impending shock.
   C. Neurological: Note changes in consciousness, e.g., fear, hysteria. Neurological evaluation is important.
   D. Skin: Temperature changes (cold), peripheral circulation other than burn site (refer to Table 33-1).
   E. Cardiorespiratory:
      1. Lung changes indicative of inhalation injury: rales or cough (if productive, note color and amount of sputum), cyanosis, labored breathing (dyspnea), stridor, singed nasal hairs. Tracheostomy or endotracheal tube may be inserted (refer to Chap. 27).
      2. Cardiac status: blood pressure, pulse (arrhythmias, signs of failure), alterations in circulation due to shifting fluid, cyanosis, capillary refill.
   F. Musculoskeletal. Decreased mobility, check for fractures. Observe for deformity secondary to immobility, observe for exposure of muscle tissue and bone structure.
   G. Urogenital: Urinary output decreased in fluid-shock phase, increases as fluid shifts after the first 24 to 36 h. Hematuria indicates renal stress.
   H. Gastrointestinal: Head and mouth injuries, check for edema, nausea, and vomiting. Observe stomach contents for blood, indicative of stress ulcer. Assess bowel sounds and abdominal distension. Patient usually has a nasogastric tube placed while in the emergency room. Observe for paralytic ileus and bleeding of the internal organs. (Refer to Chap. 29.)
   I. Observe for signs of infection, including prevalent drainage, increased body temperature.

TABLE 33-1 / ASSESSMENT OF BURNS

Degree	Skin Involvement*	Health History	Assessment
First degree	Epidermis	Complaints of tingling, throbbing, hyperesthesia, pain	Skin red; area blanches with pressure Slight edema may be present Scabbing may appear as wound heals; peeling may be seen Recovery will be complete
Second degree (superficial) Second degree (deep)	Tissue destruction occurs up to dermis Dermis affected	Often result of burn from boiling/hot water Complaints of pain, hyperesthesia Clothing burns may be the causative agent	Blistering, edema and redness may occur Blistering, edema, and redness may occur Skin may be broken and may weep liquid (usually clear) Recovery in 2–3 weeks; scarring may be present Infection may occur
Third degree	Complete tissue destruction, including subcutaneous tissue	Painless Symptoms of shock, depending upon severity and extent of damage Exposure of tissue may be noted	Dry, pale, or brownish leathery appearance Edema, with skin broken; fat tissue may be observed Hematuria Loss of shape and function of a limb
Fourth degree	Full thickness, tissue destroyed, plus underlying structures	Exposure of tissue may be prolonged	Deep electrical burns may result in charring (black) of skin; may produce harmful toxins Signs of hypovolemic shock may accompany this problem

*Depends on depth of burn, intensity, and duration.
Source: Adapted from E. R. Crews, *A Practical Manual for Treatment of Burns,* Charles C Thomas, Publishers, Springfield, Ill., 1964.

    J. Complete assessment of pain or lack of it. Accurate reporting of pain duration, intensity, quality, location, etc., important throughout the care of each patient.

    K. Behavioral assessment, including verbal and nonverbal responses, assessment of memory, judgment, level of consciousness, and orientation to time and place, are important parameters.

IV. Diagnostic tests.

    A. Serum electrolyte to evaluate fluid loss: potassium increases, sodium chloride decreases.

    B. Blood gases: assess arterial oxygen level (refer to Chap. 27).

    C. Hematocrit, hemoglobin: assess blood loss.

    D. Blood urea nitrogen, creatine: assess renal function.

    E. Hourly urine for amount, pH, protein, sugar, acetone, specific gravity, blood.

    F. Leukocyte and sedimentation rate: evaluate inflammation.

Problems

    I. Fluid shift, fluid loss.

    II. Hypovolemic shock: potential.

    III. Tissue destruction.

    IV. Infection: potential, secondary to break in skin.

    V. Respiratory distress: potential.
   VI. Pain.
  VII. Stress: anxiety, fear.
 VIII. Anemia.

Diagnosis

     I. Body fluids: depletion, secondary to impaired skin function and fluid shift.
    II. Impaired mobility, secondary to immobilization after injury.
   III. Nutritional alteration: less than required.
   IV. Self-concept: altered body image secondary to tissue destruction.
    V. Alteration in comfort: pain, moderate to severe.
   VI. Anxiety: moderate to severe, life-threatening situation.
  VII. Dysrhythm of sleep-rest pattern.
 VIII. Loss of privacy, invasion of territorial space; secondary to immobility and dependency.
   IX. Altered ability to perform self-care activity.
    X. Grieving: acute, delayed; secondary to physical loss, dependency.
   XI. Impairment of significant others' adjustment to illness.
  XII. Sensory perception: altered due to disruption in normal body rhythms and sensory stimulation.
 XIII. Thought process impaired: potential.
 XIV. Cardiac output: potential.
  XV. Alteration in socialization: potential secondary to physical appearance.

Goals of Care

 I. Immediate.
   A. Stabilize condition.   **E.** Decrease stress.
   B. Identify cause of burn.   **F.** Restore skin integrity.
   C. Prevent infection, shock. **G.** Reduce anxiety.
   D. Relieve pain.   **H.** Maintain self-esteem.
II. Long-range.
   A. Complete healing of the affected area.
   B. Prevent contractures.
   C. Preserve body integrity.
   D. Prevent recurrence.
   E. Help patient cope with physical changes, alteration in body image.
   F. Help patient cope with long-term rehabilitation.

Intervention

  I. Emergency care (refer to Chap. 44).
 II. *Acute stage:* first 24 to 36 h.
   A. Monitor fluid replacement to counteract the fluid loss of intravascular and extravascular fluid into the burn wound. Various formulas are utilized for the initial replacement therapy. Medical authorities do not agree on the proportion of colloids and elctrolyte fluid needed.
   B. Brooke formula. First 24 h: *colloid* (plasma dextran), 0.5 mL/kg times percentage of body surface burned; *electrolyte* (0.9% normal saline or Ringer's lactate), 1.5 mL/kg times percentage of body surface burned; *water requirement,* 2000 mL of 5% dextrose in water. The total of the estimated fluid requirement is divided so that one-half is given in the first 8 h, one-fourth in the second 8 h, and one-fourth in the third 8 h. It is important to start calculations of replacement from the time the burn injury occurs. Consider only second- and third-degree burns in determining the burn area.
   C. In applying the formula to burns covering more than 50 percent of the total body area, the formula is calculated as though only 50 percent of the total body area was burned. The maximum fluid requirement in the first 24 h is 10 L. The second 24-h fluid requirement: continue colloids and electrolytes at about one-half to one-fourth the amount used in the first 24 h.
   D. Evaluate and observe urinary output (amount, specific gravity), signs of transfusion

reaction, mental status, central venous pressure, gastric contents, peripheral circulation, vital signs.

E. Urinary output maintained at 30 to 50 mL/h in order to prevent congestion in the renal tubules. Oliguria may be present at first after burns. After the first 36 h, fluid shifts from the extravascular spac back to the vascular systems.

F. As urinary output increases, intravenous intake should decrease.

G. *Central venous pressure* catheter should be inserted in order to monitor the effects of fluid replacement. Readings should be taken frequently (e.g., every 1 to 2 h) to assure adequate blood volume without causing fluid overload. A pulmonary wedge catheter may also be used. See discussion of shock in Chap. 44.

H. Routine indwelling catheter care needed for continuous recording of urinary output (see Chap. 28 for discussion of catheter care).

I. Oral hygiene, care of nasogastric tube important. Intake of oral fluids as tolerated.

J. Administration of prophylactic penicillin to prevent group A betahemolytic *Streptococcus,* especially where there are multiple skin breaks.

K. Administration of multivitamins to facilitate tissue growth.

L. Provide physical comfort and emotional support. Observe patient's reaction to condition. Discuss changes, fears, and anxiety openly.

M. Administer pain medication, e.g., morphine sulfate. Observe the patient response to medication. Prevent drug dependency.

N. Establish open communication with patient and family. Help prevent social isolation, especially if reverse isolation is being used.

O. *Wound care* begins once antishock treatment is established, with the patient in isolation. Most fresh burns require aseptic care. After 48 to 72 h, gram-negative and gram-positive organisms begin to grow. *Staphylococcus aureus* and *Pseudomonas aeruginosa* are the most common types of infections. Necrotic tissue is a source of infection and therefore must be debrided (removed) before topical medication is applied. Initiate treatment as prescribed; bactericidal and bacteriostatic ointments are used. The type depends on the extent of the injury, plus the organism cultured from the wound.

  1. *Sulfamylon cream,* 10% (mafenide acetate), penetrates eschar and requires exposure to the air. No dressing is used. Patient needs turning to prevent maceration.

  2. *Silver sulfadiazine ointment,* 1% (water-soluble base), is smeared over the burn area. The use of this drug is still under investigation. It does not appear to cause acid-base imbalances and is not painful to apply. Cutaneous sensitivity can occur.

  3. *Gentamicin sulfate* (Garamycin Creme, 0.1%) is an antibiotic specifically effective against gram-negative bacteria, including many strains of *Pseudomonas*. The ointment spreads easily and is painless to apply. There is a tendency for the organism to develop resistance, so the medication is reserved for life-threatening situations.

  4. *Silver nitrate solution,* 0.5% (nonallergenic), increases sodium loss through the burn. Large supplements of sodium are required in the diet to replace this loss. The drug is applied with wet dressings. The area is covered with circular gauze bandages, moisture-retaining stockinets, and Ace bandages. A stockinet alone is used in the first 36 h due to edema. Patient must be covered with dry blankets to assure a warm environment around the wet dressings and to minimize heat loss by evaporation. This drug stains anything it comes in contact with, and care should be used during administration. The injured parts should be covered by sterile sheets.

P. Reduce anxiety. Distinguish irritability, restlessness, and discomfort due to pain from hypoxia due to hypovolemia. Listen and explain procedures carefully. Administer pain medication before painful procedures. Encourage patient to verbalize positive and negative feelings. Answer questions, explain clinical course, guide patient's expectations. (Use of other interventions to reduce pain, e.g., distraction, white noise, etc., may be used.)

Q. Reduce social isolation. Teach family the rationale for medications and procedures. Encourage visitors as allowed, and encourage patients to continue outside interests. Encourage touching to decrease sensory deprivation and physical isolation.

R. Promote self-esteem by providing opportunities for the patient to make choices and participate in self-care.

S. Encourage patient and family, pointing out progressive stages of healing.

T. Refer both patient and family for counseling as necessary.

U. Provide therapeutic diet. After removal of nasogastric tube, diet gradually increased from clear liquid to high protein. Administer oral fluids slowly so tolerance can be observed. Be alert for signs of Curling's ulcer (refer to Chap. 29); incidence is in proportion to extent of burn. Appetite needs to be encouraged. Avoid painful procedures around meal times. When appropriate, select those foods which are nutritious and enjoyed by the patient.

V. Provide environment that helps patient stay oriented to counteract sensory deprivation and disturbed body rhythms. Use clocks, colors, pictures, television, radio, and visitors.

W. Control edema and prevent decubiti by positioning the patient in supine semi-Fowler's position. Change position often.

X. Lower extremities should be extended and elevated with slight abduction and external rotation of the hips and heels off the bed. Upper extremities are elevated and abducted, with supination of the hands and external rotation of the humerus. This positioning facilitates respiration and decreases risk of contracture but limits the mobility of the patient.

Y. Further prevention of contractures is obtained by a footboard; have the patient feed self; splint hands at night only.

Z. Constant observation and reassessment of physical and psychological needs as patient progresses from the acute stage.

Evaluation

I. Reassessment.
   A. Assess progress of intervention.
   B. Reappraise the degree of impairment (healing).
II. Complications.
   A. Infection.
      1. Assessment.
         a. Culture the wound.
         b. Note any change in symptoms.
         c. Note increased restlessness.
         d. Check vital signs.
         e. Watch for fever.
      2. Intervention: administration of medication (antibiotic) specific to organism.
   B. Stress ulcer or Curling's ulcer (refer to Chap. 29).
      1. Assessment.
         a. Distension.
         b. Bleeding.
         c. Abdominal pain.
         d. Hemoptosis.
         e. Guaiac-positive stools.
         f. Change in vital signs.
      2. Intervention (see discussion of ulcers in Chap. 29).
   C. Respiratory changes: Pneumonia or respiratory distress.
      1. Assessment.
         a. Rate.
         b. Sound.
         c. Quality of respirations:
            (1) Dullness on palpation.
            (2) Decreased chest excursion.
            (3) Rales and ronchi.
         d. Stridor.
         e. Labored breathing.
         f. Cough.
         g. Hoarseness.
         h. Increased temperature.
         i. Cyanosis.

    2. Intervention (refer to Chap. 27).
       a. Observe for change.
       b. Have a tracheostomy set ready.
       c. Have oxygen equipment easily accessible.
   D. Shock (refer to Chap. 44).
   E. Depression.
    1. Assessment.
       a. Change in sleep.   *c.* Alteration in appetite.
       b. Activity.   *d.* Changes in affect.
    2. Intervention (refer to discussion of depression in Chap. 36).
   F. Contractures.
    1. Assessment: limitation of mobility.
    2. Intervention.
       a. Range-of-motion exercises: first passive, then active.
       b. Whirlpool.
       c. Footboard.
III. Intervention: surgery.
   A. Skin grafting: use of hemografts, heterografts over burn area to facilitate tissue regrowth.
   B. Eschar removal: incisions made into burn to release tissue and facilitate movement, e.g., chest.
   C. Bone reconstruction following formation of contractures.
   D. Additional care (refer to Chap. 31).

DEGENERATIVE DISORDERS

Syphilis

Definition   *Syphilis* is a serious, contagious, venereal disease caused by the motile spirochete *Treponema pallidum.* The course of illness can be fatal without adequate treatment. Syphilis is spread primarily by sexual contact but can also be the result of congenital transmission and accidental inoculation. The incubation period of syphilis is anywhere from 9 to 90 days, with an average incubation of 3 to 4 weeks. Generally syphilis is classified according to stages. Treatment and transmission of the disease depends upon the stage being observed.

   I. *Primary stage.* During this stage a painless chancre (indurated) appears with a roughly circular shape. It may appear as papule, vesicle, or ulcer. Usually it is observed at the point of entry of the spirochete, 9 to 90 days after sexual contact (see Fig. 33-9). In the female, the chancre can go unnoticed if it is located on the cervix or vaginal wall. In homosexual males the chancre is often located in the rectum or the mouth. A chancre can appear at any site of sexual contact, including penis, lips, labia, oral cavity, or anus. Lymphadenopathy may be found in the node that drains the affected site. Without treatment, the chancre heals by itself in 1 to 5 weeks. However, the disease continues to develop and remains transmissible.

   II. *Secondary stage.* During this stage a generalized skin rash appears along with flulike symptoms. This is often noted within 6 months following the date of exposure. The description of rash varies, and can be visualized as erythematous papules on face, shoulders, upper arms, chest, back, abdomen, palms of the hands, and soles of the feet. These papules turn coppery brown and gradually fade away. The rash is generally nonpruritic (see Fig. 33-10). A rash on the palms and the soles of the feet is significant, since few rashes manifest at these sites. *Condylomata lata* form in warm, moist areas. These are moist papules, pink or greyish, which contain serous fluid and are highly infectious. Mucous patches are greyish white with dull red borders that can appear in mucous membranes of mouth or tonsils, perhaps resulting in a sore throat. Rash may be accompanied by a feeling of malaise, headache, nausea, constipation, anorexia,

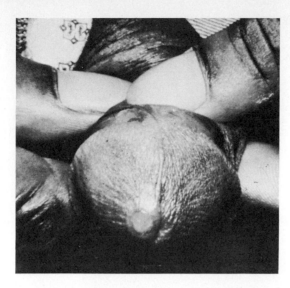

FIGURE 33-9 / Primary chancre.
[*From T. B. Fitzpatrick et al. (eds.),
Dermatology in General Medicine,
McGraw-Hill Book Company, New
York, 1971.*]

pain in long bones, alopecia, and low-grade fever. Without treatment symptoms usually
disappear in 2 to 8 weeks, but secondary relapse can occur during latent stage.

III. *Latent stage.* Syphilis is symptomatic, but gives a positive serology and negative spinal
tap. The patient may experience a relapse of secondary symptoms during the first 2
years of latent syphilis. Within 2 to 4 years patient is no longer infectious to sexual
partners.

IV. *Tertiary syphilis.* There are three types.
   A. *Benign late,* which affects skin, muscles, digestive organs, liver, lungs, eyes, and
   endocrine glands. The characteristic lesion is a gumma, which occurs in any tissue
   and results in necrosis.
   B. *Cardiovascular effects:* blood vessels and heart. The characteristic lesion is an aortic
   aneurysm.
   C. *Neurosyphilis* involves the meninges, brain, and spinal cord. Today, symptoms of
   tertiary syphilis are rarely seen, since screening and treatment methods currently in
   use pick up the disease much sooner. Patients suspected of having syphilis are often
   found in a local clinic or emergency room. Cases are reported to local health
   department. Contacts should be treated.

Assessment

I. Data sources (refer to "Skin Tumors").
   A. Patient.
   B. Previous medical record.
   C. Information presented concerning contacts.
II. Health history.
   A. Age: highest incidence is 20 to 40 years; next highest, 15 to 19 years.
   B. Sexual preference: recent sexual contacts.
   C. History of a painless chancre or symptoms of secondary syphilis and the dates they
   occur.
   D. History of last and previous contact, sites of exposure, and names of steady partners.
   E. General physical health should be explored.
   F. Life-style.
   G. History of allergies.
III. Physical examination: Observable signs discussed in "Definition." Patient should have
complete physical examination and thorough medical history should be taken.
IV. Diagnostic tests.
   A. Dark-field microscopic examination visualizes spirochete.

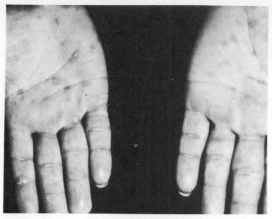

(a)

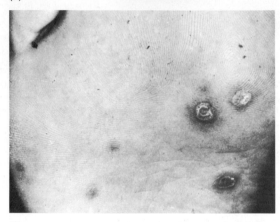

(b)

FIGURE 33-10 / Secondary syphilis. [*From T. B. Fitzpatrick et al. (eds.), Dermatology in General Medicine, McGraw-Hill Book Company, New York, 1971.*]

B. *Serology tests* for screening: a blood test (reagin antigen tests) designed to detect reagin in the blood. Less expensive than treponemal tests. If patient shows a positive reaction on initial screening, treponemal test and qualitative titer are done to determine extent of the reaction. False positives may occur with patients who have mononucleosis, malaria, hepatitis, vaccinia, and collagen diseases (lupus erythematosus, rheumatoid arthritis), and in heroin users. In the case of biological false positives, reactive, rapid plasma reagin (RPR), with negative fluorescent treponemal antibody (FTA), often cannot document the cause.

C. Commonly used blood tests are:
    1. Venereal Disease Research Lab (VDRL).
    2. RPR. If the RPR screening test is returned positive or reactive, then automatically, qualitative RPR and the fluorescent treponemal antibody absorption test (FTA–ABS) should be done.

D. *Treponemal test for diagnosis.* Blood test to detect specific syphilis antibodies is the FTA-ABS. Done following all positive RPRs.

E. Spinal tap: fluid sent for RPR (refer to Chap. 23).

Problems
    I. Potentially seriously ill patient with minor symptoms.
    II. Sexually transmissible disease.
    III. Anxiety.
    IV. Fear of social stigma.

Diagnosis   I. Impaired skin integrity: potential.
II. Patient is of high risk to self and others: transmissible disease.
III. Anxiety: mild to moderate.
IV. Alterations in self-concept, secondary to social stigma of syphilis.

Goals of Care   I. Immediate.
    A. Prevent transmission.
    B. Arrange for public health associate to perform contact interview to obtain information regarding sexual partners and to increase patient's awareness of the disease.
II. Long-range.
    A. Restore skin integrity.
    B. Long-term follow-up to prevent reinfection and treat early to prevent the progressive stages.

Intervention   I. Explain illness, course, rationale for treatment, importance of follow-up of patient and contacts. Be supportive to the patient, as discussion of the problem is often difficult and embarrassing.
II. Administration of penicillin. Check carefully for allergy. Treatment schedule for syphilis is presently under revision by the Center for Disease Control in Atlanta, Georgia. Suggested treatment as of 1976 was parenteral penicillin G as the drug of choice for the treatment of syphilis, since there is no evidence that *Treponema pallidum* is becoming resistant to the drug. For primary and secondary syphilis, and for latent syphilis with negative spinal fluid, 10 days treatment with parenteral penicillin G is recommended. A single injection of benzathine penicillin G (4.8 million units) may be given; some clinics give one or two additional injections at weekly intervals. Oral penicillins have not been adequately evaluated for treatment of syphilis and should not be used. Tetracycline or other antibiotics may be used if an allergy to penicillin is noted. Bedamid (oral drug) may be given prior to the antibiotic to enhance the effectiveness of the antibiotic.
III. Encourage follow-up. Serology (RPR) should be repeated monthly for a year, then every 3 months until negative. In cases of primary syphilis, if RPR is not negative within a year, reevaluate and re-treat. In cases of secondary syphilis and latent syphilis, allow 2 years.
IV. Identify and refer patients to public health associate at the state level who will gather information regarding contacts. Primary contacts are those within the past 3 months plus the duration of the chancre. Secondary contacts are those within 6 months plus the duration of the secondary symptoms.
V. Discuss prevention. Encourage washing areas of sexual contact with soap and water following sexual activity. Routine serological, physical, and gynecological examinations are important.
VI. Supportive counseling. Sexually transmitted disease carries moral implications for some patients. Be objective and informative; encourage patients to ask questions and verbalize positive and negative feelings toward the problem.
VII. Reportable disease. For the procedure in your local area, contact the state health department. Usually requires a phone referral and written report.
VIII. Instruct patient to abstain from sexual contact until treatment completed.
IX. Use caution when handling specimen for laboratory. Also, if chancre is present, culture may be necessary.

Evaluation   I. Reassessment.
    A. Evaluate the effectiveness of treatment by the status of serology.
    B. Note the stage of syphilis and related symptoms.
    C. Observe for signs of reinfection.
    D. Evaluate compliance by the successful remission of symptoms and lack of new symptoms.

II. Complications.
  A. Anaphylaxis reaction or procaine reaction.
    1. Anaphylaxis.
      a. Assessment.
        (1) Subjective.
          (a) Fear of impending death.   (d) Immobility.
          (b) Apprehension.   (e) Paresthesia.
          (c) Chest constriction.
        (2) Objective.
          (a) Syncope.   (e) Wheezing.
          (b) Seizure.   (f) Cyanosis.
          (c) Decreased blood pressure.   (g) Thready pulse.
          (d) Urticaria.
      b. Intervention.
        (1) Administer epinephrine.
        (2) Maintain patent airway.
        (3) Assist with fluid replacement for shock.
        (4) Administer antihistamines, steroids, oxygen.
    2. Procaine reaction.
      a. Assessment.
        (1) Subjective.
          (a) Fear of impending death.   (d) Restlessness.
          (b) Apprehension.   (e) Faintness.
          (c) Auditory and visual hallucinations.
        (2) Objective.
          (a) Syncope.   (d) Cyanosis.
          (b) Seizure.   (e) Strong pulse.
          (c) Increased blood pressure.
      b. Intervention.
        (1) Reassure patient.
        (2) Restrain if necessary.
        (3) Symptoms transitory; stay with patient.
        (4) Administer phenobarbital, observe.
    3. Neurological: paresthesia, tabes dorsalis, dementia, meningitis, Charcot's joint (refer to Chap. 23).
    4. Optic atrophy: result of late syphilis.
    5. Cardiovascular: aortitis, scarring of vessel lining, (e.g., intima), aneurysm or aortic heart block (see Chap. 26).
    6. Congenital syphilis (refer to Chap. 19).

BIBLIOGRAPHY

Arndt, Kenneth: *Manual of Dermatologic Therapeutics*, Little, Brown and Company, Boston, 1971. Excellent, concise reference manual of dermatologic problems most frequently seen in an ambulatory setting.

Bhantooa, Dhurmadut: "Fluid Replacement with Special Reference to Burned Patients-Management During Infusion," *Nursing Times*, **73**:337–338, March 1977. Good reference; discussion of nursing care relevant.

Brunner, Lillian, and Doris Suddarth (eds.): *The Lippincott Manual of Nursing Practice*, J.B. Lippincott Company, Philadelphia, 1974. Comprehensive reference manual, in outline form, of current nursing practice. Excellent resource.

Fears, Thomas, Joseph Scotto, and Marion Shneiderion: "Skin Cancer, Melanoma and Sunlight," *American Journal of Nursing*, **66**:461–464, May 1976. A good discussion of skin cancers and possible causes of the problem, e.g., sunlight.

Friberg, T.: "Assessment: Could That Itching Be Scabies?" *Nursing Update*, **7**:1–4, August 1976. Discussion and assessment of scabies.

Glasser, J.: "Psoriasis: Trends in Therapy," *Nursing Care,* **9:**12–15, August 1976. Discussion of the problem of psoriasis and current treatment.

Grant, Marcia: "The Kidney and Fluid and Electrolyte Imbalances," in D. Jones, C. Dunbar, M. Jirovec (eds.), *Medical-Surgical Nursing: A Conceptual Approach,* McGraw-Hill Book Company, New York, 1978, pp. 493–524. Excellent resource for complete nursing care of first-, second-, and third-degree burns. Photographs of burn injuries inside the back cover help provide the reader with a complete in-depth picture of all the parameters involved when caring for a patient who sustains a burn injury.

Keane, E.: "Atopic Eczema," *Nursing Times,* **71:**2013–2015, December, 1975.

Luckman, Jean, and Karen Sorensen: *Medical-Surgical Nursing: A Psychophysiologic Approach,* W.B. Saunders Company, Philadelphia, 1974. Thorough, detailed discussion of dermatologic problems, with an excellent section on burn care.

Roach, Laura: "Color Changes in Dark Skin," *Nursing '77,* **7:**48–51, January 1977. Excellent resource, with photographs depicting skin lesions and related color changes, as observed in blacks.

Sauer, Gordon: *Manual of Skin Diseases,* 2d ed., J.B. Lippincott Company, Philadelphia, 1966.

Scipien, Gladys, and Martha Barnard (eds.): "The Integumentary System," *Issues in Comprehensive Pediatrics Nursing,* July 1976. Concise coverage of the most commonly seen dermatologic problems. Specific categories, i.e., atopic dermatitis, covered in individual articles.

Walsh, T. F. (ed.): "Skin Problems: The Best Use Of Topical Therapy," *Nursing Update,* **7:**1–5, January 1976; "Skin Lesions: Watch for Common Fungal Infections," ibid., **7:**1–7, February 1976; "Finding the Cause of Contact Dermatitis," ibid., **7:**3–6, April 1976. Three-part series includes excellent practical aspects of physiology and nursing intervention.

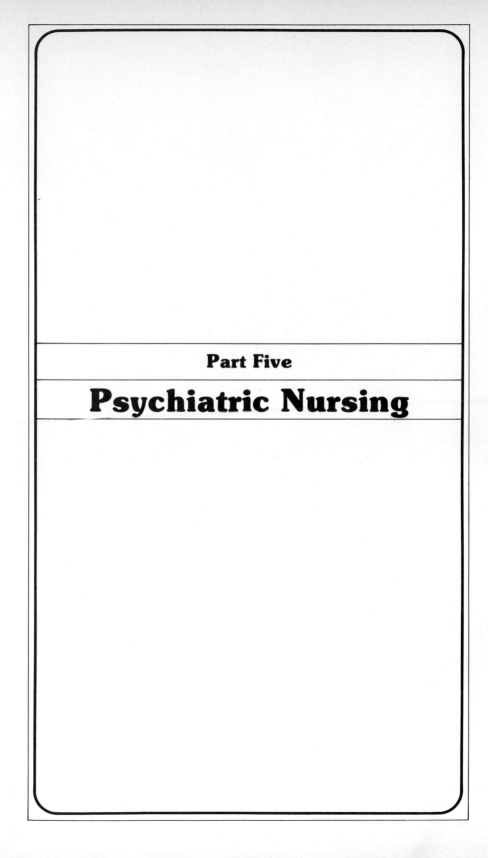

Part Five

Psychiatric Nursing

People who suffer from mental health problems constitute a large segment of hospital populations. Nurses who practice in psychiatric units face a tremendous challenge to provide appropriate nursing care for large numbers of patients.

Much is written about the human attributes such as empathy and concern that nurses who care for psychiatric patients are expected to possess. It is also necessary that the professional nurse utilize the nursing process in a cognitive sense so that the wish to help is translated into the helping act. Part 5, therefore, has as its purpose the presentation of the use of the nursing process in response to a representative group of clinical problems which are frequently presented by psychiatric patients in hospital settings. Typical dysfunctional behavioral patterns observed in both adults and children are presented. Concepts and principles related to the functioning of groups have also been included because the psychiatric inpatient is a part of a special kind of group while in the hospital. The common use of milieu therapy in hospitals makes these concepts timely and germane to nursing practice with psychiatric patients.

ANA STANDARDS OF PSYCHIATRIC–MENTAL HEALTH NURSING PRACTICE[1]

1. Data are collected through pertinent clinical observations based on knowledge of the arts and sciences, with particular emphasis upon psychosocial and biophysical sciences.
2. Clients are involved in the assessment, planning, implementation, and evaluation of their nursing care program to the fullest extent of their capabilities.
3. The problem-solving approach is utilized in developing plans of nursing care.
4. Individuals, families, and community groups are assisted to achieve satisfying and productive patterns of living through health teaching.
5. The activities of daily living are utilized in a goal-directed way in work with clients.
6. Knowledge of somatic therapies and related clinical skills is utilized in working with clients.
7. The environment is structured to establish and maintain a therapeutic milieu.
8. Nurses participate with interdisciplinary teams in assessing, planning, implementing, and evaluatiing programs and other mental activities.
9. Psychotherapeutic interventions are used to assist clients to achieve their maximum development.
10. The practice of individual, group, or family psychotherapy requires appropriate preparation and recognition of accountability for the practice.
11. Nurses participate with other members of the community in planning and implementing mental health services, which include the broad continuum of promotion of mental health, prevention of mental illness, treatment, and rehabilitation.
12. Learning experiences are provided for other health care personnel through leadership, supervision, and teaching.
13. Responsibility is assumed for continuing educational and professional development, and contributions are made to the professional growth of others.
14. Contributions to nursing and the mental health field are made through innovations in theory and practice and through participation in research.

[1] Reprinted with permission from the *American Nurses' Association Standards of Psychiatric and Mental Health Nursing Practice. Copyright © 1974 by the American Nurses' Association.*

34

Mental Health Problems in Children

Faye Gary Harris and Lucille Bright Wilson

The following thoughts may be useful for the nurse therapist who works with children and their families.

I. Therapy should be planned with the child's phase-specific maturational achievements in mind.

II. The nurse should be knowledgable about growth and development theory, and should have the ability and skill to apply theory to the clinical setting.

III. Generally speaking, one can categorize children in groupings of 4 to 7 years and find some similarities of frequencies in behaviors.

IV. Another categorization may be constructed with children from about 8 to 11 or 12 years. Each of the age groupings is different and should be perceived that way.

V. Children are usually brought to treatment by parents. The therapist should evaluate the entire family and assess the role function activities of the identified patient (child who is being brought to treatment).

VI. The nurse should encourage and support "family therapy concept" through assessment and evaluation for further therapy.

VII. The nurse should be aware of indications and contraindications of therapeutic treatment modalities and the applicability to the specific presenting family-child-milieu problems of the various modes.

VIII. After an initial family system assessment and experimental encounter, a rule to follow is to separate child from family. Each subsystem has its own therapist(s).

IX. The "need" or motivation for treatment may well rest upon how troubled the parents are about the child.

X. The "need" or motivation for treatment may also rest upon how troubled the child is and the intensity of troubled feelings that is transmitted to the parents.

XI. The nurse should like the child, it being felt that genuine feelings are difficult to develop and maintain if some transference and useful countertransference is not established.

XII. The nurse should assess the "willingness" of the parents to be in treatment. This may include:

A. Monetary adjustment.
B. Time from work and home.
C. Transportation issues.
D. Exposure of other siblings.
E. Exposure of family secrets.
F. Familial realignments, etc.

XIII. Can the family endure an image of having a sick child?

XIV. Does the family system have the necessary components essential for treatment? Each treatment center may have a different assessment of what these components are.

XV. Can the staff handle this type of child?

XVI. Clarify the priority issues in the treatment regimen.

XVII. Set and reevaluate goals of care whenever appropriate.

XVIII. The nurse and staff should assess variations in cultural, religious, and sociopolitical orientations and the impact of these upon the child-family system.

XIX. Treatment nuances may reflect the community values, constraints, and sociopolitical postures. Thus, when appropriate, nurse and staff need to know what these are.

XX. The nurse should be comfortable with own self.

XXI. The nurse should have worked through own childhood, family relations, and community influences.

XXII. The nurse should have the skill, the security, and the ability to "enter the child's world," to participate in the metaphor, and to abandon that role in seconds.

XXIII. The nurse should have the ability and skill to evaluate cognitively and affectively the meaning of the child's play, dreams, and/or fantasies.

XIV. The nurse should feel secure with ambiguities and the unknown.

XV. The nurse should possess the ability to use clinical data for heuristic purposes.

THE HYPERACTIVE CHILD

Definition

Hyperactive children have a history of sleep disturbance and an abundance of energy. They tend to be fidgety and cannot keep still in structured situations for any length of time; they talk incessantly and cannot seem to refrain from touching or (sometimes at school) hitting others. There are manifest problems with attention span; day dreaming or other types of fantasies occupy their time. They have difficulty tolerating environmental stimuli.

Impulsiveness in these children varies in degree, but may frequently be life-threatening, for example, running after a ball into a busy street without looking first. A milder example would be telling family secrets to house guests. Temper tantrums and poor frustration and conflict management make it difficult for these children to have harmonious relations with family and peers. School performance is usually poor. The community at large perceives these children as destructive, difficult to control, and as "brats." These perceptions can be internalized by the child, who frequently responds with more maladaptive behaviors.

Assessment

This assessment framework incorporates many of the guidelines presented in the mental status examination of children suggested by Simmons (1).

I. Data sources.
  A. Observations of child and parent(s).
  B. Play session with child and parent(s).
  C. Interview session with child and parent(s).
  D. Interview with other family members individually together with identified patient, and without identified patient.
  E. Appearance of child, to include conformity or nonconformity to social mores and folk ways.
  F. Appearance of each of the family members, to include conformity or nonconformity to folk ways and social class.

II. Health history (when appropriate, ask both child and parents or significant other).
  A. Age.
  B. Sex.
  C. Grade in school.
  D. Address.
  E. Occupation of parents.
  F. Description of any type of physical problems believed to have existed, treated or untreated.
  G. A listing of community agencies that are used by parents and child.
    1. A parental evaluation of the agency and agent in terms of how their needs were met or not met.
    2. The child's evaluation of the agency and agent in terms of how their needs were met or not met.
  H. Describe parents' manner of handling themselves in stressful situations.
  I. Describe parents' manner of handling stress generated by children.
  J. Have parents describe strong points and weak points about their personalities.
  K. Have parents describe strong points and weak points about their child or children.
  L. Describe the ways in which the parents express their aggression.

    M. Describe the ways in which the child expresses aggression and sexual impulses.

    N. Describe the mood or affect (predominant feelings) manifested by the parents.

    O. Describe the mood or affect (predominant feelings) manifested by the child.

    P. Describe the mood or affect of the child when in the presence of parents or when child is alone with the interviewer.

    Q. Observe and record the specific defense mechanisms used by the child during:

        1. Interview.

        2. Periods of play.

        3. Communication with parents. (It is of importance that the interviewer record descriptions of the child's behavior in precise terms, thus omitting global psychiatric terminology which may only serve to confuse the reader.)

    R. Observe and record the child's usage of senses: taste, sight, touch, hearing, smell.

    S. Neuromuscular integrative activities should be observed and recorded. Examples include:

        1. Gross motor coordination.

        2. Fine motor coordination.

        3. Eye-hand movement and coordination. Specifics:

            a. Can child skip, bounce a ball?

            b. Can child complete activities that require a crossing of midline, i.e., write name on chalkboard?

III. Thought processes.

    A. Observe and record the appropriate or inappropriate usage of words.

    B. Observe and record the overall vocabulary.

    C. Observe and record the content and affect for patterns and themes in thought process.

    D. Observe for any preoccupations.

    E. Observe for perservation (repeating same words or acts, difficulty in shifting from one thought and/or act to another).

    F. Observe and record the manner in which the child organizes thinking (time, facial expressions, motor movements, affect, and method of verbal delivery).

IV. Fantasy.

    A. Record description of dream materials.

    B. Record description of drawings (the nurse interviewer should have crayons, papers, and pencils in interview room).

    C. Describe and record wishes. The nurse interviewer can say "Tell me, [name of child], what are three wishes that you have in your head most of the time?"

    D. Describe and record storytelling. The nurse interviewer can begin by saying "Once upon a time there was a little [sex of child] who had a mother, a father, and three sisters [use content appropriate for child's situation]." The child then completes the story.

V. Self-perceptions. Does the child perceive self as:

    A. Good or bad?

    B. Meek or strong?

    C. Short or tall?

    D. Ugly or pretty?

    E. Looking like mother or father?

    F. Acting like mother or father?

    G. Some day wanting to be like mother or father? Ask why.

VI. Supportive documents.

    A. An assessment of academic functions from school officials.

    B. A list of impending stresses that the child may encounter.

    C. A list of crises or stressful periods experienced by the child.

    D. Variations: Always assess for information pertaining to the child's and family's level of comfort in relation to these variables:

        1. Religious.   **3.** Socioeconomic.

        2. Sociocultural.   **4.** Geographic (rural, urban, etc.).

VII. The affective and cognitive responses of the professional and nonprofessional staff to the child, i.e.:
   A. Do they like child, feel anger, indifference, shame and/or guilt, embarrassment, helplessness and hopelessness? Is the situation workable?
   B. Is the staff experiencing a rescue fantasy about child? Is it realistic?

Problems

Impulsivity with Aggression

I. Child makes "cutting" statements about staff to other staff without provocation.
II. Child touches staff frequently and often inappropriately.
III. Child cannot delay a comment or observation.
IV. Milieu rules and regulations are consistently and continually broken by child.
V. Child asks questions incessantly (frequently these questions are same ones asked earlier).
VI. Child cries and lies on floor screaming when immediate demands for food are not met.
VII. Child eats food in a hurried, unsocialized manner.
VIII. Child cannot sit still in *structured* play activities.
IX. Child manages better when in unstructured, solitary play type situations (for as long as 45 min).
X. Child hits peers.
XI. Child fights and demands books or toys from peers.
XII. Child uses profane language.
XIII. Child destroys property when expressing anger and/or having a temper tantrum.
XIV. Child cannot complete a task (paper and pencil) within a designated time period.
XV. Child monopolizes conversation, changes topic, and then physically leaves the environment when a discussion is uncomfortable to him.
XVI. Child, on occasion, is encopretic and enuretic (patterns of behavior may be related to tantrums and anger with staff).
XVII. Child will not attempt to complete any academic work assigned by teacher in the milieu.
XVIII. Child regurgitates medications in commode and then flushes commode.

Goals of Care

I. Immediate.
   A. Child will control enuretic and encopretic behaviors.
   B. Child will develop more acceptable sublimatory channels through which impulsivity can be controlled.
   C. Child will decrease frequency of inappropriate touching and hitting others.
   D. Child will decrease frequency and duration of temper tantrums.
   E. Child will decrease duration and frequency of making "cutting" remarks about staff to other staff.
   F. Child will decrease frequency and duration of using profane language.

   Note Professional nurses must be sensitive to their own feelings, thoughts, and reactions when a hyperactive child with a multitude of impulse control deficits is in the milieu. The immediate goals in this situation are structured from analyzing the most provocative and stressful behaviors that the child manifests. Consequently, the staff can get "a handle on things" and proceed with the total treatment plan.

II. Long-range.
   A. Child will develop a positive relationship with nurse therapist.
   B. Child will articulate frustrations and conflicts in an acceptable manner.
   C. Child will learn to recognize the feeling states accompanying impulsive acts.

D. Child will learn to identify thoughts and affective sensations that precede impulsive acts.

E. Child will learn to "program in" acceptable control devices that delay, preclude, and prevent the intensity, duration, and frequency of impulsive acts.

F. Child will recognize and articulate anger but decrease frequency and duration of destroying property.

G. Child will gain insight into behavior through reviewing videotape and discussing behaviors.

H. Child will develop basic socialization skills, such as eating properly, waiting for one's turn, and engaging in conversations with peers in an acceptable manner.

I. Child will increase the duration and frequency of engaging in tasks that can be completed and/or mastered.

J. Child will learn to wait for gratification of needs.

Intervention

Specific interventions are explicitly or implicitly related to "Problems" and "Goals of Care." A categorization has been implemented to provide for clearer organization and synthesis.

Physical Assertion

I. Identify the specific behavior pattern.

II. Record ecological conditions under which behavior occurs.

III. Observe, recognize, and record duration and frequency of touching behaviors.

IV. Solicit the nurses' (especially the nurse therapists') feelings about the touching behaviors.

V. Explore with child the meaning and utility of the milieu rules and guidelines.

VI. Identify specific situations when child touches staff and other children.

VII. Review with child "before" fighting thoughts and feelings.

VIII. Explore with child thoughts and feelings "during" the fighting period.

IX. Explore with child thoughts an feelings "after" the fighting.

X. Discuss the "taking away" of toys, books, and games from other children.
- **A.** Feelings, thoughts.
- **B.** Power, control.
- **C.** Reputation and status in relation to peers and teachers.
- **D.** Anger, guilt, shame.
- **E.** Hopelessness and uselessness.

XI. Assist child in recognizing cause-and-effect relationships that arise from each identifiable physical impulsive act.

XII. Explore alternative methods of releasing anger: consider play activities, bag punching, running, and then talking with nurse.

XIII. Video tape temper tantrum behaviors, hitting behaviors, or any other intimidating (to staff) behaviors.

XIV. Review and discuss video tape with child, assisting recall of thoughts and feelings during the identified activity.

XV. Solicit from child a reason for the specific behavior(s).

XVI. Elicit behavioral alternatives.
- **A.** Direct approach:
  1. "What could you have done to express yourself without [whatever the identified behavior may be]?"
  2. "What were you thinking about when you [whatever the identified behavior may be]?"
- **B.** Indirect approach:
  1. "I am here to talk with you as soon as you are ready."
  2. "Throwing chairs is frightening, isn't it?"

    XVII. State to child that nurse and other staff will provide controls when child is unable to provide controls.

    XVIII. All staff will model constructive methods of expressing inner feelings.

Verbal Impulsivity

    I. Assist child in articulating anger in a socially acceptable manner.

    II. Pinpoint those specific behaviors in the child's speech that are unacceptable.

    III. Collect baseline data concerning these behaviors that are pinpointed.

    IV. Record the duration and frequency of the pinpointed speech behaviors that are unacceptable.

    V. Review these data with child, and solicit a commitment to behavioral change.

    VI. Audiotape the verbally unacceptable behavior for purpose of presenting to child in a one-to-one session.

    VII. During one-to-one session, present verbally unacceptable behaviors and encourage or solicit:
- **A.** Explanations.
- **B.** Clarifications.
- **C.** Rationale for such behaviors.

    VIII. Therapist should then think in terms of unmet needs and therapeutic program methods of meeting specific needs identified.

    IX. Teach or reorient child to appropriate basic language skills in an effort to provide a verbal rather than muscular method of communicating frustrations, conflicts, and needs.

    X. When child has had a successful period (hours, days, or weeks) of appropriate and acceptable verbal interchange with people in milieu, *reward.*

    XI. Teach the child the use of sublimatory channels to express feelings, thoughts, and behaviors.

    XII. Provide immediate feedback to child when attempts at sublimation are appropriate.

    XIII. Teach behavior substitution.

    XIV. Recognize fantasies—daydreams, dreams, thoughts, feelings, and mental pictures—as being powerful sensations and images for the child.

    XV. Articulate to child that these cognitive and affective experiences are understood by nurse (staff), and reassure child that nurse (staff) will teach:
- **A.** Judgement.
- **B.** Timing.
- **C.** Delay.
- **D.** Sophistication relative to verbal expressions.

    XVI. Engage in behavior rehearsal with child, addressing specific content identified and reviewed in audiotape review of verbal impulsivity.

    XVII. State to child the effects that verbal impulsivity has upon:
- **A.** Peers.
- **B.** Staff.
- **C.** Milieu.

    XVIII. Engage in behavior rehearsals with child to address difficult interpersonal situations:
- **A.** Nurse assumes attributes of significant others as assigned by child.
- **B.** Child and nurse role play.
- **C.** Reverse situation: child assumes attributes or behaviors of significant other, and nurse assumes attributes or behaviors of child.
- **D.** Discuss, clarify, and identify thoughts, feelings, sensations, and behaviors in each of the above situations, emphasizing *adaptive* responses.
- **E.** Encourage child to evaluate the manifest behavior.

Self-care Disturbances

    I. Identify and discuss with child encopresis and enuresis as methods of expressing resentment and anger.

    II. Discuss and encourage alternative methods for expressing anger.

    III. Assist child in identifying feelings and thoughts subsequent to acts of encopresis and enuresis.

IV. Discuss with child the importance of accepting and swallowing medications.

V. Assess behavior in terms of identified feelings and thoughts child has concerning medications.

VI. Solicit questions from child concerning medications, their real or perceived side effects, functions, untoward reactions, etc.

VII. Teach child to state directly the feelings of dissatisfaction about taking medications.

VIII. Provide one-to-one milieu when beginning a regimen for child that aids in socially acceptable eating habits.

    A. Provide food that child likes.

    B. Structure specified periods of time for eating certain food on plate. ("For the next five minutes eat three bites of peas, two bites of hamburger, and three mouthfuls of fries. Here, follow me.") Then nurse models this behavior in socially close proximity.

IX. Nurse verbally states above request in a rhythmic, pacing fashion.

X. Touch child's arm in an acceptable manner, thus pacing eating activities and modeling appropriate touch behaviors.

XI. Speak firmly to child when eating activities require immediate alterations.

XII. Provide encouraging remarks for a behavior related to eating that is appropriate and acceptable.

XIII. Structure frequency of encouraging remarks based on child's ability to modify and/or change aberrant behaviors.

XIV. Reward child for having accomplished a behavior(s) with an activity that allows the child to excel or master.

XV. Teach child to take care of personal hygiene needs.

XVI. Teach and review with child the milieu rules and guidelines.

XVII. Discuss with child the need for having the milieu rules and guidelines, and solicit a commitment of cooperation with milieu.

XVIII. Provide child with opportunities for appropriate expression related to asking questions and ventilating feelings and thoughts about milieu and its guidelines.

XIX. Meet the child's requests and wishes whenever they are appropriate.

XX. When requests and wishes are not appropriate, say so, and discuss the issue.

Play Activities   These interventions are especially useful for children from 3 to 7 or 8 years of age.

I. Observe and record child's actions and verbalizations in play situations.

II. Enter the play situation, and encourage verbalizations and activities.

III. Encourage child to express conflictual feelings by "structuring" the play situation and assess:

    A. The use of specific defense mechanisms.

    B. The role of "self" in play activites (good, bad, helpless, confused, etc.).

    C. Family relations as power points, pressure points, themes of aggression, and methods of sublimation.

IV. Provide tasks that child can successfully complete; increase the complexity over time.

V. Provide activities in the structured situation that child can master; reward with verbal or nonverbal approval.

VI. Use nonstructured play as a reinforcer for completing academic tasks.

VII. Design a list of positives (things child likes to do) that can be used as reinforcers.

VIII. Structure play situations by assigning to staff family roles pertinent to child's experiences.

IX. Observe for affective changes by identifying:

    A. Associated content.

    B. Length of time into the session.

    C. Motor movements.

    D. Facial expression.

    E. Eye contact or lack of eye contact.

    F. Kinesis.

X. Ask for clarification when behaviors or verbalizations are not understood.

XI. Solicit and encourage positive talk from child about self.

XII. Provide situations whereby child can successfully interact with peer group.

Parents and Community

I. Assess and record parents' images of themselves and their perceptions of the identified child (patient) as opposed to other sibling(s).

II. Assess and record parents' perception of child as opposed to other children in the larger social system.

III. Assess whether parents are likely to facilitate a therapeutic collusion between child and therapist.

IV. Explore parents' feelings and thoughts about therapy: useful, hopeless, mystical, etc.

V. Explore parents' feelings and thoughts about child being mentally sick.

VI. Assess whether parents are feeling harassed, embarrassed, humiliated, or rejected by community because of child's difficulties.

VII. Explore with parents the formal and informal support system within their community; encourage and assist parents in mobilizing these resources.

VIII. Provide parents with appropriate therapeutic modalities.

IX. Assess the cultural, religious, socioeconomic, ethnic, sociopolitical, and geographical values and conflicts pertinent to parents, child, family, and community.

X. Assess the degree of comfort or harmony expressed by parents in relation to these values and conflicts.

XI. Identify those cultural, religious, socioeconomic, ethnic, sociopolitical, and geographical values and conflicts pertinent to self; then, look for possible opportunities for misinterpretation of conflicts when involved in therapeutic process with child or family.

Evaluation

I. Reassessment: When working with children, evaluation of treatment should be done by the team working with the child and family. In addition, a detailed assessment of the daily intervention methods employed should be carefully evaluated. The nurse should consider the following when evaluating intervention:

A. Is the nurse comfortable with the intervention?

B. Does the nurse have the support of the treatment team?

C. Has the nurse communicated appropriately with other members of the care team?

D. Are there patterns in child and family's responses to specific treatment modalities?

E. Does the nurse feel that the child and family are worthy of the time and energy required for treatment?

II. Follow-up and reevaluation.

A. Make referral to appropriate community agency by providing a summary of therapy, treatment modalities, and progress. Specify any unique and/or unusual attributes of child and family.

B. Terminate treatment with child and parents, providing them with lists of agents and agencies where professional help can be attained.

C. Collaborate with other agencies and institutions that child will, through normal course of development, encounter. The school is probably the most important institution to be considered.

    1. Intervention methods may be shared with teacher and school psychologist.

    2. Rationale for intervention is also helpful and provides a base for consistency and continuity of those techniques that facilitate the child's and family's positive growth.

    3. Identify self as a resource person available for consultation to school personnel.

D. When necessary, coordinate referrals to other community agencies, such as welfare departments, protective services, special medical services, etc. Determine the content of clinical summary to be included in each type of referral. The agency receiving the referral and the purpose of the referral will govern the content included.

THE DEPRESSED CHILD

Definition

A clinical definition of *depression* in children would include characteristics of dysphonia in mood and affect, a history of recent sleep disturbance, a general loss of interest, a low energy level, weight loss and little interest in eating, preoccupations with losses or death, and decreased cognitive functioning. These children will appear shy and withdrawn. Frequently, motor activities will include pacing, shouting, swinging or twisting hands, and pulling at hair, clothing, and objects in the environment. The motor retardation of depression is manifested, however, with characteristics such as inability to concentrate, slowed body movements, inaudible and affectless speech, or slow, controlled, and sometimes pressured speech which may or may not create a congruent thought process. Feelings of self-inadequacy and internalized anger may easily produce guilt, or it may be provoked by the slightest failure. Interpersonally, the child isolates self and shows little or no interest in surroundings.

The clinician should observe for acting out, drug usage, hostile, and agitated-type phobic reactions, and running away, if it is felt that these types of behaviors are "forerunners" or "masking" maneuvers against impending depression.

These children report feelings of hopelessness and hopefulness. Academic performance takes a marked downward turn. Real or perceived losses in the environment can usually be documented. Remember that if a *loss* is documented, one then must accept the assumption that there was a "significant other" and at one time a meaningful relationship did exist.

Problems

I. Withdrawal- and isolation-type behaviors.
  A. Child cries without provocation.
  B. Child is not interested in play activities.
  C. Child does not eat.
  D. Child would rather be alone and withdraws from all social situations.
  E. Child may physically withdraw from staff and choose not to participate in child-adult types of care-giving activities.
  F. Child has feelings of impending castastrophic situations.
  G. Child does not present eye contact behaviors.
  H. Child's speech is inaudible, pressured, monotonous, and labored.
  I. Child perceives self as "dumb" and incapable of success.
  J. Child perceives condition as "fate" in that a sentence has to follow a terrible sin that was committed.
  K. Child has mental pictures of dying, the process of actually ceasing to breathe, with significant others at his or her side.
  L. Child refuses to eat except for certain foods prepared in a specific manner.
  M. Progressively, the child refuses to eat anything (a different degree of the same noneating problem).
  N. Child may manifest encopresis and enuresis at night and during waking hours.
  O. Child is reluctant to "invest" in other children or adult staff because of the fear of rejection (sometimes there is a history of rejection).
  P. Child rejects other children and/or adults because she or he feels unworthy of attention, love, or caring.
  Q. Child has a poor academic record.
  R. Child has difficulty sleeping.
  S. Child generalizes feelings of apathy.
  T. Child cries when demands are placed upon him or her.
  U. Child sleeps for long periods of time.

II. The depressive equivalents (2): The theoretical model describes the child as having had internalized evil and unacceptable feelings about the self, with subsequent manifestation of delinquent and antisocial behaviors.

A. Child runs away from home for long periods of time.

B. Child engages in sporadic runaway behaviors.

C. Child manifests angry outburst of physical violence, aggression.

D. Child manifests angry outburst through verbal attack.

E. Child manifests general irritability through pacing, throwing things, laughing out loud.

F. Child has experienced school failure.

G. Child is clumsy or accident prone.

H. Child has made attempts to destroy self or parts of self, such as setting hair on fire, pulling out fingernails.

I. Child engages in drug ingestion to feel good and to feel free.

J. Child vacillates between periods of overeating and periods of starvation.

K. Child spends long hours listening to music alone.

L. Child is restless, irritable and sometimes weepy.

M. Child is demanding when needs are not met immediately.

Goals of Care

I. Immediate.

A. The child will recognize that *life situation* can be altered.

B. The child will verbalize to one of the staff the mental pictures about dying.

C. The child will maintain an adequate nutritional intake.

D. The child will involve self in gratifying activities that can be successfully completed.

E. Child will recognize "feeling state" and be able to express these feelings of hopelessness, powerlessness, etc., in play, storytelling, drawings, and in one-to-one talk situations.

F. Child will play with peers and communicate with staff without fear of reprisals from fate.

G. Child will perceive the environment as safe and secure.

H. Child will verbalize feelings of impending hostilities and disappointments.

I. Child will articulate those feelings that are experienced during the runaway episodes.

J. Child will control outbursts of physical violence.

K. Child will not engage in self-destructive-type behaviors.

L. Child will articulate angry and aggressive feelings and recognize that acting out these feelings is unacceptable in the treatment milieu as well as the larger society.

II. Long-range.

A. The child will learn to articulate needs, fears, and frustrations to adults and peers.

B. The child will recognize that negative feelings and thoughts resulting in running away or destroying self can be reworked and changed.

C. Child can develop a more positive and healthy image of self through collected appraisals.

D. Child will articulate thoughts and recognize feelings of the good self versus the bad self.

E. Child will learn new sublimatory channels by which aggression can be expressed.

F. Child will develop satisfactory relations with peers and adults.

G. Child will experience mastery and competency in an identified interpersonal situation with peers and adults.

H. Child will learn to express feelings and thoughts that are engendered immediately before behavioral manifestations of withdrawal, agitation, restlessness, refusal of food, etc.

I. Child will develop independent and autonomous functioning in areas of life in which she or he can have mastery and competency.

J. Child will learn to express and clarify feelings of "I am bad" or "I am good."

K. Child will learn to evaluate these feelings in relation to other people in the environment.

L. Child will develop a method by which he or she can more accurately separate and identify those actions and consequences for which he or she is directly responsible, as opposed to those actions and consequences where there was no control.

Intervention

Intervention strategies are performed in an effort to ameliorate the problems and meet the outlined goals. A categorization is provided for clarity and synthesis.

Depression:
Withdrawn Type

I. One-to-one therapeutic arrangement should be provided.

II. Assist the child at meal times with feedings; talk and maintain eye contact during meal.

III. Record amount of food child eats and drinks.

IV. Help child identify feelings associated with thoughts of worthlessness and helplessness.

V. Provide situations for child that she or he can master.

VI. Praise child verbally, through touch, and with eye contact for a task done well.

VII. Assist child in seeking out peer contacts; nurse should monitor own behavior here and withdraw from peer interactions once they are established.

VIII. Nurse should observe and record child's behaviors and verbal content when with other children.

IX. Identify and record type of children this child seeks out in the milieu.

X. Talk with child about specific incidents and experiences that have created feelings of despair.

XI. When child is observed alone in the milieu, nurse should approach child an provide opportunities for child to discuss:

A. Inner thoughts.

B. Feelings of loneliness.

C. Body sensations.

D. Mental pictures that are present at the moment.

E. Reflection about significant others.

XII. Discuss with child his or her dreams and include:

A. People in dream.

B. Their significance to child.

C. Content in specific terms.

D. The frequency of this dream.

E. The duration of this dream.

F. The awakening reactions to the dream:

1. Frightening.

2. Enjoyable.

3. "Just like real life."

4. "Would rather dream than be awake."

XIII. Observe and record sleep behaviors.

XIV. Discuss with child those events that occurred in the dream, and observe for content, addressing *loss,* self-deprecating behaviors, self-blame, parental rejection, difficulties with authority figures (police, teachers).

XV. Provide child with a variety of activities only when he or she is able to make a decision.

XVI. Provide a safe milieu that is free of contrabands and hazards.

XVII. Observe child at all times for possible suicidal attempts. This is a major task with which all staff should assist.

XVIII. Discuss with child the differences between emotional and physical emptiness as experienced:
- A. Where is this emptiness?
- B. When do you feel very, very empty?
- C. Do you sometimes feel the emptiness leaving you; when, where, and who are you with?
- D. What does food do in relation to this emptiness?
- E. Are there certain foods that fill up this emptiness?
- F. What do you think can fill up this emptiness?
- G. Who can provide this (name what child has identified) substance, thing?
- H. What can you (nurse) provide the child?
- I. Does child feel that her or his life will get better? How is a "better life" related to "emptiness"?

XIX. Assist child in articulating disappointments; help child to identify what they are and their importance.

XX. Who does child blame or want to blame for real or imagined loss?

XXI. Assist child in identifying and describing the lost object:
- A. Physical description.
- B. Habits.
- C. Nuances of the relationship with the child.
- D. How the lost object treated the child.
- E. Punishment.
- F. Fun things during time spent together.
- G. The specific circumstances or situation that produced the loss.

XXII. Nurse and staff should carefully observe and record affect, body movements, eye behavior when talking with child about lost objects.
- A. Video tape sessions when inquiries such as those in points XIX to XXI are being made.
- B. Code tapes for voice changes, restless movements, eye contact, lack of eye contact, downward gazing, tearing, wringing of hands, etc.

XXIII. Nurse should also correlate content and affect when viewing tapes.

XXIV. Nurse may elect to show child portions of video taping when there is a therapeutic value inherent in the viewing.

XXV. When discussing death of a loved one, nurse should recognize that the subject is difficult and may further elect to do the following:
- A. Observe child carefully after session.
- B. Identify and clarify with child if *promises* were made with person before death (may be associated with self-destructive thoughts and acts).
- C. What is the significance of these promises?
- D. Help child name, identify, and clarify these promises.
- E. Help child identify the consequences believed to be impending if promises are not fulfilled.
- F. Identify child's feelings associated with this promise:
  1. It is just fate.
  2. Happy feelings about promise.
  3. Frightening feelings about promise.
  4. Hopelessness, helplessness, doomed feeling.

XXVI. Explore areas in child's life that cause guilt feelings.
- A. Does child feel that her or his behaviors before death or loss of significant other were *not* "nice"?
- B. What would child do differently, in terms of behaviors, if situation could be re-created?

XXVII. Explore with child the specific feelings and thoughts he or she might have in relation to causing or not stopping certain events.

    A. Is this thinking realistic?

    B. Are there some who do blame the child?

    C. Does the child conceptualize a certain time period that is directly associated with the guilt feelings?

    D. Will guilt go away after this "penance" period?

XXVIII. Assist and encourage child to participate in active recreation.

XXIX. Assist child in participating in age-related task (recreational, social, and academic), with the goal being mastery of these tasks.

XXX. Provide opportunities for child to discuss perceptions of the relationship with the nurse.

XXI. Assess and evaluate the child's perceptions of that relationship:

    A. Has child invested in nurse?

    B. Is the relationship fostering dependency?

    C. Is there evidence of autonomous functioning or the development of autonomy?

    D. Does child express feelings and thoughts freely and without pressure?

XXXII. Does the nurse have a clear therapeutic regimen, and is this regimen for the child's care acceptable and supported by other staff and professionals?

XXXIII. The nurse should review therapeutic interventions and evaluations and own responses, feelings, and thoughts concerning therapeutic treatment process at least once each week with a well-trained nurse or other interested professional. (This may serve as a criterion for identifying who the nurse therapist should be.)

XXXIV. The nurse should continuously evaluate own actions and feelings about the child.

XXXV. The nurse should seek validation concerning own actions and communication styles when with the child.

Depressive Equivalents

I. Provide activities for talking about anger and resentment associated with loss.

II. Provide physical recreational opportunities for the expression of negative emotions.

III. Provide for space in the milieu for pacing and restless-type behaviors.

IV. Provide space for child to have privacy and "time out," when appropriate.

V. List alternative methods of expressing anger and disappointments other than through temper tantrums, throwing, and other types of acting-out behaviors.

VI. When child begins brooding, identify this type of behavior, and in here-and-now situation discuss with child:

    A. Behavior.

    B. Alternatives.

    C. Thoughts and feelings associated with the behavior.

    D. Direct feedback about how this behavior is not congruent with age, situation, or getting needs met.

    E. Direct feedback about how this specific behavior affects the therapist, other children, and the total milieu.

VII. Discuss with child behaviors in relation to school, and help child identify those necessary components that would make school pleasant. This information is of particular importance when planning for discharge and interface into the community.

    A. Is there a record of school failure?

    B. Is there evidence of a good relationship with one or more teachers?

    C. What academic subjects does the child excel in?

    D. Is there an identifiable person in the school who likes the child?

VIII. Does the child have a particular talent or gift that could help in resocializing process (singing, dancing, drawing, athletics)? This information is of particular importance when planning for discharge and interface into the community.

IX. Assess how the child feels about individual separation from parents.

X. Assess how the parents perceive individual separation from child.

XI. Does child expect punishment, complete directions, and guidance at all times from therapist?

XII. Does child appear to be more dependent and regressed in behaviors when with therapist than when with other adults and peers?

The Runaway   Specific intervention strategies for children whose impending depression is manifested through running away:

    I. Is this behavior a part of a youth counterculture?

    II. Help child specify what needs are satisfied through participating in this culture.

    III. Is running away a method of separating from family? (Why does the child feel a need to separate?)

    IV. Explore with child peers involved in the child's decision to run away.

    V. Does child verbalize a history of leaving home for hours after a family argument? Where does child go?

    VI. Explore with child the experiences engendered when "on the run":
        A. Drugs, alcohol, and sex activities.
        B. Means and methods by which child supported self.
        C. Fears, anger, guilt associated with running away.
        D. Was there a need to contact parents? Why/why not?

    VII. Explore with child and assess if parents are going through some traumatic or transitional functions in the home.

    VIII. Explore with child if family relations are entrapping and devastating.

    IX. The nurse should assess if child is having difficulty with family identity:
        A. Is child ashamed of family?
        B. Does mother's or father's behavior disturb, enhance, or humiliate the child?
        C. Is child comfortable with the "self," who he or she is in spite of parents' behaviors (perceived as good or bad)?

    X. The nurse and staff should try and assess whether the runaway behavior is:
        A. Delinquent.
        B. A healthy endeavor.
        C. A plea for help
        D. A method of forcing separation with parents.
        E. Premature autonomy.

    XI. More specific strategies for planning a regimen with runaways would specifically depend upon the home situation, the parental dynamics, and the child's perceived entrapment.

    XII. For example, if child feels running away is a method of forcing separation, nurse therapist must consider:
        A. Age.
        B. Mastery and competence level.
        C. Judgement ability.
        D. Methods family has utilized to cement child to family.
        E. Consequences for family and child should they become uncemented.
        F. Does child have necessary tools to live apart from family?
        G. Specifically, what is child running from?
        H. The level and intensity of pathology present in family and its effects upon child.

    XIII. Evaluate with child where loyalties exist: peer group, family, kind and gentle neighbor, others.

    XIV. Explore with child any contacts with police or other authority figures and agencies.

    XV. Reinforce the idea that thoughts and feelings can be expressed and verbalized, and that these thoughts and feelings will be heard by staff. Thus, running away is not necessary.

    XVI. Teach, if appropriate, methods by which negative and distasteful feelings and thoughts can be verbalized.

    XVII. Reassure child that staff can handle impulsive behaviors.

    XVIII. Solicit child's cooperation when identifying feelings and making plans to run away. Then:
        A. Help child assess the interpersonal conflicts being experienced.
        B. Explore with child the alternatives to running away.
        C. Answer what it is specifically about running away that makes this method of apparent problem solving more attractive to child.

D. Consider if the child perceives the milieu too controlling and/or too parenting in nature.

E. Consider the role of peer group members in their relations with the child.

XIX. Can child substitute "acting" for "talking"?

XX. Encourage and solicit lexical experiences about total life gestalt.

XXI. The nurse should explore own inner conflicts, frustrations, and disappointments concerning the child.

Evaluation

I. Reassessment.

A. What behaviors did the child manifest initially in the treatment milieu?

B. What are the behaviors occurring now?

C. Has the milieu changed since child first entered it? How?

D. Identify the feelings nurse and other staff have engendered through working with child.

E. Were suicidal precautions adequate?

F. Were behaviors indicating self-destruction appropriately and adequately observed, identified, and worked through?

G. Is there splitting among the staff as a result of the therapeutic regimen implemented with the child?

H. How does the treatment team feel about family?

I. Was the treatment regimen a waste of professional time and energy? Why?

J. Were nurse and staff adequately prepared to deal with specific problems child and family manifested?

K. Were resources available for further in-depth understanding?

L. Would staff "willingly" accept another child who manifests problems similar to those of child under investigation?

M. Specifically, were the "Goals of Care" listed above accomplished (the crux of the issue in evaluation)?

    1. Why were they accomplished?

    2. Who (name) facilitated this goal achievement?

    3. What in the milieu forestalled goal accomplishment?

    4. What are some facilitating learning experiences that the staff is able to identify from having had contact with the specific child?

N. Identify those components of the treatment regimen that would and should be altered.

II. Follow-up and reevaluation.

A. Make referral to appropriate community agency by providing a summary of therapy, treatment modalities, and progress. Specify any unique and/or unusual attributes about child and family.

B. Terminate treatment with child and parents, providing them with lists of agents and agencies where professional help can be obtained.

C. Collaborate with other agencies and institutions that child will, through normal course of development encounter. The school is probably the most important institution to be considered.

    1. Intervention methods may be shared with teacher, school psychologist.

    2. Rationale for intervention is also helpful and may provide a base for consistency and continuity of those techniques that facilitate the child and family's positive growth.

    3. Identify self as a resource person available for consultation to school personnel.

D. When necessary, coordinate referrals to other community agencies such as welfare departments, protective services, special medical services, etc. Determine the content of clinical summary to be included in each type of referral. The agency receiving referral and the purpose of referral will govern the content included.

REFERENCES

1. J. Simmons, *The Psychiatric Examination of Children,* 2d ed., Lea & Febiger, Philadelphia, 1974.
2. J. M. Tollan, "Depression in Children and Adolescents," *American Journal of Orthopsychiatry,* **32:** 404–412, 1962.

BIBLIOGRAPHY

Simmons, J.: *The Psychiatric Examination of Children,* 2d ed., Lea & Febiger, Philadelphia, 1974. This book provides an excellent method of organizing clinical materials.

Tollan, J. M.: "Depression in Children and Adolescents," *American Journal of Orthopsychiatry,* **32:** 404–412, 1962. The article deals with clinical issues concerning depression. It does identify and discuss the equivalents to depression, and it has use for the clinician who works with children/adolescents.

Usdin, Gene (ed.): *Depression,* Brunner/Mazel Publishers, New York, 1977. This book presents a variety of materials that address depression from a clinical, biological and psychological orientation. Its greatest utility is in defining and conceptualizing depression in children.

35
Interpersonal Problems

Rhoda L. Moyer

Difficulty in interpersonal relationships is the central factor in persons who have mental health problems. All other problems relate directly to these difficulties. Because of the significance of interpersonal relationships in both the causation and solution of mental health problems, psychiatric–mental health nursing practice includes both the scientific use of theories of human behavior and masterful, artistic use of the self. The therapeutic use of the self is considered such an absolute and essential part of nursing care for *all* patients that it will not be included in any one specific area as an intervention. General aspects of using the self therapeutically include:

1. Developing interpersonal trust.
2. Helping to increase the person's self-esteem and autonomous functioning.
3. Promoting the person's ability to maintain him- or herself interdependently with meaningful and satisfying human relationships.
4. Providing a therapeutic milieu which develops the sociopsychological aspects of the person's environment.
5. Accepting and appropriately using the surrogate parental role.
6. Assisting with the here-and-now living problems the person experiences.
7. Teaching emotional health patterns.
8. Behaving as a social agent to improve and promote the person's recreational, occupational, and social competence.
9. Operating within a contractual framework with the person.

MANIPULATION

Definition

Manipulation is an interpersonal behavioral process designed to meet one's own needs or goals by exploiting and/or controlling the behavior of others without regard for their rights, needs, or goals. It can be either consciously or unconsciously motivated. Usually, an unidentified, misinterpreted, or unmet social need arouses increasing degrees of anxiety which trigger the behavioral patterns known as manipulation. Significant factors which increase the potential for manipulative behavior include low self- esteem and low esteem of others, feelings of insecurity and powerlessness, inadequate social learning, and immature personality development.

Manipulation, as a clinical problem, does not include constructive forms such as assertiveness, teaching, selling, guiding, and socializing with other persons. The various forms of destructive manipulation include aggressive, hostile behaviors directed against or toward others and/or oneself; passive, covert behavior to control others or get needs met indirectly; and self- deprecation or deprecation of others.

In interpersonal relationships, manipulation may be observed as a single behavior or group of behaviors. As a symptom, it can be a part of the clinical picture of almost any of the psychiatric diagnoses.

Assessment

This general assessment format will be followed in subsequent sections, with areas of specific emphasis noted in each section.

I. Data sources.
   A. Observation and interview of patient.
   B. Interview with family and significant others, and observation of communication patterns with and about patient.
   C. Psychiatric and other medical and physical history.
   D. Social history.
   E. Staff's response to patient during interaction.
II. Health history.
   A. Age.
   B. Sex.
   C. Socioeconomic data.
      1. Educational level and experience.
      2. Occupation and work history.
      3. Community relationships.
      4. Available and accessible human and material resources.
   D. Patient's perception of met and unmet needs.
   E. Patient's usual coping behaviors and support system—effective and ineffective—and strengths.
   F. Patient's usual responses to stress, anger, sadness, failure, losses, frustration, success, illness, and threatening situations.
   G. Identification of current and potential stresses in personal life.
   H. Patient's present level of anxiety: mild, moderate, severe, panic level.
   I. Patient's social and interpersonal relationships, including patterns, type, quality, and quantity.
   J. Alterations and strengths in patient's ego functioning, especially thought, speech, affect, perception, mobility, judgement, and reality-testing abilities.
   K. Family history, including health problems, constellation, ways of dealing with stress or threats, interpersonal relationships, early childhood memories, and significant losses.
   L. Formulation of growth and developmental level of patient.
   M. Description of performance of activities of daily living.
   N. Any physical or intellectual problems or limitations.
III. Emotional responses of nurses and other staff members to patient's behavior, such as anger, anxiety, defensiveness, embarassment, frustration, helplessness, withdrawal, indifference, guilt, sympathy, overprotectiveness.
IV. Strengths and weaknesses of nurses and other staff members in own interpersonal relationships, such as attitudes and feelings related to specific types of patients based on factors including racial, socioeconomic, cultural, religious, national, and sexual identity, and type of illnesses.

Problems

I. Aggressive type.
   A. Patient organizes other patients to defy or minimize staff authority.
   B. Patient makes frequent demands or requests.
   C. Patient threatens others, either patients, staff, or family.
   D. Patient deliberately breaks rules, routines, procedures, or contracts.
   E. Patient requests special attention and/or privileges.
   F. Patient attempts to gain power and control in clinical setting.
   G. Patient pressures others into meeting requests.
   H. Patient reports another patient's personal confidential information.
   I. Patient attempts to use others' weaknesses against them.
   J. Patient derogates others.
   K. Patient acts up when demands are not met or a situation is displeasing.
   L. Patient coerces others by secreting articles.

    M. Patient forces others to respond by bargaining with them.
- II. Passive type.
  - *A.* Patient procrastinates or dawdles when required to do something.
  - *B.* Patient mumbles and/or avoids direct conversation.
  - *C.* Patient changes the subject or activity.
  - *D.* Patient breaks a treatment contract jointly established by nurse and patient.
  - *E.* Patient responds to confrontation with tears and/or helpless behavior.
  - *F.* Patient monopolizes the conversation in social and/or therapy situations.
  - *G.* Patient is ingratiating or overly solicitous.
  - *H.* Patient complies to gain approval or recognition.

Goals of Care

- I. Immediate.
  - *A.* The patient will recognize specific manipulatory patterns.
  - *B.* The patient will gain insight into unfulfilled needs which promote manipulatory behavior.
  - *C.* The patient will delay immediate need gratification when appropriate.
  - *D.* The patient will decrease attempts to manipulate others as measured by a behavior modification tool. [See tool utilized by Justice and Justice (1).]
- II. Long-range.
  - *A.* The patient will assume responsibility for expressing needs directly in here-and-now situations.
  - *B.* The patient will develop self-control and independence.
  - *C.* The patient will develop constructive, appropriate outlets for aggressive needs.
  - *D.* The patient will be self-aware and autonomous in relationships.
  - *E.* The patient will cooperate, compromise, and collaborate in mutually respectful relationships with others.
  - *F.* The patient will recognize how and where manipulatory patterns of behavior were learned (in primary family) and will recognize and develop new options to meet needs as an adult.

Intervention

Refer to "Problems" and "Goals of Care" above. Specific actions refer to goals previously outlined. These actions will be performed by nurse to meet goals and eliminate problems.
- I. Recognize when patient is utilizing a manipulative behavior, pattern, or game.
- II. Identify own feelings, thoughts, and actions in response to specific behaviors of patient.
- III. Identify patient's tendency to recreate similar manipulations among staff as previously done at home with parents and siblings.
- IV. Recognize the patient's attempt to intimidate staff members.
- V. Assess patient's unfulfilled needs which he or she is trying to meet through manipulation.
- VI. Assist the patient in identifying own patterns of manipulative behavior.
- VII. Assist the patient in recognizing interpersonal conflicts.
- VIII. Promote idea within patient that attainment of self-control is the responsibility of the patient.
- IX. Assist patient in identifying consequences of inappropriate behavior.
- X. Explore with patient possible reasons for inappropriate behavior.
- XI. Encourage patient to explore and express feelings verbally without acting upon them.
- XII. Encourage patient to identify alternative methods of behavior to meet needs appropriately.
- XIII. Teach patient how to use direct ways to communicate needs.

XIV. Teach patient the differences between aggressive, assertive, and passive approaches to meet needs.

XV. Demonstrate by role playing in specific situations the differences between direct, indirect, adaptive, and manipulative communication.

XVI. Invite patient to help identify real needs if you do not know what is being sought.

XVII. Teach patient to recognize differences between needs which require immediate gratification and those which can be delayed, sublimated, or substituted.

XVIII. Teach and reinforce the idea that experiencing all feelings is okay, but it is not always appropriate to act upon them.

XIX. Set limits on inappropriate or self-defeating behaviors.

XX. Use selective behavior modification program to decrease manipulation. [See tool utilized by Justice and Justice (2).]

XXI. Give direct messages to patient.

XXII. Use verbal and nonverbal reinforcement when patient functions within prescribed limits.

XXIII. Point out patient's behavior when it is manipulative.

XXIV. Prevent patient from manipulating one staff member against another by adhering to agreed-upon limits.

XXV. Permit freedom within prescribed limits.

XXVI. Avoid demonstrating hostility, negative attitudes, or aggressive or passive behaviors toward patient when she or he is being manipulative.

XXVII. Assign consistent staff to patient.

XXVIII. Develop a plan for dealing with manipulative behavior, and communicate to all staff involved in patient's care.

XXIX. Provide opportunities for the patient to explore and test alternative behaviors.

XXX. Explore with patient situations in which need is not satisfied.

XXXI. Identify situations in which patient lacks control, and point these out.

XXXII. Identify situations in which patient demonstrates self-control and independence, and point these out.

XXXIII. Teach patient to seek out relationships in which he or she is liked and accepted.

XXXIV. Utilize peer pressure to modify manipulative behavior.

XXXV. Provide experiences which build self-control and increase independence.

XXXVI. Listen to patient's requests and give reasons when requests cannot be met.

XXXVII. Allow patient an opportunity to verbalize annoyance at restrictions or disappointments.

XXXVIII. Teach assertive techniques to handle frustrating experiences.

XXXIX. Provide opportunity to experience a variety of methods to express aggression, and evaluate their usefulness with the patient.

XL. Teach patient how to verbalize "I" statements.

XLI. Teach patient the difference between "I" and "you" statements in asking for satisfaction of needs or expressing feelings.

XLII. Be alert to signs of developing anxiety or anger.

XLIII. Give consistent feedback regarding interpersonal behavior patterns; give positive reinforcement for all positive, constructive reactions.

Evaluation

I. Reassessment: Manipulative behavior needs constant evaluation to see if the nursing interventions are effective in decreasing such behavior, as it is especially resistant to change. The nurse should evaluate the behavioral changes against a specific set of criteria (expected outcomes). If patient behaviors are not changing, it is necessary to reevaluate the entire process of nursing care, paying particular attention to the priorities of care. It is also essential to be sure that the nurse's goals and the patient's goals are mutually agreed upon. Renegotiation of the initial agreement may be required if expected behavioral changes are not forthcoming.

II. Follow-up and reevaluation.
   A. Refer to a community agency and/or outpatient setting, such as a day treatment program, for further evaluation of progress toward goals.
   B. Communicate verbally and/or in writing the plan of care and summary of progress to agency or person who will follow patient.
   C. Set up methods to monitor any medication(s) continued on an outpatient basis.

WITHDRAWAL

Definition

Withdrawal is a process in which persons retreat from relationships and contacts with the external world into a world of their own. Thre is a reduction of external stimuli and an increase in internal stimuli. Usually, this process is a defense against the anxiety related to increased threat or increased stress. Withdrawal may range on a behavioral continuum from the unconcern or indifference about others observed at times in "normal" people to the profoundly withdrawn individual who is actively hallucinating.

Dysfunctional withdrawal behaviors are a way of coping with threat or stress. Behaviors may include aloofness, detachment, disinterest, active or passive removal of self from others, decreased spontaneity in planning and/or initiating things with others, inability to mingle with others and communicate freely, overt or covert avoidance of others in the environment, use of monosyllables, mutism, working independently rather than cooperatively, and loss of goal-directed behavior. In severe cases, a form of regression in which social relations and external perceptions are eliminated, resulting in hallucinations and delusions, may be observed. Specific behaviors may include refusing to talk with the nurse, being late for or avoiding appointments, answering only when asked direct questions, "forgetting" appointments, remaining in a group to avoid individual contact with the nurse, and verbally or nonverbally engaging in an activity to avoid exploring significant issues with the nurse.

Withdrawal may be observed as either a symptom or a syndrome in both acute and chronic forms of dysfunction. In its less severe forms, it may be demonstrated by persons experiencing a crisis, such as loss of a significant person.

Assessment (Refer to "Manipulation")

I. Data sources (refer to "Manipulation").
II. Health history. Note especially:
   A. Interpersonal and social relationships.
      1. Number and type of relationships.
      2. Length of time knowing friends.
      3. Patterns, quantity, and quality of friendships.
      4. Sudden changes or recent losses.
      5. Recreational interests and pursuits.
      6. Relationship patterns during childhood and adolescence.
III. Staff reaction to contact with patient. Note:
   A. Feeling of talking with a shell or an uninhabited house.
   B. Sense of not being heard or of having little or no emotional exchange.
   C. Sense of approach avoidance in the relationship.
   D. Experience being "swallowed up" or inappropriate feelings and responses from patient.
   E. Fear of being close to patient (due to patient's projections of fear or anger).

Problems

I. The patient speaks in an inaudible voice.
II. The patient does not speak or answer questions or respond to verbal stimuli.

III. The patient uses symbolic or unintelligible language.
IV. The patient's affect is altered:
    A. Inappropriate to external stimuli in environment.
    B. Flat or dull.
    C. Depressed.
    D. Affect and words and behavior are dissonant.
    E. Hostile or violent mood.
    F. Silly.
V. The patient's judgment is altered.
    A. Impulsive acts against self, others, or environment.
    B. Inappropriate social behavior, e.g., uses obscene language, plays with feces, publicly masturbates or urinates.
    C. Aggressive, hostile, or violent acts against self or others.
VI. The patient does not take care of own activities of daily living, e.g., eating, dressing, bathing, etc.
VII. The patient's thoughts are altered:
    A. Exhibits delusions of persecution, omnipotence, grandiosity, nihilism, etc.
    B. Thoughts are retarded, blocked, or loosely associated.
VIII. The patient's perceptions are altered:
    A. Hears, sees, smells, tastes, or feels things which are not there.
    B. Projects own feelings and fears onto the external world.
    C. Misinterprets events or peoples' interactions with him.
IX. The patient refuses to talk with the nurse or other staff.
X. The patient remains with other people when the nurse attempts to initiate a scheduled patient interaction.
XI. The patient initiates activities to avoid intimacy.
XII. The patient hides from the nurse during the scheduled interview time.
XIII. The patient "forgets" or is late for scheduled appointments.
XIV. The patient responds only with single words or short, routine phrases.
XV. The patient does not interact with others on unit.
XVI. The patient does not participate in activities with others.
XVII. The patient remains in own room or sleeps during the day.
XVIII. The patient exhibits behavior which is meaningful only to himself.
XIX. The patient is suspicious and mistrustful of others.
XX. The patient is shy and reserved.

Goals of Care

I. Immediate.
    A. The patient will respond appropriately to here and now situations.
    B. The patient will regain some ability to meet activities of daily living (e.g., sleep, food, hygiene, elimination, etc.).
    C. The patient will establish a positive relationship with one other person.
    D. The patient will increase contacts and relationships with others.
    E. The patient will not harm self or others.
II. Long-range (some patients will not be able to achieve *all* of the following).
    A. The patient will develop meaningful relationships with others, characterized by trust, acceptance, and closeness.
    B. The patient will be able to meet own activities of daily living and meet basic needs in an independent manner.
    C. The patient will understand own withdrawal behavior, how and why it was useful, situations which increase anxiety, how to reduce the anxiety, and will be able to choose selectively to be close to others.
    D. The patient will maintain self-control over behavior.
    E. The patient will describe self in a positive way.
    F. The patient will demonstrate increased ability to communicate with others.

Intervention

Refer to "Problems" and "Goals of Care" above. These actions will be performed by the nurse to meet the goals and eliminate the problems.

I. Point out and explore situations which increase patient's anxiety.

II. Assist patient to identify behaviors used when anxious.

III. Assist patient to identify thoughts and feelings in here-and-now situations, and to correlate behaviors used to express these.

IV. Point out inappropriate or incongruent behavior.

V. Define and stress reality to patient in here-and-now situations.

VI. Assist patient in naming and exploring feelings and behavior when hallucinating or delusional.

VII. Listen carefully to patient and indicate when you do and do not understand what is said.

VIII. Introduce an element of doubt instead of arguing regarding a delusional idea.

IX. Use distractions and changing subject to decrease delusional ideas.

X. Observe for and explore with patient the stimuli that trigger inappropriate responses.

XI. Observe for and chart behaviors and environmental stimuli that precipitate or relate to patient withdrawing into fantasy.

XII. Administer medications, e.g., phenothiazines or antidepressants, as prescribed, and observe for side effects and effect of medications on the patient.

XIII. Observe patient for areas in which assistance is needed to meet basic needs, e.g., eating, drinking, elimination, exercise, sleeping, bathing, dressing, and provide necessary assistance.

XIV. Assess level in areas of functioning day by day, and be flexible as patient progresses or regresses in ability to care for self.

XV. Suggest and encourage specific physical care measures to assure maintenance of physical well-being.

XVI. Provide instructions in step-by-step, concrete terms when patient is unable to make decisions about personal care.

XVII. Give positive reinforcement for increased self-care activities and good grooming.

XVIII. Teach patient importance of medication and of taking regularly, inform patient of side effects and toxic effects, and shift responsibility to patient as there is improvement.

XIX. Observe and record fluids and diet consumed daily.

XX. Teach patient about dietary needs in areas identified.

XXI. Observe and record general physical condition each day.

XXII. Plan with patient ways to maintain all areas of self-care after discharge, e.g., caring for clothes, transportation, food shopping and preparation, recreation, work, school, and social needs.

XXIII. Assist and support patient in setting own schedule and plans for self-care.

XXIV. Discuss with patient and family how to recognize symptoms of increasing illness and develop a plan that patient and/or family will follow in case symptoms reoccur.

XXV. Use silence; share with patient that you are willing to be together without talking if that is the patient's wish.

XXVI. Acknowledge and respond to patient's experiences and feelings when they are expressed.

XXVII. Acknowledge your lack of understanding and wish to understand when patient's messages are confused or symbolic.

XXVIII. Support patient with words and your presence during experiences and activities she or he finds frightening or difficult.

XXIX. Teach patient communication skills, e.g., how to approach people, how to use topics of interest, etc.

XXX. Provide opportunity to practice communication skills in a supportive environment.

XXXI. Broaden patient's contacts to include other person(s) besides the staff.

XXXII. Assist patient to check out perceptions and clarify distortions.

XXXIII. Identify with patient areas and situations which cause stress and difficulties in relating to others.

XXXIV. Role play new or difficult situations with patient.

XXXV. Provide opportunities to develop sensual, feeling-type awareness, such as clay modeling, dancing, or music.

XXXVI. Provide opportunities to do simple, creative tasks, such as games and crafts in a group setting.

XXXVII. Assess patient's suicidal tendencies.

XXXVIII. Assess patient's homicidal tendencies.

XXXIX. Set appropriate limits, e.g., tell patient that he or she cannot hurt self or others.

XL. Ask patient to make a contract with you not to hurt self accidentally or on purpose; in case of suicidal feelings, patient will ask for protection or will contact a staff member.

XLI. Ask patient to make a contract with you not to hurt someone else accidentally or on purpose; in case of feelings of anger or violence, patient will ask for contact with staff member or for protection, e.g., seclusion.

XLII. Protect patient and others when patient is unable to control self by using appropriate means:
  A. Seclusion, to reduce stimuli.
  B. Medication, to reduce anxiety level.
  C. Remove harmful objects from environment.

XLIII. Teach patient and significant others as needed about medications taken as preparation for discharge.

XLIV. Use the nurse's relationship with the patient as a protection for patient against hallucinations and delusions by spending time together, telling patient no one will hurt him or her while with nurse, etc.

XLV. Reassure patient of your concern for her or his physical safety.

XLVI. Explore thoughts and feelings regarding situations and people from which patient withdraws.

XLVII. Discuss alternative responses and actions to deal with feelings and needs other than withdrawal.

XLVIII. Assist patient in identifying own strengths and weaknesses in interpersonal relationships.

Evaluation

I. Reassessment: Withdrawal behavior requires constant reassessment and evaluation to determine effectiveness of interventions, e.g., whether the patient is interacting more or is less involved in active living. The nurse must determine whether there are new factors which alter the patient's adaptation to and interaction with the environment and/or people. As the patient is able to assume increasing levels of responsibility for her or his own personal needs and relationships, the nurse must be willing to relinquish the nurturing role with the patient to assure full development. It is also important to assess accurately the patient's potential and to accept the patient's right to decide on a level of wellness such that unrealistic expectations are decreased.

II. Follow-up and reevaluation.
  A. Refer to community agency and/or outpatient setting, such as a day treatment program, or public health nurse for further support and progression toward goals.
  B. Communicate verbally and/or in writing the plan of care and summary of progress:
    1. To agency or person who will follow patient.
    2. To significant others in patient's life when patient requests this.

C. Set up methods to monitor any medication(s) continued on an outpatient basis.
  1. Ask specific questions to assess patient's method and regularity of taking medications and attitudes about taking them.
  2. Questions include: How many? What time of day? What does patient do if a dose is forgotten? Does patient ever cut down on the amount? Is patient afraid of becoming dependent on drugs? Does taking medications worry patient in any way?
D. Upon discharge from hospital or after-care agency, be sure patient:
  1. Has a list and schedule of medications, can verbalize importance of taking as scheduled, knows potential side and/or toxic effects, and knows how to obtain refills.
  2. Has an appointment for follow-up with doctor, clinic, or mental health center, and knows how and when to contact them, if needed, prior to appointment.
  3. Has a plan for maintaining self daily, including adequate diet, personal grooming, and social-interactional needs.
  4. Knows importance of simple communication techniques to facilitate communication and understanding, and to receive support from others.
  5. Has one significant other who is aware of patient's communication problems and can work with patient during difficult times.

COMPULSIVE-RITUALISTIC BEHAVIOR

Definition

Compulsive-ritualistic behaviors are involuntary activities performed by a person either to avoid anxiety or to cause an involuntary, irrational, recurring thought to disappear. These behaviors are repetitive, stereotyped, and compelling, even when the individual does not wish to perform these behaviors. Both the obsessive thoughts and the compulsive-ritualistic acts are an attempt to cope with anxiety arising from conflicts that are out of awareness and are often related to hostile, aggressive, or other unacceptable impulses which are in opposition to adult functioning.

Behaviors which are compulsive-ritualistic may range from mild forms which are viewed as normal and healthy and permit the person to function well in situations requiring orderliness, frugality, and neatness, to those which are severe and cause almost total incapacitation of one's ability to function. Developmentally, these behaviors are normally observed in the stage where autonomy over one's bodily functions and control over one's world are mastered. Compulsive-ritualistic behaviors become a problem in later life when there is restriction of one's creativity, intimacy with others, and ability to experience joy and spontaneous thought, feelings, and actions.

Examples of compulsive-ritualistic behaviors include excessive handwashing or cleaning; returning to one's home to see if the door is locked or lights off; performing tasks in a rigid, never-changing manner; rituals related to activities of daily living; walking, or behaving in certain prescribed ways; and avoiding or relating to persons, situations, or things in a stereotyped, repetitive, and compelling manner. These behaviors may constitute either a symptom or a syndrome in combination with other problem behaviors related to interpersonal dysfunction. These actions may be observed in several diagnostic categories.

Assessment (Refer to "Manipulation")

I. Data sources (refer to "Manipulation").
II. Health history, note especially:
  A. Description of usual responses to stress, anger, sadness, losses, successes, failures, illnesses, hostility, aggression.

    B. Primary concern and/or feelings related to rituals and compulsive behavior, including description of usual patterns.

    C. Statement of health goals and concerns related to the problem.

III. Staff's emotional responses to patient's behavior, including pity, disgust, anger, sympathy, empathy, increased anxiety, withdrawal, frustration, and intense discomfort.

Problems

    I. Patient performs activities of daily living in a rigid, repetitive manner.

    II. Patient reports having recurring thoughts that cannot be controlled or forgotten.

    III. Patient becomes severely anxious when repetitive behavior is interrupted or interfered with.

    IV. Patient relates to people or objects in a rigid, stereotyped manner.

    V. Patient is unable to meet basic physical needs due to time invested in complex rituals.

    VI. Patient harms self and/or others by performing compelling acts against own will.

    VII. Patient avoids people or objects consistently due to obsessive thoughts or fears.

    VIII. Patient performs activities in a compelling manner, against own wishes.

    IX. Patient has compelling thoughts about killing or harming someone.

Goals of Care

    I. Immediate.

        A. The patient's defenses, such as rituals will be protected.

        B. The patient will maintain good physical health.

        C. The patient will control self- or other-destructive patterns.

        D. The patient will utilize substitute activities to control anxiety whenever possible.

        E. The patient will recognize feelings of anxiety and self-defeating behaviors.

    II. Long-range.

        A. The patient will gain some insight into the meaning of own behavior.

        B. The patient will resolve the dynamic issues by owning and accepting hostile-aggressive impulses and maintaining control of self and world.

        C. The patient will give up obsessive-compulsive-ritualistic behavior.

        D. The patient will develop new patterns of behavior that enhance well-being and increase quality of relationships and capacity for intimacy, while maintaining autonomy, e.g., control over self and world.

Intervention

    I. Provide adequate time and an appropriate place for patient to perform compulsive behavior. *if necessary*

    II. Assign a patient, tolerant nurse to remain with patient.

    III. Remain with patient during ritualistic activity.

    IV. Protect patient from ridicule of other persons.

    V. Administer antianxiety medications as prescribed.

    VI. Provide satisfying channels for substitutions, whenever possible.

    VII. Protect patient from harming self or others with hostile, aggressive behavior.

    VIII. Encourage physical activity which utilizes gross motor movements.

    IX. Rotate staff to prevent exhaustion from dealing with their own feelings about patient's behavior.

    X. Provide gloves and/or hand lotion for dermatitis.

    XI. Ensure adequate rest by permitting adequate time for pre-retiring rituals and/or administering sedative medications.

XII. Observe and record patient's activities of daily living to ensure adequacy of meeting physical needs.

XIII. Provide for nutritional needs of patient.

XIV. Discuss problem behavior with patient immediately following completion of ritual, when anxiety level is lowered.

XV. Encourage patient to discuss feelings and thoughts about ritualistic behaviors.

XVI. Point out the self-defeating nature of the behavior.

XVII. Support and accept patient when anger, hostility, and rage is expressed.

XVIII. Encourage patient to verbalize intense anger instead of acting it out symbolically.

XVIX. Provide protection and limits for safety as patient experiences intense rage.

XX. Explore the purpose the behavior fulfills in patient's life.

XXI. Provide information about the meaning of ritualistic behavior: to reduce anxiety and deal with conflict.

XXII. Identify situations which increase anxiety and increase use of rituals.

XXIII. Teach patient alternative ways of coping with anxiety, such as verbalizing and physical activity.

XXIV. Provide examples of appropriate and effective ways to handle anger.

XXV. Teach patient how to recognize changes in self that indicate impending loss of control.

XXVI. Teach patient to talk about feelings to someone trusted at times of upset.

XXVII. Introduce change slowly.

XXVIII. Encourage patient to identify strengths, as well as weaknesses.

XXIX. Assist patient to increase tolerance of differences, by discussing differences in people as unique strengths.

XXX. Encourage patient to develop a sustained interest and enjoyment of a hobby.

Evaluation

I. Reassessment: Compulsive-ritualistic behaviors are usually severe when they come to the attention of the nurse. Therefore, long-term therapeutic intervention is often required, and it is helpful to measure behavioral changes against a baseline in order to appreciate small changes. A flow chart can be used to indicate the number of times per day or per hour a particular ritualistic behavior occurs. Nurses must frequently evaluate their own responses and feelings to be sure their behavior is not interfering with the treatment or increasing the patient's anxiety. Nurses may need supportive relationships with colleagues to deal with their own anger and frustration. Reassessment should go on continually to assure quality care of this challenging patient.

II. Follow-up and reevaluation.

A. Refer the patient to a community agency or therapist for continuing support, if patient so desires.

B. Provide the agency or therapist with either a written and/or verbal plan of care and summary of progress while hospitalized, so there is continuity of care.

C. Assist the patient in developing a plan of action prior to discharge to meet personal needs and continue growth.

D. Teach the patient to recognize increasing problematic symptoms early and to know where to go for assistance before incapacitation occurs.

E. Provide for follow-up and supervision if patient is on medications at time of discharge.

DEPENDENT BEHAVIOR

Definition

Dependent behavior is a symptom or syndrome in which a person exhibits difficulty in making independent decisions; a marked tendency to lean on others for support, protection, permission, guidance, and advice; and a compulsive need to unite with a stronger person in order to face life's problems. Increased anxiety is felt when the needed person or object is not available or threatens not to be available. The dependent person may also act or behave in such a manner as not to threaten or disrupt the relationship in order to be taken care of by the significant other.

Initially, a person's survival as an infant depends on the life-sustaining relationship between self and mother in which basic needs for mothering, love, affection, shelter, protection, security, warmth, and food are met without a specific request by the infant. If this normal symbiotic relationship continues, either overtly or covertly, into later years, the person depends on another person as the source of his or her own feeling, thinking, and acting. Therefore, the behavior is such that the person depends upon others or objects for exploitation and the satisfaction of neurotic needs, rather than engaging in cooperative mutual support and affection. This dependency, or dysfunctional symbiosis, may be a result of premature separation from parents, a lack of responsiveness on the parents' part, neglect, or overprotection.

Such dependent persons constantly seek someone or something to meet their needs because they believe they are unable to meet their own needs and *must* be taken care of by someone or something other than themselves. They deny their own ability to meet their needs directly and demand that someone else meet them. These demands are passive in nature, consisting of several types of behavior:

1. Mobilizing energy to not think or do anything for themselves when a problem arises, solving the problem according to someone else's expectations rather than their own.
2. Performing an activity which is non-goal-directed to relieve tension but which avoids solving the problem.
3. Refusing to assume responsibility for themselves and their own decisions, behaviors, feelings, and thoughts.

Dependent behavior includes two main types: (1) dependency on people (referred to as symbiosis), and (2) dependency on drugs. Dependency on drugs is the psychic craving for, habituation to, or addiction to a chemical substance; such dependency creates a life-style in which individuals arrange their lives, in whole or in part, to revolve around the need to achieve a specific effect of one or more chemical agents on their mood or state of consciousness. Drug dependency is viewed as the result of altered or ineffective parenting relationships or stagnant family relationships. Drug-dependent individuals experience feelings of being cheated of rightfully deserved parenting within their family of origin. They utilize their drug dependence as a means of separating from relatedness to family members and as a means of escaping from physical and psychosocial stresses. Both types of dependent behavior—on people and on drugs—are in part the result of inadequate symbiotic relationships and cause further relational dysfunction and stagnation. (See also "Compromised Decision Making.")

Assessment (Refer to "Manipulation")

I. Data sources: people-dependent symbiosis (refer to "Manipulation").
II. Health history: people-dependent symbiosis (refer to "Manipulation"). Note especially:
   A. Family history, including health problems, constellation, ways of dealing with stress, any present or recent crises, especially losses, early childhood memories, relationship patterns within family, extended family members with drinking problems.
   B. Patient's description and perception of health status, reasons for hospitalization, expected outcomes of treatment, nutritional patterns.
   C. Patient's usual responses to stress, anger, sadness, loss, frustration, success, failure, illness.
   D. Patient's perception of coping patterns and interpersonal relationships, e.g., quality, quantity, type, feelings about these.

    E. Patient's perceptions of dependence and independence, including people, decision making, daily living experiences.

    F. Patient's ego function alterations, especially judgment, defense mechanisms (e.g., denial), reality testing, perceptions.

    G. Patient's report of present and potential stresses in personal life.

    H. Use of drugs and/or alcohol in daily life.

III. Data sources: drug-dependent symbiosis (refer to "Manipulation"). Note especially laboratory workup:

    A. Blood alcohol levels.   **D.** X-rays of abdomen.

    B. Blood chemistry.   **E.** Urine analysis.

    C. Liver function tests.

IV. Health history: drug-dependent symbiosis (refer to "Manipulation"). Note especially:

    A. Family history, including health problems; constellation; ways of dealing with stress; any present or recent crises, especially losses; early childhood memories; relationship patterns within family; extended family members with drinking or drug problems.

    B. Patient's description/perception of health status, reasons for hospitalization, expected outcomes of treatment, nutritional patterns.

    C. Use of drugs and/or alcohol in daily life.

    D. For alcohol users, assess the following areas in depth:

        1. *How often* does the patient use alcohol: daily, weekly, weekends, holidays, special occasions?

        2. *How* is alcohol used: time of day, to get started or to complete a task, to socialize, mood when drinking, to relax and ease tension, alone or with others, to celebrate an occasion (or is it *the* occasion)?

        3. *How much* does the patient drink: type and ounces of liquor, mixed or straight, more or less than friends, daily amount? Has drinking increased or decreased over the past 5 years?

        4. The patient's definition of alcoholism ("drinking problem" is often more acceptable to patients).

        5. Relationship problems: who is included as family, description of a typical day?

        6. Work problems: has time been lost and why, how often have there been job changes, does patient have salable skills, is patient in a vulnerable occupation?

        7. Health problems: any existing physical problems, what relationship exists between drinking and the health problem?

        8. Physical depenence or addiction, measured by tolerance to alcohol and withdrawal symptoms during abstinence: general physical condition, malnutrition status, presence of seizures, amnesia episodes, blackouts, tremors, anxiety, diaphoresis, anorexia, nausea, vomiting, or hallucinations within 3 days of alcohol abstinence.

    E. For drug users, assess the following areas in depth:

        1. How does the patient view the world and self in relation to it?

        2. What assets or liabilities does patient have in holding a job, handling responsibility, and in maintaining meaningful interpersonal relationships?

        3. Has patient ever been, or is patient now, involved in criminal and judicial systems?

        4. How does patient defend self from making behavioral changes? (Typical patterns include denial, projection, and manipulation.)

        5. What factors in the patient's life support the addiction and what factors bring the patient for help?

        6. Is the patient currently on drugs, and if so, what kind and how much?

V. Staff's responses related to dependent patient.

    A. Feelings, thoughts, behaviors, regarding patient: typical negative responses include anger, rejection, punitiveness, frustration, wish to rescue or save the patient from problems, taking charge, "doing for" the patient, making decisions or setting goals for the patient, fear, helplessness, and approach-avoidance behaviors.

    B. Attitudes related to alcoholism or drug addicts, use of drugs to cope with life.

C. Personal assessment of strengths and limitations. (This self-evaluation is extremely critical in working with drug abusers in order to protect oneself.)
   1. Motivation for helping role.
   2. Level of growth and development (resolution of identity and authority issues).
   3. Self-concept.
   4. Personal resources (recreational outlets and socio-familial relationships).
   5. Past experiences (professional and drug-related).
   6. Philosophy about individual choice, accountability, and responsibility for behavioral change.
   7. Level of knowledge about alcoholism, drug addiction, and psychological issues of giving-receiving, victim-victimizer, dependence-independence.

Problems

I. Patient is verbally and/or nonverbally compliant to others.
II. Patient lacks initiative.
III. Patient has inability to make simple decisions.
IV. Patient has a lack of problem-solving skills.
V. Patient is unable to meet own needs independently or without drugs or other people.
VI. Patient uses drugs or alcohol to provide order to life.
VII. Patient uses drugs or alcohol to plan his future.
VIII. Patient uses drugs or alcohol to experience joy and pleasure in life.
IX. Patient's view of self and body is extremely negative.
X. Patient perceives self as inadequate.
XI. Patient's ability to see world realistically is greatly impaired.
XII. Patient's ability to reality test is greatly impaired.
XIII. Patient has physical withdrawal symptoms after a binge.
XIV. Patient has no job due to drinking or use of drugs.
XV. Patient's mate has threatened to leave if patient does not seek help for drinking problem.
XVI. Patient misses work due to hangovers.
XVII. Patient leans on others compulsively.
XVIII. Patient lacks social skills.
XIX. Patient has a criminal record or is involved in the judicial system.
XX. Patient aligns self with a "deviant" subculture, e.g., drug users, problem drinkers, or others.
XXI. Patient lacks a broad repertoire of coping behaviors.
XXII. Patient has a low frustration tolerance.
XXIII. Patient demands immediate gratification of needs and wants.
XXIV. Patient makes many demands upon others.
XXV. Patient expresses feelings of isolation and rejection.
XXVI. Patient overadapts to others' wishes.
XXVII. Patient uses violence or agitation to meet needs.
XXVIII. Patient expresses idea that he or she cannot survive alone (without drugs or others).

Goals of Care

I. Immediate.
   A. The patient will decrease dependent behaviors.
   B. The patient will increase independent behaviors.
   C. The patient will ask for help and assistance when it is needed or desired.
   D. The patient will recognize own responsibility and choice for the problem behavior and for making behavioral changes.

E. The patient will contract to meet realistic, attainable goals.

F. The patient's physical needs, including safety, will be met satisfactorily to promote and/or maintain health.

II. Long-range (not all dependent patients will be able to meet *all* of these).

A. The patient will decrease dependent behaviors.

B. The patient will increase independent behaviors.

C. The patient will develop the ability to think and to feel simultaneously without projecting or manipulating.

D. The patient will develop social skills.

E. The patient will increase self-esteem and self-awareness.

F. The patient will give up self-destructive, maladaptive behaviors.

G. The patient will maintain a drug-or alcohol-free environment.

H. The patient will be responsible for meeting own needs in health-promoting, socially acceptable ways.

I. The patient will develop and maintain a meaningful support system of interpersonal relationships, apart from drug or alcohol users and in addition to family.

J. The patient will be responsible for making own decisions.

K. The patient will experience joy and pleasure in here-and-now living without drugs or alcohol.

L. The patient will obtain and maintain a job.

M. The patient will maintain adequate physical health, as measured by an adequate daily intake of food and adequate sleep.

N. The patient will develop insight into dependent behaviors and decide to change these behaviors.

Intervention

Refer to "Problems" and "Goals of Care" above.

I. Observe for impending delirium tremens in first 24 to 48 h after hospitalization. Symptoms include extreme agitation, fear, and auditory hallucinations. (See also Chap. 38.)

II. Treat delirium tremens (see Chap. 46).

A. Provide protective setting.

B. Provide measures to maintain rest and sleep.

C. Orient to person, place, and time.

D. Acknowledge fright.

E. Keep room lighted and prevent shadows.

F. Provide sufficient staff to administer prescribed treatments with minimal stress.

G. Provide simple explanations for tests and procedures.

H. Provide adequate nutrition and fluid intake including prescribed intravenous fluids.

III. Administer prescribed tranquilizer, e.g., Valium or Librium, for acute brain syndrome of addicted drinker, if ordered.

IV. Administer polyvitamin therapy, especially vitamin B complex, if ordered.

V. Administer oral fluids for dehydration and electrolyte imbalance.

VI. Provide high-protein, high-carbohydrate diet.

VII. Observe for symptoms of depression and suicidal ideation or behavior (see Chaps. 36 and 37).

VIII. Begin detoxification program.

IX. Provide gradual reduction of drug dosage, if prescribed.

X. Observe drug-taking behavior closely.

XI. Begin methadone maintenance program, or go "cold turkey" if prescribed.

XII. Reassure the patient regarding withdrawal symptoms.

XIII. Treat infections and/or physical complications from drug or alcohol use.

XIV. Provide protective, drug-controlled environment.

XV. Observe and record patient's clinical status and signs of drug or alcohol withdrawal.

XVI. Evaluate ability to perform self-care activities.

XVII. Encourage physical exercise.

XVIII. Assist patient to become aware of her or his social and physical deterioration.

XVIX. Educate patient regarding physiological and psychological effects of drug abuse.

XX. Assist patient to recognize that responsibility for behavior and choices lies with him or her alone.

XXI. Initially, nurse may need to *share* responsibility with patient; later relinquish it.

XXII. Provide information about having a variety of options and choices from which patient can choose.

XXIII. Assist patient to explore chosen behavior and its consequences.

XXIV. Avoid critical, punitive, or moralistic attitude.

XXV. Ask the patient to describe personal expectations for outcome of hospitalization.

XXVI. Ask the family and/or significant others to describe their expectations for the patient during hospitalization.

XXVII. Assist the patient to clarify own issues and concerns.

XXVIII. Assist the patient in selecting and setting specific goals to work toward attaining.

XXIX. Ask patient to contract not to hurt self accidentally or on purpose, e.g., overdose or suicide.

XXX. Ask patient to contract not to perform self-mutilative acts accidentally or on purpose.

XXXI. Explore with patient how her or his basic needs for affection, control, responsibility, and mastery are met.

XXXII. Encourage verbalization of needs, feelings, thoughts, and wants; help to find ways to act on these appropriately.

XXXIII. Teach how to use "I" messages.

XXXIV. Direct patient to cut out or stop a self-defeating or socially disruptive action.

XXXV. Set limits on unrealistic or inappropriate behavior.

XXXVI. Communicate expectations and goals to patient and staff so all have a clear understanding of what is to be done.

XXXVII. Assist patient in developing a specific plan to decrease dependency on others and increase ability to meet own needs independently of others, e.g., get own apartment, learn to drive a car, get job, etc.

XXXVIII. Develop a reinforcement system to reward independence, and ignore or punish dependent behaviors.

XXXIX. Discuss with patient your observations of ways in which he or she manipulates others.

XL. Permit appropriate dependency.

XLI. Reinforce successful behavior with comment, acknowledgment, and encouragement.

XLII. Prepare patient to deal with anxieties about opinions of others regarding hospitalization.

XLIII. Teach patient knowledge and skills of assertiveness training.

XLIV. Never give money or drugs to a patient who is a drug user.

XLV. Assist patient in identifying strengths in area of social functioning, e.g., sense of humor, hobby or special interest, appearance.

XLVI. Explore patient's feelings, thoughts, and behaviors related to specific social situations.

XLVII. Assist patient in improving grooming and personal hygiene by teaching, demonstrating, and discussing problem areas.

XLVIII. Assist patient in improving social manners and courtesy.

    A. Teach patient how to introduce self to another person.

    B. Demonstrate how to introduce self to a group.

    C. Explore topics and subjects that patient can use in social interactions.

    D. Teach patient how to walk and carry self.

    E. Teach patient socially approved eating habits.

XLIX. Role play problematic social situations with patient to improve or develop skills.

L. Encourage patient to interact with and relate to other people.

LI. Encourage participation in a group for former drug or alcohol abusers.

LII. Prevent and intervene in the patient's discussion of poor self-concept for secondary gains by refocusing conversation.

LIII. Provide opportunities for success experiences for patient.

LIV. Assist patient in grieving about giving up drugs, alcohol, or dependent behaviors.

LV. Encourage patient to explore life situation and need for drugs and alcohol.

LVI. Counter patient's negative interpretation or opinion regarding destructive life patterns with a constructive alternative point of view.

LVII. Encourage and support patient's ability to think and solve problems.

LVIII. Invite patient to identify and differentiate between feelings, thoughts, and behaviors.

LIX. Use a variety of treatment modalities to teach patient to think and feel, e.g., group, milieu, poetry, dance, other creative activities, occupational and recreational therapy, bibliotherapy, fantasies, gestalt techniques, individual therapy.

LX. Assist patient in improving judgments and decision making by exploring alternative choices and outcomes for specific decisions.

LXI. Provide support when patient voices independent opinions and decisions.

LXII. Encourage patient to make independent decisions in noncritical areas, such as dress, structuring of time, attendance at meetings and activities.

LXIII. Provide opportunities to redevelop work habits, perseverance, and job skills on ward.

LXIV. Use the milieu to develop patient's responsibility, and provide feedback about performance of tasks for patient.

LXV. Assist patient in identifying problems which hinder, limit, or prevent her or him from getting a job.

LXVI. Role play applying for a job with patient, and give feedback to patient.

LXVII. Explore with patient resources and methods to solve problems related to obtaining and/or maintaining job, such as completing high school diploma, vocational counseling and testing.

Evaluation

I. Reassessment: Dependency is a problem which requires long-term follow-up and continuous evaluation of the effectiveness of the treatment plan. Discharge planning with specific treatment outcomes established should begin at the time of the patient's admission to decrease the potential for depending on the staff and hospital setting and deriving secondary gains from hospitalization. The patient's ability to meet his or her own basic needs, maintain a relatively stable physical status, and follow through on a community referral are essential factors in preventing the occurrence of the "revolving door" syndrome. Behavioral outcomes of treatment should be evaluated on a regular basis, with goals and plans modified according to the patient's status and response to treatment. Relapses of alcohol or drug users should be handled in a matter-of-fact, exploratory manner.

II. Follow-up and reevaluation.

A. Refer to community agncy. It is crucial that alcohol- or drug-dependent patients be referred for long-term follow-up care in the community, such as Alcoholics Anonymous, a day-treatment program, community mental health center, alcoholic rehabilitation unit, or public health nurse. In addition, drug addicts need a new group with which to identify and relate in order to combat the severe problem of loneliness most drug addicts face. Group therapy can be the supportive link if care is carefully structured. Drug users and nonusers should be in separate groups. The nurse's main role may be as a facilitator or coordinator, rather than as primary therapist.

B. Assist with socioeconomic and family problems. Because the behavior of drug-dependent patients has far-reaching effects and is affected by all those in their system, family therapy is an effective tool for long-term care. This can be initiated prior to the discharge of patients. Other social and economic factors, such as jobs and new social ties, should also be planned in long-term care if patients are to be rehabilitated. Of course, some patients do not choose to follow through with these long-range plans.

C. Monitor prescribed medications.
  1. Alcoholics may be maintained on Antabuse or a minor tranquilizer after discharge. These patients should be followed and observed regularly for their responses to the medications, and the plan for follow-up should be clearly defined, understood, and agreed upon by the patient. Also, in case problems develop prior to the initial follow-up visit, the patient should know whom to see at what location prior to discharge.
  2. Drug users being maintained on methadone or a narcotic antagonist should know whom to see, when, where, and for what reasons prior to discharge. Unscheduled urinary drug detection tests should be taken periodically when patient is on one of these drugs.

DEMANDING BEHAVIOR

Definition

Demanding behavior is manifested in syndromes which involve dysfunctional interpersonal relationships. It usually occurs when individuals believe themselves unable to fulfill their needs and/or have their needs met by making requests in a direct, matter-of-fact manner. Therefore, they tend to coerce others to meet their needs indirectly by making requests with forceful, manipulative behaviors. If others attempt to meet the requested needs without perceiving the real, unspoken needs, or if others attempt to avoid or ignore such patients, the demanding behavior is frequently accelerated as anxiety increases. Demanding behavior may be observed in a variety of behavioral syndromes. (See "Manipulation" and "Dependent Behavior.")

Assessment (Refer to "Manipulation")

  I. Data sources (see "Manipulation").
  II. Health history (see "Manipulation"). Note especially patient's emotional responses, including withdrawal, anxiety, feelings of being swallowed up, anger, never being able to "do enough," frustration.
  III. Observations of nurses or other staff members of patient's emotional responses.

Problems

  I. Patient makes numerous requests of others.
  II. Patient asks others to do what could be done by him- or herself.
  III. Patient detains nurse or staff member in room with additional requests after initial request has been met.
  IV. Patient whines and seems helpless when making a request.
  V. Patient becomes angry when requests are not met immediately.
  VI. Patient constantly seeks attention from others.
  VII. Patient attempts to coerce others into meeting requests.

Goals of Care

I. Immediate.
  A. The patient will recognize that many demands are being made.
  B. The patient will gain insight into unfulfilled needs and wants that cause demanding behavior.
  C. The patient will decrease demands.
II. Long-range.
  A. The patient will ask directly for what is needed or wanted.
  B. The patient will develop a variety of options to meet needs.
  C. The patient will be self-aware and autonomous in relationships.

Intervention

Refer to "Problems" and "Goals of Care," above. These actions will be performed by the nurse to meet goals and eliminate problems.
  I. Identify situations in which patient is demanding.
  II. Reflect patient's behavior back to assist her or him in identifying patterns.
  III. Share own responses to patient's behavior with him or her in a matter-of-fact way.
  IV. Assess the unfulfilled needs that patient is trying to meet via demanding behavior.
  V. Identify with patient the basic needs he or she believes unmet, and decide together how these will be met (by patient or others, at what times, etc.)
  VI. Point out when patient's anxiety is increasing.
  VII. Identify and point out consequences of inappropriate behavior.
  VIII. Encourage patient to explore and express feelings without acting upon them.
  IX. Assist patient in developing new options for meeting needs effectively.
    A. Encourage patient to ask directly for what is wanted.
    B. Invite patient to use "I" messages for feelings, wants, and needs.
    C. Encourage patient to explore feelings if and when demands are not immediately met.
    D. Role play alternative ways to communicate needs other than demanding.
    E. Reinforce appropriate behaviors, e.g., when patient asks directly and is independent.
  X. Provide safe, consistent limits for behavior.
  XI. Explain to patient clearly defined expectations that are total-staff decisions.
  XII. Explore patient's strengths and liabilities with patient.

Evaluation

I. Reassessment: It is helpful to use a flow sheet or tool to evaluate the number of times and kinds of situations in which the patient is demanding in order to evaluate behavioral changes and the effectiveness of the interventions. Changes should be monitored and evaluated against baseline data developed when the plan is begun. Basic needs—physical, emotional, and social—must be met, while the patient is encouraged to achieve both independence and interdependence in meeting the needs. Be sure entire staff is consistent in its expectations and interventions with the patient. If behavior does not significantly change within a specified period (no less than a week of consistent care), reevaluate all steps in the nursing process.
II. Follow-up and reevaluation: To assure positive reinforcement and continuous growth of the patient, it may be helpful to establish a plan with the patient for "spot" checks (e.g., monthly) within the community following discharge. Referral to a community mental health center or public health nurse, with patient's consent, is recommended. If referral occurs, the plan of care and earlier progress should be shared with the person

or agency for continuity of care. The patient should also be taught prior to discharge to recognize when additional assistance may be needed and how, where, and from whom to obtain it.

COMPROMISED DECISION MAKING

Definition

Compromised decision making is a clinical problem in which patients demonstrate a lack of ability to make decisions independently, or to choose between two or more alternatives, or who tend to make choices based on the wishes or desires of other individuals regardless of his or her own wishes or desires. Such patients may agonizingly deliberate over decisions, but be unable to use effectively the ego functions of thinking, reality testing, judgment, and affect to sort out the pros and cons of particular choices and decisions. Such behavior results in ineffective relationships and a lack of ability to assume responsibility for oneself in an adult world, as these require constant decision making. Such patients are frequently aware of their difficulty and experience low self-esteem, poor interpersonal relationships, and extreme anxiety as a direct result. Severe anxiety, such as occurs in crisis situations, may also trigger compromised decision making.

The tendency to suffer from compromised decision making frequently begins in early childhood when the developmental task of autonomy versus shame and doubt must be addressed. This clinical problem is present in a variety of psychiatric diagnoses and even in normal life situations in which intense anxiety is present. In addition, it may present as a symptom of acute or chronic organic brain syndrome with physical, emotional and developmental components.

Assessment (Refer to "Manipulation")

    I. Data sources (see "Manipulation").
   II. Health history (see "Manipulation"). Note especially estimate of intellectual abilities.
  III. Observations of nurses and other staff members and their response to patient's behavior, including confusion, frustration, inability to get an answer to a question, sense of uncertainty.

Problems

      I. Patient is unable to choose between two or more alternatives.
     II. Patient bases decisions on the opinions and wishes of others rather than on own opinions and wishes.
    III. Patient lacks ability to make independent decisions.
    IV. Patient depends on other people to make decisions for her or him.
     V. Patient lacks information necessary to make decisions.
    VI. Patient denies that a problem exists.
   VII. Patient denies the significance of a problem.
 VIII. Patient is unable to see more than one solution to a problem.
    IX. Patient lacks confidence in own ability to solve problems.
     X. Patient denies that a problem has a solution.

Goals of Care

    I. Immediate.
       A. The patient will recognize his or her specific difficulties related to decision making.

    B. The patient will alter perceptions of self or the problem to facilitate the decision-making process.

    C. The patient will begin to make simple decisions.

II. Long-range.

    A. The patient will improve ability to consider alternatives for specific situations.

    B. The patient will improve decision-making skills.

Intervention

Refer to "Problems" and "Goals of Care," above. These actions will be performed by nurse to meet goals and eliminate problems.

    I. Identify issues or areas of life in which patient has difficulty making decisions.

    II. Explore with patient attitudes about self which help or hinder the ability to make decisions.

    III. Assess patient's intellectual abilities, level of knowledge, attention span, and physical or organic problems which affect decision making.

    IV. Explore goals, values, and life purpose with patient to provide a framework for decision making in specific situations.

    V. Teach patient how to test reality and validate perceptions as a part of decision making.

    VI. Identify and point out previous experiences where patient made decisions successfully.

    VII. Direct patient to resources to find necessary information about the problematic situation.

    VIII. Correct misinformation about the problem situation.

    IX. Teach patient how to identify necessary steps to meet activities of daily living and other decisions.

    X. Direct patient to write down or verbalize to a trusted person the pros and cons related to each decision that must be made.

    XI. Assist patient to identify a variety of alternatives for each decision.

    XII. Explore with patient the consequences of each alternative.

    XIII. Assist patient to focus attention on one problem at a time.

    XIV. Teach patient assertiveness techniques.

    XV. Reinforce patient in making a decision or voicing independent opinions or ideas.

    XVI. Assure patient that it is all right to make mistakes.

    XVII. Teach patient that it is okay for one to think and feel for oneself, based on what one wants and needs and not on other's expectations.

    XVIII. Permit patient to make choices about personal hygiene and dress, attendance at meetings, punctuality, structuring free time.

    XIX. Assist patient in transferring learning to new, more complex areas of decision making.

Evaluation

    I. Reassessment: Evaluation of both the goal being attained and the progress being made in the decision-making process are essentially continuous. It may be necessary to alter the goals or to select new ones as patients gain confidence in their ability to make decisions and develop new skills. Careful evaluation of the process should include both subjective and objective assessments of the patients' ability to make increasingly more complex decisions based on their life goals, values, and needs.

    II. Follow-up and reevaluation.

        A. Refer to community agency or public health nurse, especially if patient has a physical or organic limitation for long-term follow-up. Also, refer if patient or family requests such support.

        B. Provide agency or person referred to with a summary of progress, plan of care, accomplishments, and goals being worked toward.

    C. Teach patient prior to discharge about community resources that might be pursued independently for assistance in meeting long-term goals.

COMPROMISED ABILITY TO CARRY OUT ACTIVITIES OF DAILY LIVING

Definition

Compromised ability to carry out activities of daily living is a clinical problem in which a person is unable to be self-directed in the ordinary tasks of eating, drinking, bathing, hygiene and grooming, sleeping, exercising, and eliminating, and in which the assistance of another person to meet these basic needs is required. This compromised ability may be the result of a variety of factors, either physical and/or social-emotional. Many disorders and normal crises may be accompanied by an alteration in the ability of the person to carry out activities of daily living. It may be among the earliest symptoms to appear in a developing emotional disorder, and it may be part of a syndrome which combines several clinical problems, such as manipulation, dependency, severe anxiety, secondary gains of neurosis, disorientation, and loss of memory. Frequently, compromised ability to carry out activities of daily living is a result of temporary or permanent regression and/or lack of motivation and socialization skills in patients who have been hospitalized or socially isolated for a long period of time. The problem further decreases the patient's ability to interact socially with others and move out into the community.

Assessment (Refer to "Manipulation")

    I. Data sources (see "Manipulation").
    II. Health history (see "Manipulation").
    III. Observations and emotional responses of nurses or other staff to the patient's behavior, especially related to social functioning and ability to understand instructions and reinforcement.

Problems

    I. The patient is mute and does not interact with others.
    II. The patient stands, sits, or lies on floor for long hours without moving.
    III. The patient does not eat or eats with fingers in a messy manner.
    IV. The patient is incontinent of urine or feces.
    V. The patient does not dress by self or dresses inappropriately.
    VI. The patient refuses to keep clothes on.
    VII. The patient has poor personal hygiene habits.
    VIII. The patient takes little interest in own personal appearance.
    IX. The patient sleeps most of the day.
    X. The patient is socially inept and appears to be unaware of customary social behaviors.

Goals of Care

    I. Immediate.
        A. The patient will improve personal habits related to activities of daily living:
            1. Remain continent of feces and urine.
            2. Take interest in grooming, hygiene, and appearance.
            3. Improve eating habits.
            4. Dress self in own clothes appropriately.
            5. Sleep appropriate number of hours.
        B. The patient will develop social interests outside of self.

    II. Long-range.

        A. The patient will perform his or her activities of daily living in socially acceptable ways.

        B. The patient will develop interest in and identification with a group of patients.

        C. The patient will relate to other people in planned activities.

        D. The patient will have the minimum necessary social skills and abilities to function in the community.

Intervention

    I. Take incontinent patient to toilet according to a rigid routine, e.g., upon rising, after breakfast, prior to lunch, after lunch, before dinner, after dinner, and at bedtime.

    II. Ask socialized patients to assist with care of unsocialized patients.

    III. Instruct, remind, or assist patient in:

        A. Bathing.   **E.** Combing, washing, and styling hair.

        B. Caring for nails.   **F.** Changing underwear frequently.

        C. Use of deodorant.   **G.** Selection of clothes and appropriate attire.

        D. Brushing teeth regularly. **H.** Laundering and ironing clothes.

    IV. Teach female patient appropriate use of cosmetics.

    V. Encourage male patient to shave regularly.

    VI. Discuss with patient how to purchase clothing.

    VII. Note appearance when dress and grooming are appropriate.

    VIII. Arrange for patient to go to hospital beauty salon or barber.

    IX. Refer patient to dentist if necessary.

    X. Assist patient in setting up routine schedule to meet grooming, dressing, and personal hygiene needs.

    XI. Teach patient to observe proper manners while eating: how to sit, chew with mouth closed, chew a little at a time, eat with utensils properly.

    XII. Teach patient how to improve orderliness and neatness of room and personal possessions.

    XIII. Reward all appropriate behaviors with verbal recognition and acknowledge with parties, prizes, or desired trips.

    XIV. Introduce simple topics, simple presentations, and simple questions to a group of patients for remotivation.

    XV. Utilize remotivation techniques to encourage group interactions, including use of food to reinforce pleasure of socializing.

    XVI. Identify group projects and goals with patient participation.

    XVII. Take patients on trips, shopping expeditions, or walks outside hospital ward as patients are ready. (Obtain permission from administration prior to offering a group trip to patients.)

    XVIII. Plan group sport activities and social activities, such as dances or parties, when patients are ready.

    XIX. Teach the patient how to use money properly.

    XX. Encourage individual participation and responsibility in planning and implementing group activities.

    XXI. Assist patient in developing and/or expanding interests and skills.

    XXII. Assist patients to hold and participate in ward meetings.

    XXIII. Offer work assignments on unit to increase patient pride and sense of accomplishment.

    XXIV. Provide remuneration for work accomplished to teach adjustment to outside world.

    XXV. Provide opportunities for patients to care for other objects or people, e.g., plants, animals, less socialized patients.

    XXVI. Provide opportunities for patients to improve their physical environment through group activities.

Evaluation

    I. Reassessment: Since compromised ability to carry out activities of daily living is usually a long-term problem, the carefully developed plan will need continuous reassessment and modification to meet the needs and progress of individual patients. Staff will need support and reinforcement from one another and their leaders to assure continued motivation to intervene with patients with chronic regressed patterns of interaction. The goal is to move such patients back into the community as soon as they are able to function self-sufficiently an present minimal levels of social adequacy.

    II. Follow-up reevaluation: Patients should be prepared to deal with real life situations of work, family life, social interactions, and own daily care prior to discharge. If minimally competent, referral to an active day treatment program in a mental health center or half-way house or group home where they can receive support and build their knowledge, skills, and self-confidence is very valuable. A public health nurse could also provide support, on-going treatment, and be a resource for newly discharged patients.

DISORIENTATION

Definition

Disorientation is a clinical problem which involves an impaired ability to understand temporal, spatial, or personal relationships. Such individuals lose their awareness of the position of themselves in terms of time, space, or other people. They usually appear confused and perplexed and are unable to concentrate on here-and-now situations; they may be unable to identify the date, the place where they are, or who they are.

Disorientation as a clinical symptom is presented in several psychiatric disorders, e.g., whenever there is severe anxiety or as a result of an emotionally traumatic experience such as a situational crisis. Disorientation may also be part of a syndrome involving alterations of memory, judgment, affect, reality testing, and perception, such as occurs in organic brain syndrome. In all cases, there is a related disruption in interpersonal processes.

Assessment (Refer to "Manipulation")

    I. Data sources (see "Manipulation"). Note especially:
        A. Psychological examination.
        B. Laboratory work-up related to physical history and findings of examination.
        C. Staff observations and responses to patient.

    II. Health history (see "Manipulation"). Note especially alterations and strengths in patient's ego functioning (including any abrupt changes): in thought, recent and remote memory, perception, judgment, reality testing, affect.

Problems

    I. Patient cannot recall recent events of own life.
    II. Patient cannot state correctly the day, month, year, and/or season.
    III. Patient cannot state correctly present location, including address, city, state, country.
    IV. Patient cannot identify self correctly.
    V. Patient cannot identify other significant people around him or her, such as staff or family.
    VI. Patient makes up information due to anxiety related to inability to remember.
    VII. Patient experiences confusion about time, place, person, or surroundings.

Goals of Care

    I. Immediate.
        A. The patient will be safe and protected while disoriented.
        B. The patient will be supported by nursing measures while diagnostic and treatment procedures are followed to identify and correct physical (medical) problems.
        C. The patient will be assisted to improve orientation.
    II. Long-range.
        A. The patient will improve orientation to time, place, and/or person.
        B. The patient will adjust to any permanent disability.

Intervention

Refer to "Problems" and "Goals of Care," above. These actions will be performed by the nurse to meet goals and decrease problems.

    I. Supervise closely to prevent patient from hurting self, wandering off, or exhibiting inappropriate behavior.
    II. Decrease agitation and frustration with comforting, relaxing measures, such as warm bath, well-lighted room, soft music.
    III. Repeat orienting information frequently.
    IV. Use kind, quiet tone of voice with patient.
    V. Give simple, short explanations.
    VI. Use a night-light in patient's room during the night.
    VII. Avoid administering barbiturates and bromides to patients who have chronic brain syndrome.
    VIII. Observe patient carefully and provide assistance in self-care when it is needed.
    IX. Do not physically restrain patient.
    X. Listen carefully to what patient says and correct gently, in a nonpunitive manner, if information is confabulated.
    XI. Place calendars with large print and clocks with large numbers and hands in patient's living area.
    XII. Label areas such as bathroom, nurse's station, and patient's bedroom with large-lettered signs.
    XIII. Address patient by name frequently.
    XIV. Introduce self to patient each time nurse is with patient.
    XV. Wear clearly labeled name tags with correct title.
    XVI. Carefully orient patient to environment.
    XVII. Keep furniture and possessions in same place.
    XVIII. Maintain a regular routine and provide a printed schedule of activities for patient to follow.
    XIX. Assist patient to correct inappropriate behavior or learn a necessary task.
    XX. Permit patient to practice skills in a familiar environment.
    XXI. Tell patient when you do not understand her or him.
    XXII. Permit patient to bring familiar objects from home to keep with her or him.
    XXIII. Place personal items in an area which is easily accessible to patient.
    XXIV. Teach patient to use lists and appointment books to minimize forgetfulness of schedules, people, activities.
    XXV. Tape list of activities of daily care next to patient's bathroom mirror.
    XXVI. Correct patient immediately after inappropriate behavior takes place.
    XXVII. Provide consistent routine and structure for patient; introduce change slowly.
    XXVIII. Encourage patient to wear and use watch and to use a pocket calendar.
    XXIX. Prevent overstimulation from people or environment.
    XXX. Permit patient to wear own clothes.
    XXXI. Encourage as much independence as possible.
    XXXII. Teach family safety measures and principles of care.

Evaluation

I. Reassessment and modification of the plan to meet the needs of patients must be continuous and constantly adjusted to their level of functioning. The physical and medical condition of these patients should also be carefully monitored to assure maximum functioning in all spheres of activity.

II. Follow-up and reevaluation.

A. Prepare patients for any alterations in their environment by giving them simple explanations and by keeping them in contact with familiar people and objects.

B. Have public health nurse visit patients in hospital prior to their discharge to familiarize them with nurse. Provide nurse with summary of progress and treatment plan at time of patient discharge.

C. Teach patients and their family members principles of care prior to discharge, including the need for medical checkups and the taking of medication, what to expect as a result of the medication, and what to report to the public health nurse and/or physician.

D. Referral to a day treatment program in a mental health center may be helpful for patient.

E. Family therapy after patient discharge should be recommended.

REFERENCES

1. Blair Justice and Rita Justice, *The Abusing Family,* Human Sciences Press, New York, 1976, pp. 115–117.
2. Ibid.

BIBLIOGRAPHY

"An Alcohol Abuse Manual for Hospital Doctors," *Resident and Staff Physician,* **22:**9–133, February 1976. Sixteen articles related to diagnosing and treating patients who have alcohol problems. Interdisciplinary, broad community-based treatment focus, including articles on alcoholism in industry and a list of resources with addresses, for additional information and help for patients with a drinking problem.

Arieti, Silvano (ed.): *American Handbook of Psychiatry,* vol. III: *Adult Clinical Psychiatry,* 2d ed., Basic Books, Inc., Publishers, New York, 1974. A classic text on the diagnosis, symptomatology, and treatment of the syndromes of adult psychopathology from a medical point of view.

Arnold, Helen M.: "Working with Schizophrenic Patients," *American Journal of Nursing,* **76:**941–943, June 1976. An article which focuses on the therapeutic factors in working with withdrawn patients.

Berne, Eric: *Games People Play,* Grove Press, Inc., New York, 1964. Describes and analyzes from both social and psychological positions 120 games that are frequently played in human transactions. Also presents the "anti-game" for each.

Burgess, Ann Wolbert, and Aaron Lazare: *Psychiatric Nursing in the Hospital and the Community,* 2d ed., Prentice-Hall, Inc., Englewood Cliffs, N.J., 1976. A comprehensive approach to psychiatric–mental health nursing in a variety of settings. Specific strengths include its focus on the nursing process; inclusion of standards of psychiatric–mental health nursing practice; integration of medical, behavioral, psychological, and social aspects; and sections on differentiating feelings, thoughts, and behaviors, and drug and alcohol abuse. Recommended for the advanced learner.

James, Muriel, and Dorothy Jongeward: *Born to Win: Transactional Analysis with Gestalt Experiments,* Addison-Wesley Publishing Company, Inc., Reading, Mass., 1971. Presents the theoretical concepts of transactional analysis as a rational method for analyzing and understanding behavior, both in ourselves and in our patients. Excellent tool for developing self-awareness, responsibility, and autonomy.

Justice, Blair, and Rita Justice: *The Abusing Family,* Human Sciences Press, New York, 1976. Excellent source of knowledge on diagnosing, planning care, intervening, and follow-up care for abusing families, using a psychosocial systems model. Explains the concept of symbiosis and use of the goal attainment guide.

Kneisl, Carol Ran, and Holly Skodol Wilson (eds.): *Current Perspectives in Psychiatric Nursing,* Vol. I: *Issues and Trends,* The C. V. Mosby Company, St. Louis, 1976. A sourcebook providing a collection of articles related to the practice and theoretical framework of the psychiatric–mental health nurse. Includes material on new modes of treatment, including behavior modification, transactional analysis, gestalt therapy, and family mental health.

Meldman, Monte J., Gertrude McFarland, and Edith Johnson: *The Problem-Oriented Psychiatric Index and Treatment Plans,* The C. V. Mosby Company, St. Louis, 1976. Using the nursing history and process as guidelines, this book describes and explains a system for use in health care agencies operating on the problem-oriented record. It is helpful for developing specific written treatment plans for clients experiencing emotional problems.

Morgan, Arthur James, and Judith Wilson Moreno: *The Practice of Mental Health Nursing: A Community Approach,* J. B. Lippincott Company, Philadelphia, 1973. Focusing on clinical practice in the community, the authors have included descriptions and nursing implications for a number of treatment modalities. Written in simple style, it includes an excellent chapter on psychopharmacology, as well as chapters on chronic brain syndrome and drug and alcohol addiction.

Payne, Dorris B.: *Psychiatric-Mental Health Nursing,* Medical Examination Publishing Company, Inc., Flushing, N.Y., 1974. A number of socio-environmental patient problems are described in terms of etiology, dynamics, nursing assessment, and intervention in a simple basic format. Has a section on the nurse's functions and responsibilities to the patient.

Robinson, Lisa: *Psychiatric Nursing as a Human Experience,* 2d ed., W. B. Saunders Company, Philadelphia, 1977. A humanistic approach to nursing patients who have psychosocial problems. Provides an eclectic conceptual basis. Special features include material on transactional analysis applied to nursing situations, care of patients in a large state hospital, alcohol and drug addiction, and organic problems.

Snyder, Joyce Cameron, and Marge Foltz Wilson: "Elements of a Psychological Assessment," *American Journal of Nursing,* **77**:235–239, February 1977. Describes 10 factors which should be included in each psychological assessment, presented as an eclectic approach.

Trail, Ira D. (ed.): "Symposium on Alcoholism and Drug Addiction," *The Nursing Clinics of North America* **11**(3), September 1976. A group of eight articles sharing new knowledge and treatments. Applies a problem-solving approach to nursing individuals and families who are coping with the stress of alcoholism and drug addiction.

Wiley, Patricia L.: "Manipulation," in L. T. Zderad and H. C. Belcher (eds.), *Developing Behavioral Concepts in Nursing,* Southern Regional Education Board, Atlanta, Ga., 1968. Excellent application of the nursing process to the clinical problem of destructive manipulation in behavioral terms.

36
Affective Disorders

Ruth Dailey Knowles

The purpose of this chapter is to describe the implementation of the nursing process for patients with dysfunctional affective states, i.e., anxiety, depression, and elation. These affective states (particularly anxiety and depression) are associated, in varying degrees, with all illnesses and are experienced by most patients regardless of medical diagnosis.

The nurse can be the key person to use appropriate interventions in anxiety or mild to moderate depression; nurses can often be catalysts in helping patients to avoid serious depressive or high-anxiety states through knowledgeable intervention at early stages of illness or other stress.

Nursing goals, interventions, and evaluations in this chapter are oriented toward all patients whether hospitalized or at home and should expand the repertoire of meaningful nursing interventions of all nurses in dealing with the most common affective disorders. Nurses caring for patients in any clinical area can utilize selected principles reflected in this chapter. Useful behavioral techniques are described fully in the text, and pertinent annotated books and articles are listed in the bibliography.

ANXIETY

Definition

Anxiety is a feeling of apprehension evoked by a threat to some value which the individual holds essential to his or her existence as a personality; it includes a feeling of impending doom, dread, and uneasiness. Some anxiety is necessary for normal functioning, but when anxiety reaches high proportions, it narrows perceptions and interferes with functioning. High anxiety, in addition to other stresses (whether physical or emotional), can lead to aberrant behavior and immobility.

Assessment

    I. Data sources.
       A. Patient.
       B. Family.
       C. Significant others.
       D. Charts of previous hospitalizations or treatments.
       E. Observation of the patient.
       F. Observation of patient and communication patterns with family and others about the patient.
       G. Attention to discrepancies between patient and family report.
    II. Health history. This outline of a health history (including psychosocial history) is oriented toward the outpatient, regardless of presenting symptoms. It should be modified for inpatient use, as it is designed to elicit pertinent information from the verbal and cooperative patient, i.e., the patient presenting symptoms of anxiety.

       The following information should be obtained from the patient on first interview, and will provide a basis for construction of the nursing care plan. Additional comments for an expanded assessment are included under point C, below. This expanded health history section can be completed at a later date when anxiety is lower and the patient is better able to provide information and plan ways to meet personal goals. The nursing care plan should be appropriately revised to incorporate the additional information.

This is a comprehensive assessment with emphasis on psychosocial aspects, particularly those dealing with anxiety and the affective disorders. Use of indirect questions is recommended, and the assessment is designed to move from simple to complex, general to specific, and from less threatening to more intimate aspects of the person's life situation.

A. General patient information to be secured prior to the nursing interview.
    1. Name.
    2. Home address.
    3. Home phone number.
    4. Today's date.
    5. Age and birth date.
    6. Marital status.
    7. Place of employment.
    8. Business address.
    9. Business phone.
    10. Social security number.
    11. Insurance company name.
    12. Height.
    13. Weight.
    14. Vital signs: temperature, pulse, respiration, blood pressure.

B. Initial nursing interview.
    1. Chief complaint.
    2. Medical diagnosis (if applicable and known).
    3. History of present illness or symptoms.
        a. Duration of symptoms.
        b. Date of symptoms.
        c. Manner of onset and predisposing factors.
            (1) What happened immediately before onset?
            (2) What does the patient think is causing this situation?
            (3) How often do the symptoms occur?
    4. Treatment.
        a. Has the patient sought treatment before?
        b. How is the patient's health in general?
        c. Prescribed medications used.
        d. Nonprescribed medications used.
        e. Effectiveness of prior or ongoing treatment.
    5. Review of systems.
        a. Respiratory.   ***e.*** Musculoskeletal.
        b. Cardiovascular.   ***f.*** Integumentary.
        c. Gastrointestinal.   ***g.*** Genitourinary.
        d. Neurological.   ***h.*** Eyes and ears.
    6. Past history.
        a. Allergies.
            (1) Drugs.
            (2) Foods.
            (3) Respiratory (seasonal or perennial).
        b. Major illnesses and dates.   ***d.*** Hospitalizations and dates.
        c. Major operations and dates.   ***e.*** Prostheses or appliances used.
    7. Habits.
        a. Smoking (include amount).
        b. Drinking of alcoholic beverages (include amount).
        c. Hard drugs (include amount).
        d. Soft drugs (include amount).
    8. Psychosocial history.
        a. Current feelings (i.e., about chief complaint and predisposing factors).
        b. Worries.

c. Recent life-change evnts within the family.

d. Recent changes in mental status (i.e., confusion, irritability, mental fatigue, depression, inability to motivate self to get work done, etc.).

e. Previous coping skills used with similar problems.

(1) How is stress handled at home?

(2) How is stress handled at work?

(3) How does this differ from manner of handling stress before presenting symptoms?

(4) What does the patient do when angry, sad, frustrated, anxious?

f. Support systems.

(1) To whom is the patient closest?

(2) Does the patient feel that family members can be helpful at this time? Which ones?

g. Thoughts.

(1) Are there thoughts that are disturbing to patient?

(2) What are some of the "not helpful" thoughts experienced?

h. Why does the patient want treatment at this time?

(1) What does the patient see as the goal of treatment?

(2) What are some of the patient's expectations for treatment?

C. Additional health history data that can be used to augment the initial health history are derived as the patient first comes into contact with the health care system. Information gained from these questions can be used to revise the nursing care plan and make it even more specific to the individual patient.

1. Family history.

a. Current members of family (age, name, health status, occupation).

b. Financial status.

c. Hereditary illnesses.

d. Ethnicity.

e. Religion.

f. Sibling order in original family.

2. Language.

a. English preferred?

b. Other language(s) preferred?

3. Activities of daily living.

a. Eating.

(1) When?

(2) How often?

(3) Appetite.

(4) Types of foods preferred.

(5) Types of foods avoided.

(6) Changes in eating patterns.

(7) Symptoms associated with foods.

b. Fluids.

(1) Amount per day.

(2) Changes in drinking patterns.

c. Elimination.

(1) Bowel movement frequency, characteristics, difficulties, abnormalities.

(2) Current changes in elimination patterns.

(3) Times voided per day.

d. Sleep.

(1) Number hours per night.

(2) Usual time for retiring.

(3) Usual time for arising.

(4) Number of pillows used.

(5) Nighttime awakening pattern (i.e., has trouble falling back to sleep if awakened in night).

(6) Changes in nighttime sleeping pattern.
(7) Daytime rest periods.
  e. Mobility, exercise, and recreation.
    (1) What is patient's normal means of transportation? (Drives, takes bus, depends on friends?)
    (2) Assistance needed in walking?
    (3) Dependence on others for mobility?
    (4) Active or sedentary habits.
    (5) Recent changes in mobility, exercise, and recreation.
    (6) In what activities does patient engage during the normal day?
    (7) Recreational activities.
    (8) Forms of exercise.
    (9) Limitations in exercise.
  f. Living environment.
    (1) Description of neighborhood.
    (2) Type of living accommodations.
    (3) Number of individuals living with patient.
  g. Educational level.
    (1) Has patient met educational goals set for self?
    (2) How were grades when in school?
  h. Employment.
    (1) How does patient feel about job?
    (2) How long has patient been employed?
    (3) How long does patient expect to be employed there?
  i. Support systems.
    (1) Does the patient have close friends with whom to talk honestly?
    (2) Can this person provide the support the patient needs?
    (3) What is the patient's relationship with coworkers?
    (4) How does the patient respond in social situations?
    (5) How does the patient feel about self in social situations?
    (6) How does the patient feel about self in work situations?
    (7) What problems are there in the family that inhibit their support?
    (8) What are sources of support within the family?
    (9) What organizations, clubs, groups does the patient belong to, and how significant are they to the patient?
    (10) Are there other people, pets, activities on which the patient relies for support?
D. Nursing judgments based on health history information.
  1. Appearance.
    a. Posture.
    b. Gait.
    c. Gestures.
    d. Affect and facial expressions.
    e. Nonverbal behavior.
    f. Tension-relieving behaviors.
      (1) Nail biting.   **(3)** Fidgeting.
      (2) Finger picking.   **(4)** Tapping.
    g. Spontaneity.
    h. Congruence of words and nonverbal behavior.
    i. Thought processes.
      (1) Association of ideas.
      (2) Appropriate linking.
      (3) Speed of answers.
      (4) Comprehensiveness of response.
      (5) Logic.
      (6) Presence of delusions, illusions, flight of ideas.

       (7) Ideas of reference.

       (8) Incoherence.

   j. Thought content.

       (1) Factual information.

       (2) Subjective information.

       (3) History corroboration.

   k. Emotional state.

       (1) Affective expression.   **(3)** Nature of moods.

       (2) Emotional display.   **(4)** Change in moods.

   l. Handling of feelings.

       (1) What resistances are obvious?

       (2) What blocks to communication are present?

       (3) What topics of conversation cause patient to change the subject?

       (4) What does the patient refuse to discuss?

       (5) What subjects stimulate anxious nonverbal behavior?

       (6) Is patient able to express feelings?

       (7) How does patient handle feelings after she or he is aware of them?

       (8) Is expression of feeling congruent with the feeling?

       (9) What does the patient do when experiencing:

          (a) Anger?   *(d)* Happiness?

          (b) Frustration?   *(e)* Anxiety?

          (c) Sadness?

  m. Motivations.

       (1) Are needs expressed as maintenance needs or as growth-oriented needs?

       (2) What motivations does the patient have toward attaining goals?

       (3) Does the patient have hope?

       (4) What is the patient's motivation for dealing with illness or problem and cooperating in treatment?

       (5) Does patient seem willing and able to take responsibility for own behavior?

       (6) Would involvement of the spouse be supportive for treatment?

       (7) Does patient appear to have appropriate self-esteem? Is image of self inflated or deflated?

   n. What are targets for modification? List behaviors to be modifid.

III. Physical and behavioral assessment. The human organism is not meant to exhibit the symptoms and behaviors listed below except at rare times where "fight or flight" is needed. Individuals who are perennially anxious may have permanent physical changes which can include hypertension, coronary artery disease, arthritis, ulcers, colitis, skin problems, asthma, etc. Moderate to high anxiety, even for a few minutes, narrows one's perceptions, clouds judgment, produces irritability, and interferes with communication.

  A. Cardiovascular system.

    1. Increased pulse rate.

    2. Palpitations (extrasystoles) which are transient and not relieved by rest or cessation of exercise.

    3. Chest pain.

    4. Vasomotor flushing.

  B. Respiratory system.

    1. Increased respiratory rate.

    2. Hyperventilation.

    3. Transient respiratory distress, i.e., wheezing or inability to take a deep breath.

    4. Sighing.

  C. Gastrointestinal system.

    1. Diarrhea or constipation.

    2. Nausea.

3. "Butterflies" in stomach.
4. Spasm of cardiac or pyloric sphincter of the stomach.
5. Hyperchlorhydria.
6. Intestinal irritability.
7. Anorexia or excessive eating.
8. Dry mouth.
9. Indigestion.
10. Abdominal cramps.
   D. Musculoskeletal system.
1. Weakness.
2. Tremors.
3. Tense posture.
   E. Integumentary system.
1. Sweating.   3. Itching.
2. Pallor or grey tone.   4. Hives.
   F. Other physical symptoms.
1. Vertigo and/or fainting.
2. Dilated pupils.
3. Urinary frequency.
   G. Other anxiety-related behaviors.
1. Fidgety movements.   6. Downcast eyes.
2. Nail biting.   7. Strained or uneven voice; "break" in voice.
3. Finger drumming.   8. Sleeplessness.
4. Foot swinging.   9. Time urgency.
5. Toe tapping.

Problems

I. Immobilization and panic.
II. Periodic occurrence of anxiety attacks.

Goals of Care

I. Immediate.
   A. The patient will learn how to "level" anxiety (see "Special Modes of Intervention").
   B. The patient will level anxiety several times a day, particularly before and after using behavioral techniques to lower anxiety.
   C. The patient will learn progressive relaxation (see "Special Modes of Intervention").
   D. The patient will practice progressive relaxation twice per day.
   E. The patient will learn thought stopping (see "Special Modes of Intervention").
   F. The patient will practice thought stopping on not helpful thoughts.
   G. The patient will decrease use of tranquilizing drugs.
   H. The patient will identify precur or of anxiety.
   I. The patient will begin to determine repertoire of coping behaviors.
   J. The patient will begin to determine activities in which to engage to decrease anxiety.
   K. The patient will expand relationships with others (family, friends).
II. Long-range.
   A. The patient will verbalize feelings freely.
   B. The patient will associate thoughts with consequent feelings.
   C. The patient will eliminate all psychoactive drugs.
   D. The patient will control anxiety when it begins through habitual use of relaxation or other behavioral techniques.
   E. The patient will eliminate not helpful thoughts, i.e., self-deprecation, decreased hope and faith in self, worries.

F. The patient will become a generally relaxed person.

G. The patient will make assertive requests and responses.

H. The patient will express hostility and anger appropriately.

I. The patient will measure reality in thoughts and not allow one thought to generalize to negative feelings.

J. The patient will expand coping behaviors.

K. The patient will identify anxiety-supporting behaviors on the part of the family members.

L. The patient will show congruence between words and affect.

Intervention

General Intervention

These constitute good nursing practice for all patients, regardless of presenting symptoms or diagnosis, and are listed separately from specific interventions for the anxious, depressed, or elated patient.

I. Seek out patient and call by name.

II. Spend time with patient, even when patient does not verbalize. Provide quiet companionship.

III. Listen to patient and encourage catharsis where appropriate.

IV. Speak in a slow, soft, well-modulated voice.

V. Remove as many stresses as possible from the environment (including physical and psychological stresses).

VI. Present an attitude of acceptance.

VII. Encourage patient to talk about feelings.

VIII. Encourage patient to expand social contacts.

IX. Be a catalyst to relationships between patient and others.

X. Be consistent. If promises are made, they must be kept.

XI. Encourage patient to increase recreational activities.

XII. Encourage patient to increase physical exercise.

XIII. Expect good results; expect patient to follow regimen of care.

XIV. Encourage and reinforce use of coping behaviors.

XV. Encourage healthy and appropriate expression of anger, frustration, and hostility.

XVI. Observe for suicidal ideation. Inquire about details when patient confides suicidal thoughts.

XVII. Avoid reassuring patient. Express realistic hopes and expectations.

XVIII. Reinforce all positive, growth-oriented behavior.

XIX. Employ comfort measures that are pleasing to patient.

XX. Present reality; avoid agreeing with negative self-statements made by patient.

XXI. Assist patient to understand that he or she has rights and responsibilities.

XXII. Encourage patient to increase positive self-statements and to decrease negative self-statements (see "Special Modes of Intervention").

XXIII. Encourage patient to continuously evaluate own progress.

Specific Intervention

What follows relates specifically to the anxious patient.

I. Teach the patient to level anxiety (see "Special Modes of Intervention").

II. Teach the patient progressive relaxation (see "Special Modes of Intervention").

III. Teach the patient to use thought-stopping techniques (see "Special Modes of Intervention").

IV. Teach the patient to give self suggestions to support nonanxiety.

V. Teach patient to monitor thoughts which are precursors of feelings.

A. Ask patient to describe anxiety-provoking event(s).

B. Determine what the event has to do with the patient's worth from the patient's point of view.

C. Determine whether the event was an isolated event.

> **D.** Point out that one event does not mean that the patient has a reactive characteristic to that kind of event.
>
> *Example* If a girl turns a boy down for a date, this does not mean that he is unloveable any more than it means that he is the world's most loveable person.

VI. Have patient keep a diary of all activities. Each activity should be rated concerning the patient's degree of accomplishment, mastery, or pleasure.

VII. Encourage patient to complete tasks related to anxiety for the purpose of gaining feelings of accomplishment.

VIII. Encourage patient to use behaviors (according to a hierarchy from lowest anxiety producer to highest) that engender anxiety, in conjunction with progressive relaxation.

IX. Direct patient to postpone large decisions until in a less anxious state.

X. Have patient make a list of positive self-statements to use when anxious, e.g., "I have been anxious before and I got over it," "This feeling is temporary," "Nothing actually happens to me when I get anxious," "What is the worst thing that can happen to me in this situation?"

XI. Have patient list strengths and talents, and encourage patient to find opportunities to use them.

XII. Assist patient in identifying threats or stresses in personal environment that might be removed.

XIII. Teach appropriate assertive behavior.

XIV. Provide a role model of assertive behavior.

XV. Do role playing with patient related to situations calling for assertive behaviors.

XVI. Be available to patient or advise patient of whom to contact during periods of high anxiety.

XVII. Provide anticipatory guidance for future anxiety situations.

Special Modes of Intervention

LEVELING ANXIETY

Most of the time, individuals are not aware of their level of anxiety. They can recall relaxed times, and they can recall panic times. The nurse can teach patients to become more aware of their level of anxiety. This leads not only to increased identification of rising anxiety, but also to documentation, in the minds of patients, that they can reduce anxiety levels.

Have patients identify on a scale of 0 to 10 their anxiety levels (0 = asleep, 10 = absolute panic). During interviews the nurse may periodically ask patients to identify or "level" their anxiety and to report it to the nurse. Before teaching any relaxation or thought-stopping techniques, the nurse should ask the patient to level the anxiety. Immediately after participating in behavioral exercises, patients should be asked again to identify the level of anxiety. In most cases, patients will identify alowered level; hence this is an indication to them that they can affect anxity levels and exert control, to some degree, over this discomfort. Encourage patients to level their anxiety frequently. Whenever their anxiety reaches the level of 5 or 6 they should engage in an anxiety-reducing behavior. This reporting of the level of anxiety is also helpful to the nurse in identifying content areas that produce tension in the patient, since frequently anxiety may be disguised. When patients report a level of increased anxiety, both they and the nurse are objectively able to incorporate this information for therapeutic purposes.

PROGRESSIVE RELAXATION TRAINING

Relaxation is a normal and natural activity of the body, but under most circumstances we are not usually very relaxed. Anxiety and tensions promote the nonrelaxed state, but excess anxiety and tension can be reduced through conscious relaxation of body parts. Since tension and relaxation are incompatible, relaxation can be used to overcome tension.

The nurse may wish to practice relaxation for the purpose of learning how to relax by lowering his or her own anxiety or tension level. Only after the nurse has become adept at self-relaxation and has become knowledgeable of the ramifications of relaxation from the literature (see the bibliography at the end of this chapter for references related to progressive relaxation training) should the nurse teach relaxation to others. Practice on friends and family will help the nurse to refine relaxation-teaching techniques before these are taught to patients.

To teach relaxation, the nurse will have the patient assume a comfortable position with shoes off, contact lenses out, tight clothing loosened, bladder emptied, eyes closed, and all body parts supported. A quiet, private, slightly darkened room will facilitate relaxation.

Relaxation can be achieved by either of two methods: the tension-relaxation method or the relaxation-alone method. For the tension-relaxation method, the nurse will direct the patient to try to get in a comfortable position, concentrate on her or his toes, tightly contract the muscles in the toes (to about three-fourths of maximum strength), hold the tension to the count of three, and then when the nurse says "Relax," to let go instantly of the tension. The discrepancy between the tensed and relaxed states heightens the patient's awareness of the feeling of relaxation. This tension-relaxation method is best used with individuals who have difficulty in relaxing.

Regardless of which method is used, the nurse will continue, using a soft, slow, somewhat monotone voice, instructing the patient to concentrate next on the ball of the foot, then the instep, the heel, and the ankle and move up the leg (paying particular attention to relaxing the muscles in the front of the leg) to the knee, upper leg, pelvic area (including sphincters), buttocks, waist, and chest and around to the back, upper chest, and shoulders. Have the patient pay particular attention to relaxing the shoulders which are usually in a perennial state of tension and need to be "pulled down" to relax. Encourage the patient to move at any time to facilitate relaxation of a body part.

Continue with relaxing the upper arms, elbows, lower arms, wrists, hands, and each finger. Statements can be made such as "Notice the difference between the feeling of your body in the relaxed state from the way it felt a few minutes ago," or "You may notice that there is some tingling in your fingers, signifying that even your blood vessels are becoming opened and relaxed."

Return to the shoulders and neck, first the front and then the back, smoothing out the large neck muscles, and then have the patient extend the relaxed state over the scalp and top of the head and "flow" down over the forehead into the eyebrows, eyes, cheeks and nose, mouth, tongue, and jaw muscles.

When the patient is completely relaxed, have her or him experience what it feels like to be relaxed all over. Allow the patient to remain relaxed at least 1 min before announcing that you will count backward from five to one. Add that, when you get to one, the relaxation will end but, having found relaxation so comfortable, she or he will probably wish to return to the relaxed state on her or his own soon. Then count slowly from five to one. When the patient's eyes are open, ask how she or he feels. Additionally, you may request that the level of anxiety be reascertained. Usually, the patient will report that anxiety is lower after relaxing than it was before. This is additional "objective evidence" to the patient that one can control to some degree her or his own anxiety level. This control on the part of the patient should be reinforced by the nurse, as it leads to independence, increased self-esteem, and acceptance by the patient that feelings and behavior are not beyond self-control.

After skill has been gained in relaxing according to one of the methods described, the patient will probably find shortcuts to the procedures, i.e., the entire legs can be relaxed at once, then the torso, arms, head, and neck. After practice, the patient should be able to relax in a matter of minutes or seconds.

Relaxation can be used in a variety of ways to decrease anxiety, overcome specific tensions, and to obtain an overall increased sense of calm and control. Relaxation may be used as a tool to lower feelings of tension in an anxiety-provoking situation, by the patient's consciously and inconspicuously relaxing legs, torso, and shoulders. If the patient feels anxiety rising to uncomfortable heights, she or he may retire to a private area to relax completely for a few minutes.

A third way to relax is to set aside one or two 10- to 15-min periods in the day to relax the body privately, gently sweeping all thoughts from the mind and attempting to concentrate only on the feeling of relaxation. While in this relaxed state, the mind is more open to suggestion, and the patient may wish to attempt, through autosuggestion, to make her- or himself feel refreshed, less irritable, less depressed, and more alert upon "awakening" from the relaxed state, almost as one would feel if one had taken a short nap.

For optimum safety and success, plus control on the part of the patient, relaxation should be taught as something that the patient does for her- or himself and not as an activity imposed by another. Encourage the patient to practice relaxing until it is an easy activity and until parts of the body can easily be relaxed on command.

In public situations, patients may wish to use a variation of the relaxation technique. They should take a moderately deep breath, hold it for a count of three or four, and then as they slowly exhale tell themselves subvocally to relax. This may be repeated only twice, as more than a total of three times may lead to hyperventilation and subsequent reinstitution of the anxiety state.

For patients who frequently find themselves in very high states of anxiety, to the degree that they cannot think of what to do, the nurse may suggest that they carry with them a card that lists, in order of helpfulness to them, all the things they can do to reduce their anxiety, e.g., take deep breath and hold, then relax; tell self that the anxiety has always gone away and it will go away this time; find a place to do progressive relaxation; call a friend who is a calming individual; engage in physical activity; knead some clay (kept handy for the occasion); do thought stopping, etc.

All anxiety and tension cannot be alleviated on each occasion by the use of behavioral techniques, but patients should discover that use of the techniques usually decreases the anxiety or makes it manageable. Since these techniques are taught to patients to prescribe for themselves *and use,* they should eventually come to believe that they have increased control over their anxiety and tensions.

THOUGHT STOPPING

Many individuals, healthy or not, have repeated thoughts that might be classified as "not helpful" thoughts," i.e., worries, thoughts of low self-worth, obsessions, and ruminations. It is possible to control to some degree the thoughts that one has by utilizing the thought-stopping technique. To teach this to the patient, the nurse should first instruct the patient to identify in his or her mind two or three situations or remembrances that bring pleasurable thoughts. When the patient has sufficiently identified these remembrances to him- or herself (they need not be shared with the nurse), the nurse should instruct the patient to list, in written form, all not helpful thoughts and then to reorder these thoughts in priority of how disturbing they are and how frequently they occur.

The nurse should select one not helpful thought that occurs the most frequently or is the most disturbing to the patient. The nurse will ask the patient to begin to think this thought and to visualize it vividly. When the patient signals that he or she is strongly aware of the not helpful thought, the nurse should shout, *"Stop."* Of course, the patient will be startled, but should be immediately asked, "Are you still thinking the not helpful thought?" The patient will invariably report no, whereupon the nurse should point out that the patient has evidence of being able to stop not helpful thoughts, having just done so. The patient should be instructed to use this behavioral technique every time he or she is aware of thinking a not helpful thought, by either shouting stop verbally or shouting it only in his or her head (particularly useful in public!) To further reinforce this ability to stop a thought, the patient should be instructed to immediately think of the pleasurable situation identified earlier as soon as stop has been said. If the not helpful thought returns, it should be stopped again. Many individuals find that after stopping a thought repeatedly, the frequency of the occurrence of the thought decreases.

ESTEEM ENHANCING

Although many individuals think that feelings and thoughts are separate, it does take a thought to initiate a feeling. Our personalities and self-concepts are formed by the "self-statements" we give ourselves. If our parents told us that we were bad, we incorporated this as a self-statement and experienced a subjective feeling of distress associated with this thought. Over time, perception of negative statements about the self are telescoped into an almost instantaneous feeling, usually resulting in feelings of lowered self-esteem. We bypass the statement, i.e., "I am ugly; therefore no one likes me; therefore I am worthless," and we have feelings of depression and anxiety when we identify ourselves as ugly.

The nurse can help the patient to methodically identify the self-statements given to the self in an attempt to replace negative statements with positive ones. This may be done as:

Thought: I am ugly.
Replaced thought: My face has character and is different.

or

Thought: I am ugly.
Replaced thought: Although I am ugly, I have a fantastic personality.

Have patients list the negative thoughts they have that affect their self-esteem, and then have them write beside these negative thoughts the correlative positive thoughts to insert into their consciousness whenever the negative thoughts appear.

A second self-enhancing technique to use is to instruct the clients or patients to purchase a hundred 3- by 5-in index cards, number them, and then write one statement on each card that represents something they like about themselves, e.g., "I am smart," "I am kind to others," "I have good posture," "I can play the violin," "I am interested in improving myself." These cards should be placed in a frequently visited location (such as near the telephone, in the bathroom, or in the glove compartment of the car), and should be reviewed several times per day. Frequent review of these positive self-statements will help replace or partially negate negative self-statements.

Evaluation

I. Reassessment.
  A. Has patient met immediate goals? To what extent have these been met?
  B. Has patient met long-range goals? To what extent have these been met?
  C. Which goals have not been met?
    1. Were these goals realistic?
    2. Why were these goals not met?
    3. What additional interventions might be tried in order to meet these goals?
  D. How does the patient feel with regard to meeting or not meeting these goals?
  E. What additional goals does the patient wish to address?
  F. What suggestions does the patient have that might assist her or him in meeting these goals?
II. Follow-up and reevaluation.
  A. See psychotherapist or counselor regularly as indicated.
  B. Provide patient with written instructions for dealing with anxiety if this kind of assistance is requested.
  C. Give patient phone number and address of crisis center or emergency referral agency.
  D. Expect that patient will be able to handle anxiety with minimal assistance from others.
  E. Determine and identify other community resources that patient believes to be appropriate as a source of help.

DEPRESSION: SEVERE

Definition

Depression is characterized by a feeling of sadness, lowered self-esteem, and a mood stage of melancholy, inactivity, and self-deprecation. Depression may vary in intensity, ranging from "Monday morning blues" to psychotic depression when the patient is out of touch with reality. As the most common psychiatric condition, depression increases with age and is found to some degree in most psychiatric disorders. It is generally related to situations, i.e., life-change events, isolation, loss or threatened loss, disrupted interpersonal relationships, and chronic frustrations. Dynamically, depression has been seen as the turning of anger in toward the individual rather than expressing it in more mentally healthy ways. In severe depression, the patient may be mute, immobilized and suicidal.

Assessment

   I. Data sources (refer to "Anxiety").
  II. Health history (refer to "Anxiety").
 III. Physical and behavioral assessment.
    A. Physical observations or complaints reported by the patient may include:
       1. Crying.
       2. Neglect of grooming.
       3. Bowed posture when sitting.
       4. Limited verbal communication.
       5. Anorexia.
       6. Loss of weight.
       7. Decreased movements and/or slow deliberate movements.
       8. Sad facies.
       9. Disturbed sleep patterns, i.e., goes to sleep early, awakens early, and is unable to go back to sleep.
     10. Sleeplessness.
     11. Constipation.
     12. Abdominal pain.
     13. Nausea.
     14. Headaches; pressure band around head.
     15. Poor concentration; slowed thoughts.
     16. Fatigue; tired and unrefreshed after period of sleep.
     17. Gastrointestinal upsets.
     18. Back pain (may be related to stooped posture).
     19. Palpitations unrelated to exercise.
     20. Dizziness.
     21. Flushing.
     22. Withdrawal.
    B. General feelings reported or implied by patient may include:
       1. Sad and miserable.
       2. Pessimistic.
       3. Self-blaming, filled with guilt.
       4. No interest in sexual or other activities.
       5. Depersonalization.
       6. Worthlessness.
       7. Unloved and unloveable.
    C. Other behavior related to severe depression and reported by, or observed in patient. For example:
       1. Awakens at 4 A.M. every morning and is unable to return to sleep.
       2. Cries approximately one-half of each therapeutic session.
       3. Complains of nausea at mealtimes.
       4. Refuses to eat, stating she or he is not worthy of eating.

Problems

   I. Patient feels sad, worthless, and hopeless.
  II. Patient's thought, speech, and actions are slow.
 III. Patient ruminates about worthlessness, sadness, and pessimism.
 IV. Patient is unable to express anger directly; patient smolders with hostility.

V. Patient's flow of communication is blocked; there is a paucity of detail.

VI. Patient is indecisive.

VII. Patient smiles when she or he expresses suicidal ideation.

VIII. Patient is compulsive.

IX. Patient is beset with phobias (tend to occur in middle years).

X. Patient feels unable to cope with life.

XI. Patient's self-esteem is low; this may manifest as self-injurious, self-destructive activities.

XII. Patient is neglectful of self-care and self-maintenance.

Goals of Care

I. Immediate.

   A. The patient will be protected from carrying out destructive acts toward self or others.

   B. The patient will begin to eat small quantities of food and increase nutritional status.

   C. The patient will implement medication regimen.

   D. The patient will increase verbalization with nurse.

   E. The patient will decrease self-deprecating statements (baseline data taken on first day in hospital).

   F. The patient will report suicidal thoughts.

   G. The patient will stay in room no more than a total of 1 h during daytime hours.

   H. The patient will talk briefly with other patients.

   I. The patient will engage in simple tasks assigned by the nurse.

   J. The patient will engage in occupational therapy that involves nonverbal release of tension.

   K. The patient will dress self in morning.

   L. The patient will drink at least 1500 mL of fluids per day.

   M. The patient will walk at least every 2 h.

   N. The patient will improve grooming.

II. Long-range.

   A. The patient will seek out staff and other patients with whom to talk.

   B. The patient will show congruence between words and affect.

   C. The patient will identify situations in life which seem to precipitate depression.

   D. The patient will identify individuals who can be most supportive to patient.

   E. The patient will accomplish tasks assigned.

   F. The patient will engage in recreational activities of the unit.

   G. The patient will gain insight into precursors of depression in self.

   H. The patient will recognize when he or she is starting to become depressed.

   I. The patient will identify level of anxiety (see "Special Modes of Intervention" under "Anxiety").

   J. The patient will lower anxiety through use of behavioral techniques (see "Special Modes of Intervention" under "Anxiety").

   K. The patient will identify when he or she is feeling sad, angry, frustrated, or anxious.

   L. The patient will begin to express hostility appropriately.

   M. The patient will begin to make assertive requests and responses.

   N. The patient will relate appropriately to staff, patients, family.

   O. The patient will identify ways of appropriately relieving stress or tension.

   P. The patient will be able to think about and work on painful aspects of self.

   Q. The patient will engage in recreational activities and hobbies enjoyed previously.

   R. The patient will remain reality-oriented.

   S. The patient will make positive statements about self and others.

   T. The patient will decrease use of antidepressant drugs.

   U. The patient will accomplish activities of daily living without assistance from others.

      1. The patient will eat a nutritional diet.

      2. The patient will eliminate regularly.

      3. The patient will dress appropriately.

    4. The patient will stand more erectly.

    5. The patient will sleep throughout the night.

V. The patient will report decrease in all physical symptoms.

Intervention

General Intervention	See "Anxiety."

Specific Intervention

The following interventions are to be used with the severely depressed patient hospitalized on a psychiatric unit.

    I. Use short, declarative sentences when talking with patient.

    II. Talk about neutral topics initially.

    III. Allow patient time to respond.

    IV. Avoid undue cheerfulness with patient.

    V. Encourage patient to stay out of bed and out of bedroom.

    VI. Encourage others to talk with patient.

    VII. Give brief explanation of treatments and procedures.

    VIII. Encourage patient to postpone major decisions (i.e., divorce, separation, quitting jobs, selling house) until after depression lifts.

    IX. Encourage patient to engage in small tasks that can be accomplished.

    X. Encourage use of strengths. Have patient list strengths and assets (see "Special Modes of Intervention" under "Anxiety").

    XI. Encourage replacement of negative thoughts with positive ones (see "Special Modes of Intervention" under "Anxiety").

    XII. Environment should be made conducive to decreasing depression.

    XIII. Have patient room with another patient who is verbal but not intrusive toward others.

    XIV. Provide sparse furniture, softly colored walls and furnishings; avoid bright colors in room if possible.

    XV. Assign room near enough to the nurses' station that patient can be observed frequently.

    XVI. As patient becomes less depressed, suicidal potential increases. Observe for and listen for signs of suicidal ideation (see Chap. 37).

    XVII. Remove all objects from room and environs that could potentially be used by patient to injure self.

    XVIII. Inquire of any suicidal thoughts when interviewing patient.

    XIX. Do not leave patient alone in bath or shower.

    XX. Food and fluids.

        A. Food intake should be kept nutritionally adequate.

        B. Help patient find place to eat among others.

        C. Eat with patient to assist and encourage intake.

        D. Assist patient in preparing tray.

        E. Suggest first bite and first drink.

        F. Assume patient will eat, and convey this expectation.

        G. Record accurate intake.

        H. Provide soft, easily chewed, but nutritious foods.

        I. Provide small amounts of food frequently during the 24 h.

        J. Ascertain and provide patient's food preferences.

        K. Provide hand foods if use of utensils is too difficult for the patient.

       L. Use tube feeding or IV fluids as a last resort.

       M. Provide at least six glasses of fluids per day.

    XXI. Elimination.

        A. Record accurate output.

        B. Force fluids if urine output is low.

C. If no bowel movements for 3 days:
   1. Increase passive and active exercise.
   2. Increase raw and bulky foods in diet.
   3. Ask physician for order for stool softener.
   4. Check for impaction.
   5. Enema may be given if necessary.
D. Check for diarrhea. If present:
   1. Consider request for medication to slow intestinal motility.
   2. Check for impaction (remember, diarrhea can also mean impaction). Remove impaction.

XXII. Be alert for gastrointestinal or upper respiratory infections.
   A. Take temperature once per day if fluid intake is markedly rstricted.
   B. Take vital signs once per day unless indicated or ordered more frequently.
   C. Be sure patient has adequate clothing, and covering.

XXIII. Hygiene.
   A. Administer mouth care if fluid intake is restricted. Encourage mouth care by patient.
   B. Encourage a bath every day only if this seems to be pleasing to patient; otherwise, bathing may be every 2 to 3 days if agitation occurs with bath.
   C. Shave male patients or allow patient to shave self every day.
   D. Provide sanitary needs for female patients during menses.

XXIV. Observe skin for signs of dryness, edema, reddened bony prominences.
   A. Observe for pedal edema.
   B. Encourage increased activity; walk with patient.
   C. Arrange for patient to prop up feet while sitting.
   D. Encourage increase in fluids and decrease in natural sodium and salts in diet.
   D. Apply lanolin to skin, especially vulnerable areas.

Therapeutic Intervention

I. Begin therapeutic sessions with discussion of neutral topics, and progress to feeling topics and then to insight-oriented topics as patient progresses and can cope with this.
II. Require longer verbalizations as patient improves.
III. Avoid cheerfulness and reassurances that reassure the nurse, not the patient.
IV. Avoid agreement with self-deprecating statements of patient.
V. Continue to reinforce worth and rights of patient.
VI. Reinforce grooming efforts.
VII. Avoid arguing with patient or making light of self-statement .
VIII. Reinforce increased number of positive statements about self and others.
IX. Encourage the patient to engage in activities that may increase self-esteem, e.g., writing to friends, making objects for family, beginning relationships with others.
X. Present increasingly more complex decisions for the patient to make as depression lifts.
XI. Ensure that reinforcing statements are honest and not overcomplimentary.
XII. As depression lifts, help patient to understand that depression is relatively temporary.
XIII. Assist with activities of daily living only as needed.
XIV. Provide regular but not rigid schedule of activities.
XV. Encourage activities that can be completed in a relatively short period of time, i.e., one occupational therapy session, to give patient a sense of accomplishment.
XVI. Provide progress from passive activities to more active ones.
XVII. Encourage activities that are noncompetitive, e.g., walks, puzzles, simple projects. These may progress toward more competition and complexity as patient improves.
XVIII. Arrange occupational therapy sessions that emphasize activities which involve release of body tension and expression of hostile feelings in a nonverbal (hence, less threatening) manner, e.g., pounding, hammering, sanding, rubbing, repetitive actions.

Teaching Intervention

Teaching is focused upon helping the patient who has come out of or is in the process of coming out of a depression, to learn from the situation. Teaching also provides the opportunity for the nurse to assess the patient's understanding of his or her treatment, and enlists the patient as a partner in this care. Teaching includes anticipatory guidance to help the patient learn how to prevent or minimize futur occurrences of depression

I. Suggest that verbalization to carry individuals is helpful and should be utilized early.
II. Teach progressive relaxation (see "Special Modes of Intervention" under "Anxiety").
III. Instruct in behavioral techniques, i.e., thought stopping, leveling of anxiety, and methods that assist in raising self-esteem (see "Special Modes of Intervention" under "Anxiety.")
IV. Encourage patient to identify individual precipitating factors of depression.
V. Help patient to monitor feelings and to learn to determine if there is congruence between feeling experienced and affect.
VI. Teach tools of self-monitoring and self-control.
VII. Teach assertive behavior by using role-playing exercises.
VIII. Teach management of medications.
IX. Discuss activities and skills to use when confronting anxiety situations.
X. Discuss positive self-statements that the patient has identified, and encourage patient to use these positive statements to help reverse negative statements.
XI. Discuss appropriate expression of tension and hostility.
XII. Discuss appropriate diet, dress, activities, etc.

Evaluation

I. Reassessment.
  A. Has patient met immediate goals? To what extent have these been met?
  B. Has patient met long-range goals? To what extent have these been met?
  C. Which goals have not been met?
    1. Were these goals realistic?
    2. Why were these goals not met?
    3. What additional interventions might be tried in order to meet these goals?
  D. How does the patient feel about meeting or not meeting these goals?
  E. What additional goals oes the patient wish to address?
  F. What suggestions does the patient have that might assist her or him in meeting these goals?
II. Follow-up and reevaluation.
  A. See psychotherapist, physician, and/or counselor regularly.
  B. Have first outpatient appointment set up before discharge from hospital.
  C. Have medications labeled with name, dosage, time, and precautions.
  D. Provide written information as cues to patient, i.e., cards that list what he or she can do to control anxiety and depression, and to release frustrations.
  E. Give patient phone number and address of crisis center or emergency referral agency.
  F. Expect that the patient will take medications, use what has been learned in the hospital, and seek natural support systems in own environment.
  G. Provide anticipatory guidance; role play potentially stressful situations that are likely to arise after patient leaves hospital. Focus on strengths and new coping skills of patient.

DEPRESSION: MILD TO MODERATE

Definition

Mild to moderately depressed patients are reacting to frustrations in their life situation, i.e., losses or threatened losses, anger turned inward, physical illness or disability, etc. Such patients are sad and indecisive, have little zest for living, look on the dark side of many things, and have lowered self-esteem but do not require hospitalization. Activities of daily living are carried out, but with diminished enjoyment of living. These patients may have suicidal thoughts or may actually be suicidal. They continue to plod through their days but lack joy and enthusiasm in living. Mild to moderate depression may become a permanent life-style.

Assessment

    I. Data sources (refer to "Anxiety").
  II. Health history (refer to "Anxiety").
 III. Physical and behavioral assessments.
    A. Physical observations or complaints reported by the patient may include:
        1. Crying.
        2. Slightly less well groomed than usual.
        3. Stooped posture when sitting or standing.
        4. Sad facies.
        5. Decreased verbalizations.
        6. Eats less or may eat much more.
        7. Recreational activities limited.
    B. General feelings reported or implied by patient include:
        1. Sadness.
        2. Miserable.
        3. Decreased enjoyment in living.
        4. Decreased self-esteem.
        5. Decreased motivation for activities that are customarily reinforcing to patient.
        6. Constipation.
        7. Nausea.
        8. Headaches.
        9. Tiredness and fatigue.
    C. Other behavior related to mild to moderate depression and reported by, or observed in patient. For example:
        1. Cries if frustrated when talking with employer.
        2. Has stopped visiting friends.
        3. Eats approximately 4000 cal per day.
        4. Is constipated.

Problems

     I. Patient feels hopeless about the future.
    II. Patient is indecisive.
   III. Patient's verbalization is decreasing.
   IV. Patient entertains suicidal ideation.
    V. Patient's self-esteem is low.
   VI. Patient feels hostile.
  VII. Patient feels unable to cope with life situations.

Goals of Care

  I. Immediate.
    A. The patient will decrease self-deprecating statements.
    B. The patient will interact with others at least once per day.

C. The patient will engage in previously reinforcing behaviors, whether or not she or he is in the mood to do so.

D. The patient will release tensions through sports, physical exercise, or physical work.

E. The patient will finish tasks that have been started.

F. The patient will make positive statements about self and others.

G. The patient will identify situations in life that precipitate depression.

H. The patient will identify when he or she is feeling sad, angry, frustrated or anxious.

I. The patient will identify ways of appropriately relieving tension and anxiety.

J. The patient will express hostility appropriately and interpersonally.

K. The patient will report reduced incidence of suicidal ideation.

L. The patient will be able to level anxiety (see "Special Modes of Intervention" under "Anxiety").

M. The patient will be able to use progressive relaxation (see "Special Modes of Intervention" under "Anxiety").

N. The patient will be able to use thought stopping as necessary (see "Special Modes of Intervention" under "Anxiety").

O. The patient will use esteem-enhancing behavioral techniques (see "Special Modes of Intervention" under "Anxiety").

II. Long-range.

A. The patient will associate thoughts with consequent feelings.

B. The patient will measure reality in thought, and not allow one thought to generalize to negative feelings.

C. The patient will show congruence between words and affect.

D. The patient will become a generally relaxed person.

E. The patient will expand meaningful social contacts.

F. The patient will eliminate all psychoactive drugs.

G. The patient will control anxiety when it begins rather than allowing it to turn into depression.

H. The patient will expand coping behaviors.

I. The patient will eliminate not helpful thoughts, i.e., self-deprecating, hopeless, worrying thoughts.

J. The patient will make assertive requests and responses.

K. The patient will express hostility appropriately.

L. The patient will engage in activities previously enjoyed.

M. The patient will identify more behaviors to be used in coping with crisis situations that might lead to depression.

N. The patient will gain insight into own behavior.

O. The patient will be growth-oriented.

Intervention

Refer to "Anxiety."

Evaluation

Refer to "Anxiety."

ELATION

Definition

The *elated* patient exhibits a euphoric affect, is hyperactive in movement, and may engage in bizarre, grandiose, and extravagant behaviors. Such patients must be protected from harming themselves, not as much through suicidal ideation as though lack of attention to their own safety. They must also be protected from acting on their poor judgment at this time, i.e., making decisions to give away all their money. Elated behavior is seen as an affective defense against a corresponding depression. It is a flight from depression. Patients may be depressed for a short period of the day, but elated the rest of the day.

Assessment

    I. Data Sources (see "Anxiety").
   II. Health history (see "Anxiety").
  III. Behavioral assessment: elation-related behavior reported by, or observed in, patient. For example:
      A. Refuses to go to cafeteria to eat.
      B. Sleeps only 2 h per night.
      C. Frequently gets into fights with other elated patients.
      D. Is losing approximately 1 lb per day.

Problems

      I. Patient is quick moving.
     II. Patient's speech is quickened (skips words).
    III. Patient is overly self-confident.
    IV. Patient is overly optimistic.
     V. Patient is domineering.
    VI. Patient is meddlesome.
   VII. Patient is grandiose.
  VIII. Patient is overactive.
    IX. Patient is flighty.
     X. Patient changes topic frequently.
    XI. Patient is uninhibited.
   XII. Patient exhibits keen wit.
  XIII. Patient begins tasks but usually does not finish them.
  XIV. Patient has poor judgment and is unrealistic.
   XV. Patient has delusions of grandeur.
  XVI. Patient jokes, puns, laughs hilariously at trivia.
 XVII. Patient is promiscuous.
XVIII. Patient is almost sleepless, but may sleep 2 to 4 h per night.
  XIX. Patient is losing weight.
   XX. Patient does not take time to eat.
  XXI. Patient is sensitive to interpersonal hurts.
 XXII. Patient sustains many minor physical injuries.
XXIII. Patient may be irritable, demanding, or hostile.
XXIV. Patient may be clinging, compliant, and seek approval.
 XXV. Patient has exalted opinion of self.
XXVI. Patient exhibits behavior associated with change.

Goals of Care

  I. Immediate.
    A. The patient will take in calories in proportion to increased activity.
    B. The patient will extend sleeping time to at least 5 h per night.
    C. The patient will find appropriate outlets for hostility.
    D. The patient will verbalize to the nurse for short periods of time.

    E. The patient will remain in his or her bedroom for short periods of time.

    F. The patient will refrain from destroying property.

    G. The patient will occasionally talk with other patients.

    H. The patient will engage in tasks assigned (involving much acitivity).

    I. The patient will go to recreational therapy, remaining in the yard without incident.

    J. The patient will attend occupational therapy for a short period of time.

    K. The patient will wear only necessary items of clothing.

    L. The patient will use only one cosmetic at a time.

    M. The patient will drink at least 2500 mL of fliids per day.

    N. The patient will be protected from self-inflicted injuries.

  II. Long-range.

    A. The patient will dress appropriately.

    B. The patient will report decrease in minor physical injuries.

    C. The patient will sleep at least 6 h per night.

    D. The patient will express hostility and frustration appropriately and interpersonally.

    E. The patient will be assertive (not aggressive) with others.

    F. The patient will identify ways of appropriately relieving stress and tension.

    G. The patient will reestablish relationships with family and friends.

    H. The patient will learn how to identify level of anxiety (see "Special Modes of Intervention" under "Anxiety").

    I. The patient will learn how to accomplish progressive relaxation (see "Special Modes of Intervention" under "Anxiety").

    J. The patient will be able to lower anxiety through utilization of behavioral techniques.

    K. The patient will gain insight into elation and will understand when it occurs, following what situations, etc.

    L. The patient will be able to sit and talk about feelings.

    M. The patient will show congruence between words and affect.

    N. The patient will identify life situations which precipitate elation.

    O. The patient will begin and finish tasks or projects assigned or chosen by self.

    P. The patient will remain reality oriented at all times.

    Q. The patient will decrease use of psychoactive drugs.

    R. The patient will eat a nutritionally adequate diet.

    S. The patient will remain in psychotherapy and seek therapeutic assistance when stress mounts.

    T. The patient will learn to seek intervention early when depressed behavior begins.

Intervention

General Intervention

  I. Use slow, soft, clear speech, speaking at a slower rate than that used customarily.

  II. Whisper to patient occasionally.

  III. Avoid becoming entangled and affected by patient's hyperactivity.

  IV. Provide calm, pleasant, but firm psychological environment.

  V. Avoid participating in patient's nonreality.

  VI. Firmly place limits on patient to avoid destructive behaviors.

  VII. Divert patient's attention from destructive to constructive activities as much as and as quickly as possible.

  VIII. Use postponement and substitution to encourage appropriate behavior.

  IX. Avoid reasoning or arguing with the elated patient.

  X. Attempt to establish a situation in which the patient is not the center of attention all the time.

  XI. Give short explanations.

  XII. Consider all reasonable requests.

  XIII. Minimize loud noises and loud talking around the elated patient.

  XIV. Provide only one cosmetic to use at a time, preferably in subdued shades. More cosmetics and brighter colors may be given when the patient uses them appropriately.

  XV. Keep elated patients away from each other.

Environment

   I. Assign the patient a single room, away from the hub of activity of the unit.

  II. Furnishings should be pale or monotone in color.

 III. Remove all breakable objects from the room.

 IV. Request that patient's valuables be put in a place of safekeeping to avoid their being broken, lost, or given away.

  V. Limit radio, television, magazines, and newspapers, as they provide further stimulation of the elated patient.

 VI. Keep the elated patient from remaining the center of attention on the unit.

VII. Instruct visitors concerning the patient, stressing the importance of not breaking rules for the patient.

VIII. Establish close relationship with visitors, toward the purpose of their understanding and being helpful, not hurtful, to the patient.

 IX. Limit visitors to one close family member, who can advise the rest of the family of the patient's activities and progress.

  X. Read letters written by patient before they are mailed, to avoid having the patient giving away his property or getting himself into difficulties because of his poor judgment.

 XI. Provide slow, rhythmical music as a soothing factor for patient.

*Physical
Measures*

   I. Provide the patient with a high-calorie, high-protein diet.

  II. Use plastic dishes, utensils, and cups.

 III. As the elated patient may not be able to sit and eat, provide hand foods such as a banana, apple, protein bar, sandwich, etc.

 IV. Provide the patient with fluids of her or his choice. Suggest that patient take at least one drink of water each time a water fountain is passed. Keep a specially marked cup that is always filled with juice, etc., for her or him to pick up and carry.

  V. Weigh patient at least once a week to determine weight loss or gain.

 VI. Inspect patient's body frequently for minor cuts, bruises, and joint injuries.

VII. Observe for objective signs of illness, as patient may not complain even if in pain.

VIII. Insist on at least minimal mouth hygiene. Use oil or lip pomade for cracked lips.

 IX. Encourage use of a gargle for hoarseness.

  X. Observe the elderly, elated patient for signs or symptoms of congestive heart failure, pneumonia, joint injuries, etc.

 XI. Expect the patient to eat, drink, and eliminate; convey this expectation to the patient.

XII. Provide a warm bath before retiring.

*Therapeutic
Intervention*

   I. Attempt to establish a one-to-one relationship with the patient, but postpone psychotherapy until the patient has progressed through the highly elated stage.

  II. Observe patient for swings from elation to depression, at which time suicidal ideation may arise (see Chap. 37).

 III. Encourage patient to speak openly to nurse, as one of the best deterrents to suicide is a relationship in which the patient can confide these thoughts.

 IV. Provide instruction for patient if electroconvulsive therapy is ordered.

  V. If patient is ordered lithium, check blood studies frequently, and provide a high-sodium, high-fluid diet.

 VI. Postpone entrance into group psychotherapy until the high state of elation has passed.

VII. Listen to and attempt to interact with patient.

VIII. Encourage the patient to engage in physical activities, e.g., tearing strips of rags for rag rugs, fingerpainting, painting murals, pounding or sanding objects, etc.

 IX. Assign the elated patient tasks, e.g., folding linen, raking leaves, digging in the garden, washing walls or floors, etc.

  X. Emphasize the use of continuous action of large muscle groups, avoiding activities that require discrimination or fine muscle activity.

 XI. Keep patient occupied for extended periods of time writing life history, a diary of experiences in the hospital or elsewhere, suggestions for improving the activities on the unit, etc.

Evaluation

Refer to "Depression: Severe."

BIBLIOGRAPHY

Almeida, Elza M., and Arthur H. Chapman: *The Interpersonal Basis of Psychiatric Nursing,* G. P. Putnam's Sons, New York, 1972. Practical and comprehensive treatment of depression and the manic-depressive psychosis, with emphasis on nursing interventions.

Arieti, Silvano: "Manic-Depressive PVSYCHOSIS," IN Silvano Arieti (ed.), *American Handbook of Psychotherapy,* vol. I, Basic Books Publishers, New York, 1960. Classic treatment of manic-depressive psychosis with emphasis on psychodynamics and etiological factors.

Baer, Ellen D., Madeline N. McGowan, and Diane O. McGivern: "How to Take a Health History, *American Journal of Nursing,* **77:**1190–1193, July 1977. Succinct but comprehensive overview of the health history with emphasis on and examples related to indirect questions and psychologically oriented responses.

Beck, Aaron, and Maria Kovacs, "A New, Fast Therapy for Depression," *Psychology Today,* **10:** 94–102, January, 1977. Description of cognitive therapy which uncovers the patient's distortions in thinking and subsequent feeling, minimizing misinterpretation of isolated events.

Bernstein, Douglas A., and Thomas D. Borkovec: *Progressive Relaxation Training: A Manual for the Helping Professions,* Research Press, Champaigne, Ill., 1973. Comprehensive explanation of progressive relaxation training with accompanying audiorecording.

Brown, Martha M., and Grace R. Fowler: *Psychodynamic Nursing: A Biosocial Orientation,* W. B. Saunders Company, Philadelphia, 1971. Concise overview of depression and elation with nursing interventions.

Burgess, Ann W., and Aaron Lazare: *Psychiatric Nursing in the Hospital and the Community,* Prentice-Hall, Inc., Englewood Cliffs. N.J., 1976. Basic text on psychiatric nursing which can be used as a reference for interventions dealing with depressed, elated, or suicidal patients.

Cline, Foster W: "Dealing with Depression," *Nurse Practitioner,* **2**(3):21–24, January–February 1977. Emphasis on medications used in depression.

Crary, Gerald C., and William G. Crary: "Depression," *American Journal of Nursing,* **73:**472–475, March 1973. Clarifies behavioral differences between anxiety and depression.

Davidson, Park O: *The Behavioral Management of Anxiety, Depression and Pain,* Brunner/Mazel Publishers, New York, 1976. Deals with behavioral prevention and management of anxiety, depression, expression of anger, and pain. Several rating scales, outlines of interventions, and behavioral techniques are presented. For the professional who is knowledgeable of behavior therapy.

Diran, Margaret O: "You Can Prevent Suicide," *Nursing '76,* **6:**60–64, January 1976. Contemporary overview of suicide, incidence, and predisposing factors, plus numerous nursing interventions.

Drake, Ronald E., and Joseph L. Price: "Depression: Adaptation to Disruption and Loss," *Perspectives in Psychiatric Care* **13:**163–169, October–December 1975. Philosophically and dynamically oriented article dealing with patients' perceptions of the meaning of depression and their responses to various nursing interventions.

Eggland, Ellen T: "How to Take a Meaningful Nursing History," *Nursing '77,* **7:**22–30, July 1977. Summary of health history with rationale and sample history.

Gutheil, Emil A: "Reactive Depression," *American Handbook of Psychotherapy,* vol. I, Basic Books Publishers, New York, 1960. Classic and psychodynamic overview of nonpsychotic depression.

Horsley, Jo A., and Maxine E. Loomis: *Interpersonal Change: A Behavioral Approach to Nursing Practice,* McGraw-Hill Book Company, New York, 1974. Excellent summary of behavioral management, with many applications to general patient care. Useful basic book specifically related to incorporating behavior modification in planning and implementing nursing care.

Parrino, John J., and Barry A. Tanner: *Helping Others: Behavioral Procedures for Mental Health Workers,* E-B Press, Eugene, Ore., 1975. Simple overview of behavioral techniques that are applicable to psychiatric nursing and general nursing. Includes relaxation training, thought stopping, etc. Interventions are leveled to the education and experience of the helper.

"Programmed Instruction: Helping Depressed Patients in General Nursing Practice," *American Journal of Nursing* **77:**1007–1038, June 1977. Programmed instruction with vignettes of depressed patients and varying nursing approaches. Includes test of competency. Excellent review of general approaches to the depressed patient.

Robbins, Jhan, and Dave Fisher: *How to Make and Break Habits,* Dell Publishing Co., New York,

1973. Oriented toward the lay person, this book is particularly valuable for the chapter on relieving of tension, wherein explicit instructions on progressive relaxation are presented. Also covered are suggestions on behavioral techniques to use in breaking habits of overeating, smoking, excessive drinking, disruptive behavior, etc.

Snyder, Joyce C., and Marge Foltz Wilson: "Elements of a Psychological Assessment," *American Journal of Nursing,* **77:**235–239, February 1977. Organization of the psychological assessment according to various psychological theories. Actual questions to use under categories of the assessment are presented.

37

Threats to Survival

Imogene Stewart Rigdon and Karolyn Lusson Godbey

The purpose of this chapter is to describe the nursing process for (1) the suicidal patient who is a threat to her or his own survival and (2) the violent patient who is a threat to the survival of others. Awareness of the impact of the patient's threat on the family, significant others, and the nurse is considered to be a part of this process.

A threat is defined as a verbal and/or physical expression of the intention to hurt, destroy, or punish self or others. The patient's threat, whether it is self-directed or other-directed, arises out of the patient's feelings of hopelessness and helplessness. The patient resorts to destructive behaviors in a desperate attempt to obtain relief from these feelings.

When faced with the patient's threat, the family and/or significant others are often overwhelmed by their own responses. They are in need of and deserve the attention of a nurse.

Intervening with the threatening patient is an anxiety-producing experience for the nurse. The nurse needs to be aware of his or her personal response, as well as any conflict between personal and professional responses.

At any point in time the threat of destruction may become an actuality and would then be considered a psychiatric emergency. Such psychiatric emergencies would include situations in which:

1. The nurse responsible considers the situation beyond his or her control.
2. An actual suicide attempt has been made (such as, patient has taken a bottle of pills or cut wrists).
3. The patient has a lethal weapon on her or his person (such as a loaded gun or a knife).
4. A direct physical assault on a person has been made.

Such emergencies will not be dealt with in this chapter. See Chap. 46.

Both suicidal patients and violent patients may be encountered in every clinical area of nursing. This chapter is designed primarily for the nurse in the hospital but can be adapted for use in other areas. It is our hope that the nursing process presented in this chapter will help the nurse to begin to meet the needs of these patients, their significant others, and themselves.

THE THREAT OF SUICIDE

Definition

Suicide is a continuum of self-destructive behaviors that without intervention would result in death. This continuum ranges from habitual self-inflicted, life-threatening behaviors to isolated acts that could result in instant death. For the purposes of this section, the suicidal patient is one who (1) is thinking about committing a self-destructive act, (2) is expressing the intent to commit a self-destructive act, or (3) has recently attempted or committed a self-destructive act. The patient who has actually committed a self-destructive act requiring immediate intervention is considered a psychiatric emergency. The nursing process for this patient can be found in Chap. 46.

Assessment

I. Data sources.
A. Patient.

    B. Patient's significant others, including both family and friends.

    C. Police report.

    D. Emergency room staff.

    E. Intensive care staff.

    F. Health care personnel previously and presently associated with the patient (e.g., crisis intervention center).

    G. Past health and family history.

    H. Observation of patient's behavior, both verbal and nonverbal.

II. Observation of the patient's interaction with family, friends, and others.

III. Health history (see the initial nursing interview detailed under "Anxiety" in Chap. 36). Give special attention to the psychosocial history. Suicide rate increases with persons who have or believe they have a serious and/or chronic illness.

IV. Sociocultural clues to suicide.

    A. Age.

        1. Committed suicide increases with age.

        2. Suicide is increasing among adolescents, especially college students.

    B. Sex.

        1. Men are 3 times more likely than women to commit suicide.

        2. Women are 3 times more likely than men to attempt suicide.

    C. Precipitating events or stresses must be evaluated from the patient's point of view. Some stresses to be considered are:

        1. Loss of significant person by death, giving special attention to:

            a. Recent loss.

            b. One-year anniversary of the loss.

        2. Loss of significant person by divorce or separation.

        3. Loss of job, prestige, or status.

        4. Loss of health through illness, surgery, or accident.

        5. Threat of prosecution or criminal exposure.

    D. Support systems.

        1. Suicide risk is higher in the absence of available support systems. Resources to be considered are:

            a. Family.

            b. Friends.

            c. Neighbors.

            d. Physician.

            e. Clergy and church members.

            f. Lawyer.

            g. Employers and coworkers.

            h. Police.

            i. Social work agencies.

            j. Recreational and social organizations.

        2. Evaluate support systems in terms of their ability to give emotional support, since some, such as families and friends, may actually be relying on the patient for support.

    E. Life-style. The suicide rate is higher in persons with an unstable life-style, which would include such things as:

        1. Inconsistent work history.

        2. Unstable or disruptive family relationships.

        3. Unstable or disruptive marital relationships.

    F. Family.

        1. Risk of suicide is higher in divorced or single than in married persons.

        2. Risk of suicide is higher in smaller than in larger families.

        3. Risk of suicide is increased if persons in the patient's nuclear or extended family have attempted or comitted suicide.

    G. Race.

        1. Suicide rate is higher in the white than in the black population.

2. Suicide rate is increasing for black males and American Indian males.
H. Occupation.
  1. Suicide rate is highest among professionals, especially psychiatrists and lawyers.
  2. Suicide is the second most common cause of death in college students.
I. Time.
  1. Rate of suicide is higher in the early morning hours (2 to 5 A.M.), associated with the early morning awakening of the depressed patient.
  2. More suicides are committed on Monday and Tuesday than on any other days of the week.
  3. More suicides are committed in the spring than in any other season of the year.
V. Behavioral clues to suicide.
  A. Suicide plan: ask the patient directly about her or his plan (e.g., "*How* do you plan to kill yourself?"). Assess:
    1. Lethality of method: hanging, jumping from high places, and method involving use of a gun are more lethal and involve higher risk than taking pills or cutting wrist.
    2. Availability of method (e.g., does patient have the gun in hand or must it be purchased?).
    3. Specificity of details:
      a. Preparation made.
      b. Time set.
      c. Bizarre details are less threatening, unless the patient is psychotic.
  B. Previous suicide attempts. The person who has made a previous suicide attempt is likely to resort to the same behavior again.
  C. Communication that indicates patient is thinking of suicide.
    1. Verbal:
      a. Direct statements such as, "I'm going to kill myself!"
      b. Indirect statements such as, "There isn't any point in going on!" or "Take these golf clubs; I won't be needing them anymore."
      c. Cessation of verbal communication, especially with family and significant others.
    2. Nonverbal:
      a. Writing letters to ask forgiveness, to forgive others, or to say goodbye.
      b. Writing a will.
      c. Unexpectedly buying a life insurance policy.
      d. Changes in attitudes toward personal possessions.
        (1) Refusal to spend money for new possessions.
        (2) Giving away possessions.
      e. Sudden changes in behavior that are uncharacteristic, such as taking walks at midnight, staying in room alone for hours.
  D. Depression (see "Depression: Severe" in Chap. 36).
    1. Change in sleep patterns, especially awakening in early morning (2 to 5 A.M.), insomnia.
    2. Loss of appetite.
    3. Weight loss.
    4. Social withdrawal.
    5. Despondency.
    6. Apathy.
    7. Severe feelings of helplessness and hopelessness.
    8. Physical and psychological exhaustion.
    9. Deepening of depression: may indicate patient has given up all hope.
    10. Lessening of depression: patient has more energy to actually carry out a self-destructive act.
    11. Overtly cheerful behavior for no apparent reason. The decision to kill oneself may be followed by relief and unexplained lessening of depressive symptoms.
  E. Some conditions may precipitate impulse acts to obtain relief from anxiety. These

conditions warrant special consideration because there may be no other clues to the self-destructive act.

    1. Extreme fear and anxiety.

    2. Hallucinations that are verbally persecutory and self-accusatory or visually tormenting. Patient may respond to voices' command to kill self. Patient may attempt suicide in an effort to silence or get away from threatening, unfriendly voices. (See Chap. 38.)

    3. Delusional thinking that is threatening in content (see Chap. 38).

F. Determination. Patient who must maintain control over environment, no matter how anguished or incapacitated he or she may seem, could implement suicidal plan even when it seems impossible. A determined patient who seems too apathetic to get out of bed, for example, may jump from the window during a change of shifts.

G. Dependency. Being dependent on others usually necessitates much manipulation of others and, at the same time, results in hostility toward others. This is seen in statements such as, "I'll take a whole bottle of pills. Then my parents will be sorry they weren't nicer to me!"

H. Beliefs about life after death, e.g., the patient who believes he or she will go to hell may be deterred.

I. Strengths: the inner resources of the patient.

    1. Ability to respond by accepting directions.

    2. Ability to reach out.

    3. Improvement in mood and thinking during course of conversation.

    4. Past history of success in interpersonal relationships.

VI. Emergency assessment. In emergency situations, when a complete assessment of suicidal risk cannot be accomplished, the nurse should assess:

A. Suicidal plan. Ask patient directly about the plan (e.g., "How do you plan to kill yourself?"). Assess:

    1. Lethality of method: hanging, jumping from high places, and method involving use of a gun are more lethal and involve higher risk than taking pills or cutting wrist.

    2. Availability of method. Does patient have gun, pill, etc., with her or him?

    3. Specificity of details.

        a. Preparation made.

        b. Time set.

        c. Bizarre details are less threatening, unless patient is psychotic.

B. Previous suicide attempts. The patient who has made a previous suicide attempt is more likely to resort to the same behavior again.

C. Age: risk increases with age.

D. Sex: men are more likely than women to commit suicide; women are more likely than men to attempt suicide.

E. Precipitating events or stress must be evaluated from the patient's point of view. Some stresses to be considered are listed under point **IV** C, above. Ask patient questions such as, "What about life seems so intolerable that you want to kill yourself?"

F. Immediately available support systems. Who is with the patient now? Who is available to stay with the patient? Who is close to the patient?

Problems

    I. Life-threatening thoughts and gestures.

   II. Feelings of despair and hopelessness.

  III. Impaired self-esteem.

  IV. Impaired communication with significant others.

   V. Potential loss of control over present life situation.

Goals of Care

I. Immediate.
   A. The patient will be protected from self-destruction until she or he is able to assume this responsibility.
   B. The patient will report suicidal thoughts and/or hallucinations.
   C. The patient will engage in easily accomplished tasks assigned by the nurse.
   D. The patient will participate in diversional activities that provide nonverbal release of tension.
   E. The patient will make simple decisions such as what to eat, wear, and watch on television.
   F. The patient will begin to verbally identify feelings of anger.

II. Long-range.
   A. The patient will recognize when he or she is becoming suicidal.
   B. The patient will identify stresses in life which seem to precipitate suicidal thoughts.
   C. The patient will verbalize alternative behaviors to suicide.
   D. The patient will reestablish relationships with friends and family or establish new relationships when none are present.
   E. The patient will identify individuals who can be most supportive.
   F. The patient will verbalize one positive statement about self each day.
   G. The patient will list strengths and talents.
   H. The patient will verbalize one reason for living each day.
   I. The patient will identify life situation which he or she would like to change.

Intervention

All nursing interventions for the suicidal or self-destructive patient are based on the belief that the patient is ambivalent, that is, she or he wants to live *and* wants to die.

I. Intervention during hospitalization (*see* also specific interventions discussed under "Depression: Severe" in Chap. 36).
   A. General intervention. Interpersonal relationships are the greatest deterrent to suicide. A sense of someone listening and caring is essential to human survival. The nurse is a temporary lifeline. From the first contact with a suicidal person, plan for the establishment or the continuance of the usual social relationships.
   B. Specific intervention.
      1. Have one nurse on each shift establish a one-to-one relationship with the patient.
      2. Do not leave patient alone.
      3. As suicide risk decreases, decrease observations to frequent, irregular intervals (every 5 to 10 min).
      4. Search patient's personal belongings.
      5. Remove dangerous objects such as razor blades, drugs, nail files, glass objects, cords, belts, panty hose, and neckties.
      6. Explain why personal belongings are removed and that they will be returned.
      7. Give the patient a semiprivate room near the nurse's station.
      8. Notify the family or significant others that the patient is suicidal.
      9. Do not agree to keep secret the patient's reported thoughts or plans of suicide.
      10. Give medication in liquid form.
      11. Supply nourishment and physical care as needed.
      12. Instruct the patient warmly and emphatically of the necessity of always delaying any self-destructive impulse and of calling for help.
      13. Approach the patient with a hopeful attitude. Avoid overly cheerful attitude.
      14. Encourage tasks the patient can successfully accomplish in a short period of time.

15. Encourage diversional activities that can be an outlet for angry feelings, such as pounding copper in occupational therapy, bowling, working out on a punching bag, and throwing a medicine ball.

16. Avoid contact sports that could provoke the release of stored-up fury and competitive activities that could lead to a sense of failure.

17. Help the patient to participate gradually in group activities to prevent isolation and withdrawal.

18. Permit the patient to make suicidal threats whenever she or he has a need.
    a. Do not ignore or argue about threats.
    b. Take statement seriously; it is communication, not an idle gesture. The idea that people who talk about suicide will not commit suicide is a myth.
    c. Validate the patient's feelings.
    d. Do not share interpretation of the meaning of the patient's suicidal behavior with her or him.

19. Remind patient that suicide is one alternative and that there are other alternatives available.

20. Help the patient's family and significant others to identify and share their feelings. Feelings which they may experience are embarrassment, guilt, anger, self-doubt, and confusion.

21. Help patient's family and significant others identify support systems that can be useful to them.

22. Observe circumstances under which suicidal behavior occurs.

23. Help patient identify the early signs and symptoms of suicidal behavior.

24. Help patient identify specific stresses precipitating suicidal behavior.

25. Help patient identify alternative solutions, other than suicide, to stresses he or she identifies, and elaborate on them.

26. Have patient list strengths he or she may use in coping with stress.

27. Reinforce positive actions and responses to stress.

28. Avoid confronting the patient with the observation that he or she seems to be improving. Allow the patient to identify improvement in self. Confronting patient with improvement before he or she is ready to acknowledge it may precipitate suicidal response.

II. Telephone intervention. The nurse on a psychiatric inpatient unit or in the emergency room may receive a telephone call from a patient threatening suicide or self-destructive acts. The following interventions are designed to help the nurse meet this situation.

A. Establish caring and firm relationship with the suicidal person.
   1. Listen carefully.
   2. Talk and respond. Do not simply reflect feelings.
   3. Make direct, hopeful statements, e.g., "It sounds as if you do want to live, and I can and will help you."

B. Obtain basic information.
   1. Who are you?
   2. Where are you?

C. Complete emergency assessment of suicidal risk can be found above, under "Assessment" (point V).

D. Assist the person to identify and clarify the focal problem as she or he perceives it. What is making life intolerable at this moment? Why is patient calling at this time?

E. Be directive, and make decisions for the person, e.g., "I am going to send someone to your house now. You keep talking to me."

F. Involve significant others and all possible support systems. Who is with the patient now? Who is next door? Who can the nurse contact to stay with the patient? Do not rely on patient to contact this person.

G. Make contact with appropriate resource for follow-up care. Ask patient for preference. Options available are crisis center, community mental health center, police, private therapist, private doctor, doctor on call.

III. Nurse's feelings and responses. The nurse needs to be aware of her or his own response to the suicidal patient, especially the patient who has already attempted suicide. The nurse may:

A. Experience anxiety when faced with a suicidal patient, since this brings to consciousness the thoughts or fantasies of suicide which everyone has at one time or another.

B. Feel anger because the nurse was able to control own impulse to escape through suicide and the patient was not.

C. Feel burdened by the responsibility for preventing self-destructive behavior, which in turn causes tension and anxiety.

D. Feel frustrated and drained from the dependency of the patient on the nurse.

E. Have fantasies of rescuing the patient all alone.

F. Feel angry and incompetent if the patient attempts suicide in spite of her or his interventions.

G. Judge the patient's behavior in the context of her or his own life (e.g., a patient who attempts suicide to escape marriage is judged harshly by a nurse whose spouse is dead). Other peers and team members are a potential support system that the nurse has for sharing and dealing with these feelings. It is important for the nurse to utilize this support system.

IV. Involuntary hospitalization. All states provide for some form of involuntary hospitalization for the patient who is considered an imminent danger to himself or herself. The nurse needs to be familiar with state mental health legislation.

Evaluation

I. Reassessment.

A. Does the ongoing assessment of the patient's suicidal and/or behavioral clues indicate that the danger of suicide is more or less imminent?

B. What is the behavioral evidence that the patient has met the immediate goals?

C. What is the behavioral evidence that the patient has met the long-range goals?

D. How does the patient feel with regard to meeting or not meeting these goals?

E. How does the nurse feel with regard to his or her meeting or not meeting these goals?

F. Which goals have not been met, and what interfered?

1. Was the goal shared by the patient?
2. Was the goal stated so broadly or vaguely as to be immeasureable?
3. Was the goal unrealistic?
4. What other interventions might be more effective in achieving these goals?

G. Do the goals need to be changed?

H. Do the problems need to be discontinued because goals have been attained?

I. What new or additional goals can be identified?

1. What new or additional goals woul the patient like to achieve?
2. What new or additional goals can the nurse identify for the patient to achieve?
3. Are these goals shared?

II. Follow-up and reevaluation.

A. Be certain that patient has reestablished at least one personal tie.

B. Determine that living arrangements are such that the patient will not be alone.

C. Teach significant other the behavioral clues to suicide.

D. Teach significant other, without alarming her or him, that the first month after discharge is a critical period of suicide risk.

E. Have patient and significant other consider the choice of family therapy, if indicated.

F. Reassess with patient and significant other their possible support systems in the community: friends, neighbors, relatives, clergy, community mental health center, police, visiting nurses, nurses in college and university health services, emergency referral agencies, social work agencies, legal counsel.

    G. Review with the patient the early signs and symptoms of suicidal behavior.

    H. Review with the patient the alternative ways she or he has of dealing with stress other than suicide.

    I. Encourage patient to see an outpatient therapist before discharge and to continue with the same therapist.

    J. Set up the first appointment for outpatient visit with therapist.

    K. Give the patient the telephone number and address of the suicide prevention center or emergency referral agency.

THE THREAT OF VIOLENCE

Definition

Violence is a continuum of physically destructive behaviors that without intervention would result in injury, damage, or destruction to other persons or property. This continuum ranges from minor property damage to murder. Violence toward persons demands a life-risking response from the nurse. In violence toward property, the nurse accepts the reponsibility of controlling it only when there is no life-threatening risk. Violence by the hospitalized patient rarely occurs but, understandably, the fear among nurses is that it will occur. Both the patient's behavior and the responsibility of the nurse are frightening.

For the purposes of this section, the violent patient will be defined as one who is either (1) thinking about committing violence or (2) expressing verbally or physically the intent to commit a violent act. The nursing process will be developed for hospitalized patients who are threatening violence, and its focus will be the prevention of violence itself. Feeling confident in this process may lessen the nurse's fear and increase his or her effectiveness. The patient who is actually committing a physically destructive act requiring immediate intervention is considered a psychiatric emergency. The nursing process for this patient can be found in Chap. 46.

Assessment

  I. Data sources.

    A. Patient.

    B. Patient's significant others, including family and friends.

    C. Past health history.

    D. Observation of the patient's behavior, both verbal and nonverbal.

    E. Other patients' reported observations.

    F. Nurses's intuition: "gut reaction" of fear and danger.

  II. Health history (see the initial nursing interview detailed under "Anxiety" in Chap. 36). Give special attention to the psychosocial history.

  III. Behavioral clues.

    A. General.

      1. Verbalizations.

        a. Threats such as, "I'm going to hit you."

        b. Apprehension, fear, or concern about losing control such as "I'm going to blow up," or "I'm afraid I'm going to hit someone."

        c. Indirect threats such as, "I hate you."

      2. Affect.

        a. Intensity is marked.   **d.** Labile: rapid fluctuation to extremes.

        b. Angry facial expression.   **e.** Belligerent.

        c. Tense facial expression.

    B. Psychotic disturbances due to either functional or organic states may precipitate impulsive acts of violence. These conditions warrant special consideration because there may be no other clue to the violent act.

    1. Acute organic brain syndrome (see also Chap. 46).
        a. Illnesses in which general toxemia occurs.
        b. Intoxication and/or withdrawal from alcohol and/or other drugs.
        c. Trauma.
    2. Functional psychotic disturbances (see also Chap. 38).
        a. Delusional thinking that is threatening in content.
        b. Hallucinations that are verbally persecutory or visually tormenting.
        c. Manic depression, manic state (see also Chap. 36).
  C. Nonpsychotic.
    1. The antisocial personality who has no concern for others.
    2. The docile person approached in an aggressive, hostile way who may react with violence.
    3. Motor activity.
        a. Agitation: inability to sit still, pacing.
        b. Sudden cessation of activity: uneasy, tense stillness.
        c. Intensity: pounding, slamming, stomping.
        d. Jumpiness.
        e. Rigid, tense posture.
    4. History of previous destructive behaviors or violence. At what point and under what conditions does she or he lose control?
    5. Refusing medications and treatments.
IV. Situation in which threat occurs is usually one in which the patient perceives the threat of annihilation either through destruction of physical self, or perhaps, even more frightening, through destruction of self-esteem. The patient's threat is a desperate attempt to defend self against this threat of annihilation.
  A. Where is the patient?
  B. Who is with the patient?
  C. How lethal is the situation?
  D. Is the situation obviously provoking the patient to threaten violence, and can the situation be changed? Patient, e.g., is being harassed by roommate, who can be moved to another room until the two of them are able to resolve the problem.
  E. How does the patient perceive the situation?
  F. What is the patient's relationship to others? To whom does this patient relate best?
  G. Are alcohol and/or more serious drugs present on the unit?

Problems

I. Potential loss of self-control.
II. Perception of threat to self.
III. Feelings of fear and helplessness.

Goals of Care

I. Immediate.
  A. The patient will maintain self-control.
  B. The patient will be prevented from harming others.
II. Long-range.
  A. The patient will identify and report feelings of losing control.
  B. The patient will examine situation and identify stresses that are seen as perceived threats to self.
  C. The patient will identify stresses which seem to precipitate fear of loss of control.
  D. The patient will consider the consequences of losing control.
  E. The patient will verbally identify alternative behaviors to loss of control.

Intervention

I. Administrative intervention. Nursing administration has an important responsibility in the control of violent behavior on the nursing unit. This responsibility includes:

  A. The establishment of a therapeutic milieu staffed by well-trained and caring personnel.

  B. The establishment of a standard plan of action, with stated expectations for staff responses to violent behavior.

  C. Designating one person on each shift as leader/coordinator of the plan of action whose orders must be followed immediately and without question.

  D. Educating the staff to the plan of action and to therapeutic interventions in the prevention and control of violence.

  E. Providing a "quiet room," a specific room with provisions for privacy, decreased stimulation, and safety.

  F. Holding a staff meeting to review staff responses to the threat of violence.

II. Specific intervention.

  A. Take the threat of violence seriously.

  B. Remove others who may be in danger as quickly as possible.

  C. Look for immediate stresses that could be provoking the threat, such as another person arguing with the patient.

  D. Allow distance. Touch may be the final threat to loss of control.

  E. Speak to patient in a calm, firm, reassuring manner.

  F. Call patient by her or his name.

  G. Explain clearly and directly that the patient is expected to control herself or himself, e.g., "Now calm down. You can control yourself."

  H. Verbally acknowledge patient's dangerous potential, e.g., "Look, you could really have hurt someone with that pool cue." This confirms the patient's stance and reduces her or his need to be defensive.

  I. Verbally set limits on behavior, e.g., "I'm not going to let you hit anyone with that pool cue. Put it down and let's talk." Talking is an effective way of helping patient to regain self-control.

  J. Verbally acknowledge patient's feelings, e.g., "You seem very frightened."

  K. Offer medication. If patient refuses, offer again at a later time. If patient becomes violent, and medication must be given despite refusal, the nurse needs to be aware of state mental health legislation governing the administration of medications without consent.

  L. Do not threaten the patient with the use of force, e.g., "If you don't do as I say, I'll lock you up." The threat of force may:

    1. Be seen as a challenge, and thus create a power struggle.

    2. Increase the patient's fear, and escalate the threat of violence into a violent act.

    3. Decrease the patient's confidence in the nurses's ability to control the environment if the nurse is not capable of carrying out the threat.

    4. Result in patient's viewing the use of force as a punishment rather than an adjunct to self-control.

  M. Give patient the opportunity to go to the "quiet room" with one staff member, preferably one to whom the patient best relates. Other team members should be alerted and prepared to initiate the predetermined plan of action if the need arises.

  N. Do not leave the patient alone.

  O. Help the patient to identify and discuss feelings concerning the incident.

  P. Explore with patient past feelings and/or events of violence that may have been similar to the present incident.

  Q. Help the patient identify early signs of losing control.

  R. Help patient identify specific stresses that precipitate loss of control.

  S. Help patient to identify the consequences of violent behavior.

T. Help patient identify alternative solutions other than violence to stresses he or she identifies.

U. Provide constructive physical outlets for the expression of feelings, e.g., brisk walks, gardening.

V. Use physical force only if the patient is actually violent toward another person. The need for the use of physical force may be greater with the psychotic patient who is less likely to respond to the verbal intervention of the nurse. When the use of force is necessary it needs to be carried out as swiftly as possible, avoiding physical pain and undue humiliation to the patient.

W. Apply mechanical restraints only if absolutely necessary. The patient fearing loss of control occasionally requests the use of mechanical restraints. This request needs to be respected. The restraints are perceived by the patient as providing the control he or she is seeking. On the other hand, the nurse needs to be familiar with state mental health legislation before restraining the unwilling patient.

X. Use seclusion as an alternative to restraints. The seclusion room is stripped of all furnishings except a mattress. There should be no exposed light bulbs or glass and no access to the bathroom. Ideally, the room is a neutral or calming color, such as green.

Y. Notify the patient's family or significant others; they may be able to calm the patient.

III. Nurse's feelings and responses.

A. The nurse's fear of personal injury is a natural response to the patient's threat of violence. The degree of fear will be different for each nurse, depending on how life-threatening he or she considers the patient's threat. Feelings of fear can be paralyzing, or they can signal the presence of danger and the need for intervention with the patient. Fear can also evoke a variety of responses from the nurse. The nurse may:

1. Have the impulse to run away. A wise nurse may leave temporarily to seek the assistance of others. This is not running away.
2. Feel anger and outrage at the patient's threat, and threaten the patient in return, e.g., "If you do that, I'll lock you up," or, "I'll take your privileges away." Such threats of retaliation create a power struggle which no one wins.
3. Acquiesce to the patient's demands even when it is not safe to do so.
4. Be judgmental and rejecting since the patient's behavior is contrary to his or her values.
5. Feel anxious that he or she will not be able to control the situation and that actual violence will occur.
6. Be concerned that peers or supervisor will not approve of the way he or she intervened.
7. See in the patient own potential for losing control.

B. Being in touch with one's own unique responses to the threat of violence is a prerequisite to effective intervention. Other peers and members of the health team are a potential support system that the nurse has for sharing and dealing with his or her responses.

Evaluation

I. Reassessment.

A. Does the ongoing assessment of the patient's behavioral clues indicate that the danger of violence is more or less imminent?

B. What is the behavioral evidence that the patient has met the immeidate goals?

C. What is the behavioral evidence that the patient has met the long-range goals?

D. How does the patient feel with regard to meeting or not meeting these goals?

E. How does the nurse feel with regard to meeting or not meeting these goals?

F. Which goals have not been met, and what interfered?

1. Was the goal shared by the patient?

2. Was the goal stated so broadly or vaguely as to be immeasureable?
3. Was the goal unrealistic?
4. What other interventions might be more effective in achieving these goals?

G. Do the goals need to be changed?

H. Do the problems need to be discontinued because goals have been attained?

I. What new or additional goals can be identified?
1. What new or additional goals would the patient like to achieve?
2. What new or additional goals can the nurse identify for the patient to achieve?
3. Are these goals shared?

II. Follow-up and reevaluation.

A. With the patient. The follow-up care for the patient who threatens violence is dependent on the underlying problem, e.g., alcoholism, manic depression, elevated blood urea nitrogen (BUN) level, etc. The nurse will need to identify this problem in order to provide follow-up care for the patient.

B. With the patient's family or significant others:
1. Help them to identify and share their feelings, e.g., guilt, embarrassment, fear of having the patient return home.
2. Help them identify support systems that can be useful to them.

C. With the other patients. Follow-up with patients against whom the threat was directed, or those who witnessed the threat, is primary. If the incident creates general agitation among other patients they would, also, be included in the follow-up.
1. Verbally reassure them that the danger is over and that they are safe.
2. Encourage discussion of their feelings and reactions to the incident.
3. Validate their feelings concerning the incident.

D. With staff:
1. Discuss and evaluate what happened and why.
2. Discuss and share their feelings surrounding the incident.
3. Discuss questions such as:
   a. Did the staff threaten the patient with physical force?
   b. Was the nurse involved in a power struggle?
   c. Was physical force used as a last resort?
   d. Was force meant to be punitive or therapeutic?
   e. What interventions were most successful?

BIBLIOGRAPHY

Almeida, Elza M., and Arthur H. Chapman: *The Interpersonal Basis of Psychiatric Nursing,* G. P. Putnam's Sons, New York, 1972. Basic text on psychiatric nursing. Gives practical nursing interventions with suicidal and hostile patients.

Anderson, Nancy P.: "Suicide in Schizophrenia," *Perspectives in Psychiatric Care,* **11**(3):106–112, 1973. Fear of the recurrence of mental illness, sudden onset of psychosis, and remission of psychotic symptoms are clues to high suicidal risk for the schizophrenic. This article deals with the nursing process in the care of a suicidal schizophrenic patient.

Bailey, David S., and Sharon O. Dreyer: *Therapeutic Approaches to the Care of the Mentally Ill,* F. A. Davis Company, Philadelphia, 1977. Basic textbook for mental health workers. Concepts of communication are stressed. Interventions with suicidal patients are very specific, and a suicide intervention rating scale is provided. Has helpful chapter on interventions with aggressive patients.

Bircher, Andrea U.: "On the Development and Classification of Diagnosis," *Nursing Forum,* **14**:11–29, 1975. Explains what nursing diagnosis is, its dangers and its values, and proposes Maslow's hierarchy of human needs as an organizing principle from which a relevant, exhaustive classification of nursing diagnosis can be derived.

Bower, Fay Louise: *The Process of Planning Nursing Care: A Model For Practice,* The C. V. Mosby Company, St. Louis, 1977. Addresses the core of nursing practice, the nursing process. Presents a theoretical framework for holistic planning of nursing care.

Burgess, Ann Wolbert, and Aaron Lazare: *Psychiatric Nursing in the Hospital and the Community,* 2d ed., Prentice-Hall, Inc., Englewood Cliffs, N.J., 1976. The central focus of this book is humanistic.

It is especially helpful by devoting attention to stalls in the therapuetic process and a look at the humanness of the nurse. It discusses management of suicidal patients.

Davitz, Lois J., and Joel Davitz: "How Do Nurses Feel When Patients Suffer," *American Journal of Nursing,* **75**(9):1505–1510, September 1975. Looks at the problems that nurses face as they deal with both the professional and the human side of nursing. The authors ask many provocative and unanswered questions.

Farberow, Norman L.; and Edwin I. Schneidman: *The Cry for Help,* McGraw-Hill Book Company, New York, 1965. Focuses on the message of anguish and the plea for help that is expressed by and contained within suicidal behaviors. It discusses both community and psychotherapeutic responses to that cry for help.

Fawcett, Jan: *Dynamics of Violence,* American Medical Association, Chicago, 1971. Provides a world view of violence, some research investigations, and clinical problems with individual violence.

Feldman, Marvin J., et al.: *Fears Related to Death and Suicide,* MSS Information Corporation, New York, 1974. A collection of articles previously published on psychological theories on death and attitudes toward death in suicidal persons.

Flynn, Gertrude: "Interference or Intervention," *Perspective in Psychiatric Care,* **7**(4):170–186, 1960. Gives analysis of five patient-centered situations, including assessment, interventions, rationale, and possible outcomes. The situations include verbally abusive and physically violent patients. Gives excellent guidelines to therapeutic communication with violent patients.

Frederick, Calvin J.: "The Role of the Nurse in Crisis Intervention and Suicide Prevention," *Journal of Psychiatric Nursing and Mental Health Services,* **11**(1):27–31, January–February, 1973. Concise synopsis of symptoms of self-destructive behavior and the nurse's response.

Grace, Helen K., Janice Layton, and Dorothy Camilleri: *Mental Health Nursing,* Wm. C. Brown Company Publishers, Dubuque, 1977. Theoretical framework integrates social systems, social-psychological perspectives, growth and development, and crisis concepts. Views suicidal behavior as a severe restriction in the effectiveness of a person's problem-solving ability.

Grosicki, Jeanette P. (ed.) and the Committee on Research in Clinical Nursing of VA Hospital, North Little Rock Arkansas Division: *Nursing Action Guides,* U.S. Government Printing Office, Washington, D.C., 1970. Focuses on nursing interventions and their rationale. Identifies problems which interfere with the accomplishment of goals.

Haber, Judith, Anita Leach, Sylvia Schudy, and Barbara Flynn Sideleau: *Comprehensive Psychiatric Nursing,* McGraw-Hill Book Company, New York, 1978. An excellent, truly comprehensive book on psychiatric nursing. Develops the nursing process with both suicidal and violent patients.

Joel, Lucille A., and Doris L. Collins: *Psychiatric Nursing: Theory and Application,* McGraw-Hill Book Company, New York, 1978. Nursing theory and process are developed for working with patients, individually, in groups, and in the family. Crisis intervention and community theory are also included.

Jourard, Sidney M.: "Suicide, An Invitation to Die," *American Journal of Nursing,* **70**:269–275, February 1970. Proposes that a person destroys himself in response to an invitation originating from others that he stop living and that a person lives in response to the repeated invitation to continue living.

Leon, John R., Lawrence B. Levenberg, and Robert E. Strange: "Restraining the Violent Patient," *Journal of Psychiatric Nursing and Mental Health Services,* **10**(2):9–11, March–April 1972. Explains succinctly the interventions used in the care of a violent patient.

Loomis, Maxine E.: "Nursing Management of Acting Out Behavior," *Perspectives in Psychiatric Care,* **8**(4):168–173, 1970. Discusses the teaching-learning process with the patient regarding the feelings he is acting out.

McLean, Lenora: "Action and Reaction in Suicidal Crisis," *Nursing Forum,* **8**(1):28–40, 1969. Describes telephone intervention with a person who is threatening suicide.

Penningroth, Philip E.: "Control of Violence in a Mental Health Setting," *American Journal of Nursing.* **75**:606–609, April 1975. Focuses on primary intervention in the care of violent patients. Views physical restraints as a last-resort measure for control.

Schneidman, Edwin S.: *Suicidology: Contemporary Developments,* Grune & Stratton, Inc., New York, 1976. Currently active suicidologists contributed essays to this book concerning contemporary problems in suicide.

——— (ed.): *Death: Current Perspectives,* Mayfield Publishing Company, Palo Alto, Calif., 1976. A compilation of selected contemporary literature on the subject of death and dying from the cultural, societal, interpersonal, and personal perspectives. Profound.

———, Norman L. Farberow, and Robert E. Litman: *The Psychiatry of Suicide,* Science House, New York, 1970. This book is a collection of writings by the three men who initiated, organized, and administered the first suicide prevention center, the Los Angeles Suicide Prevention Center. It is a wealth of information derived from the authors' personal experiences and research.

38

Disruptions of Perceptual and Cognitive Functions

M. Josephine Snider

The perceptual and cognitive functions of the acutely ill psychiatric patient are affected in a plethora of ways. These dysfunctions constitute a wide array of clinical problems and require creative and flexible approaches by nursing staff. The most commonly encountered dysfunctions of perception and cognition are hallucinations and delusions. The two often present simultaneously in patients who are seriously disturbed. The interventions suggested for these clinical problems can be adapted to the individual patient and can provide guidelines for dealing with other related problems. It is important to recognize that delusions and hallucinations are highly individualized in content and are directly related to intense psychological needs and to attempts to explain disturbing personal experiences. The hallucinatory and delusional behaviors presented are always purposeful and have meaning to the patient.

AUDITORY HALLUCINATIONS

Definition

Hallucinations are subjective experiences of sensory perceptions for which there are no corresponding external stimuli. These perceptual experiences may involve any sensorial sphere and usually occur in the presence of a clear consciousness. Perceptual images from the auditory, visual, kinesthetic, olfactory, tactile, and gustatory spheres may be projected onto the environment; that is, the patient associates these perceptions as coming from outside the self. The hallucinatory process may characterize patients with sensory deprivation, brain lesions, oxygen deficiency, the chemical effects of psychoactive drugs, insufficient REM sleep, and psychoses. The hallucinatory process in patients with organic etiologies is briefly discussed in Chap. 35.

The auditory sphere is most commonly affected in patients suffering from the group of syndromes known as schizophrenia. While visual hallucinations are not rare, they usually occur in concert with hallucinations affecting other spheres. *Auditory hallucinations* may take the form of noise, voices which converse with the patient, and voices which converse about the patient. Voices may be accusatory, critical, comforting, or advising. The patient may be able to identify the voices, or the voices may seem to be unfamiliar. Auditory hallucinations may occur occasionally or often at any time during the waking state. The onset of the process may follow a real or fantasized loss of a significant other. Often, the onset may be accompanied by anxiety and be of considerable distress to the patient.

The primary stimulus for the hallucinatory experience is the need for psychological self-protection from painful feelings related to guilt, loneliness, anger, fears of abandonment by loved ones, and uncontrollable ego-alien impulses, thoughts, and feelings. In general, anything which seriously threatens self-esteem and the integrity and unity of the familiar self has significance to the process and content of hallucinations. Threats to self-esteem and the integrity of the familiar self result in high levels of anxiety. As anxiety increases, the ability to sort out and organize perceptions and recognize the differences between thoughts and feelings that are generated by the self decreases. Ambiguity of meaning and source increase, and rational processes lose effectiveness. It becomes increasingly difficult to determine which auditory stimuli come from one's own mind and which come from one's environment.

Assessment

I. Data sources.
   A. Patient history.
   B. Family interview.
   C. Observation of patient in the milieu.

II. Health history (See Chap. 36 for format). Note especially the following:
   A. Patient's memory of onset of sounds not validated by others.
   B. Circumstances surrounding onset.
   C. Possible relationships between perceptual (hallucinatory) experiences and cognitive (delusional) experiences.
   D. Changes in the nature of the auditory experiences, e.g., from critical to comforting, from noise to voice, from familiar to unfamiliar sounds.
   E. Related changes in the patient's life.

Problems

I. Marked anxiety associated with conversation with unobserved others.
II. Panic or fear reactions unassociated with validated environmental stimuli.
III. Complaints by the patient that strangers are talking to him or her.
IV. Complaints by the patient that she or he hears own thoughts or that thoughts have been stolen and verbalized by others.
V. Complaints by the patient that he or she sees visions, people, or objects not seen by others.
VI. The presentation of the listening attitude without appropriate stimuli.

Goals of Care

I. Immediate.
   A. Decrease in the number of hallucinatory experiences.
   B. Decrease in the anxiety level that leads to hallucinations.
   C. Identification of needs served by the hallucinatory experience.
   D. Increase in the ability to test reality at the onset of a hallucination.

II. Long-range.
   A. Cessation of hallucinatory experiences.
   B. Able to intervene in the process without the aid of others.
   C. Understand the needs that provoke hallucinatory experiences.
   D. Meet interpersonal needs in ways that are more productive.

Intervention

I. Assist the patient in increasing interpersonal competence through a one-to-one relationship.
II. Arrange a daily schedule with the patient so that specific needs are met in a predictable fashion.
III. Teach the patient to test reality through seeking consensual validation for perceptual experiences.
IV. Indicate doubt as to the reality of a hallucinatory experience.
V. Offer alternative explanations for concrete conclusions that the patient develops in support of hallucinations.
VI. Indicate in a direct fashion that the hallucination may seem real to the patient but is not shared by the nurse.

VII. Avoid reflective responses, such as, "You hear voices telling you to run away?"

VIII. Do use declarative responses when discussing feelings evoked by the hallucinatory experience, e.g., "It must be scary to hear voices that no one else can hear."

IX. Utilize directive responses when the patient hallucinates while talking with you, e.g., "Listen to me, look at me, do not pay attention to the so-called voices right now!"

X. Observe the relationship between evidence of increasing anxiety and the onset of hallucinations. Intervene in the anxiety immediately. (See Chap. 36 for additional ways of dealing with anxiety.)

XI. Provide regular physical activity that requires the use of large muscle groups and necessitates concentration.

XII. Direct the patient to notify staff when he or she fears that an experience of hearing the so-called voices is imminent.

XIII. Anticipate the situations that seem most likely to evoke hallucinatory behavior.

XIV. Teach the patient to intervene in the hallucinatory experience by active interdiction ("Go away," "You are not real").

XV. Observe for side effects of psychoactive drugs. Assess the lowest effective dose that will help diminish hallucinations and related symptoms.

Evaluation

I. Reassessment.

A. Help the patient assume increasing amounts of responsibility for intervening into the hallucinatory process as he or she becomes less anxious. Focus less and less on the problem as the anxiety level becomes manageable and as interpersonal needs are met in more appropriate ways.

B. Provide the opportunity for group-oriented activities as soon as the anxiety level is consistently below the level evocative of hallucinatory behavior.

C. Reevaluate the entire plan of intervention, particularly in regard to the assessment of self-esteem levels, if elaboration of hallucinatory experiences occurs in terms of the number of affected sensorial spheres and/or if a related delusional system becomes more global and fixed.

II. Follow-up and reevaluation.

A. Provide for continuity of intervention through a mental health clinic.

B. Help develop plans for appropriate social outlets in the community.

C. Provide for consistent monitoring of psychoactive drug regimen.

DELUSIONS

Definition

Delusions are fixed, false beliefs that are maintained regardless of objective evidence and logical argument presented contrary to that belief. Further, the belief is not shared by others of similar educational and sociocultural background. These beliefs are developed to protect the patient from anxiety and insecurity. The trends and themes represented are idiosyncratic in that they are determined by the patient's problems and needs. Delusions are considered to be extreme deviations in thought content, although there is some adjustment value in the process.

The varieties of delusion include those of control or influence, persecution, grandeur, guilt, body disorders, or absence of body parts. Delusions of persecution are frequently observed among seriously ill psychiatric patients, as are beliefs regarding control and influence.

It is important to recognize the fixed character of delusions, and to understand that the process is representative of attempts to deal with the problems and stresses of the life situation. The stimuli which evoke the delusional system may be concealed by symbolization, though occasionally the sources may be surmised through the patient's anamnestic report. The situations which combine along some common denominators appear to contain highly affective factors. The responses to these affective factors carry an irrational flavor. It is important to take advantage of any shift in the degree of fixity or elements of doubt which the patient presents in regard to delusions.

Assessment

I. Data sources.
  A. Patient's history.
  B. Periodic interview with other staff.
  C. Family or extrafamilial significant others.
  D. Observation of patient's interaction with others.
II. Health history (see Chap. 36 for format; also, see "Auditory Hallucinations"). Also include the patient's description rather than her or his interpretation of the onset and contextual factors related to onset of delusions. Note the presence of hallucinatory processes.

Problems

I. The patient expresses a persistent belief that others are trying to harm her or him, although there is an absence of corroborating data.
II. The patient expresses the persistent belief that she or he is famous or capable of remarkable powers without presenting substantiating data to that effect.
III. The patient persistently expresses the belief that he or she is controlled by others or by objects such as the television set without presenting substantiating data to that effect.
IV. The patient is unable to consider alternative interpretations of selected phenomena in a logical fashion.
V. The patient is unable to listen to disagreement with own interpretations without presenting evidence of marked anxiety and/or hostility.
VI. The patient is preoccupied with delusional system to the extent that the subject is broached in almost all interactions with others.
VII. The patient acts in concert with the delusional system without regard for reality.

Goals of Care

I. Immediate.
  A. The patient will interact with the nurse without discussing delusions.
  B. The patient will consider an alternative interpretation of a situation without undue anxiety or hostility.
  C. The patient will express doubt as to the rationality of her or his delusions.
  D. The patient will bring logical thought processes to bear on decisions regaring his behavior.
II. Long-range.
  A. The patient will consider alternative interpretations about phenomena that have personal meaning.
  B. The patient will consensually validate interpretations about phenomena that have personal meaning.
  C. The patient will recognize the interpersonal needs met by the delusional system and will use more appropriate ways to get needs met.
  D. The patient will give up the beliefs that cannot be consensually validated.

Intervention

I. Avoid the use of logic in an attempt to prove the delusion false.

II. Tell the patient that you do not share his or her interpretation (delusion).

III. Focus on parts of content that are real.

IV. Avoid ignoring the patient's verbalization of the delusional material.

V. Explain facts and data about phenomena when appropriate, though not in an argumentative manner.

VI. Identify the feelings presented when the patient discusses the delusion.

VII. Identify the theme represented by the delusional system.

VIII. Direct the patient to describe rather than interpret phenomena related to the delusion.

IX. Set limits on the number of times in an interactional session that the patient may discuss or present the delusional system.

X. Direct the patient to identify the persons to whom pronouns are attributed.

XI. Actively shift conversation from delusional system to another topic when patient exceeds limits allowed for discussion of delusions. Tell the patient why you are shifting topics.

XII. Schedule activities that will be likely to provide increased self-esteem through interaction and cooperation with others.

XIII. Avoid actively soliciting a discussion of delusional content.

XIV. Avoid argument, and inform the patient that you will not argue about her or his beliefs.

XV. Observe for side effects of psychoactive drugs.

XVI. Avoid putting medication in food.

XVII. Provide a brief and honest explanation for changes in milieu or treatment.

XVIII. Support actively any expression of doubt that the patient presents in regard to the delusional system.

Evaluation

I. Reassessment: Acutely ill patients are likely to respond to appropriate psychoactive drugs in approximately 2 weeks following the first dose. Delusions may then lose much of the bizarre, fixed character that was previously observed. Such patients may begin to express doubt and concern regarding the untenable conclusions they reached during the early stages of the disorder. The recognition that one has been "crazy" for a time can have a crisislike effect and may increase anxiety and lower self-esteem. It is crucial that the nurse help patients cope with these feelings so that a return to the delusional system is avoided. Timing is a central factor in assessing whether the status of these patients is supportive of an explanation of their previous need to use delusions for adjustment purposes. A key to the decision to speak directly with them seems to be their own request to do so. In the event that they provide cues that they are ready to attempt to understand their delusional framework, a different set of interventions should be developed. This plan should be geared toward helping them learn to intervene or seek intervention should the problem recur.

II. Follow-up and reevaluation.

A. Refer to mental health clinic for periodic visits.

B. Refer to an outpatient therapy group.

C. Arrange with after-care personnel for transfer to one person who will consistently handle the medication regimen.

D. Family therapy is an option that should be discussed with patient and family. At the least, the family should know the importance of the medication regimen and the group therapy experience.

BIBLIOGRAPHY

Clack, Janice: *Nursing Care of the Disoriented Patient,* Monograph 13, The American Nurses' Association, New York, 1962, pp. 16–26. An early description of phases of the hallucinatory process in schizophrenic patients. Based on Sullivanian concepts. General approaches to nursing intervention included.

Collins, Doris I.: "Some Specific Considerations in the One-to-One Relationship," in Lucille A. Joel and Doris I. Collins (eds.), *Psychiatric Nursing: Theory and Application,* McGraw-Hill Book Company, New York, 1978, pp. 155–167. Clinical cases illustrating concepts, including hallucinations and delusions. Provides operational definition of auditory hallucinations. Good presentation of intervention.

Freedman, Alfred M., Harold I. Kaplan, and Benjamin J. Sadok: *Modern Snyopsis of Comprehensive Textbook of Psychiatry/II,* 2d ed., The Williams & Wilkins Company, Baltimore, 1976, pp. 426–458. Etiology, clinical features, and symptoms of schizophrenia described. An authoritative work.

Gravenkemper, Katherine H.: "Hallucinations," in Shirley F. Burd and Margaret A. Marshall (eds.), *Some Clinical Approaches to Psychiatric Nursing,* The Macmillan Company, New York, 1963, pp. 184–188. One of the earliest presentations of the application of Sullivanian concepts to the understanding of the hallucinatory process. Brief discussion of case examples presented.

Grosicki, Jeanette P., and Marguerite Harmonson: "Nursing Action Guide: Hallucinations," *Journal of Psychiatric Nursing and Mental Health Services,* **7:**133–135, May–June 1969. Development and use of format in planning nursing intervention for hallucinated patients. Some specific approaches suggested.

Kalkman, Marion E: "Psychoses," in Marion E. Kalkman and Anne J. Davis (eds.), *New Dimensions in Mental Health –Psychiatric Nursing,* 4th ed., McGraw-Hill Book Company, New York, 1974, pp. 300–335. Good presentation of clinical problems and nursing care with psychotic patients. Helpful, though brief, section on hallucinations and delusions.

Keup, Wolfram: *Origin and Mechanisms of Hallucinations,* Proceedings of the 14th Annual Meeting of the Eastern Psychiatric Research Association, New York City, November 14–15, 1969, Plenum Press, New York, 1970. Research papers related to hallucinations and hallucinosis. A through coverage of etiology and process.

Kolb, Lawrence E.: *Modern Clinical Psychiatry,* 8th ed., W. B. Saunders Company, Philadelphia, 1973, pp. 308–356. Excellent discussion of the schizophrenias, including psychodynamics, etiology, symptoms, and treatment.

Salzinger, Kurt: *Schizophrenia: Behavioral Aspects,* John Wiley and Sons, Inc., New York, 1973. Presentation of research findings and current theories of schizophrenia. Good illustration of studies pertinent to all aspects of the group of disorders.

Schwartzman, Sylvia T.: "The Hallucinating Patient and Nursing Intervention," in Barbara A. Backer, Patricia M. Dubbert, and Elaine J. P. Eisenman, (eds.), *Psychiatric/Mental Health Nursing: Comtemporary Readings,* D. Van Nostrand Company, Inc., New York, 1978, pp. 140–164. Presentation of Sullivanian concepts related to hallucinations with use of case examples and discussion of intervention from several other sources.

39

Group Work in Inpatient Settings

Ann Cain

We are all born into groups and remain a member of a group until our death. Groups influence our interpersonal relationships all through life. In fact, much of our success in life depends on how successful we are in groups.

Man's first or primary group is the family. . . . It is these early experiences that directly influence and determine a person's behavior in groups, his attitudes toward the leader and group members and the kinds of interpersonal relationships he establishes in general (1).

DEFINITION

A *group* is a congregation of three or more people who can communicate with one another to accomplish common goals. An essential feature is that the members have something in common, and this holds them together. There is interaction between members, and each is influenced by the behavior and characteristics of the others and by the mood or climate present in the group.

Group dynamics are the forces in the group situation which determine the behavior of the group and its members. One needs to remember that group dynamics are not something that may or may not occur in a group. *Every group* has its own dynamics, its own pattern of forces. Sometimes certain of these forces seem to be at a very minimum in some groups, but their potentiality exists in *any* group situation. "Bad" groups can be examined as productively as "good" groups: one can learn as much about group dynamics from one as from the other. Anytime that three or more people meet, there are interactions, interpersonal relationships, group goals, problems of communication, and many other forces. These forces exist in varying degrees, but they are potentially present in all groups.

ASSESSMENT

I. Data sources.
   A. Observation.
   B. Group participation.
II. Distinguishing characteristics of groups. Knowles and Knowles (2) point out that a group must have a definable membership, a group consciousness, a shared purpose, interaction of some type, and the ability to act in a unitary way. Some other distinguishing characteristics that they suggest are the following:
   A. Group background. In every group situation, there is a history to the group before it even starts. A new group coming together for the first time will have to devote much of its early energy to getting acquainted with one another, with the group's task, and with establishing ways of working together. A group that has met together before will know each other better and will know what to expect from one another, but it may have developed habits that interfere with its efficiency, such as arguing, dividing into factions, or wasting time. Each member comes to the group with expectations or a "mental set" with reference to the group. They may be looking forward to the meeting or they may be dreading it; they may be deeply concerned about the group's task or indifferent to it. *All* these feelings affect the behavior of the participants and consequently, influence the group's behavior.
   B. Group participation patterns. In every group situation, people are participating in

1205

one way or another. There is a distinctive pattern of interaction that is particular to that one group. In some groups certain members overparticipate and dominate the group, and in other groups the leaders do all the talking. Sometimes all group members may talk to the leader directly, or all members may talk to each other, and a real sharing of ideas and opinions may occur. These patterns may tend to be very consistent in any given group, or they may vary over time. Usually, the broader the participation among members of a group, the deeper the interest and involvement will be.

C. Group communication patterns. These demonstrate how well members understand one another and how clearly they communicate their ideas, values, and feelings. Sometimes group members "speak past" each other or attempt to impress one another with elaborate vocabularies. Many feelings are communicated nonverbally; these involve body postures, facial expressions, and gestures.

D. Group cohesion. This is the strength of the bonds that bind the individual members into a unified group. It refers to the morale, the team spirit, and the strength of attraction of the group for its members. High cohesion is present when members of a group can work effectively in a cooperative situation in which all individuals have certain independent responsibilities but are at the same time interdependent. High cohesiveness in a group is evidenced when:

1. Conflict between members is appropriate and can be tolerated and resolved.
2. Support is given to members who are being attacked or criticized.
3. Feelings of "we-ness" are evident; when members speak in terms of "we" and not just "I."
4. Productivity is high, and agreement concerning new tasks is obvious.

E. Group atmosphere. This is sometimes called the social climate, and it refers to the informality or the freedom of the group situation. Members have certain feelings about the group, and these are reflected in the degree of spontaneity of their interactions. The desirable kind of group atmosphere is one in which members feel free to speak when they have something to say.

F. Group standards or norms. These are the code of ethics by which acceptable behavior is judged within the group. These are ways of behaving that emerge, that can be seen, and that are typical of a certain group. Which subjects may be discussed, which are taboo; how openly members can express their feelings; how long members can talk; whether interruptions are permitted—all these and many other dos and don'ts are part of the group's standards. If standards are clear to group members, group functioning is more effective and members neel freer to participate. Standards are either implicit or explicit, with most groups operating on implicit standards which are rarely shared openly. Group members rust know what they are.

G. Sociometric pattern. In any group situation, subgroups of one kind or another will develop. These subgroups are sometimes determined on the basis of friendship or common agreement about a particular issue, or they are sometimes determined on the basis of a common dislike of certain persons or situations. These patterns quickly show that certain members begin to identify certain other members they like more than others.

H. Group structure and organization. These can be both visible and invisible. Visibly, there are officers, appointed leaders, or committees. Invisibly, there are behind-the-scene arrangements of members according to prestige, power, seniority, ability, etc.

I. Group procedures. These are the ground rules and procedures by which the work of the group is accomplished. Frequently, these are informal, but sometimes very formal procedures such as *Robert's Rules of Order* are followed.

J. Group goals. These are sometimes clearly defined and at other times are quite vague and general. Members may be wholly, partially, or not committed at all to these goals.

III. Differences between primary and secondary groups.

A. *Primary groups* are characterized by warm, intimate, personal ties with one another.

Usually these groups are small and are face-to-face, with interpersonal behavior devoted to mutual ends. Examples of a primary group would be the family or the close friendship group like a high school gang. Earliest experiences in social unity come from the family, therefore, primary groups become the springboards for both individual and social institutions.

B. *Secondary groups* are characterized by cool, impersonal, and more formal relationships, where the group is not an end in itself but a means to other ends. These groups are usually large and members have only intermittent contacts. Examples of a secondary group would be social clubs or professional organizations (3).

IV. Difference between group content and group process.

    A. *Group content* refers to the "what." It is what the group is talking about, what they are saying.

    B. *Group process* includes all the events and interconnecting forces that occur at any given moment in a group. It refers to the "how." It is how the group handles its communication and how members are interacting with each other, i.e., who talks how much and to whom? Looking at process means to focus on what is going on in the group and to try to understand what is going on in terms of other things that have previously occurred in the group.

V. Roles of group members. Members play many roles in groups and these greatly influence group life. (4).

One thing to remember is that in groups no specific role is assigned to anyone. Inividuals move from one role to another in groups and there may be much shifting around.

    A. *Functional roles* are roles that are helpful in carrying out a group task or that help strengthen and maintain group life and activities. They can be broken down into two kinds: (1) task roles and (2) building and maintenance roles.

        1. *Task roles* are those functions required in selecting and carrying out a group task or purpose. Some task roles are:

            a. Initiating activity. Proposing solutions; suggesting new ideas, new definitions of the problem, new attack on the problem, or a new organization of material.

            b. Seeking information. Asking for clarification or suggestions; requesting additional information or facts; seeking relevant information about the group concern.

            c. Seeking opinion. Looking for an expression of feeling about something from the members; seeking clarification of values, suggestions, or ideas.

            d. Giving information. Offering facts or generalizations; relating one's own experiences to the group problem to illustrate a point.

            e. Giving opinion. Stating an opinion or belief concerning a suggestion or one of several suggestions, particularly concerning its value rather than its formal basis.

            f. Elaborating. Clarifying; giving examples or developing meanings; trying to envision how a proposal might work out if adopted; clearing up confusion.

            g. Coordinating. Showing relationships among various ideas or suggestions, trying to pull ideas and suggestions together; trying to draw together activities of various subgroups or members.

            h. Summarizing. Pulling together relatd ideas or suggestions; restating suggestions after the group has discussed them; offering a decision or conclusion for the group to accept or reject.

            i. Testing feasibility. Making application of suggestions to real situations; examining practicality and workability of ideas; preevaluating decisions.

            j. Consensus tester. Sending up trial balloons to see if the group is nearing a conclusion; checking with the group to see how much agreement has been reached.

        2. *Building and maintenance roles* are those functions required in strengthening and maintaining group life and activities. They deal with the interpersonal and emotional aspects of group life. Some building and maintenance roles are:

a. Encouraging. Being friendly, warm, and responsive to others; praising others and their ideas; agreeing with and accepting contributions of others.

b. Gate-keeping. Attempting to keep communication channels open; facilitates the participation of others, i.e., "We haven't heard from Jim yet." Suggesting procedures for sharing opportunities to discuss group problems; bringing a blocked member into the group.

c. Standard setting. Expressing standards for the group to use in choosing its content or procedures or in evaluating its decisions; reminding the group to avoid decisions which would conflict with group standards.

d. Following. Going along with decisions of the group; somewhat passively accepting ideas of others; serving as an audience during group discussion and decision making.

e. Expressing group feeling. Summarizing what group feeling is sensed to be; describing the reactions of the group to ideas or solutions.

3. Roles seen as both task and group maintenance roles are:

a. Evaluating. Submitting group decisions or accomplishments to comparison with the group standards; measuring accomplishments against goals.

b. Diagnosing. Determining sources of difficulties and the appropriate steps to take next; determining the main blocks to progress.

c. Mediating. Harmonizing; attempting to reconcile disagreements and reduce tension; getting people to explore their differences.

d. Compromising. Offering to compromise one's own position; admit own error in order to maintain the group's cohesion.

e. Relieving tensions. Draining off negative feeling by jesting or pouring oil on troubled waters; putting a tense situation into broader context.

B. Any group can be viewed from the point of view of what its purpose or function seems to be. When a member says something, certain questions can be asked:

1. Is he or she primarily trying to get the group's work accomplished (task) or is he or she trying to improve or patch up some relationships among the members (maintenance)? Every group needs both kinds of behavior and needs to work out an adequate balance of task and maintenance activities.

2. There is another question to ask when a member says something in a group. Is he or she primarily meeting some personal need or goal without regard for the group's problem?

VI. Group growth chart (Table 39-1). This is useful to consult when trying to evaluate how any group is functioning. In a new group, interaction is usually relatively superficial, anxiety is fairly high, and the interchange is often stilted and unspontaneous. In a new group, ideas and suggestions are often not followed through. Individuals often seem to see and hear relatively little of what is really going on.

Usually, as groups work together, relationships in the group become more free and open. There is less threat or fear present, and there is a greater probability that the skills and resources of the group members will be utilized effectively. Group members how greater openness to information, opinions, and new ideas. Less energy is tied up in protecting and hiding themselves. This energy is freed for constructive group activity, and there is a greater likelihood of finding involvement and satisfaction in the group.

PROBLEMS

So far, the group processes described deal with the group's attempt to work, but there are many forces active in groups which disturb work. They represent a kind of emotional underworld or undercurrent in the stream of group life. These underlying emotional issues produce a variety of emotional behaviors which interfere with or are destructive to effective group functioning. These are called the *nonfunctional roles*. They cannot be ignored or wished away. They must be recognized, their causes understood, and as the group develops,

TABLE 39-1 / GROUP GROWTH CHART

Conditions in Groups Ordinarily Contributing toward:

Negative Growth	Positive Growth
Communication	
1. Superficial, irrelevant.	1. Purposeful, relevant.
2. Differential or specialized language; common meanings not achieved.	2. Understandable language; common meanings achieved.
3. Differences kept hidden or expressed agressively.	3. Different ideas and points of view expressed freely and positively.
4. Feelings hidden and expressed indirectly through ideas.	4. Feelings expressed directly when essential.
Goals	
1. Individualistic unshared goals.	1. Parallel or commonly shared goals.
2. Use of group for ego satisfaction.	2. Use of group for growth; growth purposes clarified and/or understood.
3. A single group goal is defined and held to at all costs.	3. Both group and individual goals are permitted and encouraged.
Atmosphere	
1. Aggressive, hostile, or overfriendly, demanding.	1. Friendly, accepting, but unrealistic.
2. Prestige seeking.	2. Collaboration seeking.
3. Authorities demanded and accepted.	3. Authorities analyzed and utilized.
4. Hostile to change.	4. Supportive and encouraging of change.
Responsibility and Involvement	
1. Group discourages or denies individual's responsibility for growth; demands dependence.	1. Group allows and encourages individual to take responsibility for own growth.
2. Individual is not personally identified with the group—"It's just another group."	2. Individual is personally identified with the group—its continuance and/or function are important to her or him.
Internal Processes	
1. Group sets up a standard ritual (like "We must always be democratic" or "The leader tells us what to do").	1. Group changes its methods of operation freely and flexibly as needs arise and group development and growth continues.
2. Group sets up demands for a constant and continuing level of productivity.	2. Group varies its tempo of work and allows itself periods of relaxation.
3. Group does not allow any expression of mood other than polite friendliness.	3. Group feels free to express its moods—excitement, enthusiasm, concern, tension, etc.
Standards	
1. Only leader or resource persons help others.	1. Everyone in the group serves as resource to help group and each other.
2. Differences must be kept "out of sight."	2. Differences which are present in the group are useful.
3. Clearly defined and fixed roles are assigned to particular members.	3. Roles defined, but may easily move from member to member.
4. Member given no opportunity to test out her or his new insights or skills.	4. Member has chance to try out her or his new insights or skills in the group.

Source: David H. Jenkins, "Planning Conditions for Personal Growth," *Adult Leadership,* February 1954, pp. 16–21.

conditions must be created which permit these same emotional energies to be channeled in the direction of group effort.

One thing to guard against is the tendency to blame any person (whether it is self or others) who falls into this nonfunctional category. It is much more useful to regard this kind of behavior as a symptom that all is not well with the group's ability to satisfy individual needs through group-centered activity. As the group grows and as member needs become integrated with the group goals, there will be less of this type of behavior. It is useful to remember that each person interprets things differently. For example, what may appear as "blocking" to one person may seem to be "testing feasibility" to another.

I. Some nonfunctional roles are:
   A. Being aggressive. Working for status by criticizing or blaming others; showing hostility against the group or some individual; deflating the ego or status of others.
   B. Blocking. Interfering with the progress of the group by going off on a tangent, citing personal experiences unrelated to the problem, arguing too much on a point, or rejecting ideas without consideration.
   C. Self-confessing. Using the group as a sounding board, expressing personal, non-group-oriented feelings or points of view.
   D. Competing. Vying with others to produce the best ideas, talk the most, play the most roles, or gain favor with the leader.
   E. Seeking sympathy. Trying to induce other group members to be sympathetic to one's problems or misfortunes; deploring one's own situation or disparaging one's own ideas in order to gain support.
   F. Special pleading. Introducing or supporting suggestions related to one's own pet concerns or philosophies; lobbying.
   G. Horsing around. Clowning; joking; mimicking; disrupting the work of the group.
   H. Seeking recognition. Attempting to call attention to one's self by loud or excessive talking, extreme ideas, or unusual behavior.
   I. Withdrawing. Acting indifferently or passively; resorting to excessive formality, day dreaming, doodling, whispering to others, or wandering from the subject.

II. What are some of the basic issues or causes of this nonfunctional behavior? These are all questions group members are trying to answer. Nonfunctional behavior is produced in response to these problems and can be destructive to group functioning. These basic issues are perceived by group members as:

   A. The problem of *identity*. Questions asked are: Who am I in this group? Where do I fit in? What kind of behavior is acceptable here?
   B. The problem of *goals and needs*. Questions asked are: What do I want from the group? Can the group goals be made consistent with my goals? What have I to offer to the group?
   C. The problem of *power, control, and influence*. Questions asked are: Who will control what we do? How much power and influence do I have?
   D. The problem of *intimacy*. Questions asked are: How close will we get to each other? How personal? How much can we trust each other and how can we achieve a greater level of trust (5)?

GOALS OF CARE

I. Types of groups and goals. The psychiatric nurse, as well as all other nurses, works with many kinds of groups. This varied range of groups can include administrative groups, consultative groups, counseling and therapy groups, psychodrama, therapeutic communities, ward meetings, educational or discussion groups, social groups, and many others.

Groups have the potential to promote positive change in people. While no one knows exactly what makes groups work, certain catalysts are almost always present in successful groups. The most significant of these is the willingness of the group members to share themselves with others—their thoughts, ideas, feelings, and perceptions. The attitudes of group members can make or break any group!

Groups can be thought of as falling into three general categories:

A. Task groups. These are work-oriented and have specific tasks or goals to accomplish.

B. Psychosocial groups. These focus on the emotional and social needs of people and include social gatherings and therapy groups.

C. Combinations or variations of both.

II. Definition and goals of group therapy. Group therapy is often selected as the method of treatment for many patients. We all live in groups, and these groups influence our interpersonal relationships. If people are having problems with their interpersonal relationships, it stands to reason that part of thehealing process could also occur in a group.

A. There are three things that groups can accomplish that individual therapy cannot:

1. The group supplies warmth and cohesion similar to family solidarity with which the individual can identify.

2. The group itself exemplifies forms of social adaptation, such as love and friendly competition, which can be directly carried over to larger groups.

3. Groups can give the individual the experience of giving as well as receiving help. There is a direct and fundamental fulfillment in being capable of directed love and support controlled by the individual for the benefit of the other group members. This is ego building (6).

B. In addition to these the group is:

1. A laboratory in which to observe the member's behavior (a new milieu).

2. A place where members can try out new forms of behavior.

3. A place where the facade of defenses can be lifted.

4. A place where early unpleasant experiences with groups can be replaced with more pleasant experiences.

5. Designed to play up the healthy parts of the personality.

6. A place where members can develop a feeling of belonging and increased self-esteem.

7. A place where the member gets some validation of feelings, learning that he or she is not alone and that his or her feelings are not unique.

8. Preparing people for handling other situations such as home situations involving parents, brothers, sisters, spouses, etc.

9. A natural mode of treatment since all humans have a social hunger—they all want to belong.

C. There are various types of group therapy (7):

1. Didactic groups. Thse are based on educational material presented by the leader. Any form of structured activity can be used, such as lectures, movies, talks on mental health, anxiety, etc. The emphasis is placed on developing intellectual insight.

2. Repressive-inspirational groups. A wide variety of groups fit in here. These frequently have a planned activity and then a discussion in which members ventilate and realize that other people have similar problems. The emphasis is on morale building and supporting defenses. An example would be Alcoholics Anonymous.

3. Therapeutic social clubs. These can be both in and out of the hospital. They can be very structured or very informal and can range from social activities to group discussion of member's problems. They can be organized either by patients or staff. These are social interaction groups that increase the member's skill in social participation.

4. Psychodrama. This kind of group utilizes role playing to act out certain situations. Participants play a part, may switch roles, and then discuss what happened. Can be used with patients both in and out of the hospital.

5. Free-interaction groups. These encourage interaction in an atmosphere conducive to free expression of feelings. They are problem-centered with no specific activity planned.
   a. Group analysis makes use of the same techniques as in individual analysis but in a group situation, i.e., dreams, transference, resistance, free association, etc. This is conducted primarily with neurotics by analysts in private medical practice.
   b. Group psychotherapy. This is

   the process which takes place whenever people are gathered together for the consideration of personal emotional problems with the purpose of relieving them, in the presence and with the aid of an individual skilled in both the understanding of the individual personality and the patterns of human interrelationships and group interactions (8).

6. Combination of types. Usually a small group of six to eight members conducted by a psychologist, social worker, psychiatric nurse, etc. The purpose can be varied: it may be an admission group, a predischarge group, or a patient-government group. It may be conducted by cotherapists depending on preference.

D. Groups can also be classified as open and closed groups (9).
   1. *Open groups* are groups in which there is a rapid turnover of members, and new members replace the old members when vacancies occur. Certain themes, especially the so-called "birth theme," arise more rapidly in open groups. The kinds of anxieties and hostilities that emerged when a new baby was born, or a step-parent entered the family circle, are reexperienced by members in the group. The addition of a new member must be carefully timed to reduce the disruption of the therapeutic process. It will inevitably increase the member's anxiety, and this will be reflected in the group sessions. In most instances the emergence of unconscious material and underlying conflicts is hindered by the presence of a stranger. Open groups have some specific features:
      a. In theory, these groups may perpetuate themselves indefinitely. They are never dissolved. Members who finish their treatment or leave for various reasons are replaced.
      b. Changes can be made to achieve a composition that will facilitate therapeutic movement. Members may be added or transferred at the therapist's discretion.
      c. These groups can be started with only a few members. New members can be added as needed.
   2. *Closed groups* are defined as having a constant membership, as members are only expected to leave at a definite time. The specific qualities of closed groups almost inevitably lead to specific responses. Separation anxiety and the death theme are very evident. Some of this separation anxiety can be viewed as the primary neurotic problem of separation from the maternal figure. Separation from any important figure, whether it be in the nuclear family, in marriage, or in treatment, may bring back many of these original feelings. The group is compelled to work through the theme that no one is indispensable, and termination is another expression of this inevitability. Carried to its extreme, separation anxiety is a fear of death as the ultimate departure. A member's leaving may be symbolically perceived by the group as a final leavetaking. Closed groups can be broken down into three main types:
      a. Constant membership. Members are not permitted to leave at will, but are expected to serve the group's need for a definite period of time. The time is stipulated at the start of treatment.
      b. Family prototype. Members leave one by one when they are ready. They detach themselves as if from their nuclear families. Since no replacements

are made, the group goes out of existence when all its members have dropped out.

    c. Occasionally reopened. Members may be added or transferred according to the group's need.

INTERVENTION

  I. Types of leadership in groups. Group leaders are only as effective as the group members they are leading. The success of any group does not depend on the leader alone; it depends on each individual group member. The following is a description of six different types of leadership (10). The leader's behavior is described in relation to the group with which he or she is interacting.

    A. Authoritarian leadership. This type of leadership is characterized by power and domination. These leaders value discipline and control of the group. They have no confidence or trust that group members will act independently; consequently, group members act with fear and submission. These leaders discourage interaction and communication between members. They do not assume the responsibility for their own actions and hold the group responsible for any failures. Such groups can only be effective if the members permit their leader to have all the power. When this occurs, the group feels helpless, powerless, and dependent, and there is a low degree of satisfaction among group members. Amazingly, although this type of leadership meets the needs of the individual leader rather than the needs of the group, the task accomplishment of this group is usually highly productive.

    B. Democratic leadership. These leaders encourage members to participate in group activities that enhance group goals. They do not dominate the group but participate as members. They have confidence in, trust, and encourage communication between group members. They share the power of their position and distribute responsibilities to the group. They are friendly, involved, and meet the needs or goals of the group members rather than their individual needs.

    C. Laissez-faire leadership. These leaders facilitate communication among group members and are good listeners who reflect group thoughts back to the group. They are passive, essentially noninvolved, and function somewhat like observers apart from, rather than as a part of, the group. Morale is usually high in such groups; group goals can be achieved in this type of group if the group members are strong enough to collectively achieve them. Essentially, the leadership role is taken over by group members.

    D. Bureaucratic leadership. This type of leadership is characterized by rigidity and inflexibility due to the focus on carrying out the inherent rules of the bureaucracy. These groups are immobilized to define or achieve their own goals, as the group goals must be the rules of the bureaucracy. These leaders are impersonal, aloof, objective, and lack initiative. They do not have to assume the responsibility for their own actions, as they can always blame the rigidity or the rules of the bureaucracy.

    E. Charismatic leadership. These leaders are seen to have supernatural traits, attributed to them by the group members. They must prove themselves to their followers. These groups depend on followers who surrender themselves to the will of their leader.

    F. Shared leadership. These leaders stimulate and facilitate the interaction process among members. All members participate in and share group roles. In this sense, each time a member speaks in a way that facilitates group goals or group process, he or she assumes the leadership role at that point in time. Members ar listened to and respected by the group, and there is much interdependence between members. This type of leadership involves all members, facilitates a high degree of group cohesion, and is personally satisfying to group members. This style of leadership does not free leaders from the responsibility of defining and clarifying the group goals initially or whenever needed during the group experience. This group usually has high morale and high productivity.

II. Functions and interventions of group leaders. Gwen Marram (11) has written about the kinds of things group leaders or therapists do in groups. She has separated functions and interventions and has emphasized the difference. A *function* is the purpose of the leader in the group. An *intervention* is the specific act or set of activities that leaders employ to accomplish their purpose in the group.

The following functions and interventions apply to leadership in any type of group. Group leaders strive to provide an atmosphere in which group members can express their thoughts and feelings freely, without fear of judgment or retaliation.

A. Leadership functions.
1. The group leader facilitates the natural benefits of group membership. Leaders assist members in meeting their needs for security, belonging, and companionship.
2. The group leader maintains a viable group atmosphere. Members are free to be present, free to talk about what concerns them, and free to experiment with new behaviors without severe threat.
3. The group leader oversees group gowth. Most groups have goals. Whatever the goals of the group are, the leader has a direct responsibility to assist the group in meeting those goals. In the role of observer of group growth, the leader keeps members' attention on the goals, clarifies issues in terms of how they relate to goals, and evaluates the group's progress toward the goals periodically and with the assistance of the group members.
4. The group leader regulates individual member's growth within the group setting. Individual group members progress at different rates. Sometimes the leader will be concerned with one member's growth so as to further the progress of the total group, i.e., help one member catch up so the entire group can proceed together. Therefore, at times, the leader's interventions may be more individualized and will not be directed solely at the group.

B. Leadership interventions. These actions are carried out both by group leaders and group members.
1. Outlines and interprets group objectives. Members need to have an understanding of what is expected of them.
2. Manipulates physical and structural arrangements of the group. This includes dealing with numbers of members, room, length of group, duration, etc.
3. Increases interaction between members. Uses basic interviewing and communication skills and assists group members to share and learn from each other.
4. Encourages the sharing of common problems. This helps to develop group cohesion.
5. Employs strategies with individuals. Plans the use of techniques and experiences to further growth of group members.
6. Reduces undue anxiety. The leader is aware of the group's anxiety level and maintains it at a constructive level. Prolonged high anxiety in a group can result in group disintegration and disorganization.
7. Summarizes the group's progress toward its goals. This occurs to some extent at the end of each group session and continually throughout the life of the group.

EVALUATION

I. Reassessment: common problems in groups.
A. Conflict resolution. *Conflict* is an emotional disturbance resulting from a clash of two opposing forces in operation simultaneously. Conflict is a process, and it is a

necessary part of group life; it is unpleasant, full of tension, hostility, and opposing interests.

Conflict in a group requires at least two members involved in direct interaction with each other. They are involved in a struggle over something that is scarce; there is apparently not enough to go around to satisfy the contending members. This scarcity may apply to material resources, power, status, or values. Those involved usually assume that what their opponents get, they will lose.

Conflict is normal in groups and is an opportunity for growth rather than something to be avoided at all costs. In the course of dealing with conflict, group members can be helped to see problems and situations in new ways, to call on strengths within themselves which have been dormant, and can develop a set of attitudes and skills which will make a tremendous contribution to their future functioning as mature people. If group leaders grasp these potentialities, they can help their group to realize them and will not be intent upon discouraging all conflicts in the group.

1. There are two kinds of conflict: realistic and nonrealistic.
    a. Realistic conflicts arise from frustration of specific demands within the relationship and from estimates of gains by each of the members, involving a specific result or issue. Examples would be two members struggling for leadership in the group or members with opposing views as to how to achieve group goals.
    b. Nonrealistic conflicts do not arise from rival ends or clear issues. They arise from the need for tension release, and they may be directed against members with whom there is no issue. This sort of thing is sometimes at work in scapegoating, i.e., it may not be safe to vent feelings against the appropriate person and, therefore, they are directed against a weaker, less threatening person.
2. There are particular patterns of conflict resolution (12):
    a. Elimination. Members may combat each other, each seeking to win, and if necessary to rid the group of the opposing faction.
    b. Subjugation. The strongest subgroup or individual may force the others to accept its point of view and thus dominate the opposition.
    c. Compromise. Negotiations take place among competing members or subgroups. Both parties give up something in order to get something else in return. It is essentially a bargaining approach in which costs and rewards are weighed and eventually balanced.
    d. Alliance. Subgroups or individuals may maintain their independence, but combine to achieve a common goal.
    e. Integration. The group as a whole may arrive at a solution that not only satisfies every member but is better than any of the contending solutions. This is considered the highest achievement in group life.
3. There is another framework that focuses more on how the conflict is handled by group members rather than on its outcome. It can be thought of as a series of levels:
    a. Physical violence. This is the attempt to beat the opponents into submission.
    b. Verbal violence. This is the attempt to belittle opponents in order to make them look ridiculous and to turn the feelings of the group and others against them.
    c. Subtler verbal contention. This is the attempt to belittle and undermine the position of opponents without violently attacking them. It often involves cleverly citing associated or even irrelevant factors.
    d. Finding allies. This is the attempt to line up others to support one's position. This tends to be a power play. Various motives can be presented to potential allies, but the main point is to gain strength which is greater than that of one's opponents.

      e. Seeking an authoritative decision. This is the attempt to find someone, probably the leader, who will say definitively who is right and who is wrong.

      f. Creating diversions and delay. This is the attempt to displace attention on something other than the conflict.

      g. Respect for differences. There is a desire to understand how the opponent sees the situation, to collect the needed facts, and to attempt to think rationally about the conflict. This level is the highest in the hierarchy. There is a willingness to go beyond the clash of individuals and the desire to win: to be interested in facts, drawing reasonable conclusions from them, and to listen carefully to one's opponents.

    4. Group leaders play an important role in dealing with conflict. They try to:

      a. Fully understand the situation and the opposing views.

      b. Relate to the group as a whole without taking sides. However, they can and should give their opinion without alienating either side.

      c. Help sort out the issues and clarify areas of agreement and disagreement in the group.

      d. Formulate a strategy for change which includes thinking ahead to anticipate the consequences of each line of possible group action.

B. Decision making. This is a necessary and inherent part of group process, as there must be some mode of operation by which a group can make decisions. It is essential that the group structure be such that the members have the privileges and responsibilities of the management of their own group affairs. A collection of individuals will not develop the characteristics of a productive group unless they have the right and the ability to make decisions that are significant to their own group life.

    Every person in his or her own life is faced with making choices presumed to be based on available alternatives. To make a choice essentially means to select from available alternatives and then to implement that selection. The only "real" alternatives available are those that are within an individual's perceptual field. These are based on personal background, the characteristics of one's own personality, and the social and cultural experiences that have shaped one's personality.

    Decision making ought always to be a rational process, but it is not. Unconscious factors are powerful forces in restricting people from making rational choices. Group leaders need to help members to understand the decision-making process and to assist them in becoming more skillful and rational in arriving at their decisions.

    There are some basic steps in decision making (13). These steps do not necessarily occur in the order or sequence listed, but they do indicate a process which is inherent in decision making.

    1. Becoming aware of the problem. This includes arriving at a definition of the problem and breaking it down into component parts.

    2. Clarifying and evaluating proposed solutions. This is delineating the alternatives available and evaluating the possible consequences.

    3. Reaching a decision. This is choosing one alternative to the exclusion of all others and evaluating it as to the probable consequences.

    4. Acting upon the decision that has been reached. This is implementing the decision andevaluating the choice.

    5. Examining the results of implementing the decision. This is examining the consequences of a decision and recognizing that the consequences could be quite unanticipated.

C. Adolescent groups. These can present some special problems. One area that can give group leaders difficulty is that of developing realistic expectations of the adolescent. In this age group it is important to keep in mind that the boundaries between normal and abnormal behavior are shifting, often fluid, and frequently a matter of judgment. One may anticipate many swings such as from rebellion to submission in a relatively short period of time.

1. It is essential to have a concept of the developmental tasks of adolescence (14). These include:
   a. Emancipation from parental attachments.
   b. Development of satisfying and self-realizing peer attachments, with ability to love and appreciate the worth of others as well as oneself.
   c. An endurable and sustaining sense of identity in the family, social, sexual, and work-creative areas.
   d. A flexible set of hopes and life goals for the future.
2. Some important goals for adolescent groups are listed as follows (15):
   a. To support assistance and confrontation from peers.
   b. To provide a miniature real-life situation for study and change of behavior.
   c. To stimulate new ways of dealing with situations and tostimulate the development of new skills in human relationships.
   d. To stimulate new concepts of self and new models of identification.
   e. To decrease feelings of isolation.
   f. To provide a feeling of protection from the adult while undergoing changes.
   g. To allow the swings of rebellion or submission, which will encourage independence and identification with the leader.
   h. To uncover relationship problems not evident in individual therapy.
3. Everything written previously in this chapter also occurs in adolescent groups, sometimes with a little more intensity. Anyone working with adolescents will have more success if they develop the qualities of empathy, patience, trustfulness, tactfulness, and sensitivity. It is a real challenge to work with this age group and to watch the adolescent moving in the direction of maturity. Adolescence is truly both "the best of times" and "the worst of times."

II. Follow-up and reevaluation. Group members are carefully evaluated and referred to community agencies and/or outpatient settings if further treatment or group participation is believed necessary and useful.

The interaction among members of all groups have many similarities—the same basic group dynamics occur in *all* groups. Frequently their intensity differs in group therapy, but the basic patterns are the same. Conducting group therapy is a specialized skill that requires additional preparation, training, and experience. The therapist needs a theory base in group therapy and a body of knowledge in group dynamics. Clinical practice with groups and supervision of that experience are additional indispensable requirements.

REFERENCES

1. Dolores McManama, "Working With Groups," in Lisa Robinson (ed.), *Psychiatric Nursing As A Human Experience,* W. B. Saunders Company, Philadelphia, 1977, p. 275.
2. Malcolm Knowles and Hulda Knowles, *Introduction to Group Dynamics,* Association Press, New York, 1972, pp. 39–50.
3. Michael Olmstead, *The Small Group,* Random House, New York, 1959, pp. 17–19.
4. K. D. Benne and P. Sheats, "Functional Roles of Group Members," *Journal of Social Issues,* **4:**41–49, Spring 1948.
5. "The Tool Kit," *Adult Leadership,* January 1953, pp. 17–23.
6. Gardner Murphy, "Group Psychotherapy in Our Society," in Max Rosenbaum and Milton Berger (eds.), *Group Psychotherapy and Group Function,* Basic Books, Inc., New York, 1963, p. 33.
7. Florence Powdermaker and Jerome Frank, "Group Psychotherapy," in Silvano Arieti (ed.), *American Handbook of Psychiatry,* vol. II, Basic Books, Inc., New York, 1959, pp. 1326–1363.
8. J. E. Neighbor et al., "An Approach to the Selection of Patients for Group Psychotherapy," in Max Rosenbaum and Milton Berger (ed.), *Group Psychotherapy and Group Function,* Basic Books, Inc., New York, 1963, p. 413.
9. A. L. Kadis et al., *A Practicum of Group Psychotherapy,* Harper & Row, Hagerstown, 1974, pp. 101–104.

10. Hubert Bonner, *Group Dynamics: Principles and Application,* Ronald Press, New York, 1959, pp. 163–198.
11. Gwen D. Marram, *The Group Approach in Nursing Practice,* The C. V. Mosby Company, St. Louis, 1973, pp. 129–145.
12. G. Wilson and G. Ryland, *Social Group Work Practice,* Houghton Mifflin Company, New York, 1950.
13. Louis Lowy, "Decision-Making and Group Work," in Saul Bernstein (ed.), *Explorations in Group Work,* Boston University School of Social Work, Boston, 1965.
14. Sugar, Max (ed.): *The Adolescent in Group and Family Therapy,* Brunner/Mazel, Publishers, New York, 1975, p. 3.
15. Ibid., p. 22.

BIBLIOGRAPHY

Beukenkamp, Cornelius: *Fortunate Strangers,* Grove Press, Inc., New York, 1958. An actual report of what happened to eight patients and a doctor during group treatment. Beautifully written, this book conveys the actual human experience of group therapy in a very authentic way.

Johnson, James: *Group Therapy: A Practical Approach,* McGraw-Hill Book Company, New York, 1963. A significant and practical guide to group therapy and its techniques. Although written some years ago, this book continues to be a clear, concise, down-to-earth description of group therapy. It sets forth a very workable model for anyone using the group method. Dr. Johnson's style of writing is direct, open, and readily understandable.

Kadis, Asya, et al.: *Practicum of Group Psychotherapy,* Harper & Row, Hagerstown, Md., 1974. Excellent reference. This book covers every aspect of group psychotherapy, from starting a group and its first meeting, through the group's life cycle and its termination. This provides a very useful overview of the group therapy field.

Knowles, Malcolm, and Hulda Knowles: *Introduction to Group Dynamics.* Association Press, New York, 1972. A classic writing in group dynamics. This is an excellent primer on group dynamics, what it is, its main ideas, and its practical applications to all groups. It is an easily understood theory-and-practice introduction useful to anyone participating in groups.

Luft, Joseph: *Group Processes: An Introduction to Group Dynamics,* The National Press, Palo Alto, Calif., 1966. Presents a very useful introduction to group dynamics. Discusses the basic issues in group processes and presents the research in the field. This small text includes an excellent explanation of the Johari window, a graphic model of awareness in interpersonal relations, that is helpful in developing an understanding of groups.

Marram, Gwen: *The Group Approach in Nursing Practice,* The C. V. Mosby Company, St. Louis, 1973. A well-written book applying the group approach specifically to nursing practice. The author discusses the functions and interventions of group leaders, and these can be applied to any type of group one is leading or participating in.

McManama, Dolores: "Working With Groups," in Lisa Robinson (ed.), *Psychiatric Nursing As A Human Experience,* W. B. Saunders Company, Philadelphia, 1977, pp. 275–285. A well-written and concise presentation of the important aspects of working with groups, including the purposes of specific groups, the group contract, and the phases of group development.

Yalom, Irvin: *The Theory and Practice of Group Psychotherapy,* Basic Books, Inc., New York, 1975. This is a comprehensive, thoroughly up-to-date handbook on group therapy. It contains an excellent bibliography at the end of each chapter and is a very useful guide for the training of group therapists. Also includes a discussion of encounter or sensitivity training groups and their interface with therapy groups.

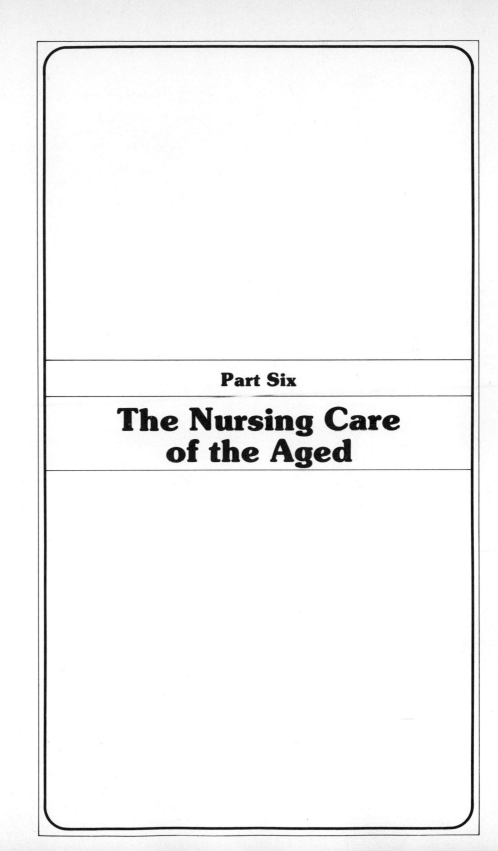

Part Six

The Nursing Care
of the Aged

The number of elderly people living in the United States has increased significantly in the last few years. This change has resulted in greater utilization of health care facilities by the elderly and has required that health care providers become more sensitive to their needs. Nurses as a group must assume a more dominant role in organizing and coordinating the care of the aged.

The way an individual ages is dependent upon many variables. Frequently, the overall impact of life crises and the manner in which they were handled have a significant influence on one's response to the aging process. Developmental changes associated with normal aging must be carefully understood by the health care provider before appropriate health care can be rendered.

Nurses working with the aged must be familiar with the physiologic as well as the psychosocial changes associated with "normal" aging. In addition, behavioral responses to losses must be recognized in order to provide comprehensive care to the elderly in health and in illness. The following chapters explore the concept of normal aging, review physiologic as well as psychosocial changes that accompany aging, examine the concept of loss and its impact on aging, and explore common health problems that affect the elderly. In Chap. 42, common health problems affecting the elderly are discussed. Since many of these problems have already been addressed in Part 4, "The Nursing Care of Adults," the content of this chapter is limited to the differences that affect the health care of this age group.

ANA STANDARDS OF GERIATRIC NURSING PRACTICE[1]

1. The nurse demonstrates an appreciation of the heritage, values, and wisdom of older people.
2. The nurse seeks to resolve her or his conflicting attitudes regarding aging, death, and dependency so that she or he can assist older persons and their relatives to maintain life with dignity and comfort until death ensues.
3. The nurse observes and interprets minimal as well as gross signs and symptoms associated with both normal aging and pathologic changes and institutes appropriate nursing measures.
4. The nurse differentiates between pathologic social behavior and the usual life-style of each aged individual.
5. The nurse supports and promotes normal physiologic functioning of the older person.
6. The nurse protects aged persons from injury, infection, and excessive stress and supports them through the multiplicity of stressful experiences to which they are subjected.
7. The nurse employs a variety of methods to promote effective communication and social interaction of aged persons with individuals, family, and other groups.
8. The nurse together with the older person designs, changes, or adapts the physical and psychosocial environment to meet his or her needs within the limitations imposed by the situation.
9. The nurse assists the older person to obtain and utilize devices which help him or her to attain a higher level of function and ensures that these devices are kept in good working order by the appropriate persons or agencies.

[1]Reprinted with permission from the *American Nurses' Association Standards of Geriatric Nursing Practice.* Copyright © 1973 by the American Nurses' Association.

40
Physiologic and Psychosocial Effects of Normal Aging

Hazel R. Mummah[1]

Individuals "age" at different rates, influenced by inherited genes, life-style, emotional well-being, physiologic health, nutritional status, and many other features. *Aging* commences when we emerge from the uterus and continues until death.

Historically, old age was certainly not known; it was simply uncommon. The average life expectancy at birth in 1000 B.C. is reported to have been about 18 years. Today, average life expectancy ranges anywhere from 70.1 to 75 years of age.

As we grow old, normal physiologic, psychologic, and social changes accompany the aging process. These changes, however, are not uniform, but are unique to each individual. The following pages will examine thoee components of the "normal" aging process as they occur in the older adult. Coping successfully with these changes will make aging a time of personal fulfillment and satisfaction.

I. Theories of aging. Researchers theorize as to the physical causes of aging. Among current hypotheses being studied are:

   A. Limited cell replications point out that the potential for cellular proliferation is limited by the number of times cells have divided, thus giving an aged organism less potential for new cell growth than a similar organism at a younger age.

   B. Error accumulation theory states that cellular reproduction is not perfect and that defective cell components may occasionally be generated due to inaccuracies within the synthesis processes. Assuming that these defective parts are stable and passed on to subsequent generations, eventual buildup of impairment of function is thought to result.

   C. Autoimmune theory postulates that there is growing evidence that autoimmune responses increase with age. These immune bodies attach to cells and lead to the destruction of healthy tissues. Related pathologies supporting the autoimmune theory include pernicious anemia, Addison's disease, and chronic thyroiditis.

   D. Irreversible decrement theory claims that aging is a fact of life and there is in fact a progressive decline in one's bodily functions that cannot be terminated.

   E. Adaptation view states that even though a decline does occur, we should be able to cope with changes and adapt accordingly. Researchers of this theory are also investigating whether aging results from intrinsic or environmental factors.

   F. Genetic theory suggests that mutations occur within the cell, especially changes related to DNA and RNA. These mutations result in physiologic manifestations of aging.

II. Physiologic effects of aging. Aging bodies differ almost as much from those of young adults as do those of small children. Geriatric research published before 1970 was almost nonexistent when compared to other specialties. It is only in the last decade that physiologists and biologists have begun to probe into the causes and effects of aging on cells, body structure, and function during the later decades of human development.

   A. Changes in perception and coordination.

     1. Alteration in perception and coordination occurs due to increased cell loss from brain tissue, especially the temporal and frontal lobes.

[1]The sections "Assessment" and "Diagnosis" and parts of the section "Intervention" were contributed by Dorothy A. Jones.

2. Alteration in sleep patterns occurs, with less deep sleep required. Older people tend to dream less and have increased periods of wakefulness.

B. Muscular and skeletal changes.

1. The most visible physiologic changes in aging relate to the decrements in body tissue.
2. There is a widespread decrease in bone mass, frequently resulting in increased stress on weight-bearing areas that become predisposed to fracture.
3. Height decreases, and kyphosis sometimes develops. There is thinning or even collapse of intervertebral disks.
4. Joints lose elasticity, and preosteoarthritic degeneration is found in joint cartilage, making the joint less flexibl.
5. Muscle size and strength both diminish with age. Muscle tone and strength peaks between ages 20 and 30 with gradual decline thereafter. While regeneration of muscle tissue is still possible in the older person, muscle mass does decrease, gradually but steadily.
6. Decreased muscle strength, increased fatigue due to decreased adenosine triphosphate (ATP) and lactic acid production.
7. Alteration in coordination may contribute to disturbance in gait. Fine motor movements may also diminish.
8. Bones becomes more brittle and tend to break more easily.

C. Sensory changes.

1. There is a decrease in efficient function of all senses with time.
2. The lens of the eye thickens.
3. The pupil aperture narrows, and the muscles in the eye function less efficiently.
4. The ability of the eye to accommodate light diminishes, as well as the inability of the individual to distinguish between various intensities of light.
5. Proprioception, the perception of one's position and relatedness in and to space, is impaired.
6. Adults in their forties and early fifties become aware of difficulties in focusing distance and submit to wearing reading glasses.
7. Hearing also changes. The ability to hear high tones declines with age; as a result, less auditory information is available.
8. The skin loses its elasticity, and the sense of touch is diminished.
9. About two-thirds of the taste buds die by the time the individual reaches age 70.
10. Other changes include decrease in perception of temperature and vibration and an increased pain threshold.
11. The decline in sensory input usually occurs gradually. The ultimate composite loss of sensory input may affect one's capacity in awareness and internalization of environmental stimuli, resulting in a decrease in responsivity and adaptation.
12. Response to pain sensation and reaction to temperature changes decreases. Decreased fever defense reaction noted.
13. Reaction time decreases and reflexes alter. Slowness to respond to situations may be influenced by the muscular and skeletal intactness.

D. Respiratory changes.

1. With increasing age there is a measurable reduction in breathing efficiency. Bronchopulmonary movement is decreased due to an increase in fibrous connective tissue and lymphoid elements; both factors lead to a rigid bronchopulmonary tree (1).
2. The exchange of air between lungs and environment is reduced due to the obstruction of the pulmonary airway and restriction in pulmonary expansion and contraction.
3. Vital capacity decreases, residual air increases, and the respiratory gas exchange functions are diminished.
4. Bronchoelimination is decreased due to a diminished cough reflex and lessened effectiveness of the ciliary mechanism.

     5. With a decrease in bronchopulmonary function, the oxygen supply needed for cell respiration and assimilation is diminished.

     6. Poor posture may decrease the capacity of the thoracic cavity and affect overall oxygenation.

E. Cardiovascular changes.

     1. Cardiac pathology is the number one cause of mortality in the aged (see Chap. 42).

     2. The normal physiologic changes in cardiac function result in the heart having to work harder to accomplish less.

     3. Peripheral resistance and circulation time, as well as systolic and diastolic blood pressure, increase with age.

     4. Physiologic changes related to the heart include the following:

          a. Cardiac output decreases approximately 30 percent by the age of 65.

          b. Prolongation of the period of contraction occurs.

          c. Increased rigidity of valves is observed.

          d. Increased cardiac output caused by exercise results in a rise in arterial blood pressure.

          e. Aortic elasticity diminishes considerably with advancing age (2).

     5. Decreased cardiac efficiency and arteriosclerotic and atherosclerotic changes in blood vessels are prime factors in diminished circulation to all parts of the aging body.

     6. Increased irritability of the cardiac muscle may result in alterations in rhythm.

     7. Tachycardia may occur in response to stress.

F. Changes in blood vessels.

     1. There is a decreased elasticity of blood vessels.

     2. Normal calcification of blood vessels (e.g., aortic arch) occurs.

     3. Athrogenesis secondary to the aging process is present.

     4. Decreased capillary permeability occurs due to sluggish exchange of blood in the capillary bed.

     5. Alteration in the vasopressor control mechanism contributes to orthostatic hypertension. Thse changes may result in dizziness, weakness, and fainting.

G. Metabolic changes.

     1. Malnutrition is epidemic in the aged population. Decreased food budgets due to poverty, faulty life-style food habits, and psychologic reactions to aging are partially responsible.

     2. In the middle late years, the resorption of gum and bony tissue surrounding the teeth is the prime factor in dental changes. This resorption of bone of the mandible and maxilla leads to a shortening of the distance between the chin and nose and a pulling inward of the lips, affecting nutrition.

     3. Loss of teeth and/or poorly fitting dentures can lead to malnutrition.

     4. Dryness of the mouth as a result of diminished saliva flow and decreased acuity in the senses of smell and taste tend to decrease the variety and selection of foods eaten. Decreased sensitivity to thirst may lead to decreased fluid intake and contribute to constipation.

     5. Nervous system changes related to metabolism include reduced hypothalamic efficiency affecting appetite and thirst responses; parasympathetic changes alter intestinal motility; and loss of cortical inhibition may contribute to diarrhea and incontinence.

     6. Gastric secretions are decreased by about 50 percent by the time the individual reaches 70. With the limited availability of digestive enzymes, some of the nutrients in the food pass through the digestive system and are not metabolized, rendering them unavailable to the body's use. Alterations in the pH of stomach acids occur and atrophy of the salivary glands contributes to alterations in metabolism.

7. Delays in emptying the esophagus are commonly seen in aged individuals and may lead to inflammation.
8. Often, insufficient high-bulk foods are ingested because of the difficulty involved in chewing them. Bulky foods help to maintain tonicity of the tract wall, but many people are unaware of this beneficial effect.
9. Obesity may be a problem for women and men over age 50. This may be due to:
   a. Diminishing exercise patterns without the altering of caloric intake.
   b. Attempts to compensate for psychologic loss with sweets.
   c. Life-style and established food habits.
   d. Poverty level; use of food often high in carbohydrates.
   e. Hormonal changes, especially in women.
10. Weight losses in the elderly may be indication of malnutrition.
11. Loss of glycogen deposits and unavailable glycogen stores are present due to an alteration in the basal metabolic rate, interfering with the body's ability to produce heat.

H. Renal changes.
1. With increasing age there is a gradual diminution in renal function caused by reduced rate of glomerular filtration and reduced effective plasma flow.
2. The primary factor involved in decreased renal function is vascular changes which result in hypertension. Vessels within the kidneys are affected by aging. Changes in the arterial system result in disturbances in tissue nutrition and ischemia.
3. Diminished neuromuscular stimulation of the bladder frequently results in incomplete emptying. Frequently, older females particularly are subject to urinary infections.
4. Prostatic enlargement is present in some degree in three-fourths of males 65 and over.
5. A reduction in fluid intake results in reduced kidney function. This can cause an electrolyte imbalance in the aged person with symptoms of fatigue, dizziness, nausea, and vomiting.

I. Skin changes.
1. Among the major changes in the skin associated with aging are the thinning of epithelial and subcutaneous fatty layers.
2. Loss of fatty tissue progresses gradually after age 45 until little subcutaneous fat is seen over the legs, forearms, and face, even in the presence of abundant abdominal and hip fat.
3. There is loss of fat padding over bony prominences, predisposing the elderly immobilized persons to decubitus ulcers.
4. Blood vessels are often prominent, observable through thinned tissue.
5. Collagen, elastic fibers, and the epithelial layer also shrink in thickness.
6. Sweat and sebaceous glands decrease in number, and the result is thin, dry, inextensible skin.
7. Loss of sweat glands causes important changes in body temperature regulation.
8. Pigmentation of the skin tends to lighten due to cellular losses of melanocytes.
9. Greying of the hair occurs due to a loss of pigmentation cells.
10. In general, there is a major thinning of scalp hair and a loss of axillary and pubic hair.
11. Wrinkling of skin develops because of frequent, repetitious use of muscles. Atrophic changes in subcutaneous tissue also contribute to the wrinkling of skin.
12. "Aging spots," due to a pigment called lipofuscin, mark the skin of aging individuals. The color ranges from yellow to brown.
13. There is a decreased ability of the body to rid itself of heat via evaporation.

This may contribute to the fact that older patients can be predisposed to heat strokes.

   J. Changes in immunity.

      1. Allergic responses appear to increase with aging, particularly in response to drugs.

      2. There is marked decrease in the aging liver and kidney functions which delay the elimination and detoxification of chemicals (e.g., medications and allergens).

      3. The immune capacity appears to break down with age, as evidenced by the fact that cancer is the number two cause of mortality in people over 65.

      4. Studies suggest that infectious processes occur which lymphocytes would have eliminated in persons of younger age (3).

   K. Endocrine changes.

      1. Gonadal hormones decrease with aging in both males and females. This decline produces slow involutional changes in genital tissue and a reduction and finally a loss in fertility. Loss in libido often does not occur.

      2. Frequency of intercourse, intensity of sensation, speed in attaining erection, and force of ejaculation are all reduced in the aging male.

      3. In women, thinning vaginal walls may provoke some pain upon intromission of the penis.

      4. Interest and capacity of sexual activity persist through old age. However, activity declines due to illness or unavailability of a suitable mate.

      5. For additional hormonal changes refer to Table 40-1.

III. Psychologic effects of normal aging. How aged individuals perceive themselves and adjust to physical, social, and environmental changes varies significantly from person to person. The attitudes and problem-solving mechanism of a 65-year-old will vary from person to person. Financial resources, increments of physical and mental decline, loss of the support of significant others, and life-style coping patterns affect self-concept and self-esteem in the aged.

   A. Role changes. Retirement results in a shift of focus from that of productivity to that of increased use of leisure time. Retirement may be viewed as something positive for many people because they now have an opportunity to finally do all the things they wished to. For others, mandatory retirement may mean a loss of self-esteem and personal identity as a child rearer or household provider.

   B. Changes in relationships with significant others. This occurs frequently with advancing age. It is not uncommon to see a wife, who has been the subordinated person in the household, suddenly become responsible for financial arrangements and leadership roles, or the husband, who never participated in household chores, become responsible for the cooking, cleaning, and laundry.

   C. Loss. There are a multiplicity of losses that the aged person must face. These include physical, psychologic, financial, and social losses. Probably the most devastating loss endured by the aged is the loss of significant others, usually a spouse. For the elderly the loss of significant others can include separation from children. This often contributes to a change in attitudes and emotional responses. (A complete discussion of loss is found in Chap. 41.)

   D. Changes in interactions with others. Diminished reaction time occurs with normal aging and can make the interactions with extended family members or friends strenuous and unrewarding. In a clinical setting care must be taken to plan activities that can be accomplished while the aged person is sitting or that expend little energy to accomplish. Children can be very stimulating (but exhausting) for the aged. Care must be taken not to exhaust the elderly with overstimulation.

   E. Isolation.

      1. Inability to move about freely, whether inside the home or out, is a source of frustration to the elderly. Physical limitations, denial of a driver's license, or financial losses may limit mobility and activity and result in depression and anxiety in many aged persons.

      2. Bus transportation is frequently inadequate in many areas, and physical limitations

TABLE 40-1 / KNOWN HORMONE CHANGES IN THE AGED*

Hormones and Controlling Factors	Normal Action	Age Change
Adrenal Cortex		
Cortisol ACTH	Stimulates protein catabolism, stimulates liver uptake of amino acids and their conversion to glucose, is permissive for stimulation of gluconeogenesis by other tissues, inhibits glucose uptake and oxidation by many body cells	Secretion somewhat decreased in proportion to decreased muscle mass
Aldosterone Angisterin plasma K$^+$ concentration	Stimulates Na reabsorption, specifically by distal tubules, stimulates transport of Na by other epithelia in the body, e.g., sweat glands, is an "all-purpose" stimulator of Na retention	Young people have been found to have secretion rates for aldosterone that are more than twice as high as those of elderly subjects; metabolic clearance rates and calculated plasma concentrations of aldosterone are also decreased
Gonads		
Ovaries: Estrogen FSH LH	Maintains the entire female genital tract and the breasts, is responsible for body hair distribution and the general female configuration, is required for follicle and ovum maturation, permits ovulation, and onset of menses	Loss of germinal cells causes decrease in levels of estrogen, which is associated with increase in pituitary activity and a decrease in estrogen levels; source of estrogen in postmenopausal women, adrenal cortex (primarily)
Progesterone FSH LH	Present only in significant amounts during luteal phase of menstrual cycle, has an effect on the endometrium, breasts, oviducts, and uterine smooth muscle	A decrease of 50% of pregnanediol (a byproduct of progesterone breakdown) in urinary excretion of women between 30 and 80
Testes: Testosterone LH	Spermatogenesis, needed for the morphology and function of the entire male duct system, development and maintenance of normal sexual drive and behavior in men, development of secondary sexual characteristics	Is not as abrupt or sudden as in female; loss of geminal cells also occurs when pituitary is functioning at high level
Pancreas		
Insulin Plasma Glucose concentrations	Stimulates the facilitated diffusion of glucose into certain cells (muscle and adipose), stimulates protein synthesis, affects liver synthesis	Response of elderly person to insulin is decreased
Kidneys		
Renin	Catalyzes the reaction in which angiotensiogen becomes angiotensin	Suggested slower response but no evidence
Angiotensin	Profound stimulator of aldosterone, secretion is the primary input into the adrenal gland, which produces aldosterone	Suggested slower response but no evidence
Erythropoietin	Stimulates erythrocyte and hemoglobin synthesis	Suggested slower response but no evidence

TABLE 40-1 / KNOWN HORMONE CHANGES IN THE AGED* (continued)

Hormones and Controlling Factors	Normal Action	Age Change
Posterior Pituitary		
ADH: Blood volume Blood pressure Electrolyte levels	Antidiuretic effect on kidney, keeps water permeability of latter nephron segments up, so H_2O reabsorption is able to keep up with Na reabsorption	Kidney (increased) response time
Thyroid Gland		
Thyroxine TSH	An iodine-containing amino acid, influences metabolic rate. O_2 consumption, and heat production in most body tissues	From 25 years onward there is a slow gradual decline in thyroid activity (until eighth decade)

*Developed by Catherine Kopac, R.N., M.N.
Source: D. Jones, C. Dunbar, and M. Jirovec, *Medical-Surgical Nursing: A Conceptual Approach,* McGraw-Hill Book Company, New York, 1978, p. 81.

of aging may make the use of this form of public transportation either fearful or impractical.
  3. Crime rates in ghetto areas, where many aged persons are forced to seek housing because of financial deprivation, further tend to reduce mobility of aged citizens. The aged are easy targets for crimes, especially if they live alone or are physically disabled.
  4. The aging person can be isolated and passive, melancholy, sad, or contemplative. They tend to withdraw from those around them and store their energy for a significant other(s) (see Chap. 41).
F. Changes in reaction to stress.
  1. Physiologic, as well as psychologic and social, changes occur throughout the life cycle. In the absence of pathophysiologic changes, the overall functioning of the body slows.
  2. An individual's ability to respond to stressful situations and return to a prestress state is maintained but may be delayed in many situations. According to Shock (4), an individual can survive (under particular conditions) with less than 49 percent of the liver, fractions of stomach and intestines, one lung, and one kidney.
  3. During stress, decreased recognition of stresses, diminished relaying information, and decreased endocrine response affects the body's response to stress (5).
IV. Sociocultural effects of aging.
  A. The elderly live with the knowledge of the reality of impending disease and death.
  B. Fear of institutionalization and of pain associated with illness are present.
  C. The elderly are concerned with the quality of life during illness. Death is often reflected in their conversations.
  D. Lack of the proximity of loved ones to support the individual during this time, public disregard for long-term care facilities, and soaring costs of hospitalization compound fears associated with hospitalization.
  E. Aged immigrants, who do not comprehend English well, face multiple problems when they age that may intensify anxiety.
  F. The inability to communicate needs, both physical and psychosocial, to the care provider causes insurmountable difficulty in adequate care delivery for all elderly persons.
  G. "Right to die" laws have been enacted in several states. The possibility of the right

to refuse to be kept alive when there is no prognosis for recovery has been eagerly requested by many aged persons. Social issues concerned with health care delivery as related to the patient's autonomy in dying are receiving much public consideration.

H. Because of physical limitations and alterations in visual and other sensory perceptions, the elderly are often victims of crimes.

I. Approximately 20 percent of the aged are impoverished (6). Substandard housing, inadequate food budgets, and the absence of luxuries constitute a burden for this age group.

J. Middle-class aged persons with modest accumulated savings to provide for retirement years find inflation and exaggerated costs of living a threat to security.

K. The frustration of abandoned travel plans, for example, are a source of deprivation to some aged individuals.

L. The industrialization of this country decreases satisfying alternative life-styles for the aged. The generation now over 65 is the first to witness the mass mobility of their children and grandchildren to transcontinental areas for employment.

M. Homes tend to be smaller and apartments are a new way of life. In a larger percentage of middle-aged families, both the husband and wife work. This has a significant impact on role definition and life-style.

N. The decrease in the number of extended family structures and the decrease in house size limit the possibility of shelter for the aged adult.

O. Many of the aged ethnic immigrants have failed to integrate into the American culture. They are frequently housed in isolated, near-ghetto urban areas where native language and cultural accoutrements are available. Retirement is often affected in these areas.

ASSESSMENT

I. Data sources.
   A. Family
   B. Patient
   C. Friends
   D. Significant others.

II. Health history.
   A. Obtain a diet history; question appetite and eating habits. Evaluate loss of appetite, and identify onset.
   B. Assess the individual's ability to eat; learn who prepares meals and how meals are cooked; assess physical limitations related to eating.
   C. Evaluate daily activity schedule. Identify rest periods and sleep habits, as well as number of hours an individual sleeps.
   D. Identify sensory changes: e.g., does the individual have visual disturbances or wear glasses; is there a hearing loss; does the person wear a hearing aid? Assess responses to pain and temperature change.
   E. Assess bowel habits (daily) and pattern of elimination. The use of laxatives and stool softeners should also be noted.
   F. Question urination pattern; assess for dysuria, nocturia, dribbling, etc. Evaluate fluid intake and output; question the presence of edema.
   G. Assess communication patterns. If language barrier is present, identify language used.
   H. Assess pattern of interaction with significant others (e.g., spouse, children, grandchildren) and mobility (including mode of transportation).
   I. Elicit history-related significant health problems, the presence of infection, chronic illness and allergies.
   J. Identify individual's occupation, retirement plans, current housing, financial support, and medical insurance.
   K. Assess personality traits. Evaluate coping patterns used to handle stress in previous encounters; evaluate patterns used to handle loss (see Chap. 41).

> *L.* Identify physical limitations, *e.g.*, shortness of breath, numbness and tingling in extremities, cyanosis, edema, complaints of dizziness, palpitations, etc. Analyze mobility and assess tolerance.

III. Physical assessment (see Table 40-2). Additional information to be included in the assessment should include:

> *A.* Changes in body weight may be noted. Both obesity and/or significant weight loss may be observed due to eating and activity habits.
>
> *B.* Neurological changes may include diminished response to pain, heat, and cold; decreased reflexes may be observed; and alteration in gait may be present. Kyphosis may also be present.
>
> *C.* Because of muscle changes, overall muscle strength, size, and tone may be affected. Coordination and fine motor movement may be disturbed with age. Tremors may be present.
>
> *D.* Peripheral pulses may be diminished. Slowed capillary refill may also be noted. Peripheral edema should be assessed.
>
> *E.* The mouth should be examined for lesions, breakdown, teeth and gum irritation, and denture fit.
>
> *F.* Fecal and urinary incontinence should be identified, along with identification of skin breakdown.
>
> *G.* Presence of calluses or other related foot problems should be identified. Shoe fit should be evaluated.
>
> *H.* Breast examination is important (refer to Chap. 30).

PROBLEMS

Potential or actual problems encountered during "normal aging":

I. Malnutrition.
II. Obesity.
III. Dehydration.
IV. Diarrhea, constipation, and incontinence.
V. Diminished energy, slowness.
VI. Isolation (friends and family).
VII. Decreased perceptional reactions.
VIII. Increased threat to safety.
IX. Alterations in sleep patterns.
X. Loss.
XI. Decreased mobility.
XII. Increased predisposition to skin breakdown.
XIII. Role change (retirement, life-style).

DIAGNOSIS

I. Nutritional alteration: malnutrition (potential), secondary to decreased intake, poor dentures, or loss of appetite.
II. Nutritional alteration: obesity (potential), secondary to increased intake, decreased metabolism, or diminished mobility.
III. Urinary elimination: incontinence (potential).
IV. Alteration in bowel elimination: diarrhea or constipation (potential).
V. Dysrhythm of sleep-rest activity (potential).
VI. Impairment of mobility, secondary to gait impairment, decreased muscle tone, and decreased energy level.
VII. Impairment of skin integrity (potential), secondary to decreased skin turgor, decreased muscle tone, dehydration, and increased fat deposits.

TABLE 40-2 / AN OVERVIEW OF PHYSICAL ASSESSMENT FOR THE ELDERLY*

Organ or System	Important Physical Symptoms	Cause of Symptom
General	Diminished pain sensation, lack of febrile response to disease, confusion	Normal changes in autonomic nervous system; normal change in thermoregulatory response; general symptom meaning "something is wrong," e.g., hypoxia, infection, dyspnea, drug toxicity, sensory deprivation, overstimulation, etc.
Skin	Loss of elasticity, dryness, pressure areas, breast lumps, poor indicator of hydration status	Normal age changes in connective tissue, oil gland atrophy, poor circulation, neoplasms, cystic disease
Eyes	Decreased visual acuity	Normal aging change, senile macular changes (vascular), cataracts, glaucoma, retinal detachment
Ears	Gradual decreased auditory acuity, sudden hearing loss	Normal aging changes or prebycusis, wax accumulation, decreased blood supply to the organ of Corti, neurological diseases
Mouth, throat	Hoarseness	Laryngeal pathology
Head, neck	Rigidity, lymphadenopathy elevation of left jugular pulse, arterial bruits	Cervical spondylosis, Parkinson's disease, arthritis, infection (always of pathologic origin), elongated aortic arch and obstruction, obstruction in carotids, heart murmurs
Cardiovascular	Irregular radial pulse, increased systolic and diastolic pressure, systolic and diastolic murmurs	Ectopic beats, atrial fibrillation, arteriosclerotic changes in arterial system (usually ejection type and not pathologic), significant cardiac pathology
Respiratory	Breathing pattern disturbance, deviation of trachea, limited expansion	Lung pathology, neurologic disease, kyphosis, scoliosis, normal age changes in rib cartilage
Gastrointestinal	Changes in bowel habits, nonrigid peritoneum in acute abdomen	Normal age changes in connective and muscle tissues, drugs, infection, organic brain disease, depressive illnesses, diverticulitis, cancer, diet changes, weak abdominal muscles
Genitourinary	Frequency, dysuria, incontinence	Capacity of bladder decreases to about 250 mL, benign prostatic hypertrophy, cancer, drugs, habitual overdistension, neurological disease, weakened pelvic muscles
Musculoskeletal	Slightly flexed posture, enlarged, stiff joints with crepitation, fractures, tremors, gait changes	Normal aging change, osteoarthritis, osteoporosis, falls, demineralization, infections, lung disease, Parkinson's disease, neurological disease, drug induced, corns, calluses, fractures (hip), neurological disease)
Central nervous system	Sudden onset of symptoms; progressive, slow onset	Vascular or epileptic diseases, degenerative or neoplastic diseases

*Developed by Deborah Downey, R.N., M.S.
Source: D. Jones, C. Dunbar, and M. Jirovec, *Medical-Surgical Nursing: A Conceptual Approach,* McGraw-Hill Book Company, New York, 1978, p. 77.

    VIII. Alteration in self-concept, secondary to physical and psychosocial loss.
    IX. Alteration in socialization patterns, secondary to loss of significant others, financial insecurity, isolation, or decreased sexuality.
    X. Anxiety: mild to moderate, secondary to fear of loss, institutionalization, lack of security, or separation.
    XI. Alteration in comfort: discomfort (potential), secondary to increased respiratory rate, tachycardia, or emotional stress.
    XII. Alteration in cardiac output: fatigue or dyspnea (potential).
    XIII. Alteration in sensory perception: visual changes, loss of hearing, or decreased pain perception (potential).

GOALS OF CARE

    I. Immediate.
        A. Prevent disruption in health and maintain the individual's optimal health.
        B. Increase activity and maximize mobility by improved ambulation.
        C. Improved nutritional status as demonstrated by maintaining weight within normal limits.
    II. Long-range.
        A. Maintain optimal functioning of the aged individual as evidenced by the ability to sustain and perform activities of daily living.
        B. Identify potential problems that may interrupt the healthy state, and select interventions to reduce their continued threat.

INTERVENTION

    I. Nutrition.
        A. Good dental care, gum care, and use of properly fitting dentures are essential to increased nutrition.
        B. Dentures should be in place, especially at meals. Plastic linings can be easily and inexpensively applied to poorly fitting dentures by a dentist.
        C. When it is impractical to obtain dentures, foods chopped in a blender are more appetizing than canned baby foods.
        D. Eye glasses facilitate seeing and the enjoyment of food service.
        E. Blind patients need to be oriented to the location of food on the plate. The simple instruction of, "Your potatoes are at twelve o'clock, the peas at three o'clock, etc.," will help the sightless person to enjoy the meal and to become more independent.
        F. Scheduling activities of daily living so that a short rest period is observed prior to mealtimes will help to conserve the patient's physical energies for eating.
        G. When loneliness is a deterrent to appetite, companionship and socialization at mealtimes helps to reduce depression and ensure appetite. If the patient is physically unable to feed self, the nurse should use the time required for hand feeding in a meaningful way. Socialization helps to make mealtimes happily anticipated.
        H. Teaching should center around helping the elderly person plan a daily menu that will be both nutritional and pleasing to the appetite and will fit within the individual's budget.
        I. Small, frequent meals and a bedtime snack should be encouraged, as this may help maintain the individual's healthy state and prevent abdominal discomfort.
        J. Eating meals prepared by others (such as meal clubs or "meals on wheels") may also help improve nutrition, especially if the preparation of meals is a problem for the patient.

K. The use of alcohol (wine, brandy) prior to eating may help to stimulate the appetite.

II. Sensibility and perception.

A. When hearing changes occur, the nurse should speak slowly, avoid shouting, face the patient when speaking, and encourage the use of a hearing aid.

B. The use of large print will help visual competence when vision is altered. Frequent eye testing and proper use of glasses should be encouraged.

C. Alterations in sleep patterns may require support and reassurance from the nurse. Naps can be taken, while the use of caffeine or other stimulants prior to bedtime is discouraged. Warm milk prior to retiring may prove to be relaxing and help promote sleep.

D. A quiet, relaxed atmosphere for older patients to decrease sensory overload and the potential for confusion and/or anxiety should be planned.

E. Individuals should be protected from alteration in temperature change (e.g., hot packs). Examination of the body parts for skin breakdown (e.g., feet) which may go unnoticed because of changes in pain perception is critical.

F. Individuals should be taught the dangers of smoking, especially in bed. Teaching patients to use visual senses to avoid those things they cannot feel is critical (e.g., teach patient to compensate for visual losses by turning head to obtain view; have others use a full view).

III. Safety.

A. If patients have visual and auditory changes, they may have to change their driving habits. If driving is stressful, it should be avoided or stopped altogether.

B. Family members as well as patients should be sensitive to patient's diminished reaction time. Patient should have enough time to perform activities in a slowed, unhurried environment. Continued support by the nurse and the family is very important.

C. Individuals should be adequately prepared for new situations, e.g., diagnostic procedures, hospitalization, etc., in order to decrease confusion and disruptions in sensory intake.

D. To compensate for alterations in blood pressure which may accompany aging, patients should be taught to adjust to this new situation by changing positions slowly. They should be encouraged to rest if they feel dizzy, until the uncomfortable feelings pass.

E. Elderly individuals should be encouraged to remove throw rugs from their environment to avoid falling. Rugs on stairs should be securely tacked down.

F. Care should be taken to prevent falls in the bathroom. Special handrails should be installed in the bathtub to prevent injury.

G. Elderly patients should be encouraged to avoid walking on ice. Special spikes can be put into boots to help prevent falls. Rubber-soled firm boots should be worn in the winter.

H. The fragility of aging bones makes them inordinately vulnerable to fractures. Care should be taken to prevent the risk of bone injuries.

I. Depressive reactions to the combination of severely debilitating diseases coupled with many of the normal losses resulting from the aging process tend to immobilize patients (see Chap. 41).

J. The installation of handrails in hallways enables the elderly person to ambulate safely at an individualized pace.

K. Teaching of proper transfer techniques, range-of-motion exercises, and body positioning is necessary to increase overall patient mobility and maintain safety.

L. Geriatric chairs, well padded, with detachable trays, are acceptable safety devices. Prosthetic ambulatory devices such as pickup or rolling walkers can assist the patient in independent ambulation.

IV. Activity.

A. Encourage the elderly individual to plan daily activities as tolerated. Routine daily exercise activities which increase muscle tone and improve cardiac and ventilatory status should be stressed. Aging patients can be encouraged to engage in sports as tolerated.

B. Consistent exercise will improve joint mobility and patient independence. When joint movement becomes impaired, patients can be taught new skills which will increase activity.

C. With all activity, rest periods should be planned as needed to avoid overexertion and fatigue.

V. Elimination.

A. Adequate intake of fluids is essential for normal metabolism and elimination. Keep a glass of water within the patient's reach, offer water with medications, and encourage fluids between meals, e.g., coffee, tea, or juices as tolerated.

B. Care should be taken to help avoid dehydration which may accompany episodes of diarrhea or acute infection. Early restoration of electrolyte and fluid balances is essential.

C. Improved nutrition, balanced diet, and adequate intake help relieve constipation. Stool softeners (e.g., Colace) may be used daily. Patients should be advised to avoid straining at stool.

D. At times, a modified squatting position created by placing feet on a stool may help improve defecation (7).

E. Formalized bowel retraining programs are based upon the restoration of previous bowel efficiency using natural stimuli. They include the assessment of past bowel habits, identification of current problems, and monitoring the effectiveness of interventions. Cooperation of the staff in the bowel retraining program is essential.

F. The dietician should be consulted for bowel retraining. Often, the addition of bulky foods and fluids to the diet will aid bowel functioning, as will the addition of bran (in such foods as cooked cereals) and prune juice. Fresh vegetables and fruits, finely chopped, are acceptable in most soft diets and also provide extra bulk.

G. Patients should be told to avoid excessive intake of fluids prior to going to bed in order to avoid nocturia.

VI. Skin care.

A. The daily bath ritual is contraindicated for aged patients as it further reduces natural skin oils. The hands, face, and perineal area require daily cleansing. Complete baths should be limited to once or twice a week.

B. Nonalcoholic lotions applied frequently to skin surfaces prevent drying, promote circulation, and satisfy the psychologic needs for cleanliness.

C. Depilatories may be used to remove excess facial hair.

D. Wigs can be used to compensate for excessive hair loss and to improve overall appearance.

E. Nonallergic or paper tape is less apt to tear the skin of aged patients. When applying dressings, use elasticized gauze dressings rather than tape when possible.

F. Application of a protective ointment to the perineum of incontinent patients following cleansing helps to prevent irritation.

G. Immobilized, aged patients with diminished circulation may be predisposed to skin breakdown. Frequent turning is essential. Pressure-relieving devices such as foam pads, alternating air mattresses, or sheepskins further reduce the possibility of skin breakdown.

H. The nurse should encourage all attempts made by the patient to improve and/or maintain personal appearance. Hair care, interest in clothes, etc., should be supported.

VII. Environment.

A. Color.

1. To minimize effects of normal aging, it is imperative that the environment be structured to provide maximum amounts of sensory stimulation. The off-white or subtle coloring of most hospital settings provides very few visual cues and

contributes to, rather than diminishes, mental disorientation. Blue tends to be calming, soothing, and restful.

2. It has been noted that for persons of any age, the ability to adapt to new situations decreases as competence diminishes (8). Therefore, when an elderly individual is moved into a new environment, he or she should oe adequately prepared for the undertaking.

3. For the aged person who already tends to be withdrawn, passive, or depressed, red-orange (active) tones as a basis for decor rather than blue-green (passive) tones are more appropriate.

4. Normal aging results in changes to the lenses of the eye and in changes of light perception, which cause older people to perceive dark colors, neutral colors, and blue-greens less effectively. The use of such colors is contraindicated in the interest of patient safety and because of their effect on the patient's mood.

B. Light.

1. Light is an integral part of the environment. Light can affect mood, orientation, and functional ability. Areas for reading and craft work should be well illuminated for the elderly to maximize visual competence.

2. Variation in the light intensities is advisable. Softer lighting promotes relaxation and socialization processes. Maximum illumination in working areas such as physical therapy areas, game areas, and hallways enhances physical potential.

3. Most institutions require installation of lighting systems so that corridors can remain lighted at night. Curtains should be pulled sufficiently to prevent these bright lights from disturbing patients and to eliminate glare which may be potentially confusing to the elderly.

4. Landmarks familiar to the individual should be visible in order to orient them to the environment.

5. Differences in hall colors or brightly painted doors are other ways of cuing patients' memories. Name plates, clearly visible, also aid in orientation.

6. Blind patients require special environmental accoutrements to maximize their independence. Room numbers of raised, textured materials can be obtained from hardware stores. They should be at least 3 in high and placed on the doorway. Door handles leading to stairs or exits may be covered with a knurled substance as an alert to the possible dangers beyond.

7. Removal of wheelchairs or similar obstacles in walkways of blind or visually handicapped persons will help ensure physical safety. Careful orientation to surrounding environment is critical.

C. Life space.

1. The life space of aged persons (that area which they can call their own and in which they function for a great portion of their day) may shrink to very small proportions when they move to a small apartment or are confined to a health car facility.

2. Frequently this diminished life space implies lessened proprietary rights. If an individual is in a nursing home or other such facility, artifacts from home, e.g., clock and calendars or photos of family, help to establish identity, decrease loneliness, and aid in orientation.

3. Recognition of personal privacy and respect for an individual's life patterns, e.g., sleep and eating habits, will help maintain an individual's self-esteem and personal control over the aging process.

4. The nurse must identify significant others within the patient's environment and facilitate interpersonal relationships between the patient and family members, regardless of the setting.

D. Textures.

1. House plants and wooden or ceramic art pieces, as well as pictures, provide textural variety.

2. Mobiles hung from the ceiling make a welcome diversion from staring at a painted wall. When purchasing bedspreads, the choosing of a variety of

complimentary colors instead of one standard color helps to decrease the feeling of "institutionalization" (see Fig. 40-1).

E. Temperature.
   1. Temperature changes can directly affect the older patient.
   2. Patients should be encouraged to avoid drafts. Layered clothing may be used to conserve heat.
   3. A room which is too warm or too cold can cause discomfort, infection, anxiety, or dehydration. Adjusting thermostats to maximize the patient's physical and emotional well-being will help facilitate patient's overall comfort.

VIII. Psychosocial needs.
   A. Support of the family members is critical during aging. Frequently children seem to give the elderly a sense of great comfort and enjoyment. Frequent visits from children are important (Fig. 40-2).
   B. Family members tend to remain the primary significant others in the patient's life when care plans are structured to enable them to do so. Should hospitalization be necessary, a preadmission interview with the family establishes a communication basis and makes hospitalization less traumatic.
   C. Sexual needs for each individual should be discussed freely and supported by the nurse.

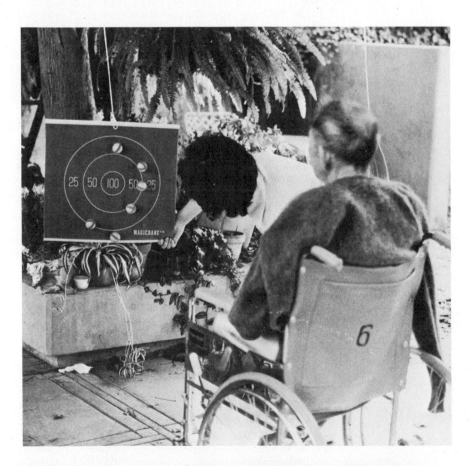

FIGURE 40-1 / A patio with its greenery and slatted sun roof provides a proper environment for restorative activities. (*Photograph by Tom Higgins.*)

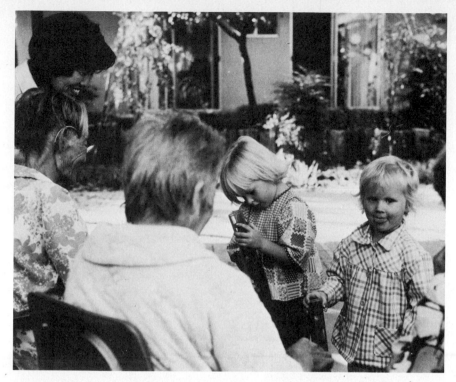

FIGURE 40-2 / Small children provide delightful stimuli to aged patients when activities are thoughtfully structured. (*Photograph by Tom Higgins.*)

D. Psychosocial interventions should be aimed at reducing depression in aged clients. Remotivation group therapies appropriately conducted by geriatric nurses aid in lessening depression and increase the patient's willingness to exert the mammoth efforts required to recover from debilitating disease (refer to Chap. 41).

E. An individual's control over the environment and participation in making choices is critical to one's self-concept and self-esteem. Attempts should be made by all health providers to allow the aged to participate in health care decisions so as to avoid disrupting an individual's life-style.

F. Changing societal attitudes towards the aged have been promoted by such organizations as the Grey Panthers, which increases the visibility of the aged.

G. Institutions are admitting aged students to and continuing education programs. Mass media is also recognizing the aged and is devoting more time and space to their concerns and interests. Large companies and colleges are conducting seminars aimed at grooming attitudes to accept the positive values of recreation and retirement.

H. Financial support, Medicare, Medicaid, Social Security, and other insurance policies should be selected for each individual as needed. When necessary, a social worker should be utilized to help the aged population.

I. Emotional stability is often based upon life experiences and successful coping patterns. During crisis, the individual may resort to coping patterns used in the past.

J. Elderly people often enjoy talking about the past (life review). Supportive listening and interest shown by the nurse will give the patient a sense of belonging.

K. Retirement settlements are developing throughout the country and are supporting independence in the elderly.

EVALUATION

    I. Reassessment.
        A. Appropriate adjustment to physiologic as well as psychosocial changes that accompany aging.
        B. Maximization of all individuals' potentials in order to optimize the quality of their lives.
    II. Complications (refer to Chap. 42).

REFERENCES

1. Oscar Balchum, "The Aging Respiratory System," in *Working With Older People,* vol. 4, U.S. Department of Health, Education and Welfare, Washington, D.C., 1971, pp. 115–118.
2. June C. Abbey, "Physiological Aspects of Aging" (unpublished manuscript), delivered in lecture at Ethel Percy Andrus Gerontology Center, University of Southern California, Los Angeles, 1973.
3. Y. Makinodan, E. H. Perkins, and M. G. Chen, "Immunologic Activity of the Aged," *Advances in Gerontological Research,* 3:171–198, 1971.
4. N. W. Shock, "Physiological Theories of Aging," in M. Rockstein et al. (eds.), *Theoretical Aspects of Aging,* Academic Press, New York, 1974.
5. Cheryl K. Ahern, Nancy Diekelmann, and Carol L. Panicucci, "Developmental Patterns of Interaction," in D. A. Jones et al. (eds.), *Medical-Surgical Nursing: A Conceptual Approach,* McGraw-Hill Book Company, New York, 1978, pp. 78–80.
6. United States Census Bureau, Washington, D.C., 1970.
7. Ahern et al., op. cit., p. 80.
8. Robert J. Newcomer and Michael A. Caggiano, "Environment and the Aged Person," in I. Burnside (ed.), *Nursing and the Aged,* McGraw-Hill Book Company, New York, 1976, pp. 559–569.

BIBLIOGRAPHY

Brotman, H.: "The Fastest Growing Minority: The Aging," National Agricultural Outlook Conference, February 24, 1972. Good perspective on the aged population and the national impact this group has upon society.

Burnside, Irene Mortenson: *Nursing and the Aged,* McGraw-Hill Book Company, New York, 1976. Excellent resource on nursing and the aged. References current and up to date. Excellent bibliography. Approaches to caring for the aged and identification of health problems dealt with in depth.

Hayward, D. G.: "Psychological Factors in the Use of Light and Lighting in Buildings," in J. Lang et al. (eds.), *Designing for Human Behavior,* Dowden, Hutchinson and Ross, Stroudsburg, Pa., 1974. Descriptive discussion of the effect of light on the behavior of the aged person. Helpful in terms of institutionalization of the aged person.

Weg, Ruth B.: *Aging: Scientific Perspectives and Social Issues,* D. Van Nostrand Company, New York, 1975, pp. 229–253.

———: *Psychological Needs of the Aged,* Ethel Percy Andrus Gerontology Center, University of Southern California, Los Angeles, 1973, p. 9.

41

Behavioral Responses to Aging

Jane Ann LaVigne

The manner in which individuals react to the process of aging varies. If a person has experienced incapacitating physical or emotional illness, poverty, or isolation, the stress of the additional losses associated with aging can be overwhelming. The person in good health, with adequate finances and intimate family ties, has the resources to adjust to the losses of aging. Often, people reach their fullest potential in later years and are able to balance the losses of old age by continuing to lead full, active, independent lives, while maintaining a sense of self-worth and high positive regard. This chapter discusses the concept of loss and the related behavioral responses to the aging process.

DEFINITION

Loss

The experience of loss is universal in its impact upon the individual's progression through life's stages. The ability to cope with loss is essential to the normal process of growth and development from infancy to old age and death. The process of birth itself can be considered as one's first experience with separation and loss. The loss of the passive in utero position and the awareness of physical discomfort are balanced by the gains of the mother's warm presence, the growing awareness of the world of objects, and other pleasurable sensations. The infant begins to learn about human interaction by signaling the need for food, warmth, and comfort and by being responded to in a loving, consistent way by parents or other caring persons. This balance between loss and gain must continue to be maintained and mastered for a forward progression of growth and development.

As normal growth and development proceed, loss of the pleasures of childlike dependency and the gaining of increased mastery over the self and the world occur. Children are most often prepared slowly and gradually to separate, individuate, and function in an independent manner. However, if there is limited preparation for aging, the introduction to the life of retirement, the death of a loved one, the loss of income, or the decline of health often seems abrupt and unplanned. Helping the individual plan for aging and the many physical, as well as behavioral changes that accompany this process, will result in healthy development of coping mechanisms.

Psychologic Coping and the Aging Process

Individuals cope with aging often in a pattern similar to the way they handled previous crises of growth and development. Bellak states that, "In the absence of major catastrophe or physical disaster, the personality traits of an aging person can be predicted from those that are evident in middle age. . . . There is no inevitable winding down, withdrawal, or inability to deal with life situations" (1).

Economic security, ability to enjoy leisure time, satisfying interpersonal relationships, and a positive outlook in life seem to be some insurance for coping with the losses of aging. Adequate preparation and planning for the change of life-style, should include financial planning, cultivation of varied interests at an earlier age, and provision for loss of spouse and separation from children.

The losses and stresses of aging (as with other stages of growth and development) can precipitate *neurotic* or *psychotic behavior.* This may interfere with an individual's ability to cope with developmental losses. Busse and Pfeiffer state that the psychologic disturbances of old age are most often direct reactions to stressful circumstances. They cite the most frequently used defenses of this age group as withdrawal, denial, projection, and somatization (2). *Personality changes* which sometimes occur in the elderly can be understood as ways of coping with loss and as a defense against the anxiety of growing old. Bellak describes some of these behaviors, which might be seen in the older patient as compartmentalization, preoccupation with the body, bizarre accusations, childlike clinging, denial of reality, regression, selfishness, and repetitive behavior (3).

Compartmentalization is a way of rigidly organizing thoughts an tasks so that only one thing at a time is given attention. The older patient seems to need more time to complete tasks or respond to new situations. It is likely that such an individual will be overwhelmed with an attempt to do too much at once. By doing only one thing at a time, patients gain reassurance, knowing they still have some control over the environment.

Signs of *hoarding* of pieces of food or bits of clothing and the unwillingness of the patient to share belongings with others often reflect the fear the patient has of being neglected, forgotten, or abandoned. Patients sometimes fear being left alone and becoming dependent on others for their well-being. It is a comfort for them to hoard things which they feel they may need at a later time.

The elderly often tend to repeat familiar stories over and over again to the same people. Such *repetition* is a way of maintaining contact with reality and of reminding oneself of a more pleasant past. If older patients have decreased memory for recent events, it becomes reassuring to remember the more remote occurrences of their lives.

Hypochondriasis, denial, projection, regression, and *depression* are additional mechanisms discussed later under "Intervention."

Personality changes can be understood as attempts on the part of the aged person to maintain order and regularity in the environment, to decrease anxiety, to be taken care of, to retain some amount of control, and to block out painful realities of the present. Often, the personal fears and anxieties of the aged manifest behavior that creates disruption or multiple demands of time and attention of others and can create negative responses from family and friends.

The Significance of Loss

As one grows, there is a change in the meaning of objects to oneself and a difference in the impact of the loss of valued objects. As the growth and maturational process occurs, the forces which regulate a person's sense of security and well-being become internalized and autonomous. The growing child becomes more self-sufficient and independent and learns to interact with adults and peers other than the parents and siblings. As aging continues, the meaning of loss shifts from the dangers of a survival threat in infancy, to the potential injury or loss of positive regard and/or loss of self-esteem. To accomplish the developmental tasks of each stage of growth and development, the child must relinquish the intensity of attachment to earlier objects and tolerate developmental losses in order to have psychic energy available to invest in new objects. The satisfactory or unsatisfactory resolution of these early object attachments and separations has an impact on the adult's ability to deal with subsequent issues of separation and loss.

   I. Types of losses. Losses vary in type and in their significance and meaning to the individual. There are several types of loss: developmental loss, concrete loss, symbolic loss, external loss, and object loss.

      A. Developmental loss. The predictable losses of growth and development, such as weaning and displacement by siblings, are instrumental in the development of gratifying interpersonal relations and are considered to be developmental losses.

      B. Concrete loss. The loss of an important person in one's milieu is one of the most intensely felt and major losses a person will encounter in life. Loss through death is an example of a concrete loss.

      C. Symbolic loss. Other losses, such as loss of self-esteem, confidence, or pride, are less tangible and considered to be symbolic losses. How one feels about the self is related (to a degree) to the way one views the self functioning in the world. To lose one's health, physical attractiveness, a spouse or loved one, a job, or a portion or extension of the self affects one's positive feelings about the self. Those issues that result in the loss of a positive feeling about the self differ from one person to the next.

D. External loss. The loss of valued objects such as a home, money, or treasured belongings is called external object loss. This is particularly difficult for aged people to handle, as there is often little chance of regaining material belongings. Such loss can create a further state of dependency upon others and force the aged individual to make unanticipated changes, e.g., moving into their children's home.

E. Object loss. This refers to a loss through death, a separation, or the incapacitating illness of important and valued persons in one's life. Separation from a loved one through death is a particularly painful loss to the aged person and a fearful reminder of the person's own mortality. Grief is a normal emotional response to such loss and is expressed in the process of mourning.

II. Response to loss.

A. There are many responses that an individual may have to loss. Each individual's reaction is unique and often based upon how a person has handled losses throughout life. Typical responses include the following:

  1. The experience of loss creates feelings of anxiety which serve to mobilize efforts to cope with the crisis.

  2. Loss has a disruptive effect upon a person's sense of equilibrium and well-being.

  3. The anxiety and sense of disequilibrium created by a crisis situation have potential for stimulating further growth or may cause regression to former levels of satisfaction and security.

  4. The individual's response to loss depends on such variables as:

  a. Type of loss.

  b. One's past experience with loss.

  c. The quality of one's physical and emotional health.

  d. The stability and meaning of interpersonal relationships.

  e. Investment in other valued objects and roles.

B. Grief and mourning.

  1. Freud describes *mourning*, in part, as the reaction to the loss of a loved *person* (4). He further cites the features of grief and mourning as:

  a. Painful dejection.

  b. Loss of interest in the outside world.

  c. Loss of the capacity to reinvest in a new love object.

  d. Inhibition in participating in activity.

  2. Behavioral characteristics of grief and mourning.

  a. In the normal work of mourning, there is a temporary *withdrawal* of investment in external activities because emotional energy is being utilized to reconcile the hurt, anger, guilt, and despair felt over the loss within the self.

  b. Initially, the reaction to death of a loved one is *shock,* since it is difficult to accept the fact that the dead person will no longer be there.

  c. There is a *preoccupation* of thoughts and feelings with the lost object. The preoccupation centers around not only pleasant thoughts and memories, but also the less positive and unpleasant feelings which were part of the relationship.

  d. There is a sense of *regret* and *sorrow* about the past arguments and negative feelings and the inability to do anything now about such things.

  e. Regret lingers as the bereaved person has a sense of not having done more positive things while there was still time to do so. The mourner expresses *despair* over not being able to relive the relationship in a more satisfactory way.

  f. *Anger* may be another aspect of grief work. The person can feel angry at the lost individual for being left behind and for having to deal with all these feelings. In a healthy resolution of the mourning process there is a working through of anger and a focusing on the good and pleasurable aspects of the lost person.

g. *Reminiscences* and *conversations* about the dead person can occur without marked feelings of despair or guilt.

h. The *acceptance* of the reality of the death and the continuation of one's own life are part of the *resolution* of the mourning process. Bellak describes the resolution of the mourning process as the slow withdrawal of love investment from the lost object and its reinvestment in other people, in one's job, and in daily life (5).

i. The lost person is remembered with good thoughts and feelings and with an appropriate degree of sadness. The mourner is able to rsume the activities and pleasures of daily life without experiencing undue feelings of guilt or shame.

3. Delayed grieving.

a. When the process of grieving is delayed, absent, or inhibited, the result is often a *chronic state of depression.*

b. Persons who are unable to grieve may have strong *negative feelings* toward the lost person which they feel too guilty to express.

c. Persons unable to grieve are often *unable to reinvest* in other people or activities without feelings of *self-reproach, guilt,* and *diminished self-esteem.*

d. There is a decreased ability to interact satisfactorily and pleasurably with the environment and expression of an unconscious need for *self-punishment* for having the negative feelings towards the lost person.

e. If the person is given the opportunity to express these feelings in a positive relationship with a warm, accepting person, the depression will usually improve, and the process of mourning can continue to a healthy, adaptive resolution.

C. Death and dying. One aspect of object loss especially noted during the ag is the preoccupation with one's own death. The fear of death for the elderly revolves around fears of loneliness and isolation and loss of control over oneself and external events.

1. Pattison (6) describes some of the fears of the dying person as fears of:

a. The unknown.
b. Loneliness.
c. Loss of family and friends.
d. Loss of the body or body part.
e. Loss of self-control.
f. Pain.
g. Loss of identity.
h. Regression.

2. In today's culture, dying is most often an impersonal, lonely, and undignified process. Death usually occurs away from home, the family, and familiar surroundings. In the rush and routine of the hospital setting, the special needs of the aged person who faces death are sometimes forgotten.

3. Bellak (7) states that the main fact to remember in helping those who will soon die is to make them feel certain that they will not be alone in the process of dying and will not be forgotten in death.

4. Kübler-Ross (8) describes the process by which the dying patient copes with the knowledge of impending death. She divides the process of dying into five specific stages, namely, denial and isolation, anger, bargaining, depression, and acceptance. Related behaviors and feelings observed in the patient and/or families are also described.

a. Denial and isolation. These are coping mechanisms utilized by most persons as an immediate response to the knowledge of impending death. Initially, there is a feeling of disbelief upon hearing that one's time is limited and that death is near. While death is an inevitable prospect for everyone, individuals do not focus their thoughts on death. Old age and death are rarely dwelt upon. Fantasies of immortality occurring in the face of reality indicate that the concept of death is foreign to the unconscious. In its fullest intensity, denial is a temporary defense but one which is used to a lesser degree in coping with death. On occasion, a person may need to retreat temporarily from the reality of the impending death. Denial and fantasies of continued life are ways of dealing with the despair and sadness over the potential loss of one's life.

b. Anger. After an initial period of denial, the person begins to feel anger at the thought of giving up the prospect of continued life. This anger can be directed at other people (such as family or nursing staff), since they will live on and continue to be part of the world the dying person must leave behind. Kübler-Ross points out that the fear of being forgotten and alone in death is often difficult for the person to verbalize and can precipitate hostile and demanding behavior toward others. Therefore, by making constant demands for time and attention from others, the patient gains reassurance that she or he will not be forgotten and left alone. Such demanding behavior may indicate the patient's resentment toward those who seem so healthy and alive.

c. Bargaining. Patients attempt to control the circumstances of their fate by bargaining for freedom from pain and for more time in return for some type of good behavior. The bargain, most often made with God, can also be for continued life until some significant event or point in future time has been reached. Individuals continuously believe that if they had more time they could correct their wrongdoings, relieve their guilt, complete tasks, and fulfill dreams. Bargaining for time will help individuals ready themselves for death.

d. Depression. As the individual begins to realize that death is inevitable, feelings of depression occur. Patients as well as families begin to react with sadness to the many physical, financial, and interpersonal losses they face. The patient begins to grieve the loss of valued and important persons, including the loss of oneself. The profound realization that one is about to lose contact with all those things that are cherished and loved creates a mood of silent reflection and thought.

e. Acceptance. Kübler-Ross states that the stage of acceptance is neither a stage of giving up nor one of joy, but rather a time of peaceful and quiet expectation of death. Patients no longer express strong feelings about their fate, and there is often little verbal communication during this period. The patient desires few visitors, and the level of interest in the environment decreases. Kübler-Ross emphasizes how much patients need the quiet presence of someone who is able to sit close by and communicate nonverbally to them, relieving the loneliness as they wait for the end.

5. The stages of coping with death and dying are not experienced by all patients in exactly the same order or at the same time. There is not necessarily a system of closure involved with each stage in the process. Patients will bargain, express anger or denial, or feel depressed throughout the process of coping with what is happening to them. The important thing to understand is the need being expressed by the patient's behavior as he or she moves toward acceptance of death.

D. Behavioral responses to physical losses of aging. The physical losses of aging (discussed in detail in Chap. 40) include such things as decreased activity, decreased perceptual abilities, decreased motor strength, loss of youthful appearance, increased dependence on others, changes in memory, and decreased ability to adapt to stress.

1. The changes experienced that affect bodily appearance and strength may be major physical losses and can precipitate further *losses in areas of self-esteem, security, interpersonal relationships,* and *behavioral reactions.* An elderly patient who begins to lose eyesight might become disoriented, confused, paranoid, and uncooperative in response to sensory deprivation.

2. *Memory loss* for recent events can occur while memory for past occurrences seems to remain intact. Weinberg points out the protective aspects of such

memory loss by describing loss of memory for recent events as a way of blocking out current losses from awareness while retaining past memories as a way of holding on to past pleasures an accomplishments (9).

3. *Losses in intellectual functioning* are difficult to assess, as they may be attributed to the aging process itself or result from serious illness or cultural and social deprivation. Bellak asserts that it is not necessarily true that intellectual functioning decreases with age (10). He points out that the aging of the intellect corresponds to the paucity of opportunities available for the aged to continue educational growth. The aged need continuous stimulation and adequate resources to continue growth and development of intellectual functioning.

4. *Loss of flexibility and adaptability,* along with a decreased ability to reason or problem solve, tends to accompany aging. The older person tends to adhere to known and safe routines and ways of coping with problems. It seems to be difficult for the aged to learn new ways of accomplishing tasks or solving problems. *Rigidity* can be viewed as a defense against painful loss and an attempt to maintain constancy in the environment and control over external events.

5. Sexual activity continues into old age as long as available partners are present and there is adequate opportunity for expression of sexual needs. Bellak states that the availability of a satisfactory partner is the single most important factor in the maintenance of an enjoyable sex life into advanced age (11).

   Loss of potency and *loss of sexual attractiveness* are threats to the aged, but the need for and enjoyment of sexual relationships does not cease as one grows older. Meaningful sexual relationships meet needs for intimacy, affection, eroticism, stimulation, tension release, warmth, and pleasure. These needs are just as great in the elderly as they are in any other age group.

   Older people need the recognition from others that there is nothing bizarre, unusual, or perverse in the desire to satisfy adult sexual impulses in privacy and peace. Sexual relationships can be at their fullest in terms of human intimacy and tenderness during this time. Sexual satisfaction during old age tends to reflect the individual's level of sexual adjustment and fulfillment throughout life.

E. Behavioral responses to socioeconomic losses. Social losses of the aged occur in the areas of job, status, role, and independence.

1. The *loss of job* can occur because of occupational retirement policy, ill health, or the voluntary desire to have more leisure time. Retirement is somewhat easier to deal with if it is a free choice rather than an enforced policy. Work provides one with a sense of productivity, accomplishment, and structure and contributes to one's self-image and self-esteem.

2. *Economic loss* is often concurrent with job loss. Lack of adequate finances in old age further aggravates the problem of diminished functioning in society, and may contribute to isolation and withdrawal.

3. The *loss of role* in one's life can be felt as a result of job retirement or because children have grown up and have moved away from home. The loss of an important and vital role can cause one to feel useless, unmotivated, and without a purpose in life. Since much of the parents' time and energy become invested in the job of raising children, they often experience a sense of emptiness and loneliness when the children leave home or are separated by distance due to long-range moving.

4. The losses suffered in functional areas may result in *loss of independence*. For the elderly, the return to a dependency state after years of independence and self-sufficiency is particularly painful and dehumanizing.

5. This *loss of control* and mastery over one's environment leads to feelings of anger, worthlessness, helplessness, fear, and isolation. The aged, consciously and unconsciously, begin to seek out in others the nurturance and care that was once provided by parental figures. Such dependency strivings have the purpose of reassuring aged persons that they will be taken care of by someone seen as stronger, more capable, and independent.

ASSESSMENT

To plan effective nursing care for the aged patient, the nurse must be aware of and understand the meaning and impact of loss upon the patient. Continuous assessment of loss is essential to planning effective nursing care of theaged. Not all patients experience similar losses or react to losses in identical ways. Patients will not always volunteer information about losses being suffered or behave in a predictable manner in reaction to their losses. Recognition of the stages of normal grief work, the absence of prolonged grief, and maladaptive responses to loss should be pursued by the nurse.

I. Data sources.
   A. The patient.
   B. The family, if the patient is unable to answer questions.
   C. The patient's past record.
   D. Significant others (e.g., a close friend).

II. Health history.
   A. Identification of a recent loss; note type, duration, intensity, and significance. Note other similar losses in a patient's lifetime, and isolate useful coping strategies used in the past.
   B. Patients may complain about periods of insomnia.
   C. Alteration in eating habits (usually loss of appetite) may be noted.
   D. The person is often preoccupied with the self, tending to focus upon bodily complaints, such as minor aches and pains and somatization.
   E. If the patient has been grieving it is important for the nurse to identify the stage of grieving and isolate the mourning period. (Refer to the discussion of grief and mourning under "Definition.")
   F. Responses which indicate loss of self-esteem or feelings of worthlessness and hopelessness should be identified.
   G. Complaints of memory loss and inability to concentrate for a significant period of time should be carefully evaluated.
   H. Adjustment to new situations should be described, and responses, e.g., anxiety or fear, should be noted.
   I. Recent loss of financial support, job, and/or separation from family members or friends should be noted.
   J. Alteration in sensory perceptions (e.g., hearing and/or vision) should be identified. Behavioral changes which may accompany these changes should be identified.
   K. Identification of the individual's role perception is important.
   L. Physical losses and current health status should oe described (refer to Chap. 40).

III. Behavioral assessment.
   A. Regression to childlike behaviors may be observed.
   B. Decreased sensory input may result in decreased social participation. Decreased auditory input (i.e., hearing loss) may lead to paranoid behavior.
   C. Withdrawal from friends and family may be noted. Depression may accompany these changes.
   D. Denial of a loss may be present, manifested by actions that can result in physical injury.
   E. Expressions of guilt may be heard, accompanied by feelings of worthlessness.
   F. Anxiety, manifested by physiologic as well as behavioral expressions, may occur, especially in response to overwhelming external demands from family, friends, or the environment as a whole.
   G. Physical loss, changes in the environment, or movement to an unfamiliar setting (e.g., hospitalization) may contribute to confusion and alteration in orientation to time and place.
   H. Physical appearance manifested by a sad, dejected look, lack of interest in personal appearance, changes in posture, and lack of eye contact may contribute information about the individual's overall response.

    I. Verbalizations which give evidence of rigid unchanging behavior may be a response to sensory overload (e.g., fear of the unknown or anxiety).

    J. Disinterest in the environment and decreased interaction with others may accompany isolation and withdrawal. Threats of suicide may be expressed and should be further explored.

    K. Stages of dying and coping mechanisms being utilized should be identified and explored.

PROBLEMS

    I. Loneliness.
    II. Confusion.
    III. Withdrawal, depression.
    IV. Separation: loss of family, friend, spouse.
    V. Increased leisure time.
    VI. Role change (retirement).
    VII. Increased dependence.
    VIII. Denial of reality.
    IX. Paranoid behavior.
    X. Inability to deal with life situations.
    XI. Altered self-concept: loss of self-esteem.
    XII. Hypochondriasis.
    XIII. Insomnia.
    XIV. Decreased socialization.
    XV. Anxiety, fear of the future (death, loss).

DIAGNOSIS

    I. Anxiety: mild to severe, secondary to physical loss, fear of the unknown, or psychosocial loss.

    II. Alteration in comfort, secondary to physical loss, immobility, pain, or social isolation.

    III. Confusion (potential), secondary to sensory loss, disorientation to time, place, and persons.

    IV. Grieving: acute, anticipated, or delayed, secondary to significant loss.

    V. Alteration in nutrition: less than required, secondary to grief response, loss, etc.

    VI. Alteration in self-concept, secondary to physical loss, occupational loss, socioeconomic loss, loss of self-esteem, or loss of control.

    VII. Alteration in sensory perception, secondary to physical loss and anxiety.

    VIII. Dysrhythm of sleep-rest pattern, secondary to insomnia and grief response.

    IX. Alteration in social interaction, secondary to isolation or withdrawal.

GOALS OF CARE

When planning care for the aged person, the nurse should remember that since each individual ages differently, goals and care plans will evolve differently. In formulating goals of nursing care, the nurse should keep two guidelines in mind. First, the age of the patient should be incorporated into the goals so that they will be realistic, recognizing past coping patterns. Second, avoid asking patients to relinquish certain behaviors without offering an alternative way of coping with or adapting to a new situation.

    I. Immediate.

      A. The client will express verbally beliefs about aging and individual responses to the process.

      B. The client will successfully identify personal, physical, psychologic, and/or social losses that are currently being dealt with and identify coping behaviors that will help him or her deal with these changes.

C. The client will successfully work through stages of loss and grief as evidenced by the giving up and separation from object losses.

D. The client will give evidence of decreased loneliness and increased interpersonal relationships by participating in social activities and seeking out situations that provide more social contact.

II. Long-range.

A. The client and/or family will utilize those assets available which will permit optimization of the health state at a given point in time.

B. The client and/or family will utilize all resources available (both physical and psychosocial), in order to cope effectively with the aging process.

C. The client and/or family will begin planning for aging and related role changes (e.g., retirement) in sufficient time to establish a sound financial base and selected diversionary activities.

INTERVENTION

I. Awareness of nurse's attitude toward aging.

A. Working with elderly patients can be both a challenging and a rewarding experience. Awareness of one's own attitudes towards aging (both positive and negative) is critical to the implementation of all nursing intervention.

B. Exploration of one's own feelings toward loss, one's own aging process, and the inevitability of one's own death can influence the nurse's relationship with the elderly.

C. Consideration and an open realization of one's ideas and prejudices about the role of the aged population in our society should be openly discussed to avoid stereotyping the elderly population.

II. Respect for the aged person.

A. Respect for the patient means interest and concern for the past accomplishments, present hopes, and future plans of the person who is now old.

B. Listening about the past helps the nurse find out about it by talking to the patient and the family.

C. Most older people enjoy reminiscing about their families, jobs, and accomplishments, and talking about the past to an interested listener is important as it can serve to increase the patient's feeling of self-esteem.

D. Respect also means considering the feelings of persons who might be incapacitated, confused, or suffering from disabling illness.

E. The nurse should be aware of the patient's feelings and emotions and respect the patient's need to be treated with dignity and kindness.

III. Coping with behavioral changes.

A. *Depression* is a common reaction to loss.

1. The nurse must be able to distinguish between the depressive affect of a patient who is grieving a loss and neurotic or psychotic depression reactions.

2. The nurse needs to assess changes that may indicate depression, such as a loss in appetite, diminished interest in the environment, decreased ability to interact with others, and feelings of guilt, worthlessness, hopelessness, or helplessness.

3. Because of the high risk of suicide in this age group, observation of changes in the patient's mood, verbal expressions of suicide, and other alterations in an individual's thought processes and behavior should be identified early and carefully evaluated.

4. Appropriate preventive measures against suicide should be instituted, including psychiatric consultation, antidepressant medication, and interaction with a concerned and supportive nursing staff. These measures can help the depressed patient to regain equilibrium.

5. Following these measures, the nurse should be aware of behavioral responses to an increased energy level in the depressed patient with a degree of psychomotor retardation. While the patient may appear improved, the danger of suicide still persists for the patient may now have the energy necessary to attempt suicide.

6. Encourage the individual to participate in activities of interest, and provide a means to help decrease isolation and withdrawal. Social groups and community living (housing) provide such alternatives and can be suggested to the elderly following resolution of depression.

B. *Regressive behavior* in the older patient can present difficulties in nursing care. Certain aspects of the patient's behavior might seem very childlike, but to label the patient as a "child" serves only to reinforce the regressive behavior.

1. The nurse needs to understand that at times of stress people sometimes revert to using earlier ways of seeking gratification and maintaining security.

2. The patient needs to be encouraged to utilize more adult ways of gaining pleasure and security.

3. The nurse can reinforce the patient's strengths and help the patient to gain confidence in the performance of appropriate activities in an independent manner.

4. The nurse should provide a sense of reality for the patient, with continual orientation to time and place.

5. The patient may begin to hoard food and make wild accusations about patients or staff.

6. It is important to remember that the patient has been a productive member of society in the past and may not be conscious of his or her present disruptive or hostile behavior. The nurse should attempt to understand the behaviors of the aged person within the context of aging and associated losses. This can be a useful way of meeting patient needs.

C. *Hypochondriasis,* or the focus on bodily symptoms and complaints, can be utilized as a defense against loss.

1. The nurse must be aware of the possibility of a significant health problem and carefully relate this information to the appropriate health team member.

2. It is important to understand that, even though a physical cause cannot be found for a patient's complaint, the symptom and the suffering is real to the patient. Some patients do not verbally express grief over loss, but do develop somatic complaints. Each physical complaint should be evaluated.

3. The nurse should recognize that an individual may have great difficulty with dependency, and can develop physical problems unconsciously as an acceptable way of seeking help and being taken care of by others.

4. The nurse has a dual role in helping to reduce the patient's suffering by meeting some of the depenency needs as well as by encouraging the patient to assume as much independent functioning as possible.

5. Older patients may need to talk about their worries and concerns over the physical changes which are taking place in their bodies. The nurse should provide an opportunity for open discussion and free exchange of ideas.

D. Sensory impairments can lead to a *decreased interest in activities of daily living,* such as eating and socializing.

1. Patients with failing eyesight or hearing difficulties may feel threatened and depressed about their losses and need continued support and guidance from the nurse and family members to capitalize on existing intact senses and to identify ways to supplement losses.

2. The nurse needs to keep an up-to-date assessment of the patient's sensorium as a way of detecting difficulties, correcting losses, and preventing further loss.

3. The nurse can help patients with failing eyesight to remain oriented and to achieve maximum independence by arranging the room in a way that will help the patient to move about freely, by alerting the patient to the presence of

other people, by keeping the patient apprised of the time of day, day of the week, and the weather, and by describing for patients things they are unable to see (refer to Chap. 42).

4. Procedures that must be performed and medications that must be administered should be carefully explained. Additional interventions which will help decrease the patient's fear and sense of helplessness should be encouraged.

5. Helping a patient to gain interest in food will require more than presenting the patient with a tray and describing where things are located. Often it is helpful to describe the food to the patient in some detail which makes it sound appetizing. Hopefully, this will increase the patient's desire to eat.

6. Hearing loss can increase feelings of isolation and paranoia in the older individual. The nurse should refrain from talking with others without making attempts to include the person in the conversation. Shouting is usually not helpful, but facing the person and speaking in a slow, carefully enunciated manner will improve the patient's understanding and decrease paranoia (refer to Chap. 40 for additional discussion).

7. Helping patients to gain self-confidence in their ability to socialize can be accomplished by interacting with the patient in a supportive, consistent, and encouraging manner.

8. Family members hould be taught to recognize sensory losses in older patients and to follow interventions suggested above.

9. Environmental stimulation, without overloading the patient, can be helpful to the elderly and serve to orient them to their surroundings.

E. *Denial* and *projection* are coping mechanisms used to defend against anxiety. The older patient might use either or both of these defenses in an attempt to cope with loss. Patients who deny physical losses might attempt to do things which can result in accidents or injuries.

1. The nurse needs to protect patients from potentially hurting themselves by reinforcing the real limitations of their physical conditions.

2. Projection serves to increase the patient's sense of self-esteem by blocking out the reality of limitations and attributing problems to some source other than the patient's self. However, projection can result in hostile, demanding behavior.

3. The nurse (as well as the hospital, the doctor, or the family) might be criticized and accused of doing harmful things to the patient. The nurse should not personalize, even though it is difficult.

4. The patient should be talked to and supported as much as possible during this time. If conflicts between the nurse and patient are severe and interfere with delivery of care, another nurse on the team may intervene.

5. Denial and projection must be understood as an attempt on the patient's part to decrease anxiety, maintain control over the environment, and preserve a sense of integrity and self-worth.

F. Although *delusions* and *hallucinations* can seem to be innocuous and harmless in the older patient, they frequently indicate serious underlying psychiatric disturbance, can cause suffering to the patient, and can necessitate treatment. The nurse needs to consult with health members of the team to evaluate the significance of this problem. The nurse should help the person focus on realistic occurrences within the environment and protect the patient from self-injury. If the problem is more involved, additional care will be required (see ''Evaluation'').

IV. Independence

A. The nurse should encourage the patient to participate in activities with others, or alone, as toleratd.

B. As the patient loses interest in self and environment, it is necessary to provide structure and meaning to the patient's day or week.

C. If signs of dependency are noted, the nurse can utilize dependency strivings to promote a relationship of trust and caring with the patient. Once patients feel they are being taken care of by a responsible and understanding person, it will be easier to help them make the most of strengths and cope in the best way with limitations.

V. Role change.

    A. It is important to encourage the middle-aged person to prepare for retirement by expanding interests beyond the role of parent and employee.

    B. The nurse can teach people in the community to anticipate retirement and a separation from children and to develop new interests and activities. Plans for retirement (e.g., living environment) and increased socialization with others (thereby expanding their interest groups) may help the transition to a new role.

    C. Adequate finances and cultivation of enjoyable and fulfilling use of leisure time can buffer the impact of job loss and retirement.

VI. Institutionalizations.

    A. The nurse should help the patient cope with voluntary or nonvoluntary institutionalization by allowing the patient to verbalize fears and feelings of anxiety.

    B. The family should be given support during this time and be provided with given guidelines for the selection of a nursing home or similar institution.

    C. Relocation of an individual can be threatening to the aging patient. The patient may become anxious and disoriented. Measures should be initiated during the admission process to help make the transition a smooth one. The patient should also be oriented to the new surroundings and be supported during the transition phase.

    D. The environment that an elderly individual is placed in should be carefully selected (see Chap. 40). If the patient appears to undergo behavioral changes during the period of institutionalization, a careful analysis of the setting will be necessary. Further exploration of the behavior demonstrated will need to be assessed.

VII. Grieving.

    A. The nurse should be sensitive to the person's need to temporarily *deny* the reality of death and the difference between this use of denial and the initial blocking out of reality.

    B. The nurse must be acutely sensitive to verbal and nonverbal clues from the patient in order to identify individual needs and signals which indicate a readiness to move on in the process of acceptance.

    C. The nurse needs to accept and understand the patient's need to deny inevitable loss or death.

    D. *Anger* related to the dying process is often difficult for family members and the nursing staff to cope with. Changes in the patient's behavior as manifested by anger are difficult for family and friends not to personalize. There may be a tendency to isolate and avoid interaction with the dying person, especially during this stage, because of the behavior being manifested.

    E. The nurse needs to understand the patient's reactions and help deal with the patient's anger, knowing that this response is part of grief work. It is important to maintain a consistent and positive interaction with the patient and to empathize in a nonjudgmental manner with the patient's sense of anger and loss of control over the future. Often, primary nursing care will help maintain this close patient contact and also allow the nurse to help the family deal with the impending loss.

    F. Helping the patient through the *bargaining stage* of the grieving process requires that the nurse carefully listen. It is important that the nurse recognize the patient's bargaining for more time to do one last thing, see one last person, or fulfill one last fantasy before death. The wish to prolong life, rather than the realities of the particular bargain, needs to be understood and responded to.

    G. During the *depression* stage, the nurse needs to be with the patient even though the patient might remain silent. It is important to respect the patient's request to be left alone in order to come to grips with the reality of impending death and the sense of loss.

    H. The nurse needs to indicate a willingness to spend time with the patient and a readiness to talk about loss and feelings of sadness. The patient generally does not respond favorably to cheerfulness, encouragement, or optimism during this stage.

I. The nurse does need to help the patient maintain a certain sense of hope which is realistic and which Kübler-Ross described as having to do with the sense that there is meaning in suffering.

J. It is necessary for nurses to work with family members who might have more difficulty than the patient in accepting the news that a loved one is dying.

K. The patient may express relief when the family has left at not having to pretend to be cheerful or optimistic. The patient might simply indicate a desire not to see certain members of the family. It is often up to the nurse to intervene with the family to help them understand the patient's need to express feelings of depression. The nurse usually needs to work with the family during this time, as they might feel abandoned, left out, and hurt at the patient's apparent rejection of their comfort, presence, and support.

L. The nurse needs to help the family understand the patient's need to let go of their presence and support in order to prepare for death. Families should be told that as the patient turns inward, during this time, there is little energy for interaction with others.

M. As Kübler-Ross suggests, the nurse can indicate by a touch of the hand or a comforting word or two that someone is close at hand until the end.

N. If the patient does have family present, the nurse will need to help them face these last moments as well as offer support after the patient has died.

EVALUATION

I. Reassessment.

A. The nurse needs to reassess the patient's status continuously in regard to object, physical, and socioeconomic losses.

B. The nurse must evaluate the patient's response to loss and determine if the planned interventions are helping the patient to express grief and adapt to loss.

C. The nurse has to be sensitive to changes in the patient's behavior which might indicate a need for change in the nursing care plan.

D. In evaluating the care of the aged patient, the nurse looks for indications that the patient is dealing with the realities of loss in the best possible way.

E. The nurse observes the patient's level of comfort and degree of independent functioning to determine if they are at their highest possible level.

F. The interaction of nursing staff with the patient and with family members also needs to be evaluated for potential problems in communication.

II. Complications. Functional psychiatric disorders are common in old age, but the clinical picture is complicated by complex causative factors and possible organic brain syndrome. Bellak does state that all studies of mental illness in old age indicate that less than 10 percent of the aged population suffer from *severe* mental illness (12). Inappropriate coping patterns, misuse of defense mechanisms, and prolonged grieving or mourning and depression must be recognized and psychiatric counseling implemented (refer to Part 5).

REFERENCES

1. Leopold Bellak, *The Best Years of Your Life,* Atheneum, New York, 1975, p. 98.
2. Edward W. Busse and Eric Pfeiffer, *Mental Illness in Later Life,* American Psychiatric Association, Washington D.C., 1973, p. 110.
3. Bellak, op. cit., p. 112.
4. Sigmund Freud, "Mourning and Melancholia," (1917), *Standard Edition,* vol. 14, Hogarth Press, London, 1955.
5. Bellak, op. cit., p. 251.
6. E. Hansell Pattison, "Help in the Dying Process," in Silvano Arieti (ed.), *The American Handbook*

of Psychiatry, vol. I: *The Foundations of Psychiatry,* 2d ed., Basic Books, Inc. New York, 1974, pp. 691–693.
7. Bellak, op. cit., pp. 239–240.
8. Elisabeth Kübler-Ross, *On Death and Dying,* MacMillan Publishing Company, Inc., New York, 1969.
9. Jack Weinberg, "Geriatric Psychiatry," in Alfred M. Freedman, Harold I. Kaplan, and Benjamin J. Sadock (eds.), *Comprehensive Textbook of Psychiatry,* vol. II, The Williams & Wilkins Company, Baltimore, 1975.
10. Bellak, op. cit., pp. 102–103.
11. Ibid., p. 108.
12. Ibid., pp. 113–140

BIBLIOGRAPHY

Bozzetti, Louis P., and James P. MacMurray: "Contemporary Concepts of Aging: An Overview," *Psychiatric Annals,* **7**(3):16–43, March 1977. Good discussion of unique components of aging according to current views.

Browning, Mary H. (compiled by): *Nursing and the Aging Patient,* The American Journal of Nursing Company, New York, 1974.

Busse, Edward, and Eric Pfeiffer (eds.): *Behavior and Adaptation in Late Life,* Little, Brown and Company, Boston, 1977.

Epstein, Charlotte: *Nursing the Dying Patient,* Reston Publishing Company, Inc., Reston, Va., 1975. Good discussion of grieving, mourning, death, and dying. Study questions at the end of each chapter helpful.

Schoenberg, Bernard, Arthur C. Carr, David Peretz, and Austin H. Kutscher (eds.): *Loss and Grief: Psychological Management in Medical Practice,* Columbia University Press, New York, 1970. Excellent resource on all types of loss.

42

Responses to Pathophysiologic Disturbances in the Aged

Joanne Kelleher Farley

Aging is an integral part of an individual's growth and development. When disruptions in physical as well as psychosocial components occur, alterations in a person's response to the effects of aging may result. The nurse working in all settings must be able to differentiate those observable changes that are the result of "normal" aging, from those that are caused by a major health problem.

This chapter focuses upon the impact of selected chronic health problems on the elderly. Since many of these problems are discussed in Part 4, this chapter explores the problem of chronicity and the other unique differences of common health problems in the aged. Implications for modification of the nursing process are also discussed, as relevant.

CHRONIC HEALTH PROBLEMS

Definition

Although an elderly person may experience an acute illness, *chronic, long-term health problems* are common afflictions of the aged. The Commission on Chronic Illness (1949–1956) has identified five criteria, one or more of which must exist in order for a disease to be considered chronic (1):

1. The problem must be permanent.
2. The problem must leave a residual disability.
3. The problem must be caused by a nonreversible pathologic condition.
4. The problem must require special rehabilitative training.
5. The problem must require long supervision and care.

Of persons 65 years of age or older, 45.9 percent are limited to some degree in their activity (refer to Table 42-1). The problems encountered by these individuals may preclude their pursuing a major activity except on a limited basis. [A *major activity* is defined as those activities related to work or keeping house (2).] The elderly population has a high degree of chronic health problems. The major chronic illnesses found in the aged include cardiovascular problems, hypertension, diabetes, chronic sensory impairments, organic brain syndrome, and accidents.

There are four distinct phases which the chronically ill go through as they begin to cope with a long-term health problem. They are identified as follows:

1. Denial and disbelief. The patient is told of the illness and denies the reality of its happening. Often the impact of the problem and its long-term consequences are so severe that the individual uses this coping mechanism to handle stress at this time.
2. Developing awareness. The patient ceases to deny the problem. There is a beginning realization of the consequences of a particular illness, and the patient is angry. During this period the patient may be argumentative and critical.
3. Reorganization. With the developing awareness of the chronic illness comes a need for reorganization of one's life. Environmental changes are made, and relationships with family members are adjusted. Frequent verbal support for any and all accomplishments is most important during this stage.

TABLE 42-1 / LIMITATION IN ACTIVITY IN PERSONS OVER 65

Sex	Total Population	No Limit, %	1,* %	2,† %	3,‡ %
Both	20,741	54.1	6.6	22.1	17.1
Male	8,578	50.3	4.8	15.0	29.8
Female	12,163	56.9	7.8	27.2	8.2

*Limited, but not in major activity.
†Limited in amount or kind of major activity.
‡Unable to carry on.
Source: Adapted from "Total Population and Number and Percent Distribution of Persons by Age and Sex, according to Chronic Activity Limitation Status: United States," in *Health Characteristics of Persons With Chronic Activity Limitation,* U.S. Department of Health, Education, and Welfare, Rockville, Md., 1974, p. 11.

4. Resolution or identity change. During this final stage, the patient acknowledges the changes that have occurred in the body. The patient is usually discharged from a health care facility at this time. After a very careful assessment, the patiet should be encouraged to become more self-directive until able to tolerate the withdrawal from health care.

Assessment

I. Data sources.
   A. Patient.   C. Friend or significant others.
   B. Family.   D. Previous medical or hospital records.
II. Health history.
   A. What is the patient's usual mode of living? Life-style?
   B. Identify physical activities, limitations. Identify mental diversions.
   C. Identify family resources and support systems.
   D. Elicit usual coping mechanism and patterns of handling loss (refer to Chap. 41).
   E. Identify nutritional habits.
   F. Evaluate fluid and electrolyte balances, dehydration, edema.
   G. Assess patterns of elimination and daily bowel habits. Question the presence of incontinence.
   H. Identify presence of confusion or disorientation (refer to "organic brain syndrome").
   I. Identify the health problem which is present. What is the patient and/or family's comprehension of this health problem?
III. Physical examination.
   A. Physical examination would depend on health problem (refer to specific chapters in Part 4 for a more complete assessment guide).
   B. Whatever the problem, it is critical to observe several key factors that affect daily living. These include:
      1. Physical condition.
      2. General appearance.
      3. Facial appearance.
      4. Speech pattern.
      5. Pattern of communication.
      6. Mental acuity.
      7. General muscle strength.
      8. Degree of joint mobility.
      9. Capacity for movement ROM, activity, and exercise.
      10. Dietary habits.
      11. Bowel habits.

12. Fluid intake.
13. Signs of dehydration.
14. Edema.
15. Sleep pattern.
16. Cardiac alterations (e.g., dyspnea, arrhythmias).
17. Pain.
18. Tolerance of stress.
19. Sensory and motor perception.
20. Orientation to time and place.

Problems/Diagnosis

Refer to specific chapters. The following list reflects actual or potential problems.
 I. Incontinence (see Chap. 28).
 II. Dehydration (see Chaps. 28 and 40).
 III. Dyspnea (see Chap. 27).
 IV. Cardiac alterations (see Chap. 26).
 V. Immobility.
 VI. Confusion.
 VII. Alterations in nutritional intake (obesity, malnutrition; see Chap. 40).
 VIII. Visual and auditory disturbances (see Chap. 42).
 IX. Alterations in sleep patterns and level of consciousness (see Chap. 23), secondary to the aging process.
 X. Alteration in elimination: diarrhea or constipation.
 XI. Disruption in skin integrity: skin breakdown, secondary to immobility, incontinence, etc.

Goals of Care

The major goal(s) for chronic problems include:
 I. Maintain optimal level of functioning as evidenced by prevention of deformity, good nutritional intake, maintaining activity level as tolerated, and performing activities of daily living to maximum potential.
 II. Verbal and nonverbal expression of a sense of worth as evidenced by a sense of belonging, feeling loved, being a contributor to family and society, and feeling successful in all undertakings.

Intervention

 I. Evaluate home for possible modification of environment.
 II. Support physical activity as tolerated by the patient. Encourage planned activity daily (active and passive exercises). Try to keep patient out of bed as much as possible.
 III. Encourage family members g)especially children and grandchildren or friends) to *sit down* and visit with the patient. Cards, checkers, or other games of interest may be stimulating for the patient. The use of environment (Chap. 40) along with radio and television can also be additional sources of stimulation.
 IV. Coordinate care at home with the assistance of a homemaker, visiting nurse, or permanent caretaker.
 V. Teach patient and family all necessary information about a particular health problem and selected intervention.
 VI. Provide continuous support for family members, and refer them to agencies which will help care for the elderly family member.
 VII. Monitor fluid intake, output, nutritional intake, and bowel habits on a daily basis.

Encourage fluids to prevent dehydration; small but frequent meals may be required to maintain the nutritional status.

VIII. If the patient is on bed rest, maintain range of motion (ROM) and proper body alignment; use of a bed board and foot board may be needed. Maintain patient safety and comfort at all times.

IX. Position the patient frequently. Observe skin integrity. Prevent skin breakdown by increasing planned activity, keeping patient out of bed as much as possible and preventing skin irritation caused by presence of urine or feces. Avoid pressure point(s) by using sheepskin or flotation mattress as needed.

Evaluation

I. Reassessment: Evaluate carefully the patient's overall health status and the patient's and/or family's ability to cope with specific chronic health problems.

II. Complications: Their prevention (e.g., decubiti, ulcers, dehydration, contractures, accidents, urinary tract infections) should be the continued focus of health promotion in the elderly.

CARDIOVASCULAR DISEASE

Definition

The major cause of death in the elderly as of 1975 was *cardiovascular disease.* Death rates indicate that the primary contributing health problems were alteration in cardiac function, hypertension, and cerebrovascular disease (refer to Table 42-2). The following discussion focuses upon alterations in cardiac function.

As individuals age, there are changes in heart size, endocardial tissue, and valve structure (refer to Chap. 40). These changes result in specific physiologic effects in the elderly:

1. Decreased cardiac reserve due to increased peripheral resistance and pooling.
2. Decreased cardiac output due to decreased stroke volume and slowed heart rate. Congestive heart failure may result (see Chap. 26).
3. Decreased blood flow through the coronary arteries (35 percent) and decreased utilization of oxygen, resulting in cardiac ischemia and angina.
4. Delayed recovery of myocardial contractility and irritability (secondary to a decreased amount of endogenous norephinephrine), resulting in an altered heart rate and rhythm.
5. Elevated peripheral vascular resistance due to atherosclerosis, increased blood viscosity, and/or decreased elasticity of the arteries.
6. Decrease in myocardial sensitivity due to the effects of atropine, and an increased sensitivity to carotid sinus stimulation.

The major cause of cardiac disease in the aged population is coronary *atherosclerosis* (3), which frequently results in symptomatic and asymptomatic *angina pectoris, coronary thrombosis,* and *congestive heart failure.* There is a lower incidence of angina pectoris in the extremely aged because of reduced activity and greater collateral circulation. However, coronary thrombosis should be suspected if angina persists or progresses. In acute coronary occlusion, the aged person manifests less pain with more dyspnea and congestive heart failure than a younger individual. Although the symptomatology seems to be less severe, the nurse should be aware of the significance of these differences from the younger patient (4) (refer to Chap. 26 for a complete discussion).

Assessment

Refer to Chap. 26.

Problems/Diagnosis

I. Respiratory dysfunction: dyspnea (potential).

II. Inability to cope with stress.

III. Anxiety; mild to moderate, secondary to fear of death.

IV. Alterations in nutritional intake (malnutrition, obesity) in light of restraints (e.g., decreased sodium and cholesterol intake).

V. Drug compliance: decreased because of physiologic effects of aging, e.g., lapses of memory.

VI. Alteration in comfort: pain (mild to moderate), secondary to coronary ischemia.

VII. Decreased activity secondary to decreased or impaired mobility.

VIII. Alteration in fluid balance: edema or fluid retention, peripheral pooling, congestive heart failure.

Goals of Care

Refer to "Chronic Health Problems" and Chap. 26.

Intervention

I. Activity programs should be established in view of the patient's cardiac status, overall energy reserve, and tolerance.

II. Medications and their use must be carefully discussed with the patient and compliance continuously evaluated, especially if the patient lives alone. Long-term use of medications may present problems such as misuse of the drugs (e.g., taking several doses of digitalis at one time because the patient forgot to take dose for 2 days), or eliminating the drug if patient begins to feel better.

III. Stress with the patient the need for adequate fluids to be sure drugs are adequately excreted; to prevent dehydration (as with diuretics); and to avoid straining at stool. Care should be taken to restrict fluid intake where the risk of congestive heart failure is high.

IV. Nutritional counseling to help patient restrict sodium and cholesterol intake is important. Because of the alteration in food intake that often accompanies aging, nutritional restrictions may be a problem for the elderly. Careful planning with family and nutritionist is important.

V. Encourage the person to stop smoking. This may be difficult for an elderly person who has established routines. The effects of nonsmoking must be evaluated in light of the stress created during the process of termination.

TABLE 42-2 / MAJOR CAUSES OF DEATH IN THE AGED, UNITED STATES, 1975

Age group	65–74	75–84	85+
All causes	3,189	7,359	15,188
Major cardiovascular disease:	1,716	4,670	10,940
Disease of the heart	1,324	3,281	9,282
Hypertension	10	31	79
Cerebrovascular diseases	303	1,076	2,655

Source: National Center for Health Statistics, *Vital Statistics Report, Advance Report Final Mortality Statistics, 1975,* U.S. Department of Health, Education, and Welfare, Rockville, Md., February 11, 1977.

VI. Environmental as well as personal stress should be kept at a minimum to decrease the demand on energy reserves and to prevent vasoconstriction.

VII. The perception of chest pain may be affected by aging and decreased activity on the part of the aged individual. The patient and family members should be encouraged to contact a physician if antianginal medication is not effective. Oxygen may be used when severe dyspnea is present or to relieve mild pain induced by stress or activity.

Evaluation

Refer to Chap. 26.

HYPERTENSION

Definition

Changes in peripheral resistance are the most significant causes of *hypertension* in the aged (5) (refer to Chap. 26). Although very prevalent in the elderly population, hypertension is not to be considered a normal part of aging; rather, it is a health problem which requires long-term treatment. Prolonged hypertension can be dangerous to the elderly patient. Complications include:

1. Impairment of circulation in the kidneys. This leads to ischemia of renal tissue which in turn liberates a pressor mediator that increases arteriolar constriction. (This cycle perpetuates the disorder (6) and can result in irreversible renal damage.)
2. Increased workload on the heart as the left ventricle is forced to work harder to cope with impaired nutrition and oxygenation to the myocardium.
3. Neurologic consequences resulting in cerebral apoplexy due to hemorrhage, thrombosis, or embolism, and eye injury.

Assessment

Refer to Chap. 26.

Problems/Diagnosis

I. Stress increased by fear of the unknown.
II. Altered emotional and behavioral responses due to antihypertensive medication or cerebral occlusive process.
III. Epistaxis secondary to increased blood pressure.
IV. Medication compliance: noncompliance.
V. Disturbance in fluid an lectrolyte balance (potential).
VI. Anemia.
VII. Altered nutritional intake: obesity.
VIII. Alteration in coordination due to disturbance in fine motor movement tremors.

Goals of Care

Refer to "Chronic Health Problems" and Chap. 26.

Intervention

I. Explain hypertension slowly and carefully to the patient; answer all questions. Provide the patient with information to clarify why emotional outbursts or behavioral changes are occurring.

II. Strive to maintain patient's independence and sense of self-worth.

III. Teach patient how to identify response patterns and encourage patient to avoid stressful situations.

IV. Provide nutritional counseling, especially in relation to weight reduction and low sodium intake.

V. Avoid dehydration, especially if diuretics are being taken. Be sure patient knows signs of electrolyte imbalance, e.g., hyperkalemia or hypokalemia (refer to Chap. 28).

VI. Explain nature of headaches. Teach patient to note when they occur and if they are relieved by rest, medication, etc.

VII. Prevent nosebleeds. When they do occur, be sure patient and family know how to treat them (e.g., Fowler's position, mouth breathing, pinching nostrils to create pressure). Following the episode of a nosebleed, the patient should be told to seek medical attention.

VIII. If excess bleeding is noted, blood loss should be evaluated (e.g., assess hemoglobin and hematocrit levels).

IX. The use of drugs to treat hypertension is extensive. Drugs used by the elderly are presented in Table 42-3 and their side effects are discussed. The patient should have knowledge of drug action and reactions (particularly behavioral changes) that can accompany drug use. It is important to stress the need for continued drug compliance even after symptoms of hypertension are alleviated.

X. Once blood pressure returns to a normal range, a planned exercise and rest program should be developed, based on the patient's interests and abilities. Exercises can include walking, swimming, bicycling, golf, etc.

XI. Rest periods should be planned periodically throughout the day. Sleep (7 to 8 h per night) is important. Rest after meals may be individualized as necessary.

XII. Reducing stress is critical to maintaining blood pressure levels within normal limits. Teach patient *how* to relax (e.g., mechanisms like biofeedback, yoga, etc.). The importance of continuing long-term drug compliance to keep blood pressure within normal limits should be stressed.

Evaluation

Refer to Chap. 26.

CEREBROVASCULAR DISEASE

Definition

Cerebrovascular disease is often a major complication of hypertension and is a leading cause of death in the aged (refer to Table 42-2). It is devastating to the aged person, because it threatens an individual's independence, dignity, and self-esteem.

Peripheral resistance increases as part of the process of aging. Blood pressure thereby rises, and hypertension can result. Prolonged hypertension can lead to sudden cerebral hemorrhage or infarction (refer to Chap. 26).

Although cerebrovascular accidents (CVA) are not found only in the aged population, the death rate associated with CVA of persons over 65 is 90 times that of persons 25 to 44 and 11 times that of persons 45 to 64 (7).

TABLE 42-3 / ANTIHYPERSENSITIVE DRUG TREATMENT IN THE AGED

Drug	Initial Dose (First 2 Weeks)	Indications	Side Effects
Rauwolfia preparatión:			
Reserpine	0.25 mg bid	Mild, moderate, or severe systolic or diastolic hypertension	Depression
Alseroxylon	2 mg bid	Same	Sexual impotence
Whole root	100 mg bid	Same	Parkinsonism
Syrosingopine	1 mg bid	Same	Insomnia, nasal stuffiness, and diarrhea
Diuretics:			
Chlorothiazide	250 mg tid	Same	Hypokalemia
Flumethiazide	250 mg tid	Same	Hyponatremia
Hydrochlorothizide	25 mg tid	Same	Hyperuricemia
Hydroflumethizide	2.5 mg bid	Same	Hypocalcemia
Bendroflumethiazide	2 mg bid	Same	Hyperglycemia
Trichlormethiazide	2 mg bid	Same	Dehydration
Chlorthalidone	50 mg daily (or less often)	Same	Azotemia
Guanethidine	10 mg daily	Moderate or severe diastolic hypertension	Diarrhea and postural hypertension
Methyldopa	250 mg tid	Severe diastolic hypertension	Drowsiness, fever, weakness, liver dysfunction, and granulocytopenia

Source: Reprinted with permission of Edith G. Robins, Deputy Director, Division of Long Term Care, HRA, DHEW from "Special Features of Heart Disease in the Elderly Patients," by Raymond Harris, *Working with Older People,* vol. IV, U.S. Department of Health, Education, and Welfare, Rockville, Md., 1971, pp. 81–102.

Assessment

Refer to Chaps. 23 and 26.

Problems/Diagnosis

I. Increased predisposition to complications of immobility, e.g., pulmonary infection or decubitus.
II. Alteration in body temperature (especially if hypothalamus is involved).
III. Loss of independence, decreased ability to perform activities and of daily living, secondary to disruption in sensory and motor activity.
IV. Loss of mobility, motor and sensory control, and coordination of body parts.
V. Grieving and depression, secondary to changes in body image and loss.
VI. Alteration in speech: aphasia and apraxia, agnosia, increasing communication difficulties.
VII. Increased mental confusion and disorientation to time and place.
VIII. Disruption in routine, altering stability and increasing anxiety.

Goals of Care

Refer to "Chronic Health Problems" and Chap. 26.

Intervention

Refer to Chaps. 23 and 26. Additional interventions include:

I. Provide assistance with eating; encourage small, frequent feedings as tolerated. Try to follow individual's eating patterns as closely as possible.

II. Exercise extreme caution in positioning bed properly to avoid skin breakdown. Prevention of contractures is critical. Decreased joint mobility which normally accompanies aging may be intensified with CVA. Early ROM exercise is critical.

III. Meticulous skin care is essential, especially if incontinence is a problem.

IV. Use all medications cautiously as the onset of CVA may alter an individual's reaction to a drug (e.g., analgesics).

V. As the patient begins to progress, it is important for family members to be patient. The person may be very slow in completing tasks, but when possible, it is important to encourage independent activities.

VI. Depression and grieving over the loss of body function is not uncommon (refer to Chap. 41). The nurse must be supportive of the patient and family during this time and encourage all actions that promote independence.

VII. Communications difficulties may intensify patient's frustration and lead to outbursts of anger. The patient needs to be told that speech problems are a result of the CVA and that speech will improve with time. A speech therapist should be enlisted when possible.

VIII. Stimulation within the environment, including physical therapy and occupational therapy, is important. Rearrangement of the home environment (e.g., use of firm chairs, removal of scatter rugs, bathroom supports, etc.) may be necessary.

IX. The patient should be told when he or she buys clothes to buy them one size larger, with elastic waists and front fasteners, in order to ease the process of dressing.

X. Teach patients to avoid hot baths; they dilate the cutaneous and muscular vascular bed, allowing blood to pool when patient rises from the tub (8). Also, teach patients to avoid straining at stool, as use of the Valsalva maneuver may increase stress and act as a vagal stimulus.

XI. Decrease stress within the environment, as the elderly person who has suffered a CVA will have decreased ability to cope with many of the problems of daily living.

XII. Bladder retraining and nutritional counseling should be provided, as needed.

Evaluation

Evaluation of all care is based upon selection of appropriate patient goals and defined measures to evaluate accomplishment of these goals. When changes in an individual's health status indicate reorganization of goals, appropriate revisions in the plan of care and related interventions must be made.

RESPIRATORY DISEASE

Definition

The rigidity of the lungs and reduction of muscle power are prime causes of pulmonary complications in the elderly. The two most prevalent pulmonary diseases found in this population are bronchitis and emphysema.

Chronic bronchitis is the leading pulmonary abnormality in the aged. It is clinically evidenced by the presence of persistent cough and sputum production. It specifically relates to patients who cough and raise sputum "on most days for a minimum of three consecutive months each year for at least two years" (9).

Many consider *emphysema* the result of chronic bronchitis, but results of clinical studies indicate that "emphysema appears to be a disease distinct from both chronic bronchitis and from the senile lung" (10). Emphysema increases progressively with age, reaching its highest degree of severity in the seventies. It is defined (11) as the destruction of lung parenchyma distal to the terminal bronchiole (refer to Chap. 27 for a complete discussion).

Assessment (Refer to Chap. 27)

I. Data sources (refer to "Chronic Health Problems").
II. Health history.[1]
   A. Question the history of previous respiratory diseases. (Rationale: Raising sputum from the bronchial tree becomes difficult after recurrent infection.)
   B. What is (was) patient's occupation? (Rationale: Inhaled fumes and dust are related to pulmonary problems.)
   C. Cough: kind, frequency, time, and precipitating factors should be elicited. Sputum: check frequency, amount, color, consistency, and content for blood. (Rationale: Cough and sputum are common symptoms of bronchitis. This is very serious to aged patients because, if sputum is not expectorated, obstruction of airways may result in respiratory failure and death.) The normal aged person has no persistent cough or sputum production.
   D. Breathing: Is patient short of breath at rest? With mild exercise? With exertion? (Rationale: Aged persons free from chronic respiratory symptoms are not short of breath unless moderate exertion is involved, e.g., running, fast walking, or climbing many stairs quickly.)
   E. Smoking: Does the patient smoke now? In the past? When did he or she start? What did he or she smoke? How much does (did) he or she smoke? [Rationale: Smoking is the major cause of chronic bronchitis. The frequency and severity is related to number of cigarettes smoked. Emphysema has a low incidence in nonsmokers. Smoking is the most significant "of all factors influencing lung disease in the aged" (12).]
   F. Energy level: Is patient's energy level decreasing? To what degree? How long has this been happening? [Rationale: The strength of muscular contractions decreases 15 to 35 percent with age, and the ability to maintain a sustained work output decreases. "The limiting factors for physical exertion in the aged person are in the mechanisms for oxygen transport to working muscles and in their ability to use oxygen" (13)].
III. Physical examination (refer to Chap. 27).
   A. Inspection: Diaphragmatic breathing may indicate pathology and should be investigated; dyspnea and its effects should be evaluated.
   B. Palpation: Any thoracic lumps, scars, or lesions should be examined. The degree of lung expansion and excursion should be palpated.
   C. Percussion: Hyperresonance of the lungs may be detected in aged persons, but this is not necessarily indicative of emphysema. Differential criteria are an obstructed pattern during forced expiration and a prolonged expiratory phase.
   D. Auscultation: Normal breath sounds should be heard in the elderly. Prolonged expiration should be evaluated. The intensity of breath sounds may be subdued in the elderly, but the abovementioned criteria must also be considered when assessing respiratory competence.

Problems/Diagnosis

I. Depletion of energy reserve: fatigue increases, decrease in activity.

[1] Information for the rationales is from Oskar Balchum, "The Aging Respiratory System," in *Working with Older People: Clinical Aspects of Aging,* U.S. Department of Health, Education, and Welfare, Rockville, Md., 1971, pp. 115–118, 121–122.

II. Altered lung structure and responsiveness to intervention.

III. Increased use of energy stores, metabolism, body fat stores increased, and cardiac stress increased by respiratory demands.

IV. Anxiety intensified by dyspnea and cerebral anoxia.

V. Occupation and related employment may have to be terminated.

Goals of Care

Refer to "Chronic Health Problems" and Chap. 27.

Intervention

I. Clarify problems for patient slowly and clearly, and encourage all improvements.

II. Provide quiet, cheerful, stress-free, supportive environment.

III. Medication should be administered as prescribed. Exercise special precautions with bronchodilators:

A. Ephedrine compounds may cause urinary retention in elderly men.

B. Aminophylline preparations are absorbed from gastrointestinal tract erratically in the aged (refer to "Medication and the Aged").

IV. Provide extensive instructions concerning activity, exercise, and breathing exercises (refer to Chap. 27). Plan rest and sleep activities as determined by the patient's need and tolerance.

V. Increase energy tolerance (e.g., being out of bed) through intermittent positive pressure breathing (IPPB) treatments.

VI. Avoid infections: aged person's perception of heat and cold may be altered, and therefore a fever may go unrecognized. Also, aged persons frequently have an elevation in temperature because they are often dehydrated and unable to perspire. Aged, dyspneic patients may not register a correct oral temperature reading. Patients should be instructed to contact a nurse or physician when sputum becomes yellow orgreen.

VII. Instruct patient to avoid extremes of heat and cold. Suggest that the patient stay indoors when extremes of weather occur. Avoid crowds. Recommend an air conditioner in extremely hot, humid weather.

VIII. Encourage fluids, especially in light of dehydration problem.

IX. Avoid contact with anyone, including children and family members, who has a cold or respiratory infection.

Evaluation

Refer to "Chronic Health Problems" and Chap. 27.

DIABETES

Definition

Another chronic problem of the aged is *diabetes*. Primary maturity-onset diabetes is a "chronic metabolic disease that is evidenced by above-normal blood glucose levels resulting from a deficiency of the pancreatic hormone, insulin. Primary maturity-onset diabetes develops after age 40 and pursues a mild course" (14). "Diabetes to the older person is basically the same disease as in younger persons" (15).

The incidence of diabetes increases with age and peaks between 65 and 74, occurring in 64.4 of 1000 persons. Of the aged population, 5 percent have diabetes. Risk factors in the elderly that predispose them to develop maturity-onset diabetes include (16):

1. Obesity.
2. Genetic predisposition.
3. Infection.
4. Severe mental anguish.
5. Surgical procedure.
6. Diabetogenic drugs (thiazides, cortisone).
7. Prolonged bed rest.

A complete discussion of diabetes is found in Chap. 24. Since several additional problems occur in the aged person with diabetes, the remaining discussion will focus on these important issues.

Assessment

Refer to Chap. 24. Additional areas to be covered in the assessment of the elderly diabetic include:

I. The patient's ability to learn and perform perceptual motor functions, e.g., insulin injection, urine testing.
II. Identification of physical limitations, if any.
III. What are the patient's dietary habits? Take a complete diet history, including whether the patient eats three meals a day. Note the amount of food taken at each meal. Elicit whether meals are taken at regular intervals. Does the patient have a good appetite?
IV. Identify availability of cooking facilities and refrigeration. Does the patient eat at home or are meals prepared elsewhere?
V. Does patient wear dentures? Is there difficulty noted in chewing? Do dentures fit well?
VI. Identify the patient's exercise pattern completed on a daily and weekly schedule.
VII. Assess medication program and patient's ability and motivation to comply. Evaluate past compliance patterns.

Problems/Diagnosis

I. Decreased perceptual and motor ability.
II. Decreased activity complicated by increased bed rest.
III. Alterations in nutritional intake: obesity or weight loss due to changes in appetite.
IV. Decreased compliance due to impairment of decision-making abilities and motor abilities, decreased understanding about disease and prevention of problems, and loss of vision.
V. Anxiety: mild to severe.

Goals of Care

Refer to Chap. 24. Additional goals in caring for the aged include:

I. Immediate.
   A. Perform the necessary perceptual and motor tasks, e.g., administering insulin and urine testing, or have a family member become skilled in performing tasks that the patient is unable to manage.
   B. Manage to cook food for self, as evidenced by eating meals planned according to dietary regimen, at regular intervals, or have food prepared and delivered according to dietary restrictions.
   C. Increase the amount of physical exercise through planning and implementing an activity schedule as tolerated by the patient.
II. Long-range. Cope with the problem of diabetes as it affects the individual's life-style

and incorporate these new behaviors into the way she or he handles the activities of daily living.

Intervention

Refer to Chap. 24. Additional interventions in the elderly include the following:

I. Consider all assessed changes when developing the teaching plan for an elderly diabetic.

II. Reinforce all progress made by the patient, and make use of repetition. Return demonstration should be supervised by the nurse.

III. Involve family to degree needed, and refer to Visiting Nurse Association or other community health agency to ensure long-term compliance.

IV. Begin dietary change by emphasizing the importance of three well-balanced meals taken at regularly spaced times.

V. If insulin or oral hypoglycemics are ordered, exchange or food groups will have to be taught. The following components should be considered when planning diet teaching:

A. Anorexia is common in the elderly.

B. Food preparation is often difficult for the aged, especially if they live alone or in a setting with limited facilities.

C. The choice of chewable foods may be limited for the elderly.

D. Patient's usual eating patterns should be preserved and diet planned close to personal eating habits and preferences, including foods especially liked.

VI. Exercise should be encouraged as tolerated. Explanation of the relationship between diabetes and exercise should be included in teaching plan. An exercise program should be planned around a patient's regular exercise habits. Encourage walking, as toleratd.

VII. Administer and teach patient how to self-administer all medications. Small amounts of insulin are usually preferred with aged [Lente or NPH (isophane insulin suspension) in 100-U doses]. Emphasize the importance of *exact* compliance; incorporate family into teaching program.

VIII. Have patient utilize a lighted magnifying glass or a preset syringe if visual disturbances interfere with performing the skill of administering insulin.

IX. Teach testing of urine by using a second voided specimen before any meal or bedtime. Teach the patient to keep a record of sugar and acetone daily, and have the patient increase testing of urine at each meal and bedtime should any illness occur (e.g., fever).

Evaluation

I. Reassessment.

A. Assess compliance, e.g., test blood sugar, test urine for sugar and acetone.

B. Return demonstration of skill, as needed.

C. Review diet.

II. Complications (see Chap. 24).

OSTEOARTHRITIS

Definition

Osteoarthritis is a noninflammatory deterioration of articular cartilages and overgrowth of adjacent bone. There are no systemic manifestations. Advancing age is the major predisposing factor. It is the most common type of arthritis occurring after age 50. After age 60, 15 percent of men and 25 percent of women have symptoms (17). (Refer to Chap. 31.)

Assessment

Refer to Chap. 31. Additional areas to be covered in the assessment include:
I. Increased tingling in fingertips, hands, and feet and crepitation.
II. Alteration in weight (obesity) which may aggravate bone problems.

Problems/Diagnosis

Refer to "Chronic Health Problems" and Chap. 31.

Goals of Care

I. Immediate (refer to "Chronic Health Problems).
II. Long-range.
   A. Perform activities of daily living to the best of ability.
   B. Understand the nature of the disease so as to live with it better.

Intervention

Refer to Chap. 31. Additional interventions include:
I. Establish exercise rest program with patient and family. Consider the following components in plan:
   A. Regularity and consistency of exercise.
   B. Emphasize extension rather than flexion of extremities.
   C. Utilize hydrotherapy before exercises to help decrease inflammation and tenderness and increase movement.
   D. Include active and passive exercises.
   E. Provide daily nap or rest periods as needed.
   F. Use foot board and bed board as needed, depending on the amount of time patient is resting.
   G. Provide proper alignment, preventing contractures by placing joints and limbs in the most functional position.
   H. Avoid complete bed rest whenever possible, as this can intensify the problem.
II. Encourage interest in personal appearance, e.g., maintain personal hygiene.
III. Utilize a weight reduction program as needed, explaining the need for weight control in order to reduce stress on joints.
IV. Medicate for pain, provide accurate instruction about the use and abuse of medication.

Evaluation

Refer to Chap. 31.

VISUAL DISTURBANCES

Definition

Most aged persons have fair to excellent vision (corrected with glasses). The three major geriatric ocular *problems* are: macular disease, cataracts, and glaucoma.

The macula is the center of retinal vision, and *diseases of the macula* cause loss of central vision. The cause of the disease is probably any of several vascular changes which occur with age and/or disease.

Cataracts are opaque lenses. If the opacity is near the center of the lens, vision is impaired. Throughout life, the lens grows by laying down new fibers. Compensatory shrinkage or drying of the nucleus occurs simultaneously. In the case of cataracts, the lens capsule thickens and a less permeable lens develops. This progresses with age until the nucleus is too hard and dry to transmit light efficiently (18).

Glaucoma manifests itself by increased intraocular pressure. The disease worsens with advancing age. The most common form is *chronic wide angle glaucoma*, due to failure in the facility for outflow of aqueous humor. The symptoms are insidious in onset, and the only definitive diagnosis is made with a tonometer. If the disease is undiagnosed and untreated, it will result in vision loss.

Assessment

Refer to "Chronic Health Problems" and Chap. 23. Additional characteristics to be noted include:

I. Macular disease.
   A. Inability to recognize faces.
   B. Inability to read.
   C. Inability to make out detail.
II. Cataracts.
   A. Poor peripheral vision in one or both eyes.
   B. Difficulty walking due to poor eyesight.
   C. Blurred vision in one or both eyes.
   D. Opaque lens in one or both eyes.
III. Glaucoma.
   A. Vague headaches.
   B. Tearing in one or both eyes.
   C. Increased intraocular pressure, determined with a tonometer.

Problems/Diagnosis

I. Impaired vision: secondary to visual disturbance.
II. Depression due to loss of vision.
III. Anxiety: mild to severe, secondary to fear of blindness.
IV. Loss of independence: dependence (potential).
V. Impaired ambulation.

Goals of Care

I. Immediate.
   A. Prevent further loss of sight.
   B. Help the patient to understand the process of the disease in order to be less anxious and depressed.
   C. Help the patient to understand the prognosis of cataracts and decrease the fear of blindness.
II. Long-range.
   A. Attain and maintain optimal level of sight.
   B. Maintain usual level of independence.
   C. Ambulate without injury.

Intervention

I. Macular disease. Suggest low-vision aids: magnifying devices, either hand-held (preferred by most aged patients) or in frames.

    II. Cataracts.
        A. Reinforce ophthalmologist's decision to operate or not to operate.
        B. If surgery is not indicated, instruct patient in use and purpose of prescribed miotics. Explain reason for decision to patient and family.
        C. If surgery is performed, give visual eye care.
        D. Reassure patient that an improvement in vision will occur.
        E. Allay fears by describing technical advances (which patient probably is not familiar with).
    III. Glaucoma.
        A. Administer and teach patient proper self-administration and action of eye drops. (Pilocarpine or carbachal is usually ordered.)
        B. Encourage patient to keep appointments with ophthalmologist.
        C. Teach patient and family importance of keeping condition well controlled by following instructions implicitly. A well-controlled glaucoma patient usually experiences no symptoms and has a tendency to relax on treatment.
        D. Instruct patient about the necessity of telling nurse or physician about *any* problem with vision, especially prior to surgery.
        E. Teach patient and family danger signals:
            1. Blurring of vision (especially in early morning).
            2. Halos around artificial lights.
            3. Pain in or around eyes.

Evaluation

    I. Reassessment.
        A. Has vision improved? Worsened?
        B. Does patient understand disease process? Prognosis?
        C. Is patient less depressed? Less anxious?
        D. Does the patient continue to express fear of blindness?
        E. Has independence level been maintained?
        F. Has patient suffered any injury due to poor eyesight?
    II. Complication: increased loss of vision (refer to Chap. 23).

AUDITORY DISTURBANCES

The majority of older persons develop some form of hearing deficiency (refer to Chap. 40). This results in distorted auditory perception and communication difficulties. The two most common causes of hearing loss are (1) conductive loss, and (2) sensorineural loss. *Conductive* losses are usually the result of dysfunctions of the external or middle ear and cause a reduction in loudness of speech. *Sensorineural* loss is the result of inner ear dysfunction and causes a distortion in sound, making speech unintelligible. Table 42-4 describes the more common auditory problems that affect the elerly.

Nursing care for the patient with a hearing loss is discussed in Chap. 23.

MEDICATION AND THE AGED

Definition

As the body ages, its ability to metabolize medications is altered. As has been seen, elderly persons often experience a chronic disease which requires the use of a large amount of medication. The number of drugs administered simultaneously often has a direct bearing on an individual's likelihood of experiencing an adverse drug reaction. The incidence for undesirable drug effects in persons over 60 is 2½ times as high as in those under 60. In

TABLE 42-4 / MAJOR AUDITORY DISTURBANCES OF THE AGED

External Ear	Middle Ear	Inner Ear
Partial occlusion with cerumen: This occurs frequently in the aged and interferes with optimum use of a hearing aid. The cerumen can usually be removed by saline irrigation. *Total occlusion with cerumen:* Common in the aged. Impacted cerumen cannot be removed easily by ordinary irrigation. The use of a wax softener or referral to an otologist for curetting may be necessary.	*Atrophic or sclerotic changes of tympanic membrane:* Common to the aged. Severe hearing loss only results when there is marked retraction of the tympanic membrane. *Otosclerosis:* This is the most common middle ear problem. An osseous growth occurs which fixes the footplate of the stapes in the oval window of the cochlea. A conductive hearing loss common to youth, it persists throughout life and eventually produces a sensorineutral loss in geriatric patients. *Treatment* includes: Surgical correction (refer to Chap. 23), use of a hearing aid, or both. Surgery in the elderly is frequently discouraged, but each candidate should be individually evaluated. Senturia and Price (19) present evidence supporting operative intervention in selected geriatric patients.	*Presbycusis* is the most common problem of the inner ear; it is a loss of hearing due to the aging process (refer to Chap. 40).

addition, women are twice as prone to adverse drug reactions as are men (20). The physiologic and behavioral changes that occur in elderly persons receiving medications must be carefully evaluated by the nurse.

The plasma level of a drug is directly related to its concentration at its site of action. This, in turn, governs the degree and duration of the body's response to the drug. The factors which influence plasma level and the specific differences in the aged individual are:

1. Absorption. Changes occur in the gastrointestinal tract during the aging process resulting in an impairment in drug absorption (refer to Chaps. 29 and 40).
2. Distribution. Active and functional tissue is replaced by fat as one ages. Drugs which accumulate in the fatty tissues have a more pronounced effect and a longer duration in the elderly.
3. Excretion. Because of a reduced rate of glomerular filtration and renal blood flow in the elderly, there is a delayed elimination of many drugs (refer to Chaps. 28 and 40).
4. Metabolism. Animal studies suggest there is a decrease in enzyme activity with aging which is reflected in higher blood levels and longer duration of drug activity.
5. Interaction. There is a decrease in the number of living, active cells in the aged person. Several drug problems result, including decreased activity of stimulants and enhanced activity of depressants.
6. Secondary responses. When a drug is administered for a particular purpose, the body often responds in ways other than intended in order to maintain homeostasis. Often there is a greater secondary effect and a lessened primary response in elderly persons because of the decreased ability to meet certain physiologic demands such as (21):
a. Poor adjustment to high and low temperatures.
b. Limited regulation of blood sugar levels.

    c. Decreased restoration of acid-base equilibrium.

    d. Decreased response to orthostatic stress.

The important thing to consider when administering medication to an elderly person is a summation of the above: *Elderly people have a decreased tolerance to drugs.*

Assessment

The phase of the nursing process of utmost importance in terms of the use of medications and the geriatric patient is the assessment. A complete drug assessment is critical in order to prevent complications and to identify the patient at risk to develop potentially negative drug reactions.

  I. Data sources (refer to "Chronic Health Problems").

  II. Health history.

    A. Identify *all* drugs being taken and the reason for their use (include over-the-counter drugs).

    B. List the amounts (dosages), times, and route of administration used for each drug.

    C. Elicit drugs taken in the past; identify reason for termination and any untoward response to any drug.

    D. Has the same physician prescribed all the drugs? If more than one physician is consulted, ask the patient if each doctor had been informed about the other. Aged persons will often see more than one doctor without informing the other, raising the potential for inadvertent drug reactions.

    E. Identify drug allergies; also, isolate any allergies to food, animals, etc. If an allergic reaction has occurred, identify changes noted.

    F. Assess patient's knowledge of drug action and adverse reactions to current drugs.

    G. Assess compliance: Does the patient follow nursing and medical orders? Did current medication taken have intended effect? (For example, did appetite increase? Did the stool soften? Did sleep become easier?) Does the patient take doses as prescribed and in the correct amount? If the patient forgets to take prescribed dose for 1 day, how is the situation corrected?

    H. Does the patient have any financial constraints? Can she or he afford the drug? Does the patient need financial assistance? Is there a pharmacy nearby that will deliver the medication and renew the prescription, if necessary?

    I. Does the patient have any physical limitations that may interfere with taking medication? Does the patient have a visual impairment that may interfere with reading the label clearly?

    J. Does the patient have any metabolic, gastrointestinal, or urinary tract problem that may interfere with drug absorption, distribution, or excretion and overall tolerance?

    K. Does the patient have any behavioral health problem that could be aggravated by a particular medication?

  III. Physical examination.

    A. Is the patient exhibiting any physical or behavioral manifestations of adverse drug reactions? Describe these effects.

    B. Is the patient manifesting positive physical or behavioral effects from the medications being taken? Describe these effects.

    C. Utilize components of observation, percussion, palpation, and auscultation in evaluating the aged person's action and reaction to each medication.

    D. Evaluate overall improvement of the patient's health status based on response to medication regimen.

Problems/Diagnosis

These will be based on specific data collected during the assessment.

Goals of Care

These will also be based on specific data collected during the assessment.

Intervention

Intervention is usually directed toward terminating the use of the drug, altering the dose, or developing a teaching and learning transaction for each patient. Knowledge of the patient's health problem(s) and the action and reaction of each drug is critical to implementing the teaching plan. Table 42-5 describes common drugs used by the elderly, potential adverse reactions, and points to emphasize in patient teaching. (Refer to specific chapters for discussion of particular disorders being treated.)

Evaluation

Reassessment should focus on compliance.

ORGANIC BRAIN SYNDROME

Definition

Organic brain syndrome is defined as "acute or chronic neuropsychiatric disorders caused by or associated with impairment of brain tissue function" (23). It is the most common psychiatric disorder in the elderly, occurring more commonly in women than in men. Determination of whether the patient's condition is acute or chronic is based on the cause of the problem and the prognosis. *Acute brain syndrome* is potentially reversible and may be due to infection, drugs, alcohol, trauma, circulatory disturbances, convulsive disorders, disturbances of metabolism, or neoplasms. *Chronic brain syndrome* is always irreversible and is generally due to congenital anomalies, brain injury, or multiple sclerosis (24). The most common type of chronic brain disorder is *cerebral arteriosclerosis,* which results in diffuse brain damage due to a loss in the number of neurons present in the cortex or an increase in the number of nonfunctioning neurons (refer to Chap. 23). This problem should not be confused with a single cerebral episode, such as a stroke, which causes focal damage. It is only when there are repeated cerebrovascular accidents that symptoms of chronic brain syndrome are evidenced. Cerebral thrombosis or carotid artery occlusion are also associated with chronic brain syndrome.

A common manifestation of cerebral arteriosclerosis and other organic brain syndromes is confusion. *Organic confusion* is caused by physical disturbances: electrolyte imbalance, infection, respiratory disturbances, etc. *Functional confusion* is brain disorder, resulting in organic changes in brain structures.

Assessment[2]

    I. Data sources (refer to "Chronic Health Problems").
   II. Health history (refer to "Chronic Health Problems").
  III. Physical examination.
      A. Organic confusion.
        1. Recent memory is more impaired than remote.
        2. Time disorientation occurs within own lifetime or reasonably near future.

[2] The assessment is based on Morris' and Rhodes' differentiation between organic and functional confusion (25).

TABLE 42-5 / MEDICATIONS FREQUENTLY USED BY AGED PERSON

Medication	Possible Adverse Reactions	Patient Teaching
Over the counter drugs: Aspirin or combination analgesics	Gastrointestinal upset Skin reactions Tinnitus	Many medications have aspirin added and may lead to an overdose if they are taken simultaneously with aspirin. Combination medications which include aspirin may have ingredients which are contraindicated for another condition. It is important to read label to determine all ingredients. Assess potential health problems that could be aggravated by aspirin (e.g., gastrointestinal problems).
Baking soda or other antacids	Increased pH of stomach Delayed absorption of acidic medications Possible respiratory stress for those susceptible to phenolphthalein	Sodium-containing antacids (Alka-Seltzer) are contraindicated for those who require sodium restriction. There is no need for daily bowel movement; changes in bowel habits occur or can occur with aging.
Mineral oil	Retards gastric emptying May impede absorption of some minerals and fat-soluble vitamins	Avoid straining at stool. Increase roughage, increase exercise, increase fluid intake, and increase intake of fruits and vegetables. Caution against diarrhea.
Vitamin C	1 g or more can cause diarrhea or precipitation of uric acid crystals in urine	Teach patient importance of not taking an excess of the vitamin. Stress foods with vitamin C.
Vitamin D	Large doses may cause hypercalcemia	Teach patient symptoms of hypercalcemia: weakness, nausea and vomiting, and diarrhea. Caution against taking an excessive dose.
Cardiac drugs: Digitalis	Cardiac arrhythmias, headache, vertigo, visual disturbances, disorientation, weakness, fatigue, nausea, vomiting, apathy	Teach patient side effects, including changes in pulse rate, yellow vision, nausea and vomiting. Instruct patient to report side effects to the nurse or physician immediately. (Depletion of potassium may occur, increasing sensitivity to the drug.) Teach patient to take pulse rate (refer to Chap. 26).
Anticoagulants	More likely to respond with a lowered prothrombin time	Teach importance of routine laboratory tests (refer to Chap. 26) to monitor Coumadin doses (prothrombin time as ordered). Care against bruising.
Antianginal agents	May induce tachycardia, hypotension, syncope	Emphasize importance of reporting all signs and symptoms to physician so that dose can be reduced. If problem not relieved, patient should contact medical personnel.

TABLE 42-5 / MEDICATIONS FREQUENTLY USED BY AGED PERSON (*continued*)

Medication	Possible Adverse Reactions	Patient Teaching
Diuretics	Increased possibility of elevated blood urea nitrogen (BUN) levels or alteration in bland electrolytes (e.g., decreased potassium or sodium)	Nitrates (long-acting) should be avoided in a person with glaucoma as they can increase intraocular pressure. Instruct patient about association between digitalis and thiazide diuretics: Thiazide diuretics increase urinary potassium excretion, which may result in hypokalemia. This (see Digitalis), may increase the myocardium's sensitivity to digitalis. Evaluate urinary intake and output. Teach the patient the signs of hypo- and hyperkalemia and hypernatremia (refer to Chap. 28).
Antidepressants	May induce hypotension	Monitor patient's blood pressure. Teach patient signs of hypotension. Monitor the patient's mood; assess changes in behavior.
Hypnotics and sedatives	Increased sensitivity Delirium Disorientation Forgetfullness Apprehension	Observe patient and teach family possible side effects of hypnotics and sedatives so that they may be alert to them. Evaluate behavioral change.
Narcotics	Very sensitive (especially to morphine; dose should be half that used for younger adults). May cause respiratory depression, hypotension, urinary retention in elderly who are sensitive to the drug (22).	Instruct to report to physician if she or he has ever had an untoward reaction to a narcotic.

Source: Adapted from Dorothy Lenhart, "The Use of Medications in the Elderly Population," *Nursing Clinics of North America,* **11**(1): 135–143, March 1976.

   3. Disoriented in a familiar, easily accessible place.
   4. Retains sense of self-identity, but misidentifies others (unknowns) as being familiar.
   5. Visual and vivid hallucinations, usually of animals and insects, are common.
   6. The patient will describe illusions.
   7. Expresses delusions about everyday occurrences and people.
   8. Confusion is erratic. There are moments of clearness mixed with episodes of confusion; more pronounced at night.
B. Functional confusion.
   1. No consistent difference between recent and remote memory impairment.
   2. Time disorientation may not be related to patient's lifetime.
   3. Disoriented in bizarre or unfamiliar places.
   4. Sense of self-identity is diminished.
   5. Misidentifies others based on a delusional system. (The nurse is a spy or the family member is an enemy.)
   6. Bizarre, symbolic auditory hallucinations.
   7. No illusions described.

8. Delusions expressed are bizarre and symbolic.

9. Confusion is quite consistent. There is no tendency for it to worsen at night.

Problems/Diagnosis

I. Failing memory, secondary to functional or organic confusion.

II. Time, place, person disoriented, secondary to functional or organic confusion.

III. Hallucinations, delusions, and illusions due to functional or organic confusion.

Goals of Care

I. Immediate.

    A. Identify cause of confusion, and eliminate or reduce confusion.

    B. Reorient to time and place, as evidenced by knowledge of such things as the day of the week, knowledge of present location, and accurate perception of time of day, etc.

    C. Experience no further increase in memory loss.

II. Long-range. Eliminate confusion precipitated by either function or organic causes as evidenced by an absence of illusion, delusion, or hallucination.

Intervention

I. Answer questions in short, simple phrases.

II. Continuously assess the patient's mental status in order to identify a possible cause of confusion. If medications are altered or withdrawn, changes in behavior should be noted and evaluated.

III. Evaluate fluid and electrolyte balances as alterations could potentiate confusion (refer to Chap. 28).

IV. Monitor vital signs. Be aware of signs of infection, as an elevation in temperature may contribute to confusion.

V. Do not support disorientation. Instead, encourage return to reality by providing an environment that is reality orienting. The use of clocks, calendars, familiar surroundings, and the presence of familiar faces (e.g., family) may help reduce confusion.

VI. Reduce the amount of change in an environment by keeping it constant and/or stable. Reducing the number of strangers entering the room, avoiding transfers from one environment to another, and stabilizing personnel may be some measures that can be utilized to orient the patient to reality.

VII. In order to provide a constant environment for the daily patterns, routines should be established and followed as part of daily activities. In addition, calling patients by names frequently will also remind them of their identity.

VIII. Avoid nocturnal sensory deprivation, as this may increase confusion. Provide night-light, and be sure the patient's safety needs are met, e.g., side rails, as needed.

IX. Administer and monitor medications as ordered. Carefully monitor the effects of all medications on the patient. Careful assessment of the patient's reaction to such things as stimulants, sedatives, CNS depressants is essential.

X. Provide mental stimulation (radio, conversation). Do not discuss delusional material with patient as this may support or perpetuate the undesired behavior.

XI. Encourage meaningful physical activity (making bed, setting table, etc.). Emphasize patient's capabilities when conversing.

XII. Keep patient out of bed as much as possible, as physical activity may help stimulate mental activity.

XIII. Support family. At times this is the most realistic goal to accomplish.

XIV. For added information about nursing care of the patient with delusions, hallucinations, and illusions, refer to Chap. 38.

Evaluation

I. Reassessment.
   A. Reassessment needed continuously to evaluate the individual's orientation to time, person, and place.
   B. Evaluate if hallucinations, delusions, or illusions have stopped.
   C. Has the patient's level of awareness increased? Is the patient able to identify persons, places, and things within the environment?
II. Complications.
   A. Increased mental confusion.
   B. Intensification of the initial problem.
   C. Continued follow-up counseling and referral needed.

ACCIDENTS

Definition

Accidents are a major cause of death in those persons 65 years of age or older. If death does not occur at the time of the accident, severe complications frequently result in the demise of the patient. Certain predisposing factors have been identified as related to the aged and injury caused by accidents. They include:

1. Intellectual deterioration. Memory and orientation to time, place, and person fail. There is decreased alertness, and the aged individual forgets to turn off the stove, does not remember the one step outside the door, or does not look before stepping into the street.
2. Chronic disease effects. The elderly tend to become unsteady and feeble as a result of chronic illness. Thus, they become more subject to falls. Decline in vision and hearing also contributes to the high rate of accidents in this age group. When sight fails, the older person is more susceptible to the dangers of poor lighting, glare, and decreased night vision. With progressive hearing loss, the aged individual often does not hear warning signals, such as automobiles, sirens, etc.
3. Clinging to habits and possessions of the past. There is a type of older person who saves anything and everything, either to maintain an identity with the past or just because he or she cannot let go of any possession. This type of individual is subjected to the danger of fire, falls, or the possibility of being crushed.

Most injuries to the aged are the result of accidental falls. Fractures occur most frequently in those between 75 and 85 years of age. The most common fracture in the elderly is that of the proximal end of the femur, which occurs 3 times more often in women than in men.

Intervention

Refer to Chap. 44. The focus of care should be directed toward prevention of accidents. This includes the following.
   I. Identify potential risk factors that are present in the elderly patient's home environment.
   II. Be sure adequate lighting is available (especially at bottom of stairs, etc.).
   III. Hand rails should be secure and in places where added support is necessary (e.g., bathroom, stairs).

IV. Remove all throw rugs; use only nonskid rugs.

V. Limit the use of floor wax.

VI. Remove low-lying objects such as foot stools, waste baskets, etc.

VII. Encourage use of shoes with corrugated soles. Ice grippers should be used in winter.

VIII. Encourage patient to avoid walking on snow and ice. Limit snow removal activities.

IX. Encourage patients to give themselves adequate time to complete activities to decrease need for rushing.

X. If driving is necessary, be sure eye examination has been performed. If highway driving is stressful for the patient, the use of alternate routes or other means of transportation should be selected.

XI. Because of altering perception of heat and cold, patients should be cautioned about the use of heat application or overexposure to cold.

XII. Maintain weight within normal limits, and subscribe to a daily activity program which will maximize physical fitness.

XIII. Use of hospital or low-lying beds and side rails should be used as needed.

XIV. Housing conditions (including heating, broader stairs, safety of cooking facilities, and general building safety) should be evaluated an changes made to protect the aged from injury.

Evaluation

Refer to Chap. 44.

REFERENCES

1. *Chronic Disease and Rehabilitation,* The American Public Health Association, Inc., New York, 1960, p. 36.
2. *Health Characteristics of Persons with Chronic Activity Limitation,* U.S. Department of Health, Education, and Welfare, Rockville, Md., 1976, p. 11.
3. Raymond Harris, "Special Features of Heart Disease in the Elderly Patient," *Working With Older People: Clinical Aspects of Aging,* U.S. Department of Health, Education, and Welfare, Rockville, Md., 1971, p. 91.
4. Ibid.
5. P. S. Timiras, "Disease of Aging," in P. S. Timiras (ed.), *Development Physiology and Aging,* The Macmillan Company, New York, 1972, p. 474.
6. Harris, op. cit., p. 89.
7. *Facts of Life and Death,* Public Health Service, 1967.
8. Simeon Locke, "Cerebrovascular Disorders in Later Life," *Working With Older People: Clinical Aspects of Aging,* U.S. Department of Health, Education, and Welfare, Rockville, Md., 1971, p. 56.
9. Irene L. Beland and Joyce Y. Passos, *Clinical Nursing,* The Macmillan Company, New York, 1975, p. 454.
10. Oskar Balchum, "The gaging Respiratory System," *Working With Older People: Clinical Aspects of Aging,* U.S. Department of Health, Education, and Welfare, Rockville, Md., 1971, pp. 121–122.
11. Beland and Passos, op. cit., p. 454.
12. Balchum, op. cit., p. 119.
13. Ibid., pp. 118–119.
14. Katherine P. Thomas, "Diabetes Mellitus in Elderly Persons," *Nursing Clinics of North America,* 11(1): 158, March 1976.
15. Ibid., p. 157.
16. Ibid., p. 160.
17. David Grob, "Prevalent Joint Diseases in Older Persons," *Working with Older People: Clinical Aspects of Aging,* U.S. Department of Health, Education, and Welfare, Rockville, Md.,1971, p. 163.
18. Dan Gordon, "Eye Problems of the Aged," *Working With Older People: Clinical Aspects of Aging,* U.S. Department of Health, Education, and Welfare, Rockville, Md., 1971, p. 29.

19. Ben Senturia and Lloyd Price, "Otolaryngological Problems in the Geriatric Patient," *Working With Older People: Clinical Aspects of Aging,* U.S. Department of Health, Education, and Welfare, Rockville, Md., 1971, p. 39.
20. David P. Richey, "Effects of Human Aging on Drug Absorption and Metabolism," in Ralph Goldman and Morris Rockstein (eds.), *The Physiology and Pathology of Human Aging,* Academic Press, New York, 1975, p. 62.
21. A. Douglas Bender, "Drug Therapy in the Aged," *Working With Older People: Clinical Aspects of Aging,* U.S. Department of Health, Education, and Welfare, Rockville, Md., 1971, pp. 308–310.
22. Timiras, loc. cit.
23. Irene M. Burnside, *Nursing and the Aged,* McGraw-Hill Book Company, New York, 1976, p. 149.
24. Adriaan Verwoerdt, "Clinical Geropsychiatry," *Working With Older People: Clinical Aspects of Aging,* U.S. Department of Health, Education, and Welfare, Rockville, Md., 1971, p. 67.
25. Magdalena Morris and Martha Rhodes, "Guideline for the Care of Confused Patients," *American Journal of Nursing,* **72**(9):1630–1633, September 1972.

BIBLIOGRAPHY

Burnside, Irene M.: *Nursing and the Aged,* McGraw-Hill Book Company, New York, 1976. This text is a comprehensive, multidisciplinary approach to the care of the aged. It deals with all aspects of aging and the appropriate nursing responsibilities. Nursing process is outlined.

Symposium on Gerontological Nursing, *Nursing Clinics of North America* **11**(1):115–206, March 1976. An excellent symposium dealing with a variety of needs of the aged, this reference depicts the philosophy of the writers and gives current nursing approaches to common problems of the elderly.

Working with Older People: Clinical Aspects of Aging, U.S. Department of Health Education and Welfare, Rockville, Md., 1971. *Working with Older People: The Practitioner and the Elderly,* ibid. *Working with Older People: The Aging Person Needs and Services,* ibid., 1974. *Working with Older People: Biological, Psychological and Sociological Aspects of Aging,* ibid. A four-volume publication which is concerned with all aspects of gerontology and geriatrics, it is an excellent reference for pathophysiology, epidemiology, and management of problems and diseases of the aged. It is multidisciplinary in approach. Nursing is not the focus.

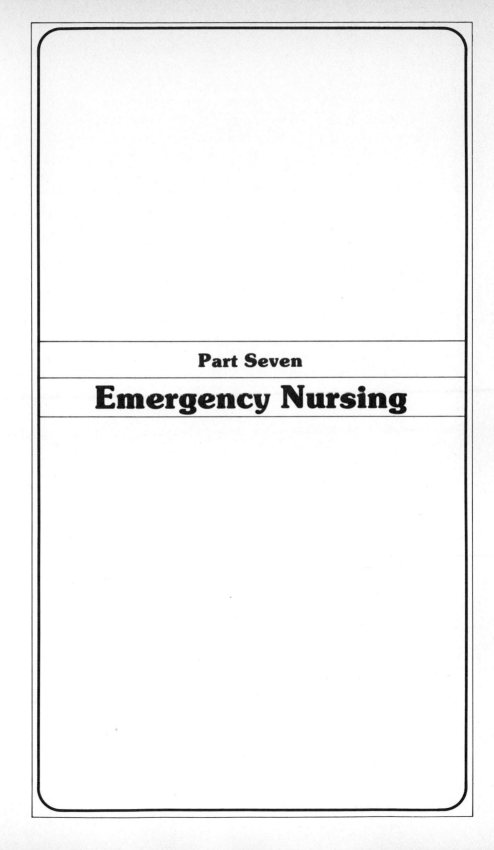

Part Seven

Emergency Nursing

espite the recent development of family medicine, utilization of emergency facilities has
continued to increase. Emergency medicine has emerged as a distinct specialty in the
attempt to meet the needs of the increased variety and complexity of problems encountered
in emergency departments.

This section of the *Handbook* is meant to be a reference for nursing personnel newly
assigned to emergency services, as well as a review and/or reference for those who have
worked in emergency situations for some time.

The section is divided into four chapters: "General Principles of Emergency Care" (Chap.
43), "Traumatic Injuries" (Chap. 44), "Medical Emergencies" (Chap. 45), and "Psychiatric
Emergencies" (Chap. 46). This classification is similar to that of most emergency references,
making it possible to refer easily to other sources when more detailed information is required.

In most instances, the following categories are used to outline the nursing plan of care
for each problem: definition, assessment, (nursing) problems, goals of care, intervention,
and evaluation. The interpretation of these categories may be modified somewhat from
problem to problem to fit the nature of the nursing plan being discussed.

Presentation of the content has been developed with the intent to reach a balance
between a general overview and specific details of the management of individual emergency
problems. With the wide variety of problems seen in emergency departments, this goal is
difficult at best. Therefore, only common emergency problems (e.g., cardiac arrest) and
regional problems that occur in relatively large numbers (e.g., snake bite) have been
included. The nursing plans of care for these problems are developed in as much detail as
space limitations permit.

The content is relevant for the management of emergency problems from the time they
are normally first encountered by emergency personnel to the time at which the patient is
usually discharged or transferred to another department. Information relative to continued
management can be found in appropriate chapters elsewhere in the book.

Although reference is frequently made to specific medications, it should be noted that the
choice of drug, route of administration, and dosage may vary from patient to patient. The
information given is meant to acquaint the reader with those medications commonly used
and with the common modes of administration, rather than to serve as an endorsement of
a particular drug or to pronounce that a particular mode of administration is *the* mode to
follow.

As in the other parts of this *Handbook*, the ANA standards of nursing practice, in this
case, of emergency nursing practice, are incorporated into each discussion of a particular
health problem. They are listed below as a guide in delineating the scope of and evaluating
emergency nursing activities.

ANA STANDARDS OF EMERGENCY NURSING PRACTICE[1]

1. The collection of data about the health status of the individual is systematic and pertinent.
   These data are recorded, retrievable, and communicated to appropriate persons.
2. Nursing diagnosis is derived from health status data.
3. Goals for nursing care are formulated.
4. The plan for nursing care prescribes nursing actions to achieve the goals.
5. The plan for nursing care is implemented.
6. The plan for nursing care is evaluated.
7. Reassessment of the individual, reconsideration of nursing diagnosis, setting of goals,
   and revision of the plan for nursing care are a continuous process.

[1]Reprinted with permission from the *American Nurses' Association Standards of Emergency Nursing
Practice.* Copyright © 1975 by the American Nurses' Association.

43

General Principles
of Emergency Care

Mary P. Wieland

Emergency department nursing is rapidly becoming a specialty in itself. The purpose of emergency nursing is to assist the patient and family in reaching the patient's maximum level of "wellness" or health. Often, these results are not seen within the emergency department or within the medical facility.

Nursing functions and responsibilities within an emergency department are determined by hospital policy and the type of facility where one is employed. However, certain *broad categories* of knowledge and skill are common to all emergency department nurses. These include:

1. The ability to perform concise but rapid focused histories.
2. Expertise in delivering basic and advanced life-support measures.
3. Knowledge of all age groups and their various health problems.
4. Rapid, thorough use of observational and assessment skills with appropriate nursing interventions.
5. Performance of a wide variety of technical and diagnostic skills in an orderly and quick fashion.
6. Ability to set priorities of care.
7. Teaching regarding health care.
8. Advocators and managers of patient care.
9. Utilization of crisis intervention techniques.

The combination of this broad nursing knowledge and skilled technical expertise contributes to the ability of each emergency department nurse to be a specialist in acute nursing care.

This chapter will present some of the basic principles involved in emergency department nursing. Emphasis will be placed on initial assessments and focused interviewing techniques. Specific nursing interventions are presented in subsequent chapters. In addition, the broad concept of triaging will be demonstrated by using a triage model.

GENERAL ASSESSMENT

I. Introduce yourself, and state your function as a health team member to each patient and family.
II. Maintain a calm, relaxed, and reassuring attitude.
III. Obtain a *"quick overview"* of the patient by utilizing observational and assessment skills.
   A. A *systematic assessment* includes:
      1. General appearance of the patient.
      2. State of consciousness.
      3. Respiratory and circulatory function.
      4. Presence of shock state or impending shock.
      5. Evidence of overt bleeding, hematomas, bruises.
      6. Ability of patient to move all extremities appropriately.
      7. Observation of obvious deformities, tenderness, suspected fractures.
IV. Realize that action and assessment may occur simultaneously in lifesaving situations.
V. Consider the ABC's of lifesaving first with each patient, prior to further evaluation (see also Chaps. 44 and 45):

    A. Airway.

    B. Breathing.

    C. Circulation.

VI. Elicit a *focused interview* or principal problem history from each patient and/or family members.

    A. Explain the purpose of this data gathering to obtain the cooperation of the patient or family.

    B. Focus on the patient's *chief complaint:* "What happened?"

    C. State this problem in the patient's own words, i.e., "My stomach hurts" does not necessarily mean that the patient is having an appendicitis attack.

    D. Elicit details regarding:

        1. Onset of the problem.

        2. The interval history.

        3. Current status or course of symptom.

    E. If possible, have the patient describe the chief complaint as to:

        1. Location and radiation.

        2. Character or quality.

        3. Influence symptom has on activities of daily living.

        4. Aggravating and relieving factors.

        5. Accompanying symptoms: see Table 43-1.

VII. In addition to the focused interview, obtain information regarding *past* history of:

    A. Allergies to medications, insect stings, pollen, food.

    B. Medications taken to relieve chief complaint and others taken on a routine basis.

    C. Cardiopulmonary disease.

    D. Diabetes mellitus.

    E. Hypertension.

    F. Stroke.

    G. Renal disease.

    H. When dealing with trauma such as lacerations and burns, elicit the date of the last tetanus toxoid booster given.

VIII. Avoid unnecessary handling and movement of the severely injured patient.

IX. Perform a thorough but rapid *head-to-toe assessment,* depending on the patient's chief complaint. This will be a general overview of the nursing assessments involved in evaluating several of the body's systems. Please refer to subsequent chapters dealing with the nursing interventions involved with specific problems.

    A. Head and spinal assessment:

        1. Observation of:

            a. Airway patency.

            b. Level of consciousness.

            c. Orientation to time, place, person.

            d. Pattern of breathing.

            e. Pupillary reaction (PEERLA, pupils equally reactive to light and accommodation).

            f. Eye movements.

            g. Obvious injury:

                (1) Bleeding.

                (2) Hematomas.

                (3) Presence of foreign objects, cerebral spinal fluid from ears, nose.

                (4) Asymmetry.

            h. Response to verbal, tactile, and painful stimuli.

            i. Spinal cord injury level (see Fig. 43-1 for summmary of brief neurological examination).

                (1) *Cervical area:*

                    (a) C5: Patient lifts elbow to shoulder height.

                    (b) C6: Bends elbow.

                    (c) C7: Straightens elbow from flexed position.

TABLE 43-1 / SUMMARY CHART FOR THE EMERGENCY REVIEW OF SYSTEMS

GENERAL
Present weight (loss or gain, period of time, contributing factors), weakness, fatigue, malaise, fever, chills, sweats or night sweats

SKIN
Pruritis, pigmentary and other color changes, tendency to bruising, lesions (location), excessive dryness, texture, character of hair and nails, use of hair dyes or other possibly toxic agents

HEAD
Headache, head injury (how, when, where), dizziness

EYES
Pain, vision, glasses, and recent change in acuity, diplopia, infection, glaucoma, cataract

EARS
Earaches, hearing, tinnitus, vertigo, discharge, infection, mastoiditis

NOSE AND SINUSES
Sinus pain, epistaxis, nasal obstruction, discharge, postnasal drip, frequent colds, sneezing

ORAL CAVITY
Toothache, recent extractions, state of dental repair; soreness or bleeding of lips, gums, mouth, tongue or throat; disturbance of taste; hoarseness; tonsillectomy

NECK
Pain, limitation of motion, thyroid enlargement

NODES
Tenderness or enlargement of cervical, axillary, epitrochlear, or inguinal nodes

BREAST
Pain, lumps, discharge, operations

RESPIRATORY
Chest pain, pleurisy, cough, sputum (character and amount), hemoptysis, wheezing (location in chest), stridor, asthma, bronchitis, pneumonia, tuberculosis or contact therewith, date of recent x-ray

CARDIOVASCULAR
Precordial or retrosternal pain or distress, palpitation, dyspnea (relate to effort), orthopnea, paroxysmal nocturnal dyspnea, edema, cyanosis; history of heart murmur, rheumatic fever (enumerate the manifestations), hypertension, coronary artery disease, last ECG

GASTROINTESTINAL
Appetite, food intolerance, dysphagia (solids, liquids), heartburn, postprandial pain or distress, biliary colic, jaundice, other abdominal pain or distress, belching, nausea, vomiting, hematemesis, flatulence; character and color of stools (bleeding, melena, clay colored, diarrhea, constipation), change in bowel habits; rectal conditions (pruritus, hemorrhoids, fissures, fistula); ulcer, gallbladder disease, hepatitis, appendicitis, colitis, parasites, hernia; date of previous x-rays

GENITOURINARY
Urinary: Renal colic, frequency of urination, nocturia, polyuria, oliguria, micturition (hesitancy, urgency, dysuria, narrowing of stream, dribbling, incontinence), hematuria, albuminuria, pyuria, kidney disease, facial edema, renal stone, cystoscopy
Male: Testicular pain, change in size of scrotum
Female: Vaginal discharge or itching; intermenstrual or postmenopausal bleeding; dysmenorrhea; dyspareunia; urinary stress, incontinence (involuntary passage of urine on coughing, sneezing,

TABLE 43-1 / SUMMARY CHART FOR THE EMERGENCY REVIEW OF SYSTEMS (*Continued*)

---

stepping off curbs, *etc.*); uterine prolapse; date and character of last menstrual period; if menopausal, date of onset

Venereal: Gonorrhea or syphilis—identify by common name and signs; note date, treatment, complications

EXTREMITIES

Vascular: Intermittent claudication, varicose veins or complications, thrombophlebitis

Joints: Pain, stiffness, swelling (note location, migratory nature, relation to known cardiac involvement); rheumatoid arthritis, osteoarthritis, gout, bursitis

Bones: Flat feet, osteomyelitis, fracture

Muscles: Pain, cramps

BACK

Pain (location and radiation, especially to the extremities), stiffness, limitation of motion, sciatica or disc disease

CENTRAL NERVOUS SYSTEM

General: Syncope, loss of consciousness, convulsions, meningitis, encephalitis, stroke

Mentative: Speech disorders, emotional status, orientation, memory disorders, change in sleep pattern, history of nervous breakdown

Motor: Tremor, weakness, paralysis, clumsiness of movement

Sensory: Radicular or neuralgic pain (head, neck, trunk, extremities), paresthesia

HEMATOPOIETIC

Bleeding tendencies of skin or mucous membrane, anemia and treatment, blood type, transfusion and reaction, blood dyscrasia, exposure to toxic agents or radiation

ENDOCRINE

Nutritional and growth history; thyroid function (tolerance to heat and cold, change in skin, relationship between appetite and weight, nervousness, tremors, results of previous basal metabolism tests, thyroid medication); diabetes or its symptoms (polyuria, polydipsia, polyphagia); hirsuitism, secondary sex characteristics, hormone therapy

---

Note: Which systems are evaluated will, of course, depend on the nature of the patient's problem. Each emergency department should be equipped with a review-of-systems form, so that the nurse can quickly determine the presence of accompanying symptoms. Medical jargon should be avoided.
Source: "Explanation Outline for Recording a History and Physical," University of Illinois Medical Center, 1972 (unpublished); reproduced from Jeanie Barry, *Emergency Nursing,* McGraw-Hill Book Company, New York, 1978, p. 186.

      (*d*) C8 and T: Hand grasps.
    (**2**) *Lumbar area:*
      (*a*) L3: Lift leg or flex hip.   (*c*) L5: Wiggle toes backward.
      (*b*) L4 and L5: Extend knee.   (*d*) S1: Push toe downward.
  2. Palpation of:
    a. Scalp, gently running fingers through patient's hair looking for:
      (**1**) Lacerations.
      (**2**) Hematomas.
      (**3**) Decompressions.
    b. Facial bones for bruising, tenderness.
    c. Spine for point tenderness.
B. Cardiopulmonary assessment.
  1. Inspection of:
    a. The color of the patient.

    b. Posture in which patient assumes the maximum use of respiratory muscles.

    c. Use of any accessory muscles for breathing.

    d. Rate, character, and depth of respirations.

    e. Bilateral movement of chest wall.

    f. Symmetry of chest wall.

    g. Neck veins.

    h. Obvious external injury.

  2. Palpate for:

    a. Deformities.

    b. Wounds.

FIGURE 43-1 / Summary chart for brief neurological examination. Starting at the cervical area, ask the patient to do the following: (1) *Lift* **the elbows up to shoulder height—C5;** *bend* **the elbow—C6;** *straighten* **the elbow from a flexed position—C7;** *grip*—**C8 and T1. (2)** *Lift* **the leg off the bed or flex the hips—L3;** *extend* **the knee—L4 and L5;** *wiggle* **the toes backwards—L5;** *push* **the toes downward—S1. The patient must be checked bilaterally. If the patient can do all these, a severe cord injury is not present. If he or she is able to bend the elbows but not extend the elbows, then one has to suspect a lesion between C6 and C7. If the arm function is intact and the chest is moving, but the patient is unable to move the legs, then the site of concern is in the upper lumbar area. If the examination shows that one arm moves well but the other arm does not, suspect a nerve root injury on the nonfunctioning side. (***From Jeanie Barry, Emergency Nursing, McGraw-Hill Book Company, New York, 1978.***)**

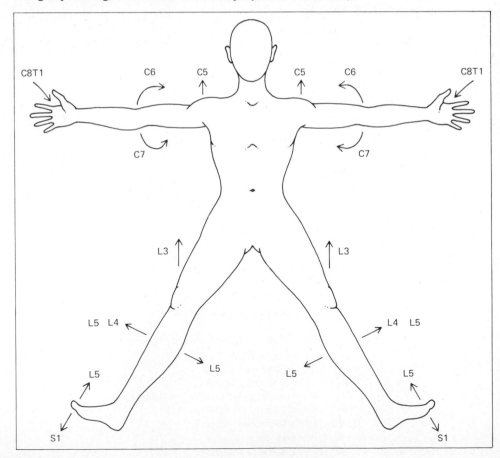

       c. Contusions.

       d. Abrasions.

       e. Scars.

       f. Tracheal deviation.

       g. Evidence of trauma, masses, lesions.

       h. Crepitus.

       i. Point of maximal intensity (PMI).

   3. Auscultate:

       a. All lung fiels for presence and equality of breath sounds.

       b. Heart sounds, noting rate and any abnormalities heard throughout the precordium.

C. Abdominal assessment.

   1. Inspection of:

       a. Texture and color of skin.

       b. Presence of lesions:

          (1) Scars.   **(4)** Striae.

          (2) Wounds.   **(5)** Bruises.

          (3) Rashes.

       c. Hair distribution.

       d. Abdominal contour (done at foot of the bed) to check for:

          (1) Symmetry.

          (2) Bulging.

          (3) Hernias.

      e Abdominal girth.

       f. Noticeable respiratory motion and/or splinting.

       g. Pulsations.

       h. Waves of peristalsis.

   2. Auscultate for:

       a. Bowel sounds, noting the quality and rate.

       b. Presence of adventitious sounds, i.e., bruits, friction rubs.

   3. Palpate for:

       a. Presence of masses.

       b. Quality of abdominal musculature.

       c. Areas of tenderness.

       d. Rebound tenderness.

       e. Costovertebral angle (CVA) tenderness.

       f. Deformity.

D. Skeletal system assessment.

   1. Utilize the five P's in your evaluation:

       a. Pain.   *d. Paralysis.*

       b. Pulses.   *e. Pallor.*

       c. Paresthesia.

   2. Inspection of:

       a. Color of extremity involved.

       b. Obvious deformities.

          (1) Swelling.

          (2) Ecchymosis.

          (3) Asymmetry.

       c. Voluntary movement.

   3. Palpate for:

       a. Quality and equality of pulses distal to injury.

       b. Areas of pain:

          (1) Tenderness.

          (2) Swelling.

          (3) Crepitus.

    X. Record all data, including:
       A. Focused history.
       B. Vital signs.
       C. Monitoring parameters.
       D. System assessments and interventions.
   XI. Relate knowledge of this data to the appropriate health care team members.
  XII. Plan appropriate crisis interventions, as needed.
 XIII. Evaluate need for health care teaching of patient and family.

TRIAGE NURSING

     I. Derived from the French word, *trier*, "to sort," "to choose."
    II. The function of the triage nurse in the emergency department is to:
       A. Obtain a rapid, concise focused history.
       B. Perform a brief quick overview of patient (see point IX under "General Assessment," above).
       C. Categorize each patient as to severity of illness.
       D. Decide proper place of treatment for each patient.
   III. *Qualities* of the triage nurse:
       A. Accurate clinical judgment.
       B. Tact and efficiency.
       C. Experience in management of patients and their health problems.
       D. Ability to conduct focused interviews with speed and accuracy.
       E. Obtain a quick overview of patient's status.
       F. Plan appropriate dispositions of patients by coding the chief complaint as:
          1. Urgent or nonurgent.
          2. Critical or routine.
          3. Emergency or nonemergency.
    IV. The major components of an *effective triage system* consist of:
       A. The nature and location of the *triage facility* to treatment areas.
       B. The *personnel* performing triage.
       C. The *rating system* used.
     V. ABCs of triage with multiple trauma patient. *Priority* order of care (see Table 43-2), modified for *any* emergency situation: airway, bleeding, consciousness, digestive organs, excretory organs, fractures.
       A. Airway.
          1. Patent airway.
             a. Hyperextend neck.
             b. "Modified jaw thrust" or "chin lift" with head and spinal injuries.
          2. Presence of foreign objects: Clear out secretions from oral cavity; nose suctioning, as necessary.
          3. Look, listen, feel for air movement.
             a. No voluntary respirations: begin rescue breathing.
               (1) Mouth to mouth.
               (2) Mouth mask.
               (3) Bag mask.
             b. Noisy respirations with open chest wound: Vaseline dressing to wound.
             c. Slow, shallow respirations: suspect possible drug overdose, metabolic disorder.
          4. Oxygen needs.
             a. Draw and evaluate arterial blood gases (ABG).
             b. Assist with:
               (1) Endotracheal intubation.   **(3)** Cricothyroid puncture.
               (2) Tracheostomy.   **(4)** Oxygen therapy.
          5. Auscultate breath sounds.
             a. Faint or absent: consider hemopneumothorax; assist with chest tube insertion.

TABLE 43-2 / SAMPLE TRIAGE MODEL OR RATING SYSTEM*

Category I (Emergency)	Category II (Urgent)	Category III (Nonurgent)
Cardiopulmonary arrests	Unexplained or severe pain	Routine laceration
Unconsciousness	Severe nausea, vomiting; diarrhea, with infants	Chronic back pain
Obstructed airway	Hemorrhage	Mild headache
Shock	Multiple lacerations	Fatigue
Multiple trauma	Burns: 15% body area with adults; 10% body area with child	Dizziness
Head injuries		Nervousness
Spinal injuries	Any burns involving face, ears, hands	Minor infection: urinary tract infection (UTI) or upper respiratory infection (URI)
	Drug overdose	Skin eruptions
	Poison ingestion	Sprains
	Respiratory distress	Strains
	Croup, with child	Hernia
	Asthma	Gastrointestinal complaints: diarrhea, constipation, hemorrhoids
	Shortness of breath (SOB)	
	Elevated temperature: 103°F with child, 101°F with adult	Dental complaints: abscess, cavities
	Gastrointestinal bleeding	
	Hematuria	
	Oliguria	
	Anuria	
	Suspected fractures of extremities	
	Attempted suicide	
	Pregnancy complications	

*Emergency = life-threatening situations; patient must be placed in treatment room immediately! Urgent = detrimental to life if not treated within 1–2 h. Nonurgent = stable conditions. This triage model is by no means complete! A triage rating system is based upon the patient's chief complaint plus the individual assessment made by the nurse.

> **b.** Adventitious lung sounds. Care of particular disease entity.
>> **(1)** Suctioning.
>> **(2)** Fluids (PO, IV).
>> **(3)** Drugs.
>
> **B.** Bleeding and shock.
>> **1.** Check carotid pulse. If absent, begin closed chest massage.
>> **2.** Areas of bleeding.
>>> **a.** Control external hemorrhage with sterile compression dressings.
>>> **b.** If wound on extremity, elevate limb.
>> **3.** Vital signs.
>>> **a.** Treat hypovolemic shock:
>>>> **(1)** Fluid replacement.
>>>> **(2)** Start peripheral IV line.
>>>> **(3)** Assist with central venous pressure (CVP) line.
>>>> **(4)** Draw and evaluate ABG, complete blood count (CBC), and hematocrit (Hct) and hemoglobin (Hb).
>>> **b.** Vasopressors, as ordered.
>>> **c.** Insert Foley catheter and/or urinary output.
>>> **d.** Evaluations every hour.

    *C. C*onsciousness.
        1. Level of awareness.
            a. Orientation to time, place, person.
            b. Describe level of consciousness:
                (1) Alert.
                (2) Lethargic.
                (3) Stuporous.
                (4) Comatose.
        2. Pupillary responses: pupils equally reactive to light and accommodation (PEERLA).
        3. Responses to tactile and painful stimuli.
            a. Movement of all extremities appropriately.
            b. Describe any abnormalities:
                (1) Decorticate.
                (2) Decerebrate.
        4. Areas of injury.
            a. Palpate scalp, ears, nose, and face for: lacerations, protrusions, blood, cerebrospinal fluid.
                (1) Apply sterile, loose dressing to wounds.
                (2) Assist with debridement of scalp laceration.
            b. Vital signs every 5 min. Consider change of increased intracranial pressure and/or metabolic disorder.
    *D. D*igestive organs.
        1. Observation for wounds, scars.
            a. Sterile dressing to site of injury.
            b. Sterile saline dressing to obtruding organs.
        2. Areas of tenderness, pain.
            a. Palpate gently tender areas last.
            b. Record the area where pain is felt or radiated to.
        3. Auscultate bowel sounds.
            a. Listen to each quadrant every 2 to 5 min.
            b. Record findings.
        4. Abdominal bleeding.
            a. Assist with peritoneal lavage and/or tap.
            b. Prepare patient for surgery and/or x-ray.
            c. Insert nasogastric tube; check for bleeding; nothing by mouth (NPO).
    *E. E*xcretory organs.
        1. Urinary output.
            a. Insert Foley catheter; evaluate urinary output every 15 min.
            b. Check for hematuria.
            c. Specific gravity every hour.
        2. Renal damage.
            a. With urethral lacerations: no catheterization; prepare for surgery.
            b. Start IV.
            c. Assist with intravenous pyelogram (IVP).
    *F. F*ractures.
        1. Five P's.
            *a. P*ain: Medicate patient, as ordered.
            *b. P*ulses: Check all pulses distal to injury.
            *c. P*aresthesia: Note movement of extremities.
            *d. P*aralysis: Immobilize fractures.
            *e. P*allor: Note color of extremities involved; deformities; swelling; asymmetry.
        2. Vital signs.
            a. Tibial fracture, can lose 2 U blood.
            b. Femur fracture, can lose 4 U blood.
            c. Pelvic fracture, can lose 6 U blood.

BIBLIOGRAPHY

Barry, Jeanie: *Emergency Nursing,* McGraw-Hill Book Company, New York, 1978. This book provides an up-to-date review of emergency nursing and provides an excellent reference for the physiology, pathophysiology, and assessment information relevant to emergency care.

Cook County Hospital Nursing Grand Rounds: "Trauma Care: Expect the Unexpected," *Nursing '76,* **6:**58–63, June 1976. A thorough presentation of the ABCs of trauma management is provided by this article.

Cosgriff, James H., and Diann L. Anderson: *The Practice of Emergency Nursing,* J. B. Lippincott Company, Philadelphia, 1975. One of the first and also one of the most comprehensive presentations of emergency nursing, this book covers all the relevant areas of emergency care, including burns.

Nelson, Doris M.: "Triage in the Emergency Suite," *Hospital Topics,* **32**(6):39–41, September 1973. The role of the emergency department nurse as a triage agent is developed in this article.

Slater, Reda R.: "Triage Nurse in the Emergency Department," *American Journal of Nursing,* **70**(1): 127–129, January 1970. This article is considered a classic in emergency nursing literature as it was probably the first publication to identify the concept of the triage nurse.

Stephenson, Hugh E.: *Immediate Care of the Acutely Ill and Injured,* The C. V. Mosby Company, St. Louis, 1974. Although relatively general in nature, this book presents a comprehensive review of trauma management.

Vayda, Eugene, and Michael Gent: "An Emergency Department Triage Model Based on Presenting Complaints," *Canadian Journal of Public Health,* **64**(3):246–253, May–June 1973. This article presents a physician's system for classification of emergency problems into categories.

Vickeray, Donald M.: *Triage: Problem-Oriented Sorting of Patients,* Robert Brady Company, Bowie, Md., 1975. This book presents the most comprehensive review of triage according to the problem-oriented medical records approach.

MUSCULOSKELETAL AND DENTAL TRAUMA

Fractures

DEFINITION
A *fracture* is a localized area of soft tissue and bone damage attended by secondary harmful effects upon adjacent regional structures and upon the patient as a whole. It usually causes a degree of immobility, and is classified according to the nature of the break, and may be *open* or *closed* (Fig. 44-1).

ASSESSMENT
I. Health history.
   A. Chief complaints concerning symptoms include:
      1. Onset.
      2. Chronology.
      3. Duration.
      4. Aggravation.
      5. Alleviation (if any).
   B. Patient's comments and interpretations, i.e., does it appear to be like any trauma of the patient's past?
   C. Degree of disability related to the complaint (1).
   D. Note type of injury and common resultant fractures.
   E. Did patient fall, receive a direct blow to affected area, have opposing forces on opposite ends of the bone tending to bend or stress it beyond a breaking point, or have a severe twist or tear on bone causing the break?
   F. Note medication allergies, especially analgesics and antibiotics.
II. Physical and behavioral assessment. Note the following:
   A. Deformity (may or may not be present).
   B. Pain, acute tenderness (may or may not be present).
   C. Loss of function and/or weight bearing; unusual mobility of area.
   D. Grating sensation of affected area; rocking of pelvis.
   E. Shortening of broken limb; muscle spasms.
   F. Discoloration and swelling, i.e., pallor, ecchymosis.
   G. Exposed bone.
   H. Injuries to associated structures with tearing and bleeding.
   I. Altered sensation or loss of sensation: e.g., fracture of humerus head or ulna may result in *altered* sensation to digits 4 and 5 or to palmar and dorsal surfaces; fracture of spinal column may result in *loss* of sensation.
   J. Decreased or absent pulses distal to injury; affected extremity colder than contralateral part.
   K. Crepitus.
III. Diagnostic tests.
   A. X-ray.
   B. Complete blood count (CBC), differential. For all multiple fracture cases, hemoglobin (Hb) and hematocrit (Hct).

PROBLEMS

I. Physiologic.
   A. Bruising or tearing of adjacent tissue if not splinted correctly.
   B. Sepsis (i.e., osteomyelitis, septic arthritis).
   C. Shock.
   D. Fat emboli.
   E. Residual impairment (peripheral nerve damage).
   F. Physical immobility: peripheral sensory deprivation.
   G. Possible surgical intervention.
II. Psychosocial.
   A. Altered body image (if immobilization or prosthetic hardware used).
   B. Pain, discomfort.
   C. Disruption of social and economic performance.

FIGURE 44-1 / Types of fractures. (From Jeanie Barry, Emergency Nursing, McGraw-Hill Book Company, New York, 1978.)

TYPE OF FRACTURE	DEFINITION
1. Transverse	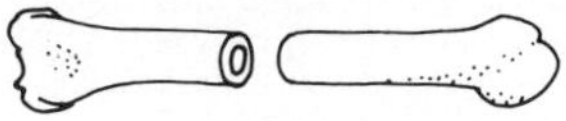 1. Usually produced by angulating force; once the fragments are aligned and immobilized, stability is assured
2. Oblique	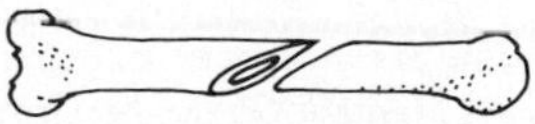 2. Fragments tend to slip by one another unless traction is maintained
3. Spiral	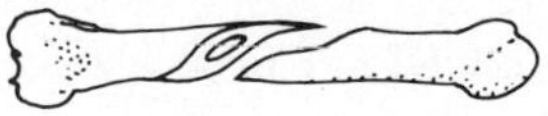 3. Produced by twisting or rotary force; reduction difficult to maintain
4. Greenstick	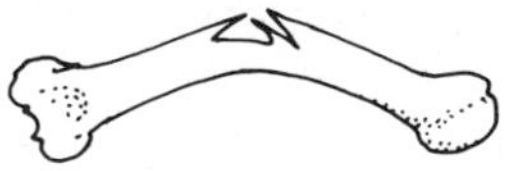 4. Caused by compression force in long axis of the bone; often seen in children under age of ten
5. Compression	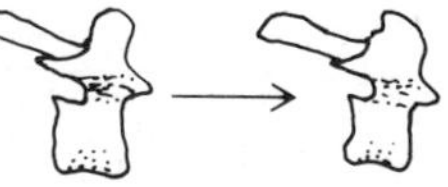 5. Usually produced by severe violence applied to cancellous bone, such as the spine
6. Comminuted	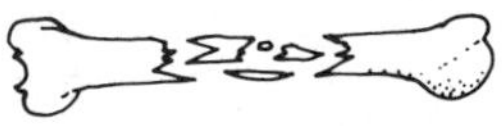 6. Always more than two fragments
7. Impacted	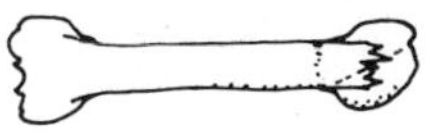 7. Produced by severe violence, driving bone fragments firmly together
8. Avulsion	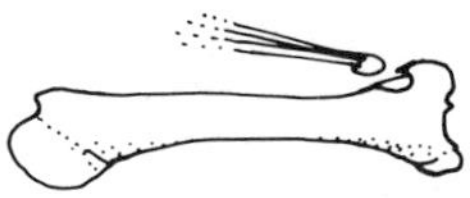 8. Produced by forcible contraction of a muscle which pulls off a fragment of bone
9. Fracture dislocation	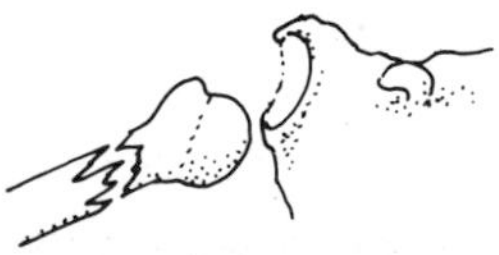 9. In addition to fracture there is a subluxation or dislocation of the joint

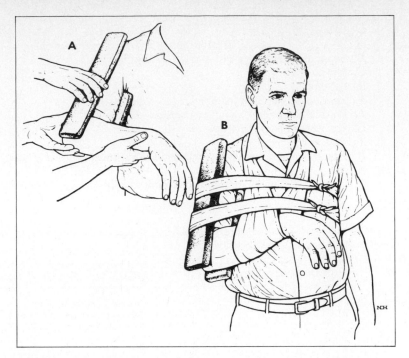

FIGURE 44-2 / Temporary splinting for broken arm, using splints and three cravats. (*From John Henderson, Emergency Medical Guide, McGraw-Hill Book Company, New York, 1978.*)

FIGURE 44-3 / Using a tongue depressor to make a finger splint. (*From John Henderson, Emergency Medical Guide, McGraw-Hill Book Company, New York, 1978.*)

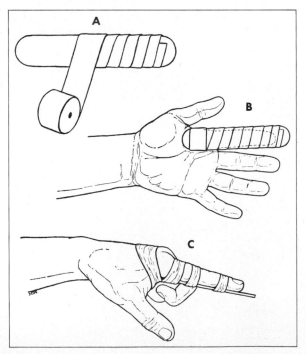

GOALS OF CARE

I. Minimize, prevent shock.
II. Immobilize in anatomical position.
III. Relieve pain.
IV. Decrease complications and further injury.
V. Restore to prefracture functional capacity.
VI. Reduce emotional stress.

INTERVENTION

I. Stop associated open bleeding with pressure or absorbent sterile dressings; estimate blood loss.
II. Remove all materials that may be difficult to remove later or that may cause constriction.
III. Apply manual traction, and realign to anatomical position if possible. (Great care must be taken not to disrupt perivasculature.)
IV. Immobilize with padded splint boards, slings and bandages, air splints, traction splints, i.e., *Thomas* splint, with or without Buck's skin traction (Figs. 44-2 through 44-5).
V. Place cold packs *around* affected area.
VI. Elevate extremity above right heart level.

FIGURE 44-4 / Improvised splinting of a fractured leg. Hold the foot and apply gentle traction while splints are being applied. (*From John Henderson, Emergency Medical Guide, McGraw-Hill Book Company, New York, 1978.*)

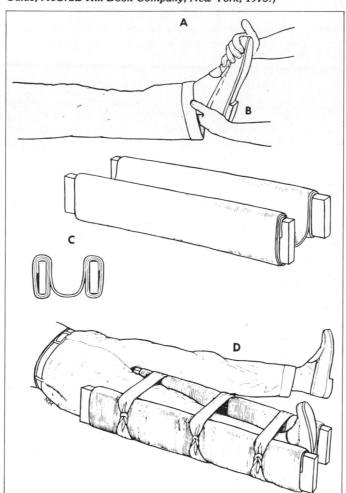

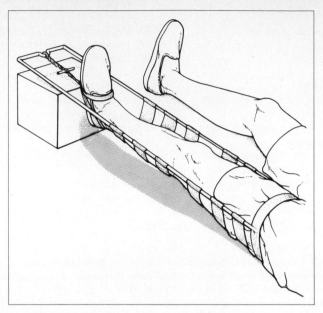

FIGURE 44-5 / Thomas splint applied. (*Adopted from Thomas Flint and Harvey Cain, Emergency Treatment and Management, 5th ed., W. B. Saunders Company, Philadelphia, 1975.*)

VII. Support extremity, and maintain traction during any repositioning.
    A. Log-roll suspected spinal fracture.
    B. Do not flex, extend, or rotate neck on any suspected cervical spine fracture.
VIII. Pad thoroughly all protuberances of joints above and below injury when immobilizing part.
 IX. Monitor extremity circulation, sensation, skin temperature and color, patient remarks about associated pain, bleeding.
  X. Withhold oral intake if surgical intervention planned.
 XI. Monitor fluid resuscitation if victim has multiple fractures.
XII. Keep airway open for all suspected or real facial fractures.

EVALUATION
  I. Decision regarding case disposition.
    A. Home with immobilization, hardware of cast, splint, crutches, sling, etc.
    B. Admit for observation, surgical intervention, further diagnostic studies.
 II. Patient teaching.
    A. Prevention and recognition of common complications.
    B. Care of splinted extremity.
    C. Knowledge of physical limitations on activity.
    D. Cast care.
      1. Keep cast dry.
      2. No autographs for 24 h; cast takes 24 to 28 h to dry.
      3. Symptoms of circulatory impairment should be reported immediately.
      4. Do not paint entire area: could cause clogging of porous material and may prevent air from circulating in the cast.
      5. Return appointment for circulation check the following day.

Maxillo-Facial Trauma

DEFINITION
Any injury to the head and/or face is potentially very serious because of possible damage to the brain or to its circulation.

ASSESSMENT
  I. Mandibular fracture.
    A. Palpate the angle of the mandible, and feel a *step-up* (see Fig. 44-6).
    B. Check for sublingual bleeding.
    C. Check for deformities of occlusion of teeth, i.e., teeth unevenly lined up, some often broken or missing.
  II. Condyle fracture.
    A. Condyle will not be felt with opening and closure of jaw, i.e., it will be pulled forward.
    B. Check for bleeding in the external auditory canal.
    C. Look for laceration of lateral wall of external ear canal.
  III. Anterior mandibular fracture or blunt trauma to face.
    A. Check airway: This fracture will occlude airway unless elevated and sustained (good technique is to use towel clip for pulling mandible out, creating open airway: no need for tracheostomy).
    B. May have open bite: malocclusion.
  IV. Maxillary fracture. Check airway: This fracture occludes airway at postnasal pharynx. Tongue must be pulled out.
  V. Zygomatic bone fracture. Check for the following:
    A. Edema of cheek and lids.
    B. Decreased or dropped prominence of cheek.
    C. Periorbital ecchymosis.
    D. Subconjunctival ecchymosis.

FIGURE 44-6 / Angles of normal and fractured mandibles.

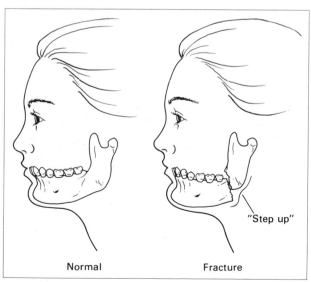

Normal   "Step up"   Fracture

    E. Unilateral epistaxis.
    F. Paresthesia of cheek, upper lip, and gingiva.
    G. Step deformity of inferior orbital margin.
    H. Diplopia and slight ptosis.
    I. Alterations of orbital level, lowering of level of globe of eye.
    J. Tenderness and limited movement.
    K. Ecchymosis of upper buccal sulcus.
    L. Comminution of lateral wall of maxilla.

PROBLEMS

  I. Physiologic.
    A. Establish an airway.   *C.* Residual impairment.
    B. Control hemorrhage into airway.   *D.* Possible surgical intervention.
  II. Psychosocial.
    A. Pain.
    B. Fear of altered body image, permanent scarring.
    C. Emotional stress from disruption of normal activities.
    D. Maintenance of pretrauma activities of daily living, especially adequate nutritional intake, appropriate meal preparation.

GOALS OF CARE

  I. Relieve pain.
  II. Immobilize.
  III. Maintain patent airway.
  IV. Minimize, prevent shock.
  V. Decrease complications and further injury.
  VI. Reduce emotional stress.

INTERVENTION

  I. Stop associated bleeding with pressure, and measure blood loss.
  II. Maintain patent airway; check for signs of respiratory difficulty at regular intervals.
  III. Immobilize with bandages and padding (Fig. 44-7).
  IV. Place cold packs around affected area.
  V. Monitor skin temperature, color, patient remarks about pain, discomfort, and bleeding.

FIGURE 44-7 / Four-tailed bandage for temporarily immobilizing a fractured jaw. *(From John Henderson, Emergency Medical Guide, McGraw-Hill Book Company, New York, 1978.)*

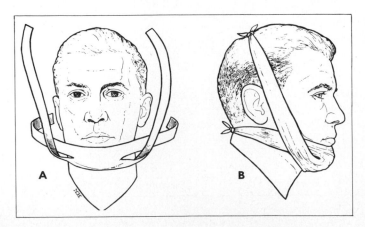

Strains

DEFINITION

A *strain* is an overstretching of a single muscle or group of muscles which results in tearing of the individual fibers or overstretching and rupturing of the related tendon. These injuries are usually due to violent, unexpected movement, i.e., wrenching.

ASSESSMENT

Note the common etiologies of this injury: associated with industrial stresses of improper lifting and carrying of heavy loads; sports (tennis, golf, basketball, squash, racket ball, etc.); vocational (acrobats, dancers, home gardeners).

I. Health history.
II. Onset and duration of injury.
    A. Characterized by sudden slight "pop" or feeling of "tearing" and associated with rigorous activity prior to injury.
    B. In older adults, leg muscle strains may have a forewarning pain a day or two prior to actual injury.
    C. Frequently described as no discomfort initially but excruciating pain with first movement after injury.
III. Physical and behavioral assessment.
    A. Severe, excruciating pain.
    B. Limited mobility (or hypermobility); stiffness.
    C. Swelling, tenderness to touch.
    D. Ecchymosis.
    E. Muscle spasms and fasciculations.
    F. "Drop" or "lag" of part.
IV. Diagnostic tests. X-ray to rule out fracture.

PROBLEM

I. Physiologic.
    A. Inflammation.
    B. Altered physical mobility.
    C. Residual impairment.
    D. Possible surgical intervention.
II. Psychosocial.
    A. Pain.
    B. Disruption of social and economic performance.
    C. Altered body image (if prosthetic hardware used or immobilized).

GOALS OF CARE

I. Reduce pain and muscle spasms.
II. Immobilize affected part.
III. Decrease further injury due to complications.
IV. Restore to prestrain functional capacity.

INTERVENTION

I. Rest the strained part in most comfortable position.
II. Elevate extremity for 2 to 3 days.
III. Immediately treat with cold until hyperemic phase and inflammatory reaction subside (12 to 24 h).
IV. Follow with heat, preferably dry and constant.
V. Give analgesics such as aspirin, dextropropoxyphene, meperidine phenylbutazone.
VI. Give muscle relaxants such as diazepam (Valium) or butazolidine.
VII. Strap injured part with adhesive tape (elastic bandage is a second choice). Start by fastening the first strip around the affected area but not joining ends; apply subsequent

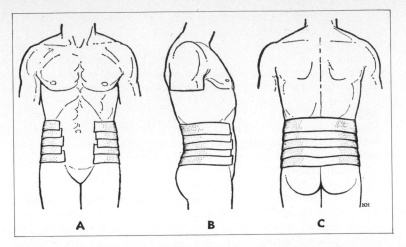

FIGURE 44-8 / Method of providing a firm adhesive tape support for injuries of lower back, particularly useful in treatment of sacroiliac strain. (*From John Henderson, Emergency Medical Guide, McGraw-Hill Book Company, New York, 1978.*)

strips parallel and slightly overlapping the preceding strip (1 to 1½ in). Continue above and below strained area until there is sufficient support. Modify for specific strains (Fig. 44-8).

VIII. Teach non-weight-bearing crutch walking if strain is in lower extremity.

EVALUATION
I. Note persistent pain and limited movement.
II. Observe for blisters resulting from taping.
III. Teach proper body mechanics using printed instructions and demonstration.
IV. Warn about repeated strains (culminating in periostitis, or myositis ossificans).

Sprains

DEFINITION
Sprains are stretching and/or tearing injuries of varying intensity involving the ligaments of a joint or the joint capsule itself. They may be minor or mild with only a small amount of ligamentous and soft tissue damage, and treatment is often not sought for 1 to 2 days after the injury. Severe sprains may be difficult to distinguish from fractures, especially avulsion fractures. This differentiation is important, especially in industrial injuries and public liability cases. A sprain may be severe enough to pull off a bone chip, e.g., some ankle injuries (sprain fracture).

ASSESSMENT
I. Health history.
A. Ascertain event(s) causing injury.
   1. Whiplash frequently accompanies auto accidents, particularly "rear-end" collisions.
   2. Common sports injury of ankle and knee: track, soccer, basketball, football (any running-leaping-twisting-type activity); of shoulder and knee: tennis, soft or hard ball, etc.
   3. Ankle sprains frequently caused by misjudging near-vision obstacles, i.e., steps, curbs, small animals, rugs, resulting in twisting and/or jerking injury.
   4. Accompanying head injuries from skiing mishaps, particularly the more recent

problems of cervical sprains from forcefully landing on a shoulder, and diving miscalculations causing blunt impact to head and neck.
   B. Onset and duration of injury. Not significantly distinguished from fractures and strains.
II. Physical and behavioral assessment.
   A. Severe pain at the site, with and without touch.
   B. Pain upon ambulation or joint movement.
   C. Swelling.
   D. Discoloration: ecchymoses in 1 to 2 days.
   E. Loss of joint function if sprain is severe.
   F. "Stiffness" or "knotted" adjoining musculature.
   G. Suspect fractare.
III. Diagnostic tests. X-ray to rule out fracture.

PROBLEMS
   I. Physiologic.
   A. Altered physical mobility.
   B. Residual weakness or impairment.
   C. Possible surgical intervention.
   II. Psychosocial.
   A. Pain.
   B. Disruption of social and economic performance.
   C. Altered body image (if immobilization or prosthetic hardware employed).

GOALS OF CARE
   I. Minimize swelling and leakage of blood into tissues.
   II. Support articulating structures by suitable immobilization.
   III. Reduce pain.
   IV. Restore joint function to preinjury status.

INTERVENTION
   I. Place sprained part at complete rest: immobilize.
   II. Elevate extremity, if possible.
   III. Use cold packs or ice bags to affected part until swelling subsides: approximately $\frac{1}{2}$ to $1\frac{1}{2}$ days.
   IV. Apply elastic bandage for support and partial immobility; check frequently (Fig. 44-9).
   V. Monitor extremity circulation, discoloration, temperature.
   VI. Tape extremity sprains according to accepted protocol and with extremity in proper anatomical alignment.
   VII. Give analgesics such as aspirin, Empirin, dextropropoxyphene groups.
   VIII. Restrict ambulation until firm strapping is applied and swelling reduced.

EVALUATION
   I. Note persistent pain upon movement of part.
   II. Watch for symptoms of strangulation with use of elastic bandage.

Dislocations

DEFINITION
Dislocation is the persistent slippage of an articulating surface at the joint site. If a ball-and-socket joint is dislocated, the ball is removed from the cup attachment and free-floats. This injury occurs as a result of a sudden twisting force, spastic muscular contraction, sudden impacted or extension force, or blunt fall where transmitted force is directly to the joint. A joint could be continually "stretched" to allow for dislocation of the articulating surface. Continual torque of joint causes "lazy" articulating surfaces.

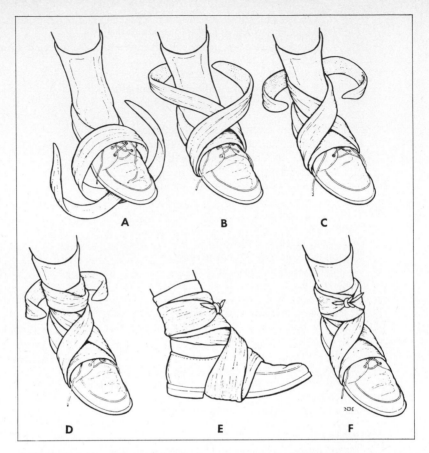

FIGURE 44-9 / Method of applying temporary support to injured ankle by using a figure-eight cravat over a shoe which has been loosened to allow for swelling. (*From John Henderson, Emergency Medical Guide, McGraw-Hill Book Company, New York, 1978.*)

ASSESSMENT

I. Health history.
   A. Obtain a description of the causative force; this helps describe the injury.
   B. Determine how many times dislocation has occurred.
II. Physical and behavioral assessment. Check for the following:
   A. An accompanying fracture of same or adjacent area.
   B. Circulation impairment distal to dislocation.
      1. Pulselessness.
      2. Pallor.
      3. Paralysis.
      4. Pain.
      5. Paresthesia.
   C. Disruption of nerve supply causing altered motor and sensory function.
   D. Muscle spasms and severe pain.
   E. Distortion of anatomical positioning and surface landmarks.
   F. Most comfortable position of affected part; usually patient prefers dislocated part "hanging" down or free.
   G. Swelling of surrounding tissue.
III. Diagnostic tests. X-ray before any attempt to reduce dislocation.

PROBLEMS

I. Physiologic.
    A. Unstable joint: residual impairment.
    B. Local circulatory compromise.
    C. Physical immobility.
II. Psychosocial.
    A. Pain.
    B. Temporary body image alteration.

GOALS OF CARE

I. Restore joint to appropriate anatomical position and physiologic function.
II. Relieve pain.
III. Reduce complications and residual damage.

INTERVENTION

Principles of reduction procedures.
    I. Grasp or hold dislocated part firmly.
    II. Apply pressure, traction until joint slips into proper position.
    III. For mandible: thumbs inside mouth, pressed downward with fingers on chin, lifting upward (Fig. 44-10).
    IV. For shoulder: with patient supine on floor, abduct arm approximately 70°, place bared foot against patient's lateral chest and pull arm until it lengthens.
    V. Immobilize reduced joint by sling, Valpcan dressing, tape, or chin strap, as appropriate.
    VI. Provide analgesics, i.e., aspirin and muscle relaxants as necessary for spasms.
    VII. Withhold oral intake if open reduction or difficult closed reduction anticipated.
    VIII. Teach patient to limit movements of torque, twist, hyperflexion, hyperextension, hyperabduction, and hyperadduction, as appropriate.

FIGURE 44-10 / Method of reducing a dislocation of the jaw by pressing downward and backward with padded thumbs. (*From John Henderson, Emergency Medical Guide, McGraw-Hill Book Company, New York, 1978.*)

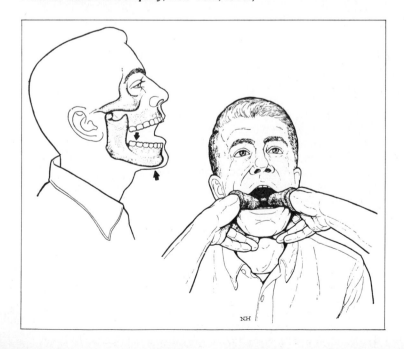

EVALUATION
I. Observe for relief of severe pain and discomfort.
II. Institute teaching regarding:
  A. Body mechanics.
  B. Accident prevention in home, business.
  C. Participation in activities of daily living with present problem.
III. Presurgery instruction, if indicated.

Subluxation

DEFINITION
Subluxation is a partial dislocation of a joint with resultant adjacent structural damage, usually caused by a sudden jerk distal to affected part. Occasional strong, constant pull on young or weakened extremity can cause same partial dislocation. It is usually a pathology of toddlers who are "lifted by hands," small children playing ball or swinging on gym bars, or older adults during square dancing maneuvers.

ASSESSMENT
I. Health history.
  A. Obtain description of physical force leading to symptoms.
  B. Note time interval when use of affected extremity was stopped.
  C. Note aggravation, alleviation of symptoms, if any.
II. Physical and behavioral assessment.
  A. Patient may treat extremity as "paralyzed," i.e., immobility of affected limb.
  B. Patient may complain of mild to severe discomfort.
  C. Note any of the following:
    1. Impairment of circulation and nerve supply.
    2. Swelling if extremity is "hanging dependent."
    3. Discoloration from impaired venous return.
    4. Distortion of anatomical position and alignment, e.g., if radial head, usually slightly flexed and pronated.
    5. Bulges, creases, "dimples," etc., on surface of affected part.
    6. Paresthesia.
III. Diagnostic tests. None; x-ray not helpful.

PROBLEM
I. Physiologic. Reduction in physical mobility.
II. Psychosocial. Pain.

GOALS OF CARE
I. Reduce swelling of affected joint.
II. Restore joint to full mobility.
III. Reduce pain, discomfort.
IV. Provide reassurance to patient and family.
V. Prevention of future occurrences through family-centered teaching; most common subluxations occur in children 1 to 4 years of age; problem often occurs as child is being "pulled along by wrist" (2).

INTERVENTION
I. Gentle traction. If radial head is partially dislocated, gently supinate and flex elbow.
II. Local or general anesthesia for more difficult reductions.
III. Allow joint to rest 12 to 24 h by using sling or appropriate bandage (Fig. 44-11).
IV. Encourage use of extremity as soon as pain subsides.
V. Provide patient teaching regarding careful "pulling" or "swinging" of younger child or geriatric person who may be a dancer, etc.

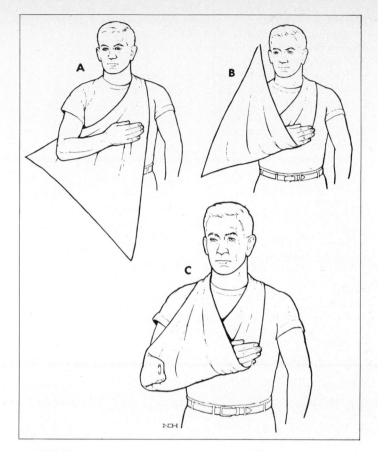

FIGURE 44-11 / Using a triangular bandage as a comfortable arm sling. (*From John Henderson, Emergency Medical Guide, McGraw-Hill Book Company, New York, 1978.*)

EVALUATION
I. Is full mobility restored?
II. Is there relief of pain?
III. Is there patient and family understanding of origin of trauma and consequences.

Dental Caries, Fractures, Traumatic or Planned Removal of Teeth

DEFINITION
Emergency concerns of the dental skeleton include pain, traumatic fractures and avulsions, and infections. Toothache may be the result of injuries, disease, or extraction.

ASSESSMENT
I. Health history. Ascertain the following:
  A. History of bleeding.
  B. Description of onset or event which caused patient to seek dental care.
  C. Regular dental caretaker, i.e., dentist, dental hygienist.
  D. Medication allergies.
  E. History of anticoagulant therapy; medications and aspirin ingestion (acetylsalicylic acid).

  F. History of medications with anticoagulant effects, i.e., steroids, muscle relaxants of the butazolidine family, etc.
II. Physical and behavioral assessment.
  A. Swelling, induration.
  B. Redness due to erythema or other discolorations.
  C. Disruption of tooth structure, alveolar ridge, or soft tissue.
  D. Hemorrhage.
  E. Distortion of facial contour.
  F. Difficulty in mastication.
  G. Speech impediment.
  H. Pain localized or general over face and head; usually sensitive to percussion.
  I. Sensitivity to heat and cold.
  J. Malodorous mouth.
  K. Febrile.
  L. Symptoms of dehydration (possible).
III. Diagnostic tests.
  A. X-ray.
  B. Dental consultants.

PROBLEMS
I. Physiologic.
  A. Feeding problem with subsequent weight loss.
  B. Choking due to possible airway obstruction.
  C. Pain.
  D. Dental extractions and complications.
  E. Sepsis.
  F. Blood loss.
II. Psychosocial.
  A. Pain.
  B. Facial, body image alteration.
  C. Fear of dental intervention.

GOALS OF CARE
I. Reduce or remove pain, discomfort.
II. Restore function of mastication, food ingestion.
III. Restore facial appearance as much like preinsult status as possible.

INTERVENTION
I. For toothache:
  A. Provide analgesic, i.e., aspirin, 0.6 g, with codeine, 30 to 60 mg, according to approved protocol. New drugs: Epiricaine or Marcaine.
  B. Apply oil of cloves or local anesthesia by ointment or viscous solution.
  C. Pack extraction site with paste of cloves and zinc oxide.
  D. Schedule for or instruct patient to seek dentist regularly. Obtain immediate dental consultation if pulp pain, pressure.
II. For trauma:
  A. Inspect mouth carefully, and remove all avulsed teeth.
  B. Hold avulsed teeth in normal saline for eventual replant.
  C. Replant partially avulsed teeth carefully, and immobilize jaw.
  D. Have patient consume soft and liquid foods until teeth firmly replanted.
  E. Provide analgesics as necessary.
  F. Teach patient not to suck, use straw, or create negative pressure in mouth.
  G. Instruct patient on careful mouth rinses after meals.
  H. Tannic acid application to bleeding extraction site or tears in gum (tea bag); this will help coagulation to occur.

I. Use a cavity varnish (Mizzy) for injuries or fractures to tooth enamel only.

J. For injuries to enamel and dentivelike chipped teeth first use calcium hydroxide compound (Dycal) and then coat with cavity varnish several times. It reduces pain and buys about 24 h of time for the tooth.

III. For abscess:

    A. Reduce acute symptoms through drainage.

    B. Administer antibiotics (usually penicillin, 250 mg qid for 7 days).

    C. Instruct patient in:

        1. Hot saline holds to localize infection.

        2. Careful mouth rinses after each meal and frequently during day.

IV. For surgical or traumatic extraction:

    A. Control bleeding by rolled gauze held firmly by clamped jaw for 30 min to 3 h.

    B. Estimate blood loss.

    C. Monitor vital signs, fluid intake and output, blood pressure.

EVALUATION

I. Evaluate relief of pain, discomfort.

II. Provide follow-up with dental personnel, or encourage patient to seek own dental care.

III. Assess patient understanding of teaching of at-home procedures regarding dental hygiene, symptoms of infection, food preparation.

ENVIRONMENTAL EXPOSURE TRAUMA

Heat Stroke

DEFINITION

Heat stroke (siriasis, sunstroke, heat hyperpyrexia) is the failure or inability to eliminate body heat due to malfunction of the sweating mechanism. It has been known to occur more frequently during July and August "dog days," when the dog star Sirius accompanies the rising of the sun: hence, siriasis. It occurs more commonly in males, elderly people, and alcohol addicts. Contributing factors also include physical exertion and high humidity. Iatrogenic causes include hospitalized patients, para-, hemi-, and quadriplegics with impaired perspiration mechanism; patients who are on medications which inhibit sweating, i.e., atropine and the phenothiazines; psychiatric patients whose behavior may camouflage signs and symptoms of impending heat stroke; surgical patients draped and under anesthesia.

ASSESSMENT

  I. Health history.

    A. Did victim collapse?

    B. Was victim found unconscious?

    C. Was victim working in extremely hot, often humid climate?

    D. Did victim's skin immediately feel abnormally hot?

  II. Physical and behavioral assessment.

    A. Hot, dry, ruddy color of skin (early).

    B. Pale to grey skin, during circulatory collapse (late).

    C. Tachycardia: full, bounding pulse (early).

    D. Bradycardia: weak, thready pulse (late).

    E. Hyperpyrexia, i.e., between 105 and 112°F or beyond 39°C.

    F. Deep, slow respirations progressing to Cheyne-Stokes pattern.

    G. Dilated pupils (usually).

    H. Malodorous body.

    I. Muscle twitching and epileptiform convulsions (early).

    J. Rise in blood pressure (early), with drop during circulatory collapse.

  III. Diagnostic tests. Body temperature measurements if fever exceeds standard thermometers.

PROBLEMS

I. Physiologic.
   A. Intravascular fluid deficit.
   B. Convulsions.
   C. Electrolyte imbalance.
   D. Set hyperpyrexia.
   E. Circulatory collapse.
   F. Permanent damage to various organs due to proteolytic changes.
   G. Rapid loss of consciousness.
II. Psychosocial.
   A. Loss of consciousness.
   B. Early, minimal pain.

GOALS OF CARE

I. Rapid restoration of body temperature to normal range.
II. Reduce residual damage to major organs.
III. Restore patient to conscious and oriented state.

INTERVENTION

I. Rapidly reduce body temperature by cold baths, ice compresses, chilled or iced saline enemas, hypothermia blankets.
II. If temperature drops to 102°F, wrap in wet, cold sheets and expose patient to forced draft (convection, evaporation).
III. Check body temperature frequently.
IV. Provide oxygen using positive pressure mask, or if inadequate ventilations present, by intubation and volumetric respirator.
V. Implement passive range-of-motion to extremities to circulate cooled blood to deeper structures.
VI. Administer cautious sedation for convulsions.
VII. Protect patient from injury during convulsions.
VIII. Judiciously use cardiac and respiratory stimulants.
IX. If known cardiac patient, place in low, semireclining position until evaluated by physician.
X. Continually monitor vital and neurologic checks throughout hospitalization.

EVALUATION

I. Prognosis guarded with 50 percent mortality in treated cases.
II. Residual mental impairment in many of the survivors.
III. Recovery based on early, rapid body temperature reduction.
IV. Convalescence slow and carefully monitored.
V. Residual unstable set and care temperatures.

Heat Exhaustion

DEFINITION

Heat exhaustion (heat prostration) is a sudden shift of blood from circulating volume to skin in an attempt to cool the body when usual mechanisms of sweating are inadequate. Condition triggered in those people: who are not accustomed to hot weather, who perspire excessively, and in women more than in men. Heat exhaustion is the result of peripheral vasomotor collapse and is less serious than heat stroke.

ASSESSMENT

I. Health history.
   A. Associated with sporadic gardeners.
   B. May resemble ordinary fainting.
   C. Note type of working quarters if industrial case.

II. Physical and behavioral assessment. Usually the patient exhibits the following symptoms:
   A. Cool or cold, moist skin.
   B. Fatigue, lassitude.
   C. Initially, fainting briefly and recurrently.
   D. Body temperature normal or subnormal (or slightly elevated).
   E. Hypotension.
   F. Tachycardia, weak, thready pulse.
   G. Nausea, vomiting.
   H. Dilated pupils (possible).
   I. Slow capillary refill times as noted by fingernail pressures.
   J. Postural blood pressure drop.
III. Diagnostic studies.
   A. None, usually.
   B. Hb, Hct if low count suspected.

PROBLEMS
I. Physiologic.
   A. Pending circulatory collapse.
   B. Dehydration from sweating, vomiting, hyponatremia.
II. Psychosocial.
   A. Headache (early).
   B. Loss of consciousness.

GOALS OF CARE
I. Reestablish normal circulating volume and distribution.
II. Assist the body in cooling as quickly and efficiently as possible.
III. Monitor vital signs, state of orientation, level of consciousness.
IV. Institute teaching for prevention of future occurrences.
V. Provide emotional reassurance.

INTERVENTION
I. Remove victim to cool and less humid environment.
II. Place patient in supine position with keees bent and feet elevated.
III. Cool body with moist, cool compresses to forehead, extremities.
IV. If patient able to swallow, give coffee; salty solutions such as soups, bouillon; sweet drinks.
V. If patient unable to take oral fluids, administer IV saline and monitor for fluid acceptance, i.e., excessive and rapid blood pressure changes, rales, neck vein distension.
VI. Use aromatic spirits of ammonia if victim does not respond rapidly.
VII. As patient recovers, do not allow him or her to sit up until compensatory mechanisms can stabilize.

EVALUATION
I. Rarely fatal condition, if treated.
II. Usually patient not hospitalized, unless case is not responsive to rest or oral fluid resuscitation, or unless victim has additional underlying pathology.

Heat Cramps

DEFINITION
Heat cramps (muscle spasms, charley horses) are sudden, painful muscle tightening due to the combination of prolonged exposure to high environmental temperatures, excessive sweating, large oral intake of water, and hence, vast body salt loss. It is a common condition

among heavy industry laborers and can also occur with people at home who engage in excessive physical work during hot weather. It is occasionally seen in heavy, active sports players.

ASSESSMENT
I. Health history.
   A. Patient describes oral intake as excessive and comprised of "free-water" liquids.
   B. Patient offers history of preceding strenuous activity (games, sports) or work.
   C. Patient describes pain as cramping, gripping, prolonged, charley horses in legs and abdomen unrelieved by stopping activity.
II. Physical and behavioral assessment.
   A. Pale, moist skin.
   B. Extreme thirst.
   C. Faintness to loss of consciousness.
   D. Normal or slightly elevated body temperature.
   E. Nausea.
   F. Tachycardia: strong, full pulse.
   G. Severe muscle cramping with palpable gastrocnemius tightening (lumping).
   H. Generalized muscle twitching (possible).
   I. Saline deficit as noted by postural blood pressure drop.
III. Diagnostic studies.
   A. Serum sodium concentration low (<140 meq/L).
   B. Urine specific gravity low (1.001 to 1.010).
   C. Serum chlorides low (<96 meq/L).

PROBLEMS
I. Physiologic.
   A. Electrolyte imbalance (saline deficit).
   B. Free-water excess.
   C. Uncontrolled muscle action, twitching.
II. Psychosocial.
   A. Pain and cramping.
   B. Work loss; associated industrial claims.

GOALS OF CARE
I. Restore fluid and electrolyte balances.
II. Eliminate pain and cramping.
III. Reduce recurrent attacks.

INTERVENTION
I. Administer salt solutions such as soups or bouillon, as nausea tolerates.
II. Reduce free-water intake in deference to saline solutions.
III. Infuse saline as circulation tolerates.
IV. Administer enteric-coated instead of plain salt tablets, to avoid nausea in some individuals.
V. Provide rest for patient in a cool environment.
VI. *Note:* Oral hypotonic salt solution may be homemade by 1 tsp table salt and $\frac{1}{2}$ tsp baking soda in 1 qt of water.
VII. Teach patient causative factors in condition and future prevention.

EVALUATION
I. Rarely need hospitalization. Assess effects of saline intake and rest on victim for relief of symptoms. Prognosis excellent.
II. Evaluate patient understanding of condition and long-term preventive measures, i.e., decrease exposure to high temperature with frequent rest periods; decrease copious fluid intake.

Hypothermia

Local Reactions: Frostbite, Chilblain, Trench Foot

DEFINITION

Frostbite, chilblain, and *trench foot* are reactions to intense cold by limited or altered blood supply and vascular change. Arteriolar vasoconstriction causes peripheral tissue anoxia, hypothermia, and eventual freezing. Upon thawing the tissue becomes hyperemic (commonly known as *flare*), and this is accompanied by intravascular fluid loss to surrounding interstitial spaces (i.e., edema). (Appears as a weal and flare response, probably due to local release of tissue histamine.) In severe cases, the thawing appears in phases with the hyperemia and interstitial edema followed quickly with a slowing of circulation due to the tissue swelling. This causes dilated vessels which become engaged with masses of erythrocytes (RBC). These may be broken up by gentle manipulation early in this phase. Later, total occlusion by thrombi occurs in arterioles.

Individuals most at risk are the elderly, very young, people with darkly pigmented skin, those having experienced previous trauma (especially cold injuries), those in previously poor physical condition, high-altitude climbers who become anoxic, hunters, those who are nervous or sweat profusely, alcoholics, and anyone with prolonged exposure to very cold weather. Occasionally, frostbite occurs in winter sports enthusiasts and with factors that cause poor tissue perfusion, i.e., arteriosclerosis, smoking, tight clothing. This injury occurs most commonly during blizzards, extreme cold, damp, and high wind-chill factor weather, and prolonged subzero temperatures. Involved tissue temperature is less than $-5.5°C$ (22°F).

ASSESSMENT

I. Health history. Patient or witnesses should provide:
   A. Description of cold exposure to determine extent of injury, including temperature plus wind-chill factor (Fig. 44-12).
   B. Description of rewarming measures employed prior to seeking medical care.
   C. History of previous cold injuries and recovery.
   D. History of smoking, if any.
   E. Past medical history for tissue perfusion abnormalities and general health.
   F. Drug history.
II. Physical and behavioral assessment.
   A. Tingling and numbness of digit and/or extremity (early).
   B. Extreme pain with or without external pressure applied.
   C. Violet, deep red hue on digits, extremities. (If untreated, digits progressively deteriorate to white, blanched appearance.)
   D. Loss of all sensation in untreated, affected tissue.
   E. During thawing, hyperemia and tissue edema in affected tissue.
   F. Visible arteriolar RBC clumping as noted by deep, red blotching over skin surface (may occur during thawing).
   G. Extreme, sharp pain in affected area during rewarming (may occur).
   H. *Note* possible clinical complications:
      1. Thrombi with infarction of affected tissue.
      2. Release of thrombi (venous) during rewarming, which become systemic risks.
   I. Development of gangrene, with eventual extended loss of function (in some cases).
III. Diagnostic tests. Arteriography: rare, and of questionable value (to ascertain extent of ischemic disease).

PROBLEMS

I. Physiologic.
   A. Circulatory disruption of exposed tissue.
   B. Complications of peripheral infarction.
   C. Loss of sensation in affected body parts.

Estimated wind speed mi/h	Actual thermometer reading, °F											
	50	40	30	20	10	0	-10	-20	-30	-40	-50	-60
	Equivalent temperature, °F											
Calm	50	40	30	20	10	0	-10	-20	-30	-40	-50	-60
5	48	37	27	16	6	-5	-15	-26	-36	-47	-57	-68
10	40	28	16	4	-9	-24	-33	-46	-58	-70	-83	-95
15	36	22	9	-5	-18	-32	-45	-58	-72	-85	-99	-112
20	32	18	4	-10	-25	-39	-53	-67	-82	-96	-110	-124
25	30	16	0	-15	-29	-44	-59	-74	-88	-104	-119	-133
30	28	13	-2	-18	-33	-48	-63	-79	-94	-109	-125	-140
35	27	11	-4	-20	-35	-51	-67	-82	-98	-113	-129	-145
40	26	10	-6	-21	-37	-53	-69	-85	-100	-116	-132	-148

(Wind speeds greater than 40 mi/h have little additional effect.)	LITTLE DANGER (for properly clothed person.) Maximum danger of false sense of security.	INCREASING DANGER Danger from freezing of exposed flesh.	GREAT DANGER

Trenchfoot and immersion foot may occur at any point on this chart.

FIGURE 44-12 / Wind-chill factor chart. (*Adapted from A. S. Earle et al., Patient Care Magazine, Copyright © 1972, Patient Care Publications, Inc., Darien, Conn. All rights reserved.*)

II. Psychosocial.
   A. Extreme pain initially and during rewarming.
   B. Loss of affected tissue sensation, i.e., sensory deprivation.
   C. Body image changes if affected tissue amputated.

GOALS OF CARE
I. Reestablish tissue perfusion, rapidly.
II. Minimize residual damage.
III. Restore total function of affected part(s).
IV. Reduce pain, discomfort.

INTERVENTION
I. Place patient in recumbent position with head of bed comfortably raised.
II. Rapidly rewarm the injured area with *moist* heat. Keep solution between 36.7 and 39°C (98 and 104°F). *Never use dry heat.*
III. Cleanse injured area carefully, and separate digits with gauze.
IV. Administer analgesics appropriately for pain: may use morphine sulfate in titrated doses IV; codeine sulfate 0.06 g, meperidine hydrochloride, 50 to 100 mg orally, or other less potent oral analgesics.
V. Protect affected tissue from further injury by using cradles for bed covers, frequent repositioning, and *no* injections into this area, etc.
VI. Administer tetanus prophylaxis; for boosters, give tetanus toxoid, 0.5 mL, or human tetanus immunoglobulin (TIG), if not vaccinated previously.
VII. May administer prophylactic antibiotics if frostbite is extensive.
VIII. Remove smoking materials from patient, and discourage this activity during hospitalization and follow-up.
IX. Keep patient warm systemically by encouraging ingestion of hot, stimulating liquids, especially coffee.
X. Do not allow weight bearing or pressure on injured parts.

XI. Provide teaching regarding care of injured areas for any future cold exposure, i.e., thermal boots and gloves; keep extremities dry, use down and waterproof external wear, etc., for protection of nose and ear lobe tips, etc.

EVALUATION

I. Possible use of low molecular weight Dextran, doses of 1 g/kg per day for tissue protection (1000 mL 6% Dextran on day of injury with 500 mL given every day for 5 days).

II. Evaluate level of patient understanding regarding teaching of care of injuries and future prevention.

III. Surgical amputation is usually withheld until line of demarcation is clear between viable and nonviable tissue.

Systemic Reaction

DEFINITION

A *systemic reaction* is caused by chilling of the whole body from therapeutic procedures, i.e., surgery and some treatment for certain poisonings, or from exposure to incremental weather. If left untreated, it progressively slows the physiologic processes, leading to death. Certain factors predict survival from this injury: length of time exposed; the innate tolerance to cold that some people have; environmental influences of altitude, barometric pressure, and humidity; the person's general physical condition, including nutritional status, previous or chronic disease(s). This condition occurs most frequently in mountain climbers who become lost or trapped without shelter, persons who have prolonged exposure in water, industrial workers in walk-in refrigerator-freezer units. Patients with core temperatures of 23.3°C (74°F) have been reported.

ASSESSMENT

I. Health history.
A. Description of exposure, including time interval and type of weather.
B. Past medical history for underlying and/or chronic disease and medication therapy.
C. Type of employment (if applicable).
D. Type of outer wear worn during insult.

II. Physical and behavioral assessment.
A. Progressive chilling.
B. Intense shivering.
C. Apathy.
D. Deterioration to unconsciousness.
E. Bradycardia.
F. Hypopnea.
G. Progressive freezing of extremities towards body.
H. Cardiac arrhythmias: at approximately 86 to 88°F, ventricular fibrillation occurs; at 82 to 86°F, asystole occurs.

PROBLEMS

I. Physiologic.
A. Cardiac arrhythmias.
B. Lowered metabolic rate.
C. Impaired renal function.

II. Psychosocial.
A. Altered level of consciousness.
B. Pain and general discomfort.

GOALS OF CARE

I. Rewarm body to normal temperature range.
II. Restore metabolic functions to preinjury state.
III. Reduce residual effects and complications.

INTERVENTION

I. Rapidly rewarm with blankets, others' body heat, hot oral liquids if victim in early stages of chilling.

II. Rewarm vigorously and rapidly, if victim's body temperature near lethal limit.

III. If body temperature is near lethal limit, carefully and with frequent monitoring apply electric blankets, warm saline enemas, hot oral liquids (if patient can swallow), warm gastric lavage, any heating device to increase room temperature, covered hot water bottles, bricks, etc.

IV. Insert Foley bladder catheter to monitor kidney function.

V. Record hourly urine output.

VI. Monitor urine pH and specific gravity.

VII. If ventilation is inadequate, establish airway and ventilation with positive pressure bag, or intubate and place on volumetric respirator.

VIII. Provide oxygen therapy to maintain arterial blood gases within normal limits (corrected for hypothermic state).

IX. Place on cardiac monitor, and observe for arrhythmias.

X. If frequent ventricular ectopy occurs, treat with Lidocaine, 50- to 100-mg bolus, then IV drip of 1 to 4 mg/min.

XI. If ventricular fibrillation occurs, treat with direct current countershock (defibrillation) and IV Lidocaine at 1 to 4 mg/min.

XII. If asystole occurs, begin cardiopulmonary resuscitation, and be ready with IV (most common) calcium chloride, 2.5 to 5.0 mL of a 10% solution (3.4 to 6.8 meq; 250 to 500 mg); calcium gluceptate, 5 mL (4.5 meq); or calcium gluconate, 10 mL of a 10% solution (4.8 meq) and IV or intracardiac epinephrine at 0.5 mg (5 mL of a 1: 10,000 solution; may repeat every 5 min).

XIII. Do not permit smoking.

EVALUATION

Patients with core temperatures of 23.3°C (74°F) have been reported.

I. *Watch for mass effects:* There are usually unpredictable medication results until patient is completely rewarmed.

II. Recheck all organ systems for ischemic damage.

III. Continue to monitor vital signs, fluid intake and output, level of consciousness, and orientation.

IV. Provide continued emotional reassurances to patient, family, and friends.

Hymenoptera and Selected Reptile Bites

DEFINITION

Insect bites involve piercing of tissue with the insect's stinger and release of venom (toxic, foreign protein antigen). The stinger may hook into the skin much like a fish hook so that it is left after the insect is brushed or flies off. The venom sac continues contracting approximately 1 to 3 min, thereby injecting additional venom. Other *Hymenoptera* leave the victim with stinger intact ready to strike again.

The principal aculeate hymenopterons are divided into four superfamilies: *Sphecoiden,* digger wasps; *Vespoidea,* true wasps; *Apoidea,* bees; and *Formicoidea,* ants. Females of all these species have an egg-laying organ (stinger) which can be used for defense or offense.

The venom of bees, hornets, wasps, and yellow jackets contains *four to six distinct chemical compounds,* each of which can provoke an allergic reaction. The exception, bumble bees, have venom more closely related to the other members of the order *Hymenoptera* (3). The venoms of all stinging hymenopterons are closely related so as to be cross-sensitizing. Of the general population, 20 percent are allergic to bee stings.

Species that live in hives are more aggressive than the solitary kind, e.g., yellow jackets which attack without provocation and hornets which are extremely protective of nests, and are especially ferocious when a person unwittingly steps on or disturbs their domain.

Most important *spider bites* are caused by the black widow and the brown recluse. These species are found everywhere in the United States except Alaska. *Scorpion bites* are common to the southwestern United States and are of two kinds: lethal and nonlethal.

Snake bites: Lethal bites are caused by pit vipers and coral snakes. Pit vipers include rattlesnakes, moccasins, cottonmouths, and copperheads. People at risk are those who work or spend much time in the less populated out-of-doors.

ASSESSMENT

I. Health history.
   A. Describe causative insect or reptile and whether envenomization has occurred (0 = no venom and 4 = very severe).
   B. Note time of incident and ensuing symptoms.
   C. Obtain past medical and drug history, especially if patient is hypertensive or diabetic or has peripheral vascular disease. There is an enhanced absorption of venom in hypertensives, a development of hypoglycemia in diabetics, and an inhibition of venom absorption in peripheral vascular disease.
   D. Specifically, obtain a past allergy history and record *all* previous antigenic agents.
   E. Note all care and medications rendered prior to hospital admission.
   F. Note if patient is at risk for tetanus.

II. Physical and behavioral assessment.
   A. Look for signs of anaphylactic reactions or angioneurotic edema.
   B. Check pulmonary functioning: may have acute cessation of ventilation.
   C. Observe for circulatory collapse, neurovasogenic type.
   D. Assess pain and itching.
   E. Note local enduration, hyperemia, erythema.
   F. *Black widow bite.* On lower extremity, symptoms are extreme pain and rigidity of abdomen; on upper extremity, pain and rigidity in chest, back, and shoulders. Patient develops fever, elevated blood pressure, leukocytosis, albuminuria, hematuria, stupor, and convulsions. The venom is neurotoxic, causing ascending motor paralysis and peripheral nerve ending destruction (4).
   G. *Brown recluse bite. Local symptoms* may not develop for 2 to 8 h after bite; area is red, painful, develops blisters and blebs surrounded by ischemia. After several days, center turns dark; after 14 days it becomes depressed, demarcated, and mummified going to a large open ulcer. *Systemic symptoms* include fever, chills, malaise, weakness, nausea and vomiting, joint pain, petechial rash, hemolysis, and thrombocytopenia (5).
   H. *Bite of pit viper. Local reactions* include intense, burning pain, swelling and copious bleeding with two puncture wounds above and below, blisters and blebs developing within 1 h, becoming extremely large and hemorrhagic. *Systemic reactions* due to general circulation absorption and the anticoagulation effects of venom, i.e., muscle fasciculations and twitching frequently around mouth, gastrointestinal bleeding, nausea, vomiting, diaphoresis, tachycardia, hypotension, syncope and coma, shallow hypopnea leading to respiratory arrest (6).
   I. *Scorpion bites. Nonlethal* bites have local swelling, pain, and occasional anaphylaxis. *Lethal* bites have *no* local effects visible; pain, hyperesthesia followed by hypoesthesia, numbness, and drowsiness; itching of nose, mouth, and throat; slurred speech, muscle spasm, generalized pain, vomiting, incontinence, and seizures. May have respiratory and circulatory collapse. Symptoms last 24 to 48 h.
   J. *Bee, hornet, wasp stings. Local reactions* include pinprick sensation, redness and wheal, local pain, itching and swelling. *Toxic reactions* include: vomiting, diarrhea, faintness, unconsciousness, edema, headache, fever, muscle spasms, and rarely seizures (see "Anaphylaxis" in Chap. 32). *Delayed reactions,* called "serum sickness," are characterized by rash, urticaria, lymphadenopathy, myalgia, arthralgia, and fever. *Unusual reactions:* nephrotic syndrome, bites around eyes may cause iris atrophy, cataracts, glaucoma, and perforation of globe.

III. Diagnostic tests.
   A. CBC, differential, coagulation screen, electrolytes, blood urea nitrogen (BUN), and blood sugar.
   B. Urinalysis.
   C. Type and cross-match blood.

PROBLEMS
I. Physiologic.
  A. Respiratory and circulatory compromise.
  B. Massive fluid shifts with resultant trapping.
  C. Anticoagulation.
  D. Elevated body temperatur g)fever).
  E. Disruption of gastric and bowel functions.
  F. Local and generalized toxic reactions.
  G. Tissue necrosis.
  H. Sensory and motor impairment.
II. Psychosocial.
  A. Pain and general discomfort.
  B. Loss of consciousness.
  C. Part or entire body disfigurement, depending on severity of bite and treatment administered.
  D. Social and financial immobilization depending on extent of bite, general symptoms, duration and course of therapy.
  E. Intense fear of insects, snakes, and scorpions.

GOALS OF CARE
  I. Neutralize or deactivate toxic substance locally and systemically.
  II. Maintain ventilations for adequate gas exchange.
  III. Reestablish a perfusing circulation.
  IV. Reduce pain, discomfort, and swelling.
  V. Return to physical mobility.
  VI. Reduce complications of hemorrhage, anticoagulation, and sepsis.
  VII. Protect patient from additional injuries, if unconscious.
  VIII. Provide emotional support for fear generated from incident.

INTERVENTION
  I. Maintain adequate airway and ventilation; provide oxygen by mask.
  II. Immediately reduce systemic absorption of venom by ice packs or cold compresses to site, reduction of activity, and placing victim at rest. Place tourniquet above bite (if on extremity); suck with syringe (without needle), *not mouth* if possible, and remove venom.
  III. Wash site with water to remove additional venom.
  IV. Carefully scrape stingers with surgical blade or razor blade until removed. *Do not* pinch, as retained venom sacs discharge residual venom.
  V. *Excise* carefully over bite area, and apply suction to remove venom.
  VI. Provide analgesics, but *not* morphine, unless prepared to support ventilations.
  VII. Fluid resuscitate with buffered isotonic solution, i.e., Ringer's, to maintain systolic blood pressure at 90 mmHg.
  VIII. Provide antivenom, if available, according to package insert recommendations.
  IX. Administer epinephrine sulfate, 0.2 to 1 mL of a 1:1000 solution, either SC or IM, preferably fastest route possible in acute reactions.
  X. Administer IV or IM antihistamines, i.e., chlorpheniramine, 10 mg IV, or 100 mg IM if symptoms persist or increase.
  XI. Administer IV corticosteroid, i.e., 100 mg of hydrocortisone sodium succinate if symptoms persist.
  XII. If antihistamines or epinephrine is not available outside of the hospital, administer cold tablets which have antihistamines and nasal decongestant components. Immediately take victim to hospital or first aid facility for additional therapy.
  XIII. Monitor vital and neurologic signs frequently for 24 h until stabilized.
  XIV. Administer a broad-spectrum antibiotic, i.e., 4 million units of aqueous penicillin IV during first 24 h, then oral penicillin.
  XV. If compartmental syndrome develops, may need to assist with fasciotomy.

XVI. If dressings required, apply bulky, fluffy; absorbent type.

XVII. Administer tetanus prophylaxis if patient at risk.

XVIII. Monitor and record prolonged bleeding times or continued hemorrhage.

EVALUATION

I. Note that antivenin therapy is controversial, and 30 to 50 percent of those receiving therapy are allergic to it (snake bite) (7). Scorpion antivenin may be obtained from Poisonous Animals Research Lab, Arizona State University, Tempe, Arizona.

II. Monitor patient cardiovascular and pulmonary functioning for signs of difficulty.

III. Assess effects of ongoing fluid resuscitation.

IV. Reevaluate relief of pain and anxiety with appropriate intervention where indicated.

Drowning and Near-Drowning Injuries

DEFINITION

Drowning and *near-drowning* involve the ingestion of fresh water into lungs and stomach by one of the following two mechanisms. The victim panics, begins to submerge, and spasmodically sucks water into trachea, which causes laryngospasm, gasps, and choking. Or, a small percentage has immediate laryngotracheal spasm causing asphyxia. A small group of the latter will have relaxation of the laryngospasm after a period of anoxia so that the lungs will partially flood with water (Fig. 44-13).

ASSESSMENT

I. Health history.

  A. Obtain description of the type of water victim inhaled.

  B. Describe where victim was found, i.e., bathtub, quarry, river, mud puddle, etc.

  C. Note time interval of anoxia, submersion, and resuscitation efforts prior to hospitalization.

  D. Obtain past medical and drug history, especially note recent respiratory diseases.

  E. Note allergy history, especially antibiotics.

  F. Question regarding accompanying injuries or causes of drowning event.

  G. Note if patient at risk for tetanus.

II. Physical and behavioral assessment. Note the following:

  A. Symptoms of inadequate gas exchange with hypoxia and acid-base derangement.

  B. Signs of acute pulmonary fluid collection.

  C. Transient neurologic symptoms of trismus, motor hyperactivity, convulsions, headache, and fear.

  D. Laryngospasm.

  E. Pink-red frothy sputum.

  F. Inability to take a deep breath.

  G. Burning sensation underneath sternum.

  H. Pleuritic pain.

  I. Hoarse, rasping cough.

  J. Signs of cardiovascular failure.

III. Diagnostic tests.

  A. Chest x-ray.

  B. CBC and differential, Hb and Hct (look for leukocytosis).

  C. Sputum cultures, if febrile or high index of suspicion regarding contaminants in inhaled fluids.

  D. Bacterial cultures on fluid samples *immediately,* as gives 24 to 72 h advance notice of probable organisms contributing to pneumonia.

PROBLEMS

I. Physiologic.

  A. Acute pulmonary edema.

    B. Sepsis.

    C. Acid-base imbalance, generally respiratory acidosis, and with secondary drowning, metabolic acidosis.

    D. Electrolyte imbalance, especially hyperkalemia and hypermagnesemia.

FIGURE 44-13 / Stages of drowning and near-drowning. (*Adapted from J. H. Modell, The Pathophysiology and Treatment of Drowning and Near-Drowning, Charles C Thomas Company, Springfield, Ill., 1971.*)

STAGES OF DROWNING

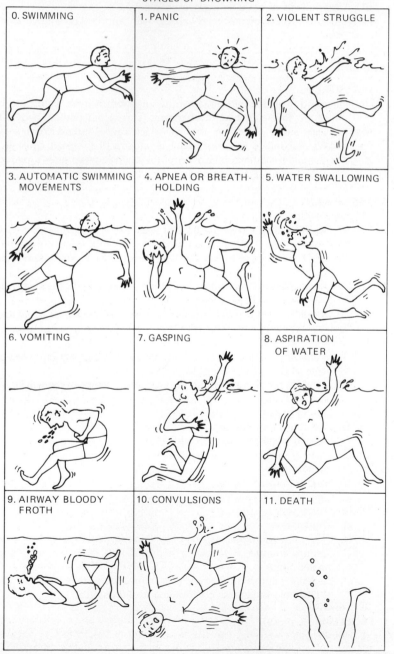

   E. Arrhythmias.
   F. Circulatory failure.
   G. Hypoxemia.
   H. Convulsions and coma.
II. Psychosocial.
   A. Fear, anxiety.
   B. Depressed level of consciousness.
   C. Cerebral anoxia with resultant memory loss and personality change.

GOALS OF CARE

   I. Establish airway patency.
   II. Establish adequate gas exchange.
   III. Return acid-base and fluid and electrolytes to normal range.
   IV. Reduce complications of sepsis and acute tubular necrosis.
   V. Minimize cardiac arrhythmias.
   VI. Reestablish circulation.
   VII. Protection of patient if unconscious.

INTERVENTION

   I. *Prior to hospitalization:* Begin cardiopulmonary resuscitation immediately.
   II. Oxygenate to maintain arterial Pa_{O_2} within normal range (greater than 80 mmHg) and acid-base in balance (pH 7.35).
   III. *In hospital:* Suction airway secretions to maintain patency.
   IV. Collect arterial blood samples frequently to ascertain changes in blood gases.
   V. Continuously monitor cardiac status via dynamic ECG.
   VI. Treat arrhythmias with prophylactic Lidocaine, 2 to 4 mg/min IV, continuous drip, and eradication of underlying cause.
   VII. Position patient with gravity flow of stomach contents to minimize aspiration of vomitus.
   VIII. Insert nasogastric tube, if stomach contents continue to threaten aspiration.
   IX. Administer appropriate IV fluids. *Fresh water drowning:* use, to keep intravenous line open, 5% dextrose in water for medication administration only. *Salt water drowning:* use 5% dextrose in saline, normal saline, or Ringer's, if no clinical electrolyte imbalances exist.
   X. Treat accompanying injuries of hemorrhage, seizures, anaphylaxis, allergic reactions, fractures, etc., with appropriate interventions.
   XI. Monitor hourly output, specific gravity, pH, and occult blood.
   XII. Administer broad-spectrum antibiotics until specific culture reports available.
   XIII. Administer tetanus prophylaxis, 0.5 mL tetanus toxoid or human immunoglobulin.
   XIV. Cleanse and dress all wounds.
   XV. Provide rapid, active rewarming for all hypothermia victims.

EVALUATION

   I. All victims should be hospitalized and observed for 24 to 48 h even if they respond immediately to resuscitation. Incidence of fulminating pneumonia and "second drowning" is extremely high, with certain mortality if untreated.
   II. All near-drowning victims should be reevaluated in 5 to 14 days for primary amebic meningoencephalitis and leptospirosis meningoencephalitis, if in endemic areas (8).

Barotrauma

Altitude and Mountain Sickness

DEFINITION

A decrease of atmospheric pressure commensurate with progressive increase of elevation over 8000 ft above sea level causes a varied symptomatology because of lesser partial pressure of oxygen in inspired air. It is common to mountain climbers who rapidly ascend past the critical level and persons not accustomed to above 17,000 ft above sea level; also, flyers and passengers in nonpressurized airplane cabins.

ASSESSMENT
I. Health history.
  A. Obtain description of environment where symptoms started.
  B. Note precautions employed by victim if seasoned mountain climber.
  C. Ascertain past medical history, including medications and allergies.
  D. Describe ascent and descent symptomatology.
  E. Record all medications administered, doses, frequency, and responses prior to reaching hospital.
  F. Note whether oxygen was administered and amount and length of time used.
  G. Describe all additional injuries or pathologies.
  H. Identify if work-related.
II. Physical and behavioral assessment. Note any of the following:
  A. Symptoms of hypoxemia with varying increases in pulse and respirations.
  B. Euphoria.
  C. Gradually decreasing mental and physical alertness.
  D. Level of consciousness.
  E. Nausea, vomiting, poor appetite.
  F. Tinnitus and deafness.
  G. Acute manifestations of pulmonary edema.
  H. Signs of thrombophlebitis.
  I. Serous effusions into the middle ear.
  J. Convulsions.
III. Diagnostic tests.
  A. Arterial blood gases.
  B. Hb and Hct (note increased Hct) and CBC (note increase in adhesiveness and aggregability of platelets).
  C. Chest x-ray.
  D. Electrolyte determinations, if vomiting persists.

PROBLEMS
I. Physiologic.
  A. Inadequate cerebral oxygenation.
  B. Potentially thrombotic or embolic due to increased hematocrit.
  C. Nausea, vomiting with electrolyte losses.
  D. Hypoxemia if left untreated.
  E. Vertigo.
  F. Anorexia.
II. Psychosocial.
  A. Disorientation and decreasing levels of consciousness.
  B. Euphoria, inappropriate coping mechanism.
  C. Impaired sensorium, making potentially irrational decisions which may be life-threatening if victim is not evacuated to lower altitude immediately.

GOALS OF CARE
I. Restore adequate fraction of inspired oxygen.
II. Return to accustomed atmospheric pressure.
III. Reestablish equilibrium and sense of balance.
IV. Restore to totally alert and oriented state.
V. Reduce complications of deafness and residual mental impairedness.

INTERVENTION
I. Supply positive pressure oxygen by face mask and rebreathing bag at 2 to 4 L.
II. Reestablish accustomed atmospheric pressure by removing victim to lower altitude or placing in pressurized compartment until transportation available.

III. Treat excessive nausea and vomiting with dimenhydrinate (Dramamine), 50 to 100 mg orally.

IV. Monitor arterialized oxygen by periodic blood gas studies.

V. Provide mild analgesia for headache; acetylsalicylic acid (aspirin), 5 to 10 g every 4 h.

VI. Obtain Hb and Hct if victim does not respond to oxygen therapy and develops thrombophlebitis.

VII. Administer nasal decongestant spray or drops to help alleviate excess middle ear fluid (ephedrine and antihistamine combinations preferred).

VIII. Orient to environment and events as patient becomes lucid.

IX. Treat acute pulmonary edema by raising head of bed 45 to 90°, 100% oxygen by mask or intranasal catheter at 8 L/min, rotating tourniquets, IV furosemide (Lasix), 40 to 80 mg over 5 min, and evacuation of victim to lower altitude immediately.

EVALUATION

I. Be aware that prognosis is excellent if victim is removed from high altitudes *immediately* upon manifesting clinical symptoms.

II. Continue to assess respiratory function for response to treatment.

III. Reevaluate at intervals patient's level of consciousness, orientation, mental and physical alertness.

Compression Air Sickness (Bends, Caisson Disease)

DEFINITION

Compression air sickness is caused by the release of nitrogen bubbles into the bloodstream during too rapid decompression from hyperbaric or greater than 760 mmHg barometric pressure, i.e., more than 1 atm of pressure. It occurs in persons who work in air locks under increased atmospheric pressure and divers who breathe compressed air or oxygen through mechanical equipment.

ASSESSMENT

I. Health history.

A. Note depth of dive and length of time in hyperbaric situation.

B. Describe if victim was scuba diving or in a helmeted deep-divingsuit.

C. Describe all therapeutic interventions prior to hospitalization.

D. Note if victim was in salt or fresh water when "bends" began.

E. Obtain past medical history, including medications and allergies.

F. Note if victim is a smoker and approximate number of packs smoked per day.

II. Physical and behavioral assessment.

A. Severe throbbing pain which shifts sites frequently from joints, muscles, and bones and may simulate an acute "surgical" abdomen.

B. Dermatologic symptoms, including intense pruritus, molting, erythema.

C. Bladder and bowel incontinence.

D. Bizarre neurologic symptoms of numbness, tingling of extremities, paresthesias, hemi-, para-, and quadriplegia, and paresis.

E. Eye manifestations of strabismus, nystagmus, diplopia.

F. Vertigo which may alter gait to appear as staggering.

G. Acute dyspnea several hours to days after successful recompression and decompression treatment.

H. Collapse and unconsciousness.

I. Hypothermia.

J. Signs and symptoms of fresh water or salt water near-drowning.

K. Rupture of tympanic membranes.

L. Some subcutaneous mediastinal emphysema.

M. Epistaxis.

N. Redness, bleb formation, and bleeding from external ear.

O. *Scuba divers:* conjunctival hemorrhages, carbon monoxide poisoning from impure air in the cylinder, and carbon dioxide poisoning.

      P. Hemoptysis.

      Q. Excessive oxygen, causing toxic effect.

      R. Pneumothorax and respiratory arrest.

  III. Diagnostic tests.

      A. Arterial blood gases.

      B. Oxygen saturation.

      C. Chest x-ray.

PROBLEMS

  I. Physiologic.

      A. Aberration in adequate blood gas exchange, with hypoxemia and free nitrogen in the blood space.

      B. Rupture bleeding of various foci, i.e., ears, nose, etc.

      C. Respiratory complications, including acute pulmonary edema and pulmonary emboli, dyspnea.

      D. Incontinence of urine, feces.

      E. Impairment of vision and eye muscle movement.

      F. Skin disruptions and discoloration.

      G. Imbalance of internal and external pressure forces.

      H. Physical immobility.

      I. Hemorrhage.

  II. Psychosocial.

      A. Disorientation, changing levels of consciousness from alert to unconscious.

      B. Alteration of sensory perception, touch, temperature.

      C. Uncontrolled motor responses.

      D. Social immobility if placed in hyperbaric and/or recompression chamber.

      E. Pain.

GOALS OF CARE

  I. Decompress or return to 1 atm pressure without complications.

  II. Reestablish airway patency, and oxygenate to normal range, i.e., Pa_{O_2}, 92 to 96 percent, or preinjury state if within safe limitations.

  III. Stop hemorrhage.

  IV. Reduce pain.

  V. Return to full sensory and motor capacity.

  VI. Protection of victim during unconscious state.

INTERVENTION

  I. Provide continuous artificial respiration by mouth-to-mouth, bag-to-mouth, or mechanical support, as feasible.

  II. Provide 100% oxygen or oxygen-helium mixture via face mask or intranasal cannula.

  III. Stop epistaxis and external ear bleeds with firm pressure against ruptured areas and equilibration of sinus pressures with barometric pressure.

  IV. Plan recompression and gradual decompression procedures.

  V. Stay with victim throughout procedure in decompression chamber to alleviate fears and help orient to reality.

  VI. Provide analgesia by narcotic, i.e., careful administration of 2 to 10 mg IV of morphine sulfate. *Watch respiratory patterns and circulation.*

  VII. Give nasal decongestants and antihistamines to reduce middle ear fluid accumulation (Actifed, a combination of triprolidine hydrochloride, 2.5 mg, and pseudoephedrine hydrochloride, 60 mg).

  VIII. Rewarm rapidly to normal body temperature range, and monitor for thermal changes over 24 to 48 h afterward.

  IX. Monitor vital and neurologic signs frequently until stabilized and victim has completed decompression procedure.

X. Minimize coughing and sneezing until internal head and thoracic pressures are normalized.

XI. Carefully observe for any signs of thrombophlebitis, and immediately treat with elevation and rest of extremity, hot, moist pack (body temperature) to affected part, anticoagulant therapy, and application of antiembolic stockings.

EVALUATION

I. Important information reducing onset time of treatment includes: knowledge of where, the shortest route to, and entrance criteria for any victim needing a decompression chamber. This information should be taught to patient and companions as well.

II. When in doubt whether to decompress or recompress, initiate procedure as it is harmless to diver and attendant (nurse).

WOUNDS

Abrasion

DEFINITION

An *abrasion* is a painful, superficial wound, scraping the epidermis and occasionally the upper levels of dermis. Frequently, it is the result of forceful, "skidding" motion. A skinned knee is an example of this type of wound. There is an excellent prognosis for complete recovery.

ASSESSMENT

I. Health history. Ascertain the following:
  A. Description of incident producing injury.
  B. Description of environmental conditions where injury occurred, i.e., gravel path, sand, cement, dirt bed, etc.
  C. Time interval from injury to request for treatment.
  D. History of tetanus immunization.
  E. Medication allergies.

II. Physical and behavioral assessment.
  A. Assess depth of destruction (superficial).
  B. Examine all elevated surfaces exposed and prone to this injury.
  C. Look for contaminants and debris ground into wound.
  D. Note any of the following:
    1. Serious, bloody drainage.   **3.** Disfigurement.
    2. Pain.   **4.** Swelling, edema.

PROBLEMS

I. Physiologic.
  A. Sepsis.
  B. Loss of body fluid (massive abrasions).
  C. Local hyperemia.

II. Psychosocial.
  A. Disfigurement.
  B. Pain.
  C. Altered sensation to temperature (massive abrasions).

GOALS OF CARE

I. Reestablish protective barrier of skin, thereby reducing infection.
II. Promote wound healing.
III. Reduce pain and discomfort.
IV. Maintain body heat within normal range.
V. Decrease chance of permanent scarring by careful removal of any foreign matter.

INTERVENTION

I. Provide anesthesia by topical ointment, sprays, jellies, or injectables. Lidocaine preferred.
   A. *Topical solution* (2 or 4%): duration of anesthesia approximately 20 min.
   B. *Ointment* (2.5, 4, and 5%); used as vehicle to remove free-floating dirt (not water soluble).
   C. *Jelly* (2.5, 4, and 5%); water soluble.
   D. *Injectable, plain* ($\frac{1}{2}$ to 2%): *do not use cardiac Lidocaine* due to deterioration of medication strength because of no preservatives).
II. Scrupulously cleanse wound with saline until dirt and particulate matter are removed.
III. Debride wound with forceps.
IV. Apply dressing.
   A. *Open:* very thin coat of petroleum-base ointment (antibiotics are acceptable but avoid Neosporin due to high incidence of sensitivity).
   B. *Closed: fine*-mesh or Owen silk gauze.
V. Tape closed dressings around and not over wound.
VI. Teach patient to care for wounds by changing dressings daily or as circumstances require and keeping areas free of moisture.
VII. Assure patient that area will be discolored for a period of time but will not scar.

EVALUATION

I. Provide for follow-up if complications arise.
II. Assess patient understanding of wound care, i.e., have patient perform return demonstration of dressing, cleansing of wound that has been taught.
III. Evaluate relief of patient pain and discomfort after treatment.

Avulsion

DEFINITION

Avulsion is the tearing away and complete loss of tissue which disallows the approximation of wound edges. It most frequently occurs with nose tip, ear lobe, and fingertip injuries.

ASSESSMENT

I. Health history.
   A. Note time of tissue loss to determine salvagability.
   B. Obtain description of forces causing tearing and removal of tissue.
   C. Ascertain if injury is job-oriented.
   D. Obtain all tissue specimens for preservation of potential replanting.
II. Physical and behavioral assessment. Note the following:
   A. Extent of tissue loss dependent on injury mechanism.
   B. Alteration in function of part affected.
   C. Any esthetic or cosmetic changes (may cause depression and fear in patient).
   D. Hemorrhage.
   E. Pain.
   F. Disfigurement.
   G. Swelling, edema.
   H. Local hyperemia.
III. Diagnostic tests.
   A. X-ray to rule out bone injury (in finger digits).
   B. If large avulsion with possible surgical intervention: CBC and differential (including Hb and Hct).

PROBLEMS

I. Physiologic.
   A. Sepsis.
   B. Incomplete wound closure.

   C. Inadequate function of underlying part at avulsion site.
   D. Body fluid and blood loss.
   E. Possible surgical intervention.
II. Psychosocial.
   A. Disfigurement.
   B. Pain.
   C. Loss of job productibility.

GOALS OF CARE
  I. Restore function of body part.
 II. Reduce pain, discomfort.
III. Rebuild avulsed area to maintain preinjury appearance.
IV. Reduce complications of sepsis.
 V. Replace body fluids to normal range.

INTERVENTION
    I. If tissue being brought from home: roll so adipose and subcutaneous tissues are inside, protect from drying by placing in airtight container with ice on outside. *Do not carry tissue in water.*
   II. Preserve all avulsed tissue in saline packs or saline solution and keep cool.
  III. Provide analgesia: topical or nerve block for wound cleaning and repair.
   IV. Cleanse avulsed area gently with free-flowing saline.
    V. Remove all dirt and contaminants with flow of fluids and/or forceps.
   VI. Do *not* soak affected tissue in antiseptic solutions.
  VII. To stop bleeding, apply gentle pressure, Gel foam, or topical thrombin.
 VIII. Dress avulsed area with fine-mesh gauze, 2- by 2-in or 4- by 4-in fluffs and tube gauze, or with gentle pressure dressing.
   IX. Provide protective devices (finger shield or guard for digits).
    X. Do *not* apply tape over injured area.
   XI. Teach patient to leave dressing intact for 10 to 14 days and to keep area dry.
  XII. Teach patient to observe for regional systemic signs of infection rather than for local symptoms.
 XIII. Provide emotional reassurance and support for patient and family.

EVALUATION
   I. Prepare patient for possibility that wound may need grafting if tissue does not fill in avulsed area.
  II. Assess teaching of wound care and of knowledge of systemic signs of infection.
 III. Arrange for reevaluation of avulsed area.
 IV. Reevaluate relief of pain, discomfort from treatment.
  V. If indicated, refer to community health nurse for home follow-up.

Contusions

DEFINITION
A *contusion* is a nonpenetrating insult to soft tissue more commonly called a "bruise." The mechanism of injury includes sharp blow to tissue causing disruption and oozing of tiny blood vessels. Small contusions resulting in mild ecchymosis are nonthreatening and resolve without intervention. Large contusions of extensive tissue mass, i.e., thigh and/or buttocks, have large pooling of blood which may infect and cause abcess formation. Victims at risk include hemophiliacs and those on anticoagulants or those who have other blood disorders characterized by bleeding.

ASSESSMENT
  I. Health history.
   A. Obtain description of injury force.

     B. Note time of injury and interval elapsed before seeking medical care.

     C. Question for past medical history and bleeding tendencies.

     D. Request medication history.

     E. Note area of bleeding entrapment, i.e., subungual hematomas.

II. Physical and behavioral assessment.

     A. Neurovascular function.

     B. Size of injured area compared to counterpart.

     C. Compartmental syndrome, i.e., pain on passive stretching of involved area, palpation tenderness, and questionable peripheral pulses and capillary filling.

     D. Subungual hematomas with pressure of trapped blood.

PROBLEMS

I. Physiologic.

     A. Hemorrhaging into interstitial areas.

     B. Infection.

     C. Swelling.

     D. Vascular disruption.

     E. Tissue compression within fascial compartment.

II. Psychosocial.

     A. Pain.

     B. Loss of extremity or digit motor function.

     C. Consequent disruption of performance in activities of daily living.

GOALS OF CARE

I. Restore vessel integrity.

II. Resolve free or trapped blood.

III. Restore motor function.

IV. Reduce pain.

V. Avoid infection.

INTERVENTION

I. Apply cold, wet compresses or ice bag or pack in fresh water ice to prevent further hemorrhage into tissues. *Do not use iced saline,* because temperature of slush is too low and tends to further damage tissues.

II. Elevate affected area, if possible.

III. Immobilize part, and place affected tissues at rest.

IV. Mark ecchymosed area to monitor continued bleeding.

V. Provide mild analgesics orally. *Avoid aspirin.*

VI. Note changes in neurovascular function, i.e., diminishing pulses or prolonged capillary refill times.

VII. For subungual hematoma, use thermolance, heated copper paper clip held on to nail just above trapped blood, or short-bevel No. 18 needle and bandaid.

VIII. After 24 h, apply heat with warm moist packs or heating pad.

IX. Incise and drain if ecchymosed area becomes infected.

X. Administer antibiotics, if infected.

XI. Administer hyabviouidose, 300 turbidity-reducing units (TRU) in 1 mL of normal saline, injected directly into hematoma, or oral proteolytics to act on entrapped blood, if indicated.

EVALUATION

I. Reevaluate effects of treatment.

     A. Decreased pain?

     B. Decreased bleeding into affected tissues?

     C. Decreased swelling?

     D. Neurovascular function stable?

II. Provide emotional reassurance and support.

Crush Wounds

DEFINITION

Crush wounds give rise to massive, generalized contusions, internal and/or external, causing gross amounts of edema, interstitial hemorrhaging, and extensive damage to a multiplicity of structures. A high incidence of this injury is found among construction workers on heavy machinery and earth-moving jobs. They also occur during traumatic events at home or during gardening which requires heavy equipment. Crush wounds are found in other occupations as well, i.e., service station operators, mechanics, press operators of various kinds. A special type of crushing occurs with wringer washer injury.

ASSESSMENT

I. Health history. Obtain the following:
   A. Description of forces causing injury.
   B. Treatment rendered prior to admission.
   C. Estimation of actual fluid and blood loss prior to admission.
   D. Description of additional injuries.
II. Physical and behavioral assessment.
   A. Arterial insufficiency due to vascular spasm, occlusion, or tears.
   B. Nerve deficits of neurotmesis, axonotmesis, neuropraxia.
   C. Loss of tendon function due to divisions or ruptures.
   D. Massive hematomas within muscles of belly.
   E. Shock symptoms.
   F. Hyperkalemia with resultant cardiac arrhythmias.
   G. Symptoms of sepsis.
   H. Accompanying fractures.
   I. "Splitting," or "explosion" lacerations.
   J. Massive discoloration of area, including ecchymoses.
   K. Extent of disfigurement.
   L. Amount of pain.
III. Diagnostic tests.
   A. Radiographic evaluation.
   B. CBC, differential, Hb, Hct, and electrolytes.

PROBLEMS

I. Physiologic.
   A. Massive fluid shifting and loss to circulating volume.
   B. Hemorrhage.
   C. Electrolyte imbalance.
   D. Sensory and motor disruption of affected part.
   E. Impaired or disrupted local circulation.
   F. Tissue hypoxia, anoxia with resultant local toxic reactions.
   G. Shock.
   H. Sepsis.
II. Psychosocial.
   A. Pain.
   B. Tactile and sensory alterations.
   C. Disfigurement.
   D. Motor rehabilitation.
   E. Body image change.
   F. Occupation rehabilitation or "retooling."
   G. Economic, emotional, social devastation due to multiple repairs and convalescence.

GOALS OF CARE

I. Restore adequate circulation.
II. Reduce complication of shock.

III. Minimize infections.
IV. Restore neuromusculoskeletal functions.
V. Reduce pain.
VI. Provide for ongoing rehabilitation, including ancillary personnel, i.e., social worker, physical therapist, occupational therapist, etc.

INTERVENTION

I. Lower affected part's temperature with fresh water ice packs.
II. Immobilize area, and place at rest (to minimize toxic products release).
III. Keep patient supine and at rest, and monitor vital signs frequently.
IV. *Small crush injuries:* Provide salty oral fluids, if conscious.
V. *Large crush wounds:* Start two large-bore central or large peripheral vein intravenous lines.
VI. Fluid resuscitate with balanced salt solutions to maintain perfusion pressure at 90 mmHg systolic.
VII. Administer packed red blood cells (PRBC) according to amount of whole blood lost.
VIII. Place patient on cardiac monitor while hyperkalemic, and observe for myocardial irritability, i.e., ventricular ectopy, multifocal ectopy, ventricular fibrillation, heart block.
IX. Periodically assess sensory functions.
X. Check appropriate pulses: circulation of part for swelling and occlusion.
XI. Prepare nor surgery for pending exploration, debridement, repair, and/or replantation.
XII. Apply light dressings until evaluated for definitive treatment.
XIII. For wringer injuries:
    A. Gently cleanse lacerations and other open wounds with antiseptic soap and water.
    B. Apply light, sterile gauze dressings, fluffs, or cotton waste, and wrap entire extremity in compression dressing from distal to proximal part.
    C. Elevate extremity to decrease blood flow and prevent further swelling.
    D. Observe all circulation and neuromuscular monitoring for 48 h.
    E. Administer tetanus prophylaxis, i.e., tetanus toxoid, 0.5 mL or human immuno-globulin.

EVALUATION

I. Continue to monitor and assess:
    A. Fluid loss.
    B. Signs of sepsis.
    C. Symptoms of shock.
    D. Signs of disruption of local circulation.
    E. Electrolyte imbalance.
    F. Myocardial irritability.
    G. Effects of treatment on pain.
II. Provide much-needed emotional support to patient and family members.

Lacerations

DEFINITION

A *laceration* is a traumatic opening of skin, mucous membranes, or parenchymal tissue which can be contused, avulsed, bevelled, straight or jagged, torn or mangled, and dirty or clean. A laceration occurs when external forces cause abrupt disruption of tissue or with incision. Occasionally, intense internal pressure of tissue will cause eruption-type laceration. Those at greatest risk include industrial workers, people in food trades, and those who handle sharp instruments. Laceration frequently accompanies trauma of all sorts, especially automobile injuries.

ASSESSMENT

I. Health history.
    A. Ascertain the mechanism of injury as it relates to management, i.e., blow to part, striking head on flat or pointed object, fall into dirt or dung, etc.

    B. Determine time of injury and interval before seeking medical care (if over 6 to 12 h old, do *not* suture, due to infection).

    C. Note past medical and drug history, including tetanus prophylaxis.

    D. Note medication allergies, especially antimicrobials.

    E. Determine if injury is work-related.

    F. If wounds are extensive, take photographs for later plastic repairs.

    G. Note what treatment was initiated prior to admission.

    H. Specifically ascertain if patient is on anticoagulants or has bleeding disorder.

II. Physical and behavioral assessment. Check for the following:

    A. Extent of hemorrhage and body fluid losses.

    B. Destruction of tissue and underlying organs relative to mechanism of injury, i.e., blunt blow causing laceration of skin may result in extensive soft tissue injury surrounding site or tear in organ parenchyma.

    C. Gross contamination of wound with foreign matter, dirt, hair, pebbles, sand, dung, etc.

    D. Irregularity and jaggedness of wound edges, with little blood supply.

    E. Healing of laceration erythema or swelling along wound edge and purulent drainage may be present.

III. Diagnostic tests.

    A. CBC, including differential.

    B. Hb and Hct.

    C. Partial thromboplastin time (PTT) and prothrombin time (PT) if patient is anticoagulated or has bleeding history.

    D. X-ray of affected part if laceration deep over bony prominence or if injury is due to fall.

    E. Wound culture and sensitivities.

PROBLEMS

I. Physiologic.

    A. Sepsis.

    B. Hemorrhage.

    C. Loss of movement due to injury or postrepair splinting.

    D. Inadequate closure due to prolonged interval before repair.

    E. Structural changes causing altered organ(s) function.

    F. Swelling.

II. Psychosocial.

    A. Pain.

    B. Body image change from scarring and/or disfigurement.

GOALS OF CARE

I. Restore tissue intactness.

II. Minimize sepsis and other complications.

III. Restore sensory and motor functions.

IV. Resuscitate to normal body fluid balance.

V. Regain mental health attitude of body wholeness (especially when there are multiple lacerations).

INTERVENTION

    I. Thoroughly prepare skin around laceration by cleansing with Betadine scrub solution: *do not put into wound.*

    II. Shave hair around laceration: *do not shave eyebrows.*

    III. Profusely irrigate wound with physiologic solutions, i.e., normal saline, *not* water. Rely on mechanical action and not on antisepsis of solution (9). Use 50 mL/in per hour.

    IV. May need to use mild soap containing butter, ointment, petroleum-base medicines found in commercial first aid kits (antiseptic solutions irritate and kill injured cells and interfere with local defense mechanism because they destroy defense cells and inhibit healing).

    V. Use jet action of irrigating, i.e., 50-mL syringe with large needle or jet lavage. *Do not use* Asepto, Toomey syringe, or IV tubing for irrigation, as ejection force is too weak for adequate mechanical action (10).

   VI. May use gloved finger and plain gauze sponges to assist in mechanical action. *Do not* use cotton-filled gauze sponges, as cotton debris left in wound causes granulomas.

  VII. *Do not use* high concentrations of anything, i.e., peroxide, as:
    A. Oxygen is used up rapidly and is not effective against anaerobes.
    B. It is painful and destroys cells. Alcohol is also painful.

 VIII. Cover wound with sterile dressings if there is a delay between cleansing and repair.

   IX. Use sterile technique from wound preparation through repair.

    X. Provide local anesthesia via infiltration or block, using one of the caines *without* epinephrine.

   XI. May need to provide anesthesia prior to cleansing, depending on severity, placement, and contamination of wound.

  XII. Debride edges and devitalized tissue to create straight edges, proper alignment, and reduced tension (11).

 XIII. Close wounds with sterile strips or appropriate suture material as indicated, so that skin edges are slightly everted, *not* inverted or wrinkled.

 XIV. Leave sterile strips 5 to 7 days, and watch for signs of infection.

  XV. Repair with smallest suture and finest needle for minimal tissue reaction and scarring.

 XVI. Use prolene or nylon monofilament on skin, wire for muscles. Avoid silk for plastic closures as it is braided and leaves holes in the skin (12).

 XVII. Dress with nonadhering covering first, then a combination of fluffs, bias mesh roller gauze, i.e., Kling, Kerlix, or tube gauze, elasticated net bandage (Surifix), and elastic-impregnated gauze, i.e., Elastoplast. *Do not use* elastic bandage (Ace) as it causes too much pressure and resultant ischemia of injured tissue (13).

XVIII. Immobilize any lacerations over joints or moving parts by casting, "wadding" dressings. Be sure immobilized part is in position of function.

 XIX. Provide tetanus prophylaxis according to patient risk.

  XX. Teach patient to observe for circulatory impairment, infection, increased pain or pressure, and when to notify physician or nurse (14).

EVALUATION

    I. Assess patient understanding regarding:
    A. Signs of circulatory impairment.
    B. Signs of increased pain.
    C. Signs of infection.

   II. Reevaluate patient pain, discomfort.

  III. Advise patient that:
    A. Repair should produce as little scarring as possible.
    B. Repaired site will remain discolored (erythema) and elevated for several weeks to 1 to 2 years, depending on severity, wound healing, and individual skin behavior.

  IV. Be aware that eventual appearance will be lighter than regular skin due to destruction of melanocytes. For dark-skinned people, final scars may take on a "pink" rather than "white" appearance.

   V. Evaluate that structures and surface contours are approximated to preinjury appearance as much as possible to reduce body disfigurement.

Punctures

DEFINITION

A *puncture* is a perforation of skin and underlying structures due to a forceful thrust or pressure from a sharp, pointed, narrow instrument or teeth. Common causes of this injury include nails, tacks, staples, "ice-pick" tools, needles and pins, and intentional or accidental stabbing with knives and daggers. Special types of punctures include animal and human bites, impaled objects, fish hooks, splinters, and needles. Disruption of tissue or organ function is relative to depth and degree of contamination. For punctures caused by hymenopterons, see "Environmental Exposure Problems."

ASSESSMENT
I. Health history.
  A. Obtain description of object causing wound and force of entry.
  B. Note tetanus immunization history.
  C. Note antibiotic allergies.
  D. Ascertain if injury is work-related.
  E. If animal bite, obtain necessary legal data of species, owner if appropriate, animal's immunization history, whether animal has been caged and under observation.
  F. If suspicious of details regarding cause of injury, obtain description of surrounding events resulting in puncture wound(s), i.e., stabbings.
II. Physical and behavioral assessment.
  A. Is foreign body retained in puncture tract, "hooked" in skin, or impaled?
  B. Is wound contaminated (this usually occurs)? Note the following:
    1. Signs of infection.
    2. Ragged wound edges (e.g., resulting from bites).
    3. Amount of pain.
    4. Amount of drainage (may be minimal, serosanguinous if superficial).
    5. Ecchymosis and discoloration of skin.
    6. Hemorrhage and deep hematomas (if chest or abdominal wounds, this may occur).
    7. Neurovascular, musculoskeletal involvement.
III. Diagnostic studies.
  A. Fluoroscopy for identification of needle or small metal objects.
  B. Culture wounds for bites (human and animal).

PROBLEMS
I. Physiologic.
  A. Sepsis.
  B. Hemorrhage (if multiple or deep wounds).
  C. Disruption of organ function if penetration wound is deep.
  D. Scarring if human or animal bites. Such scarring is due to jagged edges and inability of wounds to close.
  E. Further destruction of tissue, if foreign body difficult to retrieve.
  F. Neurovascular dysfunction.
II. Psychosocial.
  A. Pain.
  B. Anxiety and fear if due to enraged animal or intentional stabbing.
  C. Possible disfigurement.

GOALS OF CARE
I. Minimize complications of infection.
II. Remove foreign bodies.
III. Promote systematic wound healing (from lower end of tract to skin surface).
IV. Reduce pain.
V. Allay patient fear and anmiety.

INTERVENTION
I. Thoroughly cleanse and irrigate wound.
II. Debride.

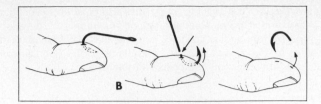

FIGURE 44-14 / **Method of removing an embedded fish hook.** (*From John Henderson, Emergency Medical Guide, McGraw-Hill Book Company, New York, 1978.*)

 III. Provide analgesia as appropriate to wound size, depth, and logistics of cleansing procedure.

 IV. If wood splinter, *do not cleanse wound with water until foreign body removed* (wood absorbs water, swells, and falls apart).

 V. Administer tetanus prophylaxis, 0.5 mL. of tetanus toxoid or appropriate dose of human hyperimmune serum.

 VI. Begin on prophylactic antibiotics depending on wound contamination.

 VII. Instruct in frequent, warm soaks, at least every other day.

 VIII. Teach patient to apply dry, sterile dressing between soaks.

 IX. *Do not use ointments on puncture wounds.*

 X. If fish hook embedded, make small incision over tip and force tip through. Cut shaft of hook with wire cutter and pull remainder out (Fig. 44-14).

 XI. Remove splinters with splinter forceps.

 XII. Leave bite wounds open initially.

 XIII. Give duck embryo vaccine (DEV) if index of suspicion for rabies is high.

 XIV. Apply bulky, fluffy, dry dressings for bites. For face bites, may use sterile strips placed loosely.

 XV. For industrial accidents extricate patient from machinery with impaled object intact.

 XVI. When transporting impaled victim, immobilize affected part and stabilize impaling object.

 XVII. Surgically remove impaling object using aseptic environment and providing for possible massive bleeding or fluid loss.

 XVIII. *Do not remove impaling object from eye:* demands opthalmologist to protect aqueous and vitreous humors.

 XIX. In emergency, remove an impaling object with thorough cleansing and withdrawing along path of entry.

EVALUATION

 I. Complete accidental injury, Workman's Compensation insurance forms as indicated in industrial accidents.

 II. Report to police and/or animal control authorities all stabbings, suspicious penetrating wounds, and animal bites, as appropriate.

 III. Be aware of necessity of retaining animal for 15 days in case of animal bites to observe for rabies.

 IV. Indicate rabies prophylaxis if animal develops symptoms of disease.

 V. Assess need for further referral to community health nurse for home follow-up and continuity of care.

Burns

Thermal **DEFINITION**

The progression of events *in thermal burning* includes: denaturization of tissue protein, especially after 45°C, causing redistribution of cellular fluid and olid components, nuclear swelling, cell membrane rupture, granulation of cytoplasm, and homogeneous coagulation of cellular contents. Cells are injured or destroyed by disruption of thermolabile enzymatic functions.

People at risk include anyone working with steam, boiling water, or objects that are fired and retain heat, i.e., bakers, kitchen workers, maintenance personnel; anyone trapped in burning material or in a burning environment; anyone trapped in hot, wet clothing; careless smokers; family involved in cooking or baking activities.

The intensity and magnitude of responses differentiate the level of burn injury. Severity of injury is related to depth and spatial distribution. Complications and alterations result from initial injury, subsequent loss of skin protection, and infection of denuded tissue. Occasionally in civilian life, fourth degree burns are encountered during intense heat from blazing structures, chemical (gasoline) fires, and molten metal in contact with victim's body.

ASSESSMENT

I. Health history.
   A. Obtain description of thermal source, i.e., dry or wet heat.
   B. Note exposure interval and approximate degree of temperature.
   C. Obtain description of events associated with injury.
   D. Determine patient age.
   E. Note past medical history and general health.
   F. Ascertain medication history and allergies.
   G. Determine possible noxious gases produced by fire and patient exposure to these.
   H. Note if fire occurred in a closed place.
   I. Ask about patient's life-style prior to accident.
II. Physical and behavioral assessment.
   A. Classify burns in first-, second-, and third-degree categories of tissue destruction.
   B. Assess depth and distribution of burns (massive disfigurement is dependent on these two factors; Fig. 44-15).
   C. Evaluate additional injuries.
   D. Note amount of pain (if first or second degree burn, pain is excruciating).
   E. Test for loss of sensations, i.e., pain, heat, cold, pressure if third-degree burn or incinerated muscle and connective tissue included. Note the following:
      1. Impairment of circulation with resultant transudation of vascular fluids.
      2. Skin integrity, alteration of protective and thermal functions.
      3. Signs of sepsis.
      4. Need for caloric and nutritional requirements (extensive usually).
      5. Erythema, blisters, edema of affected part to coagulation neurosis in third-degree burns.
      6. Systemic fluid losses.
      7. Depression, morbid state.
      8. Catastrophic fear.
      9. Cough and bronchospasm.
III. Diagnostic studies.
   A. CBC, Hb, Hct, electrolytes.
   B. Urinalysis for myoglobin and casts.
   C. Blood chemistries to include: BUN, creatinine, albumin and globulin levels, blood sugar, bilirubin and alkaline phosphatase levels, calcium and phosphorous levels, arterial blood gases, if indicated.
   D. Chest x-ray if victim of smoke or noxious gas inhalation.
   E. May obtain carbon monoxide blood level on admission.
   F. Type and cross-match blood.

PROBLEMS

I. Physiologic.
   A. Massive fluid losses depending on size and extent of burn.
   B. Alteration of body fluid composition, especially serum hyperkalemia and hypoalbuminemia.

Depth of burn	Detailed classification	Pain and pinprick sensitivity	Appearance	Healing time	End result of healing	Treatment
1°	Erythema only, no loss of epidermis	Hyperalgesia	Erythema		Normal skin	Allow to heal by natural processes. Protect from further injury and infection
2° Partial skin loss	Superficial, no loss of dermis	Hyperalgesia or normal	Erythema to opaque white blisters are characteristic	6-10 days	Normal to slightly pitted and/or poorly pigmented	
	Intermediate healing from hair follicles	Normal to hypo-algesia		7-14 days		
	Deep Healing from sweat glands	Hypoalgesia to analgesia		14-21 days	Hairless and depigmented Texture normal to pitted or flat and shiny	
3° Whole skin loss	Deep dermal Occasionally, healing from scattered epithelium	Analgesia	White opaque to charred, coagulated; subcutaneous veins may be visible	More than 21 days	Poor texture Hypertrophic Scar frequent	Elective skin grafting may save time and give better end result
	Whole skin loss Healing from edges only					
4° Deep tissue loss	Deep structure loss	May be some algesia		Never, if area is large	Hypertrophic scar and chronic granulations unless grafted	Skin grafting mandatory

    C. Extensive caloric and nutritional needs.
    D. Sepsis.
    E. Loss of sensory and motor functions.
    F. Scarring, nonviable tissue.
    G. Airway obstruction if face, nose, or mouth burned or gases inhaled.
II. Psychosocial.
    A. Pain.
    B. Body image change.
    C. Permanent disfigurement in severe cases.
    D. Sensory overload with extensive burns.
    E. Devastation of personal and public funds for exhaustive life-saving care, in severe cases.

GOALS OF CARE

I. Establish airway if indicated by type of burn or total burn severity.
II. Reduce pain.
III. Minimize fluid shifts and losses.
IV. Reduce electrolyte losses and improper shifts.
V. Avoid sepsis.
VI. Minimize complications and further tissue damage.
VII. Prevent and treat shock.
VIII. Provide emergency dressing of burns.
IX. Provide emotional support to patient and family members.

INTERVENTION

I. Establish airway and maintain respiratory support for all face, head, and neck burns, massive body surface area burns, or known closed environment entrapment or smoke inhalation. Use oxygen.
II. Combat shock by fluid resuscitation, Ringer's lactate, or another buffered, isotonic solution, based on calculation on body surface area and depth of burn. May use "rule of 9s" (modify for children; see Fig. 44-16).
III. Insert urinary bladder indwelling catheter, and attach to closed drainage system.
IV. Monitor hourly urine output.
V. Keep urine at 7.0 pH during time of great Hb and myoglobin losses, as they are more soluble in alkaline. The nurse can measure these changes with urine nitrogen paper. These values should be recorded next to the amount and specific gravity on flow sheet.
VI. Administer tetanus prophylaxis, i.e., 0.5 mL tetanus toxoid, or human immune globulin according to kilograms of body weight.
VII. Provide analgesia of 4 mg titrated IV morphine or meperidine, 20 mg, not to exceed 14 mg in 3- to 4-h period.
VIII. Administer added amounts of sodium bicarbonate via the IV to maintain desired urine pH. However, watch for other contaminant growth, as this treatment then predisposes patient to high incidence of urinary tract infections.
IX. Remove jewelry, clothing from affected or potential problem areas.
X. Gently and thoroughly cleanse burned areas with copious amounts of cooled sterile water or saline and iodophor soap.
XI. Apply fine-mesh gauze, plain or impregnated, followed with bulky, absorptive fluffs, and even compression dressing of roller gauze or Kling (bias-cut stockinette may be used over very large extremity or torso parts).
XII. Splint burned extremities involving flexor aspects in full extension position, *except* hand.

FIGURE 44-15 / **Classification of burns according to depth of burn.** (*Adapted from Carmen Sproul and Patrick Mullaney, Emergency Care: Assessment and Intervention, C. V. Mosby Company, St. Louis, 1974.*)

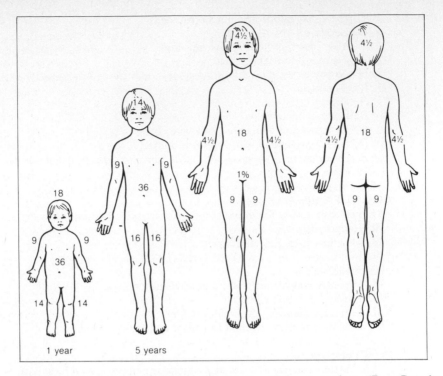

FIGURE 44-16 / Rule of 9s with modification for children and infants. (*From Dorothy Jones et al., Medical-Surgical Nursing: A Conceptual Approach, McGraw-Hill Book Company, New York, 1978.*)

XIII. Administer prophylactic antibiotic treatment of penicillin or another broad-spectrum medication.

XIV. Apply *p*-(aminomethyl)benzenesulfonamide acetate (Sulfamylon) cream after burned area has been cleansed and debrided.

XV. Keep patient's body temperature in normal range by covering with sterile sheet and light thermal blanket.

XVI. For superficial burns, reduce tissue injury and pain by packing area in iced saline or cold compresses for 20 min.

XVII. Administer oral fluids of saline, water, sugar water, juices if victim is awake and is not vomiting.

XVIII. Monitor vital signs frequently, and note orthostatic and nonorthostatic changes.

XIX. Use sterile mineral oil or bacitracin ointment to "float off" a tar deposit causing burn.

EVALUATION

I. Continue to monitor:

 A. Patency of airway.

 B. All vital signs.

 C. Signs of sepsis.

 D. Signs of shock.

 E. Extent of fluid loss, electrolyte imbalances.

 F. Relief of pain.

II. Be aware that extensive use of morphine sulfate for analgesia causes respiratory suppression and inadequate ventilation.

III. Provide continued emotional support to family and patient via direct nursing contact, and if indicated, family referral to appropriate social and clinical supportive services within institution.

Electrical

DEFINITION

An *electrical burn* is an injury affecting any tissue including bone and manifested by a local lesion which has the following characteristics: a charred black center, a middle area of gray-white coagulation necrosis, and an outer, bright red ring of partial coagulation. The coagulation areas may increase over several days after injury, due to progressive vascular thrombosis. Ischemic destruction is secondary to the intravascular thrombosis, and hemorrhage may occur hours to days after injury due to destruction of arteries. The vessels appear "friable," and hemorrhage is hard to control. Electrical injury to bone causes swelling, gradual sequestration, and discharge of devitalized areas. Neurologic injuries are broad, from paralysis of various muscle tissues to bizarre pain behavior, aphasia, and cerebellar dysfunction. Seizure activity is not uncommon. Also, posttraumatic psychoneurosis does occur. Causes of electrical burns include approximately one-fourth from lightning and three-fourths from industrial and home accidents. Extent of injury determined by current intensity and duration. The pathway of current through the body and resistance at points of contact help determine severity. Most dangerous is alternating current. Commonly termed "iceberg" injuries due to massive tissue destruction and sloughing can occur although cutaneous wound is small.

ASSESSMENT

  I. Health history.
   A. Establish who can serve as historian regarding the accident.
   B. Obtain description of voltage amounts, duration of contact, and type of electrical force.
   C. Note past medical and drug history.
   D. Ascertain whether injury related to employment.
   E. Establish if patient was unconscious and, if so, how long.
  II. Physical and behavioral assessment.
   A. Massive subcutaneous, fascia, connective tissue destruction in path of current flow.
   B. Minimal cutaneous wounds compared to underlying structure destruction.
   C. Any secondary effects of cardiac standstill, ventricular fibrillation, respiratory muscle paralysis and/or arrest.
   D. "Charred" markings at current entry site.
   E. Hemorrhage and massive fluid losses with muscle tissue injury.
   F. Fluid output amount and composition.
   G. Consciousness, orientation, and ability to conduct abstract thought.
   H. Nausea, vomiting, and paralytic ileus.
   I. Violent, tetanic state and uncoordinated muscle contractions.
   J. Signs of internal hemorrhage and perforation of intraabdominal viscus (high suspicion index with this type of injury).
 III. Diagnostic studies.
   A. Any laboratory tests associated with organs in path of injury.
   B. Urinalysis nor microscopic, myoglobin, and hemoglobin.
   C. Twelve-lead ECG.
   D. Serum potassium.

PROBLEMS

  I. Physiologic.
   A. Cardiac arrhythmias, chaos, or standstill.
   B. Selected loss of structural integrity with resultant sensory and motor changes.
   C. Impaired or lost circulatory system in affected area.
   D. Respiratory failure with resultant anaerobic respiration.
   E. Shock.
   F. Associated injuries: fractures, dislocations, lacerations, soft tissue injuries.
   G. Acidosis.
  II. Psychosocial.
   A. Loss of reality, personality changes.

   B. Catastrophic loss in economic productivity.
   C. Body image changes.
   D. Gamut of emotional responses, from extreme anxiety to depression and psychotic behavior.

GOALS OF CARE
   I. Reestablish vital functions of cardiopulmonary system.
   II. Restore body fluid balance.
   III. Reduce further injury and complications.
   IV. Prepare patient for removal of devitalized tissue and surgical repair.
   V. Provide emotional support, appropriate referral to psychosocial or community health personnel.

EVALUATION
   I. Employ both primary excision and watchful waiting.
   II. Be aware that initial injury is followed by massive tissue necrosis and sloughing along path of current flow; thus, long-term evaluation of damage extent is required.
   III. Continue to assess organ structures, as multiple organs may be included in injury and complicate recovery period.
   IV. Reevaluate patient and family emotional status with intervention, support, and referral as appropriate.

Chemical

DEFINITION
Chemical burns arise from skin contact with acid or alkali or corrosive metal. Chemicals combine progressive damage over an extended period of time. Alkalis are more dangerous than acids. This injury is most common in industries such as fertilizer production, insecticide spraying, dry cleaning, paint manufacturing, chemical processing, or whereever caustics are used. Home accidents causing chemical burns may be due to dishwasher soaps, house cleaning supplies, chlorine bleach, *etc.* School-related chemical burns occur mostly in science laboratories. *Tar burns* are a combination of chemical and thermal injury and are generally incurred during roof construction or road construction or repair.

ASSESSMENT
   I. Health history.
   A. Determine types(s) of chemical causing injury.
   B. Ascertain immediate care rendered, including attempts to neutralize chemical agent.
   C. Note if accident is work-related.
   D. Note past medical history, including drug therapy and allergies.
   E. Obtain tetanus immunization status.
   II. Physical and behavioral assessment. Note the following:
   A. Redness, erythema, severe discoloration of contacted tissue.
   B. Swelling and local hyperemia.
   C. Pain and hypersensitivity.
   D. Disruption of skin causing loss of tissue fluid by "weeping" (may be present).
   E. Affected area warm to hot by touch due to heat of chemical reactions and hyperemia.
   F. Excoriated and "raw" appearance.
   III. Diagnostic tests. Dependent upon extent of injury.

PROBLEMS
   I. Physiologic.
   A. Denuded skin or severely disrupted integrity.
   B. Hypersensitivity to temperature and pressure changes.
   C. Sepsis.
   D. Progressive reactions extending destruction of protective tissue (i.e., skin and connective tissue).
   E. Impaired mobility of affected areas, including joints and moveable parts.

II. Psychosocial.
   A. Pain.
   B. Body disfigurement and image changes.
   C. Emotional turmoil and feelings ranging from anxiety and anger to depression, depending on severity and residual effects.
   D. Financial losses depending on extent of injury and delay of return to work.

GOALS OF CARE
I. Neutralize caustic agent immediately.
II. Remove contaminating source to reduce further exposure, i.e., remove contaminated clothing.
III. Restore protective function of skin and other affected tissue.
IV. Reduce complications of sepsis and disfigurement.

INTERVENTION
I. Immediately flush area with copious amounts of water, for a lengthy time.
II. Control restlessness and pain by titrated diazepam (Valium), 1 to 5 mg IV or 2 to 5 mg orally or IM, and meperidine hydrochloride, 50 to 100 mg IM, or morphine sulfate, titrated, 1 to 5 mg IV, respectively.
III. *Tar burns:* wash with soap and warm water carefully and thoroughly or petroleum jelly to soften congealed tar, if indicated.
IV. Remove small areas of congealed tar with selected use of solvents such as skin cleanser, ether, mineral oil, or Scriptoil. Some can be removed by freezing with ice or ethyl chloride spray and then gently peeling the tar off.

EVALUATION
I. Skin grafting and further plastic repair contingent on early and rapid removal of caustic agent.
II. Prepare for hospitalization only in severe or suspected progressive destruction cases.
III. Provide patiet teaching of safety measures to reduce further incidences of chemical burns.
IV. Refer to community health nurse if home follow-up is indicated.

Radiation

DEFINITION
Radiation burns are due to radioactive, ionizing effects on all tissue exposed. May be accompanied by extreme thermal radiation, i.e., flash burns, as well as secondary burns from fission products, fall-out in contaminated water or gound, generally caused by bomb blasts or radioactive substance leaks in nuclear plants. Ionizing radiation effects are caused by one or all of the following:

1. *Alpha rays,* caused or emitted by unfissioned bomb residues of plutonium or uranium. This material may be deposited in bones and cause long-term bombardment of tissue.
2. *Beta rays,* emitted from fission products, enter body via skin, inhalation, ingestion, or break in skin. Not as penetrating as gamma rays; have similar mechanism of injury as alpha rays, i.e., localize in bone tissue and cause severe signs and symptoms. These have delayed but constant bombardment effect.
3. *Gamma rays,* liberated for very few seconds after high air burst; act like high-energy x-ray machine. Range of effect varies with size of bomb (or spray); can be lethal for several miles from explosion. Rays have extensive and tremendous penetration and are most important cause of radiation injuries.
4. *Neutrons,* formed by combination of a positively charged proton and an electron; have a short range in comparison to gamma rays. Greatest concern is the fission products formed when striking earth surface, i.e., beta and gamma rays. Victims shielded from initial blast of gamma rays may develop acute symptoms from neutron exposure.
5. *Sunburns,* are a mild type of radiation injury due to overexposure to ultraviolet radiation. Burns can be categorized into first or second degree according to depth of injury. Exposure and extent of injury determine prognosis.

Radiation exposure requires decontamination prior to triage or simultaneously with emergency treatment if rescue or aid personnel are properly protected. Triage teams may face extreme moral and emotional concerns when categorizing victims into class IV, due to lethal-dose radiation injuries.

ASSESSMENT
I. Health history.
   A. Obtain description of radiation forces, interval of exposure, and events surrounding incident.
   B. Obtain information regarding decontamination efforts and relative radioactivity still present.
   C. Ascertain from triage officer to which category of care the victim has been assigned.
   D. Note past medical and drug history, including allergies.
   E. For all hopelessly injured, seek choice of religious caretaker, i.e., minister, priest, rabbi.
II. Physical and behavioral assessment.
   A. Discoloration with initially intact skin and underlying tissue (erythema).
   B. Second degree burn with immediate blister formation accompanying the erythema (may be present).
   C. Persistent severe vomiting within 2 h after exposure (usually).
   D. High fever, diarrhea, tenesmus, and dehydration.
   E. Extreme prostration with death due to toxic effects and complete peripheral vascular collapse occurring within a few hours to days.
   F. Can demonstrate anger, frustration, anxiety, fear, and depression, depending on prognosis and speculated complications.
   G. Sunburns: dermal hyperemia, with burned surface hot to touch.
   H. Lesser degree of symptoms noted in point D, above.
   I. Severe pain unrelated to size of affected area (usually).
III. Diagnostic tests.
   A. Initially, radioactive levels as determined by beta-gamma instruments accompanied with audio amplifiers.
   B. CBC, Hb, Hct, platelet count, RBC, differentials.
   C. Urinalysis for myoglobinuria and other evidence of tissue destruction.
   D. Bone scans for radioactive elements.
   E. Electrolytes.

PROBLEMS
I. Physiologic.
   A. Massive denudation or alteration of protective tissue (skin) integrity.
   B. Fluid shifts and losses.
   C. Shock.
   D. Progressive tissue destruction and death.
   E. Alteration of blood components and normation and growth of various cells.
   F. Sepsis.
   G. High fever.
   H. Extreme fatigue and physical immobility.
   I. Sensory and/or motor impairment depending on extent of destruction.
   J. Leukopenia.
II. Psychosocial.
   A. Pain.
   B. Social restrictions until fully decontaminated.
   C. Emotional gamut of anxiety, frustration, anger, fear, and depression.
   D. Perceptions of body image change even if immediate structural disruption is delayed.
   E. Impending death with accompanying needs of religious care.

GOALS OF CARE

I. Decontaminate victim immediately.

II. Minimize complications of sepsis and fluid imbalances.

III. Support cardiopulmonary functions during shock stage.

IV. Reduce pain and discomfort, physical and emotional.

V. Establish support system(s) for terminal victims.

INTERVENTION

I. For *sunburn radiation:*

    A. Remove victim from exposure; cool affected areas with cool, moist (rotating) packs. Assist cooling by evaporation and convection methods.

    B. Reduce systemic febrile state with antipyretics, i.e., aspirin, 5 to 10 gr orally or support every 3 to 4 h, or acetaminophen, 325 to 650 mg orally every 5 h.

II. For other radiation exposure:

    A. Decontaminate immediately, remove all contaminated clothing, and properly isolate for patient and personnel protection.

    B. Provide analgesia with aspirin or narcotics according to need and extent of injury.

    C. Fluid resuscitate with amount and composition commensurate with losses, i.e.:

        1. Saline and other fluids orally if possible (1 tsp of table salt and $\frac{1}{2}$ tsp of baking soda dissolved in 1000 mL of water, give orally).

        2. IV normal saline or Ringer's, 1000 mL with caution *not* to overload the intravascular circulation.

        3. May administer sodium bicarbonate, 1000 mL of a 2% solution via rectum every day (15).

    D. Control nausea and vomiting with antiemetics such as the phenothiazines, i.e., chlorpromazine hydrochloride (Thorazine), 25 to 50 mg orally or IM; prochlorperazine (Compazine) dimaleate, 5 to 10 mg orally; or antihistamines such as dimenhydrinate (Dramamine), 50 mg orally, rectally, or IM.

    E. Support cardiovascular function with ephedrine sulfate, 50 mg orally tid, or 25 to 30 mg in 500 to 1000 mL of 5% dextrose in water or 5% dextrose in normal saline IV; or levarternol or metaraminol IM or IV (16).

    F. Keep burned areas clean, covered with sterile dressings; may be exposed if in filtered airflow rooms.

    G. Be observant for any bleeding tendencies, and notify chief of care immediately.

    H. Cautiously use IM and IV routes due to increased possibility of bleeding and lowered resistance to infection.

    I. Prepare for pending terminal state by including family, religious caretaker, and significant others in plan of care.

    J. Provide mental health support via nursing staff and consultants.

EVALUATION

I. *Sunburn radiation:*

    A. Provide patient teaching for prevention of future similar occurrences.

    B. Continue to assess relief of pain, extent of nausea, vomiting, fluid loss.

II. For other radiation burns be aware that:

    A. Survivors of initial nuclear insults must be followed throughout lifetime for possible residual effects.

    B. Tremendous societal stigma surrounds nuclear industry and particularly warfare, so that radiation victims may be isolated.

    C. Treatment and follow-up care is financially exhaustive.

    D. Genetic mutations occur in radiation victims, so that offspring are potentially mentally and physically retarded.

SHOCK

DEFINITION

Shock is a generalized state of *severe circulatory inadequacy* causing little to no tissue perfusion. Classifications proposed by Blalock in 1934 and still used today are:

1. *Hypovolemic shock,* as caused by hemorrhage and uncompensated extracellular fluid losses such as intestinal obstruction ("third space" trapping), major burns, crushing injuries, fistulas, and peritonitis. Marked by intense peripheral vasoconstriction.
2. *Cardiogenic shock,* due to inadequate cardiac pumping which accompanies pathologies such as: myocardial infarction leading to insufficiency; some cardiac arrhythmias, i.e., multifocal and salvos of premature ventricular contractions; impaired mechanical function of the heart, i.e., tamponade, papillary muscle infarction, or massive pulmonary emboli.
3. *Vasogenic shock,* sometimes referred to as neurovasogenic shock, of which septic shock is the best example. Mechanism occurs at reflex vasodilatation with decreased peripheral vascular resistance. Most commonly seen in spinal anesthesia block, fainting, insulin shock, and anaphylactic shock.

Capillary flow is impaired in all shock types, with both pre- and postcapillary sphincters constricted initially. Eventually, the precapillary sphincters relax, and blood begins to pool in the capillary bed. These events are described as ischemic anoxia progressing to stagnant anoxia. There is a marked drop in pH across the capillary beds, with stasis and backflow causing massive sequestration. Blood viscosity change in low-flow states due to catecholamine release, lowered pH, and release of lysosomal enzymes. Hypercoagulability follows low-flow states and with vasoconstriction, helps to reduce the blood loss further.

The progression of cellular events starts with reduction of aerobic metabolism, less ATP formation, influx of Na and water causing cellular edema, K^+ leaving the cell, rapid pH change to metabolic acidosis, lysosomal breakdown, destruction of cellular membranes, and bradykinin and histamine release. Activation of certain plasma polypeptides with powerful vasoactive properties, the appearance of proteolytic enzymes, and extracellular acidemia are early signs. Late results include irreversible capillary endothelial damage and intravascular coagulation.

ASSESSMENT

I. Health history.
   A. Obtain description of events leading to shock condition.
   B. Note time of onset and duration of symptoms.
   C. Obtain past medical history, including medications and allergies.
   D. Note all care administered prior to hospital admission and during receiving unit phase.
   E. Ascertain last tetanus immunization if shock is due to injury.
   F. Ascertain patient's religious faith.
   G. Note if shock is due to work-related injury.
   H. Note if patient is wearing emergency-type jewelry or tags signifying special considerations.
II. Physical and behavioral assessment.
   A. Level of consciousness.
   B. Circulatory signs of hypovolemia, hypotension, and decreased tissue perfusion.
   C. Anxiety, irritability, personality changes, fear, other emotional changes as shock worsens.
   D. Compensatory responses of:
      1. Rapid, shallow respirations.
      2. Tachycardia.
      3. Increased peripheral vascular resistance.
      4. Surge of catecholamine release.

     5. Blood glucose rises initially.

     6. Blood pressure may be variable.

  E. Warm, pink, dry peripheral tissue (septic shock) or cold, clammy, cyanotic white skin.

  F. Febrile or lower than normal temperature (with septic shock).

  G. Reduced urine output.

  H. Peripheral tissue hemostasis and intravascular coagulation.

III. Diagnostic tests.

  A. CBC and differential.

  B. Hb, Hct, BUN, blood sugar (increased BUN, increased creatinine in septic shock).

  C. Electrolytes: Na^+, K^+, Cl^-, Ca^{2+}.

  D. Arterial blood gases for acid-base and oxygenation determination (respiratory alkalosis, early, with metabolic acidosis as shock progresses).

  E. ECG, 12-lead.

  F. Blood typing.

  G. Platelet count.

  H. Coagulation screen.

  I. Fibrinogen index, FSP (fibrin split products).

  J. Blood cultures and/or other specimen cultures.

PROBLEMS

I. Physiologic.

  A. Tissue anoxia.

  B. Derangement of circulation.

  C. Reduced urinary output and increase of unexcreted toxic products.

  D. Cerebral anoxia from hypovolemia.

  E. Fever.

  F. Fluid and electrolyte imbalances.

  G. Acid-base imbalance.

  H. Hypoxemia.

  J. Bleeding and clotting abnormalities.

  J. Sepsis (septic shock).

II. Psychosocial.

  A. Loss of consciousness.

  B. Anxiety, irritability, fear, occasionally "incident" amnesia or current events amnesia.

  C. Social immobilization.

GOALS OF CARE

  I. Reestablish normal tissue perfusion.

  II. Adequately oxygenate tissue.

  III. Replace fluid and electrolyte losses.

  IV. Restore acid-base balance.

  V. Eradicate infection.

  VI. Reduce complications of intravascular hemorrhage and coagulation.

  VII. Reorient to reality and consciousness as appropriate to total well-being (avoid increasing fear and/or anxiety by recounting extensive details or announcing facts which may be misunderstood regarding the "shock" state).

INTERVENTION

  I. Place victim in supine position with legs elevated (if no head injury or predisposing contraindications; hypovolemic shock).

  II. Insure patient airway and adequate oxygenation with nasal prongs, mask, or intubation as reflected by arterial blood gas determinations.

  III. Stop all external bleeding.

  IV. Monitor vital and neurologic signs frequently and until stabilized after treatment.

V. Fluid resuscitate with balanced salt solutions, i.e., Ringer's, Dextran, Rheomucrodex, or normal saline via two large-bore intravenous lines at rapid rate and amount to maintain systolic blood pressure at 90 mmHg (hypovolemic shock).

VI. Type and cross-match for whole blood or packed RBC according to estimated blood loss and laboratory results of Hb and Hct.

VII. Obtain blood specimen for type, and cross-match (hypovolemic shock).

VIII. Frequently monitor laboratory parameters of electrolytes, cultures, and sensitivities, urinalysis, BUN, blood sugar, coagulation screens, platelet counts, creatinine, Hb and Hct, as appropriate to specific shock states.

IX. Insert Foley catheter and monitor hourly output, specific gravity, pH, and presence of hemoglobin and/or myoglobin.

X. If ordered, administer large doses of hydrocortisone preparations if victim has received appropriate replacement fluids, i.e., hydrocortisone sodium succinate (Solu-Cortef), 50 mgKg immediately into IV, or methylprednisolone sodium succinate (Solu-Medrol), 30 mg/kg given over a 10-min interval. Repeat dose once, given IV, to maximum of 1 g (17).

XI. Obtain standard 12-lead ECG.

XII. If febrile and/or toxic, obtain three to six blood cultures in rapid succession. Culture wounds, drainage, and selected specimens of urine, mucus, etc.

XIII. Administer appropriate antibiotics for septic shock as determined by causative organisms and sensitivity reports from laboratory, e.g., gentamycin sulfate, 3 mg/kg per 24 h in three doses and given IM or IV, and Cloxacillin sodium, 2 g every 4 h plus Clindamycin, 300 mg every 6 h IV or Ampicillin, 400 mg/kg per 24 h (in six doses) IV.

XIV. Administer tetanus prophylaxis if victim is at risk or injuries are massive and contaminated.

XV. Utilize vasopressors and cardiotonics (i.e., levarterenol bitartrate, 4 mg in 100 mL of 5% dextrose in water slowly, phenylephrine hydrochloride, 3 to 5 mg in 500 to 100 mL, carefully).

XVI. Monitor central venous pressure throughout resuscitation phase, and maintain between 6 and 8 cmH₂O pressure.

XVII. Auscultate lung sounds frequently during fluid resuscitation to ascertain progressive or increasing congestion.

XVIII. If patient manifesting symptoms of *cardiogenic shock,* begin IV infusion of dopamine at 2.5 μg/kg per minute, and increase dose according to package insert calculations.

XIX. Correct arrhythmias, and prevent ventricular fibrillation (may begin prophylactic Lidocaine at 1 to 4 mg min IV).

XX. Correct acid-base abnormalities with sodium bicarbonate 50 mL of 8.4% solution (50 meq) bolus.

XXI. If in *septic shock* and febrile, support with increase of calories, i.e., to 5000 cal per day depending on needs.

XXII. Administer heparin therapy if evidence of disseminated intravascular coagulation.

XXIII. Obtain clergy's and social worker's assistance for victims with grave prognosis or as requested by victim and/or family.

EVALUATION

I. Continue to monitor fluid balance.
   A. Fluid losses of 5 percent manifest clinical signs and symptoms.
   B. Fluid losses of 10 percent cause grave concern and high incidence of mortality if left untreated.

II. Follow through on blood replacement therapy as follows:
   A. With a 1- to 2-U loss of blood, electrolyte administration via a balanced salt solution will suffice, i.e., Ringer's lactate.
   B. With a 2- to 5-U blood loss, replacement consists of balanced salt solution (Ringer's) and partial amount of red blood cells.

C. With 5 U or more lost, replacement requires red blood cells and protein or reconstituted whole blood.

III. Frequently reassess treatment effects on electrolyte balance, respiratory and cardiovascular functioning, renal output, and level of consciousness.

RESPIRATORY TRAUMA

Upper Airway

DEFINITION

Upper airway trauma includes any disruption of structure or function caused by obstruction, restriction, avulsion, loss of bony or cartilaginous integrity, tears and penetrations, or by paralysis due to abrupt interruption of nerve innervation. The anatomical components considered include: nose and nasal-sinus combinations (ethmoid, sphenoid, frontal, nasal pharynx, oral pharynx, maxillary), larynx, trachea. Trauma is usually due to foreign bodies; falls; auto accidents; burns; industrial accidents; self-inflicted or homicidal acts of gunshot, stabbing, strangulation; blunt blows; accidental penetrating wounds. Foreign bodies may include: broken dentures, chewing gum, cuds of tobacco, regurgitated debris and partially digested food, blood, food bolus, mechanical items, hardware (for poisons and upper respiratory complications, see Chap. 45).

ASSESSMENT

See Table 44-1 for localization of respiratory obstructions.

I. Health history.
   A. Obtain description of mechanism or forces causing injury(ies).
   B. Note victim placement in auto, position of body during traumatic encounter.
   C. Obtain past medical history, particularly respiratory pathology, including medications and allergies.
   D. Note if injuries are work-related.
   E. Note if victim has previously been blood transfused.
   F. Ascertain if victim vomited prior to admission.
   G. Describe if victim has indicated suicidal behavior in recent past.

II. Physical and behavioral assessment.
   A. Hemorrhage, internal or external, with resultant hypotension and tachycardia.
   B. Asphyxia, dyspnea, forcible inspiratory efforts.
   C. Nasal-facial-nuchal deformity(ies), if any. Check for symmetry, depression, accessive mobility, augulations, etc.
   D. Choking, coughing.
   E. Shrill, high-pitched noises with inhalation, exhalation (foreign bodies, obstruction, restriction).
   F. "Sucking," "hissing" movement of air (through structural disruptions which have more than one passage).
   G. Stertorous respirations.
   H. Crepitus.
   I. Subcutaneous emphysema.
   J. Fractures, dislocations.
   K. Visible, nonvisible foreign bodies.
   L. Discolorations of skin and mucous membranes, cyanosis.
   M. Fractured, displaced, avulsed teeth.
   N. Edema.
   O. Presence of cerebrospinal fluid (CSF) drainage.
   P. Signs of sepsis.
   Q. Pain.
   R. Loss of sensation, gag and swallow reflexes.
   S. Loss of voice.

TABLE 44-1 / LOCALIZATION CHART: RESPIRATORY OBSTRUCTION

Sign or Symptom	Pharynx	Larynx	Trachea	Bronchi
			Level of Obstruction	
Voice changes	Slurred or thick	Hoarse or absent	Decreased volume	Decreased volume
Cough	Persistent, scratchy	Stridulous, "croupy"	Reflex irritative	Reflex irritative
Swallowing	Difficult	Difficult	Usually normal, but occasionally painful	Normal
Dyspnea	Positional	Inspiratory	Inspiratory	Often present with wheezing
Cyanosis	May be present; relieved by position changes	May be present	May be present	Often present
Intercostal retraction	Usually absent	Inspiratory	Inspiratory	If a large bronchus is blocked
Breath sounds	Normal	Roughened, coarse	Coarse rales and rhonchi	Rhonchi; absent over collapsed lung
Restlessness, excitement, apprehension	Intermittent; acute during episodes of dysphagia and dyspnea	Often acute	Rarely occur	Acute if a large bronchus is blocked

Source: Thomas Flint and Harvey Cain, *Emergency Treatment and Management,* 5th ed., W. B. Saunders Company, Philadelphia, 1975, p. 346.

    T. Thermal burns, carbon particles around mouth and nose.
    U. Emesis.
    V. Lacerations, penetrations.
III. Diagnostic tests.
    A. X-ray.
    B. Fluoroscopy.
    C. Laryngoscopy.
    D. Surgery for exploratory purposes (avulsions, foreign body discovery).
    E. Arterial blood gases for hypoxemia, respiratory acidosis, alkalosis.
    F. CBC, differential, Hb and Hct for all injuries with hemorrhage.
    G. Culture, sensitivities on CSF drainage.
    H. CSF determinations by ring test or dropping on Clinitest tablet. Type and cross-match blood for all massive wounds involving face and neck air passages.

PROBLEMS
  I. Physiologic.
    A. Inadequate airway patency.
    B. Acid-base imbalance.
    C. Edema, subcutaneous swelling.
    D. Shock.
    E. Altered vocal communication.
    F. Hemorrhage.
    G. CSF leakage.
    H. Sepsis.
    I. Aspiration complications, both upper and lower airways.
 II. Psychosocial.
    A. Pain, discomfort.
    B. Body image change if face or neck contours altered.
    C. Fear, anxiety, depression, agitation.
    D. Social immobilization with vocal or oral disruptions.
    E. Overwhelming financial costs with life-saving therapeutics.
    F. Criminal case if homicide attempt (gunshot, stabbing, etc.).

GOALS OF CARE
   I. Reestablish airway patency.
  II. Stop hemorrhage.
 III. Remove foreign body, and reduce local irritation.
 IV. Return to normal acid-base range.
  V. Oxygenate to preinjury status.
 VI. Reduce complications and residual changes.
VII. Alleviate pain, fear, other psychologic concerns.
VIII. Return to normal vocal communication pattern.
 IX. Return to preaccident face and neck structure and profile (long-term goal).

INTERVENTION
   I. Establish airway with endotracheal, nasotracheal tube, airway, patient positioning (chin lift, head tilt, unless contraindicated by cervical injury, then jaw thrust), or cricothyrotomy.
  II. Remove airway obstruction by encouraging conscious victim to forcefully cough. If unconscious, establish airway and attempt to ventilate. If unable to ventilate, provide victim with four back blows, four manual thrusts, and finger probe through mouth to remove foreign bodies before attempting next ventilation. If still unsuccessful, repeat or initiate abdominal thrusts, chest thrusts (see Fig. 44-17).
 III. Aspirate airway, and periodically suction all mucus and drainage to keep airway patent.

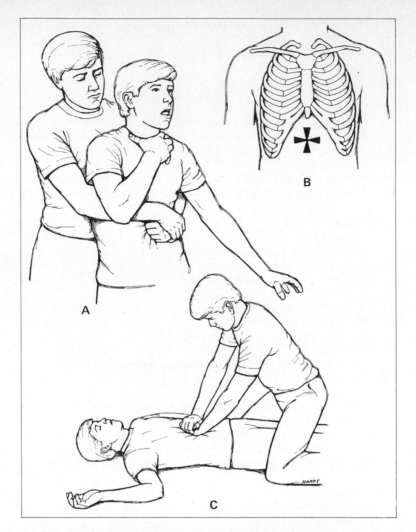

FIGURE 44-17 / The Heimlich maneuver. (*a*) The victim is grasped from behind as quickly as distress is signaled. (*b*) The rescuer's fist should be pressed into the upper abdomen at the spot marked by the cross. (*c*) Correct position of rescuer when patient is found lying face up. Note the placement of the hand, which permits a quick upward thrust. (*From John Henderson, Emergency Medical Guide, McGraw-Hill Book Company, New York, 1978.*)

IV. Provide 5 to 10 L of 100% oxygen initially, and follow arterial blood gas results for continued therapy.

V. Place on volumetric respirator if air passages are severely disrupted and high index for swelling.

VI. Administer muscle relaxant (or respiratory paralyzer) under supervision of physician, if unable to remove foreign body due to spasms. Give succinylcholine derivative according to recommended dosages on package insert. Be prepared to support victim's ventilations with positive pressure breathing bag or mechanical ventilation.

VII. Stop hemorrhage by nasal or nasopharyngeal packing, cautery, epinephrine spray, ligation of oozing vessel, treatment of underlying cause, or surgical repair, as appropriate.

VIII. Start large-bore IV line(s) for administration of medications using 1000 mL of 5% dextrose in water.

IX. Begin fluid resuscitation with large-bore IV and 1000 mL Ringer's, and continue with appropriate fluids and/or blood.

X. Cautiously administer analgesia or sedation by titrated IV route, e.g., morphine sulfate, 2 to 8 mg, depending on respiratory status, or give meperidine hydrochloride, 50 to 100 mg IM (Demerol).

XI. Begin broad-spectrum antibiotic therapy if wounds contaminated or CSF drainage noted.

XII. Monitor vital signs frequently, and in particular watch for changes in respiratory patterns and rate.

XIII. Prepare victims of penetrating neck wounds for immediate surgical debridement, exploration, and repair.

XIV. Administer tetanus prophylaxis if victim at risk.

XV. Provide emotional support to victim and family, especially if face and neck have been severely mangled.

EVALUATION

I. Monitor continuously effects of intervention on:
   - **A.** Respiratory function.
   - **B.** Control of hemorrhage.
   - **C.** Return of fluid and electrolyte balances.
   - **D.** Relief of pain.
   - **E.** Alleviation of anxiety.

II. Reevaluate antibiotic therapy when culture report available.

III. Prepare patient for transfer to intensive care unit or surgery for continued treatment.

Lower Airway

DEFINITION

Lower airway trauma includes any disruption of structure or function caused by obstruction, restriction, avulsion, loss of bony integrity, tears and penetrations, or paralysis due to abrupt interruption of neurologic innervation. Anatomical components considered include the bronchial tree (main right and left), individual lobes of the lung, alveoli, and thorax (ribs and sternum). Trauma is usually due to acceleration-deceleration forces; falls; industrial or auto accidents; blunt blows; penetrating wounds of gunshot, stabbing, and impaled objects which are accidental, suicidal, or homicidal in nature. Drivers may have "steering wheel" injuries: sudden sharp pressure changes due to a blow against the steering column can rupture the diaphragm with resultant herniation of the abdominal contents into the pleural cavity. Foreign bodies that may become lodged are essentially the same as those listed under "Upper Airway" and may have to be dislodged to a lower airway position. Cardiopulmonary resuscitation (CPR) may cause costochondral separations and rib fractures.

ASSESSMENT

I. Health history.
   - **A.** Obtain description of mechanism or forces causing injury(ies).
   - **B.** Note environmental influences altering mechanism or forces.
   - **C.** Note if injuries are work-related.
   - **D.** Ascertain past medical history, including medications and allergies.
   - **E.** If auto accident, obtain description of victim's position in car.
   - **F.** Note if victim has previously been blood transfused.
   - **G.** Ascertain if victim vomited prior to hospital admission.
   - **H.** Seek information regarding suicidal or homicidal act causing injuries.

II. Physical and behavioral assessment.
   - **A.** Signs of inadequate gas exchange, hypoxia, hypoxemia.

    B. Hemorrhage, internal or external, with resultant hypotension and tache.

    C. Asymmetry of thorax statistically and/or during ventilations.

    D. Cyanosis, central and peripheral.

    E. Sucking or hissing sounds on exhalation.

    F. Wheezing, rales, rhonchi, musical noises on inspiration and/or expiration.

    G. Signs of shock (decreased blood pressure, narrowed pulse pressure, increased pulse, weak, thready pulse, restlessness, apprehension, decreased urine output, increased ventilation).

    H. Hyperresonance (pneumothorax).

    I. Pain.

    J. Arrhythmias, including atrial flutter, fibrillation, ectopy, paroxysmal atrial tachycardia.

    K. Distant, muffled heart sounds.

    L. Dullness to no auscultate and breath sounds.

    M. Agitation, anxiety, depression of consciousness.

    N. Tracheal deviation to unaffected side.

    O. Tachycardia.

    P. Fractures, dislocations, flail chest.

    Q. Edema, swelling, crepitus, subcutaneous emphysema.

    R. Lacerations, abnormal openings to lungs and airways.

    S. Scaphoid abdomen: indication of abdominal contents herniation into chest.

    T. Excessive abdominal movement with respirations: in males may indicate chest wall damage.

    U. Hemoptysis.

    V. Mediastinal emphysema, dislocations.

    W. Bloody froth issuing from wound, e.g., tension pneumothorax from penetrating wound.

    X. Paradoxical pulse (pulsus paradox).

III. Diagnostic tests.

    A. Radiography.

    B. Bronchoscopy.

    C. CBC, differential, Hb, Hct.

    D. Type and cross-match blood if large blood loss.

    E. Arterial blood gas determinations.

    F. ECG, 12-lead, and continuous (dynamic) monitoring.

    G. Arteriovenous shunt calculations, arteriovenous extraction rates.

    H. Diagnostic tap: plunger of moistened glass syringe pushed out by increased intrathoracic pressure.

    I. Massive air leak when established on water seal drainage.

PROBLEMS

I. Physiologic.

    A. Inadequate gas exchange with resultant hypoxemia, cyanosis.

    B. Shock.

    C. Hemorrhage.

    D. Acid-base imbalance.

    E. Loss of structural integrity: thorax, cartilaginous tissue, parenchymal tissue collapse.

    F. Edema, swelling, subcutaneous and mediastinal emphysema.

    G. Aspiration complications.

    H. Sepsis.

    I. Physical immobility.

II. Psychosocial.

    A. Pain.

    B. Agitation, fear, anxiety, depressed consciousness.

    C. Body image changes.

    D. Social and financial immobility.

    E. Criminal case if homicide attempt (gunshot, stabbing, etc.).

GOALS OF CARE

I. Reestablish adequate ventilation and aerobic respiration.

II. Stop hemorrhage.

III. Support structural components of thorax until healed (fractures and separations).

IV. Reduce complications of sepsis, deformity, reduced tissue oxygenation, etc.

V. Reinflate lungs to preincident status, and stabilize.

VI. Reestablish acid-base, fluid and electrolyte balances.

VII. Alleviate pain and emotional trauma.

INTERVENTION

I. Immediately establish adequate airway patency with endotracheal or nasotracheal intubation and mechanical ventilation, positive pressure bag-mask and oxygen, or intranasal catheter and pressurized oxygen.

II. Start 100% oxygen therapy at 5 to 10 L, and continue therapy based on arterial blood gas reports.

III. Watch for signs of tension pneumothorax, especially if patient has been placed on a volumetric respirator, (i.e., absent breath sounds on affected side and deviated trachea away from tension pneumothorax).

IV. Decompress pleural space (tension pneumothorax) with No. 16 or 18 needle and 50-mL moistened syringe and plunger. Cleanse skin over area lateral to the midclavicular line in the second or third interspace on the side of tension pneumothorax. With head of bed at 60 to 90°, insert needle and attached syringe. Allow increased intrapleural pressure to force plunger out of syringe. Withdraw plunger and let air escape. When hissing noise stops, withdraw needle and cover puncture site with dry dressing.

V. Continue to monitor vital signs frequently, particularly rate, depth, and pattern of respirations.

VI. Intubate and bag victim with a flail chest who is having respiratory difficulty.

VII. Stabilize a flail chest with sandbag, tape, and padding (position victim on affected side); sterile towel forceps and slight traction; prepare for surgical repair.

VIII. Auscultate chest frequently to ascertain adequacy of ventilations and stasis of secretions.

IX. Further support flail by intubation and continuous mandatory ventilation with positive end expiratory pressure (PEEP) or intermittent mandatory ventilation with continuous positive airway pressure (CPAP). Avoid insertion of chest tube with victim in supine, flat position, as this increases risk of diaphragm injury.

X. For stabbing and gunshot wounds, protect evidence of clothes particles, carbon dust on skin, smoke residue, or other debris as site is cleansed. Lightly scrape specimens into sterile containers before introducing cleansing agents. *Avoid irrigating gunshot, stabbing wounds of chest.*

XI. Cover sucking wound with Vaseline-impregnated gauze during end of exhalation.

XII. Prior to insertion of water seal or negative pressure chest drainage, for atelectatic lung, ask patient to deep-breathe in, then forcefully exhale against a closed glottis, and quickly cover or stabilize wound with a dry sterile dressing and occlusive dressing. May reinflate atelectatic segment and buy time.

XIII. Administer analgesics by IV titration: morphine sulfate, 2 to 8 mg. Avoid respiratory depressants if victim is not supported with mechanical ventilator. May use meperidine hydrochloride, 50 to 100 mg IM. Closely observe victim responses.

XIV. Stop any external bleeding with pressure dressings and rib belt. Note downward changes in blood pressure with stabilized respiratory to indicate internal bleeding.

XV. Start fluid resuscitation; get blood typed and cross-matched, Hb and Hct; and prepare for exploratory surgery.

XVI. Assess all victims who have received CPR for fractured ribs, costochondral separations, and adequate expiratory effort.

XVII. Massive dose and early administration of methylprednisolone may be given.

XVIII. Protect skin and soft tissue from further injury when edematous, filled with subcutaneous emphysema, ecchymotic, i.e., careful consideration of pressure areas.

XIX. Administer appropriate broad-spectrum antibiotics if victim has aspirated or has high index of suspicion for infection.

XX. Administer tetanus prophylaxis if victim at risk.

XXI. Insert a nasogastric tube to decompress stomach and reduce pressure on diaphragm, hence lungs.

XXII. Place on cardiac monitor for careful observation of arrhythmias and cardiac arrest.

EVALUATION

I. Be aware that early or immediate reduction of an air leak and pneumothorax space will reduce complications of emphysema and bronchopleural fistula.

II. Reevaluate possible diaphragm injuries; these injuries are easily missed; all drivers of autos should be carefully reexamined for "steering wheel" marks.

III. Watch use of high ventilating pressures to inflate lungs. Following penetrating chest wounds may cause air emboli and resultant systemic complications.

IV. Continue to monitor respiratory function control of bleeding, return of fluid and electrolyte balances, relief of pain and anxiety.

CARDIAC AND GREAT VESSEL TRAUMA

DEFINITION

This type of trauma is a disruption of structure and/or function caused by penetration, avulsion, contusion, rupture, or tearing of cardiac muscle and/or vessels, arteries, and veins in the heart, superior and inferior vena cava, aorta, and pulmonary, subclavian, and femoral arteries. The most frequent causes of this trauma include high-speed automobile and motorcycle accidents, heavy industrial equipment accidents, and accidental, suicidal, and homicidal acts. The mechanism involved may be a direct blow, transmitted blow, compression, deceleration, blast overpressure, or combinations of these.

ASSESSMENT

I. Health history.

A. Describe mechanism or forces causing injury(ies).

B. Note if victim was driver, wearing shoulder strap or pelvic seat belt, placement in auto, position of body during traumatic encounter.

C. Obtain past medical history, particularly if cardiac pathology, including medications and allergies.

D. Note if injuries are work-related.

E. Note if victim has received CPR prior to admission.

F. Ascertain if victim on anticoagulant therapy: look for Medic-Alert or similar medical jewelry on victim.

G. Note if victim has received blood transfusions previously.

H. Note if victim has indicated suicidal behavior in recent past.

I. Ascertain tetanus immunization record.

II. Physical and behavioral assessment.

A. Hemorrhage: external and internal, with resultant hypotension and tachycardia.

B. Changes in cardiovascular system:

1. Arrhythmias; ventricular fibrillation; sinus tachycardia; coarse atrial fibrillation, flutter, gallop rhythms; extra sounds of S_3 or S_4; new conduction defects.

2. Asystole.

3. Distant, muffled, "mushy" heart sounds.

4. Mechanical alternans, pulsus paradoxus, pulsus alternans.

5. Asymmetry of upper and/or lower extremity blood pressures, e.g., rupture of aorta, hypertension of upper extremities and hypotension in lower extremities.

6. Narrowing pulse pressure.

7. Enlarged and/or displaced (point of maximal impulse) PMI.
8. Distension of jugular veins when the head of the bed is raised more than 45°.
9. Visible "atrial kick."
10. May have friction rub from traumatic pericarditis.
11. Sudden onset aortic regurgitation, mitral regurgitation.
12. Murmurs; bruits (e.g., systolic murmur over precordium or on the back medial to the left scapula with rupture of aorta).

C. Precordial, substernal, diffuse pain; back and subscapular pain (with ruptured aorta).
D. Hoarseness due to hematoma pressure on left recurrent laryngeal nerve.

III. Diagnostic tests.
   A. Serial ECGs.
   B. Radiography. Look for:
      1. Widened mediastinum on anteroposterior x-ray.
      2. Enlarged cardiac silhouette.
   C. Arterial pressure monitoring.
   D. Hb and Hct, CBC with differential; type and cross match blood.
   E. Arterial blood gases.
   F. Arteriography.

PROBLEMS

I. Physiologic.
   A. Alteration of electrophysiology.
   B. Disrupton of myocardial (muscle) contractibility.
   C. Hemorrhage.
   D. Loss of circulation or perfusion pressure from conduit rupture or tear or cardiac event.
   E. Hypoxemia.
   F. Physical immobilization.
II. Psychosocial.
   A. Pain.
   B. Catastrophic insult to psyche, including fear, anxiety, moroseness.
   C. Social and financial immobility with prolonged loss of work, insurance claims, etc.

GOALS OF CARE

I. Reestablish electromechanical cycle which generates normal cardiac ejection pressure.
II. Stop hemorrhage: tamponade.
III. Reestablish adequate circulating volume and components.
IV. Maintain pretrauma arterial oxygenation and saturation.
V. Reestablish adequate tissue perfusion.
VI. Resume activities of daily living.
VII. Eliminate pain.
VIII. Develop a healthy mental attitude and coping mechanism to deal with the associated emotional trauma.

INTERVENTION

I. Immediately establish patent airway with endotracheal tube with adequate ventilation. Subsequently administer 100% oxygen until arterial blood gas results available.
II. Insert two lines with large needles, No. 16 or 18, for IV fluids and medications.
III. Obtain blood type, and cross match immediately.
IV. Provide fluid resuscitation with Ringer's lactate, normal saline, colloid solutions, blood, and/or blood component therapy commensurate with losses. Be sure massive or exsanguinating bleeds are replaced by fresh whole blood with retained clotting factors/or cryoprecipitate.
V. Obtain arterial blood gases every 30 to 60 min until oxygen saturation is maintained within normal limits.

VI. Obtain electrolytes every 4 to 8 h, Hb, Hct; coagulation screen including PT, PTT, platelet count when blood replacement passes 10 U of banked blood.

VII. Immediately assist with pericardiocentesis. *Be sure treatment of fluid resuscitation has begun.*

VIII. Constantly monitor vital signs with comparisons of bilateral blood pressures and pulses.

IX. Establish arterial line, and monitor to keep systolic greater than 90 mmHg unless victim was a known hypertensive prior to accident, then keep systolic between 130 and 140 mmHg.

X. Obtain frequent chest x-rays for comparison.

XI. Compare apical and radial pulses for narrowing pulse pressure.

XII. May monitor central venous pressure (CVP) if no arterial lines available. Maintain pressure between 10 and 12 cmH$_2$O.

XIII. Insert nasogastric tube to low, intermittent suction (decompress stomach). Calculate fluid and electrolyte losses; monitor pH of gastric contents every 4 to 8 h.

XIV. Insert Foley bladder catheter, and monitor output every hour, specific gravity, and pH.

XV. Obtain chest x-ray only if victim's condition is stable.

XVI. Prepare for immediate surgical intervention in the operating room in cases of penetrating cardiac trauma or rupture of aorta.

XVII. Place victim on continuous cardiac monitoring.

XVIII. If victim has blunt cardiac trauma, treat much like acute myocardial infarction with arrhythmia monitoring, minimal activity level, and bed rest, serial enzymes, appropriate drugs.

EVALUATION

I. Continue to monitor the following until appropriate transfer to surgery or intensive care unit is accomplished:

A. Cardiovascular function.
D. Respiratory function.
B. Renal function.
E. Level of consciousness.
C. Fluid and electrolyte balances.
F. Relief of pain.

II. Be aware that:

A. Penetrating wounds of aorta have more serious prognosis than cardiac stab wounds due to:

1. High pressure sustained in the aorta.
2. Thinner aortic wall that does not seal as well as the myocardium.
3. Mediastinum less resistant to the egress of blood than an intact pericardium.
4. Delayed rebleeding of aorta is more common.
5. Survivors of the initial aortic insult are at higher risk for future problems of false aneurysm or arterior venous fistula.

B. Prognosis for cardiac contusion is excellent.

ABDOMINAL TRAUMA

DEFINITION

Abdominal trauma includes any disruption of structure and/or function caused by penetration, rupture, tear, contusion, avulsion, or ingestion of corrosive agents or foreign bodies, which involves the abdominal viscera or wall.

The anatomical components considered are liver, small bowel, stomach; colon; mesentery and omentum; spleen; diaphragm; pancreas; duodenum; biliary system, including liver and gallbladder; pancreas; retroperitoneal structures and kidneys. Other lesser structures of uterus, sciatic plexus, urinary bladder, ovary, adrenals, vagina, and muscles. The trauma may be due to high-velocity auto and motorcycle accidents, causing sharp and blunt injuries; seat belt syndrome; penetrating wounds of stabbing, gunshot, and shotgun, knives, glass, scissors, screw drivers, pencils, automobile radio antennae, bicycle spokes; crush injury;

blast injury from air or immersion which usually affects air-filled organs more severely; corrosive gastritis from hydrochloric, nitric, trichloracetic, sulfuric, and carbolic acids or alkalis affecting the esophagus; ingested foreign bodies. Many iatrogenic causes for abdominal injury include endoscopy with biopsy; external cardiac compression, CPR; paracentesis or thoracentesis; peritoneal dialysis; rupture from inhalation therapy; barium enema; sigmoidoscopy; peritonealoscopy; liver biopsy; radiation therapy with corrosion to bowel or specific organ. Mechanisms of iatrogenic problems can be categorized into two major areas: extra- and intraperitoneal perforations and radiation injuries. Mortality is generally correlated with the number of abdominal organs injured and the relative destruction of each.

ASSESSMENT

I. Health history.
  A. Obtain description of mechanisms or forces causing injury(ies).
  B. Note if driver of auto and/or passengers wearing seat belt and what type.
  C. Describe speed or abruptness of onset of symptoms.
  D. Note previous medical history, including medications, allergies, and abdominal surgical history.
  E. Describe drinking history, cultural mores.
  F. Note if injuries are work-related.
  G. Note if victim has received blood transfusions previously.
  H. Note if victim received CPR prior to admission.
  I. Ascertain additional and/or associated injuries.
II. Physical and behavioral assessment.
  A. Hemorrhage.
  B. Symptoms of hypovolemic shock with resultant compensatory mechanisms of tachycardia, hypotension, oliguria, peripheral vasoconstriction, increased circulating catecholamines, increased blood glucose, normal range Hb and Hct progressing to hemodilution, tissue ischemia leading to total organism death.
  C. Signs of sepsis.
  D. Pain: diffuse; burning; peristaltic; rebound tenderness; referred.
  E. Findings on abdominal examination:
    1. Absence of bowel sounds; abnormal location; bruits with major vessel disruption.
    2. Rigid and guarded abdomen.
    3. Spillage and loss of intraluminal contents, i.e., bile, gastric juices, proteolytic enzymes.
    4. Abdominal mass(es).
    5. Tympany of abdomen.
    6. Girth size increases rapidly.
  F. Degrees of unresponsiveness.
  G. Loss of dullness over major organs (percussion).
  H. Less common signs: priapism, testicular pain.
  I. Kehis sign (left shoulder pain).
  J. Associated rib fractures: posterior (left), 9 to 12 (spleen injury).
III. Diagnostic tests.
  A. Culdocentesis.
  B. Vaginal and bimanual examinations.
  C. Rectal examination.
  D. Hb, Hct, CBC, including WBC and differential, serial Hct.
  E. Radiography.
  F. Peritoneal lavage with laboratory analysis of RBC, WBC, bile, amylase and bacteria; paracentesis.
  G. Radionuclide photo images (spleen injuries).
  H. Serum albumin, prothrombin, serum transaminases, lactic dehydrogenase (LDH), serum bilirubin, serum amylase, BUN, blood glucose.
  I. Electrolytes.
  J. Urinalysis.

   K. Radiography: flat plate of abdomen and kidneys, ureter, and bladder, then for free air, dilatation, and extravasation of contrast media.

   L. Liver and spleen scans.

PROBLEMS

  I. Physiologic.
    A. Circulating volume deficit (saline losses).
    B. Hypotension and shock.
    C. Fluid and electrolyte imbalances.
    D. Acid-base derangement.
    E. Hemorrhage.
    F. Oncotic pressure losses and third spacing.
    G. Massive tissue devitalization and necrosis.
    H. Sepsis.
    I. Physical immobilization.

  II. Psychosocial.
    A. Pain.
    B. Prolonged loss of work.
    C. Emotional responses ranging from anger and frustration to depression.
    D. Cultural implications of odiferous gut contents spillage.

GOALS OF CARE

   I. Establish patent airway and adequate ventilation.
   II. Restore preinjury circulating volume balance.
  III. Stop hemorrhage.
   IV. Reestablish normal fluid and electrolyte balances.
   V. Reestablish normal acid-base range.
   VI. Restore patency of gastrointestinal tract.
  VII. Progressively return digestion, absorption, and elimination processes.
 VIII. Prevent infection.
   IX. Relieve pain and discomfort.
   X. Provide emotional reassurance; referral to ancillary support services, if indicated.

INTERVENTION

   I. Establish patent airway with intubation, and provide adequate ventilation to maintain arterial oxygenation at $P_{O_2} = 80$ mmHg.

   II. Insert two large-bore needles, No. 16 or 18, to administer IV fluids and medications.

  III. Provide fluid resuscitation with Ringer's lactate, normal saline, colloid solutions, blood and/or blood component therapy, commensurate with losses. Be sure massive or exsanguinating bleeds are replaced by fresh whole blood with retained clotting factors or cryoprecipitate.

  IV. Obtain blood type, and cross-match immediately.

   V. Insert Foley bladder catheter to straight drainage, and monitor hourly until output stable.

  VI. Insert nasogastric tube, and connect to intermittent suction drainage.

 VII. Continue to obtain serial electrolytes, BUN, Hb, Hct, and arterial blood gases.

VIII. Establish a CVP line and/or pulmonary wedge pressure monitoring.

  IX. Establish careful intake and output records.

   X. Mark abdomen at greatest girth size, and measure for baseline data.

  XI. Stabilize associated injuries, i.e., pneumothorax, hemothorax, disruption of cardiac function which is life-threatening.

 XII. Obtain baseline weight.

XIII. Administer electrolyte therapy to begin one-half correction of losses plus regular basic allowances. This should be a 24-h plan.

XIV. Assist with peritoneal lavage by obtaining trochar and/or knife handle and blades of varying sizes and shapes, peritoneal dialysis catheter, and 1 L of normal saline or balanced salt solution for flush; tape and dry dressings.

XV. Provide analgesia by IV titration and careful observation of victim if pending or is in shock or has respiratory insufficiency.

XVI. Administer tetanus prophylaxis if victim is at risk.

XVII. Monitor vital signs with blood pressure in supine and relative standing (bed change) positions until stable at more than 90 mmHg systolic.

EVALUATION

I. Carefully reassess for abdominal injuries: this is in lieu of other more prominent and obvious trauma.

II. Reevaluate at regular intervals patency of airway, fluid and electrolyte balances, signs of cardiovascular problems, symptoms of shock, relief of pain and discomfort.

NEUROTRAUMA

DEFINITION

Neurotrauma is a disruption of structure and/or function caused by penetration, avulsion, contusion, concussion, rupture, shearing or tearing of dura, brain parenchymal tissue, vessels, spinal cord, and peripheral nerves leaving or entering spinal column; also, penetration and/or fracture of bone skull.

Anatomical components from most cerebral to caudal include: *cerebral hemispheres,* including sensory and motor strips, basal nuclei, and lateral ventricles; *diencephalon,* with thalamus, hypothalamus, pineal body, and foramen of Monroe connecting to third ventricle; *mesencephalon* (midbrain), which includes cerebral aqueduct of Sylvius, cerebral peduncles, oculomotor (III) cranial nerves, and trochlear (IV) cranial nerves, and corpora quadrigemina (which are reflex centers for visual, auditory, and tactile impulses); *pons,* a bridge between cell bodies, the pontine nuclei, and each half of the cerebellum. Included are nerve roots of the trigeminal (V) cranial nerve. At the pons base, abducens (VI), facial (VII), and acoustic or auditory (VIII) cranial nerves. *Medulla* includes the reticular formation, the glossopharyngeal (IX), vagus (X), accessory (XI), and hypoglossal (XII) cranial nerves, *brain coverings* of Dura mater, arachnoid mater, pia mater; *vessels of importance,* middle meningeal arteries, circle of Willis, including arteries of: anterior cerebrals, anterior communicating, middle cerebrals, posterior communicating arteries, then arteries of: basilar, vertebrals, and internal carotids: veins of superior sagittal sinus and transverse sinuses; *spinal cord,* particularly cervical C2 to C6, thoracic T1 to T12, and lumbar L1 to L12.

The trauma usually results from high-speed automobile and motorcycle accidents; falls; heavy industrial equipment accidents; accidental, suicidal, and/or homicidal acts.

The mechanisms of injury include acceleration-deceleration; blunt blows; crushing; penetration by bullets, stabbings, impaling objects; torquing with subsequent shearing, tearing, or rupture; "whiplash" of cervical spine (acceleration); cord compression with associated mechanical distortion of neural tissue and local cord ischemia and contusion; vascular insufficiency which complicates contusion and some fractures; and combinations of above.

Most common types of fracture types are basal, temporal, parietal, occipital, and frontal with associated sinus disruptions.

ASSESSMENT

I. Health history.

A. Obtain description of mechanism or forces causing injury(ies), i.e., speed, impact.

B. Note victim's initial complaints and level of consciousness, particularly prehospital if there is a reliable historian.

C. Note if motorcyclist(s) wore helmet(s).

D. Ascertain if victim was thrown from car, how many feet, the position in which victim was found.

    E. Ascertain if victim was wearing seat or shoulder belt.

    F. Obtain past medical history, including medications and allergies. Note particularly if victim has known drug or alcohol abuse.

    G. Ascertain if victim has recently had:

        1. Ingestion, inhalation, injection of drugs or alcohol.

        2. Hypoglycemic state or other physical disruption of arrhythmia, myocardi infarction.

        3. Cessation of respiration for any reason.

        4. Fainting.

        5. Abrupt onset of neurologic or special sensory deficit.

    H. Obtain description of victim's cultural, educational, social background.

    I. Note if victim wears glasses or contact lenses.

    J. Ascertain tetanus immunization record.

    K. Look for medical tag or identification.

    L. Note if injuries are work-related.

    M. Note if victim has indicated suicidal behavior in recent past.

II. Physical and behavioral assessment.

    A. Hemorrhage.

    B. Respiratory patterns commencing with normal rate, depth, and rhythm and progressing from cerebral to caudal fashion:

        1. Epileptic respiratory inhibition.

        2. Apraxia for breath holding or deep breathing.

        3. Cheyne-Stokes (slow hypnea-apnea; suprastentorial).

        4. Posthyperventilation apnea.

        5. Central neurogenic hyperventilation (localizing in midbrain and brainstem pons; excessive, rapid hypnea); *Biot's* respirations.

        6. Periodic apneustic (arrest of respiration during inspiration; upper pons).

        7. Ataxic (unregulated; medulla or pontomedullary junction).

        8. Agonal.

    C. Levels of consciousness: may be awake and alert to time and date, surroundings, people of family, and lastly self, with coma on the other end of continuum.

    D. Other signs of neurologic deficit:

        1. Orientation, disorientation.

        2. Speech: aphasia-type.

        3. Pupillary reflexes: round, level, and properly placed; briskly reactive to light; consensual agreement, accommodation to no response; fixed and dilated, nystagmus. Extraocular muscles of lateral medial; dolls' eyes; corneal reflex may be absent: wisp cotton gently over cornea or eyelashes to produce "blink," "sunset" eyes; "cat's eyes;" pinpoint pupils of pons lesions; photophobia, diplopia.

        4. Motor reflexes:

            a. Pyramidal or motor tract responses, upper motor neuron:

                (1) Babinski, positive.

                (2) Clonus, sustained or intermittent, unsustained.

            b. Deep tendon reflexes:

                (1) Equal response (symmetry).

                (2) Hyperactive (increased).

                (3) Hypoactive (decreased).

        5. "Frontal lobe" release signs (elicit by tapping upper lip):

            a. Rooting, snorting.   *c.* Teeth grinding.

            b. Sucking.   *d.* Cortical thumb.

        6. Ciliospinal reflex: pinch sternocleidomastoid muscle, and eyes (pupils) jerk to side of stimulus.

        7. Deep pain. Melnick triad: response to pressure of examiner's knuckles on sternum, against optic nerve as it courses through a foramen-medial supraorbital ridge; and pinch of testicle or nipple. May have violent headache with diffuse irritation of meninges (if awake to tell examiner); may respond with nuchal rigidity.

8. Decorticate posturing (rigidity): flexion of upper extremities; extension of lower extremities with "toeing in."
9. Decerebrate posturing (rigidity); extension and internal rotation of upper extremities; extension of lower extremities and "toeing in."
10. Areflexic: no response to any stimuli (flaccidity).
11. Weakness of muscle strength which progresses from normal motion. Decreased motion against gravity, slight contractility to no contractility.
12. Drifts of extended extremities.
13. Battle's sign: bleeding into mastoid sinus with obvious ecchymosis due to fracture through temporal bone.
14. Dermatographia. Fingernail over abdominal skin: raised, welted line which shows the victim has lost sympathetic nervous system innervation.
15. Altered pain, pressure, touch and thermal sensations.
16. Altered body temperature control.

E. Systolic blood pressure and falling diastolic blood pressure.
F. Hemorrhage; open through wounds, as space-occupying lesions, into orbital space, ear canal, nose, etc.
G. Cerebral spinal fluid rhinorrhea or otorrhea as noted by spot test: bloody center with peripheral clear ring or drop on glucose test strip with positive result.
H. Cushing triad:
   1. Projectile vomiting.
   2. Papilledema.
   3. Vital sign changes.
I. May have "traumatic" diabetes insipidus with copious urine output of very low specific gravity (1.001).
J. Lateralizing signs.
K. Crepitance, false motion, and tenderness over cervical spine fracture.
L. Pain and/or selected loss of sensation; loss of voluntary movement with spinal injury.
M. Loss of bladder, bowel control; priapism.
N. Extreme agitation, restlessness, depression with head trauma.
O. Pain: headache.
P. Movable fractures, dislocations, and physical changes.
Q. Edema, swelling of injured cervical, thoracolumbar muscles.
R. Rigidity and splinting of neck and back muscles with spinal fractures.
S. Initial loss of consciousness, followed by lucid interval with rapid deterioration as arterial bleed progresses (epidural bleed).

III. Diagnostic studies.
A. Radiography: most common types are anteroposterior, lateral skull; Towne (half-axial view); cervical views including the odontoid for C1 to C2 fractures. Note pineal gland shifts of greater than 2 mm from midline.
B. Cerebral angiography to identify intracranial space-occupying lesions.
C. Trephine-Burr holes to locate subdural hematomas (craniectomy).
D. Computerized axial tomography (CAT scan).
E. Twist drill (through cranium) to locate hematoma.
F. Radioactive scan (may diagnose intracerebral hematoma, subdural and/or extradural hematoma).
G. Echoencephalography (ultrasound technique) to determine presence of midline shift.
H. Questionable use or relevance of EEG (electroencephalogram).
I. Questionable use or relevance of ventriculography or pneumoencephalography.
J. Lumbar puncture: *Rarelh or never use with head injury due to herniation risk.*
K. Urinalysis.
L. CBC, differential, Hb, Hct, electrolytes.

    M. Blood cultures.

    N. Secretion cultures for pyrogens gaining entrance through breaks into dura and/or cranial vault.

PROBLEMS

  I. Physiologic.

    A. Cerebral hypoxia, ischemia.

    B. Changing intracranial pressure.

    C. Altered cerebral circulation.

    D. Loss of physical control, i.e., disrupted sensory and motor function.

    E. Edema, hemorrhage, sepsis.

    F. Fluid and electrolyte imbalances (if diabetes insipidus).

    G. Open and/or communicating wounds.

    H. Spinal shock.

    I. Incontinence: involuntary release of rectal sphincter.

    J. Gastric and bowel immobility.

  II. Psychosocial.

    A. Loss of consciousness or varying degrees thereof.

    B. Possible change of orientation to complete disorientation.

    C. Immobility: social, emotional, financial with prolonged loss of work.

    D. Pain.

    E. Sensory deficits of touch, pressure, thermal, verbal.

    F. Catastrophic psychic disruption to "lose time"; fear, anxiety, depression, anger.

    G. Concern over residual deficits, i.e., paresis, paralysis, impaired thought, learning, reasoning functions (integrative).

GOALS OF CARE

  I. Establish airway and adequate ventilation.

  II. Stabilize vertebral column.

  III. Reestablish cerebral circulation and tissue perfusion.

  IV. Restore fluid volume.

  V. Minimize sepsis and residual complications.

INTERVENTION

  I. Immediately establish patent airway (with intubation as necessary), and adequately ventilate based on serial arterial blood gases.

  II. Immediately triage for cervical spine injury, immobilize with back board, collar, sand bags or any material which keeps neck and head from moving.

  III. Prevent aspiration or obstruction by careful suctioning and positioning to encourage gravity drainage.

  IV. Stop or reduce hemorrhage of all external wounds by packing and pressure dressings. Note increasing ecchymosis of mastoid area, orbital space, etc., and report.

  V. Thoroughly assess neurologic (especially levels of consciousness) vital signs; cardiac rhythm; physical signs of CSF drainage or ecchymoses, position and extent, and record every 15 min until stable. *Watch for signs of increasing intracranial pressure.*

  VI. *Carefully* administer *isotonic* IV fluids to maintain blood pressure and urine output. *Limit* intake to keep patient "on dry side."

  VII. Maintain *careful* recording of intake and output. *Prevent fluid overload.*

  VIII. Obtain serum electrolytes and Hct as needed, at least every 24 h.

  IX. Maintain quiet, reality-oriented environment. *Avoid or limit stimulation and hyperactivity.* Do not allow patient to initiate Valsalva maneuver.

  X. Elevate head of bed 30° to aid in venous return, or maintain preset height if ventriculostomy tube in place.

XI. Observe for bladder and gastric detention if catheter and nasogastric tubes are not in place.

XII. Monitor hourly urines for amount, specific gravity, and pH in any serious head injury. Note change indicating traumatic diabetes insipidus.

XIII. Watch for any occlusion of jugular venous return (e.g., occlusive, tight dressings, tape).

XIV. Carefully observe acid-base balance to avoid hypercarbia (i.e., ventilate by bagging a tidal volume which does not reduce venous return from the head).

XV. Watch and protect victim against neurologic deficit pressure areas, and position and reposition to avoid skin breakdown. If patient is placed on "egg carton" mattress or low-pressure mattress, touch contact parts of body to stimulate dinferent sensation. (Keeps patient from becoming "weightless" and sensory deprived and "floating out of reality.")

XVI. Maintain anatomical positions of function for feet, wrists, and hands by placing bolsters, foot board, or supports to feet. Provide passive range-of-motion four times a day between regular bath or bedtime care. Keep body properly aligned.

XVII. Provide mental health consultation and/or psychosocial, emotional, spiritual support to patient and family.

XVIII. If victim is on circle bed, Bradford frame, or other special bed, constantly orient and protect patient.

XIX. Meticulously monitor all rhinorrhea or otorrhea, and maintain reverse isolation to avoid sepsis.

XX. May administer diuretics (osmotic-type such as mannitol area), of limited use except to "buy time" when cerebral edema present.

XXI. May administer corticosteroids for cerebral edema (dexamethasone, 4 to 12 mg, depending on physician preference).

XXII. May assist with internal decompression (partial temporal lobe resection) for cerebral edema refractory to conservative treatment.

XXIII. In cerebral edema, hyperventilate to keep P_{CO_2} approximately 30 to 32 to promote cerebral vasoconstriction.

XXIV. Administer prophylactic diphenylhydantoin (Dilantin), 100 mg bid, tid, or at level satisfactory to avoid seizure activity. (Necessary for victims with trauma, including disrupted dura.)

XXV. For excessive febrile states, place patient on hypothermia mattress and gradually decrease temperature to approximately 100°F (38°C).

XXVI. For febrile states, may administer acetaminophen (Tylenol) or acetylsalicylic acid (aspirin) orally or by suppository.

XXVII. Medicate with appropriate antibiotics according to culture and sensitivity reports. Initially, may anticipate contaminating organism and begin broad-spectrum antibiotic *after* first cultures are obtained.

XXVIII. Keep hyperchlorhydria to minimum by administering antacids via nasogastric tube, with clometidine to maintain gastric pH greater than 6. Check gastric contents for positive guaiac.

XXIX. Observe victim carefully for signs of complications, including: *neurogenic pulmonary edema and inappropriate ADH release* (antidiuretic hormone) causing expanded extracellular and intracellular volume leading to decreased aldosterone output. This causes urinary salt loss, known as "cerebral salt wasting."

XXX. If oral intake possible, five Tegretol; if not, administer Pitressin for traumatic diabetes insipidus.

XXXI. Carefully maintain ventrivulostomy tube and any intracranial pressure monitor probes in exact degree to head of bed and ventricles.

XXXII. Constantly orient patient to surroundings, procedures, time, date, and personnel. Be sensitive to patient's unspoken and uncommunicated needs. Consult with social worker and mental health personnel for special or financial needs.

XXXIII. Administer tetanus prophylaxis if at risk.

CHILD ABUSE

DEFINITION
The term "child abuse" includes any problem resulting from a lack of adequate or reasonable care and/or protection of children by their parents, guardians, or other care providers (18). It is especially important to diagnose possible cases of abuse and/or neglect within the first 6 months of life, because of the increased risk of a fatal outcome if such a diagnosis is not made. Types of abuse include:

1. Physical, e.g., bruises, fractures, burns, head injuries, or any nonaccidental trauma inflicted by a caretaker (19).
2. Nutritional neglect, e.g., failure to thrive, malnutrition, dehydration.
3. Emotional neglect or abuse, e.g., scapegoating, terrorizing of a child, locking child in closet, basement.
4. Sexual abuse, e.g., vulvitis, vaginitis, or venereal disease in prepubertal child should arouse suspicions of sexual abuse.
5. Neglect of medical care, e.g., not following through on prescribed treatment for a chronic disease, withholding insulin from a child diabetic.

ASSESSMENT
I. Health history.
   A. Obtain time, place, situation surrounding child's injury; usually there is an implausible or vague explanation given.
   B. Note any discrepancies between histories offered by two parents or during two separate interviews.
   C. Obtain child's innoculation history, medical records, history of allergies.
   D. Note if any delay in seeking medical care for injury (very common).
   E. Obtain child's dietary history, i.e., formula preparation, amounts given and retained, etc., if nutritional neglect suspected.
II. Physical and behavioral assessment. Note any of the following:
   A. Bruises, welts, scars at multiple stages of healing.
   B. Fingerprints on arms (from grabbing child).
   C. Lash and/or choke marks.
   D. Human bite marks: crescent-shaped areas of hyperpigmentation with light centers.
   E. Burns (especially from cigarettes on palms and soles).
   F. Acute hyphema, dislocated lens, detached retina.
   G. Coma, convulsions (suspect subdural hematoma).
   H. Recurrent vomiting with abdominal distension.
   I. Absent bowel sounds.
   J. Localized abdominal tenderness.
   K. Paucity of subcutaneous tissue (failure to thrive), e.g., pinched face, wasted buttocks, prominent ribs.
   L. Recurrent subluxations (especially of elbows, shoulders).
III. Diagnostic tests.
   A. Bleeding time, platelet count, prothrombin time.
   B. Failure to thrive indicated by:
      1. CBC.
      2. Erythrocyte sedimentation rate.
      3. Urinalysis and culture.
      4. Stool pH.
      5. Serum electrolytes.
      6. Calcium level.
      7. BUN.
   C. Appropriate x-rays for trauma, i.e., long bones, skull, ribs, and pelvis (look for multiple bone injuries at different stages of healing).

PROBLEMS

Dependent on extent of injury:

I. Decreased respiratory function.
II. Decreased cardiovascular function.
III. Coma, convulsions.
IV. Pain.
V. Emotional trauma of victim.
VI. Fractures, bruises, burns, possible complications with residual impairment, possible sepsis.
VII. Possible hemorrhage.
VIII. Fluid and electrolyte imbalances.

GOALS OF CARE

Dependent on extent of injury:

I. Maintain respiratory function.
II. Relieve pain, discomfort.
III. Maintain cardiovascular function: stop hemorrhage.
IV. Monitor neurologic status: assist with control of convulsions.
V. Treat fractures, bruises, burns appropriatelh.
VI. Maintain fluid and electrolyte balances.
VII. Provide emotional support, comfort to child and family members.

INTERVENTION

I. Assist respiratory function as indicated, i.e., CPR if needed, administration of oxygen placement on mechanical ventilator, etc.
II. Assure adequate cardiovascular function with cardiac monitoring, vital sign and blood pressure check at frequent intervals, auscultation of heart regularly, intravenous insertion for medication administration and fluid replacement.
III. Monitor neurologic status of patient (see Chap. 23).
IV. Relieve pain with appropriate medications, e.g., Tylenol, Demerol (IM), as indicated.
V. Control hemorrhage, and provide for fluid replacement if needed: ascertain regular serum electrolytes, accurate fluid intake and output, urine specific gravity.
VI. See "Fractures," "Contusions," and "Burns" for specific interventions appropriate to each.
VII. Institute ongoing support with appropriate referral to social, supportive agencies or individuals for victim *and* parents.

EVALUATION

I. Report to local protective services agency. This is required by law.
II. Consider referral to public health nurse for home services to family, home assessment of other siblings, and environmental conditions.

REFERENCES

1. Walter F. Ballinger, Robert Rutherford, and George Zaidema, *The Management of Trauma*, W. B. Saunders Company, Philadelphia, 1973, p. 2.
2. Jeanie Barry, *Emergency Nursing*, McGraw-Hill Book Company, New York, 1978, p. 336.
3. Howard Rapaport, "Disarming Insect Stings," *Drug Therapy*, **5:** 272–277, May 1975.
4. Ibid.
5. Ibid.
6. Ibid.
7. Ibid.
8. Barry, op. cit., p. 385.
9. Judie Wischman and Peggy McMahon, "The Patient with Surface Trauma" (unpublished).
10. Ibid.
11. Ibid.

12. Ibid.
13. Ibid.
14. Ibid.
15. Jeffrey Jahre et al., "Medical Approach to the Hypertensive Patient and the Patient in Shock," *Heart and Lung*, **4:** 577–587, July–August 1975.
16. Ibid.
17. "Therapeutic Considerations in Critical Care Medicine," Upjohn Publication H-5891-4, 1977, p. 31.
18. Victor Vaughn, James McKay, and Waldo Nelson, *Nelson Textbook of Pediatrics*, W. B. Saunders Company, Philadelphia, 1975, p. 107.
19. Ibid.

BIBLIOGRAPHY

Barry, Jeanie (ed.): *Emergency Nursing*, McGraw-Hill Book Company, New York, 1978. Excellent nursing text dealing with the basics in emergency care. Good review of systems initially tied into discussion of pathophysiology throughout rest of book. Very concise tables throughout text that pinpoint signs and treatment required for various emergency care situations.

Flint, Thomas, and Harvey Cain: *Emergency Treatment and Management*, 5th ed., W. B. Saunders Company, Philadelphia, 1975. Basically a treatment manual for common emergency care situations. Very concise, accurate accounting of problems and the immediate *medical* intervention required.

Henderson, John: *Emergency Medical Guide*, McGraw-Hill Book Company, New York, 1978. In-depth section on some outdated material, individual poisons, relevant symptoms, and appropriate treatment in basic and advanced life support, but a fairly good source for information about poisons, drug abuse, and musculoskeletal trauma.

Primary Care Nursing: A Manual of Clinical Skills, F. A. Davis Company, Philadelphia, 1977. This is an outstanding compilation of solid intervention techniques, developed from a curriculum devised for nurses who practice in the remote areas of Canada. Much of the information can be readily adapted for nursing use in emergency situations inside or outside a major institution.

45
Medical Emergencies
Marilyn de Give and Annalee Oakes

POISONINGS

Drug Abuse: Overdose

Definition   An *overdose* is any intoxication created by a greater than therapeutic level of medication: ingested, inhaled, injected, or otherwise consumed without prescription or under the supervision of medical personnel. The act of administering a medication with the ultimate result of toxic and/or greater than normal range levels and for other than therapeutic reasons may be accidental or intentional. Therefore, the victim may also have committed a misdemeanor, and *the nurse is legally required to report all incidences of drug overdoses where certain drugs are identified.* The most common overdosed medications include salicylates, narcotics, sedatives, tranquilizers, mood elevators, and antipsychotics.

Assessment   I. Health history.

   A. Ascertain victim's drug abuse previously, and the type. What drugs are available to the patient? If victim is a poor historian, telephone neighbors, ask relative or police to search premises for drugs.

   B. Ascertain multiple doses and kinds for combination effects.

   > ***Example***   A person ingested large amounts of Dilantin, atropine, aspirin, Nembutal, thyroid extract, and Percodan. He was apneic, comatose, hyperthermic, and hypertensive.

   C. Ascertain initial symptoms which may provide clues as to type of drug involved and/or which suggest additional pathologic processes (diseases).

   > ***Example***   A young woman was thought to have an aspirin overdose, until friends reported the victim had a sudden onset of excruciating headache and immediately ingested a large amount of aspirin; the diagnosis was subarachnoid hemorrhage.

   II. Physical and behavioral assessment.

   A. Initially note respirations and blood pressure, and treat if these vital signs are falling.

   B. Do a careful general and neurologic examination. Pay particular attention to the following:
   1. Levels of consciousness.
   2. Pupil responses.
   3. Eye movements and extraocular movements.
   4. Corneal reflexes.
   5. Optic fundi.
   6. Gag reflex.
   7. Response to pain.
   8. Deep tendon reflexes (DTR).
   9. Evidence of focal weakness.

   C. Beware of diseases that are masquerading as "overdoses," such as subdural hematoma, meningitis, subarachnoid hemorrhage, and brain tumor; particularly look for head trauma

   D. Watch for the associated, additional pathology accompanying the patient with drug intoxication:
   1. Aspiration pneumonia.
   2. Pulmonary edema.
   3. Cardiac arrhythmias.
   4. Hepatitis.
   5. Stabbing or gunshot wounds.
   6. Subacute bacterial endocarditis.
   7. If female, is she pregnant?

    E. Note: Pressure neuropathies and myopathies are common in patients who have not moved for several hours.

    F. Document all evidence of skin lesions, trauma, ecchymoses, and apparent neuropathies (for medicolegal purposes).

III. Diagnostic tests. Routine studies include:

    A. Hematocrit (Hct).

    B. White blood count (WBC).

    C. Urinalysis.

    D. Electrolytes.

    E. Liver function tests.

    F. Blood sugar.

    G. Arterial blood gases.

    H. Electrocardiogram (ECG).

    I. Chest x-ray.

    J. Send blood for appropriate toxicology studies. Since common screen includes only aspirin and barbiturates, must request others for suspected overdosed drug. Provide any information to laboratory regarding drug categories or specificity of amounts, etc.

    K. Send specimen samples of urine and gastric contents for toxicology screen.

Problems

I. Compromise of respiratory function.

II. Fluid-electrolyte imbalance.

III. Loss of consciousness, coma.

IV. Derangement of cardiovascular system.

V. Decline of renal function.

VI. Residual neurologic deficits.

VII. Emotional, social disruption.

Goals of Care

I. Reestablish ventilation; maintain patent airway.

II. Restore to pretrauma fluid and electrolyte balances.

III. Monitor level of consciousness.

IV. Reestablish adequate circulation: monitor and assess cardiac arrthymias (common with drugs such as Elavil and Mellaril).

V. Assist with return of renal function via dialysis or forced diuresis.

VI. Monitor neurologic status persistently for change.

VII. Provide emotional and social resources via direct intervention and appropriate referral for patient and family.

Intervention

I. Do *not* discharge patient if in doubt about consciousness or orientation status.

II. Intubate if shallow respirations, cyanosis, or absent gag reflex noted, or if prognosis indicates respirations may deteriorate.

III. *Do not* perform spinal tap if patient has obvious head trauma, papilledema, or focal neurologic signs.

IV. *Do* perform spinal tap if patient is comatose, has elevated temperature, and/or nuchal rigidity.

V. Obtain skull films for all patients presenting with one or more of the following signs (look for pineal shifts):

    A. Coma.

    B. Lethargy.

    C. Confusion.

    D. Signs of head trauma.

    E. Papilledema.

    F. Focal neurologic findings.

VI. Use syrup of Ipecac or gastric lavage as follows:

    A. Ipecac is useful in purging drugs from stomach only if administered *before* they are absorbed. *Use judiciously* with adequate oral fluids to allow for "flushing" of stomach. Guard against aspiration of contents during vomiting. *Never* administer Ipecac to victim who is known to have ingested fast-acting depressant (e.g., Valium), as patient will produce obtundation as he or she begins to vomit. *Do not* administer Ipecac to patient if:

1. Patient is lethargic.
2. Patient has absent reflex.
3. Patient has ingested hydrocarbon-type compounds.

B. Lavage should be performed on all obtunded and comatose drug intoxication victims. Should be done even several hours after ingestion. Procedure of choice:

1. Insert into stomach large-bore, red rubber tube with multiple holes at gastric end.
2. Place head lower than waist.
3. Initially *intubate* if comatose or gag reflex absent.
4. Use copious amounts of normal saline with 100 to 200 mL at a time (intermittent flow and drainage).
5. Do not cool normal saline in order to avoid lowering body temperature.
6. Continue lavage intil return is clear, which may require 10 L or more (usually 2 to 5 L is sufficient).
7. Visually inspect gastric contents for drug particles.
8. Send sample (20 to 50 mL) of gastric contents to toxicology laboratory for analysis.

VII. General management for any drug intoxication should include:

A. Frequent observation at 15- to 30-min intervals, to note changes in:

1. Levels of consciousness.   3. Pupils.
2. Vital signs.   4. Signs of focal neurologic deficit.

B. Postural drainage of secretions, frequent tracheal suctioning (provision for meticulous airway care and patency).

C. Intravenous (IV) line with 5% dextrose in water for medications and fluid resuscitation.

D. Turning and repositioning of patients at frequent intervals (at least every 2 h) to reduce pressure areas and neuropathies.

E. Protective eye care if unconscious (i.e., methylcellulose eye drops and taping of lids).

F. Cardiac monitoring if risk of cardiac arrhythmia (i.e., with drugs such as Elavil and Mellaril).

VIII. The question of *hypoxic brain damage* should not be a determining factor in emergency room treatment. Certain drugs may produce fixed pupils and cause neurologic depression bordering death, and the victims may fully recover. Only after several days have passed and drug levels dropped to zero, if neurologic deficits persist, then hypoxic brain damage may be a factor (1).

IX. Assist with dialysis or forced diuresis.

A. *Dialysis* is life-saving in ethylene glycol poisoning and when deep coma is prolonged (e.g., phenobarbital or Placidyl).

B. *Diuresis* (forced) and alkalization of the urine is of little value generally and may be dangerous, especially in patients with renal or heart failure. *May be helpful in aspirin intoxications.*

X. *Withdrawal syndrome* may follow acute intoxication, which is manifested in many by only slight agitation and brisk tendon reflexes, progressing to gross delirium and convulsions resembling alcohol withdrawal. Look for other causes of delirium such as electrolyte imbalance and infection (elevated temperature). May need to treat withdrawal with intravenous fluids, restraints, and sedation.

XI. If patient's signs worsen after initial 24 h, look for another cause of coma.

XII. Obtain *psychiatric consultation* for all drug intoxication patients. Patients should be restrained until it is determined they are not an immediate danger to self or others (2).

XIII. Obtain neurology consult on all people in stupor or coma.

Commonly
Abused Drugs

The following is a categorical listing of drugs which are commonly abused. Key concepts of the most notorious drugs, selected laboratory data, and accepted management are provided as general guidelines for the nurse who delivers early and emergency care to the drug-intoxicated patient.

I. Sedatives, hypnotics, and tranquilizers.

    A. Long acting: phenobarbital. Intermediate acting: secobarbital, pentobarbital, Tuinal (secobarbital and amobarbital).

        1. Key concept. Produce profound CNS depression of several days' duration. Onset is relative to drug, i.e., the intermediate acting have a more rapid onset and shorter duration of action. The longer acting may have a gradual progression of lethargy to coma.

        2. Assessment.

            a. Absent DTR (some patients occasionally have DTR).

            b. Respiratory arrest.

            c. Hyperactive reflexes.

            d. Hypotension.

            e. Hypothermia.

            f. May lose brainstem reflexes (doll's eyes, corneals, cold calorics).

            g. Patients may have an early period of "paradoxical agitation."

        3. Intervention.

            a. Intubation.

            b. Mechanical ventilation.

            c. Intravenous saline for hypotensives if heart and kidneys can tolerate load.

            d. Give vasopressors in severely depressed cases, i.e., dopamine or Levophed to help support blood pressure to 90 mmHg systolic.

            e. Dialysis if in prolonged coma and if barbiturate level is high.

    B. Placidyl (ethchlorvynol), chloral hydrate.

        1. Key concept. Obtundation and sweet breath (Juicy Fruit).

        2. Assessment.

            a. Chloral hydrate and alcohol with "Mickey Finn" may cause:

                (1) Sudden loss of consciousness.   **(3)** Liver damage.

                (2) Irritation of gastric mucosa.   **(4)** Renal cell damage (3).

            b. Placidyl has in addition:

                (1) Associated respiratory depression.

                (2) Hypotension.

                (3) Hypothermia.

                (4) Bradycardia of seizures: exacerbated by alcohol.

            c. Both have withdrawal phenomena.

        3. Intervention.

            a. Basically supportive.

            b. May need dialysis.

    C. Quaalude (methaqualone).

        1. Key concept. A "fashionable drug" with college, university, and some high school populations ("heroin for lovers").

        2. Assessment.

            a. Stupor, coma, and death in similar manner to barbiturates.

            b. Pulmonary edema.

            c. Cutaneous edema.

            d. Hypotension.

            e. Liver and renal damage.

            f. Bleeding disorders.

         3. Intervention. Basically supportive.

    D. Valium (diazepam), Librium (chlordiazepoxide).

        1. Key concept. Valium may produce loss of consciousness in 10 to 30 min, with Librium having a slower reaction and obtundation lasting several days.

2. Assessment. Initial symptoms:
   a. Drowsiness.
   b. Ataxia.
   c. Slurred speech.
   d. Nystagmus.
   e. Respiratory depression, frequently combined with alcohol to cause synergistic effect.
3. Intervention.
   a. Supportive respirations.
   b. Gastric lavage, if early (relative to each drug).
   c. Do not use Ipecac with Valium.

II. Opiates.
   A. Heroin, methadone, codeine, morphine.
      1. Assessment.
         a. Severe respiratory depression, cyanosis.
         b. Pinpoint, nonreactive pupils.
         c. "Railroad tracks."
         d. Pulmonary edema (may be due to contaminants).
         e. Atrial fibrillation.
         f. Other associated complications (endocarditis, hepatitis).
         g. Look for other drug-mixing symptomatology: strychnine, which may have been used to dilute the powder and can produce hyperthermia and convulsions.
      2. Intervention.
         a. Intubate, and support respirations as necessary; use oxygen.
         b. Administer appropriate dose of Naline (nalorphine), i.e., 5 mg IV to produce pupillary dilation and improved respirations.
         c. May have to repeat Naline in 20 to 30 min. Do not use unless quite sure this is an opiate overdose, as Naline causes respiratory depression.
         d. Narcan (Naloxone) is a morphine antagonist at 0.4 mg IV but can also produce primary respiratory depression.
         e. Pulmonary edema and atrial fibrillation usually resolve spontaneously (4).
   B. Darvon (propoxyphene). Member of opiate family; treat accordingly.
      1. Assessment.
         a. Stupor progressing to coma plus respiratory depression.
         b. Pupils pinpoint, unreactive.
         c. Convulsions.
         d. Metabolic acidosis.
      2. Intervention.
         a. Narcan (see above).   d. Intubate if necessary.
         b. Naline (see above).   e. Sodium bicarbonate if necessary.
         c. Oxygen.

III. Stimulants.
   A. Amphetamines: Ritalin (methylphenidate).
      1. Assessment.
         a. Produces agitated hyperactivity progressing to syndrome like heat stroke.
         b. Tremulousness.
         c. Flushing.
         d. Tachycardia.
         e. Mydriasis.
         f. Hypertension.
         g. Hyperactive tendon reflexes.
         h. Vivid, threatening, visual hallucinations.
         i. Muscular twitching.
         j. Dry mouth, nausea, vomiting, abdominal cramps.

    κ. Convulsions, hyperthermia, coma.

    l. Coagulopathies.

> *Note* Look for other drugs which may be complicating situation, i.e., barbiturates and strychnine (amphetamine abusers use barbiturates to "level out the highs"). Watch known amphetamine abusers who present in depressed state as they may have inadvertently overdosed on barbiturates. Monoamine oxidase (MAO) inhibitors may increase severity of amphetamine-induced hyperthermia and hypertension.

  2. Intervention.

    a. Supportive care.

    b. Cooling blanket for hyperthermia.

    c. May judiciously use sedatives; monitor level of consciousness.

    d. May use thorazine carefully.

    e. Ice baths and packs if febrile past 106°F.

    f. May administer antihypertensives in hypertensive crises.

IV. Hallucinogens.

  A. LSD.

    1. Assessment.

      a. May present anticholinergic state, i.e.:

        (1) Agitation.   **(3)** Delirium.

        (2) Hot, flushed.   **(4)** Hallucinations (last 12 to 18 h).

      b. Cardiovascular shock and death when combination of LSD, phenothiazines, and some other hallucinogen taken.

    2. Intervention.

      a. Support observation.

      b. *Very cautiously* provide sedation with diazepam or chlordiazepoxide (Valium or Librium) *only when absolutely* necessary.

  B. Phencyclidine (angel dust).

    1. Key concept. A veterinary anesthetic; "on the street" it can be popped, dropped, or shot.

    2. Assessment.

      a. Agitated or depressed.

      b. Respiratory failure.

      c. Pinpoint pupils which do not respond to Naline or Narcan.

      d. Effect lasts 2 to 4 days with paradoxical excitement in various stages of withdrawal.

      e. Overdose facilitated by alcohol.

      f. If taken IV, may cause sudden death.

    3. Intervention. Support and observation.

V. Anticholinergics (Atropinics): Cogentin, Kemadrin, Artane, over-the-counter sleeping pills (e.g., Sleep-Ez, Compose, Cope).

  A. Assessment.

    1. Delirious.   **6.** Seizures.

    2. Flushed.   **7.** Urinary retention.

    3. Hyperthermic.   **8.** Paralytic ileus.

    4. Dilated pupils and poor accommodation.   **9.** Tachycardia

    5. Absent perspiration.

> *Note* Psychotic patients on phenothiazines are often taking anticholinergics for their antiparkinsonian effects.

  B. Intervention.

    1. Cooling blanket.

    2. Ice baths, ice packs, for hyperthermia more than 106°F.

    3. Avoid sedatives unless *absolutely* necessary.

    4. Insert Foley bladder catheter.

    5. Support with intravenous fluids as necessary.

VI. Psychotherapeutic drugs.

    A. Thorazine (chlorpromazine), Stelazine (trifluoperazine), Mellaril (thioridazine), Compazine (prochlorperazine), Haldol (haloperidol, α-butyrophenone), Trilafon (perphenazine).

        1. Assessment.

            a. Lethargy.

            b. Hypotension (orthostatic).

            c. Stupor and frank hypotension.

            d. Pulmonary edema.

            e. Cardiac arrhythmias (Mellaril).

            f. Lowered seizure threshold (all phenothiazines).

            g. Urinary retention.

            h. Hyperthermia.

            i. May produce idiosyncratic extrapyramidal symptoms of rigidity, dystonic movements, opisthotonus, oculogyric crises.

            Note Patients taking these drugs usually have a baseline psychotic personality.

        2. Intervention.

            a. Observation, supportive care.

            b. Administer intravenous fluids for hypotension (usually normal saline if heart and kidneys can tolerate it).

            c. Must remain flat in bed until hypotension resolved.

            d. Intravenous Lidocaine or Dilantin (diphenylhydantoin) with Mellaril-induced cardiac arrhythmias.

            e. Provide Benadryl, 50 mg IV, for extrapyramidal symptoms.

    B. Tricyclics ("mood elevators"): Elavil (amitriptyline), Tofranil (imipramine), Norprimin (desipramine), Triptil (prototriptyline), Aventyl (nortriptyline).

        1. Assessment.

            a. Cardiac arrhythmia and sudden death.

            b. Arrive excited with progression to lethargy, obtundation with tachycardia, and hypotension.

            c. ECG changes show marked conduction defects with alterations of terminal phase of the QRS-T complex.

            d. Atrial and ventricular arrhythmias.

            e. Variable degrees of atrioventricular block.

            f. Seizures.

            g. Hyperthermia.

            h. Hypotension or hypertension.

            i. May have anticholinergic or extrapyramidal effects.

        2. Intervention.

            a. Constant ECG monitoring.

            b. ECG changes require Dilantin coverage [250 mg diphenylhydantoin given *slowly* intravenously every 15 to 30 min to total of 1 g, then 300 mg orally per day for 1 week (5); intravenous Dilantin can cause hypotension].

            c. Monitor blood pressure carefully.

            d. *Do not use phenobarbital to counteract seizures* as it exacerbates the effect of tricyclics.

    C. Triavil (perphenazine and amitriptylene).

        1. Key concept. A combination of a phenothiazine and a tricyclic (Elavil).

        2. Assessment.

            a. Obtundation.

            b. Hypotension.

            c. Cardiac arrhythmias.

            d. Seizures.

            e. Hyperthermia.

            f. Anticholinergic and extra-pyramidal symptoms.

     3. Intervention.
       a. Same as above.
       b. Dilantin therapy for arrhythmias may aggravate hypotension.

VII. Aspirin.
  A. Key concept.
     1. Produces metabolic acidosis an respiratory alkalosis.
     2. Blood levels of greater than 40 to 50 mg per 100 mL are considered serious. Blood level may not peak for several hours after ingestion.
  B. Assessment.

     1. Tinnitus.
     2. Headache.
     3. Nausea.
     4. Hyperventilation.
     5. Increased perspiration.
     6. Thirst.
     7. Lethargy.
     8. Agitation.
     9. Delirium.
    10. Convulsions.
    11. Coma.
    12. Hyperthermia.
    13. Petechiae (usually not serious hemorrhage).

  C. Intervention.
     1. Intubate as necessary.
     2. Gastric lavage with normal saline.
     3. Administer syrup of Ipecac, if early.
     4. Assist with forced diuresis, including acetuzolimide, bicarbonate, sodium chloride, and potassium, may be useful. *Do not overcorrect the metabolic acidosis.*
     5. Frequently monitor arterial blood gases and aspirin levels.
     6. Place patient on cooling blanket.

VIII. Alcohol: ethanol, methanol (methyl alcohol metabolized to formaldehyde and formic acid); ethylene glycol (antifreeze, metabolized from ethylene glycol to oxalic acid, which then combines with calcium to form an insoluble calcium oxalate which precipitates in kidneys).
  A. Assessment.
     1. Ataxia.
     2. Slurred speech.
     3. Nystagmus.
     4. Agitated state.
     5. Stupor, respiratory depression (which is associated with cold clammy skin and hypothermia).
     6. While awake, may have increased pain threshold.
     7. Watch for associated head trauma, pneumonia, meningitis, liver failure.
     8. Onset of blurred vision, headache, delirium, nausea, vomiting, and abdominal pain (methyl alcohol).
     9. Optic disks hyperemic (methyl alcohol leads to irreversible retinal and optic nerve damage).
    10. Elevated serum amylase with associated pancreatitis.
    11. Coma with hyperventilation and profound metabolic acidosis.
    12. Pulmonary edema, followed by renal failure (ethylene glycol).
    13. Seizures and hypocalcemia (ethylene glycol).
    14. Oxalate crystals on microscopic urinalysis (ethylene glycol).
  B. Intervention.
     1. Supportive, with respiratory assistance as necessary.
     2. *Rapid intervention to correct acidosis* with intravenous bicarbonate and intravenous ethyl alcohol to block metabolism of methanol by alcohol dehydrogenase (methanol abuse), i.e., titrate a 10% solution of ethanol to maintain blood level at approximately 100 to 150 mg per 100 mL.
     3. Treat ethylene glycol poisoning as methanol poisoning with the following addition: provide supplemental calcium as necessary.

    C. Evaluation: complications (withdrawal).
        1. Assessment. There are generally separate phases for minor withdrawal and major withdrawal.
            a. Minor withdrawal usually begins at zero after intoxication and lasts approximately 40 to 45 h. May peak in 20 to 25 h with symptoms of:
                (1) Tremor.
                (2) Mild
                (3) Hallucinations.
                (4) Convulsions.
                (5) Minimal disorientation.
                (6) Rising blood pressure.
                (7) Increased heart rate, increased respiration.
                (8) Nystagmus, which is a fine movement in lateral gaze.
                (9) Increased temperature.
            b. Major withdrawal (delerium tremens) has onset approximately 30 h after being intoxicated, peaks between 70 and 90 h after "drinking binge," and may last to 130 h or 4½ days after intoxication with symptoms of:
                (1) Psychomotor activity.
                (2) Tremors.
                (3) Autonomic activity with profuse sweating.
                (4) Hallucinations (e.g., cannot tell he or she is whole, loss of reality, becomes psychotic).
                (5) Grand mal convulsions.
                (6) Profound disorientation.
        2. Intervention.
            a. May include careful and judicious use of Valium, Librium, etc.
            b. Watch respirations and support airway ventilation.

Food Poisoning

Definition

Botulism occurs 18 to 36 h after eating improperly processed canned foods. Time lapse can be longer in some instances. Prognosis is dependent upon the amount of toxin ingested in relation to body weight (6).

    Bacterial food poisoning occurs 2 to 6 h after ingestion of staphylococcic enterotoxins; from streptococcic contamination, in 2 to 12 h. From organisms themselves, i.e., *salmonella,* with symptoms coming on 8 h or more after ingestion.

    Chemical food poisoning results from ingestion of acid foods that were placed in containers lined with antimony, cadmium, lead, or zinc. From eating unwashed fruits or vegetables sprayed with preparations containing the metal salts listed above; also from food preservatives, sugar and salt substitutes (7).

Assessment

    I. Botulism. Symptoms include:
        A. Gastrointestinal upset.
        B. Dimness of vision, double vision.
        C. Drooping of eyelids.
        D. Decreased blood pressure.
        E. Afebrile.
        F. Difficulty in talking, swallowing.
        G. Shortness of breath.
        H. Paralysis of throat muscles (late).
        I. Coma and death from respiratory paralysis.
    II. Bacterial food poisoning. Signs and symptoms include:
        A. Vertigo.   *C.* General malaise.
        B. Weakness.   *D.* Salivation.

        E. Nausea, vomiting.   *H.* Diarrhea.
        F. Gastric pain.   *I.* Muscular cramps.
        G. Tenesmus.   *J.* Shock.

III. Chemical food poisoning. Signs and symptoms include:
    A. Nausea, vomiting.
    B. Diarrhea.

Problems

I. Inadequate ventilation.
II. Fluid and elctrolyte imbalances.
III. Coma, convulsions.
IV. Shock.
V. Pain, discomfort.
VI. Lack of knowledge involving food preparation and/ or handling.

Goals of Care

I. Maintain respiratory function.
II. Restore fliid and electrolyte balances.
III. Monitor neurologic status.
IV. Treat shock, if imminent.
V. Relieve pain, discomfort.
VI. Provide emotional support.
VII. Institute teaching for future prevention of similar episodes.

Intervention

I. Assist with ventilating effort as appropriate, i.e., nasal cannula with oxygen, cardiopulmonary resuscitation (CPR), mechanical ventilation.
II. See discussions of coma (Chap. 23) and shock (Chap. 44) for appropriate interventions.
III. Treatment of individual types of food poisoning as follows:
    A. Botulism.
        1. Hospitalize at once for treatment with trivalent botulinum antitoxin.
        2. Symptomatic and supportive care as indicated.
        3. Emetics and lavage of little value after 12 to 100 h have elapsed since ingestion (8).
        4. Stimulants and oxygen therapy are isually indicated.
    B. Bacterial food poisoning (9).
        1. Empty stomach at once by emetics and gastric lavage followed by activated charcoal.
        2. Castor oil, 30 mL, or 0.2 g Calomel (mercurous chloride) by mouth.
        3. Control pain with morphine sulfate. Administer subcutaneously; intramuscular and intravenous administration is also effective.
        4. Relieve tenesmus, diarrhea with 1 g bismuth subcarbonate or 7.5 g PO of Kaolin. Paregoric (tincture of opium), 4 to 8 mL, may be given orally after each loose bowel movement.
        5. Hospitalize if severe shock or dehydration is present.
    C. Chemical food poisoning.
        1. Emetics, followed by gastric lavage (if profuse vomiting has not taken place).
        2. Activated charcoal in water by mouth.
        3. Saline cathartics.
        4. Atropine sulfate, 0.5 mg SC.
        5. Bismuth subcarbonate by mouth.
        6. Specific treatment as outlined under specific metals (10).
IV. Teach victim and family appropriate food storing, preparation, foods likely to be contaminated (e.g., poultry, frankfurters in *Salmonella*, etc.).

Evaluation

I. Public health nurse follow-up is indicated at patient's home for reinforcement of teaching and assessment of patient recovery if he or she is not hospitalized.
II. All cases of food poisoning should be reported to the local department of health.

Carbon Monoxide Poisoning

Definition

Carbon monoxide poisoning is caused by inhalation of the colorless, odorless gas, carbon monoxide, resulting from incomplete combustion. Such inhalation may take place in the presence of improperly functioning or inadequately vented equipment; burning, heating, or illuminating gas; from automobile exhaust fumes; or also, with the use of open circuit-diving apparatus (11).

Assessment

I. Health history.
    A. History of exposure.
    B. Note length of time exposed, immediate treatment given.
    C. History of depression, suicide attempts.
    D. Note previous medical history, use of medication, allergies.
II. Physical assessment. Common findings include:
    A. Cherry red color to lips (may be absent or transient).
    B. Peaceful expression.
    C. Facial twitchings.
    D. Elevated temperature.
    E. Pale skin.
    F. Brownish red strippling on arms or trunk may be present.
III. Diagnostic studies.
    A. Arterial blood gases.
    B. CBC with differential.
    C. Serum electrolytes.

Problems

I. Inadequate ventilation requiring resuscitation.
II. Fluid-electrolyte imbalance
III. Possible myocardial irritability.
IV. Possible residual neurologic damage.
V. Coma, convulsions.
VI. Emotional problems, perhaps long-term, if carbon monoxide poisoning is due to suicide attempt.

Goals of Care

I. Restore ventilatory function.
II. Maintain fluid-electrolyte balance.
III. Prevent and treat if myocardial irritability occurs.
IV. Monitor neurologic status.
V. Provide emotional support; refer to appropriate psychiatric, supportive services where indicated.

Intervention

I. Institute immediate expired-air respiration after removal from exposure and determining that the airway is clear (12). Provide 95 to 100% oxygen under positive pressure using endotracheal catheter or face mask.
II. Insert IV line: use dextrose solution (50%), 100 mL, slowly.
III. Prevent chilling, excitement.
IV. Hospitalize for observation, supportive treatment (including transfusions).
V. Consider induction of hypothermia in *severe* cases.
VI. *Do not:*
    A. Give methylene blue solution intravenously.
    B. Administer cardiac stimulants unless there is no recourse.
    C. Give morphine, atropine sulfate, or synthetic narcotics.
    D. Let the patient go home after recovery from the immediate postexposure phase. There are myocardial and neurologic effects that are delayed and may be life-threatening (13).

ENDOCRINE EMERGENCIES

Insulin Insufficiency–Glucagon Excess

Definition
 Hypoglycemia and *hyperglycemia* are (chronic) systemic diseases respectively characterized by disorders of intermediary metabolism of carbohydrates, proteins, and fats, and microangiopathy of blood vessels due to too little or no production and release of insulin from beta cells, islands of Langerhans, from the tail and head of pancreas. The number of granules in the beta cells parallels the insulin content of the pancreas. These same cells also contain antiinsulin antibodies. Insulin is regulated by circulating blood sugar and several hormones which all act on the opposite end of spectrum.

The proposed theory of insulin action is as follows. Insulin activates a receptor which probably couples with a "controller" within the cell. It is not understood how the system relays the message from the receptor to one or more controllers. Possibly, one controller is cyclic AMP which affects multiple events of glycolysis, glycogen synthesis, lipolysis, and protein synthesis. Glucagon is produced by alpha cells in the pancreas. Insulin facilitates glucose via permeability of membrane in skeletal muscle and adipose tissue.

Insulin insufficiency is specific organ system destruction:

I. Pancreas.
    A. Reduction in size and number of islets.
    B. Beta cell degranulation.
    C. Glucagon accumulation within beta cells.
    D. Amyloid replacement of islets.
    E. Leukocytic infiltration of the islet.
II. Vascular system: microangiopathies and destruction of cell membrane, particularly of heart, aorta, and small capillaries.
III. Kidneys—Diabetic nephropathy.
    A. Glomerular lesions.
    B. Renal vascular lesions (arteriosclerosis).
    C. Pyelonephritis (includes necrotizing papillitis).
    D. Glycogen and fatty changes in tubular epithelium.
IV. Nervous system.
    A. Peripheral, symmetric neuropathy.
    B. Microchanges of brain parenchyma.
V. Eyes.
    A. Retinopathy.
    B. Cataract formation.
    C. Glaucoma.
VI. Other organ systems.
    A. Liver.
        1. Changes in intermediary metabolism pathways, synthesis and storing of glucose, proteins, lipids.
        2. Scar tissue and atrophic changes.
    B. Skin.
        1. Atrophic.   3. Loss of connective tissue elasticity.
        2. Keratosis.   4. Dryness.

Assessment
I. Health history.
    A. Obtain description of onset of symptomatology, i.e., slow, gradual, progressive, or abrupt and acute.
    B. Obtain past medical history, including medications, allergies.
    C. Obtain information regarding recent surgery, other stress events.
    D. Note family history regarding endocrine disturbances.
    E. Where did incident (symptoms) occur, and what were immediate treatments?
    F. Note recent ingestion of food, drugs, alcohol, other substances.
    G. Note if patient is juvenile or adult onset diabetic and specific oral hypoglycemics.

II. Physical and behavioral assessment (see Table 45-1). Specific symptoms:
  A. Hyperosmolar. Change of personality due to osmotic effect of water leaving parenchymal cells and causing brain "shrinkage," may present in coma.
  B. Insulin excess. Catecholamine release to stimulate gluconeogenesis and glycolysis with following associated responses: sweating, pallor, anxiety, weakness, tachycardia, irritability, headache, slow cerebration, feeling of vagueness, mental confusion, respiratory arrest, death.
  C. Somogyi effect. Nighttime drop of blood pressure and onset of hypoglycemia which cause "nightmares," followed by mobilization of glucagon to increase blood sugar: 400 mg per 100 mL by early morning.
III. Diagnostic tests.
  A. Blood sugar: taken at various times and in response to various stimulations, i.e., postprandial, serial, fasting.
  B. Urinalysis.
  C. Electrolytes (blood and urine).
  D. Blood urea nitrogen (BUN).
  E. Hct.
  F. ECG.
  G. Serum osmolarity, osmolality.
  H. Serum acetone.

Problems

I. Physiologic.
  A. Airway and ventilation inadequacy.
  B. Fluid and electrolyte imbalances.
  C. Microcirculation destruction.
  D. Associated organ dysfunction (whichever is relative).
  E. Acid-base derangements.
  F. Physical immobilization (depending on degree of loss of consciousness).
II. Psychosocial.
  A. Loss of consciousness.
  B. Pain.

TABLE 45-1 / ENDOCRINE EMERGENCIES: INSULIN INSUFFICIENCY–GLUCAGON EXCESS (INCLUDES INSULIN REACTIONS)

	Insulin Insufficiency–Glucagon Excess		
	Ketoacidosis	*Hyperosmolarity*	*Insulin Excess*
Duration of diabetes	Variable	Recent onset	Uncontrolled, variable
Precipitating events	Infection, stress	Burns, steroids, stress, diuretics, particularly chlorthiazides	Recent insulin injection / Timed or second rush of insulin release
Age	All ages	Fifth to seventh decades	All ages, particularly insulin-dependent patients
Dehydration	Variable	Severe	Not primary problem
pH	Low	Normal	Low: lactic acidosis and anaerobic metabolism
Acetone	Present	Absent	Absent at onset
Breathing	Kussmaul	Normal	Shallow, absent
Blood sugar	400–800 mg per 100 mL	900+ mg per 100 mL	20–50 mg per 100 mL
Mortality	<5–10%	>50%	>80%

C. Social and financial immobility if drug- and diet-dependent; insurance and driver's license identifiable.

D. Anger, anxiety due to disease chronicity.

Goals of Care

I. Reduce crisis states.

II. Reduce residual complications: sepsis, loss of circulation; immobility.

III. Increase feeling of physical productivity.

IV. Restore optimum physiologic condition.

Intervention

I. Insure airway patency and adequate ventilation with oral airway and oxygenation, or in more severe respiratory depression, intubation and mechanical ventilation.

II. Fluid resuscitate immediately (use large intravenous No. 16 to 18 needles) with normal saline for extracellular fluid deficit and 5% dextrose in water for cellular water deficit.

III. Cautiously administer potassium replacement when kidney function established, i.e., 5 meq per kilogram of body weight in intravenous fluids. *Watch cardiac and vessel reactions.*

IV. Administer small intravenous doses of regular insulin (10-U increments), and monitor blood sugar every hour until within 250 to 350 mg per 100 mL (insulin insufficiency; *watch insulin sticking to IV tubing and glass bottle*).

V. Administer intravenous glucose, 50 mL of 50% glucose, to maintain blood glucose over 100 mg per 100 mL or 300 g carbohydrate daily (insulin excess).

VI. Monitor acid-base imbalance by arterial blood gases every 30 min during rapid resuscitation and every 4 h until stable.

VII. Monitor serum electrolyte levels every 4 h until fluid and electrolyte balances remain relatively stable (usually within 24 h).

VIII. May administer one sodium bicarbonate ampule in 1 L of water over 3 to 4 h and discontinue when serum bicarbonate level is 15 meq/L.

IX. Obtain urine specific gravity, sugar and acetone testing every hour until patient has stable acid-base status, then every 4 h until blood sugar within 250 to 350 mg per 100 mL.

X. Monitor vital signs and neuromuscular checks everh hour.

XI. Auscultate breath sounds, and observe ventilatory patterns every hour until acid-base balance returns to compensated, normal range.

XII. Immediately and frequently assess level of consciousness and mentation status.

XIII. Insert Foley bladder catheter, and attach to straight drainage.

XIV. Carefully monitor intake and output, with urine measured every hour.

XV. Institute meticulous skin protection and care.

XVI. Reestablish insulin coverage according to individual needs.

XVII. If patient is unconscious, insert nasogastric tube and attach to low intermittent suction.

Evaluation

I. After the crisis, patient should be reassessed for understanding of diabetic control.

II. Begin patient education regarding precipitating factors in triggering another crisis episode, i.e., alcohol intake, other drugs, medications, insulin dosage, and activity levels, etc.

Adrenal Insufficiency

Definition

Adrenal insufficiency is caused by the inability or depressed state of adrenal gland to produce catecholamines and steroids. It generally occurs in patients who have been on large doses of glucocorticoids and have been discontinued. May be due to idiopathic atrophy or infection of adrenals (tuberculosis or fungus). Precipitating stress is usually present.

Assessment

I. Health history.
  A. Past medical history, including medications and allergies.
  B. Note recent high-stress events.
II. Physical and behavioral assessment.
  A. Hypotension, due to aldosterone insufficiency, Na, obligatory water loss.
  B. Anorexia, due to cortisol insufficiency.
  C. Vomiting, due to cortisol insufficiency.
  D. Abdominal pain.
  E. Apathy and confusion.
  F. Extreme weakness.
  G. Tachycardia.
III. Diagnostic studies.
  A. Blood sugar and cortisol levels.
  D. Serum and urine electrolytes.
  E. Urinalysis.

Problems

I. Physiologic.
  A. Saline deficit and volume depletion: possible circulatory collapse.
  B. Defenselessness in stress or crisis situations.
  C. Weight loss and anorexia.
  D. Physical immobility.
II. Psychosocial.
  A. Lassitude and fatigue.
  B. Poor mentation.
  C. Depression.

Goals of Care

I. Maintain vascular volume and electrolyte balance.
II. Reduce stress.
III. Prevent complications of cachexia, sepsis, mental dullness.
IV. Reestablish adrenal gland functions.

Intervention

I. Maintain airway patency and adequate ventilation.
II. Administer normal saline with 5% dextrose to maintain vascular volume.
III. Administer hydrocortisone (intravenous) 300 mg over 24 h, in divided doses.
IV. Identify and treat underlying cause(s).
V. Keep supine until orthostatic blood pressure stable at 90 to 110 mmHg systolic.

Evaluation

I. May need periodic replacement of corticosteroids if adrenals are permanently injured or damaged.
II. Patient teaching regarding stress precipitators, i.e., infections.

Thyrotoxicosis ("Thyroid Storm")

Definition

Thyrotoxicosis is an excessive outpouring of thyroid hormone and catecholamine release. It is usually precipitated in individuals who have high levels of thyroxine and are subject to stress (14). Thyroid storms are indicated by:

1. Pulse greater than 120 per minute.
2. Temperature greater than 100°F.
3. Confused mental status.

Assessment

I. Health history.
  A. Previous medical history, with medications and allergies included.

        B. Precipitating factors to present condition.

        C. Ingestion of other over-the-counter medications, street drugs, alcohol, etc.

    II. Physical and behavioral assessment.

        A. Febrile over 100°F (38°C).

        B. High-output failure syndrome: widening pulse press.

        C. Heart rate over 130 beats per minute.

        D. Dysfunctions of CNS, cardiovascular, and gastrointestinal systems.

        E. Sticky, hot, moist skin over inner aspect of arms.

        F. Face flushed.

        G. Muscle jerking and uncontrolled "jitters."

        H. Obtundation and coma.

        I. Enlarged thyroid gland.

        J. Exophthalmos.

   III. Diagnostic studies.

        A. Thyroid scan.

        B. Serum electrolytes.

        C. Thyroid levels (blood chemistries): T_3 or T_4.

Problems

    I. Physiologic.

        A. Hypermetabolism.

        B. Neurologic deficits.

        C. Cardiovascular collapse.

    II. Psychosocial.

        A. Extreme "nervousness" and agitation.

        B. Social immobility due to uncontrolled behavior.

Goals of Care

    I. Reduce thyroid hormone emission to normal range.

    II. Protect cardiovascular system.

   III. Reduce complications of exophthalmos, fluid and electrolyte imbalances, and excessive febrile states.

   IV. Support all organ systems.

Intervention

    I. Correct underlying cause, e.g., sepsis with appropriate antibiotics, etc.

    II. Suppress hormone production orally or with nasogastric tube: propylthiouracil, 80 to 120 mg daily in three divided doses or methimazole (Tapazole), 80 to 120 mg daily in three divided doses.

   III. Block hormone release: 30 min after antithyroid drugs have been started, begin sodium iodide, 1 g in 1000 mL 5% dextrose in water or normal saline over 8 to 12 h. May give Lugol's solution 10 gtt PO, tid, as an alternative.

   IV. Block adrenergic response by administration of following: reserpine, 2.5 mg IV every 4 to 6 h to deplete catecholamine discharge; guanethidine, 100 to 150 mg IV or PO in a single dose to block catecholamine discharge (may cause orthostatic hypotension); or, propranolol (Inderal), 1 to 5 mg IV or 20 to 80 mg PO every 4 h (use cautiously, especially in patients with congestive heart failure, diabetes mellitus, or asthma).

    V. Meet metabolic needs, i.e., provide carbohydrates, calories, and vitamin replacement.

   VI. May use peritoneal dialysis for refractory cases.

Evaluation

    I. Patient education regarding disease entity, effects of stress, avoidance, or better management of stressful situations. Long-term management involves surgery or radioactive iodine (15).

    II. Continue to evaluate effects of three major aspects of therapy:

        A. Supplying of fluid lost by evaporation, i.e., maintenance of fluid and electrolyte balances.

        B. Supporting the increased energy loss [result of hypermetabolic state (16), i.e., cooling blanket for increased temperature].

C. Decreasing the production of thyroxine and thus decreasing its peripheral effects (i.e., administration of antithyroid drigs via nasogastric tube).

CARDIOVASCULAR EMERGENCIES

Definition *Cardiovascular emergencies* include angina pectoris, myocardial infarction, congestive heart failure, and cardiogenic shock. *Angina* is characterized by impaired blood flow through coronary arteries due to atherosclerosis and/or arteriosclerosis. It is precipitated by exertion, causing disparity between oxygen consumption and availability. Angina is most common in individuals with predisposing risk factors of familial history, high cholesterolemia and lipidemia, smoking history, hypertension, and associated diseaes, i.e., diabetes mellitus.

Myocardial infarction is the interruption of the blood supply to a localized portion of the heart muscle. It is precipitated by the same causes as angina, with the addition of:

1. No exertion.
2. Electrical abnormalities.
3. Stress events within relatively short time period to incident.
4. Unknown precipitation.

Congestive heart failure can be characterized by insufficiency of contractile power coupled with inadequate blood flow. Increasing left ventricular end diastolic pressure with resultant "back" pressures causes systemic venous pressure increase. Ultimately, there is venous pooling and occlusion with resultant systemic engorgement, edema, and hypertension.

Cardiogenic shock is ultimate contractile deficit with little or no perfusion of cardiac or systemic tissue.

Assessment
I. Health history.
   A. Obtain precipitating events, history.
   B. Note past medical history, medications, and allergies.
   C. Obtain description of life-style, especially for myocardial infarction patient.
   D. Note any treatment instituted before patient brought to hospital.
II. Physical and behavioral assessment.
   A. Disparities of electromechanical cycle.
   B. Hypertension or hypotension.
   C. Pain: precordial, chest, jaw, left arm, neck (left side).
   D. Fatigue, lassitude, weakness.
   E. Diaphoresis.
   F. Pallor, ashen skin color.
   G. Venous engorgement: distended neck veins.
   H. Narrowing pulse pressure.
   I. Arrhythmias.
III. Diagnostic studies.
   A. Twelve-lead ECG and dynamic monitoring.   **D.** Chest x-ray.
   B. Serum electrolytes.   **E.** Digitalis level.
   C. Cardiac enzymes: isoenzymes.   **F.** CBC with Hb, Hct, differential.

Problems
I. Physiologic.
   A. Inadequate tissue perfusion.   **D.** Medication toxicity.
   B. Arrhythmias.   **E.** Reduced activity levels.
   C. Fluid and electrolyte imbalances.
II. Psychosocial.
   A. Catastrophic psychic shock.
   B. Social and financial immobility if prolonged work loss.
   C. Depression, anger, denial; may be agitated and anxious.

Goals of Care
    I. Preserve cardiovascular integrity.
    II. Reduce complications of arrhythmias and failure.
    III. Return patient to highest level of organ function (i.e., daily activities and work performance).
    IV. Develop healthy coping mechanisms to progressive disease state.

Intervention
    I. Angina.
        A. Administer glyceryl trinitrate (NTG), 0.3 to 0.6 mg, repeated every 5 min (sublingual lozenges). If three doses do not cause marked relief of symptoms, suspect myocardial infarction.
        B. Place patient at rest, seated or supine as tolerated.
        C. Start intravenous (No. 16 to 18 needle) infusion of 5% dextrose in water for medications.
        D. Obtain 12-lead ECG and look for ischemic changes.
        E. Monitor vital signs every 15 min until stable.
    II. Myocardial infarction.
        A. Establish adequate airway and ventilation, usually with endotracheal intubation.
        B. Administer external cardiac compression if victim is pulseless (see Tables 45-2 and 45-3 and Figs. 45-1 and 45-2).
        C. Provide oxygen via intubation tube, positive pressure bag, or mechanical ventilation.
        D. Place electrodes for monitoring, and assess cardiac rhythms.
        E. Defibrillate with 400 W/s if ventricular fibrillation or ventricular tachycardia present and if patient is symptomatic (unresponsive).
        F. Start intravenous (No. 16 to 18 needle) infusion of 5% dextrose in water for medications.
        G. Provide lidocaine; 4 mg/min, for unstable irritability, i.e., ventricular ectopy.
        H. Keep supine, provide bed rest.
        I. Administer morphine sulfate, 5 to 15 mg IV in 2- to 5-mg aliquots; meperidine hydrochloride (Demerol), 50 to 100 mg in 25-mg aliquots; hydromorphone (Dilaudid), 2 to 4 mg in 1-mg doses. *Watch respirations and hypotension.*
        J. Monitor vital signs and mentation every 30 to 60 min until stable.
        K. Record *carefully* intake and output.
        L. Obtain serial ECG and enzymes every 3 days.
        M. Pace on continuous cardiac monitoring.
    III. Congestive heart failure: Note for myocardial infarction.
        A. Provide furosemide (Lasix), 40 to 80 mg IV, and watch for diuresis responses.
        B. Keep upright (head of bed at 90°) or in position of comfort with legs dangling.
        C. Phlebotomize (bloodless) with rotating tourniquets serially to proximal portions of three of the four extremities with periods of release of one tourniquet at a time for 15 min. *Obstruct venous return and not arterial flow.* Generally inflate to 60 to 80 mmHg, and use blood pressure cuffs for equal pressure distribution. May phlebotomize 200 to 500 mL, especially if patient has polycythemia vera.
        D. Digitalize (for previous undigitalized) with 1.5 mg Digoxin and start with intravenous dose, 0.25 to 0.5 mg, 4- to 8-h intervals.
        E. Use Swan-Ganz pressure monitoring.
        F. Listn to heart sounds for appearance of gallops or murmurs.
    IV. Cardiogenic shock: Note for myocardial infarction.
        A. Use vasopressor agents to maintain blood pressure. Dopamine (drug of choice) according to prescribed (individual) doses and based on blood pressure, urine output responses. Use IVAC or drip-monitoring regulators.
        B. Administer inotropic agents such as digitalis (according to medication levels prescribed in congestive heart failure).
        C. Maintain meticulous intake and output records.
        D. Watch peripheral circulation and tissue oxygenation: arterial blood gases. Protect skin and pressure areas with sheep skin and turning.

TABLE 45-2 / BASIC LIFE SUPPORT PROCEDURES INCLUDING UNWITNESSED CARDIAC ARREST (ONE OR TWO RESCUERS)

Time Required for Preparation	What to Do First	General Procedures	Remarks
4–10 s	Make sure victim is unconscious and not breathing	Turn victim face up; shout at victim to see if he or she responds	Make sure victim is not suffering from some disease that does not require resuscitation (simple fainting, diabetes, coma, etc.)
7–15 s	Establish patent airway	Place one hand under neck, other hand on forehead in order to tilt head back and extend neck	In this way, neck can be extended, nostrils closed, and jaw jutted forward for mouth-to-mouth inflation
10–20 s	Give four quick inflations	Make sure nostrils are pinched off, neck is extended, mouth seal is tight	Volume of each inflation should be about 800 mL, enough to give a quick supply of oxygen; check chest for expansion
15–20 s	Check for presence or absence of carotid pulse on each side	This is most easily found in the groove just to one side of the larynx	Time is of the essence, and sometimes pulse may be weak and difficult to find
75–90 s	Start cardiac pulmonary resuscitation in the ratio of 15 compressions to two inflations	Make sure you and the victim are properly positioned and in trying to do two things at once there is no air leakage	During compression it is particularly important that both hands and arms be correctly positioned. When there is a single rescuer, try to give 80 compressions per minute; with two rescuers, use 60.* Two very fast lung inflations are given after each 15 chest compressions
80–100 s	Determine if breathing and pulse have returned	Continue efforts, if necessary, until a satisfactory CPR function is established	The pupil size (beginning contraction) will give a good hint of returning function

*When two rescuers are available, one should do inflation and the other cardiac compression. Functions may be switched as fatigue requires; it is important not to get in each other's way or interfere with either rhythm. When a second rescuer arrives on the scene, the change in rhythm to 60 compressions per minute is accomplished as follows: Rescuer No. 1 says: "One-one thousand, two-one thousand, three-one thousand, four-one thousand, five-one thousand," and so on until the second person is ready. Then Rescuer No. 1 says "We switch on next breath." The inflator takes over at the count of three-one thousand and the new compressor begins and picks up the count without pause. Rescuer No. 1 then quickly checks for pulse and pupils.

Source: John Henderson, *Emergency Medical Guide,* McGraw-Hill Book Company, New York, 1978, p. 143; reproduced in condensed form from the *Instructors' Manual of Basic Cardiac Life Support.*

TABLE 45-3 / INFANT RESUSCITATION*

Time Required for Preparation	What to Do First	General Procedures	Remarks
3–5 s	Make sure infant is unconscious	Place infant in horizontal position	Make sure that cardiac arrest has taken place
6–10 s	Establish patent airway	Do not overextend the neck	Simply tilt head gently backward
9–15 s	Give four gentle puffs into mouth	In infants do not breathe as forcefully as in adults	Horizontal position facilitates cardiac massage, if necessary
14–25 s	Determine lack of pulse	Use carotid or precordial pulse	Overextension of head may block airway (collapsed trachea) rather than help it
44–55 s	If cardiac arrest is present, begin cycles of five compressions to one inflation	Use two fingers for compression—gently—as sternum is very flexible; pressure is exerted about midsternum, as in infants the heart lies higher than in adults; danger to liver is also greater for the same reason	In infants, rate should be 80–100 compressions per minute with rapid inflation after five compressions (this equals about five compressions every 3 s with one inflation every 3 s, i.e., 5:1 ratio.)

*Major changes in the technique of infant resuscitation will soon be advised by the American Heart Association.
Source: John Henderson, *Emergency Medical Guide,* McGraw-Hill Book Company, New York, 1978, p. 143; reproduced in condensed form from the *Instructors' Manual of Basic Cardiac Life Support.*

    E. Monitor arterial pressures and pulmonary artery, capillary wedge pressures.
    F. Auscultate heart sounds for gallops and murmurs.

Evaluation
    I. Prepare patient for transfer to cardiac unit. Be aware that patients with 40 percent or more myocardial damage are certain candidates for cardiogenic shock. They have an exceedingly poor prognosis.
    II. Myocardial infarction victims and sudden cardiac arrest victims have best morbidity and mortality when cardiopulmonary resuscitation begins immediately to 4 min after incident. Brain damage is relative to length of anoxic-anaerobic period.
    III. Standards for CPR and advanced cardiac life support may be obtained from the American Heart Association, Dallas, Texas.

ABDOMINAL EMERGENCIES

Definition
    Abdominal emergency is a general term including diverse conditions that necessitate immediate care. Such conditions may be traumatic (see Chap. 44). Examples of acute abdominal conditions include infection, torsion, or obstruction of gut; hemorrhage; peritonitis; space-occupying masses; and vascular problems (17). The etiology is usually one of the following categories:

    1. Inflammation: appendicitis, cholecystitis, diverticulitis, pancreatitis, ulcerative colitis, viral gastroenteritis.
    2. Perforation: duodenal and gastric ulcers, cancer of the colon, ovarian cyst, ectopic tubal pregnancies, appendicitis.
    3. Trauma (see Chap. 44).

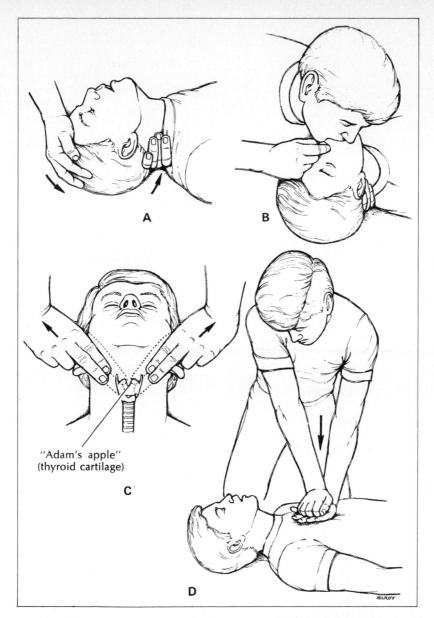

A

B

"Adam's apple"
(thyroid cartilage)

C

D

FIGURE 45-1 / Major steps in cardiopulmonary resuscitation. (*a*) Make certain the victim has an open airway. (*b*) Start respiratory resuscitation immediately. (*c*) Feel for the carotid pulse in the groove alongside the "Adam's apple" or thyroid cartilage. (*d*) If pulse is absent, begin cardiac massage. Use 60 compressions a minute with one lung inflation after each group of five chest compressions. (*From John Henderson, Emergency Medical Guide, 4th ed., McGraw-Hill Book Company, New York, 1978, p. 142.*)

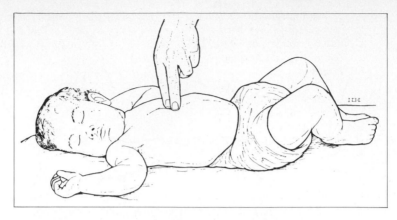

FIGURE 45-2 / For external cardiac massage in children, gentle pressure is exerted with tips of fingers rather than with the heel of hand. (*From John Henderson, Emergency Medical Guide, 4th ed., McGraw-Hill Book Company, New York, 1978.*)

4. Vascular problems: abdominal aortic aneurysms, mesenteric vascular occlusions, volvulus of the intestine (loss of circulation to part of the bowel with necrosis).
5. Obstruction: causative agents such as tumor, a torsion (volvulus), adhesions, or hernias, foreign bodies.
6. Bleeding: ulcers of upper gastrointestinal tract; tumors of stomach, colon; inflammatory disease, i.e., ulcerative colitis.
7. Other conditions: a partial list of clinical conditions which may mimic acute abdominal disease can be found in (18).

Assessment

  I. Health history.
    A. Age of patient.
    B. Sexual and menstrual history.
    C. Course of onset.
    D. Note any of the following:
      1. Bleeding.
      2. Change in bowel or digestive habits.
      3. Chronic pain.
      4. Weight loss.
      5. Anorexia.
      6. Jaundice.
    E. Past operations, illnesses, medications (especially aspirin, alcohol, or steroids).
    F. History of allergies.
    G. Bleeding tendencies.
    H. Recent exposure to hepatitis or different geographic areas.
  II. Physical and behavioral assessment.
    A. Pain, tenderness. ["The general rule can be laid down that the majority of severe abdominal pains which ensue in patients who have been previously fairly well, and *which last as long as six hours,* are caused by conditions of surgical import" (19)].
      1. Location and character of pain.
      2. Referred pain, e.g., fractured lumbar vertebra: abdominal pain.
      3. Cough tenderness.
      4. Rebound tenderness [a test for peritoneal initiation (20)].
      5. Rectal, pelvic examination (usually done last).
      6. Check for pain over flank and costovertebral angles over kidney.
    B. Distension and peristalsis.
      1. Increased bowel sounds (gastroenteritis).

    2. High-pitched bowel sounds with quiet intervals (intestinal obstruction).

    3. Decreased bowel sounds (generally peritonitis).

C. Rigidity, spasm of abdominal wall, e.g., voluntary spasm in early appendicitis, involuntary spasm of advanced disease of the abdomen.

D. Vomiting.

    1. Type, e.g., is it projectile in nature?

    2. What is vomited?

    3. Amount and frequency.

III. Diagnostic studies.

    A. CBC with differential, Hb, Hct.

    B. Urinalysis.

    C. X-ray of patient in erect and supine positions.

    D. BUN.

    E. Possible paracentesis.

    F. Possible gastrointestinal series, if indicated; gallbladder series.

    G. Serum amylase.

    H. Typing and cross match.

Problems

I. Acute pain, discomfort.

II. Fluid-electrolyte imbalance.

III. Shock (potential).

IV. Inadequate respiratory function (potential).

V. Fear, anxiety of the patient.

VI. Preparation for surgical intervention.

Goals of Care

I. Restore and maintain:

    A. Respiratory function.

    B. Fluid-electrolyte balance.

    C. Cardiovascular functioning, if impaired.

II. Prevent shock.

III. Relieve pain; provide emotional support to patient and family.

Intervention

I. For shock, see Chap. 44.

II. Insert large-gauge intravenous needle. For dehydrated patients with history of vomiting, fluid resuscitate with a balanced salt solution.

III. Assess extent (if any) of hemorrhage, have patient's blood typed and crossmatched in preparation for transfusion (a patient with hypotension, rapid pulse, and history of GI bleeding should have a minimum of 3 U of blood cross matched (21)].

IV. Insert nasogastric tube.

V. Insert indwelling Foley catheter to straight drainage. Maintain accurate input and output record. Observe urine for blood, cloudiness, etc.

VI. Prepare patient for surgical intervention, if indicated.

VII. Provide ongoing support to patient and family.

VIII. For specific drugs, treatment for individual diagnoses, an excellent resource is Chap. 13 in the *Manual of Medical Therapeutics* (22).

Evaluation

Place certain patients under observation for at least 24 h if diagnosis remains unclear. During this time, patient should be hydrated with intravenous fluids, given nothing by mouth, and observed frequently (23).

FEVER

Definition

Fever is an elevation of body temperature from the usual "normal" of 98.6°F. However, normal body temperatures range, rectally, from 97.2 to 100.4°F and, orally, from 96.5 to

99.2°F. Activity, emotion, ambient temperature, dress, etc., can all cause variations in body temperature within these normal ranges.

The causes of fever are many in children, but the usual cause is infection. Fevers may be classified according to patterns:

1. Continuous: temperature move of nearly constant level (e.g., typhoid fever).
2. Remittent: daily fluctuations of more than 2°F (e.g., septicemia, lymphomas).
3. Intermittent: drops to below normal and then rises to previous height (e.g., malaria, juvenile rheumatoid arthritis).
4. Relapsing or recurrent: initial febrile period followed by normalization for several days, only to rise again to its previous height [e.g., Pel-Ebstein fever of Hodgkin's disease (24)].

Assessment:

I. Health history.
 E. Past medical history.
 F. History of allergies.
 G. Medications, if any.
 H. Age of patient.
II. Physical and behavioral assessment.
 A. Pulse rate.
 B. Respiratory rate.
 C. General physical examination for infectious etiology, including rectal and pelvic examination on adults where indicated. *For infants under 6 months of age or newborns,* the presence of fever requires a systematic and thorough evaluation. Look for the following:
   1. Anorexia.
   2. Lethargy, especially in young children and infants.
   3. Irritability, especially in young children and infants.
   4. Rashes.
   5. Petechiae.
   6. Adenopathy.
   7. Inflamed joints.
   8. Abdominal findings.
   9. Upper and lower respiratory tract findings.
III. Diagnostic tests.
 A. CBC.
 B. Urinalysis.
 C. Erythrocyte sedimentation rate.
 D. Chest x-ray, e.g., tachypnea out of proportion to the fever in an infant may be a clue to explain presence of infiltrate on chest x-ray (25).

Problems

I. Fever.
II. Possible infectious etiology.
III. Possible seizures in young children if fever not controlled.

Goals of Care

Assist with reducing fever and accompanying symptoms with major goal of determining cause of fever.

Intervention

I. Remove unneeded clothing to allow radiation of heat.
II. Sponge patient with tepid water. *Do not* use cold water or cold, wet towels, for they produce peripheral vasoconstriction with conservation of body heat. They may also cause shivering, resulting in increased heat production (26).
III. Give aspirin (60 mg for *every year of age up to 5 years, every 4 h*). For 5- to 10-year-old child, 300 mg suffices; 600 mg suffices for older children. If vomiting occurs, give dose rectally. Acetaminophen in dropper dosage form, 60 mg per 0.6 mL, is convenient for infants and toddlers (27).

Evaluation	I. Provide for continuity of care with adequate follow-up for reevaluation of fever if patient is sent home.
	II. Institute teaching for parents, i.e., many do not know how to read a thermometer or what to do if a fever occurs.

SEIZURES

Status Epilepticus

Definition Status epilepticus is the state of prolonged seizures when two or more major seizures occur without intervening return of consciousness (28). It is associated in over 50 percent of cases with tumor, vascular disease, infection or trauma. The largest single cause is idiopathic. One must search for metabolic causes: hypoglycemia, hyponatremia, hypocalcemia, hypomagnesemia, hepatic dysfunction, uremia, and endocrine disorders.

Assessment
I. Health history.
  A. History of seizure disorder.
  B. Medications, if any.
  C. Associated illnesses, e.g., hypertension.
  D. Acute illness prior to seizure.
  E. Description of seizure:
    1. Localized, generalized.
    2. Cyanosis.
    3. Duration.
    4. Incontinence.
II. Physical and behavioral assessment.
  A. Determine adequacy of the airway.
  B. Perform brief physical examination with special attention to the neurologic system. Look for a Medic-Alert tag or identification card in the patient's wallet.
  C. Obtain vital signs.
III. Diagnostic tests.
  A. Electrolytes.   F. Carbon dioxide toxicity.
  B. BUN.   G. Toxicology screen.
  C. Blood sugar.   H. Blood lead level.
  D. Calcium.   I. Urinalysis.
  E. pH.   J. Lumbar puncture.

Problems
I. Seizures with possible hypoxia due to respiratory embarrassment, aspiration. Possible respiratory arrest.
II. Possible physical damage to patient during seizure activity.
III. Coma with possible residual neurological impairment.
IV. Social embarrassment of patient and family: fear, anxiety about underlying disorder.

Goals of Care
I. Control seizures.
II. Maintain respiratory function.
III. Prevent physical damage to patient during seizures.
IV. Monitor neurologic status.
V. Provide community contacts for patient and family: give ongoing emotional support.

Intervention
I. Assure adequate ventilation:
  A. Resuscitate, if indicated.
  B. Suctioning at regular intervals.
  C. Administer oxygen whether or not cyanosis is present.
  D. Possible early intubation because of respiratory depression due to use of anticonvulsant drugs.

II. Start a slow intravenous infusion of 5% dextrose.

III. Insert indwelling Foley catheter and monitor carefully intake and output at 15-min intervals.

IV. Administer appropriate drugs as ordered:

    A. Diazepam (Valium), 5 to 10 mg IV at a rate of no more than 5 mg/min. If seizure has not stopped within 10 min, another 5 to 10 mg may be given 10 to 20 min, after the second dose. If not controlled after 25 to 30 mg, other therapy must be considered. Monitor blood pressure and respirations *closely,* since hypotension and respiratory depression may accompany high cumulative doses of Diazepam (29).

    B. Phenobarbital: Initial dose, 150 mg (never more than 200 mg) IV, at a rate of 25 to 50 mg/min; additional increments may be given after 15 to 20 min. In patients responding to diazepam, a single dose of 150 to 200 mg phenobarbital IV at 25 mg/min. will give longer acting epileptic coverage. Also produces hypotension and respiratory depression.

    C. Diphenylhydantoin (Dilantin): Usually 750 to 1000 mg IV, plus 250 to 500 mg IM, following diazepam or other drugs (30). To avoid *cardiac toxicity,* give Dilantin in three or four 250-mg doses 1 h apart at no more than 50 mg/min. *Dilantin given intravenously may have toxic cardiac effects, slowing conduction velocity and heart rate.*

    D. Paraldehyde: Give intravenously, intramuscularly, or rectally if above drugs fail. Administer rectally in oil retention enema, 0.2 mL/kg IV; 5 mL is dissolved in 500 mL 5% dextrose in water and infused rapidly until seizures are controlled. *Respiratory depression may occur.*

V. Monitor neurologic status.

VI. Make sure patient bed is well padded with side rails up to prevent injury during seizure activity. A padded tongue blade should be placed between the teeth at the back of the mouth to prevent damage to cheeks, tongue, or teeth (31).

VII. Provide ongoing emotional support to family and patient. Call appropriate clergy if indicated.

Febrile Seizures

Definition   Three to five percent of children have febrile convulsions. Most occur after the first 6 months of age but within the first 2 to 3 years of life. These seizures merely represent an initial symptom of an acute benign febrile illness. They are self-limiting in nature. However, any child presenting with a seizure should be evaluated for the possibility of some other etiology, e.g., tetany, lead encephalopathy, hemorrhage or tumor, hypoglycemia, asphyxia, epilepsy, acute nephritis, etc.

Assessment   I. Health history.

    A. Previous attacks of similar nature.

    B. Immediately preceding symptoms, e.g., hyperirritability, headache, vomiting, dizziness, fever, poisoning of any kind.

    C. Family predisposition to seizures.

    D. Exposure to infection.

II. Physical and behavioral assessment. Complete physical examination, with special attention to features that might point to specific infectious causes for seizures, e.g., note signs and symptoms of hyperirritability and lethargy with meningitis.

III. Diagnostic.

    A. CBC with differential.

    B. Urinalysis.

    C. Chest x-ray, where indicated.

    D. Throat culture.

Problems	I. Fever.
	II. Seizures and possible respiratory embarrassment.
	III. Infection of unknown etiology.
	IV. Possible injury to child during seizure activity.
	V. Emotional problems of parents and child.

Goals of Care	I. Relieve fever.
	II. Control seizure activity.
	III. Assist with diagnosis and treatment of infection.
	IV. Protect child from injury.
	V. Support parents and child through direct intervention and appropriate referral.

Intervention

I. Begin fever control with tepid water sponging and rectal aspirin 60 mg per year of age, up to 600 mg.

II. Give as ordered:
   A. Phenobarbital: usually 2 to 3 mg/kg IV. If not effective in 10 min, give additional 2 to 3 mg/kg IM. Maximum dose of 120 mg advised. Use of intravenous phenobarbital not warranted (32).
   B. Diazepam for use with children is under investigation. It must not be used with phenobarbital.
   C. Paraldehyde: either initially or in conjunction with phenobarbital. Administer via high rectal tube, 0.3 mL/kg, up to 6.0 mL; mix with equal volume of mineral oil injected in tube and 10 mL of normal saline [used to flush mixture through tube (33)].

III. Make sure child is protected from falls and bruising during possible seizure activity.

IV. Continue to provide emotional support to parents and child.

Evaluation

I. Refer to appropriate social service agencies or public health nurse for home follow-up, further emotional support, parent teaching regarding medication, future high fevers, etc.

II. At the present time, long-term treatment of children who have experienced febrile seizures with daily phenobarbital, 30 to 60 mg at bedtime is controversial. Parents may expect this preventive treatment and may need to be reassured if it is not prescribed.

EMERGENCY DELIVERY

Definition

As is well known, all deliveries do not occur in a well-planned manner in a hospital or similar facility. All nurses should be familiar with the basic principles of emergency delivery of an infant. The illustrations in this section depict the basic steps in the delivery process with the exception of the spontaneous delivery of the placenta (see "Intervention").

Assessment

Determine if patient is in true labor:
I. Obtain history regarding duration of pregnancy.
II. Assess type, duration, strength, and frequency of uterine contractions.
III. Ask if there was bloody show; check to see if present.
IV. Ask if the membranes have ruptured.
V. Perform a pelvic exam to determine:
   A. Position of presenting part.
   B. Dilation of cervix.

Problems

I. Tearing of vaginal opening, second- and third-degree lacerations.
II. Hemorrhage.
III. Incomplete delivery of placenta.
IV. Health of the newborn.
V. Supportive care to mother during and after delivery.

Goals of Care

I. Minimize possible tearing of vaginal opening.
II. Control and prevent hemorrhage.
III. Evaluate placenta for completeness once delivered: save for physician to determine if manual removal of fragments is indicated.
IV. Assess newborn's status, and monitor condition.
V. Provide ongoing support and instruction for mother during delivery and postpartum periods.

Intervention

I. See Figs. 45–3 through 45–11 (34).
II. For delivery of the placenta:
   A. Do *not* pull the cord to facilitate delivery of the placenta. This can tear a blood vessel and lead to hemorrhage.
   B. When placenta is at the vulva, bring it out with a little gentle pressure.
   C. Usually, the placenta is expelled spontaneously 10 to 20 min after delivery of the baby. This expulsion is accompanied normally by a gush of blood.

Evaluation

I. Continue to check mother for signs of softening of uterus, possible hemorrhage.
II. Transfer mother and infant to appropriate in-hospital services.

FIGURE 45-3 / Positioning the mother on a bed, table, or other surface for emergency delivery. A soft protective pad should be under her buttocks (a thick layer of newspapers if nothing better is available), as well as a soft support for her head. (*From John Henderson, Emergency Medical Guide, 4th ed., McGraw-Hill Book Company, New York, 1978.*)

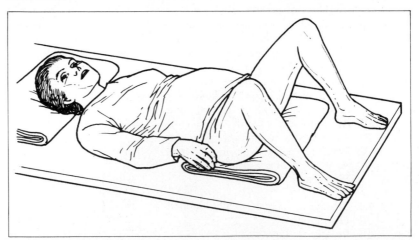

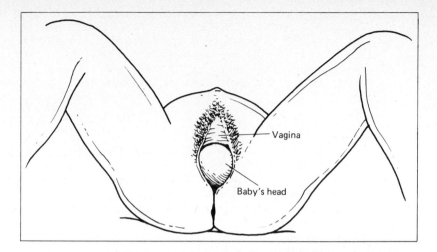

FIGURE 45-4 / The appearance of the top of the baby's head (caput) at the vulval opening shows that actual delivery is beginning to take place at this stage. *(From John Henderson, Emergency Medical Guide, 4th ed., McGraw-Hill Book Company, New York, 1978.)*

FIGURE 45-5 / Sagittal view of Fig. 45-4, showing position of the baby inside the mother at beginning of actual delivery. *(From John Henderson, Emergency Medical Guide, 4th ed., McGraw-Hill Book Company, New York, 1978.)*

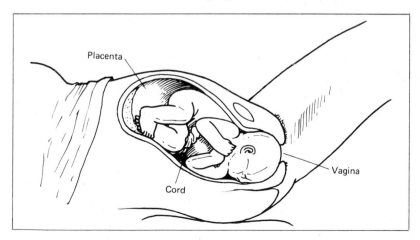

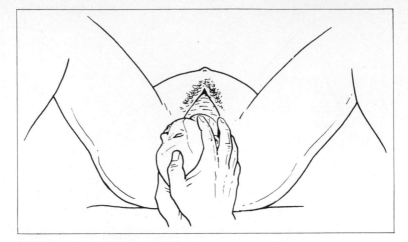

FIGURE 45-6 / Method of easing baby's head gently through the vulval opening so as to minimize the possibility of tearing the skin and deeper tissues between the vulva and anus. (*From John Henderson, Emergency Medical Guide, 4th ed., McGraw-Hill Book Company, New York, 1978.*)

FIGURE 45-7 / The baby's head is gently directed downward to help deliver the upper (anterior) shoulder, which usually is the first to emerge. (*From John Henderson, Emergency Medical Guide, 4th ed., McGraw-Hill Book Company, New York, 1978.*)

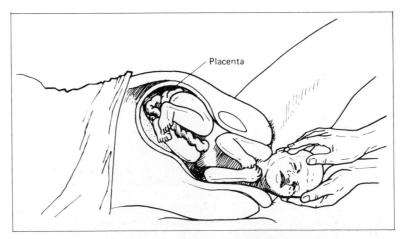

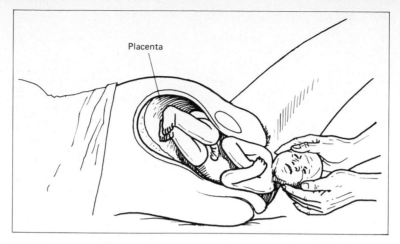

FIGURE 45-8 / The lower (posterior) shoulder is delivered by very gently directing the axis of the baby's head and neck upward. Never pull hard in an attempt to drag the baby out; this could cause permanent damage to the baby, or mother, or both. (*From John Henderson, Emergency Medical Guide, 4th ed., McGraw-Hill Book Company, New York, 1978.*)

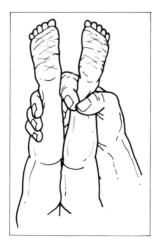

FIGURE 45-9 / Method of firmly holding the baby after delivery so that the infant cannot slip while cleansing the mouth and nose and initiating breathing. (*From John Henderson, Emergency Medical Guide, 4th ed., McGraw-Hill Book Company, New York, 1978.*)

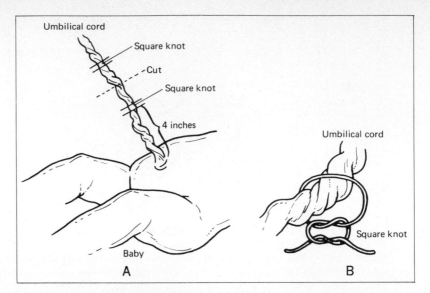

FIGURE 45-10 / The cord is firmly tied off (*a*) with two strips of tape (shoe laces will do in a pinch) and then cut between the two ties. The tie is made (*b*) using a square knot which will not slip. (*From John Henderson, Emergency Medical Guide, 4th ed., McGraw-Hill Book Company, New York, 1978.*)

FIGURE 45-11 / Position of hand for compressing the uterus (which can easily be felt somewhat like a football) to stimulate contraction and thus help to control postpartum bleeding. In the absence of drugs to keep the uterus contracted, gentle manual kneading must be maintained for at least an hour, or until medical help becomes available. (*From John Henderson, Emergency Medical Guide, 4th ed., McGraw-Hill Book Company, New York, 1978.*)

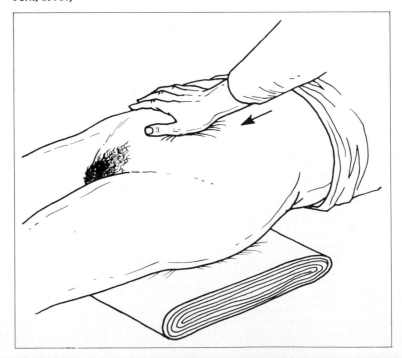

REFERENCES

1. Thomas Flint, Jr., and Harvey D. Cain, *Emergency Treatment and Management,* 5th ed., W. B. Saunders Company, Philadelphia, 1975, p. 433.
2. Ibid.
3. Ibid.
4. Ibid.
5. Ibid.
6. Ibid.
7. Ibid.
8. Ibid., p. 393.
9. Ibid., p. 433.
10. Ibid.
11. Ibid., p. 398.
12. Ibid.
13. Ibid., p. 399.
14. Jeanie Barry, *Emergency Nursing,* McGraw-Hill Book Company, New York, 1978, p. 372.
15. Ibid., p. 373.
16. Ibid.
17. Ibid., p. 300.
18. Ibid., p. 305.
19. Sir Zachary Cope, *The Early Diagnosis of the Acute Abdomen,* Oxford University Press, New York, 1968, p. 3.
20. Barry, op. cit., p. 307.
21. Charles Eckert, *Emergency-Room Care,* 3d ed., Little, Brown and Company, Boston, 1976, p. 164.
22. Edgar C. Boedeker and James H. Dauber (eds.), *Manual of Medical Therapeutics,* Little, Brown and Company, Boston, 1976, Chap. 13.
23. Eckert, op. cit., p. 165.
24. John Graef and Thomas E. Cone (eds.), *Manual of Pediatric Therapeutics,* Little, Brown and Company, Boston, 1975, p. 174.
25. Ibid., p. 175.
26. Eckert, op. cit., p. 398.
27. Ibid.
28. Boedeker and Dauber, op. cit., p. 398.
29. Ibid., p. 399.
30. Ibid., p. 400.
31. Ibid., p. 398.
32. Graef and Cone, op. cit., p. 42.
33. Ibid.
34. Henderson, John, *Emergency Medical Guide,* 4th ed., McGraw-Hill Book Company, New York, 1978, pp. 570–575.

BIBLIOGRAPHY

Boedeker, Edgar, and James Dauber (eds.): *Manual of Medical Therapeutics,* Little, Brown and Company, Boston, 1976. This text is the looseleaf "Washington Manual," a compendium of medical situations, including both medical and neurologic emergencies, their diagnosis, appropriate laboratory tests, signs and symptoms, and immediate treatment. A very clear, concise set of guidelines for the practitioner in medical-surgical and emergency nursing.

Cope, Sir Zachary: *The Early Diagnosis of the Acute Abdomen,* Oxford University Press, London, 1968. This is the classic textbook on the acute abdomen. If none of the rest of the book is read, the first four chapters alone would give the practitioner the necessary skills and knowledge to assess the patient with an abdominal emergency. Varied, individual entities are also described in detail in subsequent chapters, ending with diseases which may simulate the acute abdomen presentation.

Graef, John, and Thomas Cone, *Manual of Pediatric Therapeutics,* Little, Brown and Company, Boston, 1975. A looseleaf reference book dealing with the management and assessment of pediatric diseases and emergencies. Etiology, evaluation, treatment, follow-up, and prevention of each entity is handled concisely throughout the text. An excellent resource for immediate information needed to assess pediatric patient situations.

46
Psychiatric Emergencies
Sherry W. Honea and Beverley H. Durrett

ACUTE DRUG-RELATED PROBLEMS

Definition

The patient may present in coma or delirium, in a panic with extremely hyperactive and/or paranoid behavior, or in convulsions. There are often no immediate clues to assist in identification of the toxic substance ingested; the patient may come in alone or be brought in by police or a rescue squad. (For information on symptoms associated with ingestion of specific types of drugs, refer to Chap. 45.)

Assessment

It is essential to rule out the possibility that the patient's symptoms are due to cerebral trauma, hyper- or hypoglycemia, or other organic abnormality.

I. Data sources.
   A. Patient interview (if possible) may reveal type of substance ingested. Patient's personal effects may reveal empty pill bottles or other clues.
   B. Interview of family or others accompanying patient should focus on identifying details such as when and where patient was found, time of onset of symptoms, clues in the patient's environment, such as pill bottles and/or suicide note.
II. Physical examination.
   A. Note vital signs, particularly respiration and blood pressure.
   B. Note state of consciousness: is patient euphoric, stuporous, or comatose?
   C. Check reaction of pupils; assess status of deep tendon reflexes.
   D. Particularly note any signs of physical trauma and obvious signs of drug use, such as needle "tracks."
III. Diagnostic tests.
   A. Blood and urine screen for drugs and alcohol.
   B. Blood glucose level
   C. Electrolytes.

Problems

I. Maintenance of vital functions.
II. Protection of patient from accidental or self-inflicted injury.
III. Protection of others in the environment if the patient is physically aggressive.

Goals of Care

I. Immediate.
   A. Stop progression of symptoms.
   B. Stabilize vital signs.
   C. Prevent seizures.
II. Long-range. Provide education regarding effects, side effects, physical sequelae of drugs.

Intervention

If the specific substance(s) ingested has been identified, refer to Chap. 45, for management. If the substance(s) is not identified, the patient will have to be managed symptomatically.

I. Coma, with the major symptom of respiratory depression, requires:

    A. Provision of adequate airway: clear respiratory passages of foreign matter, extend head and neck, insert airway if necessary.

    B. Institution of mouth-to-mouth or mechanically assisted ventilation if patient still unable to adequately ventilate by him- or herself; cardiopulmonary resuscitation may be necessary.

    C. Continuous monitoring of vital signs and determination of arterial blood gases.

    D. Provision of intravenous route for administration of drugs; physician will likely decide to place a central venous catheter. Make certain essential supplies are at hand.

    E. Correction of acidosis; physician's decision to administer sodium bicarbonate will be based on assessment of blood gases and success in improving ventilatory exchange. Make certain sodium bicarbonate is available. Naloxone (Narcan), a narcotic antagonist which does not cause respiratory depression, should also be available.

    F. In the deeply comatose patient, resuscitative measures may need to be followed by the insertion of a cuffed endotracheal tube and performance of gastric lavage.

II. Panic, hallucinations, and other hyperactive behavior can be controlled most effectively in the following manner.

    A. Reduce external stimuli; place the patient in a quiet room.

    B. Allow a familiar person to stay with patient, to "talk him down." A staff member should perform this function if patient presents alone.

    C. Keep communication simple: explain all procedures; avoid sudden movements; avoid whispering about patient to another person as this may unnecessarily increase suspicion and anxiety in the patient.

    D. Avoid use of sedative drugs if possible; depressants are contraindicated. If extreme agitation or psychotic thinking is present, diazepam (Valium) or a phenothiazine drug may be ordered; the major side effects to be observed for are hypotension and extrapyramidal symptoms.

III. Convulsions require:

    A. Prevention of injury to patient by placing in bed with side-rails, if possible, or, at the least, positioning patient in manner to prevent injury to head and limbs.

    B. Maintenance of airway, using padded tongue blade or other suitable instrument to hold tongue forward.

    C. Administration of intravenous diazepam (Valium) in convulsion does not spontaneously terminate within a short period of time.

Evaluation

I. Once respiratory function has been stabilized in the comatose patient, it is often necessary to undertake measures to remove the offending substance from the gastrointestinal tract and the bloodstream. These measures will be determined by laboratory identification of the offending substance(s).

II. Hyperactivity and panic caused by ingestion of hallucinogens will usually subside within 4 to 16 h with no further treatment.

III. Detailed history taking following stabilization of the hallucinating patient may indicate need for more intensive psychiatric management.

IV. Further management of the convulsive patient will depend on drug ingestion and medical history. Hospitalization may be indicated to adequately evaluate etiology and initiate appropriate therapy.

ASSAULTIVE BEHAVIOR

Definition

Although proportionately rare in occurrence, *assaultive episodes* are perhaps the most disturbing and disruptive situations encountered by emergency room personnel. The individual who is or has been actually harmful to others is often identified by law enforcement personnel and comes into the emergency room already physically subdued, at least to some extent. The more difficult situation to deal with is the person who goes out of control after arriving at the emergency room; this person may be presenting for treatment himself or may have accompanied someone else for treatment. (Factors contributing to violent behavior are enumerated in Chap. 37.)

Assessment

Due to the life-threatening nature of this situation, it may be necessary to take immediate action, then assess the situation. Factors to be considered immediately include:

I. Is the individual wielding a weapon?
II. Are sufficient personnel available to subdue the individual?
III. Are others in the environment in imminent danger?

Problems

I. Immediate threat to life.
II. Arousal of anxiety, fear, and anger for all involved in the situation.

Goals of Care

I. Immediate.
  A. Protect lives and property from harm.
  B. Assist individual in regaining control of behavior.
II. Long-range. Assist all involved in dealing with emotional responses to the incident.

Intervention

I. Call for any needed additional help.
II. Talk with the violent individual, and keep talking throughout management of the situation. Often, conveying the expectation that the situation is under control and that the patient will behave well is sufficient to end the crisis.
III. If there is immediate danger to the violent individual or others, staff must intervene, regardless of personal risk; if violence is destructive only to property, staff should intervene when this can be done at no personal risk.
IV. As quickly as possible, remove from the situation any others who may be in danger.
V. If initial attempts at verbal intervention are not sufficient, move quickly to bring physical measures to bear on the situation. Gather as much physical force as would be necessary to subdue the patient (at least four people for an adult male). This "show of force" is frequently all that it takes to subdue the patient.
VI. When it is obvious that physical control is necessary, limit the patient's range of movement and work him or her into a corner if possible.
VII. Throwing a blanket over the patient's head or pinning him or her to the wall with a lightweight mattress are very effective ways to immobilize him or her, especially if the individual is wielding a weapon.

VIII. After immobilizing the patient, bring him or her to the floor so that he or she is in a face-down position.

IX. Medications (most often phenothiazines) may be administered to effect control. Physical restraint should be maintained until medication takes effect. Close monitoring of vital signs should be maintained; hypotension is a frequent side effect of phenothiazines.

X. Mechanical restraints should be used only if medication does not sufficiently control the patient's behavior. If restraints are necessary, the following precautions should be observed:

A. Protect skin from abrasion by using padded restraints.

B. Constant attendance of patient is preferred. If this is not possible, he or she should be observed at least every 15 min.

C. Check circulation of extremities frequently; loosen or reposition restraints as necessary.

D. If the patient is maintained in restraints for more than 2 h, provision must be made for exercise of extremities. Remove restraint from one extremity at a time, provide range-of-motion exercises, replace restraint, and repeat procedure for other extremities. If the patient is still fighting restraints, at least two staff should be present when even one extremity is removed from restraint. Repeat every 2 h.

E. Provide skin care and change position, if necessary, when the range-of-motion exercises are performed.

F. Offer fluids frequently but in small amounts. To prevent aspiration, assist patient to sitting position, if possible, before offering nourishment.

G. Offer urinal and/or bedpan at frequent intervals.

H. The decision to remove restraints should be based on careful assessment of patient's physical and mental status. Calming of physical activity and verbalization of intent to cooperate *may* indicate that the patient may be released from restraints. Sufficient personnel should be available to control unpredictable behavior before restraints are removed. Assist the patient to ambulate slowly; postural hypotension may cause initial dizziness and unsteadiness.

XI. Seclusion may be necessary to remove the individual from stimuli with which he or she cannot cope. If seclusion is utilized, the following precautions should be observed:

A. The room should be "safe," i.e., minimal or no furnishings, protected electrical outlets, recessed light fixtures, and a smooth, non-toxic finish on walls and floors. If this environment is not available, the patient must be constantly attended.

B. Frequent or constant observation of the patient is essential, minimally *every* 15 min.

C. Staff should never enter the seclusion room alone, even after the aggressive behavior has subsided.

D. Food and fluids should be served in nonbreakable, preferably paper, dishes.

E. The decision to allow the patient to come out of the seclusion room to use the toilet will depend on its location. Initially, it may be advisable to use a portable commode chair or urinal. If the patient is allowed to go to the toilet, he or she must be constantly attended. *Providing privacy is not appropriate at this point.*

F. After giving care, always check the room before leaving to be sure you are taking all equipment with you.

G. When the decision is made to allow the patient out of seclusion, he or she should be constantly attended until assessment is made of his or her ability to handle additional stimulation.

Evaluation

I. When the individual's behavior is brought under control, further assessment of the situation is in order. This should include:

A. Interview of patient, if appropriate, to identify precipitating events. If a significant other is available, he or she may be able to provide this information.

      B. Review of health history for:
        1. Previous record of assaultive behavior.
        2. History of alcohol or drug abuse.
        3. History of psychiatric illness, such as schizophrenia, antisocial personality, or paranoid state.
        4. Symptoms suggestive of temporal lobe epilepsy and/or cerebral lesion.
        5. Difficulties in interpersonal relationships such as explosive personality, domestic quarreling, generalized social maladjustment.
      C. Assessment of the potential for future incidents of violence. Is he or she going back into the same situation which precipitated the current episode? Is he or she experiencing command hallucinations of a homicidal nature?

II. Further treatment will depend on the findings of the assessment. Alternatives may include:
      A. Admission to an inpatient facility for psychiatric and/or medical evaluation.
      B. Referral for treatment of alcohol or drug abuse.
      C. Referral for psychotherapy on an outpatient basis.

III. For all involved in the life-threatening situation, it is essential to provide time for discussion of their reactions to the incident. Staff, as well as other patients, need an opportunity to ventilate their feelings of fear, anger, and frustrations generated by such situations.

RAPE

Definition

Rape is most often defined as sexual intercourse with a female without her consent; intercourse may be effected by force or intimidation, or she may be too young or without sufficient intelligence to give consent. While most rape victims are young women, the elderly and the pregnant woman are also frequent victims, as well as children of both sexes and men. For all victims, rape is an encounter with life-threatening violence. It is not necessarily perceived as primarily a sex crime. Although physical trauma is frequently seen, psychological trauma is usually far more devastating to the victim. Emotional responses include shock, anger, guilt, shame, and fear of rejection by friends and family. Lasting impairment of sexual functioning may be a frequent result of unresolved psychological trauma.

Assessment

I. Physical examination.
      A. Particularly note bruises, lacerations, general condition of victim's clothing and body.
      B. Vaginal examination should be performed with water-moistened speculum, noting any evidence of trauma to external or internal genitalia.

II. Psychological assessment.
      A. Note mental status.
      B. Identify major concerns.
      C. Identify social supports available to victim (spouse, family, friends).

III. Diagnostic tests.
      A. Provide for immediate examination of smears from vulva and fornix for presence of motile sperm.
      B. Culture for *Neisseria* and *Treponema*.
      C. Take fingernail scrapings.
      D. Comb pubic hair for free hairs.

Problems

    I. Physical trauma.

    II. Psychological trauma.

    III. Possible venereal disease.

    IV. Possible pregnancy.

Goals of Care

    I. Immediate.

        A. Treat physical trauma.

        B. Provide support in coping with psychological trauma.

    II. Long-range.

        A. Preserve physical evidence for use in court.

        B. Assist patient to deal with possible physical sequelae (pregnancy, venereal disease).

Intervention

    I. Make certain that victim is not left alone. If she comes to the agency alone, stay with her until arrangements are made for a friend, relative, or rape crisis counselor to be with her. (Know how to contact a rape crisis center in your community.)

    II. Encourage verbalization. Assist in identifying feelings, fears, available social supports.

    III. Explain physical examination; stay with victim, repeating explanations as necessary.

    IV. Emphasize need for preservation of physical evidence in case of prosecution. Do not allow bath or shower before examination.

    V. Assist victim in explanation to family or friends if they are available.

    VI. Provide full information on prophylaxis available for prevention of pregnancy and venereal disease.

    VII. Arrange escort home. If available, rape crisis counselors provide this service.

    VIII. Make certain that all findings are accurately recorded in the medical record, including results of the physical examination, description of the victim's appearance and responses, and a description of the assault in the patient's own words.

Evaluation

    I. Before discharge from your facility, make arrangements for follow-up. A phone call or a home visit within a few days to evaluate victim's coping and need for further assistance is appropriate.

    II. Counseling may be indicated for the victim and family as they attempt to integrate the experience into their lives. Problems with resuming sexual functioning are common.

    III. Long-term therapy may be indicated for the victim who develops phobic reactions, persistent sexual dysfunctions, chronic anxiety, and depression.

SUICIDE

Definition

The term *suicide* is applied to all cases of death resulting directly or indirectly from a positive or negative act of the victim himself which he or she knows will produce this result. An "attempt" is an act so defined but falling short of actual death. The patient who either presents a suicidal risk or who has actually made a suicidal attempt is the most common emergency in psychiatric practice.

The patient may present her- or himself to a health agency requesting help in dealing with suicidal impulses or stating she or he has ingested a potentially lethal substance such as pills, household chemicals, pesticides, poison. She or he may be brought into an emergency facility in coma or with self-inflicted physical trauma from any number of causes.

A number of factors are positively correlated with high suicide risk. Depression is the most common of these factors. Also included are a history of previous suicide attempts or violent episodes, recent real or perceived loss of personal significance, chronic medical illness, alcohol or drug abuse, and chronic lack of resources such as people, money, or purpose. (For a more detailed discussion of factors associated with suicide risk, see Chap. 37.)

Assessment

I. Physical examination.
   A. Trauma.
   B. Level of consciousness.
   C. Vital signs.
II. Psychological assessment (if patient's condition permits).
   A. Expressed intent. Did he or she want to die? Was he or she using the gesture as a cry for help?
   B. What are his or her feelings about outcome of attempt? Is he or she glad to have been found? Does he or she express wish to have died?
   C. What are his or her plans for future? Does he or she talk about "doing a better job" next time? Can he or she voice any hope?
III. Medical and psychiatric history (may have to be obtained by interviewing family or friends).
   A. Previous suicide attempts.
   B. Previous episodes of violence.
   C. Chronic medical or psychiatric illness.
   D. Alcohol or drug use.
   E. Prescribed medications (some which may cause depression as a side effect include steroids, hormones, antihypertensives).
IV. Social assessment.
   A. Marital status.
   B. Living arrangements.
   C. Job situation.
   D. Financial status.
   E. Tangible losses.
   F. Blows to self-concept.
   G. Friends.

Problems

I. Immediate treatment of physical results of suicide attempt.
II. Assessment of continued suicide risk.
III. Provision of appropriate follow-up.

Goals of Care

I. Immediate.
   A. Stabilize physiologically.
   B. Provide protection from further self-harm.

  C. Provide opportunity to express feelings.

  D. Assist in identifying alternatives to harming self.

 II. Long-range. Establish ongoing supportive relationship with professional person or organization.

Intervention

 I. *Do not leave patient alone.*

 II. Treat physical trauma as indicated (suturing, lavage, setting fractures, oxygen, prepare for surgery, etc.).

 III. Encourage ventilation of feelings.

 IV. Provide care in a manner to enhance self-esteem. Provide privacy, listen, acknowledge the feelings of hopelessness and despair.

 V. Assist in identifying strengths and resources.

 VI. Assist in identifying situations which precipitate suicidal ideation, consequences of self-destructive behavior, and more positive alternative coping behaviors, based on identified strengths and resources.

 VII. Avoid guilt-inducing statements, such as, "But you have so much to live for," or, "Don't you care anything about how your family (friends) feels?"

 VIII. Prepare for dealing with the responses of significant others, which are likely to be anger, guilt, feelings of responsibility for causing the act.

 IX. In the case of the completed suicide, the family or friends of the victim are likely to need supportive care.

  A. Do not leave them alone when they are given the news of the death.

  B. Encourage verbalization of feelings.

  C. Acknowledge difficulty in dealing with grief, anger, and sense of responsibility for the death.

  D. Provide assistance in making arrangements for disposition of the body.

Evaluation

 I. Hospitalization is indicated for management of the continuing high-risk patient. Commitment may be necessary and can be effected on the basis of "imminent danger to self" in all jurisdictions.

 II. If discharge is planned when physiologically stable, provision must be made to insure patient is not alone; family, friends, YWCA, YMCA, Salvation Army are all possible resources.

 III. Confirm plans for follow-up before releasing patient, such as referral to personal physician or mental health center.

 IV. Educate patient on availability of emergency services in the community such as hot-line or suicide prevention service.

 V. Explore possibility of family therapy.

 VI. Assist in identifying social outlets in the community such as clubs, church groups, volunteer work.

ACUTE ALCOHOLIC INTOXICATION

Definition

Alcoholic intoxication may be defined as a state in which the ingestion of alcohol has resulted in noticeable impairment of speech and coordination or alteration in behavior. The acutely intoxicated patient often presents in the emergency room because the impairment in his or her behavior has resulted in accidental injury or has brought him or her to the attention of law enforcement agents. (For a more complete description of the stages of intoxication, refer to Chap. 35.)

Assessment

It is important to rule out other medical conditions which may result in behavior which "looks like" acute intoxication. Assuming that an individual who is disoriented or uncoordinated and smells of alcohol is "drunk" may result in a tragic outcome for individuals suffering from such conditions as subdural hematoma, other cerebral trauma, hypoglycemia, hepatic failure, diabetic coma, barbiturate overdose, toxic psychosis secondary to mixing alcohol and other drugs.

I. Physical examination.
   A. Vital signs: close monitoring of respiratory rate and depth is essential.
   B. Reaction of pupils.
   C. Reflexes.
   D. Evidence of physical trauma such as bruises, abrasions, or lacerations.
II. Health history (may have to be obtained from family or friends).
   A. Chronic medical or psychiatric illness.
   B. Other drugs ingested or available.
   C. History of falls, head trauma.
III. Drinking history (may have to be obtained from family or friends).
   A. Description of this episode. When did drinking start? How much alcohol was consumed? Was there any concomitant food intake?
   B. What is his or her usual behavior when drinking?
   C. Are any situational factors associated with excessive drinking?
IV. Diagnostic tests.
   A. Blood alcohol level.
   B. Blood sugar.
   C. Blood urea nitrogen.
   D. Urine screen for drugs.

Problems

I. Maintenance of vital functions.
II. Protection of patient from accidental or self-inflicted injury.
III. Protection of others in environment from hostile or aggressive behavior.

Goals of Care

I. Immediate.
   A. Control disruptive behavior.
   B. Treat physical trauma, medical complications.
II. Long-range. Provide patient education:
   A. Effects of alcohol: how much, how fast body can handle lithout toxic effects.
   B. Alternate methods of dealing with anxiety and tension.

Intervention

I. Treatment of trauma, acute medical problems, as indicated.
II. Control disruptive behavior.
   A. Nonstimulating environment.
   B. Soft restraints.

C. Tranquilizing drugs are indicated only in otherwise unmanageable situations. Diazepam (Valium) or chlordiazepoxide (Librium) would be the drug of choice. Potentially synergistic depression of vital functions requires close monitoring of vital signs.

III. Antiemetics may be ordered parenterally for nausea.

IV. Nonjudgmental attitude is essential on part of care providers. Avoid labeling patient as "just another drunk," as the needs for care are legitimate.

V. Attempts at "reasoning" with patient are likely to be ineffective during intoxicated state. Act to bring situation under control as quickly as possible and then talk with patient.

VI. When patient is sober, attempt to provide information on effects of alcohol, other medical problems, and other alternatives for dealing with anxiety and tension, such as meaningful leisure-time activities, psychotherapy.

Evaluation

I. Hospitalization is indicated if there are serious medical problems.

II. Release to family or friends is first choice if not hospitalized; refer to community facilities, such as YWCA, YMCA, or Salvation Army if no personal resources.

III. Jail may be appropriate if a crime has been committed while under the influence of alcohol or if he or she poses a threat to society.

IV. Arrange follow-up appointment with health professional or mental health agency to assess extent of alcohol problem and need for long-term therapy.

ACUTE GRIEF REACTION

Definition

For purposes of this discussion, an *acute grief reaction* is one following a sudden, unexpected loss of a significant person or persons in one's life. This is likely to be encountered by emergency room personnel as a result of death by trauma, as in an automobile accident, or sudden death from natural causes such as myocardial infarction or cerebral hemorrhage. The grief reaction may be manifested by any number of behaviors, ranging from no apparent emotional reaction to hysteria. Feelings of anger and guilt are often expressed in self-blaming, such as, "If only I hadn't . . . ," or blaming health care personnel, such as, "Why wasn't there a doctor here sooner? Wasn't there anything else you could do? Don't you care at all?"

Assessment

I. Is the bereaved individual alone?

II. Is the individual openly expressing grief?

III. What was the individual's relationship with the deceased? How close was the emotional attachment?

IV. Is any information available on the physical condition of the bereaved individual?

V. What social supports are immediately available?

Problems

I. Providing support and acceptance in expression of grief.

II. Encouraging ventilation of feelings.

III. Maintaining objectivity on part of staff.

Goals of Care

Facilitate expression of feelings in the initial phase of shock and grief reaction.

Intervention

I. Do not leave the bereaved individual alone. Staff should leave only if other family members are present and request to be left alone.

II. Provide privacy: take the bereaved away from the mainstream of hospital activity. If a hospital chapel is available, it is ideal. If not, any quiet area can be used.

III. Acknowledge the feelings of sadness, loss, guilt, and anger. Avoid personalizing blame, if this is occurring. Remain as objective as possible, as it is difficult to be helpful if you are overly involved emotionally.

IV. Encourage expression of feelings through verbalization and/or crying.

V. Allow and encourage the bereaved to view the body of the deceased. This may later be a significant aspect of accepting the reality of the loss of the significant other.

VI. If requested, call a minister and/or relatives. If not requested, ask the bereaved if there is anyone he or she wishes to have called.

VII. Assist with arrangements for disposition of the body: explain an autopsy if one is required or requested; call the mortician chosen by the bereaved.

VIII. Often medications such as sedatives and hypnotics are given to assist the bereaved to cope with intense feelings. If this is so, watch for immediate side effects such as oversedation and hypotension; monitor vital signs.

Evaluation

I. Do not allow the individual to leave alone if this can be avoided. If family, friends, or minister are not available, or the bereaved is a stranger to the area, contact local social service agencies to provide immediate arrangements for companionship, lodging, and food.

II. Reassess physical condition, particularly if any medical or psychiatric problems are known to exist. Treat any exacerbation of symptoms.

III. Assess suicide risk. This is particularly important if the bereaved is alone and/or is showing little apparent reaction to the loss. If there is significant suicide risk and there is no one to stay with the bereaved, hospitalization is indicated.

IV. Provide appropriate information to the individual about the use and side-effects of drugs prescribed to be taken at home. If drugs are given, caution the individual against driving.

BIBLIOGRAPHY

Ciuca, Rudy, Carol S. Downie, and Magdalena Morris: "When a Disaster Happens," *American Journal of Nursing*, **77**:3, March 1977. This is an excellent article, well worth reading for its objective treatment of an emotion-laden occurrence. It emphasizes the need for every hospital to have a workable disaster plan which includes a mental health team, since emotional support for survivors is as important as medical care for victims. The role of the mental health team is described as one of crisis intervention in the initial phase of shock and grief reactions, with the primary goal being to facilitate the emotional expression of grief.

Findeiss, J. Clifford: "Drug Abuse Today: Recognition and Emergency Management," *Emergency Medical Care*, International Medical Books, New York, 1974, pp. 111–112. This takes some of the guesswork out of diagnosing drug abusers in the emergency room, by presenting some of the more common manifestations of abuse and overdose. Presenting symptoms are succinctly enumerated, and alternatives for intervention are suggested. The article points out medical complications as well as emotional consideration of drug abuse.

Lindemann, Erich: "Symptomatology and Management of Acute Grief," *American Journal of Psychiatry*, **101**:141–148, September 1944. This article, a classic of its kind, is as relevant today as when it was written in 1944 by Dr. Lindemann, a pioneer in the study of bereavement. His theoretical formulations on grief and crises intervention have been of invaluable assistance to counselors in understanding and treating patient's grief responses, both normal and abnormal. A basic premise is that abnormal grief may be transformed to normal grief through the use of appropriate techniques or preventive intervention. This inquiry has encouraged other investigators to test and observe and has stimulated a rich succession of studies on crisis.

Slaby, Andrew E., Julian Lieb, and Laurence R. Tancredi: *Handbook of Psychiatric Emergencies*, Medical Examination Publishing Company, New York, 1975. This is a fairly complete guide for handling psychiatric emergencies, especially those occurring in the emergency room. Although written for physicians, it is easily adaptable for use not only by nurses, but also by allied health personnel. It is particularly helpful to the inexperienced emergency room worker, since it pinpoints some of the more common fears and suggests prompt and decisive interventions.

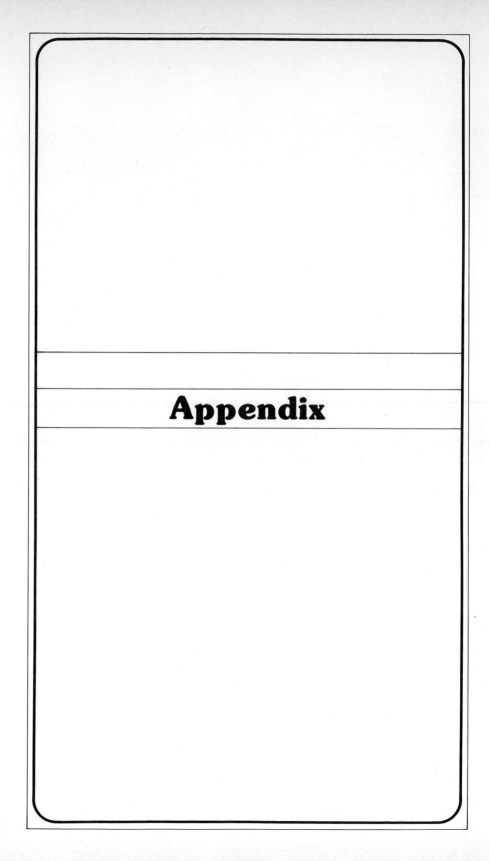

Appendix

COMMUNICABLE AND INFECTIOUS DISEASES

Name	Incubation period	Period of communicability	Mode of transfer
Amebic dysentery (amebiasis)	2–4 weeks	During period of passing of feces contaminated with protozoan cysts; may continue for years	Food or water contaminated with the feces of infected persons
Anthrax	2–5 days, at least within 7 days	No evidence of transmission from person to person; articles and soil contaminated with spores may remain infective for years	Skin contact with tissue, wool, hides, and hair of infected animals and with soil contaminated by infected animals; inhalation of spores; ingestion of contaminated undercooked meat
Bacillary dysentery (shigellosis)	Usually less than 4 days, range 1–7 days	During acute infection and until infectious agent no longer present in feces (usually within 4 weeks of illness)	Fecal-oral transmission from infected individual or carrier, either by direct contact or contamination of food, water, or fomites; spread of contaminated feces by flies
Brucellosis	5–21 days, occasionally several months	No evidence of communicability from person to person	Contact with body fluids, tissues, aborted fetuses, and placentas of infected animals; ingestion of milk and dairy products from infected animals; inhalation of infectious agent
Candidiasis (moniliasis, thrush)	Variable, 2–5 days for thrush	While lesions persist	Contact with excretions from mouth, skin, vagina, and with feces of patients or carriers; during birth via contact with vaginal secretions; contact with contaminated bladder catheters and IV tubing
Chancroid	3–5 days, up to 14 days; can be as short as 24 h if mucous membranes not intact	While infectious agent present in original lesion or in discharging regional lymph nodes; can last for weeks	Sexual contact with discharges from open lesions or buboes; may be asymptomatic infection in women
Chickenpox (varicella) shingles (herpes zoster)	13–17 days; may extend to 21 days	As long as 5 days before eruption of chickenpox and not more than 6 days after last crop of vesicles	Spread of respiratory secretions of infected persons by direct, droplet, or airborne route; indirect spread by fomites freshly soiled with discharges from vesicles and mucous membranes of infected persons; scabs are not infective; susceptible persons may contract chickenpox from individuals with herpes zoster
Cholera	2–3 days; range from a few hours to 5 days	Not definitely known, presumed to last for duration of stool-positive carrier state which lasts for a few days after recovery	Ingestion of food or water contaminated with feces or vomitus of infected persons or with feces of carriers
Coccidioidomycosis	1–4 weeks	Not directly transmitted from persons or animals to man	Inhalation of spores from soil or culture media
Common cold	24 h; range 12–72 h	24 hours before onset to 5 days after onset	Direct oral contact or spread by droplet Fomites freshly soiled by nasal and oral discharges of infected persons
Dengue fever	5–6 days; range 3–15 days	Not directly transmitted from person to person	Bite of infective mosquito

COMMUNICABLE AND INFECTIOUS DISEASES (continued)

Name	Incubation period	Period of communicability	Mode of transfer
Diphtheria	2–5 days	Usually 2 weeks or less, but seldom more than 4 weeks Until virulent bacilli are no longer present in discharges and lesions Carrier may disseminate organisms for 6 months or longer	Contact with droplets from mouth, nose, or throat of infected person or carrier Rarely by articles soiled with discharges from lesions of infected person
Encephalitis Mosquito-borne	5–15 days	Not directly transmitted from person to person	Bite of infective mosquito
Tick-borne	7–14 days	Same as above	Bite of infective ticks, milk from certain infected animals
Flukes Blood (schistosomiasis)	4–6 weeks after infection systemic manifestations usually begin	Usually 1–2 years or as long as eggs are discharged in urine or feces of infected person; may be 25 years or longer	Penetration of skin by free-swimming larvae
Intestinal (fasciolopsiasis)	Approx. 7 weeks from ingestion of infective larvae; eggs found in stool 1 month after infection	As long as viable eggs are discharged by patient: not directly transmitted from person to person	Ingestion of uncooked freshwater plants and snails containing the encysted larvae
Liver (clonorchiasis)	Undetermined; flukes reach maturity within 16–25 days after person ingests encysted larvae	Viable eggs may be passed by infected individual for up to 30 years, not directly transmitted from person to person	Ingestion of freshwater fish containing encysted larvae
Food Poisoning Botulism	Usually 12–36 h, sometimes several days	Not directly transmitted from person to person	Ingestion of improperly processed and inadequately cooked foods (usually from cans or jars) containing the toxin
Clostridium perfringens	10–12 h; range 8–22 h	Same as above	Inadequately heated meats containing feces or soil in which organism has multiplied
Salmonellosis	12–36 h; range 6–72 h	Several days to several weeks; occasionally a temporary carrier state continues for months, but rarely for over 1 year	Ingestion of food contaminated by feces of infected man or animals; inadequately cooked meat, poultry, and egg products; pharmaceuticals made from animal products
Staphylococcal	2–4 hours; range 1–6 h	Not directly transmitted from person to person	Ingestion of contaminated food in which toxin-producing staphylococci from humans or cows have multiplied; food left standing before serving
German measles (rubella)	18 days; range 14–21 days	1 week before and at least 4 days after onset of rash	Droplet spread or direct contact with nasopharyngeal secretions of infected persons or with articles freshly soiled with discharges from nose and throat; may also be spread by urine, blood, and feces of infected persons
Giardiasis	Variable, usually 6–22 days	Entire period of infection	Water contaminated by feces; hand-to-mouth transfer of cysts from feces of infected persons

COMMUNICABLE AND INFECTIOUS DISEASES (continued)

Name	Incubation period	Period of communicability	Mode of transfer
Gonorrhea	Usually 2–5 days, may be as long as 9 days	Months or years if untreated, especially in females who are often asymptomatic	Sexual contact with exudate from mucous membranes of infected persons
Granuloma Inguinale	Unknown, presumably 8–80 days	Unknown; presumably during period of open lesions on skin and mucous membranes	Sexual contact with lesions
Hepatitis Infectious (type A)	28–30 days; range 15–50 days	From latter half of incubation period to a few days after onset of jaundice	Person to person transmission via fecal-oral route; ingestion of contaminated food and water containing infective human feces, blood, or urine; parental administration of infected blood or blood products
Serum (type B) (homologous serum jaundice)	60–90 days; range 45–160 days	From several weeks before onset of symptoms through clinical course of disease; carrier state may last for years	Parenteral administration of infected blood and blood products; contaminated needles, syringes, and IV equipment
Herpes simplex	Up to 2 weeks	Up to 7 weeks after recovery from stomatitis for HSV type 1	HSV Type 1: Direct contact with virus in saliva of carriers HSV Type 2: Sexual contact
Histoplasmosis	10 days; range 5–18 days	Not usually transmitted from person to person	Inhalation of spores on dust particles
Infectious mononucleosis	2–6 weeks	Unknown	Spread from person to person via oral-pharyngeal route
Influenza	1–3 days	3 days from onset	Direct contact, droplet infection, or contact with articles freshly contaminated with discharges from nose and throat of infected persons
Keratoconjunctivitis, epidemic	5–12 days	From late in incubation period until 14 days after onset	Direct contact with eye secretions of infected persons or with instruments or solutions contaminated with these secretions
Leishmaniasis, visceral (kala azar)	2–4 months; range 10 days–2 years	While parasite remains in circulating blood or skin of mammalian reservoir host	Bite of infective sandflies; direct transmission from person to person and via blood transfusion has been reported
Leptospirosis	10 days; range 4–19 days	Direct transmission from person to person is rare	Contact with water, moist soil, or vegetation contaminated with urine of infected animals; direct contact with infected animals
Lymphogranuloma venereum	5–30 days	Variable; while active lesions persist; may be weeks or years	Sexual contact with open lesions; indirect contact with articles contaminated by discharges

COMMUNICABLE AND INFECTIOUS DISEASES (continued)

Name	Incubation period	Period of communicability	Mode of transfer
Malaria			*For all:* Bite of infective female anopheline mosquito; injection or transfusion of blood of infected person; use of contaminated syringes
Benign Tertian (vivax malaria)	14 days	1–3 years	
Quartan	30 days	Indefinitely	
Malignant tertian (falciparum malaria)	12 days	Not more than one year *For all:* patient infective for mosquitoes for as long as plasmodia gametocytes are present in blood	
Measles (rubeola)	10 days; range 8–13 days from exposure to onset of fever; 14 days until rash appears	From beginning of prodromal period until 14 days after rash appears	Droplet spread or direct contact with nose and throat discharges or urine of infected persons; less commonly transmitted by fomites freshly soiled with nose and throat secretions or by airborne spread
Meningococcal meningitis	3–4 days; range 2–10 days	Until organisms no longer present in secretions from nose and mouth; communicability ceases within 24 h after start of appropriate chemotherapy	Droplet spread and direct contact with discharges from nose and throat of clinically infected persons and carriers
Mumps	18 days; range 12–26 days	Height of communicability occurs approximately 48 h before swelling begins; virus has been found in saliva from 6 days before salivary gland involvement to 9 days after	Droplet spread and direct contact with saliva of an infected person
Paratyphoid fever	1–10 days for gastroenteritis, 1–3 weeks for enteric fever	1–2 weeks or as long as organism exists in excreta	Direct or indirect contact with urine or feces of patient or carrier; commonly spread by milk products or shellfish contaminated by hands of a carrier
Pediculosis	Eggs of lice hatch in 1 week under optimal conditions; sexual maturity is reached in 2 weeks	While lice remain alive on infested person or in clothing and until eggs in hair and clothing have been destroyed	Direct contact with an infested person, indirect contact with clothing, linen, and headgear on which lice or eggs exist
Plague	2–6 weeks	Bubonic plague not directly transmitted from person to person; pneumonic plague highly communicable in conditions of overcrowding	Bubonic plague transmitted by bite of oriental rat flea (*Xenopsylla cheopis*) and by contact with tissues of infected animals; pneumonic plague spread by airborne droplets from respiratory tract of an infected person
Pneumonia			
Pneumococcal and Other Bacterial	1–3 days	While infectious agent present in oral and nasal discharges	Spread by droplet or direct oral contact; indirect transmission through articles freshly soiled with respiratory discharges of infected persons
Primary atypical (mycoplasmal)	14–21 days	Usually less than 10 days; occasionally may last longer with persisting fever	Same as above
Poliomyelitis	7–12 days; range 3–21 days	7–10 days before and after onset of symptoms	Direct contact with feces or secretions from pharynx of infected persons

COMMUNICABLE AND INFECTIOUS DISEASES (continued)

Name	Incubation period	Period of communicability	Mode of transfer
Q Fever	14–21 days	Direct transmission from person to person is rare	Inhalation of the rickettsiae in dust particles contaminated with excreta of infected animals; direct contact with infected animals and associated materials such as straw, fertilizer
Rabies	2–8 weeks	In biting animals for 3–5 days before onset of symptoms and throughout course of the disease	Virus transmitted in the saliva from the bite of an infected animal
Ringworm			
Body (tinea corporis)	4–10 days	While lesions present on body and viable spores exist on fomites	Contact with skin lesions of infected persons and animals and with contaminated furniture, bathroom fixtures, floors, and shower stalls
Foot (tinea pedis, athlete's foot)	Unknown	Same as above	Contact with skin lesions of infected persons or with contaminated floors, shower stalls, and other articles used by infected persons
Scalp (tinea capitis)	10–14 days	Same as above	Contact with infective lesions and with articles such as seats, toilet articles, or clothing contaminated with hair from infected persons or animals
Rocky mountain spotted fever	3–10 days	Not directly transmitted from person to person; tick remains infective for life, often as long as 18 months	Bite of an infected tick which has been attached to the skin for at least 4–6 h; contamination of the skin with crushed tissue or excreta of the tick
Roundworms			
Giant intestinal roundworm (ascariasis)	Worms reach maturity about 2 months after embryonated eggs are ingested by humans	As long as fertilized female worms live in intestine; adult worm usually lives less than 10 months; embryonated eggs may live in soil for months	Ingestion of soil containing infective eggs in human feces; not directly transmitted from person to person
Hookworm (ancylostomiasis)	A few weeks to several months	Potentially for several years if infected person not treated	Penetration of skin (usually of foot) by larvae in moist soil contaminated with feces
Pinworm (enterobiasis)	Life cycle of worm is 3–6 weeks	As long as gravid females remain in intestine; frequently reinfection by self or family members occurs	Direct transfer of eggs from anus to mouth by unwashed hands; indirect transfer of eggs via food, clothing, bedding, toilet seats Inhalation of eggs on dust particles
Threadworm (strongyloidiasis)	Indefinite and variable	As long as living worms remain in intestine	Penetration of skin (usually of foot) by larvae in moist soil contaminated with feces
Trichinosis	9 days after ingestion of infective meat; range 2–28 days	Not directly transmitted from person to person	Ingestion of insufficiently cooked pork containing encysted viable larvae
Whipworm (trichuriasis)	Indefinite	Same as above	Ingestion of soil contaminated with eggs from human feces
Scabies	Several days to weeks before itching occurs	Until mites and eggs are destroyed by specific treatment	Direct contact with skin of an infected person; to a small extent by bedding and clothing used by an infected person

COMMUNICABLE AND INFECTIOUS DISEASES (continued)

Name	Incubation period	Period of communicability	Mode of transfer
Scarlet fever	1–3 days	10–21 days in untreated cases	Droplet spread by patient or carrier
Shingles (herpes zoster)	See Chickenpox		
Smallpox (variola)	10–12 days to onset of illness; range 7–17 days; 2–4 more days to onset of rash	Approx. 3 weeks; from development of first lesions to disappearance of all scabs; most communicable during first week	Direct contact with respiratory discharges, mucous membranes, and skin lesions of infected persons; indirect contact with articles contaminated by infected person; airborne spread
Streptococcal sore throat	1–3 days	10–21 days in untreated cases; transmission generally eliminated in 24 h with adequate penicillin therapy	Direct contact with respiratory discharges of an infected person; ingestion of contaminated milk or other food
Syphilis	21 days; range 10 days–10 weeks	Variable; intermittently communicable for 2–4 years during primary and secondary stages and during mucocutaneous recurrence; infectiveness ends within 24 h with adequate treatment with penicillin	Direct contact during sexual activity with saliva, semen, vaginal discharges, blood, and exudates from moist skin lesions and mucous membranes; placental transfer after 4th month of pregnancy; occasionally transferred by blood transfusion
Tapeworms			
Beef	8–14 weeks	Not directly transmitted from person to person	Ingestion of inadequately cooked beef containing the infective larvae
Fish	3–6 weeks	Same as above	Ingestion of inadequately cooked fish
Pork	8–14 weeks	Eggs remain viable for months and are discharged in feces for as long as worms live in intestines	Ingestion of inadequately cooked pork containing infective larvae; direct transfer of eggs in feces to mouth; ingestion of food or water containing eggs
Tetanus (lockjaw)	10 days; range 4–21 days	Not directly transmitted from person to person	Tetanus spores enter body via puncture wounds contaminated with soil which contains the feces of infected persons or animals
Trachoma	5–12 days	While active lesions are present in conjunctivae and surrounding mucous membranes	Direct contact with discharges from the eye and possibly discharges from nasal mucous membranes of infected persons; contact with articles contaminated with these discharges
Trichomoniasis	7 days; range 4–20 days	While infection persists	Sexual contact with vaginal and urethral secretions of infected persons; during birth via contact with vaginal secretions
Tuberculosis	4–12 weeks from infection to primary lesion	As long as infectious tubercle bacilli are discharged in sputum	Airborne and droplet spread from sputum of infected persons
Tularemia	3 days; range 1–10 days	Not directly transmitted from person to person	Handling diseased animals or their hides; ingestion of undercooked infected wild rodents; bite of insects which have fed on infected animals

COMMUNICABLE AND INFECTIOUS DISEASES (continued)

Name	Incubation period	Period of communicability	Mode of transfer
Typhoid fever	7–21 days	Until typhoid bacilli no longer appear in excreta; approx. 10% of patients discharge bacilli for 3 months after onset of symptoms; 2–5% become carriers	Ingestion of food or water contaminated by feces or urine of a patient or carrier
Typhus fever Epidemic louse-borne	12 days; range 7–14 days	Not directly transmitted from person to person	Rubbing crushed lice or their feces into bitten area on skin
Flea-borne (murine)	Same as above	Same as above	Bite of infective rat fleas
Mite-borne (scrub typhus, tsutsugamushi disease)	10–12 days; range 6–21 days	Same as above	Bite of infective mites during the larval stage
Whooping cough (pertussis)	7 days, not longer than 21 days	7 days after exposure to 3 weeks after onset of paroxysmal cough	Direct contact with respiratory secretions of infected persons; droplet spread; indirect contact with fomites freshly soiled with respiratory discharges of infected persons
Yellow fever	3–6 days	Not directly transmitted from person to person; highly communicable where many susceptible persons and mosquito vectors concurrently exist	Bite of infective mosquitoes
Yaws	2 weeks–3 months	Variable; while moist lesions are present	Direct contact with exudates from early skin lesions of infected persons

FAHRENHEIT AND CELSIUS EQUIVALENTS

Fahrenheit to Celsius: $(F - 32) \times 5/9 = C$ or $C = \dfrac{F - 32}{1.8}$

F°	C°	F°	C°	F°	C°	F°	C°	F°	C°
−40	−40.0	11	−11.67	62	16.67	113	45.0	164	73.33
−39	−39.44	12	−11.11	63	17.22	114	45.56	165	73.89
−38	−38.89	13	−10.56	64	17.78	115	46.11	166	74.44
−37	−38.33	14	−10.0	65	18.33	116	46.67	167	75.0
−36	−37.78	15	−9.44	66	18.89	117	47.22	168	75.56
−35	−37.22	16	−8.89	67	19.44	118	47.78	169	76.11
−34	−36.67	17	−8.33	68	20.0	119	48.33	170	76.67
−33	−36.11	18	−7.78	69	20.56	120	48.89	171	77.22
−32	−35.56	19	−7.22	70	21.11	121	49.44	172	77.78
−31	−35.0	20	−6.67	71	21.67	122	50.0	173	78.33
−30	−34.44	21	−6.11	72	22.22	123	50.56	174	78.89
−29	−33.89	22	−5.56	73	22.78	124	51.11	175	79.44
−28	−33.33	23	−5.0	74	23.33	125	51.67	176	80.0
−27	−32.78	24	−4.44	75	23.89	126	52.22	177	80.56
−26	−32.22	25	−3.89	76	24.44	127	52.78	178	81.11
−25	−31.67	26	−3.33	77	25.0	128	53.33	179	81.67
−24	−31.11	27	−2.78	78	25.56	129	53.89	180	82.22
−23	−30.56	28	−2.22	79	26.11	130	54.44	181	82.78
−22	−30.0	29	−1.67	80	26.67	131	55.0	182	83.33
−21	−29.44	30	−1.11	81	27.22	132	55.56	183	83.89
−20	−28.89	31	−0.56	82	27.78	133	56.11	184	84.44
−19	−28.33	32	0.0	83	28.33	134	56.67	185	85.0
−18	−27.78	33	0.56	84	28.89	135	57.22	186	85.56
−17	−27.22	34	1.11	85	29.44	136	57.78	187	86.11
−16	−26.67	35	1.67	86	30.0	137	58.33	188	86.67
−15	−26.11	36	2.22	87	30.56	138	58.89	189	87.22
−14	−25.56	37	2.78	88	31.11	139	59.44	190	87.78
−13	−25.0	38	3.33	89	31.67	140	60.0	191	88.33
−12	−24.44	39	3.89	90	32.22	141	60.56	192	88.89
−11	−23.89	40	4.44	91	32.78	142	61.11	193	89.44
−10	−23.33	41	5.0	92	33.33	143	61.67	194	90.0
−9	−22.78	42	5.56	93	33.89	144	62.22	195	90.56
−8	−22.22	43	6.11	94	34.44	145	62.78	196	91.11
−7	−21.67	44	6.67	95	35.0	146	63.33	197	91.67
−6	−21.11	45	7.22	96	35.56	147	63.89	198	92.22
−5	−20.56	46	7.78	97	36.11	148	64.44	199	92.78
−4	−20.0	47	8.33	98	36.67	149	65.0	200	93.33
−3	−19.44	48	8.89	99	37.22	150	65.56	201	93.89
−2	−18.89	49	9.44	100	37.78	151	66.11	202	94.44
−1	−18.33	50	10.0	101	38.33	152	66.67	203	95.0
0	−17.78	51	10.56	102	38.89	153	67.22	204	95.56
1	−17.22	52	11.11	103	39.44	154	67.78	205	96.11
2	−16.67	53	11.67	104	40.0	155	68.33	206	96.67
3	−16.11	54	12.22	105	40.56	156	68.89	207	97.22
4	−15.56	55	12.78	106	41.11	157	69.44	208	97.78
5	−15.0	56	13.33	107	41.67	158	70.0	209	98.33
6	−14.44	57	13.89	108	42.22	159	70.56	210	98.89
7	−13.89	58	14.44	109	42.78	160	71.11	211	99.44
8	−13.33	59	15.0	110	43.33	161	71.67	212	100.0
9	−12.78	60	15.56	111	43.89	162	72.22		
10	−12.22	61	16.11	112	44.44	163	72.78		

FAHRENHEIT AND CELSIUS EQUIVALENTS:
BODY TEMPERATURE RANGE

F°	C°	F°	C°	F°	C°	F°	C°	F°	C°
94.0	34.44	97.0	36.11	100.0	37.78	103.0	39.44	106.0	41.11
94.2	34.56	97.2	36.22	100.2	37.89	103.2	39.56	106.2	41.22
94.4	34.67	97.4	36.33	100.4	38.00	103.4	39.67	106.4	41.33
94.6	34.78	97.6	36.44	100.6	38.11	103.6	39.78	106.6	41.44
94.8	34.89	97.8	36.56	100.8	38.22	103.8	39.89	106.8	41.56
95.0	35.00	98.0	36.67	101.0	38.33	104.0	40.00	107.0	41.67
95.2	35.11	98.2	36.78	101.2	38.44	104.2	40.11	107.2	41.78
95.4	35.22	98.4	36.89	101.4	38.56	104.4	40.22	107.4	41.89
95.6	35.33	98.6	37.00	101.6	38.67	104.6	40.33	107.6	42.00
95.8	35.44	98.8	37.11	101.8	38.78	104.8	40.44	107.8	42.11
96.0	35.56	99.0	37.22	102.0	38.89	105.0	40.56	108.0	42.22
96.2	35.67	99.2	37.33	102.2	39.00	105.2	40.67		
96.4	35.78	99.4	37.44	102.4	39.11	105.4	40.78		
96.6	35.89	99.6	37.56	102.6	39.22	105.6	40.89		
96.8	36.00	99.8	37.67	102.8	39.33	105.8	41.00		

CELSIUS AND FAHRENHEIT EQUIVALENTS

Celsius to Fahrenheit: 9/5 C + 32 = F or F = (C × 1.8) + 32

C°	F°	C°	F°	C°	F°	C°	F°	C°	F°
−50	−58.0	−19	−2.2	12	53.6	43	109.4	74	165.2
−49	−56.2	−18	−0.4	13	55.4	44	111.2	75	157.0
−48	−54.4	−17	1.4	14	57.2	45	113.0	76	168.8
−47	−52.6	−16	3.2	15	59.0	46	114.8	77	170.6
−46	−50.8	−15	5.0	16	60.8	47	116.6	78	172.4
−45	−49.0	−14	6.8	17	62.6	48	118.4	79	174.2
−44	−47.2	−13	8.6	18	64.4	49	120.2	80	176.0
−43	−45.4	−12	10.4	19	66.2	50	122.0	81	177.8
−42	−43.6	−11	12.2	20	68.0	51	123.8	82	179.6
−41	−41.8	−10	14.0	21	69.8	52	125.6	83	181.4
−40	−40.0	−9	15.8	22	71.6	53	127.4	84	183.2
−39	−38.2	−8	17.6	23	73.4	54	129.2	85	185.0
−38	−36.4	−7	19.4	24	75.2	55	131.0	86	186.8
−37	−34.6	−6	21.2	25	77.0	56	132.8	87	188.6
−36	−32.8	−5	23.0	26	78.8	57	134.6	88	190.4
−35	−31.0	−4	24.8	27	80.6	58	136.4	89	192.2
−34	−29.2	−3	26.6	28	82.4	59	138.2	90	194.0
−33	−27.4	−2	28.4	29	84.2	60	140.0	91	195.8
−32	−25.6	−1	30.2	30	86.0	61	141.8	92	197.6
−31	−23.8	0	32.0	31	87.8	62	143.6	93	199.4
−30	−22.0	1	33.8	32	89.6	63	145.4	94	201.2
−29	−20.2	2	35.6	33	91.4	64	147.2	95	203.0
−28	−18.4	3	37.4	34	93.2	65	149.0	96	204.8
−27	−16.6	4	39.2	35	95.0	66	150.8	97	206.6
−26	−14.8	5	41.0	36	96.8	67	152.6	98	208.4
−25	−13.0	6	42.8	37	98.6	68	154.4	99	210.2
−24	−11.2	7	44.6	38	100.4	69	156.2	100	212.0
−23	−9.4	8	46.4	39	102.2	70	158.0		
−22	−7.6	9	48.2	40	104.0	71	159.8		
−21	−5.8	10	50.0	41	105.8	72	161.6		
−20	−4.0	11	51.8	42	107.6	73	163.4		

CELSIUS AND FAHRENHEIT EQUIVALENTS:
BODY TEMPERATURE RANGE

C°	F°	C°	F°	C°	F°	C°	F°	C°	F°
34.0	93.20	35.5	95.90	37.0	98.60	38.5	101.30	40.0	104.00
34.1	93.38	35.6	96.08	37.1	98.78	38.6	101.48	40.1	104.18
34.2	93.56	35.7	96.26	37.2	98.96	38.7	101.66	40.2	104.36
34.3	93.74	35.8	96.44	37.3	99.14	38.8	101.84	40.3	104.54
34.4	93.92	35.9	96.62	37.4	99.32	38.9	102.02	40.4	104.72
34.5	94.10	36.0	96.80	37.5	99.50	39.0	102.20	40.5	104.90
34.6	94.28	36.1	96.98	37.6	99.68	39.1	102.38	40.6	105.08
34.7	94.46	36.2	97.16	37.7	99.86	39.2	102.56	40.7	105.26
34.8	94.64	36.3	97.34	37.8	100.04	39.3	102.74	40.8	105.44
34.9	94.82	36.4	97.52	37.9	100.22	39.4	102.92	40.9	105.62
35.0	95.0	36.5	97.70	38.0	100.40	39.5	103.10	41.0	105.80
35.1	95.18	36.6	97.88	38.1	100.58	39.6	103.28		
35.2	95.36	36.7	98.06	38.2	100.76	39.7	103.46		
35.3	95.54	36.8	98.24	38.3	100.94	39.8	103.64		
35.4	95.72	36.9	98.42	38.4	101.12	39.9	103.82		

LENGTH CONVERSIONS

Meters	Centimeters	Yards	Feet	Inches
1	100	1.094	3.281	39.37
.01	1	.01094	.0328	.3937
.9144	91.44	1	3	36
.0348	30.48	1/3	1	12
.0254	2.54	1/36	1/12	1

WEIGHT CONVERSIONS (METRIC AND
AVOIRDUPOIS)

Grams	Kilograms	Ounces	Pounds
1	.001	.0353	.0022
1000	1	35.3	2.2
28.35	.02835	1	1/16
454.5	.4545	16	1

WEIGHT CONVERSIONS (METRIC AND APOTHECARY)

Grams	Milligrams	Grains	Drams	Ounces	Pounds
1	1000	15.4	.2577	.0322	.00268
.001	1	.0154	.00026	.0000322	.00000268
.0648	64.8	1	1/60	1/480	1/5760
3.888	3888	60	1	1/8	1/96
31.1	31104	480	8	1	1/12
373.25	373248	5760	96	12	1

VOLUME CONVERSIONS (METRIC AND APOTHECARY)

Milliliters	Minims	Fluid drams	Fluid ounces	Pints
1	16.2	.27	.0333	.0021
.0616	1	1/	1/480	1/7680
3.697	60	1/60	1/8	1/128
29.58	480	1	1	1/16
473.2	7680	8	16	1
	128			

Liters	Gallons	Quarts	Fluid ounces	Pints
1	.2642	1.057	33.824	2.114
3.785	1	4	128	8
.946	1/4	1	32	2
.473	1/8	1/2	16	1
.0296	1/128	1/32	1	1/16

COMMONLY USED METRIC AND APOTHECARY EQUIVALENTS

Grains	Grams	Milligrams
1/300	.0002	0.2
1/200	.0003	0.3
1/150	.0004	0.4
1/120	.0005	0.5
1/100	.0006	0.6
1/60	.001	1
1/30	.002	2
1/12	.005	5
1/6	.010	10
1/4	.015	15
3/8	.025	25
1/2	.030	30
3/4	.050	50
1	.060	60
1½	.100	100
2	.120	120
3	.200	200
5	.300	300
7½	.500	500
10	.600	600
15	1	1,000
30	2	2,000
60	4	4,000

APPROXIMATE HOUSEHOLD MEASUREMENT EQUIVALENTS (VOLUME)

					1 tsp	=	5 ml
				1 tbsp = 3 tsp		=	15 ml
			1 fl oz	= 2 tbsp = 6 tsp		=	30 ml
		1 cup =	8 fl oz			=	240 ml
	1 pt =	2 cups =	16 fl oz			=	480 ml
1 qt =	2 pt =	4 cups =	32 fl oz			=	960 ml
1 gal = 4 qt =	8 pt =	16 cups =	128 fl oz			=	3840 ml

POUND-TO-KILOGRAM CONVERSION TABLE*

Pounds	0	1	2	3	4	5	6	7	8	9
0	0.00	0.45	0.90	1.36	1.81	2.26	2.72	3.17	3.62	4.08
10	4.53	4.98	5.44	5.89	6.35	6.80	7.25	7.71	8.16	8.61
20	9.07	9.52	9.97	10.43	10.88	11.34	11.79	12.24	12.70	13.15
30	13.60	14.06	14.51	14.96	15.42	15.87	16.32	16.78	17.23	17.69
40	18.14	18.59	19.05	19.50	19.95	20.41	20.86	21.31	21.77	22.22
50	22.68	23.13	23.58	24.04	24.49	24.94	25.40	25.85	26.30	26.76
60	27.21	27.66	28.12	28.57	29.03	29.48	29.93	30.39	30.84	31.29
70	31.75	32.20	32.65	33.11	33.56	34.02	34.47	34.92	35.38	35.83
80	36.28	36.74	37.19	37.64	38.10	38.55	39.00	39.46	39.91	40.37
90	40.82	41.27	41.73	42.18	42.63	43.09	43.54	43.99	44.45	44.90
100	45.36	45.81	46.26	46.72	47.17	47.62	48.08	48.53	48.98	49.44
110	49.89	50.34	50.80	51.25	51.71	52.16	52.61	53.07	53.52	53.97
120	54.43	54.88	55.33	55.79	56.24	56.70	57.15	57.60	58.06	58.51
130	58.96	59.42	59.87	60.32	60.78	61.23	61.68	62.14	62.59	63.05
140	63.50	63.95	64.41	64.86	65.31	65.77	66.22	66.67	67.13	67.58
150	68.04	68.49	68.94	69.40	69.85	70.30	70.76	71.21	71.66	72.12
160	72.57	73.02	73.48	73.93	74.39	74.84	75.29	75.75	76.20	76.65
170	77.11	77.56	78.01	78.47	78.92	79.38	79.83	80.28	80.74	81.19
180	81.64	82.10	82.55	83.00	83.46	83.91	84.36	84.82	85.27	85.73
190	86.18	86.68	87.09	87.54	87.99	88.45	88.90	89.35	89.81	90.26
200	90.72	91.17	91.62	92.08	92.53	92.98	93.44	93.89	94.34	94.80

* Numbers in the farthest left column are 10-pound increments; numbers across the top row are 1-pound increments. The kilogram equivalent of weight in pounds is found at the intersection of the appropriate row and column. For example, to convert 54 pounds, read down the left column to 50 and then across that row to 4: 54 pounds = 24.49 kilograms.

GRAM EQUIVALENTS FOR POUNDS AND OUNCES:
CONVERSION TABLE FOR WEIGHT OF NEWBORN

	Ounces																
	0	1	2	3	4	5	6	7	8	9	10	11	12	13	14	15	
Pounds																	**Pounds**
0	—	28	57	85	113	142	170	198	227	255	283	312	430	369	397	425	**0**
1	454	482	510	539	567	595	624	652	680	709	737	765	794	822	850	879	**1**
2	907	936	964	992	1021	1049	1077	1106	1134	1162	1191	1219	1247	1276	1304	1332	**2**
3	1361	1389	1417	1446	1474	1503	1531	1559	1588	1616	1644	1673	1701	1729	1758	1786	**3**
4	1814	1843	1871	1899	1928	1956	1984	2013	2041	2070	2098	2126	2155	2183	2211	2240	**4**
5	2268	2296	2325	2353	2381	2410	2438	2466	2495	2523	2551	2580	2608	2637	2665	2693	**5**
6	2722	2750	2778	2807	2835	2863	2892	2920	2948	2977	3005	3033	3062	3090	3118	3147	**6**
7	3175	3203	3232	3260	3289	3317	3345	3374	3402	3430	3459	3487	3515	3544	3572	3600	**7**
8	3629	3657	3685	3714	3742	3770	3799	3827	3856	3884	3912	3941	3969	3997	4026	4054	**8**
9	4082	4111	4139	4167	4196	4224	4252	4281	4309	4337	4366	4394	4423	4451	4479	4508	**9**
10	4536	4564	4593	4621	4649	4678	4706	4734	4763	4791	4819	4848	4876	4904	4933	4961	**10**
11	4990	5018	5046	5075	5103	5131	5160	5188	5216	5245	5273	5301	5330	5358	5386	5415	**11**
12	5443	5471	5500	5528	5557	5585	5613	5642	5670	5698	5727	5755	5783	5812	5840	5868	**12**
13	5897	5925	5953	5982	6010	6038	6067	6095	6123	6152	6180	6290	6237	6265	6294	6322	**13**
14	6350	6379	6407	6435	6464	6492	6520	6549	6577	6605	6634	6662	6690	6719	6747	6776	**14**

1 pound = 453.59 grams. 1 ounce = 28.35 grams. Grams can be converted to pounds and tenths of a pound by multiplying the number of grams by .0022.

NORMAL LABORATORY VALUES

BODY FLUIDS AND OTHER MASS DATA

Body fluid, total volume: 56% (in obese) to 70% (lean) of body weight
  Intracellular: 30 to 40% of body weight
  Extracellular: 23 to 25% of body weight
Blood:
  Total volume:
    Males: 69 ml/kg body weight
    Females: 65 ml/kg body weight
  Plasma volume:
    Males: 39 ml/kg body weight
    Females: 40 ml/kg body weight
  Red blood cell volume:
    Males: 30 ml/kg body weight (1.15–1.21 liters per m² body surface area)
    Females: 25 ml/kg body weight

$$meq/liter = \frac{mg/100\ ml \times 10 \times valence}{atomic\ weight}$$

$$mg/100\ ml = \frac{meq/liter \times atomic\ weight}{10 \times valence}$$

TABLE A-1
Atomic weights of elements commonly encountered in clinical medicine

Calcium	40.08	Magnesium	24.32
Carbon	12.01	Nitrogen	14.008
Chlorine	35.46	Oxygen	16.00
Copper	63.54	Phosphorus	30.98
Hydrogen	1.008	Potassium	39.100
Iodine	126.91	Sodium	22.997
Iron	55.85	Sulfur	32.07

CEREBROSPINAL FLUID

Cells: 5/mm³, all lymphocytes
Pressure, initial (horizontal position): 70–200 mm water
Colloidal gold test: Not more than one to two in first few tubes
Creatinine: 0.4–1.5 mg/100 ml
Glucose*: 44–100 mg/100 ml
pH*: 7.35–7.70
Protein:
  Lumbar: 14–45 mg/100 ml; gamma-globulin, < 10% of total
  Cisternal: 10–20 mg/100 ml
  Ventricular: 1–15 mg/100 ml

CHEMICAL CONSTITUENTS OF BLOOD†
(See also under Function Tests, especially Metabolic and Endocrine)

Acetone, serum: 0.3–2.0 mg/100 ml
Albumin, serum: 3.5–5.5 g/100 ml
Aldolase: 0–8 IU/liter
Alpha-amino nitrogen, plasma: 3.0–5.5 mg/100 ml
Ammonia, whole blood, venous: 30–70 μg/100 ml
Amylase, serum (Somogyi): 60–180 units/100 ml; 0.8–3.2 IU/liter

Arterial blood gases:
  HCO_3^-: 21–28 meq/liter
  P_{CO_2}: 35–45 mmHg
  pH: 7.38–7.44
  P_{O_2}: 80–100 mmHg
Ascorbic acid, serum: 0.4–1.0 mg/100 ml
  Leukocytes: 25–40 mg/100 ml
Barbiturates, serum: 0
  "Potentially fatal" level (Schreiner) phenobarbital: Approx. 8 mg/100 ml
  Most short-acting barbiturates: 3.5 mg/100 ml
Base, total, serum: 145–155 meq/liter
Bilirubin, total, serum (Mallory-Evelyn): 0.3–1.0 mg/100 ml
  Direct, serum: 0.1–0.3 mg/100 ml
  Indirect, serum: 0.2–0.7 mg/100 ml
Bromides, serum: 0
  Toxic levels: Above 17 meq/liter; 150 mg/100 ml
Bromsulphalein, BSP (5 mg/kg body weight, IV): 5% or less retention after 45 min
Calcium, ionized: 2.3–2.8 meq/liter; 4.5–5.6 mg/100 ml
Calcium, serum: 4.5–5.5 meq/liter; 9–11 mg/100 ml
Carbon dioxide–combining power, serum (sea level): 21–28 meq/liter; 50 65 vol%
Carbon dioxide content, plasma (at sea level): 21–30 meq/liter; 50–70 vol%
Carbon dioxide tension, arterial blood (sea level): 35–45 mmHg
Carbon monoxide content, blood: Symptoms with over 20% saturation of hemoglobin
Carotenoids, serum: 50–300 μg/100 ml
Ceruloplasmin, serum: 27–37 mg/100 ml
Chlorides, serum (as Cl): 98–106 meq/liter
Cholesterol:
  Total, serum (Man-Peters method): 180–240 mg/100 ml
  Esters, serum: 100–180 mg/100 ml
Cholesterol ester fraction of total cholesterol, serum: 68–72%
Complement, serum, total hemolytic (CH_{50}): 150–250 units/ml
Copper, serum (mean ± 1 SD): 114 ± 14 μg/100 ml
Corticosteroids, plasma (Porter-Silber) (mean ± 1 SD): 13 ± 6 μg/100 ml at 8:00 A.M.
Cortisol (competitive protein binding): 5–20 μg/100 ml at 8:00 A.M.
Creatine phosphokinase, serum:
  Females: 5–25 U/ml
  Males: 5–35 U/ml
Creatinine, serum: 1–1.5 mg/100 ml
Dilantin, plasma:
  Therapeutic level, 10–20 μg/ml
  Toxic level, >30 μg/ml
Ethanol, blood:
  Mild to moderate intoxication: 80–200 mg/100 ml
  Marked intoxication: 250–400 mg/100 ml
  Severe intoxication: Above 400 mg/100 ml
Fatty acids, serum: 380–465 mg/100 ml
Fibrinogen, plasma: 160–415 mg/100 ml
Folic acid, serum: 6–15 ng/ml
Gastrin, serum: 40–150 pg/ml
Globulins, serum: 2.0–3.0 g/100 ml
Glucose (fasting):
  Blood (Nelson-Somogyi): 60–90 mg/100 ml
  Plasma: 75–105 mg
Hemoglobin, blood (sea level):
  Males: 14–18 g/100 ml
  Females: 12–16 g/100 ml

---

* Since cerebrospinal fluid concentrations are equilibrium values, measurement of blood plasma obtained at the same time is recommended.

† *IU = International units.*

NORMAL LABORATORY VALUES (continued)

Immunoglobulins, serum:
  IgA: 90–325 mg/100 ml
  IgG: 800–1,500 mg/100 ml
  IgM: 45–150 mg/100 ml
Iron, serum:
  Males and females (mean ± 1 SD): 107 ± 31 μg/100 ml
Iron-binding capacity, serum (mean ± 1 SD): 305 ± 32 μg/100 ml
  Saturation: 20–45%
Ketones, total: 0.5–1.5 mg/100 ml
Lactic acid, blood: 0.6–1.8 meq/liter
Lactic dehydrogenase, serum:
  200–450 units/ml (Wrobleski)
  60–100 units/ml (Wacker)
  25–100 IU/liter
Lead, serum: <20 μg/100 ml
Lipase, serum (Cherry-Crandall): 1.5 ml N/20 NaOH (upper limit of normal). (However, values above 1.0 should be regarded with suspicion.)
Lipids, total, serum: 500–600 mg/100 ml
Lipids, triglyceride, serum: 50–150 mg/100 ml
Magnesium, serum: 1.5–2.5 meq/liter; 2–3 mg/100 ml
Nitrogen, nonprotein, serum: 15–35 mg/100 ml
5'-Nucleotidase, serum: 0.3–2.6 Bodansky units/100 ml
Nutrients, various: See Table 81-3
Osmolality, serum: 280–300 mOsm/kg serum water
Oxygen content:
  Arterial blood (sea level): 17–21 vol %
  Venous blood, arm (sea level): 10–16 vol %
Oxygen percent saturation (sea level):
  Arterial blood: 97%
  Venous blood, arm: 60–85%
Oxygen tension, blood: 80–100 mmHg
pH blood: 7.38–7.44
Phosphatase, acid, serum:
  Bessey-Lowry method: 0.10–0.63 unit
  Bodansky method: 0.5–2.0 units
  Fishman-Lerner (tartrate sensitive): <0.6 unit/100 ml (up to 0.15/100 ml)
  Gutman method: 0.5–2.0 units
  International units: 0.2–1.8
  King-Armstrong method: 1.0–5.0 units
  Shinowara method: 0.0–1.1 units
Phosphatase, alkaline, serum:
  Bessey-Lowry method: 0.8–2.3 units (3.4–9)*
  Bodansky method: 2.0–4.5 units (3.0–13.0)*
  Gutman method: 3.0–10.0 units
  International units: 21–91 U/liter at 37°C incubation
  King-Armstrong method: 5.0–13.0 units (10.0–20.0)*
  Shinowara method: 2.2–8.6 units
Phospholipids, serum: 150–250 mg/100 ml (as lecithin)
Phosphorus, inorganic, serum: 1–1.5 meq/liter; 3–4.5 mg/100 ml
Potassium, serum: 3.5–5.0 meq/liter
Proteins, total, serum: 5.5–8.0 g/100 ml
Protein fractions, serum:
  Albumin: 3.5–5.5 g/100 ml (50–60%)
  Globulin: 2.0–3.5 g/100 ml (40–50%)
    α_1: 0.2–0.4 g/100 ml (4.2–7.2%)
    α_2: 0.5–0.9 g/100 ml (6.8–12%)
    β: 0.6–1.1 g/100 ml (9.3–15%)
    γ: 0.7–1.7 g/100 ml (13–23%)
Pyruvic acid, serum: 0–0.11 meq/liter

* Values in parentheses are those found in children.

Salicylate, plasma: 0
  Therapeutic range: 20–25 mg/100 ml
  Toxic range: over 30 mg/100 ml
Sodium, serum: 136–145 meq/liter
Steroids: See under Function Tests: Metabolic and Endocrine
Transaminase, serum glutamic oxalacetic (SGOT): 10–40 Karmen units/ml; 6–18 IU/liter
Transaminase, serum glutamic pyruvic (SGPT): 10–40 Karmen units/ml; 3–26 IU/liter
Urea nitrogen, whole blood: 10–20 mg/100 ml
Uric acid, serum:
  Males: 2.5–8.0 mg/ml
  Females: 1.5–6.0 mg/ml
Vitamin A, serum: 50–100 μg/100 ml
Vitamin B_{12}, serum: 200–600 pg/ml
Zinc, serum: 120 ± 20 μg/100 ml

FUNCTION TESTS
Circulation

Cardiac output (Fick): 2.5–3.6 liters/m²/min
Circulation time: Arm to lung, ether: 4–8 s
  Arm to tongue:
    Calcium gluconate: 12–18 s
    Decholin: 10–16 s
    Saccharin: 9–16 s
Ejection fraction:
  Stroke volume/end-diastolic volume (SV/EDV), normal range: 0.55–0.78; A_1: 0.67
Left ventricular work:
  Stroke work index: 30–110 g-m/m²
  Left ventricular minute work index: 1.8–6.6 kg-m/m²/min
Pressures, intracardiac and intraarterial:
  Aorta: Systole: 100–140 mmHg
    Diastole: 60–90 mmHg
  Atrium: Left (mean): 2–12 mmHg
    Right (mean): 0–5 mmHg
  Pulmonary artery: Systole: 12–28 mmHg
    Diastole: 3–13 mmHg
    Wedge (mean): 3–13 mmHg
  Ventricle, left: Systole: 120 mmHg
    Diastole: 2–12 mmHg
  Ventricle, right: Systole: 25 mmHg
    Diastole: 0–5 mmHg
  Venous (antecubital): 70–140 mmH₂O
Systemic vascular resistance: 770–1,500 dynes-sec-cm^{-5}
Pulmonary vascular resistance: 100–250 dynes-sec-cm^{-5}
Systolic time intervals (see Table A-2)

TABLE A-2

Systolic time intervals in normal individuals (in ms)

Regression equation	SD of index
QS_2 (M) = −2.1 HR + 546	14
QS_2 (F) = −2.0 HR + 549	14
PEP (M) = −0.4 HR + 131	13
PEP (F) = −0.4 HR + 133	11
LVET (M) = −1.7 HR + 413	10
LVET (F) = −1.6 HR + 418	10

QS_2 = total electromechanical systole, PEP = preejection phase, LVET = left ventricular ejection time, HR = heart rate, M = male, F = female, SD = standard deviation of the systolic time interval index. (From AM Weissler, CL Garrard, Mod Concepts Cardiovasc Dis 40: 1971)

NORMAL LABORATORY VALUES (continued)

Gastrointestinal
(See also Stool)

Absorption tests:

D-Xylose absorption test: After an overnight fast, 25 g xylose is given in aqueous solution by mouth. Urine collected for the following 5 h should contain 5–8 g (or >20% of ingested dose). Serum xylose should be 25–40 mg/100 ml 1 h after the oral dose.

Vitamin A absorption test: A fasting blood specimen is obtained and 200,000 units vitamin A in oil given by mouth. Serum vitamin A levels should rise to twice fasting level in 3 to 5 h.

Gastric juice:

Volume: 24 h, 2–3 liters; nocturnal, 600–700 ml; basal, fasting, 30–70 ml/h

Reaction: as pH, 1.6–1.8; titratable acidity of fasting juice, 15–35 meq/h

Acid output:

Basal: Females 2.0 ± 1.8 meq/h
       Males   3.0 ± 2.0 meq/h

Maximal (after subcutaneous histamine acid phosphate 0.04 mg/kg, preceded by 50 mg Phenergan, or Histalog 1.7 mg/kg):

Females 16 ± 5 meq/h
Males   23 ± 5 meq/h

Basal acid output/maximal acid output ratio: 0.6 or less

Tubeless gastric analysis with azure A dye: Acid present if more than 0.6 mg dye is excreted in urine over a 2-h period. (CAUTION: A negative test is meaningless and requires performance of the ordinary test with a gastric tube.)

Metabolic and endocrine

Adrenal-pituitary function tests (see Chap. 93)

Adrenal steroid values, including cortisol, aldosterone, keto-steroids, renin, and angiotensin (see Table 93-1)

Corticotropin (ACTH) response tests (see Table 93-4)

Insulin tolerance test: Blood glucose usually falls to 50% of fasting level in 20–30 min and returns to normal levels in 90–120 min after IV administration of 0.1 unit crystalline insulin per kg body weight

Metyrapone test (see page 532)

Basal metabolic rate: −15 to +15% of mean standard

Catecholamines, urinary excretion (24 h):

Free catecholamines, epinephrine, and norepinephrine: Less than 100 μg

Metanephrine, normetanephrine: Less than 1.3 mg

VMA: Less than 8 mg/24 h

Estrogens, gonadotropins, and progesterone:

Estrogens, urinary (Brown method):

Females (postpubertal, premenopausal):

Estrone: 5–20; estradiol: 2–10; estriol: 5–30 μg/24 h

Females (postmenopausal):

Estrone: 0.3–2.4; estradiol: 0–14; estriol: 2.2–7.5 μg/24 h

Males and prepubertal females:

Estrone: 0–15; estradiol: 0–5; estriol: 0–10 μg/24 h

Gonadotropins (radioimmunoassay):

Females (postpubertal, premenopausal, except at ovulation):

FSH: 10–30; LH: 10–25 mIU/ml

Ovulatory surge:

FSH: 25–35; LH: 35–100 mIU/ml

Females (postmenopausal):

FSH: 40–150; LH: 30–100 mIU/ml

Males (postpubertal):

FSH: 10–30; LH 10–25 mIU/ml

Males and females (prepubertal):

FSH: 2–10; LH: 2–10 mIU/ml

Progesterone (radioimmunoassay):

Females (preovulatory): 0.2–2.0 μm/ml

Females (postovulatory): 2.0–20.0 μm/ml

Males, prepubertal and postmenopausal females: 0.2 μm/ml

Glucose tolerance test, oral: 100 g glucose or 1.75 g glucose/kg body weight. Blood sugar not more than 160 mg/100 ml "true glucose" (Somogyi-Nelson) after 1/2 h; return to normal by 2 h; sugar not present in any urine specimen.

Hyperparathyroidism, tests for (see pages 2017–2018)

Pancreatic islet cell function tests (see pages 559–560)

Plasma and urine steroids

	Plasma	Urine
Cortisol	9–24 μg/100 ml (8 A.M.)	2–10 mg/24 h (Porter-Silber) 5–23 mg/24 h (ketogenic)
Free cortisol		7–25 mg/24 h (male) 4–15 mg/24 h (female)
Testosterone	0.3–1.0 μg/100 ml (male) 0.01–0.1 μg/100 ml (female)	47–156 μg/24 h (male) 0–15 μg/24 h (female)
Aldosterone		2–10 μg/24 h

Renin test (see page 530)

Thyroid function tests:

Iodine, protein-bound: 4–8 μg/100 ml

Iodine radioactive uptake: Range 5–45% in 24 h (range and mean vary widely in specific geographic areas owing to variations in iodine intake)

Resin T_3 uptake: 25–35% (expressed as ratio to normal: 0.82–1.17)

Thyroxine (competitive protein binding): 4–11 μg/100 ml (radioimmunoassay): 5–12 μg/100 ml

Thyroxine, free concentration (dialysis or ultrafiltration): 2.4 ng/100 ml (values vary among laboratories)

Triiodothyronine (radioimmunoassay): 80–160 ng/100 ml

TSH (radioimmunoassay): 0–6 μU/ml (upper limit normal varies among laboratories)

T_3 suppression test: Measure thyroid radioiodine uptake before and after 10 days of T_3 (100 μg/day p.o.). Uptake should decrease to half of original value or into subnormal range.

Pulmonary

TABLE A-3
Normal spirometric values for seated subjects

Age	Men	Women
FORCED EXPIRATORY VOLUME IN 1 s (FEV$_1$), LITERS		
20–39	3.11–4.64	2.16–3.65
40–59	2.45–3.98	1.60–3.09
60–70	2.09–3.32	1.30–2.53

NORMAL LABORATORY VALUES (continued)

FEV_1/VITAL CAPACITY (FEV%)

20–39	77	82
40–59	70	77
60–70	66	74

MAXIMAL MIDEXPIRATORY FLOW ($MMEF_{25-75\%}$) LITERS/S

20–39	3.8	3.4
40–59	2.8	2.2
60–70	2.2	1.6

Arterial blood gas measurements in normal subjects (at sea level):
P_{CO_2} in mmHg: 38 (± 2.9 SD) seated; no change with age
P_{O_2} in mmHg: seated, $104.2 - 0.27 \times$ age in years; supine, $103.5 - 0.42 \times$ age in years

TABLE A-4
Prediction formulas* for lung volumes and spirometric tests in seated subjects

	Age, to nearest year (A)	Height, m (H)	Weight, kg (W)	Constant (C)	Residual standard deviation (RSD)
MEN					
TLC, liters		+6.92	−0.017	−4.30	0.67
VC, liters	−0.020	+4.81		−2.81	0.50
FRC, liters	+0.015	+5.30	−0.037	−3.89	0.56
FRC/TLC, %	+0.18		−0.12	+52.3	6.8
FEV_1, liters	−0.033	+3.44		−1.00	0.50
FEV%	−0.37			+91.8	7.2
$MMEF_{25-75\%}$	−0.0523			+5.85	1.00
WOMEN					
TLC, liters	−0.015	+6.71		−5.77	0.48
VC, liters	−0.022	+4.04		−2.35	0.40
FRC, liters		+5.13	−0.028	−4.50	0.41
FRC/TLC, %	+0.16		−0.08	+45.2	4.7
FEV_1, liters	−0.028	+2.67		−0.54	0.36
FEV%	−0.26			+92.1	5.4
$MMEF_{25-75\%}$	−0.0579			+5.63	0.71

* *Answer* = ($A \times$ age) + ($H \times$ height) + ($W \times$ weight) + $C \pm 2$ RSD.
Example: The normal value and lower limit for the FEV_1 are sought in a man, age forty years, height 1.77 m, and weight 76 kg. The following equation gives the normal value:
$FEV_1 = (-0.033 \times 40) + (3.44 \times 1.77) + (-1.00) = 3.77$ liters
The lower limit of normal: $3.77 - 2 \times 0.50 = 2.77$ liters
Only 2.5% of a normal population will fall below this value (2 SD below the mean).
Key: FRC, functional residual capacity; FEV_1, forced expiratory volume in 1 s; FEV%, FEV_1 expressed as percent of nonforced expiratory VC; $MMEF_{25-75\%}$, mean flow rate during the middle half of the forced expiratory vital capacity.
SOURCE: *Birath et al, Acta Med Scand 173:193, 1963; Grimby, Soderholm, Acta Med Scand 173:199, 1963.*

Renal

Clearances (corrected to 1.73 m² body surface area):
Measures of glomerular filtration rate:
Inulin clearance (C_I):
Males: 124 ± 25.8 ml/min
Females: 119 ± 12.8 ml/min
Endogenous creatinine: 91–130 ml/min
Urea: 60–100 ml/min
Measures of effective renal plasma flow and tubular function:
Para-aminohippuric acid (C_{PAH}):
Males: 654 ± 163 ml/min
Females: 594 ± 102 ml/min
Tubular maximum for *PAH*, males and females:
77.2 mg/min

Diodrast: 600–800 ml/min; 20–30% excretion in 15 min
Concentration and dilution test:
Specific gravity of urine:
After 12 h fluid restriction: 1.025 or more
After 12 h deliberate water intake: 1.003 or less
Phenolsulfonphthalein:
After intravenous injection:
Excretion in urine in 15 min: 25% or more
Excretion in urine in 2 h: 55–75%
After intramuscular injection:
Excretion in urine in 2 h: 55–75%
Protein excretion, urine: <150 mg/24 h
Males: 0–60 mg/24 h
Females: 0–90 mg/24 h
Specific gravity, maximal range: 1.002–1.028
Tubular reabsorption phosphorus:
79–94% of filtered load

HEMATOLOGIC EXAMINATIONS
(See also Chemical Constituents of Blood)

Bone marrow
(See Table A-7)

Erythrocytes and hemoglobin
(See also Table A-5)

Carboxyhemoglobin:
Nonsmoker: 0–2.3%
Smoker: 2.1–4.2%
Fragility, osmotic:
Slight hemolysis: 0.45–0.39%
Complete hemolysis: 0.33–0.30%
Haptoglobin, serum: 128 ± 25 mg/100 ml
Hemochromogens plasma: 3–5 mg/100 ml
Hemoglobin, fetal: < 2% of fetal
"Life span":
Normal survival: 120 days
Chromium, half-life ($T\frac{1}{2}$): 28 days
Methemoglobin: Up to 1.7% of total
Plasma iron turnover rate: 20–42 mg/24 h (0.47 mg/kg)
Protoporphyrin, free erythrocyte (EP):
16–36 μg/100 ml RBCs
Reticulocytes: 0.5–2.0% of red blood cells
Sedimentation rate:
Westergren: <15 mm/1 h
Wintrobe: Males: 0–9 mm/1 h
Females: 0–20 mm/1 h

Leukocytes

TABLE A-6
Normal values

	Percent	Average	Minimum	Maximum
Total number, per mm³		7,000	4,300	10,000
Neutrophils:				
Juvenile and band	0–21	520	100	2,100
Segmented	25–62	3,000	1,100	6,050
Eosinophils	3–8	150	0	700
Basophils	0.6–1.8	30	0	150
Lymphocytes	20–53	2,500	1,500	4,000
Monocytes	2.4–11.8	430	200	950

NORMAL LABORATORY VALUES (continued)

TABLE A-5
Normal values at various ages

Age	Red blood cell count, millions/mm³	Hemoglobin, g/100 ml	Vol. packed RBC, ml/100 ml	Corpuscular values*			
				MCV, fl	MCH, pg	MCHC, g/100 ml	MCD, μm
Days 1–13	5.1 ± 1.0†	19.5 ± 5.0†	54.0 ± 10.0†	106–98	38–33	36–34	8.6
Days 14–60	4.7 ± 0.9	14.0 ± 3.3	42.0 ± 7.0	90	30	33	8.1
3 mon–10 yr	4.5 ± 0.7	12.2 ± 2.3	36.0 ± 5.0	80	27	34	7.7
11–15 yr	4.8	13.4	39.0	82	28	34	
Adults:							
Females	4.8 ± 0.6	14.0 ± 2.0	42.0 ± 5.0	90 ± 7	29 ± 2	34 ± 2	7.5 ± 0.3
Males	5.4 ± 0.9	16.0 ± 2.0	47.0 ± 5.0	90 ± 7	29 ± 2	34 ± 2	7.5 ± 0.3

Note: MCV = mean corpuscular volume, MCH = mean corpuscular hemoglobin, MCHC = mean corpuscular hemoglobin concentration, MCD = mean corpuscular diameter. (Wintrobe et al: Clinical Hematology, 7th ed. Philadelphia: Lea & Febiger, 1974).
* fl = cu μm; pg = μμg.
† The range of values represents almost the extremes of observed variations (93 percent or more) at sea level. The blood values of healthy persons should fall well within these figures.

Platelets and coagulation

Bleeding time (Ivy method, 5-mm wound), 1–9 min; Duke method, 1–4 min

Clot retraction:
  Qualitative: Apparent in 60 min, complete in <24 h, usually <6 h
Coagulation time (Lee-White):
  Majority and range (glass tubes): 9–15 min, 2–19 min
  Majority and range (siliconized tubes): both 20–60 min
Prothrombin time (Quick's one stage): Comparable to normal control (with most thromboplastins, 11–16 s)
Partial thromboplastin time (PTT) (Nye-Brinkhous method): Comparable to normal control. With standard technique, 68–82 s; activated, 32–46 s
Plasma thrombin time: 13–17 s
Platelets, per mm³, Brecher-Cronkite method: 290,000 (150,000–400,000)
Whole-clot lysis: >24 h

Schilling test

Excretion in urine of orally administered radioactive vitamin B_{12} following "flushing" parenteral injection of B_{12}: 7–40%

STOOL

Bulk:
  Wet weight: <197.5 g/day (mean 115 ± 41)
  Dry weight: <66.4 g/day (mean 34 ± 16)
Coproporphyrin: 400–1,000 μg/24 h
Fat, on diet containing at least 50 g fat: <7.0 g/day when measured on a 3-day (or longer) collection (mean 4.0 ± 1.5)
  As percent of dry weight: <30.4 (mean 13.3 ± 8.07)
  Coefficient of fat absorption: >93%
Fatty acid:
  Free: 1–10% of dry matter
  Combined as soap: 0.5–12% of dry matter

TABLE A-7
Differential nucleated cell counts of bone marrow

	Normal mean %*		Range†	AGL	CGL	CLL	Multiple myeloma	Hemolytic anemia
Myeloid	56.7							
Neutrophilic series		53.6						
Myeloblast		0.9	0.2– 1.5	↑↑↑	↑			
Promyelocyte		3.3	2.1– 4.1		↑			
Myelocyte		12.7	8.2–15.7		↑			
Metamyelocyte		15.9	9.6–24.6		↑			
Band		12.4	9.5–15.3		↑			
Segmented								
Eosinophilic series		3.1	1.2– 5.3		↑			
Basophilic series		<0.1	0– 0.2		↑			
Erythroid	25.6							
Pronormoblasts		0.6	0.2– 1.3					↑↑
Basophilic normoblasts		1.4	0.5– 2.4					↑↑
Polychromatophilic normoblasts		21.6	17.9–29.2					↑↑
Orthochromatic normoblasts		2.0	0.4– 4.6					↑↑
Megakaryocytes	<0.1							
Lymphoreticular	17.8							
Lymphocytes		16.2	11.1–23.2			↑↑↑		
Plasma cells		1.3	0.4– 3.9				↑↑↑	
Reticulum cells		0.3	0– 0.9					

* Taken from Wintrobe et al: Clinical Hematology, 7th ed., Philadelphia: Lea & Febiger, 1974.
† Range observed in 12 healthy men.
Abbreviations: AGL = acute granulocytic leukemia, CGL = chronic granulocytic leukemia, CLL = chronic lymphocytic leukemia.

NORMAL LABORATORY VALUES (continued)

Nitrogen: <1.7 g/day (mean 1.4 ± 0.2)
Protein content: Minimal
Urobilinogen: 40–280 mg/24 h
Water: Approximately 65%

URINE
(See also Function Tests: Metabolic and Endocrine)

Acidity, titratable: 20–40 meq/24 h
α-Amino nitrogen: 0.4–1.0 g/24 h
Ammonia: 30–50 meq/24 h
Amylase (Somogyi): 35–260 units/h
Calcium, 10 meq or 200 mg calcium diet:
  <7.5 meq/24 h or <150 mg/24 h
Catecholamines: Less than 100 μg/24 h
Copper: 0–25 μg/24 h

Coproporphyrins (types I and III): 100–300 μg/24 h
Creatine, as creatinine:
  Adult males: <50 mg/24 h
  Adult females: <100 mg/24 h
Creatinine: 1.0–1.6 g/24 h
Glucose, true (oxidase method): 50–300 mg/24 h
5-Hydroxyindoleacetic acid (5HIAA): 2–9 mg/24 h
Ketones, total (mean ±1 SD): 50.5 ± 30.7 mg/24 h
Lactic dehydrogenase: 560–2,050 units/8 h urine
Lead: <0.08 μg/ml or <120 μg/24 h
Protein: <50 mg/24 h
Porphobilinogen: 0 μg/24 h
Potassium: 25–100 meq/24 h (varies with intake)
Sodium: 100–260 meq/24 h (varies with intake)
Urobilinogen: 1–3.5 mg/24 h
Vanillylmandelic acid (VMA): 0.7–6.8 mg/24 h
D-Xylose excretion: 5–8 g/5 h after oral dose of 25 g

SOURCE: G. W. Thorn et al.: *Harrison's Principles of Internal Medicine*, 8th ed., McGraw-Hill, New York, 1977.

FOOD AND NUTRITION BOARD, NATIONAL ACADEMY OF SCIENCES—NATIONAL RESEARCH COUNCIL, RECOMMENDED DAILY DIETARY ALLOWANCES

	Age (yr) from, up to	Weight kg	Weight lb	Height cm	Height in	Energy kcal	Protein g	Fat-soluble vitamins Vitamin A activity RE	Vitamin A activity IU	Vitamin D IU	Vitamin E activity IU	Ascorbic acid mg
Infants	0.0–0.5	6	14	60	24	kg×117	kg×2.2	420^g	1,400	400	4	35
	0.5–1.0	9	20	71	28	kg×108	kg×2.0	400	2,000	400	5	35
Children	1–3	13	28	86	34	1300	23	400	2,000	400	7	40
	4–6	20	44	110	44	1800	30	500	2,500	400	9	40
	7–10	30	66	135	54	2400	36	700	3,300	400	10	40
Males	11–14	44	97	158	63	2800	44	1,000	5,000	400	12	45
	15–18	61	134	172	69	3000	54	1,000	5,000	400	15	45
	19–22	67	147	172	69	3000	54	1,000	5,000	400	15	45
	23–50	70	154	172	69	2700	56	1,000	5,000	...	15	45
	51+	70	154	172	69	2400	56	1,000	5,000	...	15	45
Females	11–14	44	97	155	62	2400	44	800	4,000	400	10	45
	15–18	54	119	162	65	2100	48	800	4,000	400	11	45
	19–22	58	128	162	65	2100	46	800	4,000	400	12	45
	23–50	58	128	162	65	2000	46	800	4,000	...	12	45
	51+	58	128	162	65	1800	46	800	4,000	...	12	45
Pregnant	...	...	...	...		+300	+30	1,000	5,000	400	15	60
Lactating	...	...	...	...		+500	+20	1,200	6,000	400	15	60

SOURCE: B. T. Burton: *Human Nutrition*, 3d ed., McGraw-Hill, New York, 1976.

ABRIDGED CANADIAN DIETARY STANDARDS (1970)

Sex	Age, yr	Weight, lb	Activity category	Calories	Protein, g	Calcium, g
Both	0–1	7–20	Usual	360–900	7–13	0.5
Both	1–2	20–26	Usual	900–1200	12–16	0.7
Both	2–3	31	Usual	1400	17	0.7
Both	4–6	40	Usual	1700	20	0.7
Both	7–9	57	Usual	2100	24	1.0
Both	10–12	77	Usual	2500	30	1.2
Boy	13–15	108	Usual	3100	40	1.2
Girl	13–15	108	Usual	2600	39	1.2
Boy	16–17	136	B	3700	45	1.2
Girl	16–17	120	A	2400	41	1.2
Boy	18–19	144	B	3800	47	0.9
Girl	18–19	124	A	2450	41	0.9
Male	Adult	154	B	3582	47	0.5
Female	Adult	124	A	2390	40	0.5

SOURCE: B. T. Burton: *Human Nutrition*, 3d ed., McGraw-Hill, New York, 1976.

	Water-soluble vitamins					Minerals					
Folacin μg	Niacin (B₁) mg	Riboflavin (B₂) mg	Thiamin mg	Vitamin B₆ mg	Vitamin B₁₂ μg	Calcium mg	Phosphorus mg	Iodine μg	Iron mg	Magnesium mg	Zinc mg
50	5	0.4	0.3	0.3	0.3	360	240	35	10	60	3
50	8	0.6	0.5	0.4	0.3	540	400	45	15	70	5
100	9	0.8	0.7	0.6	1.0	800	800	60	15	150	10
200	12	1.1	0.9	0.9	1.5	800	800	80	10	200	10
300	16	1.2	1.2	1.2	2.0	800	800	110	10	250	10
400	18	1.5	1.4	1.6	3.0	1,200	1,200	130	18	350	15
400	20	1.8	1.5	1.8	3.0	1,200	1,200	150	18	400	15
400	20	1.8	1.5	2.0	3.0	800	800	140	10	350	15
400	18	1.6	1.4	2.0	3.0	800	800	130	10	350	15
400	16	1.5	1.2	2.0	3.0	800	800	110	10	350	15
400	16	1.3	1.2	1.6	3.0	1,200	1,200	115	18	300	15
400	14	1.4	1.1	2.0	3.0	1,200	1,200	115	18	300	15
400	14	1.4	1.1	2.0	3.0	800	800	100	18	300	15
400	13	1.2	1.0	2.0	3.0	800	800	100	18	300	15
400	12	1.1	1.0	2.0	3.0	800	800	80	10	300	15
800	+2	+0.3	+0.3	2.5	4.0	1,200	1,200	125	18	450	20
600	+4	+0.5	+0.3	2.5	4.0	1,200	1,200	150	18	450	25

Iron, mg	Vitamin A, IU	Vitamin D, IU	Ascorbic acid, mg	Thiamin, mg	Riboflavin, mg	Niacin, mg
5	1,000	400	20	0.3	0.5	3
5	1,000	400	20	0.4	0.6	4
5	1,000	400	20	0.4	0.7	4
5	1,000	400	20	0.5	0.9	5
5	1,500	400	30	0.7	1.1	7
12	2,000	400	30	0.8	1.3	8
12	2,700	400	30	0.9	1.6	9
12	2,700	400	30	0.8	1.3	8
12	3,200	400	30	1.1	1.9	11
12	3,200	400	30	0.7	1.2	7
6	3,200	400	30	1.1	1.9	11
10	3,200	400	30	0.7	1.2	7
6	3,700	. . .	30	1.1	1.8	11
10	3,700	. . .	30	0.7	1.2	7

FOOD EXCHANGE LISTS

Food product	Amount in 1 exchange
Milk Exchanges	
Whole milk products (also count as 2 fat exchanges)	
Whole milk	1 cup
Canned, evaporated whole milk	½ cup
Buttermilk	1 cup
Yogurt (unflavored)	1 cup
Low-fat milk products	
1% fat-fortified milk (also counts as ½ fat exchange)	1 cup
2% fat-fortified milk (also counts as 1 fat exchange)	1 cup
Yogurt made from 2% fat-fortified milk, unflavored (also counts as 1 fat exchange)	1 cup
Nonfat milk products	
Skim milk	1 cup
Powdered milk in dry form	⅓ cup
Canned, evaporated skim milk	1 cup
Yogurt made from skim milk (unflavored)	1 cup
One milk exchange contains 12 g carbohydrate, 8 g protein, a trace of fat, and 80 calories	

Vegetable Exchanges

Food product	Amount in 1 exchange
Asparagus	½ cup
Bean sprouts	½ cup
Beets	½ cup
Broccoli	½ cup
Brussels sprouts	½ cup
Cabbage	½ cup
Carrots	½ cup
Cauliflower	½ cup
Celery	½ cup
Cucumber	½ cup
Eggplant	½ cup
Greens (beet, chard, collards, kale, mustard, spinach, turnip)	½ cup
Mushrooms	½ cup
Okra	½ cup
Onion	½ cup
Rhubarb	½ cup
Rutabaga	½ cup
Sauerkraut	½ cup
String beans	½ cup
Summer squash	½ cup
Tomato or tomato juice	½ cup
Turnip	½ cup
Vegetable juice cocktail	½ cup
Zucchini	½ cup

The following may be used raw in any amount desired
  Chicory
  Chinese cabbage
  Endive
  Escarole
  Lettuce
  Parsley
  Radish
  Watercress
One vegetable exchange contains approximately 5 gm carbohydrate, 2 g protein, and 25 calories. (See Bread Exchange List for the starchy vegetables)

Food product	Amount in 1 exchange
Fruit Exchanges (without sugar added)	
Apple	1 small
Apple juice	⅓ cup
Applesauce, unsweetened	½ cup
Apricot, fresh	2 medium
Apricot, dried	4 halves
Banana	½ small
Berries	
Blackberries	½ cup
Blueberries	½ cup
Raspberries	½ cup
Strawberries	¾ cup
Cherries	10 large
Cider	⅓ cup
Dates	2
Figs, fresh	1
Figs, dried	1
Grapefruit	½
Grapefruit juice	½ cup
Grapes	12
Grape juice	¼ cup
Mango	½ small
Melon	
Cantaloupe	¼ small
Honeydew	⅛ medium
Watermelon	1 cup
Nectarine	1 small
Orange	1 small
Orange juice	½ cup
Papaya	¾ cup
Peach	1 medium
Pear	1 small
Persimmon	1 medium
Pineapple	½ cup
Pineapple juice	⅓ cup
Plums	2 medium
Prunes	2 medium
Prune juice	¼ cup
Raisins	2 tablespoons
Tangerine	1 medium
One fruit exchange contains 10 g carbohydrate and 40 calories	

Bread Exchange

Food product	Amount in 1 exchange
Breads	
White, including French or Italian	1 slice
Whole wheat	1 slice
Rye or pumpernickel	1 slice
Raisin	1 slice
Bagel, small	½
Plain roll, bread	1
Frankfurter roll	½
Hamburger bun	½
Dry bread crumbs	3 tablespoons
Tortilla, 6 in.	1
Cereals	
Bran flakes	½ cup
Other ready-to-eat, unsweetened cereal	¾ cup
Puffed cereal, unsweetened	1 cup
Cooked cereal	½ cup
Grits, cooked	½ cup
Rice or barley, cooked	½ cup
Macaroni, noodles, or spaghetti, cooked	½ cup

FOOD EXCHANGE LISTS (continued)

Food product	Amount in 1 exchange	Food product	Amount in 1 exchange
Popcorn, popped, no fat added	3 cups	Dried beans and peas (also counts as 1 bread exchange)	½ cup
Cornmeal, dry	2 tablespoons	One lean meat exchange contains 7 g of protein, 3 g of fat, and 55 calories	
Flour	2½ tablespoons		
Wheat germ	¼ cup	Medium-fat meats (also count as ½ fat exchanges)	
Crackers		Beef: ground (15%) fat, canned corned beef, rib eye, round	1 oz
Arrowroot	3		
Graham, 2½ in. square	2	Pork: tenderloin (all cuts), picnic shoulder, shoulder blade, Boston butt, Canadian bacon, boiled ham	1 oz
Matzoth, 4 in × 6 in.	½		
Oyster	20		
Pretzels, 3⅛ in. long × ⅛ in. diameter	25	Liver, heart, kidney, and sweetbreads	1 oz
Rye wafers, 2 in. × 3½ in.	3	Cottage cheese, creamed	¼ cup
Saltines	6	Cheese: mozzarella, ricotta, farmer's cheese, neufchatel	1 oz
Soda, 2½ in. square	4		
Beans, peas, lentils (dried and cooked)	½ cup	Parmesan cheese	3 tablespoons
Baked beans without pork, canned	¼ cup	Egg	1
Starchy vegetables		Peanut butter (also counts as 2½ fat exchanges)	2 tablespoons
Corn	⅓ cup		
Corn on the cob	1 small	High-fat meats (also count as 1 fat exchange)	
Lima beans	½ cup	Beef: brisket, corned beef brisket, ground beef (more than 20% fat), hamburger (commercial), chuck (ground commercial), rib roasts, club and rib steaks	1 oz
Parsnips	⅔ cup		
Green peas, canned or frozen	½ cup		
Potato, white	1 small		
Potato, white, mashed	½ cup	Lamb: breast	1 oz
Pumpkin	¾ cup	Pork: spare ribs, loin (back ribs), ground pork, country ham, deviled ham	1 oz
Winter squash, acorn or butternut	½ cup		
Yam or sweet potato	¼ cup	Veal: breast	1 oz
Prepared foods (also count as 1 fat exchange)		Poultry: capon, domestic duck, goose	1 oz
Biscuit, 2 in. diameter	1	Cheese: cheddar types	1 oz
Cornbread, 2 in × 2 in. × 1 in.	1	Cold cuts 4 ½ in. × ⅛ in. slice	½ in. × ⅛ in. slice
Corn muffin, 2 in. diameter	1		
Crackers, round, butter type	5	Frankfurter	1 small
Muffin, plain, small	1	**Fat Exchanges**	
Potatoes, French fried, 2 in. to 3½ in. long	8		
Potato chips or corn chips**	15	Unsaturated fats	
(also counts as 2 fat exchanges)		Margarine, soft	1 tsp
Pancake, 5 in × ½ in.	1	Avocado, 4 in. diameter	⅛
Waffle, 5 in × ½ in.	1	Oil: corn, cottonseed, olive, peanut, safflower, soy, sunflower	1 tsp
One bread exchange contains 15 g carbohydrate, 2 g protein, and 70 calories			
		Olives	5 small
		Almonds	10 whole
		Pecans	2 large whole
Meat Exchanges		Peanuts, Spanish	20 whole
		Peanuts, Virginia	10 whole
Lean meats		Other nuts	6 small
Beef: baby beef, chipped beef, chuck, flank steak, tenderloin, top round, bottom round, rump, spare ribs, tripe	1 oz	Saturated fats	
		Margarine, regular stick	1 tsp
		Butter	1 tsp
Lamb: leg, rib, sirloin, loin roast, loin chops, shank, shoulder	1 oz	Bacon fat	1 tsp
		Bacon, crisp	1 strip
Pork: leg (whole rump, center shank), ham, smoked center slices	1 oz	Cream, light or sour	2 tbsp
		Cream, heavy	1 tbsp
Veal: leg, loin, rib, shank, shoulder, cutlets	1 oz	Cream cheese	1 tbsp
Poultry: (meat without skin): chicken, turkey, Cornish hen, guinea hn, pheasant	1 oz	Salad dressings, French or Italian style	1 tbsp
		Lard	1 tsp
Fish: any canned or frozen	1 oz	Mayonnaise	1 tsp
canned salmon, tuna, mackerel, crab, and lobster	¼ cup	Salad dressing, mayonnaise-type	2 tsp
clams, oysters, shrimp, scallops	5 or 1 oz	Salt pork	¾ in. cube
sardines, drained	3	One fat exchange contains 5 g fat and 45 calories	
Cheeses containing less than 5% butterfat	1 oz		
Cottage cheese, dry or 2% butterfat	¼ cup		

SOURCE: Adapted from *Exchange Lists for Meal Planning*, prepared by Committees of the American Diabetes Association, Inc., and The American Dietetic Association, in cooperation with the National Institute of Arthritis, Metabolism and Digestive Diseases and the National Heart and Lung Institute, National Institutes of Health, Public Health Service, U.S. Department of Health, Education and Welfare.

APPROXIMATE COMPOSITION OF ORAL FLUIDS

Fluid	CHO gm/liter	Calories per liter	Na	K	HCO$_3$
				meq/liter	
Apple juice	120	480	1.3	30	
Coca-Cola	109	436	0.4	13	13.4
Gatorade	46	184	22	2.6	
Ginger ale	90	360	3.5	0.1	3.6
Grape juice	180	700	0.4	31	32
Grapefruit juice	125	500	2.0	20	22
Jello (1 box)	80	325	144	54	
Lytren	70	280	25	25	18
Milk, skim	55	375	23	43	
Milk, whole	49	670	22	36	30
Orange juice	100	400	0.4	38	38.4
Pedialyte	50	200	30	20	14
Pepsi Cola	120	480	6.5	0.8	7.3
Pineapple juice	135	540	<1.0	35	35
7-Up	102	410	7.0	0.5	0
Tea (1 bag)	0	0	<0.1	0.5	
Tomato juice	57	230	120	70	10

APPROXIMATE VITAMIN, IRON, AND CARBOHYDRATE COMPOSITION OF COMMONLY USED INFANT FORMULAS

	Vitamin A units	Vitamin D units	Vitamin C gm	Iron gm	
Standard formulas	per quart normal dil.				**Carbohydrate composition**
Baker's Inf. Form.	2500	400	50	7.5	Lactose, maltose, dextrose, dextrins
Bremil	2500	400	50	tr.	Lactose
Carnalac	1035	400	80	tr.	Lactose
Cow's Milk (undil.)	946	38	17	tr.	Lactose
Enfamil	1500	400	50	1.4	Lactose
Evaporated 1:2	800	265	—	tr.	Lactose
Formil	2500	400	50	tr.	Lactose
Human Milk	1419	95	40	tr.	Lactose
Lactum	400	400	2	tr.	Lactose, maltose, dextrins
			45	10	Lactose, maltose, dextrose, dextrins
Modilac	1500	400			
			80	8	Lactose
Optimil	2500	400	—	tr.	Lactose, maltose, dextrose, dextrins
Purevap	800	400		tr.	dextrins
			50	7.5	Lactose
Similac	2500	400	50		Lactose
SMA S-26	2500	400			
Soy formulas					
Isomil	1419	378	47	11.4	Sucrose, malto-dextrins
Mull-Soy	2000	400	40	5	Sucrose
Neo-Mull-Soy	2000	400	50	8	Sucrose
ProSobee	1500	400	50	8	Sucrose, maltose, dextrose, dextrins
Sobee	1500	400	50	8	Sucrose, maltose, dextrins
Soyalac	1500	400	30	10	Sucrose, maltose, dextrose, dextrins
CHO-Free	2000	400	52	8	
Special formulas					
Alacta (premie)				tr.	Lactose, maltose, dextrins
Dryco	2500	400		tr.	Lactose
Lofenalac	1500	400	50	15	Arrow root starch, maltose, sucrose, dextrins
Nursette Premature	1500	400	50	tr.	Lactose, corn starch, sucrose
Nutramigen (pwdr)	1500	400	30	9.5	Sucrose, arrow root starch
Olac	2500	400		tr.	Lactose, maltose, dextrins
PM 60/40 (pwdr)	2500	400	50	2	Lactose
Similac c̄ Fe 24	3000	480	60	15	Lactose

APPROXIMATE FAT, PROTEIN, CARBOHYDRATE, AND ELECTROLYTE COMPOSITION OF COMMONLY USED INFANT FORMULAS

Standard formulas	Normal dil.	Cal/oz	Fat	Protein	CHO	Na	K	Ca	P
			percentage			meq/liter			
Baker's Inf. Form.	1:1	20	3.3	2.2	7.0	17	23	42	37
Bremil	1:1	20	3.5	1.5	7.0	11	16	23	25
Carnalac	1:1	20	3.2	2.8	7.1	21	30	53	47
Cow's Milk (undil.)		20	3.7	3.3	4.8	25	35	62	56
Enfamil	1:1	20	3.7	1.5	7.0	11	16	29	25
Evap. Milk 1:2	1:2	15	2.7	2.3	3.5	18	25	44	40
Formil	1:1	20	3.5	1.65	7.0	13	18	31	28
Human Milk		20	3.5	1.2	7.0	7	14	17	9
Lactum	1:1	20	2.8	2.7	7.7	21	29	51	46
Modilac	1:1	20	2.6	2.0	7.7	15	21	38	34
Optimil	1:1	20	3.8	1.47	7.2	9	15	19	16
Purevap	1:2	20	2.6	2.3	8.0	18	25	44	40
Similac	1:1	20	3.4	1.7	6.6	13	18	32	29
SMA S-26	1:1	20	3.6	1.5	7.2	7	14	21	19

Soy formulas

Isomil	1:1	20	3.6	2.0	6.8	13	18	35	28
Mull-Soy	1:1	20	3.6	3.1	5.2	16	40	68	45
Neo-Mull-Soy	1:1	20	3.5	1.8	6.4	17	25	42	24
ProSobee	1:1	20	3.4	2.5	6.8	24	28	47	42
Sobee	1:1	20	2.6	3.2	7.7	22	33	50	32
Soyalac	1:1	20	4.0	2.1	6.0	13	22	21	21

Special formulas

Alacta (premie)	†	†	1.4	3.9	13.0	23	46	74	63
CHO-Free	1:1 c̄ 12.8% CHO sol.	20	3.5	1.8	6.4	.35	.85	.85	.6
						(g/qt)			
Lofenelac	1:2	20	2.7	2.2	8.5	25	37	47	47
Nursette Prem.	Premixed	24	3.7	2.84	9.1	20	33	50	52
Nutramigen (pwdr)	1:6	20	3.1	3.3	9.3	17	26	50	46
Olac	1:1	20	2.7	3.4	7.5	22	41	60	58
PM 60/40 (pwdr)	1:2	20	3.4	1.5	7.2	7	14	16.5	12
Portagen	1:6	20	3.2	2.7	7.7	17	33	48	46
Similac c̄ Fe 24	Premixed	24	4.2	2.12	8.0	13	27	41	36

† Plus carbohydrate to 20 cal/oz.

PRIMARY IMMUNIZATION FOR CHILDREN NOT IMMUNIZED IN EARLY INFANCY[1]

Under 6 years of age

First visit	DTP, TOPV, tuberculin test
Interval after first visit	
1 mo	Measles,[1] mumps, rubella
2 mo	DTP, TOPV
4 mo	DTP, TOPV[3]
10 to 16 mo or preschool	DTP, TOPV
Age 14–16 yr	Td,[4] repeat every 10 yr

6 years of age and over

First visit	Td[3], TOPV, tuberculin test
Interval after first visit	
1 mo	Measles, mumps, rubella
2 mo	Td, TOPV
8 to 14 mo	Td, TOPV
Age 14–16 yr	Td; repeat every 10 yr

[1] Physicians may choose to alter the sequence of these schedules if specific infections are prevalent at the time. For example, measles vaccine might be given on the first visit if an epidemic is underway in the community.

[2] Measles vaccine is not routinely given before 15 months of age.

[3] Optional.

[4] Td, combined tetanus and diphtheria toxoids (adult type) for those more than 6 years of age, in contrast to diphtheria and tetanus (DT) toxoids, which contain a larger amount of diphtheria antigen.

SOURCE: *Report of the Committee on Infectious Diseases,* American Academy of Pediatrics, 18 ed., 1977.

RECOMMENDED SCHEDULE FOR ACTIVE IMMUNIZATION OF NORMAL INFANTS AND CHILDREN

2 mo	DTP[1]	TOPV[2]
4 mo	DTP	TOPV
6 mo	DTP	TOPV[3]
1 yr		Tuberculin Test[4]
15 mo	Measles, Rubella[5]	Mumps[5]
1½ yr	DTP	TOPV
4-6 yr	DTP	TOPV
14-16 yr	Td[6]—repeat every 10 years	

[1] Diphtheria and tetanus toxoids combined with pertussis vaccine.

[2] Trivalent oral poliovirus vaccine. This recommendation is suitable for breast-fed as well as bottle-fed infants.

[3] A third dose of TOPV is optional but may be given in areas of high endemicity of poliomyelitis.

[4] Frequency of repeated tuberculin tests depends on risk of exposure of the child and on the prevalence of tuberculosis in the population group. For the pediatrician's office or outpatient clinic, an annual or biennial tuberculin test, unless local circumstances clearly indicate otherwise, is appropriate. The initial test should be done at the time of, or preceding, the measles immunization.

[5] May be given at 15 months as measles-rubella or measles-mumps-rubella combined vaccines.

[6] Combined tetanus and diphtheria toxoids (adult-type) for those more than 6 y of age, in contrast to diphtheria and tetanus (DT) toxoids, which contain a larger amount of diphtheria antigen.

Tetanus toxoid at time of injury: For clean, minor wounds, no booster dose is needed by a fully immunized child unless more than 10 y have elapsed since the last dose. For contaminated wounds, a booster dose should be given if more than 5 y have elapsed since the last dose.

Concentration and storage of vaccines: Because the concentration of antigen varies in different products, the manufacturer's package insert should be consulted regarding the volume of individual doses of immunizing agents. Because biologics are of varying stability, the manufacturer's recommendations for optimal storage conditions (e.g., temperature, light) should be carefully followed. Failure to observe these precautions may significantly reduce the potency and effectiveness of the vaccines.

SOURCE: *Report of the Committee on Infectious Diseases,* American Academy of Pediatrics, 18 ed., 1977.

DIRECTORY OF STATE BOARDS OF NURSING

Miss Betty Tomlin, Exec. Off.
Board of Nursing
State Administrative Building
Montgomery, Alabama 36104

Miss Joyce Hazelbaker, Exec. Off.
Alaska Board of Nursing
2702 Denal St., Room 206
Anchorage, Alaska 99503

Miss Elaine J. Laeger, Exec. Sec.
Arizona State Board of Nursing
1645 W. Jefferson St., Room 254
Phoenix, Arizona 85007

Mrs. Mildred Armour, Exec. Dir.
Arkansas State Board of Nursing
9107 Rodney Parham Rd.
Little Rock, Arkansas 72205

Mr. Michael R. Buggy, Exec. Sec.
Board of Registered Nursing
1020 N St., Room 448
Sacramento, California 95814

Mrs. Henrietta Walsh, Exec. Sec.
Colorado State Board of Nursing
1525 Sherman St., Room 115
Denver, Colorado 80203

Miss Anne F. McGuigan, Chief Nsg.
  Exam.
Board of Examiners for Nursing
79 Elm St., Room 101
Hartford, Connecticut 06115

Miss Frieda W. McMullan, Exec. Dir.
Delaware Board of Nursing
Cooper Bldg., Room 234
Dover, Delaware 19901

Mr. Joseph A. Richards, Administrator
Nurses Examining Board
614 H St., N.W.
Washington, D.C. 20001

Miss Helen P. Keefe, Exec. Dir.
Florida State Board of Nursing
6501 Arlington Expwy., Bldg. B.
Jacksonville, Florida 32211

Miss Genevieve Jones, Ed. Supv.
Board of Examiners of Nurses
166 Pryor St., S.W.
Atlanta, Georgia 30304

Mrs. Mary T. Sanchez, RN, Chairman
Guam Board of Nurse Examiners
PO Box 2816
Agana, Guam 96910

Mrs. Maybelle Clark, Exec. Sec.
Hawaii Board of Nursing
Box 3469
Honolulu, Hawaii 96801

Mrs. Eileen K. Merrell, RN, Exec. Dir.
Idaho State Board of Nursing
481 N. Curtis Rd.
Boise, Idaho 83704

Mrs. Annie L. Lawrence, Nsg. Ed.
  Coord.
Department of Registration and Education
55 E. Jackson St.
Chicago, Illinois 60604

Miss Emma Flinner, Exec. Sec.
State Board of Nurses Registration and
  Nursing Ed.
100 N. Senate Ave., Room 1018
Indianapolis, Indiana 46204

Mrs. Lynne M. Illes, Exec. Dir.
Iowa Board of Nursing
300 4th St.
Des Moines, Iowa 50309

Mr. Ray E. Showalter, Exec. Admin.
Kansas State Board of Nursing
701 Jackson, Room 314
Topeka, Kansas 66603

Mrs. Doris McDowell, Exec. Dir.
Kentucky Board of Nursing Education
  and Nurse Registration
6100 Dutchman's Lane
Louisville, Kentucky 40205

Miss Merlyn M. Maillian, RN, Exec. Dir.
Louisiana State Board of Nurse
  Examiners
150 Baronne St., 907 Pere Marquette
  Bldg.
New Orleans, Louisiana 70112

Miss Marion Klappmeier, Exec. Dir.
Maine State Board of Nursing
295 Water St.
Augusta, Maine 04330

Miss Rita D. Solow, Exec. Dir.
State Board of Examiners of Nurses
201 W. Preston St., State Office Bldg.
Baltimore, Maryland 21201

Miss Janet M. Dunphy, RN, Exec. Sec.
Board of Registration in Nursing
100 Cambridge St., Room 1509
Boston, Massachusetts 02202

Miss Helen Dunn, RN, Admin. Sec.
Michigan Board of Nursing
1033 S. Washington Ave.
Lansing, Michigan 48910

Miss Joyce M. Schowalter, Exec. Dir.
Minnesota Board of Nursing
717 Delaware St., S.E.
Minneapolis, Minnesota 55414

Dr. E. E. Thrash, Exec. Sec.
Board of Trustees of State Institutions of
  Higher Learning
PO Box 2336
Jackson, Mississippi 39205

Miss Vivian Meinecke, Exec. Sec.
Missouri State Board of Nursing
Box 656
Jefferson City, Missouri 65101

Mrs. Gertrude Malone, Exec. Sec.
Montana State Board of Nursing
Lalonde Bldg., Last Chance Gulch
Helena, Montana 59601

Mrs. Margaret Pavelka, Exec. Dir.
State Board of Nursing
State House Station, Box 94703
Lincoln, Nebraska 68509

Mrs. Jean T. Peavy, Exec. Sec.
Nevada State Board of Nursing
100 Vassar, Room 202
Reno, Nevada 89502

Miss Marguerite Hastings, Exec. Sec.
State Board of Nursing
105 Loudon Rd.
Concord, New Hampshire 03301

Mr. Richard E. David, Exec. Dir.
New Jersey Board of Nursing
1100 Raymond Blvd., Room 319
Newark, New Jersey 07102

Mrs. Ruth T. Dilts, Exec. Dir.
New Mexico Board of Nursing
505 Marquette Ave., N.W.
Albuquerque, New Mexico 87101

Miss Mildred S. Schmidt, Exec. Sec.
New York State Board for Nursing
State Education Dept., Office of
  Professional Education
Albany, New York 12230

Miss Mary McRee, Exec. Dir.
Board of Nursing
Box 2129
Raleigh, North Carolina 27602

Mrs. Irene E. Sage, Exec. Dir.
North Dakota Board of Nursing
219 N. 7th St.
Bismarck, North Dakota 58501

Miss Myra C. Freet, Exec. Sec.
State Board of Nursing Education and
  Nurse Registration
180 E. Broad St., Suite 1130
Columbus, Ohio 43215

Miss Frances I. Waddle, RN, Exec. Dir.
Board of Nurse Registration and Nursing
  Education
4545 N. Lincoln, Suite 76
Oklahoma City, Oklahoma 73105

Miss Beverly C. Andre, Exec. Dir.
Oregon State Board of Nursing
1400 S.W. 5th Ave., Room 575
Portland, Oregon 97201

Miss Geraldine M. Wenger, Sec.
Pennsylvania State Board of Nurse
  Examiners
Box 2649
Harrisburg, Pennsylvania 17120

DIRECTORY OF STATE BOARDS OF NURSING (continued)

Mrs. Aida C. Ferrer, Supervisor
Accreditation and Development for
 Schools of Nursing
Council on Higher Education—University
 of Puerto Rico
Rio Piedras, Puerto Rico 00931

Miss Helen E. Jones, RN, President
Board of Nurse Registration
State Office Bldg., Room 366
Providence, Rhode Island 02903

Miss Hazel Peeples, RN, Exec. Dir.
State Board of Nursing for South Carolina
1777 St. Julian Pl., Suite 102
Columbia, South Carolina 29204

Sr. Vincent Fuller, Exec. Sec.
South Dakota Board of Nursing
132 S. Dakota Ave., Suite 200
Sioux Falls, South Dakota 57102

Miss Dorothy L. Hocker, RN, Exec. Dir.
Tennessee Board of Nursing
301-7th Ave., N., Capitol Hill Bldg.,
 Room 354
Nashville, Tennessee 37219

Mrs. Margaret L. Rowland, Exec. Sec.
Board of Nurse Examiners for the State of
 Texas
7600 Chevy Chase Dr., Suite 502
Austin, Texas 78752

Mrs. Thelma C. Sawyer, RN, Exec. Sec.
Utah State Board of Nursing Dept. of
 Registration
330 E. 4th S.
Salt Lake City, Utah 84111

Miss Louise Alcott, RN, Exec. Sec.
Vermont Board of Nursing, Licensing and
 Registration Div.
130 State St.
Montpelier, Vermont 05602

Miss Ianthe Blyden, President
Board of Nursing Registration and
 Nursing Education
Charlotte Amalie
St. Thomas, Virgin Islands 00801

Miss Eleanor J. Smith, RN, Exec. Sec.
Virginia State Board of Nursing
6 N. 6th St., Room 404
Richmond, Virginia 23219

Mrs. Margaret M. Sullivan, Exec. Sec.
Washington State Board of Nursing
PO Box 649
Olympia, Washington 98504

Miss Freda Engle, RN, Exec. Sec.
Board of Examiners for Registered Nurses
1800 Washington St., E., Room 416
Charleston, West Virginia 25305

Mrs. Elaine F. Ellibee, RN, Sec.
Wisconsin State Division of Nurses
201 E. Washington Ave.
Madison, Wisconsin 53702

Mrs. Dorothy G. Randell, RN, Exec. Dir.
State of Wyoming Board of Nursing
Cheyenne, Wyoming 82002

There are no Schools of Nursing—R.N. in American Samoa and Canal Zone.

CANADIAN NURSES' ORGANIZATIONS

Canadian Nurses' Association
50 The Driveway
Ottawa, Ontario
K2P 1E2

Northwest Territories Registered Nurses Association
Box 2757
Yellowknife, N.W.T.
X1A 2R1

Registered Nurses Association of British Columbia
2130 West 12th Avenue
Vancouver, B.C.
V6K 2N3

Alberta Association of Registered Nurses
10256 - 112 Street
Edmonton, Alberta
T5K 1M6

Saskatchewan Registered Nurses Association
2066 Retallack Street
Regina, Saskatchewan
S4T 2K2

Manitoba Association of Registered Nurses
647 Broadway Avenue
Winnipeg, Manitoba
R3C 0X2

Registered Nurses Association of Ontario
33 Price Street
Toronto, Ontario
M4W 1Z2

Ontario Nurses Association
415 Yonge Street
Suite 1401
Toronto, Ontario
M5B 2E7

Order of Nurses of Quebec
4200 Dorchester Blvd.
Montreal, Quebec
H3A 1V4

New Brunswick Association of Registered Nurses
231 Saunders Street
Fredericton, N.B.
E3B 1N6

Registered Nurses Association of Nova Scotia
6035 Coburg Road
Halifax, Nova Scotia
B3H 1Y8

Association of Nurses of Prince Edward Island
41 Palmers Lane
Charlottetown, P.E.I.
C1A 5V7

Association of Registered Nurses of Newfoundland
67 Le Marchand Road
St. John's, Nfld.
A1C 2G9

Index

Index